Casarett and Doull's
TOXICOLOGY

The Basic Science of Poisons

All substances are poisons; there is none which is not a poison. The right dose differentiates a poison and a remedy.

PARACELSUS
(1493–1541)

EDITED BY

John Doull, M.D., Ph.D.

Professor of Pharmacology and Toxicology,
University of Kansas School of Medicine,
Kansas City, Kansas

Curtis D. Klaassen, Ph.D.

Professor of Pharmacology and Toxicology,
University of Kansas School of Medicine,
Kansas City, Kansas

Mary O. Amdur, Ph.D.

Senior Research Scientist, Energy Laboratory,
Massachusetts Institute of Technology,
Cambridge, Massachusetts; Associate
Professor of Toxicology, Harvard University
School of Public Health, Boston, Massachusetts

Casarett and Doull's
TOXICOLOGY

The Basic Science of Poisons

SECOND EDITION

Macmillan Publishing Co., Inc.
New York

Collier Macmillan Canada, Ltd.
Toronto

Baillière Tindall
London

Earlier edition, entitled *Toxicology: The Basic Science of Poisons*, edited by Louis J. Casarett and John Doull, copyright © 1975 by Macmillan Publishing Co., Inc.

MACMILLAN PUBLISHING CO., INC.
866 Third Avenue, New York, New York 10022

COLLIER MACMILLAN CANADA, LTD.
BAILLIÈRE TINDALL · London

Library of Congress Cataloging in Publication Data
Casarett, Louis J.
    Casarett and Doull's *Toxicology: The Basic Science of Poisons*
    Includes bibliographies and index.
    1. Toxicology. I. Doull, John, (date)
II. Klaassen, Curtis D. III. Amdur, Mary O.
IV. Title. V. Title: Toxicology.
RA1211.C296   1980   615.9   79-18632
ISBN 0-02-330040-X

Printing: 3 4 5 6 7 8   Year: 1 2 3 4 5 6

Foreword to the Second Edition

THE PUBLICATION in 1975 of Casarett and Doull's *Toxicology: The Basic Science of Poisons* was so opportunely timed, it is tempting to credit these editors with prescience. However, creating the text was not fortuitous; the driving force was the compelling desire of the late Louis J. Casarett and his wife, now Dr. Margaret C. Bruce, to give the students in a pioneering course at the University of Hawaii a source of facts and theories embracing the largely disseminated toxicologic information.

The intervening few years have witnessed a tumultuous, disorganized, and at times painful upsurge (1) in the demands for trustworthy knowledge and for able, informed toxicologists and (2) in the attempts to respond to toxic health hazards of crisis proportions, locally and nationally. Toxicologists are not created instantaneously by legislation; recruits have been drawn from many fields, e.g., clinical medicine, pharmacology, and biochemistry—but still too few to fill the urgent demands. Educational efforts lag, but are moving. Graduate courses in toxicology leading to doctorates are slowly expanding, many schools now offer master's degree programs, and recently undergraduate baccalaureates with majors in toxicology are being announced. For all of these activities, textbooks are sought; the audience for Casarett and Doull's *Toxicology: The Basic Science of Poisons* today has increased manyfold over that in 1975.

The sharp growth meantime in research output as it appears in scholarly and applied monographs and journals and the accompanying sophistication of instrumentation and methods, of ideas and hypotheses, clarify little by little our understanding of the natures, and the modes, of toxic effects. Harvesting the relevant new data and ideas and weaving them into the structure of the second edition of this textbook tax the skill of the authors and the editors. They are commended for successfully accepting these challenges.

HAROLD C. HODGE

Preface to the Second Edition

THE SECOND edition of this textbook and reference has had a change in title to *Casarett and Doull's Toxicology: The Basic Science of Poisons* to serve as a reminder to future students and practitioners that the book owes its inception to the vision and wisdom of the first editors, Louis J. Casarett and John Doull. To replace Dr. Casarett, who died during the final stages of preparing manuscript and illustrations for the first edition, two additional academic toxicologists—Curtis D. Klaassen and Mary O. Amdur—have joined Dr. Doull as coeditors of the second edition. Both Dr. Klaassen and Dr. Amdur have had a long-time relationship to the book since they served as contributors to the first edition.

Our goals in the second edition have remained those of the first edition. This volume has been designed primarily as a textbook for, or adjunct to, courses in toxicology. In the preparation of the second edition we have welcomed, solicited, and as far as possible heeded the comments of our academic colleagues who used the first edition in their classrooms. The positive response to the first edition provided convincing evidence that our primary objective reflected a current need in biomedical education, but the comments and suggestions of our colleagues who were using the book both for teaching and research indicated that we had underestimated the need outside of the classroom. The second edition should again be of interest to those not directly involved in didactic teaching of toxicology. Research toxicologists will find updated material in areas of their special or peripheral interests. The expansion of toxicology and the advent of the Toxic Substances Control Act in the United States, as well as similar legislation in other countries, have led scientists in other disciplines and those in other professions to feel the need for information on many facets of toxicology and the concepts and modes of thought that are its foundation.

Without permitting the second edition to become unwieldy in size and prohibitive in cost, we have added three new chapters: "Genetic Toxicology," "Water and Soil Pollutants," and "Regulatory Toxicology." The chapter on "Toxic Responses of the Central Nervous System" now includes material related to the peripheral as well as the central nervous system. The chapter entitled "Chemical Carcinogens" has been extensively revised and altered in its approach to the subject. With this edition, we have also instituted a policy of changing the authorship of at least 20 percent of the chapters in order to provide a broader input and coverage of the many aspects of toxicology.

While maintaining an overall framework similar to that of the first edition, we have made alterations to improve the sequence of material in the second edition. Unit I, "General Principles of Toxicology," now also contains chapters on teratogenesis, chemical carcinogenesis, and genetic toxicology. The growing importance of research and toxicology testing in these three areas made this appropriate. Unit II, "Systemic Toxicology," contains chapters that discuss the types of injury produced in specific organs or organ systems, illustrated by examples of toxic agents that produce these effects. Unit III, "Toxic Agents," contains chapters on specific classes of toxic materials. In a new Unit IV, "Environmental Toxicology," we have grouped the chapters on food additives and contaminants, air pollutants, and water and soil pollutants. Unit V, "Applications of Toxicology," addresses the ramifications of toxicology into all areas of the health sciences and includes a new chapter on regulatory toxicology. This unit is intended to provide perspective for nontoxicologists as well as for toxicologists; it should give those in other disciplines a better understanding of the activities of basic scientists, clinicians, and others engaged in various aspects of the discipline of toxicology.

The editors are grateful to the contributors, whose combined expertise made a volume of this breadth possible. We wish to acknowledge with gratitude the cooperation of contributors to the first edition for carrying out our difficult charge to "revise and update but not increase length." We also thank Susan P. Converse and Billie J. Radke for their many hours of skilled editorial assistance.

J.D.
C.D.K.
M.O.A.

Preface to the First Edition

THIS VOLUME has been designed primarily as a textbook for, or adjunct to, courses in toxicology. However, it should also be of interest to those not directly involved in toxicologic education. For example, the research scientist in toxicology will find sections containing current reports on the status of circumscribed areas of special interest. Those concerned with community health, agriculture, food technology, pharmacy, veterinary medicine, and related disciplines will discover the contents to be most useful as a source of concepts and modes of thought that are applicable to other types of investigative and applied sciences. For those further removed from the field of toxicology or for those who have not entered a specific field of endeavor, this book attempts to present a selectively representative view of the many facets of the subject.

Toxicology: The Basic Science of Poisons has been organized to facilitate its use by these different types of users. The first section (Unit I) describes the elements of method and approach that identify toxicology. It includes those principles most frequently invoked in a full understanding of toxicologic events, such as dose-response, and is primarily mechanistically oriented. Mechanisms are also stressed in the subsequent sections of the book, particularly when these are well identified and extend across classic forms of chemicals and systems. However, the major focus in the second section (Unit II) is on the systemic site of action of toxins. The intent therein is to provide answers to two questions: What kinds of injury are produced in specific organs or systems by toxic agents? What are the agents that produce these effects?

A more conventional approach to toxicology has been utilized in the third section (Unit III), in which the toxic agents are grouped by chemical or use characteristics. In the final section (Unit IV) an attempt has been made to illustrate the ramifications of toxicology into all areas of the health sciences and even beyond. This unit is intended to provide perspective for the nontoxicologist in the application of the results of toxicologic studies and a better understanding of the activities of those engaged in the various aspects of the discipline of toxicology.

It will be obvious to the reader that the contents of this book represent a compromise between the basic, fundamental, mechanistic approach to toxicology and the desire to give a view of the broad horizons presented by the subject. While it is certain that the editors' selectivity might have been more severe, it is equally certain that it could have been less so, and we hope that the balance struck will prove to be appropriate for both toxicologic training and the scientific interest of our colleagues.

L.J.C.

J.D.

Although the philosophy and design of this book evolved over a long period of friendship and mutual respect between the editors, the effort needed to convert ideas into reality was undertaken primarily by Louis J. Casarett. Thus, his death at a time when completion of the manuscript was in sight was particularly tragic. With the help and encouragement of his wife, Margaret G. Casarett, and the other contributors, we have finished Lou's task. This volume is a fitting embodiment of Louis J. Casarett's dedication to toxicology and to toxicologic education.

J.D.

Contributors

Amdur, Mary O., Ph.D. Senior Research Scientist, Energy Laboratory, Massachusetts Institute of Technology, Cambridge, Massachusetts; Associate Professor of Toxicology, Harvard University School of Public Health, Boston, Massachusetts

Autian, John, Ph.D. Professor and Director of Materials Science Toxicology Laboratories, Colleges of Pharmacy and Dentistry, University of Tennessee Center for the Health Sciences, Memphis, Tennessee

Baselt, Randall C., Ph.D. Associate Professor of Pathology, University of California School of Medicine, Davis, California

Beliles, Robert P., Ph.D. Director of Toxicology, Litton Bionetics, Kensington, Maryland

Brown, John F., D.V.M., Ph.D. Associate Professor, Veterinary Section, Animal Science Department, University of Arkansas, Fayetteville, Arkansas

Bruce, Margaret C., Sc.D., Senior Research Associate, Department of Pediatrics, University Hospitals, Case Western University, Cleveland, Ohio

Casarett, Louis J., Ph.D. Late Professor of Pharmacology, University of Hawaii School of Medicine, Honolulu, Hawaii

Corn, Morton, Ph.D. Professor and Division Head, Environmental Health Engineering, School of Hygiene and Public Health, Johns Hopkins University, Baltimore, Maryland

Cornish, Herbert H., Ph.D. Professor of Environmental and Industrial Health, University of Michigan School of Public Health, Ann Arbor, Michigan

Cravey, Robert H., M.S. Chief Forensic Toxicologist, Office of the Sheriff-Coroner, County of Orange, California

Dixon, Robert L., Ph.D. Chief, Laboratory of Environmental Toxicology, National Institute of Environmental Health Sciences, Research Triangle Park, North Carolina

Doull, John, M.D., Ph.D. Professor of Pharmacology and Toxicology, University of Kansas School of Medicine, Kansas City, Kansas

Fowler, Murray E., D.V.M. Professor and Chairman, Department of Clinical Science, University of California School of Veterinary Medicine, Davis, California

Gonasun, Leonard M., Ph.D. Assistant Director, Department of Medical Research, Sandoz Pharmaceuticale, East Hanover, New Jersey

Hammond, Paul B., D.V.M., Ph.D. Professor of Environmental Health, University of Cincinnati College of Medicine, Cincinnati, Ohio

Harbison, Raymond D., Ph.D. Associate Professor of Pharmacology and Biochemistry, Vanderbilt University School of Medicine, Nashville, Tennessee

Hobbs, Charles H., D.V.M. Assistant Director, Inhalation Toxicology Research Institute, Lovelace Biomedical and Environmental Research Institute, Albuquerque, New Mexico

Hodge, Harold C., Ph.D. Professor Emeritus of Pharmacology, University of California School of Medicine, San Francisco, California

Hook, Jerry B., Ph.D. Professor of Pharmacology and Toxicology, Michigan State University, East Lansing, Michigan

Kilgore, Wendell W., Ph.D. Professor and Chairman, Department of Environmental Toxicology, Food Protection and Toxicology Center, University of California, Davis, California

Kingsbury, John M., Ph.D. Lecturer in Phytotoxicology, New York State Veterinary College; Professor of Botany, Cornell University, Ithaca, New York

Klaassen, Curtis D., Ph.D. Professor of Pharmacology and Toxicology, University of Kansas School of Medicine, Kansas City, Kansas

Lauwerys, Robert R., M.D., D.Sc. Professor of Industrial Toxicology, Catholic University of Louvain, Brussels, Belgium

Li, Ming-Yu, Ph.D. Documentation Specialist, Department of Environmental Toxicology, Food Protection and Toxicology Center, University of California, Davis, California

Liber, Howard L., M.S. Research Assistant, Department of Nutrition and Food Science, Massachusetts Institute of Technology, Cambridge, Massachusetts

McClellan, Roger O., D.V.M. Director, Inhalation Toxicology Research Institute, Lovelace Biomedical and Environmental Research Institute, Albuquerque, New Mexico

McCutcheon, Rob S., Ph.D. Formerly Executive Secretary, Toxicology Study Section, Division of Research Grants, U.S. Public Health Service, National Institutes of Health, Bethesda, Maryland

Menzel, Daniel B., Ph.D. Professor of Pharmacology and Medicine, Duke University Medical Center, Durham, North Carolina

Menzer, Robert E., Ph.D. Professor of Entomology, University of Maryland, College Park, Maryland

Murphy, Sheldon D., Ph.D. Professor and Director, Division of Toxicology, University of Texas Medical School at Houston, Houston, Texas

Neal, Robert A., Ph.D. Professor of Biochemistry, Vanderbilt University School of Medicine, Nashville, Tennessee

Nelson, Judd O., Ph.D. Assistant Professor of Entomology, University of Maryland, College Park, Maryland

Norton, Stata, Ph.D. Professor of Pharmacology, University of Kansas School of Medicine, Kansas City, Kansas

Oehme, Frederick W., D.V.M., Dr.Med.Vet., Ph.D. Professor of Toxicology and Medi-

cine, Kansas State University College of Veterinary Medicine, Manhattan, Kansas

Peterson, Robert G., M.D., Ph.D. Assistant Professor, Pediatrics and Anesthesiology, University of Colorado Health Science Center, Denver, Colorado

Plaa, Gabriel L., Ph.D. Professor and Chairman, Department of Pharmacology, University of Montreal, Montreal, Quebec

Potts, Albert M., Ph.D., M.D. Professor and Chairman, Department of Ophthalmology, University of Louisville School of Medicine, Louisville, Kentucky

Rumack, Barry H., M.D. Director, Rocky Mountain Poison Center, Denver, Colorado; Associate Professor of Pediatrics, Medicine, and Pharmacology, University of Colorado School of Medicine, Denver, Colorado

Smith, Roger P., Ph.D. Professor and Chairman, Department of Pharmacology and Toxicology, Dartmouth Medical School, Hanover, New Hampshire

Thilly, William, G., Sc.D. Professor of Nutrition and Food Science, Massachusetts Institute of Technology, Cambridge, Massachusetts

Weisburger, John H., Ph.D. Vice President for Research, Naylor Dana Institute for Disease Prevention/American Health Foundation, Valhalla, New York; Research Professor of Pathology, New York Medical College, Valhalla, New York

Williams, Gary M., M.D. Chief, Division of Experimental Pathology, Naylor Dana Institute for Disease Prevention/American Health Foundation, Valhalla, New York; Research Professor of Pathology, New York Medical College, Valhalla, New York

Contents

UNIT I
GENERAL PRINCIPLES
OF TOXICOLOGY

Chapter 1

ORIGIN AND SCOPE OF TOXICOLOGY

Louis J. Casarett and *Margaret C. Bruce*

WHAT IS TOXICOLOGY?

In contrast to the apparent simplicity of this question, there is no simple answer. Because toxicology has evolved as a multidisciplinary field of study, definitions of toxicology often reflect the area of study from which the definition derives. For example, a pharmacologist might view toxicology as a study of drugs, a chemist might view the subject from a chemical or analytic viewpoint, whereas those with a particular interest in an organ or system might have a still different definition of toxicology. Toxicology is broader than these parochial definitions. It is more than the science of poisons. Further, the discipline of toxicology is still developing and expanding in scope, and a proper definition must include its breadth and take into account its probable future development.

An understanding of what toxicology is may be gained by considering who its practitioners are, what they do, and how they do it. Although not truly definitive, this approach is informative. There is clearly a body of scientists who designate themselves as "toxicologists." Furthermore, there are those who do not so designate themselves, but who, in fact, are engaged in activities and have points of view closely aligned with those of toxicologists. In short, there is an area of study properly called toxicology, growing numbers of scientists who can and do identify themselves as toxicologists, a toxicologic literature, and a thread of basic agreement about what toxicologists do.

The activities and contributions of toxicologists are many and varied. In the biomedical area the toxicologist is concerned with intoxications by drugs and other chemicals and the demonstration of their safety or hazard prior to their entry on the market. The recognition, identification, and quantitation of relative hazard from occupational or public exposure to toxicants comprise another major function. This relates closely to private and governmental responsibilities to assure safety of workers and the general public in their contact with industrial

and commercial products, in ensuring air and water purity, as well as the safety of foods, drugs, and cosmetics. The development of poisons with a selective toxic action on weeds, insects, and other unwanted organisms, as well as assessment of their hazard, is also the province of toxicology.

Toxicologists, whether they be academically, commercially, industrially, or governmentally employed, are called upon to make predictions. The toxicologist is charged with garnering sufficient data on the toxicity of materials and having adequate knowledge of the mechanisms by which they produce their effects to make reasonable predictions of their hazard and impact on the human population and on the environment. The assessment of hazard and the rational projection of effects in a population are such overriding functions of toxicology that an alternate definition might be "the science that defines limits of safety of chemical agents."

Some insight into the development of the scope of toxicology, and of the roles, points of view, and activities of the toxicologist, is offered by an examination of the historic evolution of the discipline.

HISTORY OF TOXICOLOGY

Antiquity

Toxicology, in a variety of specialized and primitive forms, has been a relevant part of the history of man (Figure 1–1). Earliest man was well aware of the toxic effects of animal venoms and poisonous plants. His knowledge was used for hunting, for waging more effective warfare, and, probably, to remove undesirables from the small groups of primitive society. The Ebers papyrus, perhaps our earliest medical record (circa 1500 B.C.), contains information extending back many centuries. Of the more than 800 recipes given, many contain recognized poisons. For example, one finds hemlock, which later became the state poison of the Greeks; aconite, an arrow poison of the ancient Chinese; opium, used as both poison and antidote; and such

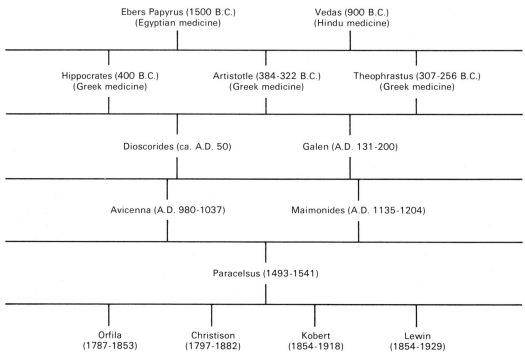

Figure 1–1. Major reference points in the evolution of toxicology as a science.

metals as lead, copper, and antimony. There is also an indication that plants containing substances akin to digitalis and belladonna alkaloids were known. Hippocrates, while introducing rational medicine about 400 B.C., added a number of poisons. He further wrote instructions that might be considered primitive principles of toxicology, in the form of attempts to control absorption of the toxic materials in therapy and overdosage.

In the mythology and literature of classic Greece, one finds many references to poisons and their use, and it was during this period that the first professional treatment of the subject began to appear. For example, Theophrastus (370–286 B.C.), a student of Aristotle, included numerous references to poisonous plants in *De Historia Plantarum*. Dioscorides, a Greek physician in the court of Emperor Nero, made the first attempt at a classification of poisons, which was accompanied by descriptions and drawings. The separation into plant, animal, and mineral poisons he used not only remained a standard for 16 centuries, but is still a convenient classification today (see Gunther, 1934). Dioscorides also dabbled in therapy, recognizing the use of emetics in poisoning and the use of caustic agents or cupping glasses in snakebite.

Poisoning with plant and animal toxins was quite common. Perhaps the best-known recipient

of a poison used as a state method of execution was Socrates (470–399 B.C.), although he was in distinguished company. Expeditious suicide on a voluntary basis also made use of toxicologic knowledge. Demosthenes (385–322 B.C.), who took poison hidden in his pen, was only one of many examples. The mode of suicide calling for one to fall on his sword, although manly and noble, carried little appeal and less significance for ladies of the day. Cleopatra's (69–30 B.C.) knowledge of natural, primitive toxicology permitted her the more genteel method of falling on her asp instead.

The Romans too made considerable use, often political, of poisons. Much legend and myth have grown out of the skill of poisoners and the occupational hazards of political life. One such legend tells of the King Mithridates VI of Pontus whose numerous experiments on unfortunate criminals led to his eventual claim that he had discovered "an antidote for every venomous reptile and every poisonous substance" (Guthrie, 1946). He himself was so fearful of poisons that he regularly ingested a mixture of 36 ingredients (Galen reports 54) as protection against assassination. On the occasion of his imminent capture by enemies, his attempts to kill himself with poison failed because of his successful concoction and he was forced to use his own sword held by a servant. From this tale comes the term "mithridatic" referring to an antidotal or protective mixture. Another term from the Greek, "theriac," also has become a synonym for "antidote" although the word derives from a poetic treatise by Nicander of Colophon (204–135 B.C.) entitled "Theriaca," which dealt with poisonous animals. Another poem, "Alexipharmaca," was about antidotes.

This search for antidotal measures or chemicals remained a preoccupation for centuries. In addition to the terms given above, others were applied such as Alexiteria and Bezoardica, the latter referring to concretions found in the goat bladder. The practice of medicine was based largely on an "antidoting" of disease, and descriptions of therapeutic agents also were so classified. For example, an early respectable forerunner of the modern pharmacopoeia was the *Antidotarium of Nicholaus*. It was not until the seventeenth century that a commission appointed by the Pope to Matthiolus opened the horizons to a search for *Antidota specifica*.

In Rome, poisoning seemed to take on epidemic characteristics, which are described by Livy as being especially distressing to the public in the fourth century B.C. It was during this period that a conspiracy of women to remove those from whose death they might profit was uncovered, and similar large-scale poisoning continued from time to time until 82 B.C., when Sulla issued the *Lex Cornelia*. This appears to be the first law against poisoning, and it later became a regulatory statute directed at careless dispensers of drugs.

The history of poisons and their use is the basis of entertaining retrospective diagnosis, as described by Meek in his essay *The Gentle Art of Poisoning* (1928) and in a book by Thompson entitled *Poisons and Poisoners* (1931). Although most poisons used during the period were of vegetable origin, the sulfide of arsenic and arsenous acid were known to be used. It has been postulated that arsenic was the poison with which Agrippina killed Claudius to make Nero the emperor of Rome. This postulate is supported by the later use of the same material by Nero in poisoning Britannicus, Claudius's natural son. The deed was performed under the direction of Locusta, a professional poisoner attached to the family.

The mixture of fact and legend surrounding that murder illustrates the practices of the times. A first attempt to poison Britannicus failed, but the illness reported contained evidence of all the symptoms of arsenic poisoning. The failure led to suspicion and the hiring of a taster. The second, and successful, attempt involved a more devious scheme. The arsenic was placed in cold water and Britannicus was served excessively hot soup. The taster had demon-strated the safety of the soup, but it was not retested after the water had been added to cool the soup.

Here superstition and legend embellish the story. Nero claimed that Britannicus had died of epilepsy and ordered immediate burial to prevent others from seeing the blackening of the body believed to occur after poisoning. As the legend continues, the corpse was painted with cosmetics to hide the deed, but, in a raging storm, the cosmetics washed off, revealing Nero's perfidy.

Middle Ages

Prior to the Renaissance and extending well into that period, the Italians, with characteristic pragmatism, brought the art of poisoning to its zenith. The poisoner became an integral part of the scene, if not as a social being, at least as a political tool and as custodian of a common social expedient. The records of the city councils of Florence, and particularly the infamous Council of Ten of Venice, contain ample testimony of the political use of poisons. Victims were named, prices set, contracts recorded, and when the deed was accomplished, payment made. The notation "*factum*" often appeared after the entry in the archives, indicating successful accomplishment of its transaction.

In less organized but more colorful ways, the citizens of Italy in the Middle Ages also practiced the art of poisoning. A famous figure of the time was a lady named Toffana, who peddled specially prepared arsenic-containing cosmetics (*Agua Toffana*). Accompanying the product were appropriate instructions for use. Toffana was succeeded by an imitator with organizational genius, a certain Hieronyma Spara, who provided a new fillip by directing her activity toward specific marital and monetary objectives. A local club was formed of young, wealthy, married women, which soon became a club of eligible young, wealthy widows, reminiscent of the matronly conspiracy many centuries earlier.

Among the prominent families engaged in poisoning, the Borgias are the most notorious. Although there is no doubt that they were among the leading entrepreneurs in the field, they probably received more credit than their due. Many deaths that were attributed to poisoning are now recognized as having occurred from infectious diseases such as malaria, which was sufficiently bad as to make Rome virtually uninhabitable during the summer months. It appears true, however, that Alexander VI, his son Cesare, and Lucretia were quite active. Aside from personal reasons, the deft applications of poisons to men of stature in the Church swelled the holdings of the Papacy, which was the prime heir.

A paragon of the distaff set of the period was Catherine de Medici. Catherine, although not so thoroughly fabled as her Borgia relatives and ancestors, was, in tune with her time, a practitioner of the art of applied toxicology. She also represented a formidable export from Italy to France. As appeared to be all too common in this period, the prime targets of the ladies were their husbands. However, unlike others of an earlier period, the circle represented by Catherine (and epitomized by the notorious Marchioness de Brinvillers) depended on direct evidence to arrive at the most effective compounds for their purposes. Under guise of delivering provender to the sick and the poor, Catherine tested toxic concoctions, carefully noting the rapidity of the toxic response (onset of action), the effectiveness of the compound (potency), the degree of response of the parts of the body (specificity, site of action), and the complaints of the victim (clinical signs and symptoms). Clearly, Catherine must be given credit as perhaps the earliest untrained experimental toxicologist.

Culmination of the practice in France is represented by the commercialization of the service by a Catherine Deshayes, who earned the title *La Voisine*. Her business was dissolved by her execution. Her trial was one of the most famous of those held by the Chambre Ardente, a special judicial commission established by Louis XIV to try such cases without regard to age, sex, or national origin. La Voisine was convicted of many poisonings, including over 2,000 infants among the victims.

During the Middle Ages and on into the Renaissance, poisoning seems to have been accepted as one of the normal hazards of living. It had some elements of sport, with a code, unwritten rules of honor, and a fatalistic attitude on the part of the selected victim. Devices and methods of poisoning proliferated at an alarming rate. The Chambre Ardente created in France was but a mild deterrent, and it remained for the rise of scientific methods in modern times to make the practice more risky for poisoners.

Another individual whose contributions to toxicology have survived through the years was Moses ben Maimon, or Maimonides (A.D. 1135–1204). In addition to being a competent and well-respected physician, Maimonides was also a prolific writer. Of particular significance was his volume entitled *Poisons and Their Antidotes* (1198), a first-aid guide to the treatment of accidental or intentional poisonings and insect, snake, or mad dog bites. Maimonides recommended that suction be applied to insect stings or animal bites as a means of extracting the poison and advised application of a tight bandage above a wound located on a limb. He also noted that the absorption of toxins from the stomach could be delayed by ingestion of oily substances such as milk, butter, or cream. A cautious and critical observer, Maimonides rejected numerous popular remedies of the day after finding them to be ineffective (e.g., the use of unleavened bread in the treatment of scorpion stings) and mentioned his doubts concerning the efficacy of others.

Age of Enlightenment

A significant figure in the history of science and medicine in the late Middle Ages was the renaissance man, Philippus Aureolus Theophrastus Bombastus von Hohenheim-Paracelsus (1493–1541). Between the time of Aristotle and the age of Paracelsus there was little substantial change in the biomedical sciences. In the sixteenth century the revolt against the authority of the Church was accompanied by a parallel attack on the godlike authority exercised by the followers of Hippocrates and Galen. Paracelsus, personally and professionally, embodied the qualities that forced numerous changes in this period. He and his age were pivotal, standing between the philosophy and magic of classic antiquity and the philosophy and science willed to us by figures of the seventeenth and eighteenth centuries. Clearly one can identify in Paracelsus's approach, his point of view, and his breadth of interest numerous similarities to the discipline we now call toxicology.

Paracelsus formulated many then-revolutionary views that remain an integral part of the present structure of toxicology. He promoted a focus on the "toxicon," the toxic agent, as a chemical entity. A view initiated by Paracelsus that became a lasting contribution held, as corollaries, that (1) experimentation is essential in examination of responses to chemicals; (2) one should make a distinction between therapeutic and toxic properties of chemicals; (3) these properties are sometimes, but not always, indistinguishable except by dose; and (4) one can ascertain a degree of specificity of chemicals and their therapeutic or toxic effects. The latter view presaged the "magic bullet" of Paul Ehrlich and the introduction of the therapeutic index. Further, in a very real sense, this was the first sound articulation of the dose-response relation, which is a bulwark of toxicology (Pachter, 1961).

Another noteworthy contribution was his volume entitled *Bergsucht* (1533–1534), the first treatise in the medical literature to provide a comprehensive description of the occupational diseases of miners. The book contains numerous clinical observations of chronic arsenic and mercury poisoning and describes in detail the asthmatic attacks and gastrointestinal symptoms of Miners' disease (Pagel, 1958).

Modern Toxicology

Often cited as the founder of toxicology is Mattieu Joseph Bonaventura Orfila (1787–1853), a Spanish physician who held a position of respect as attending physician to Louis XVIII of France and occupied a chair at the University of Paris. Orfila was the first to attempt a systematic correlation between the chemical and biologic information of the then-known poisons. Much of his contribution was based on personal observation of the effect of poisons in several thousand dogs. Among other contributions, he singled out toxicology as a discipline distinct from others and defined toxicology as the study of poisons.

Orfila also turned attention to problems combining chemistry and jurisprudence. He pointed to the necessity of chemical analysis for legal proof of lethal intoxication and he devised methods for detecting poisons, some of which are still used. A major outcome of his activity was the emergence of autopsy material for the purpose of detection of accidental and intentional poisonings. The introduction of this approach survives in modern toxicology as one specialty area, that of forensic toxicology.

The era of modern toxicology ushered in by Orfila marked the beginning of a number of analytic developments that made poisoning detectable. The close relationship between poisons and the occult that had evolved earlier began to dissipate with the advent of tests to determine whether a murder has been committed. For example, the test for arsenic by Marsh, in 1836, removed from the unknown and undetected one of the most widely used susbtances for murder.

The fascination with toxic substances was common among many leading physiologists of the eighteenth and nineteenth centuries. Francois Magendie (1783–1855) spent a significant part of his time in the study of the mechanism of action of emetine and strychnine. He was interested in "arrow poisons" used by primitive tribes and began a study of their actions (see Olmsted, 1944). Magendie transmitted this interest to his equally famous student Claude Bernard (1813–1878).

Bernard continued the study of arrow poisons and reported a classic experiment identifying the site of action of curare, confirming an earlier report of Kolliker at Würtzburg (Bernard, 1850). Bernard held and propagated the view that "the physiological analysis of organic systems . . . can be done with the aid of toxic agents." Bernard assiduously applied this principle using a number of agents besides curare, including strychnine and carbon monoxide, which he noted formed a complex with hemoglobin (Bernard, translated by Greene, 1949).

Louis Lewin (1854–1929) was a prodigious figure in toxicology. His interests were broad, leading to many publications dealing with the toxicology of methyl, ethyl, and higher alcohols, chloroform, chronic opiate use, and hallucinogenic materials contained in plants. Among his publications was a toxicologist's view of world history, and, in the year of his death, a textbook of toxicology (1920, 1929). Robert Christison (1797–1882), who studied toxicology under Orfila, produced a major work on poisons (1845). Rudolf Kobert (1854–1918), a student of Oswald Schmiedeberg and a contemporary of Lewin, also produced a textbook on toxicology (1893).

Developments in toxicology occurred rapidly in the twentieth century. On the one hand, there were many toxic and therapeutic agents that served as the starting points for fundamental studies of mechanisms, for example, the development by Rudolf Peters and colleagues (1945) of dimercaprol (BAL) as an antidote to arsenic-containing war gases and studies of the mechanism of BAL action on organic arsenicals by Carl Voegtlin and associates (1923). On the other hand, there were developments leading to discovery and understanding of toxic substances for use by man, such as the discovery and study of DDT by Paul Müller and the discovery and development of organophosphorus insecticides by Willy Lange and Gerhard Schrader. Following this refinement of analytic techniques, toxicology developed rapidly. Although the contributions are too numerous to catalog, a selective sampling of contributions to toxicology may be informative. Such a list is presented in Table 1–1.

ROLES OF TOXICOLOGY

Modern toxicology includes much more than a simple extension of the work of Orfila. In fact, the toxicologist finds himself in the midst of a formidable spectrum of interests and activities. The bewildering array of economic poisons in use today is testimony to the diligence of chemists, agronomists, botanists, and entomologists concerned with control of biologic pests by toxic agents. The same poisons represent a challenge to those concerned with maintenance of ecologic balance, with conservation of the environment, and with protection of the health of man, all objectives to which the toxicologist may contribute. The shelves of our markets bulge with edible products that are forever "new," or "improved" by addition of chemicals to keep them fresh, make them more nutritious, or provide greater appeal to the palate. The toxicologist has a key role to play in assuring

Table 1–1. SELECTION OF DEVELOPMENTS IN TOXICOLOGY

Development of early advances in analytic methods

Marsh, 1836: development of method for arsenic analysis
Reinsh, 1841: combined method for separation and analysis of As and Hg
Fresenius, 1845; von Babo, 1847: development of screening method for general poisons
Stas-Otto, 1851: extraction and separation of alkaloids
Mitscherlich, 1855: detection and identification of phosphorus

Early mechanistic studies

F. Magendie, 1809: study of "arrow poisons," mechanism of action of emetine and strychnine
C. Bernard, 1850: carbon monoxide combination with hemoglobin, study of mechanism of action of strychnine, site of action of curare
R. Bohm, ca. 1890: active anthelmintics from fern, action of croton oil catharsis, poisonous mushrooms

Introduction of new toxins, antidotes

R. A. Peters, L. A. Stocken, and R. H. S. Thompson, 1945: development of British antilewisite (BAL) as a relatively specific antidote for arsenic, toxicity of monofluorocarbon compounds
K. K. Chen, 1934: introduction of modern antidotes (nitrite and thiosulfate) for cyanide toxicity
C. Voegtlin, 1923: mechanism of action of As and other metals on the SH groups
P. Müller, 1944–1946: introduction and study of DDT (dichlordiphenyltrichloroethane) and related insecticide compounds
G. Schrader, 1952: introduction and study of organophosphorus compounds
R. N. Chopra, 1933: indigenous drugs of India

Miscellaneous toxicologic studies

R. T. Williams: study of detoxication mechanisms and species variation
A. Rothstein: effects of uranium ion on cell membrane transport
R. A. Kehoe: investigation of acute and chronic effects of lead
A. Vorwald: studies of chronic respiratory disease (beryllium)
H. Hardy: community and industrial poisoning (beryllium)
A. Hamilton: introduction of modern industrial toxicology
H. C. Hodge: toxicology of uranium, fluorides; standards of toxicity
A. Hoffman: introduction of lysergic acid and derivatives; psychotomimetics
R. A. Peters: biochemical lesions, lethal synthesis
A. E. Garrod: inborn errors of metabolism
T. T. Litchfield and F. Wilcoxon: simplified dose-response evaluation
C. J. Bliss: method of probits, calculation of dosage-mortality curves

---

safety of additives. The practicing physician faces ever more drugs; the toxicologist faces a precisely equal increase in potential problems from these drugs. With greater availability of potent drugs, the burgeoning number and complexity of intoxications are of concern to the social scientists and the law enforcement official, a concern shared by the treating physician and by the toxicologist.

In the modern enlightenment of industrial practice, there has been great concern about maintaining a safe working environment. The proliferation of new, potent, and complex chemicals and processes projects the continuing specter of industrial and occupational over-exposure. In addition, the hazard of the plant and the potential danger of its effluent spill over into the general populace.

In an attempt to cope with the ever-increasing number of chemicals to which both human beings and the environment are exposed, the U.S. Congress signed into law in 1976 the Toxic Substances Control Act (TOSCA). The act stipulates that both use of a new chemical (i.e., one not listed prior to November 1977) and new uses of existing chemicals must be reported to the Environmental Protection Agency (EPA) by the manufacturer or processor 90 days prior to use. The administrator of EPA has the responsibility for determining whether the new chemical or new use will present an unreasonable risk to health or to the environment. If there is reason to suspect that the new compound or new use might be hazardous, or if there are insufficient data to predict the health or environmental effects, TOSCA authorizes EPA to require the company to provide, at its own expense, the necessary data.

The passage of this act represents a significant effort to prevent disasters similar to those in which workers or the environment have suffered irreparable damage as a result of industrial exposure to kepone, methyl mercury, polychlorinated biphenyls, tetrachlorodibenzodioxin, and vinyl chloride, to name a select few. The act also places a tremendous degree of responsibility on the administrator of EPA and on toxicologists in general to accurately determine, on the basis of very little information and in a manner that does not "impede unduly or create unnecessary economic barriers to technological innovation," which compounds and new uses of compounds are safe and which will require further testing.

Elements of Toxicology

From the foregoing it should not be surprising that a definition of toxicology, suitably simple and inclusive, is difficult to formulate. However, there are a number of common elements to modern toxicology.

One can immediately identify three interrelated elements that are required. (1) There must be a chemical or physical agent capable of producing a response. (2) One must identify a biologic system with which the agent may interact to produce a response. (3) There must be a response that can be considered to be deleterious to the biologic system. Clearly, there also must be a means by which the agent and the biologic system are permitted to interact.

Throughout the discussion, it is clear that a central element of toxicology is the delineation of the safe use of chemicals. To use the term "poison" alone is inadequate, as any effective chemical is a poison. The word has also been used for limited legal purposes. Rather, the toxicologist has as a major part of his discipline a contribution to make to the identification of "hazard," defined as the probability that injury will result from a chemical under specific conditions, and to the establishment of limits of "safety," defined as the practical certainty that injury will not result from use of a substance under specified conditions of quantity and manner of use. These contributions may be made in many ways, most of which represent measures of "toxicity," defined as the capacity of a substance to produce injury.

In the era of development of toxicology as a discipline, another important, even essential, ingredient has been added: the "why" of the toxic response. Basic research is necessary to determine how noxious substances gain access to the biologic system and arrive at a site of action and to define the molecular events underlying the changes that occur.

It bears repeating that the science of toxicology is rapidly evolving despite clearly identifiable stable features. Because of its rapid development, one can expect further changes in those who are part of it and in the roles that toxicologists may play. It will become clear from examination of other chapters in the book that the field of study promises provocative and exciting vistas in future years.

REFERENCES

Bernard, C.: Action du curare et de la nicotine sur le système nerveux et sur le système musculaire. *C.R. Séances Soc. Biol.*, **2**:195, 1850.
———: *An Introduction to the Study of Experimental Medicine*, translated by H. C. Greene, H. Schuman, New York, 1949.
Christison, R.: *A Treatise on Poisons*, 4th ed. Barrington & Howell, Philadelphia, 1845.
Gunther, R. T.: *The Greek Herbal of Dioscorides*. Oxford University Press, New York, 1934.
Guthrie, D. A.: *A History of Medicine*. J. B. Lippincott Co., Philadelphia, 1946.
Kobert, R.: *Lehrbuch der Intoxikationen*. Enke, Stuttgart, 1893.
Lewin, L.: *Gifte und Vergiftungen*. Stilke, Berlin, 1929.
———: *Die Gifte in der Weltgeschichte. Toxikologische, allgemeinverständliche Untersuchungen der historischen Quellen*. Springer, Berlin, 1920.
Meek, W. J.: *The Gentle Art of Poisoning*. Medico-Historical Papers. University of Wisconsin, Madison, 1954; reprinted from Phi Beta Pi Quarterly, May 1928.
Olmsted, J. M. D.: *Francois Magendie. Pioneer in Experimental Physiology and Scientific Medicine in XIX Century France*. Schuman, New York, 1944.
Orfila, M. J. B.: *Traité des Poisons Tirés des Règnes Minéral, Végétal et Animal, ou, Toxicologie Générale Considérée sous les Rapports de la Physiologie, de la Pathologie et de la Médecine Légale*. Crochard, Paris, 1814–1815.
———: *Secours à Donner aux Personnes Empoisonées et Asphyxiées*. Feugeroy, Paris, 1818.
Pachter, H. M.: *Paracelsus: Magic into Science*. Collier Books, New York, 1961.
Pagel, W.: *Paracelsus: An Introduction to Philosophical Medicine in the Era of the Renaissance*. S. Karger, New York, 1958.
Peters, R. A.; Stocken, L. A.; and Thompson, R. H. S.: British anti-lewisite (*BAL*). *Nature*, **156**:616–19, 1945.
Thompson, C. J. S.: *Poisons and Poisoners. With Historical Accounts of Some Famous Mysteries in Ancient and Modern Times*. H. Shaylor, London, 1931.
Voegtlin, C.; Dyer, H. A.; and Leonard, C. S.: On the mechanism of the action of arsenic upon protoplasm. *Public Health Rep.*, **38**:1882–1912, 1923.

SUPPLEMENTAL READING

Adams, F. (trans.): *The Genuine Works of Hippocrates*. Williams & Wilkins Co., Baltimore, 1939.
Beeson, B. B.: Orfila—pioneer toxicologist. *Ann. Med. Hist.*, **2**:68–70, 1930.
Bernard, C.: Analyse physiologique des propriétés des systèmes musculaire et nerveux au moyen du curare. *C.R. Acad. Sci. (Paris)*, **43**:325–29, 1856.
Bryan, C. P.: *The Papyrus Ebers*. Geoffrey Bales, London, 1930.
Clendening, L.: *Source Book of Medical History*. Dover, New York, 1942.
DuBois, K. P., and Geiling, E. M. K.: *Textbook of Toxicology*. Oxford University Press, New York, 1959.
Gaddum, J. H.: *Pharmacology*, 5th ed. Oxford University Press, New York, 1959.
Garrison, F. H.: *An Introduction to the History of Medicine*, 4th ed. W. B. Saunders Co., Philadelphia, 1929.
Hamilton, A.: *Exploring the Dangerous Trades*. Little, Brown & Co., Boston, 1943.

Levey, M.: Medieval Arabic toxicology. The *Book on Poisons* of Ibn Waḥshīya and its relation to early Indian and Greek texts. *Trans. Am. Philos. Soc.*, **56**:Part 7, 1966.

Loomis, T. A.: *Essentials of Toxicology*, 2nd ed. Lea & Febiger, Philadelphia, 1974.

Macht, D. J.: Louis Lewin. Pharmacologist, toxicologist, medical historian. *Ann. Med. Hist.*, 3:179–94, 1931.

Müller, P.: Über zusammenhänge zwischen Konstitution und insektizider Wirkung. I. *Helv. Chim. Acta*, **29**: 1560–80, 1946.

Munter, S. (ed.): *Treatise on Poisons and Their Antidotes.* Vol. II of the *Medical Writings of Moses Maimonides.* J. B. Lippincott Co., Philadelphia, 1966.

Paracelsus (Theophrastus ex Hohenheim eremita): *Von der Besucht.* Dillingen, 1567.

Ramazzini, B.: *De Morbis Artificum Diatriba.* Modena, 1700.

Schmiedeberg, O., and Koppe, R.: *Das Muscarin das giftige Alkaloid des Fliegenpilzes.* Vogel, Leipzig, 1869.

Sigerist, H. E.: *The Great Doctors.* Doubleday & Co., Garden City, N.Y., 1958.

Chapter 2

EVALUATION OF SAFETY:
TOXICOLOGIC EVALUATION

Curtis D. Klaassen and *John Doull*

INTRODUCTION TO TOXICOLOGY

Toxicology is the study of the adverse effects of chemicals on living organisms. The *toxicologist* is specially trained to examine the nature of these adverse effects and to assess the probability of their occurrence. The variety of potential adverse effects and the diversity of chemicals present in our environment combine to make toxicology a very broad science. Toxicologists are thus usually specialized to work in one area of toxicology.

Different Areas of Toxicology

The professional activities of toxicologists fall into three main categories: descriptive, mechanistic, and regulatory. The *descriptive toxicologist* is concerned directly with toxicity testing. The appropriate toxicity tests (as described later in this chapter) in experimental animals are designed to yield information that can be used to evaluate the risk posed to man and the environment by exposure to specific chemicals. The concern may be limited to effects on man as in the case of drugs or food additives. Toxicologists in the chemical industry, however, must be concerned not only with risk posed by the company's chemicals (insecticides, herbicides, solvents, etc.) to man himself but also with potential effects on fish, birds, plants, and other factors that might disturb the balance of the ecosystem.

The *mechanistic toxicologist* is concerned with elucidating the mechanisms by which chemicals exert their toxic effects on living organisms. Results of these studies often lead to sensitive predictive tests useful in obtaining information for risk assessment, help develop chemicals that are safer, or suggest rational therapy for toxic symptoms. In addition, an understanding of the mechanisms of toxic action also contributes to the knowledge of basic physiology and biochemistry. For example, studies on the toxicity of fluoro-organic alcohols and acids contributed to the knowledge of basic carbohydrate and lipid metabolism; knowledge of regulation of ion gradients in nerve axonal membranes has been greatly aided by studies of natural and synthetic toxins such as tetrodotoxin and DDT. Mechanistic toxicologists are active in universities, in research institutes supported by the government or by private sources, and in the pharmaceutical and chemical industries.

A *regulatory toxicologist* has the responsibility of deciding on the basis of data provided by the descriptive toxicologist whether or not a drug or chemical has a low enough risk to be marketed for the described purpose. The Food and Drug Administration (FDA) is responsible for admitting drugs, cosmetics, and food additives onto the market. The Environmental Protection Agency (EPA) is responsible for regulating most other chemicals. Regulatory toxicologists are also involved in the establishment of standards for the amount of chemicals permitted in ambient air, in industrial atmospheres, or in drinking water. The philosophic aspects of regulatory toxicology are discussed in Chapter 29 and the details of the legal aspects are discussed in Chapter 30.

Two other specialized areas of toxicology are designated as forensic and clinical. *Forensic toxicology* is a hybrid of analytic chemistry and fundamental toxicologic principles. It is concerned primarily with the medicolegal aspects of the harmful effects of chemicals on man and animals. The expertise of the forensic toxicologist is primarily invoked to aid in establishing the cause of death and elucidating its circumstances in a postmortem investigation (see Chap. 27). *Clinical toxicology* designates within the realm of medical science an area of professional emphasis concerned with diseases caused by, or uniquely associated with, toxic substances (see Chap. 26). Efforts are directed at treating patients poisoned with drugs or other chemicals and at development of new techniques to treat these intoxications.

Spectrum of Toxic Dose

One could define a poison as any agent capable of producing a deleterious response in a biologic system, seriously injuring function or producing death. This is not, however, a useful working definition for the very simple reason that virtually every known chemical has the potential to produce injury or death if present in a sufficient amount. Paracelsus (1493–1541) phrased this well when he noted, "All substances are poisons;

Table 2–1. APPROXIMATE ACUTE LD50s OF A SELECTED VARIETY OF CHEMICAL AGENTS

AGENT	LD50 (mg/kg)
Ethyl alcohol	10,000
Sodium chloride	4,000
Ferrous sulfate	1,500
Morphine sulfate	900
Phenobarbital sodium	150
DDT	100
Picrotoxin	5
Strychnine sulfate	2
Nicotine	1
d-Tubocurarine	0.5
Hemicholinium-3	0.2
Tetrodotoxin	0.10
Dioxin (TCDD)	0.001
Botulinus toxin	0.00001

Based on Loomis (1974).

there is none which is not a poison. The right dose differentiates a poison and a remedy."

Among chemicals there is a wide spectrum of doses needed to produce deleterious effects, serious injury, or death. This is demonstrated by Table 2–1, which shows the dose of chemical needed to produce death in 50 percent of the dosed animals (LD50). Some chemicals will produce death in microgram doses and are commonly thought of as being extremely

poisonous. Other chemicals may be relatively harmless following doses in excess of several grams. Categories of toxicity have been devised on the basis of the wide variation in the dose of chemical needed to produce death. An example of such a classification is shown in Table 2–2, which provides a toxicity rating or class based on the probable oral lethal dose for man. Such classifications are only qualitative but they serve a practical and useful purpose, especially to a toxicologist who is asked by someone in another discipline, "How toxic is this chemical?"

Risk and Safety

In practical situations the critical factor is not the intrinsic toxicity of a substance per se but the risk or hazard associated with its use. Risk is the probability that a substance will produce harm under specified conditions. Safety, the reciprocal of risk, is the probability that harm will not occur under specified conditions. Depending on the conditions under which it is used, a very toxic chemical may be less hazardous than a relatively nontoxic one. Risk assessment takes into account possible harmful effects on individuals or on society from the use of a material in the quantity and in the manner proposed. It is important to consider harmful effects on the environment as well as more direct effects on human health.

The question of what constitutes an acceptable risk is a matter of judgment. Such decisions are multifaceted and complex and involve a balance of risk and benefit. High risks may be acceptable in the use of lifesaving drugs that would be unacceptable in the use of food additives. Some of the factors considered in determining an acceptable risk are (1) the need met by the substance, (2) the adequacy and availability of alternative substances to meet the identified need, (3) the anticipated extent of public use, (4) employment considerations, (5) economic considerations, (6) effects on environmental quality, and (7) conservation of natural resources. The overall philosophy and problems inherent in such decision making are discussed in Chapter

Table 2–2. TOXICITY RATING CHART

| TOXICITY RATING OR CLASS | PROBABLE ORAL LETHAL DOSE FOR HUMANS | |
	DOSE	FOR AVERAGE ADULT
1. Practically nontoxic	>15 g/kg	More than 1 quart
2. Slightly toxic	5–15 g/kg	Between pint and quart
3. Moderately toxic	0.5–5 g/kg	Between ounce and pint
4. Very toxic	50–500 mg/kg	Between teaspoonful and ounce
5. Extremely toxic	5–50 mg/kg	Between 7 drops and teaspoonful
6. Supertoxic	<5 mg/kg	A taste (less than 7 drops)

29 as the concept of acceptable risk is in many ways the crux of regulatory toxicology.

CLASSIFICATION OF TOXIC AGENTS

Toxic agents are classified in a variety of ways depending on the interests and needs of the classifier. In this textbook, for example, toxic agents are discussed in terms of their target organ (liver, kidney, hematopoietic system poisons, etc.), their use (pesticides, solvents, food additives, etc.), their source (animal and plant toxins), and their effects (carcinogens, mutagens, etc.). Toxic agents may also be classified in terms of their physical state (gases, dusts, metals), their labeling requirements (explosives, flammables, oxidizers), their chemistry (aniline derivatives, halogenated hydrocarbons, etc.), or their poisoning potential (extremely toxic, very toxic, slightly toxic, etc.). Classification of toxic agents on the basis of their biochemical mechanism of action (sulfhydryl inhibitors, methemoglobin producers) is usually more informative than classification by general terms such as irritants and corrosives, but the more general classifications such as air pollutants, occupation-related agents, and acute and chronic poisons can provide a useful focus on a specific problem. It is evident from the above that no single classification will be applicable for the entire spectrum of toxic agents and that combinations of classification systems or classification based on other factors may be needed to provide the best rating system for a special purpose. Nevertheless, classification systems that take into consideration both the chemical and biologic properties of the agent and the exposure characteristics are most likely to be useful for legislative or control purposes and for toxicology in general.

Historically the first attempts to classify toxic agents were based on natural sources. One of the first of these by Dioscorides divided the sources into animal, plant, and mineral poisons (Gunther, 1934). The animal sources in these early classifications included the venoms and toxins produced in the specialized organs of snakes, spiders, and marine animals. Current classifications based on this approach would need to include marine organisms since fish poisons such as ciguatera toxin are due to marine organisms in the diet of fish and there is current concern that toxic substances present in marine organisms may be concentrated in the process of preparing food or protein sources (Halstead, 1965; Rodricks, 1978). The plant sources in the early classifications included therapeutically useful agents such as digitalis, morphine, salicylates, etc., arrow poisons such as curare and strychnine, and many of the so-called social poisons such as nicotine,

caffeine, marijuana, mescaline, etc. (For information on plant poisons, see Chapter 22; for information on social poisons, the reader should consult Chapter 25 in the first edition of this book.) Modern classification systems based on source would be likely to contain lower plant forms (kingdom Protista in Haeckel's classification) since they are a source of antibiotics, fungi-produced agents such as ergot, mycotoxins such as aflatoxin, ochratoxin, and patulin, and bacterial endotoxins (*Salmonella*, *Clostridium botulinum*, etc.). Other recent additions to a source classification system might include the red tide organism (*Gymodinium brevae*), certain blue-green algae, the mycotoxins, luteoskyrin, and cyclochloratine, which produce "yellow rice" hematoma (Uraguchi, 1965).

CHARACTERISTICS OF EXPOSURE

Adverse or toxic effects in a biologic system are not produced by a chemical agent unless the agent or its metabolites or conversion products reach appropriate receptors in the system at a concentration and for a length of time sufficient to initiate the toxic manifestation. Whether or not a toxic effect occurs is dependent, therefore, on the chemical and physical properties of the agent, the exposure situation, and the susceptibility of the biologic system or subject. Thus, to fully characterize the potential hazard or toxicity of a specific chemical agent we need to know not only what type of effect it produces and the dose required to produce the effect, but also information about the agent, the exposure, and the subject. Some of the toxicity-influencing factors related to the agent (composition, vehicle, formulation, etc.) and the subject (age, sex, species, nutritional status, etc.) are discussed in Chapter 5 of this textbook, and the various kinetic factors that influence toxicity (absorption, distribution, metabolism, and excretion) are discussed in Chapters 3 and 4. The major toxicity-influencing factors related to the exposure situation are the route of administration and the duration and frequency of exposure.

Route and Site of Exposure

The major routes by which toxic agents gain access to the body are through the gastrointestinal tract (ingestion), the lungs (inhalation), and the skin (topical), and through parenteral administration. Toxic agents generally exhibit the greatest potency and produce the most rapid response when given by the intravenous route, and an approximate descending order of effectiveness for the other routes would be: inhalation, intraperitoneal, subcutaneous, intramuscular, intradermal, oral, and topical. With oral exposure the onset of symptoms and the severity of effects are usually influenced by the stomach contents since absorption tends to be more rapid and more complete from an empty stomach. The vehicle and other formulation factors can markedly alter the absorption following inges- tion, inhalation, or topical exposure, and this effect may also occur with parenteral administra- tion. Similarly, the site of administration can influence the toxicity of agents given parenterally. For example, an agent that is detoxified in the liver would be expected to be less toxic when given via the portal circulation than when given via the systemic circulation.

Industrial exposure to toxic agents occurs most frequently by inhalation and topical exposure, and accidental and suicidal poisoning occurs most frequently through oral ingestion. Com- parison of the lethal dose of an agent by different routes of exposure often provides useful informa- tion concerning the absorption of the agent. For many agents the lethal dose for topical exposure is about ten times the lethal dose for oral administration, which in turn is about ten times the lethal dose with intravenous administration. In those situations where the lethal dose for oral or topical administration is close to the lethal dose for intravenous administration, it usually means that the toxic agent is absorbed rapidly and easily. Conversely, in those cases where the lethal dose by the dermal route is several orders of magnitude higher than the oral lethal dose, it is likely that the skin can be expected to provide an effective barrier to poisoning by the agent. Toxic effects by any route of exposure can also be influenced by the concentration of the agent in its vehicle, the total volume of the agent and vehicle to which the system is exposed, and the rate at which exposure occurs. Blood level studies are often needed to clarify the role of these and other factors as well as exposure route differences.

Duration and Frequency of Exposure

Toxic effects may be produced by acute and/or chronic exposure to chemical agents. Acute exposure is defined as a single exposure or multiple exposure occurring within a short time (24 hours or less). For many agents, the toxic effects of acute exposure are quite different from those produced by chronic exposure (colic with acute exposure to lead versus wrist drop with chronic lead exposure). Acute exposure to agents that are rapidly absorbed is likely to produce immediate toxic effects, but acute exposure can also produce delayed toxicity that may or may not be similar to the toxic effects of chronic exposure. Conversely, chronic exposure to a toxic agent may produce some immediate or

acute effects with each administration in addi- tion to the long-term, low-level, or chronic effects of the agent. In characterizing the toxicity of a specific chemical agent, it is evident that information is needed not only for the single-dose (acute) and long-term (chronic) effects, but also for exposures of intermediate duration. Con- ventionally, such exposures are referred to as short term (a week or so) and subchronic (usually three months) in toxicity testing pro- grams.

The other time-related factor that is important in the temporal characterization of exposure is the frequency of administration. In general, fractionation of the dose reduces the effect. A single dose of a test substance that produces an immediate severe effect might produce less than half of the effect when given in two divided doses and no effect when given in ten doses over a period of several hours or days. Such fractiona- tion effects occur when metabolism or excretion occurs between successive doses or when the injury produced by each administration is partially or fully reversed prior to the next administration. A diagrammatic representation of these concepts is presented in Figure 2–1. It is evident that with any type of multiple dose (multiposal) the production of toxic effect is not only influenced by the frequency of administra- tion but may, in fact, be totally dependent on frequency rather than duration of exposure. Chronic toxic effects occur, therefore, when the agent accumulates in the biologic system (absorp- tion exceeds metabolism and/or excretion) or when an agent produces irreversible toxic effects or when there is insufficient time for the system to recover from the toxic effect within the exposure frequency interval. When the rate of elimination is less than the rate of absorption, the toxic agent usually does not accumulate indefinitely, but reaches a steady state where the rate of elimination equals the rate of administra- tion. For additional discussion of these relation- ships, the reader should consult Chapter 3 of this text or other references (Boyd, 1970; Goldstein et al., 1974; Loomis, 1974; Paget, 1970).

SPECTRUM OF UNDESIRED EFFECTS

The spectrum of undesired effects of chemicals is broad. Some are deleterious and others are not. In therapeutics, for example, each drug produces a number of effects but only one of these is usually associated with the primary mission of the therapy; all other effects are referred to as *undesirable* or *side effects* of that drug for that therapeutic indication. However, some of these side effects might be desired for another therapeutic indication. For example,

chemicals involved. A number of terms have been used to describe pharmacologic and toxicologic interactions. An *additive* effect is the situation in which the combined effect of two chemicals is equal to the sum of the effect of each agent given alone (example: 2 + 3 = 5). The effect most commonly observed when two chemicals are given together is an additive effect. For example, when two organic phosphate insecticides are given together, the cholinesterase inhibition is usually additive. A *synergistic* effect is the situation in which the combined effect of two chemicals is much greater than the sum of the effect of each agent given alone (example: 2 + 3 = 20). For example, both carbon tetrachloride and ethanol are hepatotoxic agents, but together they produce much more liver injury than the mathematical sum of their individual effects on the liver would suggest. *Potentiation* is the situation when one substance does not have a toxic effect on a certain organ or system, but when added to another chemical it makes the latter much more toxic (example: 0 + 2 = 10). Isopropanol, for example, is not hepatotoxic, but when isopropanol is added to carbon tetrachloride, the hepatotoxicity of carbon tetrachloride is much greater than when it is not given with isopropanol. *Antagonism* is the situation in which two chemicals, when given together, interfere with each other's actions or one interferes with the action of the other chemical (example 4 + 6 = 8, 4 + (−4) = 0, 4 + 0 = 1). Antagonistic effects of chemicals are often very desirable effects in toxicology and are the basis of many antidotes. There are four major types of antagonism: functional antagonism, chemical antagonism, dispositional antagonism, and receptor antagonism. *Functional antagonism* is when two chemicals counterbalance each other by producing opposite effects on the same physiologic function. Advantage is taken of this principle in that the blood pressure can markedly fall during severe barbiturate intoxication, and it can be effectively antagonized by intravenous administration of a vasopressor agent such as norepinephrine or metaraminol. Similarly, many chemicals, when given at toxic dose levels, produce convulsions and the convulsions can often be controlled by giving anticonvulsants such as the short-acting barbiturates (example: amobarbital). *Chemical antagonism or inactivation* is simply a reaction between two chemicals to produce a less toxic product. For example, dimercaprol (BAL) chelates with various metals such as arsenic, mercury, and lead, which decreases their toxicity. The use of antitoxins to treat various toxins is an example of chemical antagonism. The use of the strongly basic low-molecular-weight protein protamine sulfate to form a stable complex with heparin, which abolishes its anticoagulant activity, is another example.

Dispositional antagonism is the situation in which the disposition, that is the absorption, metabolism, distribution, or excretion of the chemical, is altered so that less of the toxic compound reaches the target organ or the duration at the target organ is less. Thus, the prevention of absorption of a toxicant by ipecac or charcoal and the increased excretion of a chemical by administering an osmotic diuretic or by altering the pH of the urine are examples of dispositional antagonism. If the parent compound is responsible for the toxicity of the chemical (such as the organophosphate insecticide paraxon) and its metabolites are less toxic than the parent compound, then increasing the compound's biotransformation by a microsomal enzyme inducer (like phenobarbital) will decrease its toxicity. However, if the chemical's toxicity is largely due to a metabolic product (such as the organophosphate insecticide parathion), then inhibiting its biotransformation by an inhibitor of microsomal enzyme activity (SKF-525a or piperonyl butoxide) will decrease its toxicity. *Receptor antagonism* is when two chemicals that bind to the same receptor produce less of an effect when given together than the addition of their separate effects (example: 4 + 6 = 8) or when one chemical antagonizes the effect of the second chemical (example: 0 + 4 = 1). Receptor antagonists are often termed blockers. This concept is used to advantage in the clinical treatment of poisoning. The receptor antagonist naloxone is used for treating the respiratory depression effects of morphine and other morphine-like narcotics. The treatment of organic phosphate insecticide poisoning with atropine is an example not of the antidote competing with the poison for the receptor but rather blocking the receptor responsible for the toxic effect, which is due to the excess acetylcholine produced by poisoning of the acetylcholinesterase by the organic phosphate.

DOSE RESPONSE

The characteristics of exposure and the spectrum of effects come together in a correlative relationship customarily referred to as the dose-response relationship. This relationship is the most fundamental and pervasive concept in toxicology. Indeed, an understanding of the relationship and the facile use of its dimensions constitute the essence of the study of toxic materials.

Although a full exposition of the intricacies of

dose and response entails many complexities, only a few basic assumptions form the skeleton of the relationship. In viewing data presentation such as that given in Figure 2–2, an implicit assumption of causality is made. To arrive at a quantitative and precise statement of the relation between a toxic material and an observed effect or response, therefore, one must know with reasonable certainty that the relationship is indeed a causal one. Examination of the literature readily reveals that the language and form of a dose-response relationship appear in other contexts. For example, an epidemiologic study might result in discovery of an "association" between a response (e.g., disease) and one or more impinging variables. Frequently the data are amenable to presentation in terms similar to those employed in the experimental use of

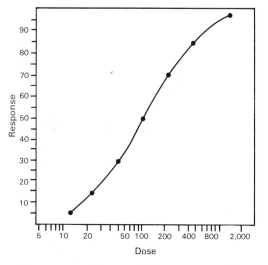

Figure 2–2.   Diagram of dose-response relationship.

"dose-response" in pharmacology and toxicology.

The use of dose-response expressions in such a study is convenient. It is also meaningful in many instances because it carries an implication that some part or all of the response may be causally related to a portion of the environment. Despite the value of such studies and despite the fact that similar terms can be used to express the data, the use of dose-response in this context is suspect. One is usually in some doubt about the identity of the specific toxic agent or the true dose to which the organism has been exposed or the site and relative specificity of the response, or all of these. In its most strict usage, then, the dose-response relationship is firmly based on the knowledge or a reasonable presumption that the effect is a result of the known toxic agent(s).

A second assumption seems simple and obvious, namely, that the response is, in fact, related to the dose. Perhaps because of its apparent simplicity this assumption is often a source of misunderstanding. The assumption is really a composite of three others that will recur frequently.

1. There is a molecular or receptor site (or sites) with which the chemical interacts to produce the response.

2. The production of a response and the degree of response are related to the concentration of the agent at the reactive site.

3. The concentration at the site is, in turn, related to the administered dose.

Thus, the numerical and graphic dimensions of the dose-response relationship include the assumptions that (1) the response is a function of the concentration at a site, (2) the concentration at the site is a function of the dose, and (3) response and dose are causally related.

In assessing the safety of a substance it is necessary to have both a quantifiable method of measuring and a precise means of expressing the toxicity. There are a great variety of criteria or end points of toxicity that could be used. The ideal criterion would be one closely associated with the molecular events resulting from exposure to the toxin. Early in the assessment of toxicity such an ideal is usually unapproachable; indeed, it might not be approachable at all even for well-known toxicants.

Failing in a mechanistic, molecular ideal criterion of toxicity, one looks to a measure of toxicity that is unequivocal and clearly relevant to the toxic effect. For example, with a new compound chemically related to the class of organophosphate insecticides, one might approach the measurement of toxicity by measuring inhibition of cholinesterase in blood. In this way one would be measuring, in a readily accessible system by a technique that is convenient and reasonably precise, a prominent effect of the chemical and one that is usually pertinent to the mechanism by which toxicity is produced.

The selection of a toxic end point for measurement is not always so straightforward. Even the example cited above may be misleading as an organophosphate may produce a decrease in blood cholinesterase, but this change may not be directly related to its toxicity (DuBois, 1961; Doull, 1972). As additional data are gathered to suggest a mechanism of toxicity for any substance other measures might be selected. Although many end points are quantitative and precise, they are often indirect measures of toxicity. Changes in enzyme levels in blood can be indicative of tissue damage such as SGOT and SGPT measurement in suggesting liver damage or cardiac dysfunction. Patterns of isozymes and their alteration may provide insight as to the organ or system that is the site of toxic effects. These measures may not be directly related to the mechanism of the toxic action.

Many direct measures of effect are also not necessarily related to the mechanism by which a substance produces its harm to the organism but have the advantage of permitting a causal relation to be drawn between the agent and its action. For example, measurement of the alteration of the tone of smooth or skeletal muscle for substances acting on the muscles represents a rather fundamental approach to toxicologic assessment. Similarly, measures of heart rate, blood pressure, electrical activity of heart muscle, nerve, or brain are examples of the use of physiologic parameters as indices of toxicity. Measurement can also take the form of a still higher level of integration, such as the degree of motor activity or behavioral change.

The measurements used as examples all assume prior information about the toxicant, such as its target organ or site of action or a fundamental effect. Such information is usually available only after toxicologic screening and testing using other measures of toxicity. With a new substance the customary starting point in toxicologic evaluation utilizes lethality as an index. Measurement of lethality is precise, quantal, and unequivocal and is, therefore, useful in its own right if only to suggest the level and magnitude of the potency of the substance. Lethality provides a measure of comparison among many substances whose mechanism and sites of action may be markedly different. Further, the lethality measure is the medium through which to obtain clues to the direction to be taken in further studies. This comes about in two important ways. First, simply recording a death is not an adequate means of conducting a lethality study with a new substance. A key element must be a careful, disciplined, detailed observation of the intact animal extending from the time of administration of the toxicant to the death of the animal. From properly conducted observation, immensely informative data can be gathered by the trained person. Second, a lethality study ordinarily is supported by histologic examination of major tissues and organs for abnormalities. From the latter observations, one can usually glean more specific information about the events leading to the lethal effect, target organ(s) involved, and often a preview of possible mechanisms of toxicity at a relatively fundamental level.

Whatever response is selected for measurement, the relation between the degree of response of the biologic system and the amount of toxicant administered assumes a form that occurs so consistently as to be considered classic and fundamental and is referred to as the dose-response relationship. This is the relationship that Trevan (1927) envisioned in his introduction of LD50. In Figure 2–2 is presented the typical sigmoid form that is found when this relationship is measured. The ordinate is simply labeled "response"; this may be the degree of response in an individual or system or the fraction of a population responding. A distinction is sometimes made between a quantal or "all-or-none" response and a "graded" response. Although the distinction may be useful for some purposes, for practical and sound conceptual reasons they can be considered to be identical. As an illustration consider the hypothetic curve in Figure 2–2 as representative of cholinesterase inhibition in the presence of an organophosphate, smooth muscle contraction with Ba^{2+}, bone marrow depression with benzene, or similar graded responses to increasing doses. Many other examples are applicable.

In toxicology the quantal dose-response is used extensively. Determination of the median lethal dose (LD50) is usually the first experiment performed with a new chemical. In practice this is experimentally determined, usually using mice or rats and using either the oral or intraperitoneal route of administration. At least ten animals are used per dose and a range of doses is used so that at least three and preferably more of the doses result in producing some deaths and some survivals, i.e., that kill less than 100 percent and more than 0 percent. If a large number of doses is used with a large number of animals per dose, a sigmoid dose-response curve is observed as depicted in the top panel of Figure 2–3. With the lowest dose given (6 mg/kg), 1 percent of the animals died. A normally distributed sigmoid curve such as this one approaches a response of 0 percent as the dose is decreased and approaches 100 percent as the dose is increased but theoretically never passes through 0 and 100 percent. However, the minimally effective dose of any chemical that evokes a stated all-or-none response is called the *threshold dose* even though it cannot be determined experimentally.

The sigmoid curve has a relatively linear portion between 16 and 84 percent, which is used to draw the line to determine the LD50 and the slope of the LD50 line. These values represent the limits of one standard deviation of the mean (and the median) in a truly normal population. However, it is usually not practical to describe the dose-response curve from this type of plot because one does not usually have large enough sample sizes to adequately define the sigmoid curve.

The middle panel of Figure 2–3 shows that

quantal dose responses such as lethality exhibit a normal gaussian distribution. This panel exhibits the frequency histogram and also shows the relationship between dose and effect. The data used to construct this histogram are the

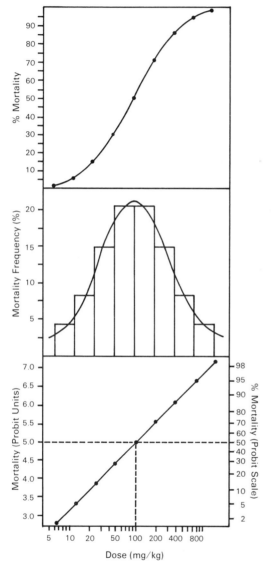

Figure 2–3. Diagram of quantal dose-response relationship. The abscissa is a log dose of the chemical. In the top panel the ordinate is percent mortality; in the middle panel the ordinate is mortality frequency; and in the bottom panel the mortality is in probit units.

same as those used in the top panel. The bars represent the percent of animals that died at each dose minus the percent that died at the lower dose. One can clearly see that only a few animals responded at the lowest dose and also a small

number at the highest dose. Larger numbers of animals responded to doses intermediate between these two extremes, and the maximum frequency of response occurred in the middle portion of the dose range. Thus, we have a bell-shaped curve known as a *normal frequency distribution*. The reason for this normal distribution is that there are differences in susceptibility among individuals to chemicals, which is known as *biologic variation*. Those animals responding at the left end of the curve are referred to as the *hypersusceptible* animals and those at the right end of the curve as the *resistant* animals.

In a normally distributed population, the mean ±1 standard deviation (SD) represents 68.3 percent of the population, the mean ±2 SD represents 95.5 percent of the population, and the mean ±3 SD equals 99.7 percent of the population. Since quantal dose-response phenomena are usually normally distributed, one can convert the percent response to units of deviation from the mean or normal equivalent deviations (NED). Thus, the NED for a 50 percent response is zero; an NED of +1 is equated with 84.1 percent response. Later it was suggested (Bliss, 1935, 1952, 1957) that units of NED be converted by the addition of five to the value to avoid negative numbers and that these converted units be called probit units. The probit, then, is an NED plus five. In this transformation a 50 percent response becomes a probit of 5, +1 deviation becomes a probit of 6, and −1 deviation is a probit of 4.

PERCENT RESPONSE	NED	PROBIT
0.1	−3	2
2.3	−2	3
15.9	−1	4
50.0	0	5
84.1	+1	6
97.7	+2	7
99.9	+3	8

The data given in the top two panels of Figure 2–3 are replotted in the bottom panel with the mortality plotted in the probit units. The data in the top panel (which was in the form of a sigmoid curve) and in the middle panel (a bell-shaped curve) form straight lines when transformed into probit units. In essence, what is accomplished in a probit transformation is an adjustment of mortality or other quantal data to an assumed normal population distribution, which results in a straight line. The LD50 is obtained by drawing a horizontal line from the probit unit 5, which is the 50 percent mortality point, to the dose-effect line. At the point of intersection a vertical line is drawn and this line intersects the abscissa at the LD50 point. It is

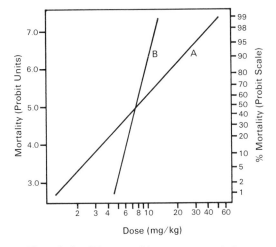

Figure 2–4. Diagram of dose-response relationships. Chemical B has a much steeper dose response than chemical A.

evident from the line that information with respect to the lethal dose for 90 percent of the animals or for 10 percent of the animals may be derived by a similar procedure. In addition to the LD50, the slope of the dose-response curve can also be obtained. Figure 2–4 demonstrates the dose-response curves for mortality to two compounds. It is evident that the LD50 for both compounds is the same (8 mg/kg). However, the slopes of the dose-response curves are quite different. At one-half of the LD50 of the compounds (4 mg/kg) less than 1 percent of the animals exposed to compound B would die, but 20 percent of the animals given compound A would die. For more information on the mechanics of determining the LD50 and the slope of line, the reader is referred to Bliss (1957), Finney (1971), and Litchfield and Wilcoxon (1949). All of these methods require a large number of animals (approximately 50) to obtain an LD50. Other statistical techniques are available to estimate the LD50 that can use a

smaller number of animals, such as the "up-and-down method" of Brownlee and associates (1953) and the "moving-average method" of Thompson and Weil (1952; Weil, 1952).

The quantal or "all-or-none" response is not limited to lethality. Similar-type dose-effect curves can be constructed for cancer, liver injury, and other types of toxic responses as well as for beneficial therapeutic responses such as sleep. While some toxic and therapeutic responses are all-or-none such as sleep, other graded responses such as blood pressure can be transformed into quantal responses. This is usually performed by quantitating that parameter (example: blood pressure) in a large number of control animals and determining its standard deviation, which is a measure of its variability. Since the mean ± 3 standard deviation represents 99.7 percent of the population, one can assign all animals that lie outside of this range after treatment with the chemical as exhibiting an effect and those lying within this range as not being affected by the chemical. Using a series of doses of the chemical, one can thus construct a quantal dose-response curve similar to that described above for lethality.

In Figures 2–2, 2–3, and 2–4, the dose has been given on a log basis. Although the use of the log of the dose is empiric, log dose plots usually provide a more nearly linear representation of the data. It must be remembered, however, that this is not universally the situation. Some radiation effects, for example, give a better probit fit when the dose is expressed arithmetically rather than logarithmically. There are other situations in which other functions (e.g., power functions) of dose provide a better fit to the data than the log function. It is also conventional to express the dose in milligrams per kilogram. It might be argued that expression of dose on a mole-per-kilogram basis would be better particularly for making comparisons of a series of compounds. Although such an argument has considerable merit, dose is usually expressed as milligrams per kilogram.

Table 2–3 COMPARISON OF DOSAGE BY WEIGHT AND SURFACE AREA (100 mg/kg) DOSE

SPECIES	WEIGHT (g)	SURFACE (cm²)	DOSE BY WEIGHT (mg)	DOSE BY SURFACE (mg)	RATIO
Mouse	20	36	2	2	1
Rat	200	325	20	14	1.43
Guinea pig	400	564	40	24	1.65
Rabbit	1500	1272	150	55	2.74
Cat	2000	1381	200	60	3.46
Monkey	4000	2975	400	128	3.12
Dog	12,000	5766	1200	248	4.82
Man	70,000	18,000	7000	776	9.08

One might also view dosage on the basis of weight as being not as appropriate as other bases such as surface area. Such a dosage term would reduce interspecies variation and even reduce variation in a single species where there is a wide variation in size, such as occurs in man. In Table 2–3 selected values are given to compare the differences in dosage by the two means. Given a dose of 100 mg/kg, it can be seen that the range of the ratio of dose by weight and dose by surface area extends from unity for the mouse to about 9:1 for man.

Figure 2–5 illustrates the quantal dose-response curve for a therapeutic effect of a chemical (ED), such as anesthesia, a toxic effect (TD), such as liver injury, and the lethal dose (LD). As depicted in Figure 2–5, a parallelism is

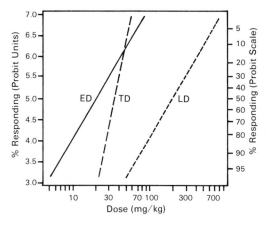

Figure 2–5. Comparison of effective dose (*ED*), toxic dose (*TD*), and lethal dose (*LD*). Plot of log dose versus percent of population responding in probit units.

apparent between the effective dose curve and the toxicity curve expression of lethality (LD). It is tempting to view the parallel dose-response curves as indicative of identity of mechanism, i.e., to conclude that the lethality is a simple extension of the therapeutic effect. While this conclusion may ultimately prove to be correct in any particular case, it is not warranted solely on the basis of the two parallel lines. The same admonition applies to any pair of parallel "effect" curves or any other pair of toxicity or lethality curves.

The hypothetic curves in Figure 2–5 illustrate two other interrelated points, viz., the importance of the selection of the toxic criterion and the interpretation of comparative effect. The concept of the "therapeutic index" introduced by Paul Ehrlich (1913) can be used to illustrate this relationship. Although therapeutic index is directed to a comparison of a therapeutically

effective dose relative to toxicity, it is equally applicable to considerations of comparative toxicity. The *therapeutic index* (TI) in its broadest sense is defined as the ratio of the dose required to produce a toxic effect to that required to produce a desired therapeutic response. Similarly, an index of comparative toxicity is obtained by either the ratio of doses of two different materials to produce identical responses or the ratio of doses of the same material necessary to yield different toxic effects.

The most commonly used index of effect, whether beneficial or toxic, is the median dose, i.e., the dose required to produce a response in 50 percent of a population (or to produce 50 percent of a maximal response). From Figure 2–5 one can approximate a "therapeutic index" using these median doses.

$$TI = \frac{LD50}{ED50}$$

The ED50 is approximately 20 and the LD50 about 200; thus, the therapeutic index is 10, a very respectable number suggesting a wide margin of safety. Obviously, such a measure of safety would be inadequate if one notes that there is actually an overlap of the populations such that a dose that is effective in one segment of the population would be toxic to another fraction of the population.

From these considerations, it is clear that (1) lethality alone cannot serve as the type of toxic effect best suited for estimation of safety, and (2) use of median figures might allow for more overlap of populations than would be desirable. A therapeutic index or a measure of comparative toxicity then is more valuable and reliable if the effect selected as a criterion is relatively basic or subtle and one uses such measures as the TD1 and ED99 to separate the populations and their responses. It should also be noted that the curve for the toxicity measurement is not parallel but intersects the line designating an "effective dose." (It also does not parallel the lethality curve.) The degree of selectivity exercised in choosing a toxic end point and the relative seriousness of the toxic effect chosen are major determinants to both the value of the comparative curves and the interpretations of the relative degree of safety.

SELECTIVE TOXICITY

Selective toxicity means that a chemical produces injury to one kind of living matter without harming some other kind, even though the two may be in intimate contact (Albert, 1965, 1973). The living matter that is injured is known as the *uneconomic form*, and the matter protected is called the *economic form*. They may be related to one another as parasite and host, or they may be two tissues in one organism. This biologic diversity interferes with the ability of the toxicologist to predict the toxic effects of a chemical in one species (man) from experiments performed in another species (laboratory animal). However, by taking advantage of the biologic diversity, it may be possible to develop an agent that is lethal for an undesired species and harmless for other species. In agriculture, for example, there are fungi, insects, and even competitive plant life that injure the crop and thus selective pesticides are needed. Also, animal husbandry and human medicine require agents that are selectively toxic to the uneconomic form but do not produce damage to the economic form of living matter.

Drugs and other chemical agents used for selective toxic purposes are selective for one of two reasons. Either (1) the chemical is equitoxic to both economic and uneconomic cells but is accumulated mainly by the uneconomic cells, or (2) it reacts fairly specifically with (a) a cytologic or (b) a biochemical feature that is absent from or does not play an important part in the host (Albert, 1965, 1973). Selectivity due to differences in distribution is usually the result of differences in absorption, biotransformation, or excretion of the toxicant. The selective toxicity of an insecticide spray may be partly because a greater surface area per unit weight causes the insect to absorb a proportionally greater dose than the mammal being sprayed. The effectiveness of radioactive iodine in the treatment of hyperthyroidism is due to the selective ability of the thyroid gland to accumulate iodine. A major reason why chemicals are toxic to one type of tissue and not another is that there are differences in accumulation of the ultimate toxic compound in various tissues due to the differences in the ability of various tissues to biotransform the chemical into the ultimate toxic reactive product. Thus carbon tetrachloride is toxic to the liver because the liver has a high capacity to biotransform the CCl_4 to the trichloromethyl free radical ($CCl_3 \cdot$). While it has been stated that one reason for selective toxicity is due to differences in accumulation of the chemical in economic and uneconomic cells, this should not be construed to mean that the target organ for toxicity is the organ that concentrates that chemical to the highest degree. For example, the chlorinated hydrocarbon insecticides, such as DDT, attain the highest concentration in the fat depots of the body but produce no known toxic effects there.

Selective toxicity due to differences in comparative cytology is exemplified by comparison of plant and animal cells. Plants differ from animals in many ways: e.g., absence of a nervous system, an efficient circulatory system, and muscles and the presence of a photosynthetic mechanism and cell walls. The fact that bacteria contain cell walls and man does not has been utilized in developing selective toxic chemotherapeutic agents, like penicillin and cephalosporins, that kill the bacteria but are relatively nontoxic to the mammalian cells.

Selective toxicity can also be a result of a difference in biochemistry of the two types of cells. For example, bacteria do not absorb folic acid but synthesize it from p-aminobenzoic acid, glutamic acid, and pteridine, while mammals cannot synthesize folic acid but absorb it from their diet. Thus, sulfonamide drugs are selectively toxic to the bacteria because the sulfonamides, which resemble p-aminobenzoic acid in both charge and dimensions, antagonize the incorporation of p-aminobenzoic acid into the folic acid molecule, a reaction that man does not carry out.

DESCRIPTIVE ANIMAL TOXICITY TESTS

Two main principles underlie all descriptive animal toxicity testing. The first is that the effects produced by the compound in laboratory animals, when properly qualified, are applicable to man. This premise underlies all of experimental biology and medicine. On the basis of dose per unit of body surface, toxic effects in man are usually in the same range as those in experimental animals. On a body weight basis, man is generally more vulnerable than the experimental animal, probably by a factor of about ten. With an awareness of these quantitative differences, appropriate safety factors can be applied to calculate relatively safe dosages for man. All known chemical carcinogens in man, with the possible exception of arsenic, are carcinogenic in some species but not in all laboratory animals. This species variation appears to be due to differences in biotransformation of the procarcinogen to the active carcinogen.

The second main principle is that exposure of experimental animals to toxic agents in high doses is a necessary and valid method of discovering possible hazards in man. This principle is based on the quantal dose-response concept that the incidence of an effect in a population is greater as the dose or exposure increases. Practical considerations in the design of experimental model systems require that the number of animals used in experiments on toxic materials will always be small compared with the size of the human populations similarly at risk. To obtain statistically valid results from such small groups of animals requires the use of relatively large doses so that the effect will occur frequently enough to be detected. For example, an incidence of a serious toxic effect, such as cancer, as low as 0.01 percent would represent 20,000 people in a population of 200 million and would be considered unacceptably high. To detect such a low incidence in experimental animals directly would require a minimum of about 30,000 animals. For this reason, we have no choice but to give large doses to relatively small groups and then to use toxicologic reason in extrapolating the results to estimate risk at low doses.

The first toxicity test performed on a new chemical is the determination of the LD50 via two routes of administration (usually orally and intravenously), one being the intended route of exposure, in several species. The species most often used are the mouse, rat, rabbit, and dog. In the mouse and rat the LD50 is usually determined as described earlier in this chapter, but in the larger species only an approximation of the LD50 is obtained by increasing the dose until serious toxic effects of the chemical are demonstrated. The number of animals that die in a 7- or 14-day period after a single dose is tabulated. In addition to mortality, periodic examination of test animals should be conducted for signs of intoxication, lethargy, behavioral modifications, morbidity, etc.

The ability of the chemical to irritate the skin and eye after an acute exposure is usually determined in the rabbit. For the dermal irritation test, the rabbits are prepared by removal of the fur on a section of their backs by electric clippers. The chemical is applied to the skin under a covered patch and usually kept in contact for a period of either 4 or 24 hours. The degree of skin irritation is scored for erythema and eschar formation, edema formation, and corrosive action. These dermal irritation observations are repeated at various intervals after the covered patch is removed. To determine the degree of ocular irritation to the chemical, the agent is instilled into one eye of each of the test rabbits. The eyes of the rabbits are then examined at various times after application.

The toxicity of the chemical after subchronic exposure is then determined. Subchronic exposure can last for different periods of time, but 90 days is the most common test duration. The subchronic study is usually performed in two species (rat and dog) by the route of intended use or exposure. At least three doses are employed (a high dose that produces marked toxicity, a low dose that produces no toxic effects, and an intermediate dose) using 15 rats of each sex per dose and four dogs of each sex per dose. Observations on the test animals include mortality, body weight changes, diet consumption, hematology, and clinical chemistry measurements. Hemato-

logy measurements usually made include hemoglobin concentration, hematocrit, erythrocyte counts, leukocyte counts, differential counts, clotting time, and prothrombin time. Clinical chemistry determinations commonly made include glucose, urea nitrogen, glutamic pyruvic transaminase, alkaline phosphatase, creatinine, bilirubin, triglycerides, and cholesterol. At the end of the experiment the gross and microscopic condition of the organs and tissues (about 15 to 20) and the weight of various organs (about 12) are recorded and evaluated. The subchronic toxicity studies not only characterize the dose-response relationship of a test substance following repeated administration but also provide data for a more reasonable prediction of appropriate doses for the chronic exposure studies.

After the acute and subchronic studies are completed on an agent and after some special studies that might be required due to known toxicity of that class of agents (and the agent is a drug), the company can file an IND (Investigational New Drug) to the FDA and, if approved, clinical trials can commence. At the same time that phase I, phase II, and phase III clinical trials are being performed, chronic exposure of the animals to the test compound can be performed in laboratory animals as well as additional specialized tests.

The long-term or chronic exposure studies are performed similarly to the subchronic studies except the period of exposure is longer. The length of exposure is somewhat dependent on the intended period of exposure in man. If the agent is a drug that is planned to be used for short periods of time, such as an antimicrobial agent, a chronic exposure of six months might be sufficient, whereas if the agent is a food additive and will be used in man for a longer duration, then a chronic study up to 1.5 to 2 years is likely to be required.

Chronic exposure studies are often used to determine the carcinogenic potential of chemicals. These studies are usually performed in rats and mice and extend over the average lifetime of the species. Thus, for a rat exposure is two years. To assure that 30 rats per dose survive the two-year study, 60 rats per group per sex are often started in the study. Both gross and microscopic pathologic examinations are made, not only on those animals that survive the chronic exposure but also on those that die early. (See Chapt. 6 for a detailed discussion of the use of the chronic test for detecting carcinogens.)

Teratogenic potential of chemicals is also determined in laboratory animals. Teratology is defined as the study of malformations induced during development from conception to birth. Teratogenic studies are usually performed in rats and rabbits with two doses of the test chemical (both of which produce no maternal toxicity). Teratogens are most effective when administered during the first trimester, the period of organogenesis. Thus, the animals are usually exposed on days 6 to 15 of gestation and the fetuses removed by cesarean section prior to the estimated time of delivery. The uterus is examined for the number of implantations, and dead and living fetuses are counted, weighed, and examined grossly. Some fetuses are examined histologically and others are cleared and stained for skeletal abnormalities. Since teratogens can produce functional as well as morphologic changes, functional changes in the offspring, such as behavioral changes, are sometimes monitored at various times after delivery of the animals.

Fertility and reproductive toxicity studies are usually performed in rats at dosage levels similar to those used for the teratology studies. In a typical reproductive study the male parent is given the agent for 60 to 80 days and the female for 14 days prior to mating. The percentage of animals that become pregnant is determined plus the number of stillborn and live offspring, their weight, growth, survival, and the general condition of the offspring during the first three weeks of life.

The perinatal and postnatal toxicities of agents are also often examined. This test is performed by administering the test agent to the rat from the fifteenth day of gestation throughout delivery and lactation and determining its effect on birth rate, survival, and growth of the offspring.

Investigation of the mutagenic potential of the chemical is becoming increasingly important. Mutagenesis is the ability of chemicals to cause changes in the genetic material in the nucleus of the cell in ways that can be transmitted during cell division. If mutations are present in the genetic material at the time of fertilization in either the egg or sperm, the resulting combination of genetic material may not be viable and death may occur in the early stages of embryonic cell division. Alternatively, the mutation in the genetic material may not affect early embryogenesis but may result in death of the fetus at a later developmental period, resulting in abortion. Congenital abnormalities may also result from mutations. Since the initiation event of chemical carcinogenesis is thought to be a mutagenic event, mutagenic tests are often used to screen for potential carcinogens. Several *in vivo* and *in vitro* procedures have been devised for testing chemicals for their ability to cause mutations. Since some mutations are visible with the light microscope, cytogenic analysis of bone marrow smears after the animals have been exposed to the test agent is used as a mutagenesis test. Since most mutations are incompatible with normal development, the mutagenic potential of a chemical can also be measured by the dominant lethal test. This test is usually performed in rodents. The male is exposed to the test compound for three months and then mated with two untreated females. The females are sacrificed before term and the number of live embryos and the number of corpora lutea determined. The mutagenic test receiving the widest attention at the present time is the reverse mutation test developed by Ames and colleagues (Ames *et al.*, 1975). This test uses a mutant strain of *Salmonella typhimurium* that lacks coding for the enzyme phosphoribosyl ATP synthetase, which is required for histidine synthesis. Thus, this strain is unable to grow in a histidine-deficient medium unless a reverse mutation has occurred. Since many chemicals are not mutagenic or carcinogenic unless they are biotransformed to a toxic product by the endoplasmic reticulum (microsomes), rat liver microsomes are usually added to the medium containing the mutant strain and the reverse mutation is then quantitated by the growth of the strain in a histidine-deficient medium.

Most of the tests described above will be included in a "standard" toxicity testing protocol since most of these tests are required by the appropriate regulatory agency. Additional tests may also be required or included in the testing protocol to provide information relating to a special route of exposure (inhalation) or to a special effect (behavior). Inhalation toxicity tests in animals are usually carried out in a dynamic (flowing) gassing chamber rather than in static chambers to avoid settling problems with particulates and exhaled gas complications. Such studies usually require special dispersing and analytic methodology depending on whether the agent to be tested is a gas, vapor, or aerosol; additional information on methods, concepts, and problems associated with inhalation toxicology are considered in Chapters 12 and 24 of this text. A similar discussion of behavioral toxicology can be found in Chapter 9 of this text. The exposure duration for both inhalation and behavioral toxicity tests can be acute, subchronic, or chronic, but acute studies are more common with inhalation toxicology and chronic studies are more common with behavioral toxicology. Other special types of animal toxicity tests include immunotoxicology, toxicokinetics (absorption, distribution, metabolism, and excretion), the development of appropriate antidotes and treatment regimes for poisoning, and the development of analytic techniques to detect residues of the test agent in tissues and other biologic materials.

PREDICTIVE TOXICOLOGY

The main purpose of the toxicity tests described in the preceding section of this chapter is to provide a data base that can be used to assess the risk (or evaluate the hazard) associated with a situation in which the chemical agent, the subject, and the exposure conditions are defined. It is evident that the ideal situation is one in which the agent, subject, and exposure conditions used for the toxicity tests are identical to those which will be encountered in the situation where the risk assessment is desired. Thus, by carrying out toxicity studies on various forms of birds, fish, and other wildlife, it is usually possible to establish with reasonable certainty a safe or no-observed-effect level (NOEL) for the species tested [also referred to as no-effect level (NEL) and no-observed-adverse-effect level (NOAEL)]. In most cases, however, there are differences between the toxicity testing situation and the "real world" situation where the risk estimate is desired that require extrapolation of the data base or prediction of the hazard in areas not covered by the data base. Changes in the formulation of the agent, the use of animal tests for estimating risk to man, changes in route, dose, duration, and frequency of exposure are all examples of situations in which predictive toxicology is employed. In most cases, predictive toxicology provides the risk portion of the risk-benefit analysis, which is the basis of regulatory toxicology (see Chapter 29 in this text).

The traditional approach for establishing safe levels or tolerances for chemical agents to which man may be exposed is to reduce the threshold dose or NOEL by a safety factor that takes into consideration both the intraspecies and interspecies variation. A safety factor of ten might be used, for example, with an agent for which there exist toxicity data in man rather than the factor of 100 (tenfold for each type of variation), which is commonly used for animal toxicity test data. Conversely, higher safety factors might be used in situations where there is increased concern about the type of adverse effect (irreversible toxicity, for example) or the quality of the data base or the relevance of the animal data to the situation in man (differences in kinetics, target organ, repair processes, etc.). Since the NOEL is by definition a subthreshold dosage level, it is evident that the safety factor approach would not be applicable for agents that produce non-threshold effects. Thus, in the case of carcinogens and mutagens, the argument that these processes have no threshold because their effect can result from a single molecule producing the initiating event (one molecule–one hit) would require that the safe level for such agents be established at less than one molecule (zero tolerance). However, most carcinogens and mutagens exhibit a dose-response relationship, and there is an "apparent" or effective threshold for at least some of these agents, which suggests that such agents should be "controlled" rather than "banned." This and similar problems have stimulated the development of alternative approaches to the hazard evaluation process and particularly to the procedures used to extrapolate the results of animal toxicity data to provide an estimate of risks in man.

One of the major alternatives to the use of safety factors is the risk estimate approach, which is derived, in part, from early attempts to provide a quantitative theory for carcinogenesis. Iverson and Arley (1950), using a mathematical model in which the probability of tumor occurrence was generally related to a polynomial function of the dose, found that in the low-dose range a linear function of dose provided a reasonable approximation. In attempting to extrapolate high-dose animal toxicity data to the low-dose region of interest, however, other mathematical dose-response relationships have been proposed, such as the log-probit method of Mantel and Bryan (1961) and various types of dichotomous response models (probabilistic, hitness, or multievent, time to tumor induction, etc.) (NAS-NRC Drinking Water Committee Reports, 1977, 1979; Crump et al., 1976; Cornfield, 1977; Hoel et al., 1975; Armitage & Doll, 1961). Each of the mathematical models proposed for use in the risk estimate approach has advantages and disadvantages, but they all share the objective of providing a method for assessing risk for nonthreshold agents. It has been suggested that the risk estimate approach may also be applicable to predicting other types of toxicity hazards for agents that exhibit thresholds, and it is likely that extrapolation models will be proposed that provide for this situation. Whether such models could substitute for the safety factor approach, which has the advantage of decades of experience and established relationships to other standards (ADI, TLV, etc.), is debatable, but it is evident that this will be an exciting and controversial area of toxicology for some time. It should be pointed out that both the safety factor approach and the risk estimate approach are risk assessment procedures. In the safety factor approach, it is assumed that the factor used reduces the risk to a negligible level, whereas the risk estimate approach requires a separate determination of what level of risk will be acceptable. It should also be pointed out that epidemiology provides another method of risk assessment that can be used in addition to or in place of predictive toxicology.

REFERENCES

Albert, A.: Fundamental aspects of selective toxicity. *Ann. N.Y. Acad. Sci.*, **123**:5–18, 1965.

Albert, A.: *Selective Toxicity.* Chapman and Hall, London, 1973.

Ames, B.; McCann, J.; and Yamasaki, E.: Methods for detecting carcinogens and mutagens with the Salmonella/mammalian microsome mutagenicity test. *Mutation Res.*, **31**:347–64, 1975.

Armitage, P., and Doll, R.: Stochastic models for carcinogenesis. Proc. Fourth Berkeley Symposium on Mathematical Statistics and Probability, 1961.

Bliss, C. L.: The calculation of the dose-mortality curve. *Ann. Appl. Biol.*, **22**:134–67, 1935.

———.: *The Statistics of Bioassay.* Academic Press, Inc., New York, 1952.

———: Some principles of bioassay. *Am. Sci.*, **45**:449–66, 1957.

Boyd, E. M.: *Predictive Toxicometrics.* Scientechnica Ltd., Bristol, 1970.

Brownlee, K. A.; Hodges, J. L.; and Rosenblatt, M.: The up-and-down method with small samples. *Am. Statist. Assoc. J.*, **48**:262–77, 1953.

Cornfield, J.: Carcinogenic risk assessment. *Science*, **198**:693, 1977.

Crump, K. S.; Hoel, D. G.; Langley, C. H.; and Peto, R.: Fundamental carcinogenic processes and their implication for low-dose risk assessment. *Cancer Res.*, **36**: 2973–96, 1976.

Doull, J.: Personal communication, 1972.

DuBois, K. P.: Potentiation of the toxicity of organophosphorus compounds. *Adv. Pest Control Res.*, **4**:117–51, 1961.

Finney, D. J.: *Probit Analysis.* Cambridge University Press, Cambridge, 1971.

Goldstein, A.; Aronow, L.; and Kalman, S. M.: *Principles of Drug Action.* John Wiley, New York, 1974.

Gunther, R. T.: *The Greek Herbal of Dioscorides.* Magdalen College, Oxford University Press, New York, 1934.

Halstead, B. W.: *Poisonous and Venomous Marine Animals of the World*, Vol. 1, *Invertebrates.* U.S. Govt. Printing Office, Washington, D.C., 1965.

Hoel, D. G.; Gaylor, D. W.; Kirschstein, R. L.; Saffiotti, V.; and Schneiderman, M. A.: Estimation of risks of irreversible-delayed toxicity. *J. Toxicol. Environ. Health*, **1**:133–51, 1975.

Iverson, S., and Arley, N.: On the mechanism of experimental carcinogenesis. *Acta Pathol. Microbiol. Scand.*, **27**:773–803, 1950.

Levine, R. R.: *Pharmacology: Drug Actions and Reactions*, 2nd ed. Little, Brown and Company, Boston, 1978.

Litchfield, J. T., and Wilcoxon, F.: Simplified method of evaluating dose-effect experiments. *J. Pharmacol. Exp. Ther.*, **96**:99–113, 1949.

Loomis, T. A.: *Essentials of Toxicology*, 2nd ed. Lea & Febiger, Philadelphia, 1974.

Mantel, N., and Bryan, W. B.: "Safety" testing of carcinogenic agents. *J. Nat. Cancer Inst.*, **27**:455–70, 1961.

National Academy of Sciences, National Research Council: *Drinking Water and Health.* Report of the Safe Drinking Water Committee, Washington, D.C., 1977, 1979.

Paget, G. E.: *Methods in Toxicology.* Blackwell Scientific Pub. Co., Oxford, 1970.

Rodricks, J. V.: Food hazards of natural origin. *Fed. Proc.*, **37**:2587–93, 1978.

Thompson, W. R., and Weil, C. S.: On the construction of tables for moving average interpolation. *Biometrics*, **8**:51–54, 1952.

Trevan, J. W.: The error of determination of toxicity. *Proc. R. Soc. Lond. (Biol.)*, **101**:483–514, 1927.

Uraguchi, K.: Chronic toxicity of "yellowed rice"—divergence and phase in its development through long-term feeding with hepatoxin. Proc. 23rd International Congress of Physiological Science, 1965, pp. 465–74.

Weil, C. S.: Tables for convenient calculation of median-effective dose (LD_{50} or ED_{50}) and instruction in their use. *Biometrics*, **8**:249–63, 1952.

Chapter 3

ABSORPTION, DISTRIBUTION, AND EXCRETION OF TOXICANTS

Curtis D. Klaassen

INTRODUCTION

The skin is the main barrier that separates man from toxic substances. However, man is not completely separated from his environment and toxicants do enter the body to produce damage. For most toxic agents, the higher the concentration of the toxicant attained in the body, the greater the damage will be. The concentration of the toxicant in the body is obviously a function of the amount of toxicant the individual comes in contact with, but also depends on the rate and amount absorbed, the distribution of the toxicant within the body, the rate of metabolism (biochemical transformation), and the rate of excretion of the toxicant. These factors are depicted in Figure 3–1 and will be discussed in detail in this chapter.

A toxicant is usually absorbed and enters the blood before it produces its undesirable effects, unless it acts topically, as, for example, a caustic agent like acid. The major routes by which toxicants enter the body are the lungs, gastrointestinal tract, and skin. Once the chemical has entered the bloodstream, it is available to go to the site in the body where it produces damage, often termed the target organ. It also may exert its toxic action directly in the bloodstream as is the case with arsine gas, which produces hemolysis. The circulatory system transports the toxicant to other organs where it may produce its toxic action. Mercury and lead produce damage to the central nervous system, kidney, and hematopoietic system, benzene to the hematopoietic system, carbon tetrachloride to the liver, and so forth. For a chemical to produce a toxic effect in a certain organ, the toxic agent must reach that organ, but the organ in which the toxicant is most highly concentrated is not necessarily the organ where most of the tissue damage occurs. For example, the chlorinated hydrocarbon insecticides attain the highest concentration in the fat depots of the body, but produce no known toxic effects there.

The toxicant is eliminated from the blood by biotransformation, excretion, and accumulation at the various storage sites. The relative importance of these processes is dependent on the physical and chemical properties of the toxicant. The kidney plays the major role in the elimination of most toxicants from the body; other organs, however, are of greater importance in the elimination of certain toxicants. An example is excretion by the lungs of a volatile agent such as carbon monoxide or the biliary excretion of a substance such as lead. Although the liver is the organ most active in the biotransformation of toxicants, enzymes in other tissues, such as the esterases in the plasma and enzymes in the kidney, lung, and gastrointestinal tract, may also metabolize the toxicant. Biotransformation is often a prerequisite for the renal excretion of a toxicant because many toxicants are lipid soluble, and these are subsequently reabsorbed by the renal tubules after filtration. After the toxicant is biotransformed, its metabolites may be excreted to the bile, as are the metabolites of DDT, or they may be excreted into the urine, as are the metabolites of organophosphate insecticides.

Cell Membranes

A toxic agent may pass through a number of barriers before achieving a sufficient concentration at the organ where it produces its characteristic lesion. These include the membranes of a number of cells such as the thick layer of cells of the skin, the thin layer in the lung and gastrointestinal tract, the capillary cell, the cells of the organ where the toxicant produces its deleterious effect, and the cells of the organs that eliminate the toxicant from the body. The plasma membranes that surround all of these cells are remarkably similar. The thickness of the cell membrane is on the order of 70 Å. Current concepts that have emerged from electron micrographic, chemical, and physiologic studies

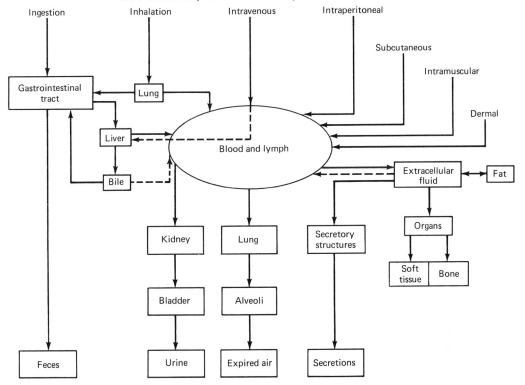

Figure 3–1. Routes of absorption, distribution, and excretion of toxicants in the body. (Courtesy of L. J. Casarett.)

visualize the cell membrane as a bimolecular layer of lipid molecules coated on each side with a protein layer (Cohn, 1971). Certain branches of the protein layer appear to penetrate the lipid bilayer and others extend all the way through. The lipid portion of the membrane consists primarily of lecithin, cephalin, and cholesterol. The fatty acids of the membranes do not have a rigid crystalline structure but at physiologic temperatures are quasi-fluid in character. The fluid character of membranes is largely determined by the structure and relative proportion of unsaturated fatty acids. When the membranes contain more unsaturated fatty acids, they are more fluid, and active transport has been demonstrated to be more rapid (Fox, 1972).

The mechanisms by which a toxicant may pass through a membrane can be divided into two general types: (1) diffusion or passive transfer of the chemical, in which the cell plays no active role in its transfer; and (2) specialized transport, in which the cell takes an active part in the transfer of the toxicant through the membranes.

Passive Transport

Simple Diffusion. Most toxicants cross body membranes by simple diffusion. This can occur for very small hydrophilic compounds by passage through aqueous channels, or more frequently by larger organic molecules that possess a certain degree of lipophilicity, by diffusing through the lipid membrane. Therefore, a lipid-soluble compound like ethyl alcohol readily passes cell membranes by simple diffusion. Ethyl alcohol is absorbed in the stomach and intestine by diffusion and then passes into the central nervous system and other organs also by simple diffusion. The rate of transfer of toxic agents across cell membranes is dependent on their lipid solubility, as measured by the lipid/water partition coefficient, and their concentration gradient across the membrane.

Many toxic chemicals exist in solution in both the ionized and nonionized form. The ionized form is often unable to penetrate the cell membrane because of its low lipid solubility, while in contrast, the nonionized form may be lipid soluble enough to diffuse across cell membranes. Diffusion is dependent on the lipid solubility of the nonionized form of the compound.

The amount of a weak organic acid or base in the nonionized form is dependent on its dissociation constant. The pK_a is an arithmetic expression (similar to pH) and is simply the negative logarithm of the acid dissociation constant. The degree of dissociation and ionization of a weak acid or base is dependent on the pH of the medium. When the pH of a solution is equal to the pK_a of a compound, half exists in the ionized and half in the nonionized state. Conventionally, the dissociation constant for both acids and bases is expressed as a pK_a. An acid with a low pK_a is a strong acid and one with a high pK_a is a weak acid. Conversely, a base with a low pK_a is a weak base and one with a high pK_a a strong base. The pK_a value alone does not indicate whether the compound is acidic or basic because a basic compound can have a pK_a less than 7 and an acidic compound can have a pK_a greater than 7.

The degree of ionization of a chemical depends on both the pK_a of the drug and the pH of the solution in which it is dissolved, a relation described by the Henderson–Hasselbalch equations:

$$\text{For acids} \quad pK_a - pH = \log \frac{[\text{nonionized}]}{[\text{ionized}]}$$

$$\text{For bases} \quad pK_a - pH = \log \frac{[\text{ionized}]}{[\text{nonionized}]}$$

pH	Benzoic Acid	% Nonionized	Aniline	% Nonionized
1	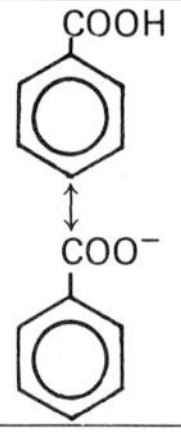 COOH	99.9	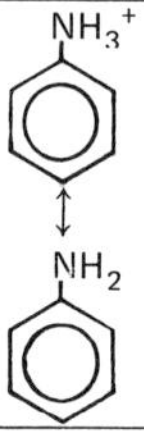 NH₃⁺	
2		99		0.1
3		90		1
4		50		10
5		10		50
6	COO⁻	1	NH₂	90
7		0.1		99

Figure 3–2. Effect of pH on the ionization of benzoic acid ($pK_a = 4$) and analine ($pK_a = 5$).

The effect that the alteration of pH has on the ionization of an acid, benzoic acid, and a base, aniline, is shown in Figure 3–2. At pH 4, 50 percent of benzoic acid is ionized and 50 percent is nonionized, since this is the pK_a of the compound. As the pH decreases, more of the compound assumes the nonionized form because it has gained a proton. Conversely, as the pH increases, less of it is nonionized since it has lost a proton (an acid is a proton donor) and has become negatively charged. For an organic base like aniline, the opposite occurs. That is, as the pH decreases, less of the chemical is in the nonionized state since it has gained a proton and thus a positive charge, and when the pH increases more of it is in the nonionized form. Since the lipid-soluble form (nonionized) of a weak electrolyte is the species that crosses cell membranes, organic acids are more likely to diffuse across membranes when they are in an acidic

environment and organic bases when in a basic environment.

Filtration. When water flows in bulk across a porous membrane, any solute that is small enough to pass through the pores flows with it. Passage through these channels is called filtration, since it involves bulk flow of water due to a hydrostatic or osmotic force. One of the main differences between various body membranes is the size of these channels. In the kidney glomeruli and the capillaries of the body these pores are relatively large (40 Å) and allow molecules smaller than albumin (molecular weight 60,000) to pass through, whereas the channels in most cells are relatively small (4 Å) and allow chemicals only up to a molecular weight of 100 to 200 to pass through (Schanker, 1962; Cohn, 1971).

Special Transport

There are a number of instances in which the movement of a compound across a membrane cannot be explained by simple diffusion or filtration because the compound is too lipid insoluble to dissolve in the cell membranes and too large to flow through the channels. To explain this phenomenon (movement), the existence of specialized transport systems has been postulated. Specialized transport systems are responsible for the transport of many nutrients such as sugars, amino acids, and nucleic acids across cell membranes as well as for the transport of some foreign molecules.

Active Transport. The following are classic properties of an active transport system: (1) chemicals are moved against electrochemical gradients, (2) at high substrate concentrations the transport system is saturated and a transport maximum (Tm) exhibited, (3) the transport system is selective, and certain basic structural requirements exist for chemicals transported by the same mechanism, and thus competitive inhibition can occur among these substances, and (4) the system requires the expenditure of energy so that metabolic inhibitors block the transport process.

Substances that are actively transported across a cell membrane are presumed to pass into the cell interior by forming a complex with a macromolecular carrier on one side of the membrane. The complex subsequently diffuses to the other side of the membrane where the substance is released, and thereafter the carrier returns again to the original surface to repeat the transport process. Active transport is especially important in toxicology for the elimination of foreign compounds from the organism after they have been absorbed. The central nervous system has two transport systems at the choroid plexus, one for organic acids and one for organic bases, to transport substances out of the cerebro-spinal fluid. The kidney likewise has two active transport systems that eliminate foreign compounds from the body, and the liver has at least three active transport systems, one for organic acids, one for organic bases, and one for organic neutral compounds.

Facilitated Diffusion. This term is applied to carrier transport that has all the properties of active transport except that the substrate does not move against a concentration gradient, and the transport process is not energy dependent. The transport of glucose from the gastrointestinal tract into the blood, from plasma into the red blood cells, and from the blood into the central nervous system is thought to occur by this process.

Additional Transport Processes. Additional forms of specialized transport systems have been proposed; however, the actual role of these processes in all parts of the body is not known at the present time. Phagocytosis and pinocytosis are processes in which the cell membrane flows around and engulfs particles. This type of transfer across cell membranes is important for removal of particulate matter from the alveoli by alveolar phagocytes and for removal of some toxic substances from the blood by the reticuloendothelial system of the liver and spleen.

ABSORPTION

The process by which the toxicant is able to pass the body membranes and enter the bloodstream is referred to as absorption. As one might suspect, no specialized system exists in mammals for the sole purpose of absorption of toxicants. The toxicant appears to penetrate the body membranes and enter the bloodstream by the same processes that are utilized for the physiologic absorption of oxygen, foodstuffs, and other nutrients. The main routes by which toxic agents are absorbed are the gastrointestinal tract, lungs, and skin. However, specialized routes of administration such as intraperitoneal and subcutaneous are often used in toxicologic studies.

Absorption of Toxicants by the Gastrointestinal Tract

The gastrointestinal tract is an important route by which toxicants are absorbed. Many environmental toxicants enter the food chain and are absorbed from the gastrointestinal tract. This route of absorption is also of interest to the toxicologist since suicide attempts frequently involve an overdose of an orally administered drug. The gastrointestinal tract is also the most common route by which children are poisoned.

The gastrointestinal tract may be viewed as a tube going through the body. Although it is within the body, its contents can be considered exterior to the body. Therefore, poisons within the gastrointestinal tract do not produce injury to the individual until they are absorbed, unless the agent is caustic or very irritating to the gastrointestinal tract. Most toxicants that are ingested by the oral route do not produce a systemic effect unless they have been absorbed into the bloodstream.

Absorption of toxicants can take place along the length of the gastrointestinal tract, even in the mouth and rectum. For example, some drugs such as nitroglycerin are administered sublingually and other drugs are administered rectally. If a toxicant is a weak organic acid or base, it will tend to be absorbed by diffusion in the part of the gastrointestinal tract in which it exists in the most lipid-soluble form. Since gastric juice is acidic and the intestinal contents are nearly neutral, the lipid solubility of a toxicant can differ markedly in these two areas of the gastrointestinal tract. By using the Henderson-Hasselbalch equation one can determine what percent or fraction of the toxicant is in the nonionized lipid-soluble form and thereby available for absorption. The percent of a weak acid (benzoic) and a weak base (aniline) in the ionized form in the stomach and intestine is indicated on the next page. The conclusions are obvious. A weak organic acid is in the nonionized lipid-soluble form in the stomach and therefore tends to be absorbed by the stomach. On the other hand, a weak organic base is not in the lipid-soluble form in the stomach but is in the intestine. Organic bases tend to be absorbed in the intestine rather than the stomach. The above equations are misleading with respect to the ability of the small intestine to absorb weak organic acids. Since only 1 percent of benzoic acid, for example, is in the lipid-soluble form in the intestine, one might conclude that the intestine has little capacity to absorb organic acids. However, as the intestine absorbs the nonionized benzoic acid, the equilibrium will always be maintained at 1 percent in the lipid-soluble form available for absorption. Moreover, because of the very large surface area of the intestine (the villi and microvilli increase the surface area approximately 600-fold), the overall capacity of the intestine for chemical absorption is magnified.

The mammalian gastrointestinal tract has specialized transport systems for the absorption of nutrients and electrolytes. There is a carrier system for the absorption of glucose and galactose, three separate transport systems for the absorption of amino acids, an active transport system for the absorption of pyrimidines, and separate transport systems for the absorption of iron, calcium, and sodium.

$$pK_a - pH = \log \frac{[\text{nonionized}]}{[\text{ionized}]}$$

Benzoic acid $pK_a \approx 4$

Stomach pH ≈ 2

$$4 - 2 = \log \frac{[\text{nonionized}]}{[\text{ionized}]}$$

$$2 = \log \frac{[\text{nonionized}]}{[\text{ionized}]}$$

$$100 = \frac{[\text{nonionized}]}{[\text{ionized}]}$$

Ratio favors absorption

Intestine pH ≈ 6

$$4 - 6 = \log \frac{[\text{nonionized}]}{[\text{ionized}]}$$

$$-2 = \log \frac{[\text{nonionized}]}{[\text{ionized}]}$$

$$\frac{1}{100} = \frac{[\text{nonionized}]}{[\text{ionized}]}$$

$$pK_a - pH = \log \frac{[\text{ionized}]}{[\text{nonionized}]}$$

Aniline $pK_a \approx 5$

Stomach pH ≈ 2

$$5 - 2 = \log \frac{[\text{ionized}]}{[\text{nonionized}]}$$

$$3 = \log \frac{[\text{ionized}]}{[\text{nonionized}]}$$

$$1000 = \frac{[\text{ionized}]}{[\text{nonionized}]}$$

Intestine pH ≈ 6

$$5 - 6 = \log \frac{[\text{ionized}]}{[\text{nonionized}]}$$

$$-1 = \log \frac{[\text{ionized}]}{[\text{nonionized}]}$$

$$\frac{1}{10} = \frac{[\text{ionized}]}{[\text{nonionized}]}$$

Ratio favors absorption

The absorption of some of these substances is complex and depends on a number of factors. The absorption of iron, for example, is dependent on the need for iron, and its absorption takes place in two steps. Iron first enters the mucosal cells, and then it moves into the blood. The first step is a relatively rapid one, and the second is slow. Consequently, iron accumulates within the mucosal cells as a protein-iron complex termed ferritin. When the iron of the blood is decreased below normal values, this element is liberated from the mucosal stores of ferritin-iron, and more iron is absorbed from the gut in order to replenish these stores. Calcium is also absorbed by a two-step process: calcium is first absorbed from the lumen and then extruded into the interstitial fluid. The first step is faster than the second, and therefore intracellular calcium rises during absorption. Vitamin D is required for both steps in transport of calcium.

Some toxicants can be absorbed by these same specialized transport systems; for example, 5-fluorouracil is absorbed by the pyrimidine transport system (Schanker and Jeffrey, 1961), thallium is transported by the system that normally absorbs iron (Leopold *et al.*, 1969), and lead may be absorbed by the system that normally transports calcium (Sobel *et al.*, 1938). Cobalt and manganese compete for the iron transport system (Schade *et al.*, 1970; Thomson *et al.*, 1971a, 1971b).

There are a few toxicants that are actively absorbed by the gastrointestinal tract; most are absorbed by simple diffusion. Although lipid-soluble substances are more rapidly and extensively absorbed by simple diffusion than are nonlipid-soluble substances, the latter may be absorbed to some degree. Upon oral ingestion, about 10 percent of lead is absorbed, 4 percent of manganese, 1.5 percent of cadmium, and 1 percent of chromium. If the compound is very toxic, this small amount of absorption can produce serious effects. An organic compound that one would not suspect to be absorbed on the basis of the pH-partition hypothesis is the fully ionized quaternary ammonium compound, pralidoxime (2-PAM), which is almost entirely absorbed from the gastrointestinal tract (Levine and Steinberg, 1966). The mechanism or mechanisms by which some lipid-insoluble compounds are absorbed are not clear.

It is interesting that even particles can be absorbed by the gastrointestinal epithelium. Particles of azo dye, variable in size but averaging several hundred Å in diameter, have been shown to be taken up by the duodenum (Barnett, 1959). Emulsions of polystyrene latex particles of 2,200 Å in diameter have been demonstrated to be picked up by the intestinal epithelium, carried through the cytoplasm within intact vesicles, and discharged into the interstices of the lamina propria where entrance is gained into the lymphatics of the mucosa (Sanders and Ashworth, 1961). The particles appear to enter the intestinal cell by pinocytosis, a process that is much more prominent in the newborn than the adult (Williams and Beck, 1969). Therefore, it seems that many types of toxicants can be absorbed to some extent by the gastrointestinal tract.

The stability of chemicals to the acid pH in the stomach, to the enzymes in the stomach and intestine, and to the intestinal flora is of extreme importance. The toxicant may be altered by the action of the acid, enzymes, or intestinal flora to form a new compound that may differ in toxicity from the parent compound. Relative to intravenous exposure, snake venom is nontoxic when administered orally because it is broken down by the digestive enzymes of the gastrointestinal tract. Ingestion of well water with a high nitrate content has produced methemoglobinemia much more frequently in infants than in adults. This is due to the higher pH of the gastrointestinal tract in the newborn and the associated presence of higher flora of certain bacteria, especially *Escherichia coli*, which convert the nitrate into nitrite. The nitrite formed by the bacterial action then produces the methemoglobinemia (Rosenfield and Huston, 1950). Also, the intestinal flora can reduce aromatic nitro groups to aromatic amines that may be goitrogenic or carcinogenic (Thompson *et al.*, 1954). The intestinal flora, more specifically *Aerobacter aerogenes*, have been shown to degrade DDT to DDE (Mendel and Walton, 1966). The formation of carcinogenic nitrosamines can also occur in the stomach when secondary amines, such as those present in fish, vegetables, and fruit juices, come in contact with nitrite, which is often used as a food additive in meats and smoked fish (see Chap. 6).

There are many factors that alter the gastrointestinal absorption of toxicants. Ethylenediaminetetraacetic acid (EDTA) increases the absorption of a number of agents (Levine and Pelikan, 1964). This effect is nonspecific in the sense that EDTA increases the absorption of strong bases, strong acids, and neutral compounds. It appears that EDTA increases the permeability of the membrane by chelating and thus removing calcium.

Alteration of gastrointestinal motility can also affect the absorption of toxicants. A decreased motility tends to increase the overall rate of absorption, whereas an increased intestinal motility tends to decrease absorption (Levine, 1970). This is due to the high absorptive capacity of the proximal segment of the small intestine; almost one-half of the total mucosal area is found in the proximal one-fourth of the small intestine. Therefore, if the toxicant remains in the proximal part of the small intestine for a longer period of time, more will be absorbed.

Experiments have shown that oral toxicity is increased for some chemicals by diluting the dose (Ferguson, 1962; Borowitz *et al.*, 1971). This phenomenon, which has been shown for many xenobiotics, may be explained by the increased rapidity of stomach emptying, which is induced by the increased dosage volume, and thus more rapid absorption in the duodenum because of the larger surface area available.

The absorption of a toxicant from the gastrointestinal tract can also be dependent on the physical properties of the compound, such as the dissolution rate. If the toxicant is relatively insoluble, the compound will have limited contact with the gastrointestinal mucosa and therefore will not be absorbed extensively. If the particle size is large, even less will be absorbed by diffusion since dissolution rate is proportional to particle size (Gorringe and Sproston, 1964; Bates and Gibaldi, 1970). This is the reason that metallic mercury is relatively nontoxic when ingested orally and that finely subdivided arsenic trioxide is significantly more toxic than coarsely powdered material, and that appreciable amounts of the latter may be eliminated in the feces without dissolving (Schwartze, 1923).

A number of other factors have been shown to alter absorption. One metal can alter the absorption of another: cadmium decreases the absorption of zinc and copper, calcium decreases the absorption of cadmium, zinc decreases the absorption of copper, and magnesium decreases the absorption of fluoride (Pfeiffer, 1977). Milk has been found to increase lead absorption (Kello and Kostial, 1973), and starvation enhances the absorption of dieldrin (Heath and Vandekar, 1964). The age of the animal also appears to affect absorption. For example, two-hour-old rats absorb 12 percent of a dose of cadmium while adult rats absorb only 0.5 percent (Sasser and Jarboe, 1977). While lead and many other heavy metals are not readily absorbed from the gastrointestinal tract, EDTA and other chelators will increase the solubility and absorption of metals, and thus it is important not to give a chelator orally while metal is still present in the gastrointestinal tract.

Absorption of Toxicants by the Lungs

It is well known that toxic responses to chemicals can result from their absorption from the lung. The most frequent cause of poisoning, carbon monoxide, and probably the most important occupational disease, silicosis, are results of the absorption or deposition of airborne poisons by the lungs. This route of absorption has even been used in chemical warfare (chlorine gas, phosgene gas, lewisite, mustard gas) and for executing criminals in gas chambers (hydrogen cyanide).

Toxicants that are absorbed by the lung are usually gases such as carbon monoxide, nitrogen dioxide, and sulfur dioxide, vapors of volatile or volatilizable liquids such as benzene and carbon tetrachloride, and aerosols such as silica.

Clouds consisting of solid particulate matter, such as smokes, dusts, or pollen, and fogs or sprays consisting of fine liquid droplets are examples of aerosols.

The site of deposition of aerosols is highly dependent upon the size of the particles. This relationship is discussed in detail in Chapter 12. Particles of 5 μm or larger are usually deposited in the nasopharyngeal region (Fig. 3–3). Those deposited in the unciliated anterior portion of the nose tend to remain at the site of deposition until they are removed by nose wiping, blowing,

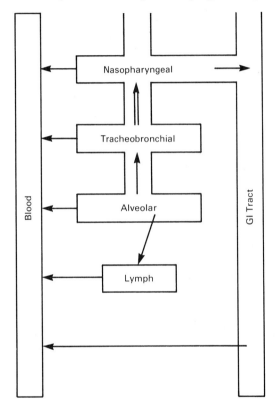

Figure 3–3. Schematic diagram of absorption and translocation of chemicals by the lung.

or sneezing. The mucous blanket of the ciliated nasal surface carries with it insoluble particles as it is propelled by the beating of the cilia. These particles as well as particles inhaled through the mouth are swallowed within minutes and pass to the gastrointestinal tract. Soluble particles may dissolve in the mucus and be carried to the pharynx or be absorbed through the epithelium into the blood.

Particles of 2 to 5 μm are deposited in the tracheobronchiolar regions of the lung where they are cleared by the upward movement of the mucus layer in the ciliated portions of the

respiratory tract. The rate of ciliary movement of the mucus varies in different parts of the respiratory tract but is a rapid and efficient removal mechanism. Measurements have shown transport rates between 0.1 and 1 mm/min resulting in half-lives between 30 and 300 min. Coughing and sneezing result in a rapid movement of the mucus and particulate matter toward the glottis. The particles may also be swallowed and absorbed from the gastrointestinal tract.

Particles 1 μm and below penetrate to the alveolar portions of the lung. They may be absorbed systemically into the blood or may be cleaned by scavenging action of alveolar macrophages.

The alveolar zone is an area of the lung where toxicants are readily absorbed. The surface area is large (50 to 100 sq m) and blood flow to the lung is high and in close proximity to the alveolar air (10 μm). Gas in the alveoli equilibrates almost instantaneously with blood passing through the pulmonary capillary bed. The concentration of the gas in the blood as it leaves the lung is dependent on the solubility of the gas in the blood, where solubility is defined as the ratio of the concentration of dissolved gas in fluid (blood) to the concentration in the gas phase, at equilibrium. This is simply another way of stating Henry's law. Using this definition, it can be shown that chloroform has a high solubility (15) and ethylene a low solubility (0.14). For a substance like ethylene that has a low solubility, only a small percentage of the total gas in the lung is removed by the blood during each respiration. Because the blood is carrying all the gas that it can, increasing the respiratory rate or minute volume would not change the transfer of the gas to the blood. However, increasing the rate of cardiac output would markedly increase the rate of uptake of the gas. Blood as a potential reservoir for an insoluble gas such as ethylene would be small and filled quickly. It has been calculated that the time for the blood and gas to come to equilibrium for a relatively insoluble gas would be 8 to 21 minutes.

For a very highly soluble gas such as chloroform, so much is transferred to the blood during each breath that little, if any, remains in the alveoli just before the next inspiration. The more soluble a toxic agent is in blood, the more of it must be dissolved in the blood to reach equilibrium and, naturally, the time required to equilibrate with body water will be very much longer than with low-solubility gases and has been calculated to take a minimum of one hour. This can be very much prolonged if the gas has a high tissue solubility (i.e., high solubility in fat) as do many of these toxic agents. With these highly soluble gases, the principal factor that limits the rate of absorption is respiration. Because the blood is already removing virtually all the gas from the lungs, increasing the cardiac output could not materially increase the rate of absorption, but the rate can be very substantially hastened by furnishing the gas to the alveoli more rapidly by increasing the rate or depth of respiration.

Thus the rate of absorption of gases is variable and dependent on the toxicant's blood:gas solubility. If the gas has a very low solubility, the rate of transfer is highly dependent on blood flow through the lung (perfusion limited) whereas for gases with a high solubility, it is highly dependent on the rate and depth of respiration (ventilation limited). Of course, there is a transition zone between the two types of extreme behavior, which centers at a blood-gas solubility of about 1.2.

Not only are gases absorbed in the alveoli but liquid aerosols and particles are often absorbed. The liquid aerosols, if lipid soluble, will readily pass the alveolar cell membranes by passive diffusion. Mechanisms responsible for the removal or absorption of particulate matter that reaches the alveolus (usually less than 1 μm in diameter) are less clearly defined than those responsible for removal of particles deposited in the tracheobronchial tree, discussed above. Alveolar removal is a slow process and is in no way comparable to the effective and rapid action of the bronchial mucociliary system. The removal of toxic agents from the alveoli appears to occur by three major routes. The first is physical removal of particles from the alveoli. It is thought that particles deposited on the fluid layer of the alveoli are aspirated onto the mucociliary escalator of the tracheobronchial region to the GI tract. The origin of the thin fluid layer in the alveoli is probably the transudation of lymph and the secretion of lipid and other components by alveolar epithelium. The alveolar fluid flows to the terminal bronchioles by some unknown mechanism, but probably is dependent on lymphatic flow, capillary action, respiratory motion of the alveolar walls, the cohesive nature of the respiratory tract fluid blanket, and the propelling power of the ciliated bronchioles. The second route of removal of particles from the alveoli is by phagocytosis. The principal cell responsible for engulfing alveolar debris is the mononuclear phagocyte or macrophage. These cells are found in large quantities in normal lungs and contain many phagocytized particles of both exogenous and endogenous origin. They then apparently migrate to the distal end of the mucociliary escalator. The third route of removal is via the lymphatics. Normally water together with electrolytes and soluble proteins up to the size of albumin passes freely back and forth from capillary to interstitial and alveolar space and back via the lymphatic system. Both free and phagocytized particles can migrate via the lymphatic system. The particulate material can remain in the lymphatic tissue for long periods of time and for this reason has been termed the dust stores for the lungs.

The overall removal of particulates from the alveolus is relatively inefficient. Within the first day only about 20 percent is removed from the alveoli, and that which remains longer than 24 hours is often very slowly removed. The rate of this clearance can be predicted by the compounds' solubility in lung fluids. The least soluble compounds are removed at a slower rate than the soluble compounds. Thus it appears that removal is probably largely due to dissolution and vascular removal. Some particles may remain in the alveolus indefinitely. This can occur when alveolar cells ingest dust particles that do not desquamate but instead proliferate and, in association with a developing network of reticulin fibers, form an alveolar dust plaque or nodule.

Absorption of Toxicants Through the Skin

The skin of man comes into contact with many toxic agents. Fortunately, the skin is not highly permeable and, therefore, is a relatively good lipoid barrier separating man from his environment. However, some chemicals can be absorbed by the skin in sufficient quantities to produce systemic effects. For example, nerve gases, such as sarin, are readily absorbed by the intact skin. Also, carbon tetrachloride can be absorbed by the skin to produce liver injury, and various insecticides have produced death in agricultural workers after absorption through the intact skin.

In order for the toxicant to be absorbed through the skin, the chemical must either pass through the epidermal cells, the cells of the sweat glands, or the sebaceous glands, or enter through the hair follicles. Although follicular pathways may enable immediate entry of small amounts of toxicants, most chemicals pass through the epidermal cells, which constitute the major surface area of the skin. The sweat glands and hair follicles are scattered throughout the skin in varying numbers but are comparatively sparse; their total cross-sectional area is probably between 0.1 and 1.0 percent of the area of the skin.

For a chemical to be absorbed by the percutaneous route it must pass through the outer densely packed layer of horny, keratinized epidermal cells, through the germinal layer of

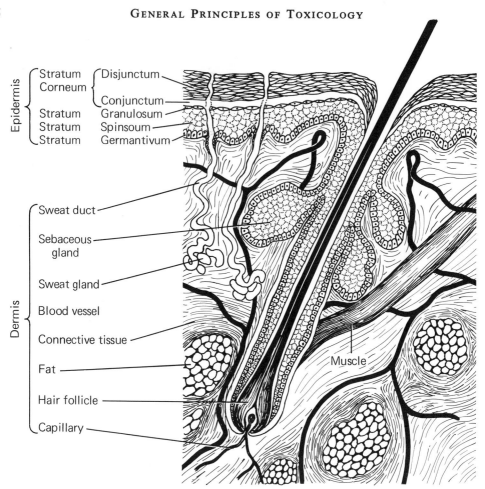

Figure 3-4. Diagram of a cross-section of human skin.

the epidermis, through the corium, and on into the systemic circulation (Fig. 3–4). Therefore, for a toxicant to be absorbed through the skin, the chemical must pass through a large number of cells. In contrast, when toxicants are absorbed by the lung and gastrointestinal tract, the chemical may pass through only two cells.

The first phase of percutaneous absorption is diffusion of the toxicant through the epidermis, and it is in this area that the rate-limiting barrier for the cutaneous absorption of toxicants exists. More specifically the barrier is the stratum corneum—the thin, cohesive, multicellular membrane that comprises the dead surface layer of the skin. Studies have shown that the stratum corneum is replenished about every two weeks in the adult. This complex process includes a gross dehydration and polymerization of the intracellular material, resulting finally in a keratin-filled, biologically inactive, dried cell layer. In the course of keratinization the cell walls apparently double in thickness due to the

inclusion, or deposition, of chemically resistant material. Thus a change in the physical state of the tissue and a commensurate change in its diffusivity occur, that is, a transformation from an aqueous fluid medium characterized by liquid-state diffusivity to a dry, semisolid, keratin membrane characterized by a much lower diffusivity.

It appears that all toxicants move across the stratum corneum of mammals by passive diffusion and not by active transport. Kinetic measurements support the postulate that polar and nonpolar toxicants diffuse through the stratum corneum by different molecular mechanisms. Polar substances appear to diffuse through the outer surface of protein filaments of the hydrated stratum corneum while nonpolar molecules dissolve in and diffuse through the nonaqueous lipid matrix between the protein filaments (Blank and Scheuplein, 1969). The rate of diffusion of nonpolar toxicants is related to the lipid solubility and inversely related to the molecular weight (Marzulli *et al.*, 1965).

In human stratum corneum there are significant differences in structure and chemistry from one region of the body to another, and these are reflected in the skin permeability. Skin from the plantar and palmar regions of the body is much different from that in other areas; the horny layer of the palms and soles is adapted for weight bearing and friction, and the membranous horny layer of the rest of the body surface is adapted for flexibility, impermeability, and fine sensory discrimination. While the stratum corneum is much thicker on the palms and soles (being 400 to 600 μm in callous areas) than on the arms, back, legs, and abdomen (8 to 15 μm), it has much more diffusivity per unit thickness. Permeability of the skin is dependent on both the diffusivity of the stratum corneum and its thickness. Thus toxicants readily cross the scrotum since it is extremely thin and has high diffusivity; toxicants cross the abdominal skin less rapidly since it is both thicker and exhibits less diffusivity; and toxicants cross the sole with most difficulty since it has such a great distance to traverse even though it exhibits the greatest diffusivity.

The second phase of percutaneous absorption is diffusion of the toxicant through the dermis, which is far inferior to the stratum corneum as a diffusion barrier. In contrast to the stratum corneum, the dermis contains a porous, non-selective, watery diffusion medium. The toxicants pass through this area by simple diffusion into the systemic circulation, which is dependent on the effective blood flow, interstitial fluid movement, lymphatics, and perhaps other factors such as combination with dermal constituents.

The absorption of toxicants through the skin varies under a number of circumstances. Since the stratum corneum plays a critical role in determining cutaneous permeability, abrasion or removal of this layer causes an abrupt increase in the permeability of the epidermis for all kinds of molecules, large or small, lipid soluble and water soluble (Malkinson, 1964). Injurious agents such as acids, alkalis, and mustard gases likewise will injure the barrier cells and increase permeability (Malkinson, 1964). Water plays an extremely important role in skin permeability. Under normal conditions the stratum corneum is always partially hydrated. Skin normally contains about 90 g of water per gram of dry tissue. This much water increases the permeability of the stratum corneum approximately tenfold over that when it is perfectly dry. Upon additional contact with water the stratum corneum can maximally increase its weight of tightly bound water three to five times, which results in an additional two- to threefold increase in permeability. Studies on dermal absorption of toxicants often utilize the method of Draize and associates (1944) in which plastic is wrapped around the animal and the chemical placed between the plastic and the skin. This hydrates the stratum corneum and enhances the absorption of the toxicant.

Various solvents such as dimethyl sulfoxide (DMSO) can also facilitate the penetration of toxicants through the skin. DMSO increases the permeability of the skin barrier layer, the stratum corneum. Little information is available concerning the mechanism by which DMSO enhances the permeability. However, it has been suggested that DMSO (1) removes much of the lipid fraction of the stratum corneum, which makes holes or artificial shunts in the membrane, (2) produces reversible configurational changes in protein structure brought about by substitution of integral water molecules by DMSO, and (3) functions as a swelling agent (Allenby et al., 1969; Dugard and Embery, 1969).

Various species have been employed in studying the absorption of toxicants, and species variation in the cutaneous permeability have been observed. The skin of the rat and rabbit is more permeable, the skin of the cat is less permeable, while the cutaneous permeability characteristics of the guinea pig, pig, and monkey are similar to those observed in man (Scala et al., 1968; Coulston and Serrone, 1969; Wester and Maibach, 1977). Species differences in the percutaneous absorption account for the fact that many insecticides are more toxic to insects than to man. For example, the LD50 of DDT is approximately equal in an insect and mammal when the insecticide is injected but is much less toxic to the mammal than to the insect when applied to the skin. This appears to be due to the fact that DDT is poorly absorbed through the skin of a mammal but passes readily through the chitinous exoskeleton of the insect and the fact that insects have a much greater body surface area in relation to weight than do mammals (Winteringham, 1957; Albert, 1965; Hayes, 1965).

Absorption of Toxicants After Special Routes of Administration

Toxic agents usually enter the bloodstream of man after absorption from the skin, lungs, or gastrointestinal tract. However, in studying chemical agents, toxicologists frequently administer these chemicals to laboratory animals by various special routes, the most common of which are (1) intraperitoneal, (2) subcutaneous, (3) intramuscular, and (4) intravenous. The intravenous route of administration introduces the toxicant directly into the bloodstream and thus the process of absorption is eliminated. The intraperitoneal route of administration of toxicants to laboratory animals is also a common procedure. This method results in a rapid absorption of toxicants due to the rich blood supply to the peritoneal cavity and to the large surface area. Compounds administered intraperitoneally are absorbed primarily through the portal circulation and, therefore, must pass through the liver before reaching other organs (Lukas *et al.*, 1971). Toxicants administered subcutaneously and intramuscularly are usually absorbed at a slower rate. The rate of absorption by these two routes can be altered by changing the blood flow to the area and by altering the solution in which the toxicant is administered. For example, epinephrine will cause vasoconstriction and decrease the rate of absorption of a toxicant. The formulation of the toxicant may also affect the rate of absorption; toxicants are absorbed more slowly from suspensions than from solutions.

The toxicity of a chemical may or may not be dependent on the route of parenteral administration. If a toxicant is injected intraperitoneally, most of the drug will enter the liver via the portal circulation before it reaches the general circulation of the animal. Therefore, an intraperitoneally administered compound might be completely metabolized or extracted by the liver and excreted into the bile and never gain access to the remainder of the animal. Propranolol (Shand and Rangno, 1972) and lidocaine (Boyes *et al.*, 1970) are two such drugs that are efficiently extracted during the first pass through the liver. Any toxicant handled in such a manner that has a selective toxicity for an organ other than the liver and gastrointestinal tract would be expected to be much less toxic when administered intraperitoneally than when injected subcutaneously or intramuscularly. The toxicity of compounds that are not metabolized by the liver or excreted into the bile would not be expected to be markedly different when administered by these three routes, unless other factors such as differences in the rate of absorption from the three routes were involved. Therefore, it is possible to obtain some preliminary information on the metabolism and excretion of a toxicant by comparing its toxicity when given by various routes.

DISTRIBUTION

After the toxicant enters the plasma water, either by absorption or by direct intravenous administration, it is available for distribution throughout the body. Distribution usually occurs rapidly, and the rate of distribution to the tissues of each organ is determined by the blood flow through the organ and the ease with which the chemical crosses the capillary bed and penetrates the cells of the particular tissue. Its eventual distribution is largely dependent on the ability of the chemical to pass the cell membrane of the various tissues and the affinity of the various tissues in the body for the chemical. The penetration of toxicants into cells depends on many of the same mechanisms discussed previously for gastrointestinal absorption. Small, water-soluble molecules and ions apparently diffuse through aqueous channels or pores in the cell membrane. Lipid-soluble molecules readily permeate the membrane itself. Water-soluble molecules and ions of moderate size (molecular weights of 50 or more) cannot enter cells easily except by special transport mechanisms.

Some toxicants do not readily pass cell membranes and therefore have a restricted distribution, whereas other toxicants readily pass through cell membranes and distribute throughout the body. In addition, some toxicants accumulate in various parts of the body as a result of binding, active transport, or high solubility in fat. While the site of accumulation of a toxicant may be its site of major toxic action, more often it is not. When the toxicant has accumulated at a site other than the site at which it produces its toxic action, the accumulation may serve as a protective mechanism by distributing part of the toxicant into a storage depot, which could keep the concentration of the toxicant in the target organ at a lower level. In this case the chemical in the storage depot is toxicologically inactive; however, since the chemical in the storage depot is in equilibrium with the free toxicant, it is slowly released into the circulation as the free toxicant is eliminated.

Volume of Distribution

The total body water may be divided into three distinct compartments: (1) plasma water, (2) interstitial water, and (3) intracellular water. Extracellular water is made up of plasma water plus interstitial water. The concentration that a toxicant will achieve in the blood after a certain exposure will depend largely on its apparent volume of distribution (V_d). For example, if 1 g of a chemical was injected directly into the bloodstream of a 70-kg man, marked differences in its plasma concentration would be observed depending on its distribution (see the next page).

A high concentration would be observed in the plasma if it distributed only in the plasma water, and a much lower concentration would be reached if it distributed in a large pool like the total body water. The distribution of a toxicant is usually not as simple as equal distribution into one of the water compartments in the body but is complicated by binding to

COMPARTMENT	PERCENT OF TOTAL	LITERS IN 70-kg MAN	PLASMA CONC. AFTER 1 g OF CHEMICAL
Plasma water	4.5	3	333 mg/L
Total extracellular water	20	14	71 mg/L
Total body water	55	38	26 mg/L

various storage sites in the body, such as fat, liver, or bone.

Storage of Toxicants in Tissues

Toxicants are often concentrated in a specific tissue. Some toxicants achieve their highest concentration at their site of toxic action, such as carbon monoxide, which has a very high affinity for hemoglobin, and paraquat, which accumulates in the lung (Sharp *et al.*, 1972). Other agents concentrate at sites other than the site of toxic action. Lead, for example, is stored in bone, while the symptoms of lead poisoning are due to lead in the soft tissues. The compartment where this toxicant is concentrated can be thought of as a storage depot. The toxicant while it is stored often does no harm to the organism. Storage depots, therefore, could be considered as protecting organs, preventing high concentrations of the toxicants from being achieved at the site of toxic action. The toxicants in these depots are always in equilibrium with free toxicant in plasma, and as the chemical is metabolized or excreted from the body, more is released from the storage site. As a result, the biologic half-life of compounds that are stored can be very long. The following are the major storage sites for toxicants.

Plasma Proteins as a Storage Depot for Toxicants

Several proteins within the plasma can bind normal physiologic constituents in the body as well as some foreign compounds. As depicted in Figure 3–5, albumin has the capacity to bind many compounds. A β_1-globulin, transferrin, is important for the transport of iron in the body. The other main metal-binding protein is ceruloplasmin, which carries most of the copper in the serum. The α- and β-lipoproteins are very important for the transport of lipid-soluble compounds such as vitamins, cholesterol, and steroid hormones. The antibody γ-globulins interact very specifically with antigens (Goldstein *et al.*, 1968).

Protein binding is usually determined by dialyzing plasma against buffer or by ultrafiltration. The fraction that passes through the dialysis membrane or the ultrafiltrate is the unbound or free fraction, and that which is retained is the total concentration, which is the sum of the bound and free fraction. The bound fraction is thus the difference of the total and free fraction.

Most foreign chemicals that are bound to plasma proteins are bound to albumin. The binding involves reversible bonds such as hydrogen, van der Waal's, and ionic bonds. The high molecular weight of the plasma protein prevents passage of the toxicant across capillary walls and tends to restrict the chemical to the vascular space. The fraction of toxicant in the plasma bound to plasma proteins is not immediately available for distribution into the extravascular space or for filtration at the kidney. However, the interaction of a chemical with plasma proteins is a rapidly reversible process. As unbound chemical diffuses from the capillaries, bound chemical dissociates from the protein until chemical in the extravascular water equilibrates with unbound chemical in the plasma. Active processes such as those in the kidney and liver are not limited by a high degree of plasma protein binding.

Many therapeutic agents have been examined with respect to plasma protein binding. The extent to which toxicants are bound to plasma proteins can vary considerably. Some, such as antipyrine, are not bound at all; others such as secobarbital, are bound about 50 percent; and some, like thyroxine, are 99.9 percent bound. The plasma proteins can bind acidic compounds like phenylbutazone, basic compounds like imipramine, and neutral compounds like digitoxin.

The binding of chemicals to plasma proteins is of special importance to toxicologists, because severe toxic reactions can result if the agent is displaced from the plasma protein. The bound form of the chemical is not available to go to the target organ to produce injury. However, it has been demonstrated that another chemical agent may displace the first from the plasma protein, making it available in the free form. In this way a second chemical can induce toxicity from the first chemical. For example, if a strongly bound sulfonamide drug is given to a patient who is taking an antidiabetic drug, it may displace the antidiabetic drug and induce hypoglycemic coma. Foreign compounds can also compete and displace normal physiologic compounds that are bound to plasma proteins. The importance of this fact was demonstrated in a clinical trial

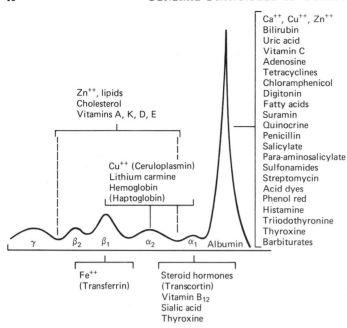

Ca++, Cu++, Zn++
Bilirubin
Uric acid
Vitamin C
Adenosine
Tetracyclines
Chloramphenicol
Digitonin
Fatty acids
Suramin
Quinocrine
Penicillin
Salicylate
Para-aminosalicylate
Sulfonamides
Streptomycin
Acid dyes
Phenol red
Histamine
Triiodothyronine
Thyroxine
Barbiturates

Zn++, lipids
Cholesterol
Vitamins A, K, D, E

Cu++ (Ceruloplasmin)
Lithium carmine
Hemoglobin
(Haptoglobin)

γ β_2 β_1 α_2 α_1 Albumin

Fe++
(Transferrin)

Steroid hormones
(Transcortin)
Vitamin B$_{12}$
Sialic acid
Thyroxine

Figure 3–5. Interactions with plasma proteins. Plasma proteins are depicted according to their relative amounts (y-axis) and electrophoretic mobilities (x-axis). Some representative interactions are listed. (From Goldstein, A.; Aronow, L.; and Kalman, S. M.: *Principles of Drug Action* [copyright © 1968, by Harper and Row; reprinted by permission of John Wiley & Sons, Inc., copyright proprietor]. Modified from Putnam, F. W.: Structure and function of the plasma proteins. In Neurath, H. [ed.]: *The Proteins*, 2nd ed., Vol. III [Academic Press, Inc., New York, 1965].)

comparing the efficacy of tetracycline and of a penicillin-sulfonamide mixture in the management of premature infants (Silverman *et al.*, 1956). It was found that the sulfonamide mixture resulted in a much higher mortality than the tetracycline. This was because the sulfonamide displaced a considerable amount of bilirubin from the albumin, and the bilirubin was then free to diffuse into the brain and produce a severe type of brain damage termed kernicterus.

Most of the research performed on the binding of xenobiotics to plasma proteins has been with drugs. Other chemicals, such as the insecticide dieldrin, also avidly bind to plasma proteins (99 percent). It is likely that chemicals other than drugs may also compete for these same binding sites and chemical-chemical interactions are likely to occur by this mechanism.

High Concentration of Toxicants in Liver and Kidney

The liver and the kidney have a high capacity to bind chemicals, and these two organs probably concentrate more toxicants than any other organ. This might be related to the fact that they are very important in the elimination of toxicants from the body; the kidney and the liver have a capacity to excrete many chemicals and the liver has a high capacity to metabolize them. Although the precise mechanism by which the liver and kidney remove toxicants from the blood has not yet been established, active transport or binding to tissue components is likely to be involved.

Active transport and protein binding have been suggested as possible mechanisms by which the liver and the kidney might remove toxic materials from the blood. Recent reports in the literature suggest that intracellular binding proteins may be important in concentrating toxicants within the liver and kidney.

A protein in the cytoplasm of the liver (Y protein or ligandin) has been demonstrated to have a high affinity for many organic acids, and it has been suggested that this protein may be important in the transfer of organic anions from plasma into the liver (Levi *et al.*, 1969). This protein also binds azodye carcinogens and corticosteroids (Litwack *et al.*, 1971). Another binding protein (metallothionein) has been found in the kidney and liver to bind cadmium (Margoshes and Vallee, 1957; Lucis *et al.*, 1970). As an example of the rapidity with which liver binds foreign compounds, 30 minutes after a single administration of lead, the hepatic concentration is 50 times higher than in the plasma (Klaassen and Shoeman, 1972).

Fat as a Storage Depot of Toxicants

Many of the organic compounds entering the environment are highly lipophylic, a characteristic that permits rapid penetration of cell membranes and uptake by tissues. Since they are highly lipid soluble, it is not surprising that they distribute and concentrate in body fat. This has been demonstrated for a number of chemicals such as chlordane, DDT, polychlorinated biphenyls, and polybrominated biphenyls.

Toxicants appear to be stored in fat by simple physical dissolution in the neutral fats. Neutral fats constitute about 50 percent of the body weight of an obese individual and about 20 percent of the body weight of a lean, athletic individual. Thus, a toxicant that has a high lipid/water partition coefficient may be stored in the body fat to a large extent, and this storage will lower the concentration of the toxicant in the target organ and thus serve as a protective mechanism. One might suspect that the toxicity of some compounds that concentrate in fat might not be as great to a fat as a lean person. However, of more practical concern is the possibility of a sudden increase in the concentration of the chemical in the blood and in the target organ should there occur a rapid mobilization of stored fat for energy. A number of studies have shown that signs of intoxication can be produced by short-term starvation of experimental animals previously overexposed to long-lived organochlorine insecticides.

Bone as a Storage Depot of Toxic Materials

A relatively inert tissue such as bone can also serve as a reservoir for compounds such as fluoride, lead, and strontium. Bone is a major site for storage for some toxicants; for example, 90 percent of the lead in the body is found in the skeleton.

The phenomenon of skeletal uptake of foreign materials can be considered to be essentially a surface chemistry phenomenon, in which the exchange takes place between the bone surface and the fluid in contact with it. The fluid is the extracellular fluid and the surface on which the exchange phenomenon takes place is that of the hydroxyapatite crystals of bone mineral. Many of these crystals are small and of such dimensions that the surface is large in proportion to the mass. Upon being brought to a crystal of bone by extracellular fluid, the toxicant enters the hydration shell of the crystal and penetrates to the crystal surface. By virtue of similarities in size and charge, F^- may readily replace OH^- and lead or strontium may replace calcium in the hydroxyapatite lattice structure by an exchange adsorption reaction.

The deposition and storage of toxicants in bone may or may not be toxic. Lead is not toxic to the bone but the chronic effects of fluoride deposition (skeletal fluorosis) and radioactive strontium (osteosarcoma and other neoplasms) are well known.

Foreign compounds deposited in bone are not irreversibly sequestered by this tissue. The toxicants can be released by ionic exchange at the crystal surface and by dissolution of bone crystals through osteoclastic activity. An increase

in osteolytic activity, such as that seen after parathormone, leads to an enhanced mobilization of the toxicant, which will be reflected by an increased plasma concentration of the toxicant.

Blood-Brain Barrier

The blood-brain barrier is not an absolute barrier to the passage of toxic materials into the central nervous system, but rather represents a site that is less permeable than most other areas of the body. Many poisons do not enter the brain in appreciable quantities.

There are three major anatomic and physiologic reasons why some toxicants have difficulty entering the CNS. First, the capillary endothelial cells of the CNS are tightly joined leaving few or no pores between the cells. Second, the capillaries of the CNS are largely surrounded by glial connective tissue processes (astrocytes), and third, the protein concentration in the interstitial fluid of the CNS is much less than elsewhere in the body. Thus, in contrast to other tissue, the toxicant has difficulty going between capillaries and has to traverse not only the capillary endothelium itself but also the membranes of glial cells in order to gain access to the interstitial fluid. Since the interstitial fluid is low in protein, it cannot use protein binding to increase the distribution to the CNS. These features together act as a protective mechanism to decrease the distribution of toxicants to the CNS and thus the toxicity.

The effectiveness of the blood-brain barrier varies from one area of the brain to another. For example, the cortex, lateral nuclei of hypothalamus, area postrema, pineal body, and posterior lobe of the hypophysis are more permeable than are other areas of the brain. It is not clear if this is due to the increased blood supply to these areas or to a more permeable barrier or both.

The entrance of toxicants into the brain, in general, follows the same principle as does transfer across other cells in the body. Only the free toxicant—that is, one not bound to plasma proteins—is free to enter the brain. The lipid solubility of a compound plays a major role in determining the rate at which it enters the central nervous system. If an agent is ionized, it will not enter the central nervous system readily because it is not lipid soluble. If it is not ionized, it will enter the brain at a rate proportional to its lipid/water partition coefficient. Therefore, a very lipid-soluble compound readily enters the central nervous system and a less lipid-soluble compound enters the brain with difficulty. Thus, methyl mercury enters the brain much more readily than does inorganic mercury. Also, since 2-PAM is a quaternary nitrogen derivative, it will not readily penetrate the brain and is quite ineffective in reversing inhibition of brain cholinesterase.

The blood-brain barrier is not completely developed at birth, and this is one reason why some chemicals are more toxic in the newborn than in the adult. For example, morphine is three to ten times more toxic in the newborn rat than in the adult because of the higher permeability of the brain of the newborn to morphine (Kupferberg and Way, 1963). Lead produces encephalomyelopathy in newborn rats but not in adults, also apparently because of differences in the development of the blood-brain barrier (Pentschew and Garro, 1966).

Passage of Toxicants Across the Placenta

For years the term "placental barrier" typified a concept that the main function of the placenta was to protect the fetus against passage of noxious substances from mother to fetus. However, the placenta has other functions such as to exchange waste, nutrients, oxygen, and carbon dioxide between mother and fetus. Most of the vital materials necessary for the development of the fetus are transported by energy-coupled specific active transport systems. For example, vitamins, amino acids, essential sugars, and ions such as calcium and iron are transported from the mother to the fetus against a concentration gradient (Young, 1969; Ginsburg, 1971). Even oxygen does not appear to cross the placenta by simple diffusion (Gurtner and Burns, 1972). On the other hand, most toxic materials pass the placenta by simple diffusion, except for a few antimetabolites that are structurally similar to the endogenous purines and pyrimides that are normally actively transported from maternal to fetal circulation.

Many foreign substances can cross the placenta. Not only chemicals but also viruses (e.g., rubella virus), cellular pathogens (e.g., syphilis spirochete), antibody globulins, and even erythrocytes (Goldstein *et al.*, 1968) traverse the placenta.

Anatomically the placental barrier is the result of a number of layers of cells interposed between fetal and maternal circulations. The number of layers varies with the species and the state of gestation and this probably affects the permeability of the placenta. Placentas in which all six layers are present are called epitheliochorial (Table 3–1), and those in which the maternal epithelium is absent are called sydesmochorial. When only the endothelial layer of the maternal tissue remains, it is called endothelialchorial; when even the endothelium is gone, so that the chorionic villi bathe in the maternal blood, they are called hemochorial. In some species, some of the fetal tissues are absent and then are termed hemoendothelial (Dawes, 1968). Therefore, one might suspect that a relatively thin placenta, such as in the rat, would be more permeable to toxic agents than the placenta of man, while a thicker placenta, such as that in the goat, would be less permeable. Within a single species, the placenta may also change its histologic class during gestation (Amaroso, 1952). For example, the rabbit at the beginning of gestation has a placenta with six major layers (epithelochorial) and at the end of gestation has a placenta of one layer (hemoendothelial). However, the relationship of the number of layers of the placenta to its permeability has not been thoroughly investigated.

As is the case in the transfer of most compounds across body membranes, diffusion appears to be the mechanism by which most toxicants pass the placenta. The same factors, especially lipid/water partition, are important determinants in the placental transfer. It is questionable if the placenta plays an important active role in preventing the passage of noxious substances from mother to fetus; however, it has been noted that triamterene is transferred from the fetus much more rapidly than to the fetus

Table 3–1. TISSUES SEPARATING FETAL AND MATERNAL BLOOD*

	MATERNAL TISSUE			FETAL TISSUE			
	Endo-thelium	Connective Tissue	Epi-thelium	Tropho-blast	Connective Tissue	Endo-thelium	SPECIES
Epitheliochoria	+	+	+	+	+	+	Pig, horse, donkey
Syndesmochorial	+	+	−	+	+	+	Sheep, goat, cow
Endotheliochorial	+	−	−	+	+	+	Cat, dog
Hemochorial	−	−	−	+	+	+	Man, monkey
Hemoendothelial	−	−	−	−	−	+	Rat, rabbit, guinea pig

* Modified from Amaroso, E. C.: Placentation. In Parkes, A. S. (ed.): *Marshall's Physiology of Reproduction*, Vol. 2. Longmans, Green & Co., London, 1952.

(McNay and Dayton, 1970) and that the placenta has drug biotransformation mechanisms that may prevent some toxic substances from reaching the fetus (Juchau, 1972). Of the substances that cross the placenta by passive diffusion, the more lipid-soluble substances will traverse more rapidly and attain a maternal-fetal equilibrium more rapidly. During steady-state conditions, the concentrations of a toxic compound in the plasma water of the mother and fetus will be the same. However, the concentration in the various tissues of the fetus will be determined by the ability of the tissue to concentrate the toxicant. For example, the concentration of diphenyl-hydantoin in the plasma of the fetal goat was found to be about one-half that found in the mother goat. This was due to differences in plasma protein concentration and binding affinity for diphenylhydantoin (Shoeman *et al.*, 1972). Also, some organs, such as the liver of the new-born (Klaassen, 1972) and fetus (Mirkin and Singh, 1972), do not concentrate some exogenous chemicals and, therefore, lower levels might be found in the liver of the fetus. On the other hand, higher concentrations of some chemicals such as lead are found in the brain of the newborn since the blood-brain barrier is immature.

Redistribution of Toxicants

The distribution of a toxic material in the body can change with time. The initial site where a chemical localizes is dependent on the blood flow to the area, the permeability of the tissue to the toxicant, and the binding sites that are immediately available. A chemical can later redistribute to less well-perfused tissues when more binding sites become available. An example of redistribution is seen with inorganic lead. Immediately after absorption, the lead is localized in the erythrocytes, liver, and kidney. Approximately 50 percent of the lead is localized in the liver two hours after administration (Hammond, 1969; Klaassen and Shoeman, 1972). The lead is later redistributed to the bone and substitutes for calcium in the crystal lattice. A month after administration 90 percent of the lead left in the body is localized in the bones.

EXCRETION

Toxicants are eliminated from the body by various routes. The kidney is a very important organ for the excretion of poisons and probably more chemicals are eliminated from the body by this route than any other (see Chapter 11). However, other routes are very important for the excretion of specific compounds; the liver and biliary system are important for the excretion of DDT and lead, and the lungs excrete gases such as carbon monoxide. All body secretions appear to have the ability to excrete foreign compounds; toxicants have even been found in sweat, tears, and milk (Stowe and Plaa, 1968).

Urinary Excretion

The kidney is a very efficient organ for the elimination of toxicants from the body. Toxic compounds are excreted into the urine by the same mechanisms the kidney uses to remove end products of metabolism from the body. These processes are passive glomerular filtration, passive tubular diffusion, and active tubular secretion.

The kidney receives about 25 percent of the cardiac output, and 20 percent of this is filtered at the glomeruli. The glomerular capillaries have large pores (40 Å), and therefore a compound will be filtered at the glomerulus unless its molecular weight is large (greater than 60,000). Most toxic agents are small enough to be filtered at the glomerulus. The degree to which a toxic material binds to plasma protein affects the rate of filtration because a bound toxic agent is too large to pass through the pores.

Once the toxicant has been filtered at the glomeruli, it may remain within the tubular lumen and be excreted, or it may be passively reabsorbed across the tubular cells of the nephron into the bloodstream. The principles governing the back diffusion of a toxicant across the tubular cells are the same ones that relate to any passive membrane transfer. Therefore, toxicants with a high lipid/water partition coefficient will be passively reabsorbed, and polar compounds and ions will be unable to diffuse and therefore will be excreted into the urine. Generally, toxicants that are bases are excreted to a greater extent if the urine is acidic, whereas acid compounds are excreted more favorably if the urine is alkaline. A practical application of this knowledge is in the treatment of pheno-barbital poisoning. Since phenobarbital is a weak acid with a pK_a of 7.2, the percentage of the drug in the ionized form in the urine can be markedly altered by changes in pH at levels obtainable in mammalian urine. Phenobarbital poisoning, therefore, can be treated by alkalinization of the urine through the administration of sodium bicarbonate, resulting in a significant increase in the excretion of phenobarbital (Weiner and Mudge, 1964). Similarly in acute salicylate poisoning, acceleration of salicylate loss via the kidney can be achieved by sodium bicarbonate administration.

Toxic agents can also be excreted from the plasma by passive diffusion through the tubule into the urine. This mechanism is probably of only minor significance. Since urine is normally acid, this process may play a role in the excretion of some organic bases because an organic base is ionized in the acidic environment of the urine. For organic acids, simple diffusion across the renal tubule plays little or no role in their excretion, because, after weak acidic compounds are filtered at the glomerulus, many are reabsorbed by passive diffusion. Thus, the excretion of weakly acidic compounds by renal mechanisms would take a very long time because after they are filtered, they are passively reabsorbed. Fortunately, however, weak acids are frequently metabolized to stronger acids, thereby increasing the percentage of the ionic forms and hindering their tubular reabsorption.

Toxicants can also be excreted into the urine by active secretion. There are two tubular secretory processes, one for organic anions (acids) and the other for organic cations (bases). p-Aminohippurate (PAH) is the prototype for an agent excreted by the organic acid transport system, and N-methylnicotinamide (NMN) is the prototypal base. These systems appear to be located in the proximal convoluted tubules, and, in contrast to filtration, protein-bound toxicants are fully available for active transport. These processes have all the characteristics of an active transport system; therefore, various compounds compete with one another for secretion. This fact was put to use during World War II when penicillin was in short supply and high demand. Since penicillin is actively excreted by the organic acid transport system of the kidney, another acid was sought whose excretion would compete with the excretion of penicillin and thereby prolong its duration of action. Probenecid was introduced for this purpose. By this same process of competition, other toxicants that are transported by the organic acid transport system can produce an increase in the plasma uric acid concentration and precipitate an attack of gout, since the organic acid transport system normally excretes uric acid.

The renal excretory mechanisms (glomerular filtration, renal secretion, renal reabsorption, or any combination thereof) usually remove a constant fraction of the toxicant in the blood delivered to the kidney. It is known that the polymeric carbohydrate inulin is neither bound to plasma proteins nor secreted into the tubule nor reabsorbed from the tubule, but enters the urine by filtration. In fact, all of the inulin filtered at the kidney is excreted into the urine, but since the kidney reabsorbs 99 percent of the water filtered, this water returns to the circulation without inulin in it. In other words, the kidney has "cleared" a large volume of plasma of its inulin by the processes of filtration of fluid and inulin with subsequent reabsorption of fluid without inulin. This volume is termed clearance

and its units are milliliters per minute. In other words, clearance is a theoretic volume of plasma from which all of the chemical was removed per unit time. Since with inulin none is reabsorbed after being filtered, its clearance (Cl_{IN}) is the same as the glomerular filtration rate (GFR).

Many substances are reabsorbed back into the circulation with the fluid after they are filtered at the glomerulus. For these substances, the volume of plasma cleared is smaller than the filtered volume ($Cl_X < Cl_{IN}$). For substances that are secreted by the kidney, the volume of plasma cleared of the substance can be greater than the GFR because theoretically all of the chemical reaching the kidney can be cleared by active secretion ($Cl_X > Cl_{IN}$), and it must be remembered that renal plasma flow (660 ml/min) is much larger than GFR (125 ml/min). Thus by comparing the renal clearance of a toxicant to that of inulin, one can determine how substances are excreted by the kidney. However, after the chemical is filtered or secreted into the tubule, the toxicant, if in a lipid-soluble form, can be passively reabsorbed. For many toxicants, more than one process is responsible for the urinary excretion of the toxicant, and the use of competitive blockers of the active transport systems and changes in acid-base balance may be necessary to fully elucidate the mechanisms of excretion. One must remember that only the portion of the toxicant that is not bound to plasma proteins is available for filtration while both bound and unbound toxicant are available for secretion.

Although clearance tells us the virtual volume of plasma cleared per minute, it tells us nothing about the rate at which the plasma concentration of the toxicant is lowered by the renal excretory process. For this we need to know the apparent volume of distribution (V_d). Clearly, the greater the volume of distribution, the more slowly the plasma level of the toxicant will fall. For example, if a toxicant is excreted solely by glomerular filtration (125 ml/min), the half-life of the toxicant would be about 16 minutes if it distributed in plasma water (3 liters) but would be about 210 minutes if it distributed in total body water (38 liters).

Because many functions of the kidney are incompletely developed at birth, some foreign chemicals are eliminated slowly and thus are more toxic in the newborn than the adult. For example, the clearance of penicillin by premature infants is only about 20 percent of that observed in older children (Barnett et al., 1949). It has been demonstrated that the development of this organic acid transport system in the newborn can be stimulated by administration of substrates that are normally excreted by this system (Hirsch and Hook, 1970). Some compounds such as cephaloridine are known to be nephrotoxic in adult animals but not in newborns. The reason for this is that cephaloridine is nephrotoxic only when high concentrations are achieved in the kidney. Since the active uptake of cephaloridine by the kidney is not well developed in the newborn, the kidney of the newborn cannot concentrate cephaloridine and thus it is not nephrotoxic. If one increases the development of the uptake mechanism in newborn animals by substrate stimulation, the newborn can take up the cephaloridine more readily and then nephrotoxicity is observed (Wold *et al.*, 1977). Similarly the nephrotoxicity of cephaloridine can be blocked by probenecid, which competitively inhibits the uptake of cephaloridine into the kidney (Tune *et al.*, 1977).

Biliary Excretion

The liver is in a very advantageous position for removing toxic materials from the blood after absorption by the gastrointestinal tract. Since the blood from the gastrointestinal tract passes through the liver before it reaches the general systemic circulation, the liver can remove compounds from the blood and prevent their distribution to other parts of the body. Also, since the liver is the site where the biotransformation of most toxic agents occurs, the metabolites may be excreted directly into the bile without reentering the bloodstream to be excreted by the kidney. A toxicant may be excreted by the liver cells into the bile and thus pass into the small intestine and remain there. However, if the properties of such a toxicant favor its reabsorption, an enterohepatic cycle may result.

Foreign compounds excreted into the bile are often divided into three classes on the basis of the ratio of their concentration in bile in comparison to that in plasma. Class A substances have a ratio of nearly 1.0 and include sodium, potassium, glucose, mercury, thallium, cesium, and cobalt. Class B substances have a bile-to-plasma ratio greater than 1.0 and usually between 10 and 1,000. These include bile salts, bilirubin, sulfobromophthalein, lead, arsenic, manganese, and many other foreign compounds. Among class C substances, which have a bile-to-plasma ratio less than 1.0, are inulin, albumin, zinc, iron, gold, and chromium. Compounds rapidly excreted into the bile are most likely to be class B substances. However, a compound does not have to be highly concentrated in bile for biliary excretion to be of quantitative importance. For example, mercury is not concentrated in bile yet bile is the main route of excretion for this slowly excreted substance.

The mechanism by which foreign substances are transported from plasma into liver and from liver into bile is not known with certainty. Little is known about the mechanism of transfer of class A and C compounds. However, it is thought that most class B compounds are actively transported across both sides of the hepatocyte by active transport processes. The liver has at least three transport systems for the excretion of organic compounds into the bile. The organic acid transport system has been studied the most thoroughly with sulfobromophthalein (BSP) as the prototype. The rate of removal of BSP has long been used as a measure of hepatic function and dysfunction. This is performed by injecting the blue dye intravenously and at a certain time thereafter (usually 30 min), a blood sample is taken and the concentration of BSP in the plasma is determined. If the liver is functioning properly, it should remove the dye from plasma and excrete it into the bile. If the concentration of BSP left in the plasma is higher in the animals receiving the toxicants than in the controls, the toxicant has probably produced liver injury.

The transport system that excretes BSP is also responsible for the transfer of bilirubin from the plasma into the bile, and thus jaundice is often observed after liver injury. The liver also has an active transport system for the excretion of bases as does the kidney; procainamide ethyl bromide (PAEB) is the prototype for this transport system. The liver also has a third transport system for the excretion of neutral compounds such as ouabain. In addition to these three transport systems for organic compounds, it appears that the liver has at least one transport system for the excretion of metals (Klaassen, 1976). For example, lead is excreted into the bile against a large bile/plasma concentration ratio (100) and an apparent biliary transport maximum exists. Whether other metals are excreted into the bile by the same or similar mechanisms, or if metals compete for biliary excretion, remains to be determined.

As with renal tubular secretion, toxic agents that are bound to plasma proteins are fully available for biliary excretion; in fact, many compounds of this type are excreted into the bile.

It is not known what determines if a chemical will be excreted into the bile or the urine. However, low-molecular-weight compounds are poorly excreted into bile, while compounds with molecular weights exceeding a minimum value (about 325 or such a value attained by a metabolic change, usually conjugation) are excreted in appreciable quantities into bile.

The relative importance of the biliary excretory route depends on the substance and species concerned. The percentage of various compounds excreted into the bile has previously been tabulated (Stowe and Plaa, 1968; Plaa, 1971). The effect of eliminating the biliary excretory route, by ligating the bile duct of rodents, on the toxicity of some chemicals that are known to be excreted into the bile is shown in Table 3–2. Bile duct ligation (BDL) had little effect on the toxicity of some chemicals; however, a number of compounds were much more toxic in BDL rats than in sham-operated rats; probenecid was 1.7, colchicine 1.8, iopanoic acid 2.2, rifampin 2.4, ouabain 3.9, digoxin 4.2, indocyanine green 5.4, and diethylstilbestrol (DES) about 130 times more toxic in BDL rats than in sham-operated rats. The marked effect that BDL has on DES toxicity has been further examined, and it appears that the biliary route is the only pathway by which DES can be eliminated from the body. When this pathway is excluded, the amount of DES in the body does not decrease with time, and the maintained high level of DES is toxic to the animal (Klaassen, 1973b).

There is a marked species variation in the rate of biliary excretion of foreign compounds into the bile, which results in species variation in the biologic half-life of a compound and its toxicity. For example, the organic acid sulfobromo-phthalein is excreted at a similar rate in the rat and rabbit but five times slower in the dog (Klaassen and Plaa, 1967). The rabbit and rat are very efficient in transporting the organic base, procainamide ethyl bromide (PAEB), from the plasma into the bile, while the dog almost entirely lacks this ability (Hunter and Klaassen, 1972). Over 50 percent of the organic neutral compound ouabain is excreted into the bile of the rat in two hours but less than 3 percent is excreted by the rabbit and dog (Russell and Klaassen, 1972); and the rabbit excretes lead into the bile at a rate one-half, and the dog at a rate one-fiftieth, of that observed in the rat (Klaassen and Shoeman, 1972). This species variation makes it very difficult to extrapolate information from laboratory animals to man.

Once a compound is excreted into the bile and enters the intestine, it can be either reabsorbed or eliminated in the feces. Many organic compounds are biotransformed into polar metabolites before excretion into the bile, and these as such are not lipid soluble enough to be reabsorbed. However, intestinal microflora can hydrolyze various glucuronide conjugates enabling the toxicant to be reabsorbed. If the xenobiotic is reabsorbed, an enterohepatic cycle results. A

Table 3–2. COMPARISON OF THE TOXICITY OF CHEMICALS IN SHAM-OPERATED RATS AND BILE DUCT–LIGATED RATS (BDL)*

	SHAM-LD50	BDL-LD50	SHAM/BDL
Amitryptiline	100	100	1.0
Azorubin	1300	950	1.4
Bishydroxycoumarin	95	70	1.4
Chloramphenicol	80	88	0.91
Colchicine	6.1	3.3	1.8
Diethylstilbestrol	100	0.75	130
Digitoxin	5.1	3.7	1.4
Digoxin	11	2.6	4.2
Erythromycin	130	180	0.7
Fluorescein	1700	1700	1.0
Glutethimide	84	71	1.2
Guanethidine	290	280	1.0
Indocyanine green	700	130	5.4
Iopanoic acid	530	240	2.2
Nafcillin	920	830	1.1
Novobiocin	400	580	0.7
Ouabain	47	12	3.9
Pentobarbital	110	130	0.8
Probenecid	420	240	1.7
Quinine	170	190	0.9
Rifampin	390	160	2.4
Sulfobromophthalein	320	260	1.2
Taurocholic acid	450	310	1.5
Thioridazine	160	160	1.0

* From Klaassen, C. D.: Comparison of the toxicity of chemicals in newborn rats to bile duct-ligated and sham-operated rats and mice. *Toxicol. Appl. Pharmacol.*, **24**:37–44, 1973.

toxicant that undergoes an enterohepatic cycle might have a very long duration in the body if it continues to undergo enterohepatic cycling, and thus it might be advantageous to interrupt the cycle to hasten the elimination of the toxicant from the body. This principle has been utilized in the treatment of methyl mercury poisoning by introducing a polythiol resin into the gastrointestinal tract that binds the mercurial and thus prevents its reabsorption (Clarkson and Magos, 1976).

If the liver is injured by disease or chemical means, the biliary excretory ability of the liver is often decreased. In fact, the clearance of sulfobromophthalein (BSP) and indocyanine green (ICG) are often used to assess hepatic function. This decrease in hepatic function results in a longer biologic half-life of the compound and can increase the toxicity of some compounds.

An increase in hepatic excretory function has been observed after pretreatment with some drugs. For example, phenobarbital has been demonstrated to increase the plasma disappearance and biliary excretion of sulfobromophthalein, bilirubin, phenol-3,6-dibromophthalein disulfonate, amaranth, indocyanine green, ouabain, procainamide ethyl bromide, and mercury (Klaassen, 1970a, 1975a). This increase in biliary excretion is not due only to an increased biotransformation, for this effect is observed with phenol-3,6-dibromophthalein disulfonate, amaranth, and ouabain, agents that are not conjugated before excretion. The increase in bile flow produced by phenobarbital (Klaassen, 1971) appears to be an important factor in increasing the biliary excretion of sulfobromophthalein (Klaassen, 1970b), but other factors such as the increase in ligandin, an intracellular binding protein (Reyes et al., 1969), increase in conjugating capacity of the liver, and increase in blood flow may also be important for the enhanced plasma disappearance and biliary excretion of some drugs after phenobarbital. Not all microsomal enzyme inducers increase biliary flow and excretion (Klaassen, 1969, 1970b); 3-methylcholanthrene and 3,4-benzpyrene have little effect.

An increase in biliary excretion can decrease the toxicity of foreign compounds. Phenobarbital treatment of laboratory animals has been shown to enhance the biliary excretion and elimination of methyl mercury from the body (Klaassen, 1975a; Clarkson and Magos, 1976). Recently two steroids that are known to induce microsomal enzymes, spironolactone and pregnenolone-16α-carbonitrile, have also been shown to increase bile production and biliary excretion of sulfobromophthalein (Zsigmond and Soly-

mose, 1972). These two steroids have been demonstrated to decrease the toxicity of a number of chemicals (Seyle, 1971), including cardiac glycosides (Selye, 1969), and mercury (Selye, 1972). These steroids protect against the toxic effects of cardiac glycosides by increasing their biliary excretion, which decreases their concentration in the heart, the target organ for toxicity (Castle and Lage, 1972, 1973; Klaassen, 1974a). The protection offered by spironolactone against mercury does not appear to be due to an increase in biliary excretion but rather an alteration in the distribution of mercury. Spironolactone is metabolized in the body to canrenone and thioacetate. The thioacetate forms a ligand with mercury in the body and reduces its concentration in the kidney, the target organ for mercury toxicity, and thus protects the animal against mercury toxicity (Klaassen, 1975b).

In contrast, the toxicity of some compounds can be directly related to their biliary excretion. For example, indomethacin has been demonstrated to produce intestinal lesions. It has been shown that the sensitivity of various species to this toxic response is directly related to the amount of indomethacin excreted into the bile and that the formation of intestinal lesions can be abolished by bile duct ligation (Duggan et al., 1975).

The hepatic excretory system is not fully developed in the newborn and is another reason why some compounds are more toxic in the newborn than in the adult (Klaassen, 1972, 1973a). For example, ouabain is about 40 times more toxic in the newborn than in the adult rat. This is due to the almost complete lack of ability of the liver of the newborn rat to remove the ouabain from the plasma. A similar relative inability of the liver of the newborn to excrete other foreign compounds has been demonstrated (Klaassen, 1973c). Enhancement of the development of the hepatic excretory mechanisms can be achieved by administering microsomal enzyme inducers (Klaassen, 1974b).

Other Routes of Excretion

Lung. Substances that exist predominantly in the gas phase at body temperature are excreted principally by the lungs. Because liquids are in equilibrium with a gas phase, they too may be excreted via the lungs. Thus, the amount of liquid excreted by the lungs is related to its vapor pressure. This principle is widely used for determining the amount of ethanol in the body. Highly volatile liquids, such as diethyl ether, are almost exclusively excreted by the lungs.

No specialized transport systems have been described for the excretion of toxic substances by the lung; they are eliminated by simple

concentration of chemical in the plasma by the volume of distribution.

Total amount in body $= C \cdot V_d$

Another pharmacokinetic parameter often calculated for a toxicant is the "total body clearance." This is similar to the concept of renal clearance except that the body as a whole is acting as a chemical-eliminating system. This clearance is the sum of the individual clearances of the chemical by the various organs and tissues of the body. Thus, in the case of a chemical that is eliminated solely by renal excretion and hepatic biotransformation, total body clearance is the sum of renal and hepatic clearance. Total body clearance (Cl_b) can be calculated by the following equation:

$$Cl_b = V_d \cdot k_{el} = \frac{\text{DOSE}_{1.v.}}{\text{AUC}_{0 \to \infty}}$$

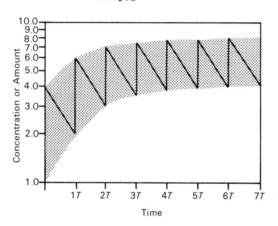

Figure 3–7. Schematic curves of accumulation with repeated exposure at constant intervals.

The concentration of a chemical in the plasma and other tissues and the amount of chemical in the body after repeated exposure or administration are obviously important factors to be considered in the toxicologic evaluation of a substance. If the half-life is small in relation to the exposure interval, the substance may be almost completely eliminated during this interval, and the amount after consecutive doses would be practically equal to that after the initial dose. When the half-life is about the same as or larger than the exposure interval, an appreciable amount of toxicant will be left in the body prior to the second and subsequent exposures, and the toxicant will accumulate (Fig. 3–7). Assuming that the first-order elimination processes following a single dose do not change, the cumulative concentration or amount in the body, as shown in Figure 3–7, fluctuates between the exposures.

The "average" concentration at the plateau, $\bar{C}_\infty$, can be determined by the following equation:

$$\bar{C}_\infty = \frac{F \cdot D}{V_d k_{el} \tau}$$

where τ is the constant time interval between administration or exposure. The "average" body burden at steady state ($\bar{X}_\infty$) is described by the following relationship:

$$\bar{X}_\infty = \bar{C}_\infty \cdot V_d$$

Often after administration of a chemical to an animal, one does not observe a monoexponential elimination of the toxicant from the body (i.e.,

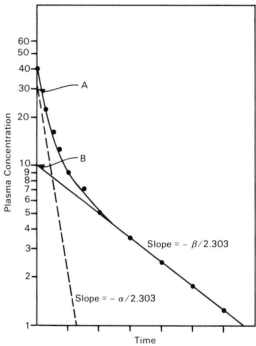

Figure 3–8. Semilogarithmic plot of concentration of chemical in plasma after intravenous injection when the body may be represented as a two-compartment, open system. The dashed line is obtained by "feathering" the curve.

the kinetic behavior is that of a single compartment system) but rather a biexponential one as shown in Figure 3–8. The disposition of the drug is said to obey a two-compartment model. If a chemical is injected intravenously, it usually takes some time before it is distributed in the body. During the distributive phase (α), concentrations of the chemical in the plasma will decrease more rapidly than in the postdistributive phase (β). The distributive phase may last for only a few minutes or for hours or days. Whether or not this distributive phase is apparent will depend on the timing of the plasma samples. If a chemical's fate can be described by a two-compartment model, the semilogarithmic plot of plasma concentration as a function of time after intravenous administration can be resolved into two exponential components. This can be done graphically, by the method of residuals (also called "feathering") as is depicted in the figure, where the β phase was extrapolated to 0 time, and the difference between the observed points and the extrapolated line were plotted to give the new line α. The slopes of the rapid and slow exponential components are designated as $-\alpha/2.303$ and $-\beta/2.303$, respectively. The intercepts on the concentration axis are designated A and B.

A biexponential decline of chemical from the plasma usually justifies, from a pharmacokinetic point of view, the representation of the body as an open, two-compartment, linear system. It is

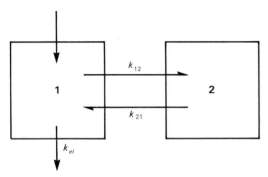

Figure 3–9. Schematic representation of the two-compartment system consisting of a central compartment (1) and a peripheral compartment (2). The numbering of the rate constants (k) indicates the originating compartment (first numeral) and the receiving compartment (second numeral).

usually assumed that the chemical is removed from the central or plasma compartment as depicted in Figure 3–9. The reason for this assumption is that the liver and kidney, the major sites of biotransformation and excretion, are well perfused with blood and thus are rapidly accessible to chemical in the central compartment. The rate constants between the two compartments and excretion are given by the following equations:

$$k_{21} = \frac{\alpha B + \beta A}{A + B}$$

$$k_{el} = \frac{\alpha\beta}{k_{21}}$$

$$k_{12} = \alpha + \beta - k_{21} - k_{el}$$

It should be noted that the elimination rate constant (k_{el}) in a two-compartment model is not the same as the terminal half-life (β) as it is in

a one-compartment model. Determination of these rate constants permits an assessment of the relative contribution of distribution and elimination processes to the chemical concentration versus time profile of the chemical.

The apparent volume of distribution (V_d) of a chemical in a two-compartment system can be calculated from the following equation:

$$V_d = \frac{D}{(\text{AUC}_{0\to\infty})\,\beta}$$

The elimination of some chemicals may be more complex than what can be described by a two-compartment model, and a multicompartment model might be necessary. Toxicants that are slowly distributed to and released from "deep" compartments such as that in fat and bones may require multicompartmental models.

CONCLUSIONS

Man is in continual contact with toxic agents. They are in the food he eats, the water he drinks, and the air he breathes. Depending on the physical and chemical properties of the toxic agents, they may be absorbed by the gastrointestinal tract, lungs, and/or skin. Fortunately, the body has the ability to metabolize and to excrete these compounds into the urine, bile, and air. However, when the rate of absorption exceeds the rate of excretion, the toxic compound accumulates to a critical concentration in the body, and toxic effects are observed.

REFERENCES

Albert, A.: *Selective Toxicity*, 3rd ed. Methuen & Co., London, 1965.

Allenby, A. C.; Creasey, N. H.; Edginton, J. A. G.; Fletcher, J. A.; and Schock, C.: Mechanism of action of accelerants on skin penetration. *Br. J. Dermatol.*, **81** (Suppl. 4):47–55, 1969.

Amoroso, E. C.: Placentation. In Parks, A. S. (ed.): *Marshall's Physiology of Reproduction*, Vol. 2, 3rd ed. Longmans, Green & Co., London, 1952, pp. 127–311.

Barnett, H. L.; McNamara, H.; Schultz, S.; and Tompsett, R.: Renal clearances of sodium penicillin G, procaine penicillin G, and inulin in infants and children. *Pediatrics*, 3:418–22, 1949.

Barrnett, R. J.: The demonstration with the electron microscope of the end-products of histochemical reactions in relation to the fine structure of cells. *Exp. Cell Res.*, (Suppl. 7):65–89, 1959.

Bates, T. R., and Gibaldi, M.: Gastrointestinal absorption of drugs. In Swarbrick, J. (ed.): *Current Concepts in the Pharmaceutical Sciences: Biopharmaceutics.* Lea & Febiger, Philadelphia, 1970.

Blank, I. H., and Scheuplein, R. J.: Transport into and within the skin. *Br. J. Dermatol.*, **81** (Suppl. 4):4–10, 1969.

Borowitz, J. L.; Moore, P. F.; Yim, G. K. W.; and Miya, T. S.: Mechanism of enhanced drug effects produced by dilution of the oral dose. *Toxicol. Appl. Pharmacol.*, 19:164–68, 1971.

Boyes, R. N.; Adams, H. J.; and Duce, B. R.: Oral absorption and disposition kinetics of lidocaine hydrochloride in dogs. *J. Pharmacol. Exp. Ther.*, **174**:1–8, 1970.

Castle, M. C., and Lage, G. L.: Effect of pretreatment with spironolactone, phenobarbital or β-diethylaminoethyl diphenylpropylacetate (SKF 525-A) on tritium levels in blood, heart and liver of rats at various times after administration of [³H] digitoxin. *Biochem. Pharmacol.*, **21**:1449–55, 1972.

———: Enhanced biliary excretion of digitoxin following spironolactone as it relates to the prevention of digitoxin toxicity. *Res. Commun. Chem. Pathol. Pharmacol.*, **5**:99–108, 1973.

Clarkson, T., and Magos, L.: The effect of oral doses of a polythiol resin on the excretion of methylmercury in mice treated with cysteine, *d*-penicillamine or phenibarbitone. *Chem. Biol. Interact.*, **14**:325–35, 1976.

Cohn, V. H.: Transmembrane movement of drug molecules. In La Du, B. N.; Mandel, H. G.; and Way, E. L. (eds.): *Fundamentals of Drug Metabolism and Drug Disposition.* Williams & Wilkins Co., Baltimore, 1971, pp. 3–21.

Coulston, F., and Serrone, D. M.: The comparative approach to the role of nonhuman primates in evaluation of drug toxicity in man: a review. *Ann. N.Y. Acad. Sci.*, **162**:681–704, 1969.

Dawes, G. S.: *Foetal and Neonatal Physiology. A Comparative Study of the Changes at Birth.* Year Book Medical Publishers, Inc., Chicago, 1968.

Dowling, R. H.: Compensatory changes in intestinal absorption. *Br. Med. Bull.*, **23**:275–78, 1967.

Draize, J. H.; Woodard, G.; and Calvery, H. O.: Methods for the study of irritation and toxicity of substances applied topically to the skin and mucous membranes. *J. Pharmacol. Exp. Ther.*, **82**:377–90, 1944.

Dugard, P. H., and Embery, G.: The influence of dimethyl sulphoxide on the percutaneous migration of potassium butyl [³⁵S] sulphate, potassium methyl [³⁵S] sulphate and sodium [³⁵S] sulphate. *Br. J. Dermatol.*, **81**, (Suppl. 4):69–74, 1969.

Duggan, D. E.; Hooke, K. F.; Noll, R. M.; and Kwan, K. C.: Enterohepatic circulation of indomethacin and its role in intestinal irritation. *Biochem. Pharmacol.*, **24**:1749–54, 1975.

Ferguson, H. C.: Dilution of dose and acute oral toxicity. *Toxicol. Appl. Pharmacol.*, **4**:759–62, 1962.

Fox, C. F.: The structure of cell membranes. *Sci. Am.*, **226** (2):30–44, 1972.

Ginsburg, J.: Placental drug transfer. *Annu. Rev. Pharmacol.*, **11**:387–408, 1971.

Goldstein, A.; Aronow, L.; and Kalman, S. M. (eds.): *Principles of Drug Action: The Basis of Pharmacology*, 2nd ed. John Wiley & Sons, Inc., New York, 1974.

Gorringe, J. A. L., and Sproston, E. M.: The influence of particle size upon the absorption of drugs from the gastrointestinal tract. In Binns, T. B. (ed.): *Absorption and Distribution of Drugs.* Williams & Wilkins Co., Baltimore, 1964, pp. 128–39.

Gurtner, G. H., and Burns, B.: Possible facilitated transport of oxygen across the placenta. *Nature (Lond.)*, **240**:473–75, 1972.

Hammond, P. B.: Lead poisoning. An old problem with a new dimension. In Blood, F. R. (ed.): *Essays in Toxicology*, Vol. 1. Academic Press, Inc., New York, 1969, pp. 115–55.

Hayes, W. J., Jr.: Review of the metabolism of chlorinated hydrocarbon insecticides especially in mammals. *Annu. Rev. Pharmacol.*, **5**:27–52, 1965.

Heath, D. F., and Vandekar, M.: Toxicity and metabolism of dieldrin in rats. *Br. J. Ind. Med.*, **21**:269–79, 1964.

Hirsch, G. H., and Hook, J. B.: Maturation of renal organic acid transport: substrate stimulation by penicillin and *p*-aminohippurate (PAH). *J. Pharmacol. Exp. Ther.*, **171**:103–108, 1970.

Hunter, A., and Klaassen, C. D.: Species difference in the plasma disappearance and biliary excretion of procaine amide ethobromide. *Proc. Soc. Exp. Biol. Med.*, **139**:1445–50, 1972.

Juchau, M. R.: Mechanisms of drug biotransformation reactions in the placenta. *Fed. Proc.*, **31**:48–51, 1972.

Kello, D., and Kostial, K.: The effect of milk diet on lead metabolism in rats. *Environ. Res.*, **6**:355–60, 1973.

Klaassen, C. D.: Biliary flow after microsomal enzyme induction. *J. Pharmacol. Exp. Ther.*, **168**:218–23, 1969.

———: Effects of phenobarbital on the plasma disappearance and biliary excretion of drugs in rats. *J. Pharmacol. Exp. Ther.*, **175**:289–300, 1970a.

———: Plasma disappearance and biliary excretion of sulfobromophthalein and phenol-3,6-dibromophthalein disulfonate after microsomal enzyme induction. *Biochem. Pharmacol.*, **19**:1241–49, 1970b.

———: Studies on the increased biliary flow produced by phenobarbital in rats. *J. Pharmacol. Exp. Ther.*, **176**:743–51, 1971.

———: Immaturity of the newborn rat's hepatic excretory function for ouabain. *J. Pharmacol. Exp. Ther.*, **183**:520–26, 1972.

———: Comparison of the toxicity of chemicals in newborn rats to bile duct-ligated and sham-operated rats and mice. *Toxicol. Appl. Pharmacol.*, **24**:37–44, 1973a.

———: The effect of altered hepatic function on the toxicity, plasma disappearance and biliary excretion of diethylstilbestrol. *Toxicol. Appl. Pharmacol.* **24**:142–49, 1973b.

———: Hepatic excretory function in the newborn rat. *J. Pharmacol. Exp. Ther.*, **184**:721–28, 1973c.

———: Effect of microsomal enzyme inducers on the biliary excretion of cardiac glycosides. *J. Pharmacol. Exp. Ther.*, **191**:201–11, 1974a.

———: Stimulation of the development of the hepatic excretory mechanism for ouabain in newborn rats with microsomal enzyme inducers. *J. Pharmacol. Exp. Ther.*, **191**:212–18, 1974b.

———: Biliary excretion of mercury compounds. *Toxicol. Appl. Pharmacol.*, **33**:356–65, 1975a.

———: Effect of spironolactone on the distribution of mercury. *Toxicol. Appl. Pharmacol.*, **33**:366–75, 1975b.

———: Biliary excretion of metals. *Drug Metab. Rev.*, **5**:165–96, 1976.

Klaassen, C. D., and Plaa, G. L.: Species variation in metabolism, storage, and excretion of sulfobromophthalein. *Am. J. Physiol.*, **213**:1322–26, 1967.

Klaassen, C. D., and Shoeman, D. W.: Biliary excretion of lead. Proceedings of the Fifth International Congress of Pharmacology (abstract), 1972, p. 757.

Kupferberg, H. J., and Way, E. L.: Pharmacologic basis for the increased sensitivity of the newborn rat to morphine. *J. Pharmacol. Exp. Ther.*, **141**:105–12, 1963.

Leopold, G.; Furukawa, E.; Forth, W.; and Rummel, W.: Comparative studies of absorption of heavy metals *in vivo* and *in vitro*. *Arch. Pharmacol. Exp. Pathol.*, **263**:275–76, 1969.

Levi, A. J.; Gatmaitan, Z.; and Arias, I. M.: Two hepatic cytoplasmic protein fractions, Y and Z, and their possible role in the hepatic uptake of bilirubin, sulfobromophthalein, and other anions. *J. Clin. Invest.*, **48**:2156–67, 1969.

Levine, R. R.: Factors affecting gastrointestinal absorption of drugs. *Am. J. Dig. Dis.*, **15**:171–88, 1970.

Levine, R. R., and Pelikan, E. W.: Mechanisms of drug absorption and excretion. Passage of drugs out of and into the gastrointestinal tract. *Annu. Rev. Pharmacol.*, **4**:69–84, 1964.

Levine, R. R., and Steinberg, G. M.: Intestinal absorption of pralidoxime and other aldoximes. *Nature (Lond.),* **209**:269–71, 1966.

Litwack, G.; Ketterer, B.; and Arias, I. M.: Ligandin: A hepatic protein which binds steroids, bilirubin carcinogens and a number of exogenous organic anions. *Nature (Lond.),* **234**:466–67, 1971.

Lucis, O. J.; Shaikh, Z. A.; and Embil, J. A., Jr.: Cadmium as a trace element and cadmium binding components in human cells. *Experientia,* **26**:1109–10, 1970.

Lukas, G.; Brindle, S. D.; and Greengard, P.: The route of absorption of intraperitoneally administered compounds. *J. Pharmacol. Exp. Ther.,* **178**:562–66, 1971.

McNay, J. L., and Dayton, P. G.: Placental transfer of a substituted pteridine from fetus to mother. *Science,* **167**:988–90, 1970.

Malkinson, F. D.: Permeability of the stratum corneum. In Montagna, W., and Lobitz, W. C., Jr. (eds.): *The Epidermis.* Academic Press, Inc., New York, 1964.

Magos, L., and Clarkson, T. W.: The effect of oral doses of a polythiol resin in the excretion of methylmercury in mice treated with cysteine, D-penicillamine or phenobarbitone. *Chem.-Biol. Interactions,* **14**:325–35, 1976.

Margoshes, M., and Vallee, B. L.: A cadmium protein from equine kidney cortex. *J. Am. Chem. Soc.,* **79**:4813–14, 1957.

Marzulli, F. N.; Callahan, J. F.; and Brown, D. W. C.: Chemical structure and skin penetrating capacity of a short series of organic phosphates and phosphoric acid. *J. Invest. Dermatol.,* **44**:339–44, 1965.

Mendel, J. L., and Walton, M. S.: Conversion of p,p'-DDT to p,p'-DDD by intestinal flora of the rat. *Science,* **151**:1527–28, 1966.

Mirkin, B. L., and Singh, S.: Placental transfer and pharmacokinetics of digoxin in the pregnant rat. Proceedings of the Fifth International Congress of Pharmacology (abstract), 949, 1972.

Pentschew, A., and Garro, F.: Lead encephalo-myelopathy of the suckling rat and its implications on the porphyrinopathic nervous diseases. *Acta Neuropathol. (Berl.),* **6**:266–78, 1966.

Pfeiffer, C. J.: Gastroenterologic response to environmental agents—absorption and interactions. In Lee, D. H. K. (ed.): *Handbook of Physiology. Section 9: Reactions to Environmental Agents.* American Physiological Society, Bethesda, 1977, pp. 349–74.

Plaa, G. L.: Biliary and other routes of excretion of drugs. In La Du, B. N.; Mandel, H. G.; and Way, E. L. (eds.): *Fundamentals of Drug Metabolism and Drug Disposition.* Williams & Wilkins Co., Baltimore, 1971, pp. 131–45.

Reyes, H.; Levi, A. J.; Gatmaitan, Z.; and Arias, I. M.: Organic anion-binding protein in rat liver: drug induction and its physiologic consequence. *Proc. N.Y. Acad. Sci.,* **64**:168–70, 1969.

Rosenfield, A. B., and Huston, R.: Infant methemoglobinemia in Minnesota due to nitrates in well water. *Minn. Med.,* **33**:787–96, 1950.

Russell, J. Q., and Klaassen, C. D.: Species variation in the biliary excretion of ouabain. *J. Pharmacol. Exp. Ther.,* **183**:513–19, 1972.

Sanders, E., and Ashworth, C. T.: A study of particulate intestinal absorption of hepatocellular uptake. Use of polystyrene latex particles. *Exp. Cell Res.,* **22**:137–45, 1961.

Sasser, L. B., and Jarboe, G. E.: Intestinal absorption and retention of cadmium in neonatal rat. *Toxicol. Appl. Pharmacol.,* **41**:423–31, 1977.

Scala, J.; McOsker, D. E.; and Reller, H. H.: The percutaneous absorption of ionic surfactants. *J. Invest. Dermatol.,* **50**:371–79, 1968.

Schade, S. G.; Felsher, B. F.; Glader, B. E.; and Conrad, M. E.: Effect of cobalt upon iron absorption. *Proc. Soc. Exp. Biol. Med.,* **134**:741–43, 1970.

Schanker, L. S.: Mechanisms of drug absorption and distribution. *Annu. Rev. Pharmacol.,* **1**:29–44, 1961.

——: Passage of drugs across body membranes. *Pharmacol. Rev.,* **14**:501–30, 1962.

Schanker, L. S., and Jeffrey, J. J.: Active transport of foreign pyrimidines across the intestinal epithelium. *Nature (Lond.)* **190**:727–28, 1961.

Schwartze, E. W.: The so-called habituation to "arsenic:" variation in the toxicity of arsenious oxide. *J. Pharmacol. Exp. Ther.,* **20**:181–203, 1923.

Selye, H.; Krajny, M.; and Savoie, L.: Digitoxin poisoning: Prevention by spironolactone. *Science,* **164**:842–43, 1969.

——: Hormones and resistance. *J. Pharm. Sci.,* **60**:1–28, 1971.

——: Mercury poisoning: Prevention by spironolactone. *Science,* **169**:775–76, 1970.

Shand, D. G., and Rangno, R. E.: The disposition of propranolol. 1. Elimination during oral absorption in man. *Pharmacology,* **7**:159–68, 1972.

Sharp, C. W.; Ollolenghi, A.; and Posner, H. S.: Correlation of paraquat toxicity with tissue concentrations and weight loss of the rat. *Toxicol. Appl. Pharmacol.,* **22**:241–51, 1972.

Shoeman, D. W.; Kauffman, R. E.; Azarnoff, D. L.; and Boulos, B. M.: Placental transfer of diphenylhydantoin in the goat. *Biochem. Pharmacol.,* **21**:1237–43, 1972.

Silverman, W. A.; Andersen, D. H.; Blanc, W. A.; and Crozier, D. N.: A difference in mortality rate and incidence of kernicterus among premature infants allotted to two prophylactic antibacterial regimens. *Pediatrics,* **18**:614–25, 1956.

Sobel, A. E.; Gawron, O.; and Kramer, B.: Influence of vitamin D in experimental lead poisoning. *Proc. Soc. Exp. Biol. Med.,* **38**:433–35, 1938.

Stowe, C. M., and Plaa, G. L.: Extrarenal excretion of drugs and chemicals. *Annu. Rev. Pharmacol.,* **8**:337–56, 1968.

Thompson, R. Q.; Sturtevant, M.; Bird, O. D.; and Glazko, A. J.: The effect of metabolites of chloramphenicol (Chloromycetin) on the thyroid of the rat. *Endocrinology,* **55**:665–81, 1954.

Thomson, A. B. R.; Olatunbosun, D.; and Valberg, L. S.: Interrelation of intestinal transport system for manganese and iron. *J. Lab. Clin. Med.,* **78**:642–55, 1971a.

Thomson, A. B. R.; Valberg, L. S.; and Sinclair, D. G.: Competitive nature of the intestinal transport mechanism for cobalt and iron in the rat. *J. Clin. Invest.,* **50**:2384–94, 1971b.

Tune, B. M.; Wu, K. Y.; and Kempson, R. L.: Inhibition of transport and prevention of toxicity of cephaloridine in the kidney. Dose-responsiveness of the rabbit and the guinea pig to probenecid. *J. Pharmacol. Exp. Ther.,* **202**:466–71, 1977.

Weiner, I. M., and Mudge, G. H.: Renal tubular mechanisms for excretion of organic acids and bases. *Am. J. Med.,* **36**:743–62, 1964.

Wester, R. C., and Maibach, H. I.: Percutaneous absorption in man and animal: a perspective. In Drill, V. A., and Lazar, P. (eds.): *Cutaneous Toxicity.* Academic Press, Inc., New York, 1977.

Williams, R. M., and Beck, F.: A histochemical study of gut maturation. *J. Anat.,* **105**:487–501, 1969.

Winteringham, F. P. W.: Comparative biochemical aspects of insecticidal action. *Chem. Ind. (London),* 1195–1202, 1957.

Wold, J. S.; Joost, R. R.; and Owen, N. V.: Nephrotoxicity of cephaloridine in newborn rabbits: role of the renal anionic transport system. *J. Pharmacol. Exp. Ther.*, **201**:778–85, 1977.

Young, M.: Three topics in placental transport: amino acid transport; oxygen transfer; placental function during labour. In Klopper, A., and Diczfalusy, E. (eds.): *Foetus and Placenta*. Blackwell Scientific Publications, Oxford, 1969.

Zsigmond, G., and Solymoss, B.: Effect of spironolactone, pregnenolone-16α-carbonitrile and cortisol on the metabolism and biliary excretion of sulfobromophthalein and phenol-3,6-dibromophthalein disulfonate in rats. *J. Pharmacol. Exp. Ther.*, **183**:499–507, 1972.

SUPPLEMENTAL READING

Alberti, R. E.; Lippmann, M.; Spiegelman, J.; Strehlow, C.; Briscoe, W.; Wolfson, P.; and Nelson, N.: The clearance of radioactive particles from the human lung. In Davies, C. N. (ed.): *Inhaled Particles and Vapours*, Vol. 11. Pergamon Press, New York and London, 1967, pp. 361–77.

Ariëns, E. J.; Simonis, A. M.; and Offermeier, J.: *Introduction to General Toxicology*. Academic Press, Inc., New York, 1976.

Asling, J., and Way, E. L.: Placental transfer of drugs. In La Du, B. N.; Mandel, H. G.; and Way, E. L. (eds.): *Fundamentals of Drug Metabolism and Drug Disposition*. Williams & Wilkins Co., Baltimore, 1971, pp. 88–105.

Barltrop, D., and Khoo, H. E.: The influence of nutritional factors on lead absorption. *Postgrad. Med. J.*, **51**:795–800, 1975.

Barth, D. S.; Black, S. C.; and Hammerle, J. R.: Chemical agents in air. In Lee, D. H. K. (ed.): *Handbook of Physiology. Section 9: Reactions to Environmental Agents*. American Physiological Society, Bethesda, 1977, pp. 157–66.

Brodie, B. B.: Distribution and fate of drugs: therapeutic implications. In Binns, T. B. (ed.): *Absorption and Distribution of Drugs*. Williams & Wilkins Co., Baltimore, 1964a, pp. 199–251.

———: Physico-chemical factors in drug absorption. In Binns, T. B. (ed.): *Absorption and Distribution of Drugs*. Williams & Wilkins Co., Baltimore, 1964b, pp. 16–48.

Brundelet, P. J.: Experimental study of the dust-clearance mechanism of the lung. I. Histological study in rats of the intrapulmonary bronchial route of elimination. *Acta Pathol. Microbiol. Scand.*, (Suppl. 175):7–141, 1965.

Butler, T. C.: The distribution of drugs. In La Du, B. N.; Mandel, H. G.; and Way, E. L. (eds.): *Fundamentals of Drug Metabolism and Drug Disposition*. Williams & Wilkins Co., Baltimore, 1971, pp. 44–62.

Cafruny, E. J.: Renal excretion of drugs. In La Du, B. N.; Mandel, H. G.; and Way, E. L. (eds.): *Fundamentals of Drug Metabolism and Drug Disposition*. Williams & Wilkins Co., Baltimore, 1971, pp. 119–30.

Casarett, L. J.: Toxicology: The respiratory tract. *Annu. Rev. Pharmacol.*, **11**:425–46, 1971.

———: The vital sacs: Alveolar clearance mechanisms in inhalation toxicology. In Hayes, W. J., Jr. (ed.): *Essays in Toxicology*, Vol. 3. Academic Press, Inc., New York, 1972.

Christensen, H. N.: *Biological Transport*, 2nd ed. W. A. Benjamin, Inc., Reading, MA, 1975.

Davidson, C.: Protein binding. In La Du, B. N.; Mandel, H. G.; and Way, E. L. (eds.): *Fundamentals of Drug Metabolism and Drug Disposition*. Williams & Wilkins Co., Baltimore, 1971, pp. 63–75.

Fingl, E., and Woodbury, D. M.: General principles. In Goodman, L. S., and Gilman, A. (eds.): *The Pharma-cological Basis of Therapeutics*, 4th ed. Macmillan Publishing Co., Inc., New York, 1970, pp. 1–35.

Gehring, P. J.; Watanabe, P. G.; and Blau, G. E.: Pharmacokinetic studies in evaluation of the toxicological and environmental hazard of chemicals. In Mehlman, M. A.; Shapiro, R. E.; and Blumenthal, H. (eds.): *Advances in Modern Toxicology*. Vol. 1: *New Concepts in Safety Evaluation*. Hemisphere Publishing Co., Washington, DC, 1976, pp. 195–270.

Gibaldi, M.: *Biopharmaceutics and Clinical Pharmacokinetics*, 2nd ed. Lea & Febiger, Philadelphia, 1977.

Gibaldi, M., and Levy, G.: Pharmacokinetics in clinical practice. 1. Concepts. *J.A.M.A.*, **235**:1864–67, 1976.

———: Pharmacokinetics in clinical practice. 2. Applications. *J.A.M.A.*, **235**:1987–92, 1976.

Green, G. M.: Pulmonary clearance of infectious agents. *Annu. Rev. Med.*, **19**:315–36, 1968.

Greenblatt, D. J., and Koch-Weser, J.: Drug therapy: Clinical pharmacokinetics. *N. Engl. J. Med.*, **293**:702–705, 964–70, 1975.

Hartiala, K.: Metabolism of foreign substances in the gastrointestinal tract. In Lee, D. H. K. (ed.): *Handbook of Physiology. Section 9: Reactions to Environmental Agents*. American Physiological Society, Bethesda, 1977, pp. 375–88.

Hatch, T. F., and Gross, P.; *Pulmonary Deposition and Retention of Inhaled Aerosols*. Academic Press, Inc., New York, 1964.

Hayes, W. J., Jr.: *Essays in Toxicology*, Vol. 3. Academic Press, Inc., New York, 1972.

Hayes, W. J.: *Toxicology of Pesticides*. Williams & Wilkins Co., Baltimore, 1975.

Jackson, M. J., and Cohn, V. H.: Determinants of xenobiotic transport at biological barriers. In Lee, D. H. K. (ed.): *Handbook of Physiology. Section 9: Reactions to Environmental Agents*. American Physiological Society, Bethesda, 1977, pp. 397–418.

Kilburn, K. H.: Clearance mechanisms in the respiratory tract. In Lee, D. H. K. (ed.): *Handbook of Physiology. Section 9: Reactions to Environmental Agents*. American Physiological Society, Bethesda, 1977, pp. 243–62.

Klaassen, C. D.: Biliary excretion of xenobiotics. In Goldberg, L. (ed.): *Critical Reviews in Toxicology*, Vol. 4. CRC Press, Inc., Cleveland, 1975, pp. 1–29.

———: Biliary excretion of metals. *Drug Metab. Rev.*, **5**:165–96, 1976.

———: Biliary excretion. In Lee, D. H. K. (ed.): *Handbook of Physiology. Section 9: Reactions to Environmental Agents*. American Physiological Society, Bethesda, 1977, pp. 537–54.

Klocke, R. A.: Pulmonary excretion of absorbed gases. In Lee, D. H. K. (ed.): *Handbook of Physiology. Section 9: Reactions to Environmental Agents*. American Physiological Society, Bethesda, 1977, pp. 555–62.

Levy, G., and Gibaldi, M.: Pharmacokinetics. In Eichler, O.; Farah, A.; Herken, H.; and Welch, A. D. (eds.): *Handbook of Experimental Pharmacology*, Vol. XXVIII/3. Springer, Berlin, 1975.

Loomis, T. A.: *Essentials of Toxicology*, 2nd ed. Lea & Febiger, Philadelphia, 1974.

Lyle, W. H.; Green, J. N.; Gore, V.; and Vidler, J.: Enhancement of cadmium nephrotoxicity by pencillamine in the rat. *Postgrad. Med. J.*, **44**, (Oct. Suppl.): 18–21, 1968.

Malkinson, F. D., and Gehlmann, L.: Factors affecting percutaneous absorption. In Drill, V. A., and Lazar, P. (eds.): *Cutaneous Toxicity*. Academic Press, Inc., New York, 1977, pp. 63–81.

Marzulli, F. N.: Barriers to skin penetration. *J. Invest. Dermatol.*, **39**:387–93, 1962.

Melmon, K. L., and Morrelli, H. F. (eds.): *Clinical Pharmacology: Basic Principles in Therapeutics*. Macmillan Publishing Co., Inc., New York, 1972.

Morrow, P. E.; Bates, D. V.; Fish, B. R.; Hatch, T. F.; and Mercer, T. T.: Deposition and retention models for internal dosimetry of the human respiratory tract. *Health Phys.*, **12**:173–207, 1966.

Morrow, P. E.; Gibb, F. R.; and Gazioglu, K.: The clearance of dust from the lower respiratory tract of man: an experimental study. In Davies, C. N. (ed.): *Inhaled Particles and Vapours*, 11. Pergamon Press, New York and London, 1967, pp. 351–59.

Munson, E. S., and Eger, E. I., II: Pulmonary disposition of drugs. In La Du, B. N.; Mandel, H. G.; and Way, E. L. (eds.): *Fundamentals of Drug Metabolism and Drug Disposition.* Williams & Wilkins Co., Baltimore, 1971, pp. 106–18.

Pfeiffer, C. J., and Hänninen, O.: Alimentary excretion of environmental agents and unnatural compounds. In Lee, D. H. K. (ed.): *Handbook of Physiology. Section 9: Reactions to Environmental Agents.* American Physiological Society, Bethesda, 1977, pp. 513–36.

Piotrowski, J. K.: Retention and excretion kinetics of chemical agents. In Lee, D. H. K. (ed.): *Handbook of Physiology. Section 9: Reactions to Environmental Agents.* American Physiological Society, Bethesda, 1977, pp. 389–96.

Rall, D. P.: Drug entry into brain and cerebrospinal fluid. In La Du, B. N.; Mandel, H. G.; and Way, E. L. (eds.): *Fundamentals of Drug Metabolism and Drug Disposition.* Williams & Wilkins Co., Baltimore, 1971, pp. 76–87.

Schanker, L. S.: Drug absorption. In La Du, B. N.; Mandel, H. G.; and Way, E. L. (eds.): *Fundamentals of Drug Metabolism and Drug Disposition.* Williams & Wilkins Co., Baltimore, 1971a, pp. 22–43.

————: Intimate study of drug action. I: Absorption, distribution, and excretion. In DiPalma, J. R. (ed.): *Drill's Pharmacology in Medicine*, 4th ed. McGraw-Hill Book Co., New York, 1971b, pp. 21–35.

Scheuplein, R. J.: Permeability of the skin. In Lee, D. H. K. (ed.): *Handbook of Physiology: Reactions to Environmental Agents.* American Physiological Society, Bethesda, 1977, pp. 299–322.

Schiller, E.: Inhalation, retention and elimination of dusts from dogs' and rats' lungs with special reference to the alveolar phagocytes and bronchial epithelium. In Davies, C. N. (ed.): *Inhaled Particles and Vapours.* Pergamon Press, New York and London, 1961, pp. 342–44.

Shaw, J. E.; Chandrasekaran, S. K.; Campbell, P. S.; and Schmitt, L. G.: New procedures for evaluating cutaneous absorption. In Drill, V. A., and Lazar, P. (eds.): *Cutaneous Toxicity.* Academic Press, Inc., New York, 1977, pp. 83–94.

Smith, F. A., and Hursh, J. B.: Bone storage and release. In Lee, D. H. K. (ed.): *Handbook of Physiology: Reactions to Environmental Agents.* American Physiological Society, Bethesda, 1977, pp. 469–82.

Street, J. C., and Sharma, R. P.: Accumulation and release of chemicals by adipose tissue. In Lee, D. H. K. (ed.): *Handbook of Physiology: Reactions to Environmental Agents.* American Physiological Society, Bethesda, 1977, pp. 483–94.

Vandam, L. D.: Uptake and transport of anesthetics and stages of anesthesia. In DiPalma, J. R. (ed.): *Drill's Pharmacology in Medicine*, 3rd ed. McGraw-Hill Book Co., New York, 1965, pp. 85–99.

Wollman, H., and Dripps, R. D.: Uptake, distribution, elimination, and administration of inhalational anesthetics. In Goodman, L. S., and Gilman, A. (eds.): *The Pharmacological Basis of Therapeutics*, 4th ed. Macmillan Publishing Co., Inc., New York, 1970, pp. 60–70.

Chapter 4

METABOLISM OF TOXIC SUBSTANCES

Robert A. Neal

INTRODUCTION

As noted by Hayes (1975), the word metabolism has more than one meaning. It may refer to the sum of the chemical reactions that serve to maintain life. On the other hand it may refer to the chemical transformation of compounds foreign to an organism by various enzymes present in that organism. This latter process is also referred to as biotransformation. The term foreign compounds, meaning nonnutrient compounds not a part of the normal metabolism of the organism, does not mean that the compounds in question are foreign to all organisms, since a number of those foreign to man and other animals may be synthesized by plants, for example. The present chapter will deal with the various ways in which foreign compounds are metabolized by animal organisms.

Foreign compounds may enter the body through ingestion in food or drink, by inhalation, or by absorption through the skin. They in turn can be excreted by way of urine, bile, feces, perspiration, vomitus, milk, hair, or expired air. The ease with which these compounds are excreted largely depends on their water solubility. Compounds that are more soluble in lipid-like materials than in water tend to accumulate in mammalian organisms. This accumulation may disrupt cellular processes, leading to a toxic response.

A number of enzymes in animal organisms are capable of metabolizing lipid-soluble compounds in such a way as to render them more water soluble and thus more easily excreted. Williams (1959) has proposed that these enzymic reactions are of two types: phase I reactions, involving oxidation, reduction, and hydrolysis; and phase II reactions, consisting of conjugation or synthesis. Phase I reactions generally convert foreign compounds to derivatives that can undergo phase II reactions. Although the enzymes carrying out phase I and phase II reactions are often referred to as detoxication enzymes, it should be emphasized that metabolism of foreign compounds is not strictly related to

detoxication. In a number of examples the metabolic products are more toxic than the parent compounds. This is particularly true of some chemical carcinogens, organophosphate insecticides, and a number of compounds that cause cell death in the lung, liver, and kidney.

The enzymes that metabolize foreign compounds are localized mainly in the liver; however, metabolism in other tissues such as the intestine, kidney, lung, brain, and skin is also known to occur.

In this chapter we have divided the discussion of the metabolism of toxic substances into two major subdivisions. The first is qualitative metabolism in which the specific enzymes involved in phase I and phase II reactions will be examined. These enzymes will be discussed from the standpoint of the cofactors required, a general example of the type of reactions catalyzed, the mechanism of the reaction, if known, the subcellular localization of the enzyme, and the importance of each enzyme in the metabolism of foreign compounds across animal species. The second major subdivision is quantitative metabolism in which we will discuss factors such as polarity, protein binding, nutritional status, enzyme induction, sex, and species differences as they relate to the rates of metabolism of foreign compounds.

Some general references to the subject of the metabolism of toxic substances are Testa and Jenner, 1976; Hayes, 1975; Gram and Gillette, 1971; and La Du *et al.*, 1971.

QUALITATIVE METABOLISM OF TOXIC SUBSTANCES

Cytochrome P-450–Containing Monooxygenases

The most important enzyme systems involved in phase I reactions are the cytochrome P-450–containing monooxygenases. These enzyme systems are composed of two enzymes, NADPH–cytochrome *c* reductase, which is also known as NADPH–cytochrome P-450 reductase, and a heme-containing enzyme, cytochrome P-450. Recent evidence indicates the presence of multiple forms of cytochrome P-450 enzymes in the livers of various mammalian species. These cytochrome P-450 enzymes differ in both the structure of the polypeptide chain and the specificity of the reactions they catalyze. The proposed scheme for cytochrome P-450 monooxygenase–catalyzed reactions is shown in Figure 4–1. In reactions catalyzed by this enzyme system the substrate (RH) combines with the oxidized form of cytochrome P-450 (Fe^{3+}) to form a substrate–cytochrome P-450 complex. Two electrons are then transferred to the substrate–cytochrome P-450 complex as it oxidizes NADPH to NADP. Although Figure 4–1 shows the simultaneous transfer of two electrons, there is evidence to support a sequential one-electron transfer to the

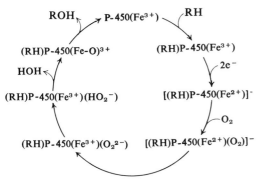

Figure 4–1. Proposed scheme for the metabolism of substrates by the cytochrome P-450–containing monooxygenases.

substrate–cytochrome P-450 complex. The reduced (Fe^{2+}) substrate–cytochrome P-450 complex combines with molecular oxygen, and, in a series of steps that are not well understood, one atom of the molecular oxygen, in the presence of two protons (not shown), is reduced to water and the other oxygen atom is introduced into the substrate. The oxygenated substrate then dissociates, regenerating the oxidized form of cytochrome P-450.

The cytochrome P-450–containing monooxygenases are localized in the endoplasmic reticulum, a complex network of membranes within the cell that is continuous with the outer nuclear membrane. When a cell is homogenized, the endoplasmic reticulum degrades to small vesicles known as microsomes. Most *in vitro* studies with the cytochrome P-450–containing monooxygenases are carried out using microsomes.

The cytochrome P-450–containing monooxygenases involved in the metabolism of

foreign compounds are found predominantly in the endoplasmic reticulum of the liver; however, kidney, lung, intestine, brain, and skin also contain measurable activities of these enzyme systems. Cytochrome P-450–containing monooxygenases are also found in liver mitochondria, in the endoplasmic reticulum and mitochondria of the adrenal cortex, and in the endoplasmic reticulum of cells from testes and ovary. However, these latter enzyme systems are rarely, if ever, involved in the metabolism of foreign compounds. Rather, they carry out specific hydroxylation reactions involving steroids. The cytochrome P-450–containing monooxygenases have been found in the hepatic endoplasmic reticulum of every animal species so far examined. The wide distribution of this enzyme system in various organs of a single species and among the various animal species, coupled with its versatility in catalyzing the introduction of oxygen atoms into foreign compounds of widely different structure, makes it, without question, the most important group of enzymes involved in the metabolism of foreign compounds.

Examples of the types of reactions catalyzed by the cytochrome P-450–containing monooxygenases are shown in Table 4–1. Aromatic hydroxylation (reaction 1) involves the addition of the oxygen atom across a double bond in the aromatic compound. The resulting epoxide is unstable and may rearrange to the corresponding phenol. Aliphatic hydroxylation (reaction 2) is best visualized as resulting from the insertion of the oxygen atom into a carbon-hydrogen bond. The dealkylation of N, O, and S alkyl compounds (reaction 3) is also thought to proceed by way of a cytochrome P-450 monooxygenase-catalyzed carbon-hydrogen insertion reaction in which the resulting hydroxyalkyl (hydroxymethyl in this case) product is unstable and rearranges with the loss of the aldehyde derivative of the alkyl group (formaldehyde in the case of a methyl group). Epoxidation (reaction 4) occurs by addition of the oxygen atom across the double bond. Desulfuration, sulfoxidation, and N-hydroxylation (reactions 5, 6, and 7) occur by the addition of the oxygen atom to an unshared electron pair on the sulfur or nitrogen atoms. In the case of desulfuration (reaction 5) the resultant intermediate is generally unstable and often rearranges with the loss of sulfur, forming the corresponding oxygen analog.

The cytochrome P-450–containing monooxygenase system is also apparently involved in reduction of azo and nitro compounds (Gillette, 1969). The reduction of azo compounds (Table 4–2) can be catalyzed either directly by NADPH–cytochrome *c* reductase or in conjunction with cytochrome P-450 in a complete monooxygenase

Table 4–1. EXAMPLE OF THE GENERAL TYPE OF OXIDATION REACTIONS CATALYZED BY THE CYTOCHROME P-450–CONTAINING MONOOXYGENASES

REACTION	EXAMPLE
1. Aromatic hydroxylation	$R-\langle\bigcirc\rangle \longrightarrow R-\langle\bigcirc\rangle-OH$
2. Aliphatic hydroxylation	$R-CH_2-CH_2-CH_3 \longrightarrow R-CH_2-CHOH-CH_3$
3. N, O, or S-dealkylation	$R-\overset{H}{(N, O, S)}-CH_3 \longrightarrow R-(NH_2, OH, SH) + CH_2O$
4. Epoxidation	$R-CH=CH-R' \longrightarrow R-\overset{O}{\overset{\diagdown}{CH}-CH}-R'$
5. Desulfuration	$R_1R_2\overset{S}{\overset{\|}{P}}-X \longrightarrow R_1R_2\overset{O}{\overset{\|}{P}}-X + S$
6. Sulfoxidation	$R-S-R \longrightarrow R-\underset{O}{\overset{\|}{S}}-R'$
7. N-hydroxylation	$R-NH-\overset{O}{\overset{\|}{C}}-CH_3 \longrightarrow R-NOH-\overset{O}{\overset{\|}{C}}-CH_3$

system. The available data suggest that the reduction of some nitro compounds, like azo compounds, requires the complete cytochrome P-450–containing monooxygenase system whereas others are reduced by NADPH–cytochrome c reductase alone.

A number of books and review articles deal with the subject of cytochrome P-450 monooxygenase–catalyzed reactions. Two of these are by Gram and Gillette (1971) and Testa and Jenner (1976).

Amine Oxidase

Another monooxygenase of lesser importance than the cytochrome P-450–containing systems is the enzyme amine oxidase. This enzyme is a flavoprotein containing the acid-dissociable co-enzyme FAD. This enzyme, which has been isolated from pig liver microsomes (Ziegler and Mitchell, 1972), can catalyze the conversion of tertiary amines to N-oxides and of secondary amines to hydroxylamine derivatives. The source of electrons for activation of oxygen by amine oxidase is NADPH. As noted previously, cytochrome P-450–containing monooxygenases can also carry out N-oxidation and N-hydroxylation reactions. A recent study (Gorrod, 1973) has indicated that the pK_a of the nitrogen in organic compounds is the primary determinant of whether the compound is metabolized by amine oxidase or the cytochrome P-450–containing monooxygenases. Thus, those compounds in which the pK_a of the nitrogen is 8 to 11 are metabolized primarily by amine oxidase, whereas those with pK_a values below 1 are metabolized

primarily by the cytochrome P-450–containing monooxygenase systems. Those compounds in which the pK_a value of the nitrogen is between 1 and 7 appear to be substrates for both cytochrome P-450–containing monooxygenases and amine oxidase. The extent to which N-oxidation of these latter compounds occurs by either enzyme is dependent on the ratio of the activities of the two enzymes present in a particular species

Table 4–2. EXAMPLES OF THE REDUCTION OF AZO AND NITRO COMPOUNDS BY NADPH–CYTOCHROME c REDUCTASE AND BY CYTOCHROME P-450–CONTAINING MONOOXYGENASES

REACTION	EXAMPLE
1. Azo reduction	$R-N=N-R' \longrightarrow$ $R-NH_2 + R'NH_2$
2. Aromatic nitro reduction	$R-\langle\bigcirc\rangle-NO_2 \longrightarrow$ $R-\langle\bigcirc\rangle-NH_2$

and the pK_a of the nitrogen atom in the compound, a lower pK_a value favoring metabolism by the cytochrome P-450–containing monooxygenase system and a higher pK_a value favoring metabolism by amine oxidase.

The amine groups in organic compounds may be either primary (RNH_2), secondary ($RNHR'$), or tertiary (RNR'R"). In compounds in which the pK_a of the nitrogen is greater than 8 (RCH$_2$NH$_2$, RCH$_2$NHR', RCH$_2$NR'R"), it is the tertiary derivatives that are most readily metabolized. The corresponding primary and secondary derivatives are only rarely metabolized to their hydroxylated derivatives. Similarly, the tertiary derivatives of those compounds with pK_a values for the nitrogen between 1 and 7 (ArNH$_2$, ArNHR, ArNRR'; Ar = aromatic) are more readily metabolized although some evidence for metabolism of primary derivatives has been noted. Those compounds with pK_a values less than 1 are most often amides (RCONH$_2$, RCONHR', RCONR'R"). The metabolism of secondary amides has been noted. In addition, some few primary amides are metabolized by the cytochrome P-450–containing monooxygenase systems. Tertiary amides are not substrates for either monooxygenase (Gorrod, 1973).

Epoxide Hydratase

As noted previously, the cytochrome P-450–containing monooxygenases can metabolize

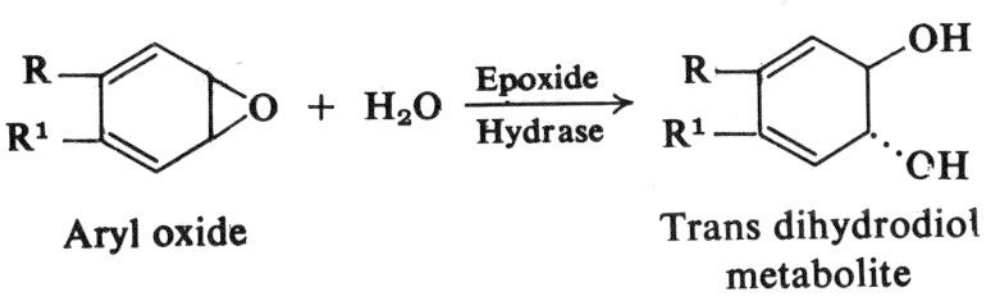

Figure 4–2. Dihydrodiol formation catalyzed by epoxide hydratase.

aromatic and olefinic compounds to their corresponding epoxides. In the case of aromatic compounds the resulting epoxides are generally unstable and rearrange to the corresponding phenols. The epoxide metabolites of some aromatic and olefinic compounds are thought to be responsible for the mutagenic and carcinogenic effects of these compounds. An enzyme, epoxide hydratase, catalyzes the metabolism of these epoxides to their corresponding trans-dihydrodiols. An example of the type of reaction catalyzed by epoxide hydratase is shown in Figure 4–2.

Epoxide hydratase activity has been detected in the endoplasmic reticulum of a number of organs and tissues but not in blood components. Epoxide hydratase appears to be closely associated with cytochrome P-450 within the endoplasmic reticulum. This may be important relative to a role for epoxide hydratase in detoxifying aromatic and olefinic epoxides. As noted above, aromatic epoxides are unstable and rearrange to

form phenols. Despite the chemical instability of aromatic epoxides, substantial amounts of these metabolites are enzymatically hydrated by epoxide hydratase to the corresponding dihydrodiols. Thus, the close association of epoxide hydratase with cytochrome P-450 may play an important role in detoxication of these reactive epoxides.

There is some evidence to indicate that more than one epoxide hydratase enzyme may be present in animal tissues. The major difficulty in resolving this question is the broad substrate specificity of epoxide hydratase. This enzyme appears to be capable of hydrolyzing the epoxides of a wide variety of structurally dissimilar compounds.

Esterases and Amidases

Mammalian tissues contain a large number of nonspecific esterases and amidases that can hydrolyze amide and ester linkages in foreign compounds. This hydrolytic cleavage of amide and ester linkages liberates carboxyl groups and an alcohol function in the case of esters and an amine or NH$_3$ in the case of amides. These carboxyl, alcohol, and amine groups may undergo a variety of conjugations (phase II reactions).

Esterases may be broadly categorized into four main classes (Testa and Jenner, 1976): (1) arylesterases, which preferentially hydrolyze aromatic esters (ArCOOR'; Ar = aromatic), (2) carboxylesterases, which hydrolyze aliphatic esters (RCH$_2$COOR'), (3) cholinesterases, which hydrolyze esters in which the alcohol moiety is choline [(CH$_3$)$_3$N$^+$—CH$_2$—CH$_2$—OOCR], and (4) acetylesterases, in which the acid moiety of the ester is acetic acid (CH$_3$—COOR'). It should be noted that there is considerable overlap in substrate specificity among these classes of esterase. For example, a carboxyl esterase may hydrolyze an aromatic ester at a detectable rate. Therefore, these classifications should not be considered to be absolute.

In contrast to esterases, amidases cannot be readily classified according to substrate specificity. In general, enzymatic hydrolysis of amides occurs more slowly than with esters. Enzyme specificity for the various amides may be partially responsible for this slower rate of metabolism. However, electronic factors are also important. Thus R groups in primary, secondary, and tertiary amides that have electron-withdrawing properties will cause a weakening of the amide bond making the amide more susceptible to enzymatic hydrolysis. Because their action exposes functional groups capable of undergoing phase II reactions, esterase and amidase activity is generally referred to as a phase I reaction.

Alcohol and Aldehyde Dehydrogenases

There are present in mammalian tissues enzymes that catalyze the oxidation of a wide variety of aliphatic alcohols to their corresponding aldehydes and ketones using NAD^+ as a cofactor, for example, the oxidation of ethanol to acetaldehyde catalyzed by alcohol dehydrogenase ($CH_3CH_2OH + NAD^+ \rightarrow CH_3CHO + NADH + H^+$). These enzymes also catalyze the reduction of aldehydes or ketones to their corresponding alcohols using NADH as a cofactor. A number of aliphatic alcohols have narcotic properties. Therefore, the metabolism of these alcohols to the corresponding aldehydes may decrease their toxicity. However, aldehydes are also toxic because of their chemical reactivity under physiologic conditions. For example, they readily form Schiff's bases with primary amine groups. Aldehyde dehydrogenases present in mammalian tissues oxidize aldehydes to their corresponding acids using NAD^+ as a cofactor, for example, the oxidation of acetaldehyde to acetic acid in a reaction catalyzed by aldehyde dehydrogenase ($CH_3CHO + NAD^+ + H_2O \rightarrow CH_3COOH + NADH + H^+$). The corresponding carboxylic acids are usually much less toxic than the aldehydes. In addition, these acids may undergo conjugation (phase II) reactions with amino acids such as glycine or glutamine.

Glucuronyl Transferases

As noted in the introduction, phase II reactions involve the synthesis of a derivative of a foreign compound (substrate) that is generally more water soluble and more easily excreted than the substrate. These phase II reactions are generally referred to as conjugation reactions. The most common and one of the most important conjugation reactions is the synthesis of glucuronic acid derivatives of various substrates, which can be either foreign or endogenous compounds such as steroids or bilirubin. The enzyme carrying out this reaction is uridine diphosphate glucuronyl transferase or UDP-glucuronyl transferase. The coenzyme for the reaction is uridine-5′-diphospho-α-D-glucuronic acid (UDPGA) (Fig. 4-3). Glucuronyl transferase activity is localized in the endoplasmic reticulum, mainly of the liver. However, activity has also been noted in the kidney, intestine, skin, brain, and spleen. There is evidence that more than one form of glucuronyl transferase exists within the hepatic endoplasmic reticulum.

Numerous chemical groups present in foreign compounds are capable of undergoing conjugation reactions with glucuronic acid. These are aliphatic and aromatic alcohols, some carboxyl groups, sulfhydryl groups, and primary and secondary aromatic and aliphatic amines. In reactions involving conjugation of these functional groups, carbon 1 of glucuronic acid, in the form of UDPGA, is activated to nucleophilic attack by the oxygen, sulfur, or nitrogen groups on substrates with uridine diphosphate (UDP) being the leaving group. In UDPGA the bond between carbon 1 of glucuronic acid and the phosphate group of UDP is of the α-configuration. During reaction with substrates there is an inversion of configurating leading to glucuronide derivatives that have a β-configuration.

Table 4-3 shows general examples of the types of products formed in UDP-glucuronyl transferase–catalyzed reactions of UDPGA with foreign compounds containing various functional groups. Reaction 1, the formation of glucuronic acid derivatives of alcohols, leads to the formation of ether-type glucuronides. Both aliphatic and aromatic alcohols (phenols) form glucuronides. Carboxylic acids form ester-type glucuronides (reaction 2). The formation of

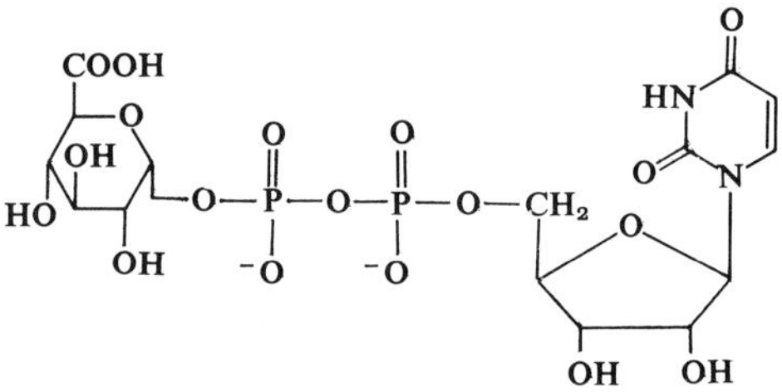

Figure 4-3. Uridine-5′-diphospho-α-D-glucuronic acid (UDPGA).

ester glucuronides is largely restricted to aromatic acids in which the carboxyl group is directly adjacent to the aromatic ring or separated from the aromatic ring by a single methylene or substituted methylene group. Both aromatic (thiophenols) and aliphatic compounds containing sulfhydryl groups (reaction 3) and aliphatic and aromatic amines form glucuronides (reaction 4). The nitrogen-containing functional groups may be either a primary or secondary amine. Of the reactions shown in Table 4-3 the formation of glucuronides of alcohols and carboxylic acids is of greatest quantitative importance.

The glucuronide derivatives of foreign compounds are excreted by way of the urine and bile. Whether the glucuronide is excreted in the urine or bile is largely dependent upon the molecular weight and polarity of the conjugate. Those compounds with a larger molecular weight (> 300 MW) and less water solubility are more often excreted in the bile.

The enzyme β-glucuronidase, which is found

in most mammalian tissues, catalyzes the hydrolysis of ether- and ester-type glucuronides to glucuronic acid and the parent compounds. The physiologic significance of this enzyme is not clear. However, it has been suggested that the enzyme may function to regulate the action of hormones by releasing the active form of these hormones from their inactive glucuronic acid derivatives (Testa and Jenner, 1976).

Glutathione S-Transferases

The glutathione S-transferases are a family of enzymes that catalyze the initial step in the formation of *N*-acetylcysteine (mercapturic acid)

Table 4-3. GENERAL EXAMPLES OF GLUCURONIDES OF ALCOHOLS, CARBOXYLIC ACIDS, SULFHYDRYL COMPOUNDS, AND AMINES

SUBSTRATE	PRODUCT
1. Aliphatic or aromatic alcohols (ROH)	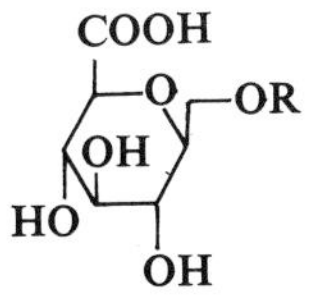 COOH / O—OR / OH / HO / OH
2. Carboxylic acids (RCOOH)	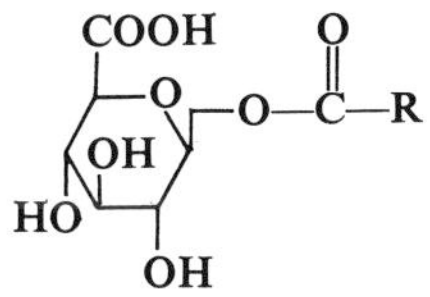 COOH / O—O—C—R (=O) / OH / HO / OH
3. Sulfhydryl compounds (RSH)	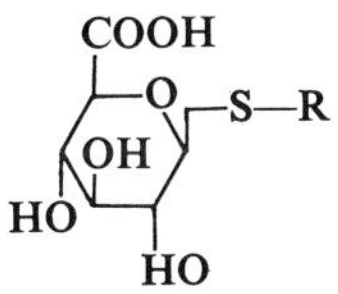 COOH / O—S—R / OH / HO / HO
4. Amines (RNH₂, RR′NH)	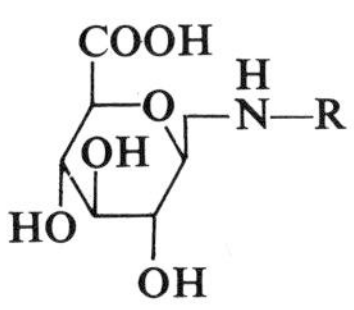 COOH / O—N(H)—R / OH / HO / OH

derivatives of a diverse group of foreign compounds. The formation of mercapturic acid derivatives is considered to be a phase II reaction. At least seven different glutathione S-transferases have been isolated from the cytosol of rat liver (Jakoby *et al.*, 1976). The cofactor for reactions catalyzed by these enzymes is the tripeptide glutathione (Fig. 4-4). The glutathione S-transferases catalyze the reaction of glutathione with compounds containing electrophilic carbon atoms forming a thioether bond between the carbon atom and the sulfhydryl group of glutathione.

There are three common features of compounds that are substrates for the glutathione S-transferases: They must be hydrophobic to some degree, they must contain an electrophilic carbon atom, and they must react nonenzymatically with glutathione at some measurable rate (Jakoby and Keen, 1977). Some examples of the general types of reactions catalyzed by the glutathione-S-transferases are shown in Table 4-4.

The glutathione (GSH) derivatives of various compounds are subsequently cleaved enzymatically to the cysteine derivatives. The α-amino group of the cysteine is subsequently acetylated to give the N acetylcysteine (mercapturic acid) derivatives of these compounds, which are readily excreted. The sequence of reactions leading to the formation of a mercapturic acid derivative is shown in Figure 4-5. The loss of glutamic acid from the glutathione conjugate is catalyzed by the enzyme glutathionase, an enzyme found mostly in the liver and kidney of animal species. However, there is considerable variation among species in the activity and location of this enzyme. Subsequently, various

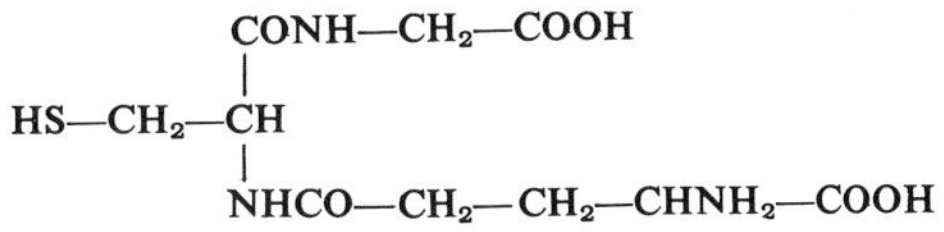

$$CONH—CH_2—COOH$$
$$HS—CH_2—CH$$
$$NHCO—CH_2—CH_2—CHNH_2—COOH$$

Figure 4-4. Glutathione.

peptidases present in kidney, liver, and pancreas catalyze the loss of glycine from the conjugate. Finally, *N* acetyl transferase enzymes present in the cytosol carry out the acetylation of the α-amino group of cysteine to form the mercapturic acid derivative. The cofactor for the acetylation reaction is acetyl–coenzyme A.

The importance of reactions catalyzed by the glutathione S-transferases has become increasingly apparent over the last few years. Man is continually exposed to reactive electrophilic compounds as constituents of the food he eats, the air he breathes, the drugs he takes, and in the work place. The glutathione S-transferase enzymes provide a means of reacting these electrophilic compounds with the endogenous low-molecular-weight nucleophile glutathione thus preventing, to a degree, the reaction of these compounds with essential constituents of the cell. In addition, in the process of the metabolism of foreign compounds, particularly in reactions catalyzed by the cytochrome P-450–containing monooxygenase, a number of highly reactive electrophilic compounds are formed. Some of these reactive intermediates can react with cellular constituents and cause cell death or

Table 4–4. TYPES OF REACTIONS CATALYZED BY GLUTATHIONE S-TRANSFERASE

REACTION	PRODUCT
1. (3-chloro-4-nitro... benzene with NO₂) + GSH* 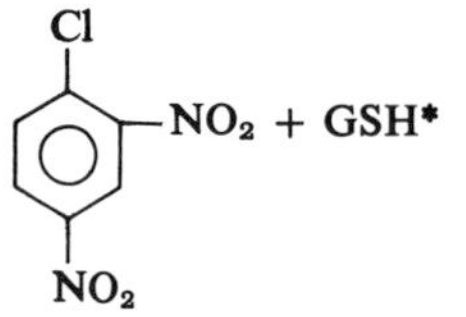 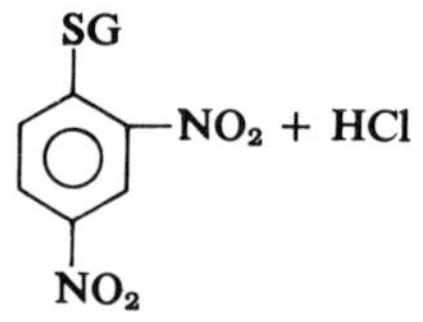	(SG-substituted) $-NO_2$ + HCl
2. $R-O-\overset{O}{\underset{\|}{C}}-CH=CH-\overset{O}{\underset{\|}{C}}-O-R'$ + GSH*	$R-O-\overset{O}{\underset{\|}{C}}-CH_2-\overset{SG}{\underset{\|}{CH}}-\overset{O}{\underset{\|}{C}}-O-R'$
3. $(RO)_2\overset{O}{\underset{\|}{P}}-O-CH_3$ + GSH*	$(RO)_2\overset{O}{\underset{\|}{P}}-OH + CH_3-S-G$
4. $R-CH_2-NO_2$ + GSH*	$R-CH_2-S-G + HNO_2$

* GSH denotes glutathione.

induce a neoplastic process. Considerable evidence indicates that glutathione S-transferases also act to prevent to a varying degree the reaction of these reactive intermediates with constituents of the cell. For example, bromobenzene is metabolized by the cytochrome

$$\begin{aligned}&\text{CONH}-CH_2-COOH\\&|\\\gtrdot C-S-CH_2-CH\\&|\\&NHCO-(CH_2)_2-CHNH_2COOH\end{aligned}$$

H_2O | glutathionase

$$\begin{aligned}&\text{CONH}-CH_2-COOH\\&|\\\gtrdot C-S-CH_2-CH\\&|\quad + HOOC-(CH_2)_2-CHNH_2COOH\\&NH_2\qquad\text{glutamic acid}\end{aligned}$$

H_2O | peptidase

$$\begin{aligned}&\text{COOH}\\&|\\\gtrdot C-S-CH_2-CH\quad + H_2NCH_2COOH\\&|\qquad\qquad\text{glycine}\\&NH_2\end{aligned}$$

Acetyl CoA | N-acetylase

$$\begin{aligned}&\text{COOH}\\&|\\\gtrdot C-S-CH_2-C\\&|\\&HN-COCH_3\end{aligned}$$

Mercapturic acid conjugate

Figure 4–5. Reaction sequence in the formation of a mercapturic acid conjugate. [$\gtrdot$C] denotes a carbon atom of a substrate subject to reaction with glutathione.

P-450–containing monooxygenase enzyme system of the liver to the corresponding epoxide (Fig. 4–6). This reactive epoxide may bind covalently to various constituents in hepatocytes causing cell death or react with GSH preventing the covalent binding to vital cellular constituents.

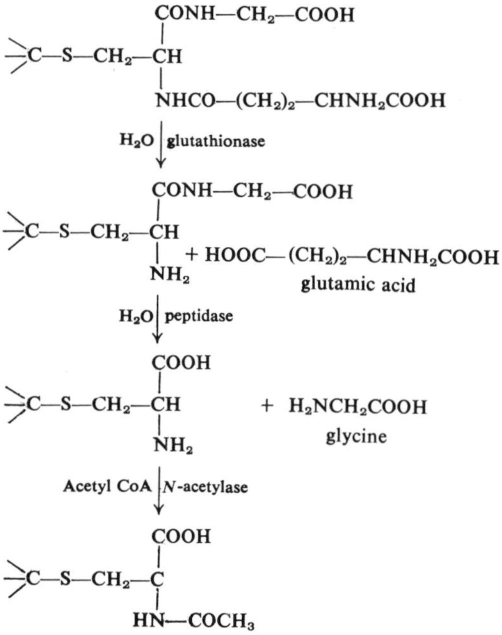

Sulfotransferases

The conjugation of foreign compounds with sulfate, another phase II reaction, is catalyzed

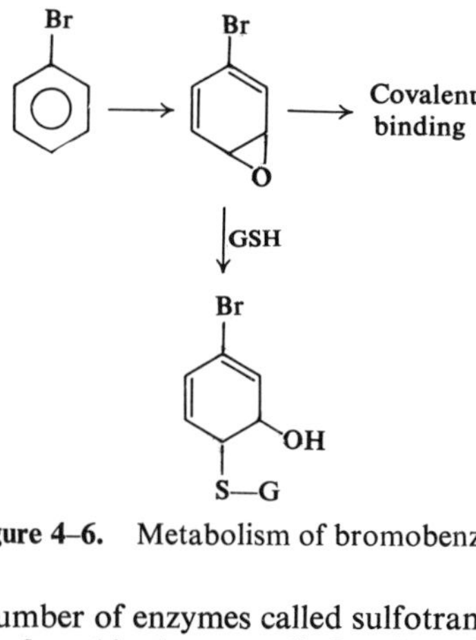

Figure 4–6. Metabolism of bromobenzene.

by a number of enzymes called sulfotransferases that are found in the cytosolic fraction of various tissues including, liver, kidney, and intestine. The functional groups that are substrates for sulfate transfer are phenols and aliphatic alcohols. In addition, the sulfation of aromatic amines (ArNH₂) to form the corresponding sulfamates (ArNHSO₃⁻) is occasionally seen. In the case of phenols and aliphatic alcohols

(ROH) the products formed are the corresponding sulfate esters (ROSO$_3$$^-$), also known as ethereal sulfates. The cofactor for these reactions is 3'-phosphoadenosine-5'-phosphosulfate (PAPS) (Fig. 4–7). In the reactions catalyzed by the sulfotransferases, the SO$_3$$^-$ group of PAPS is readily transferred in a reaction involving nucleophilic attack of the alcohol oxygen or the amine nitrogen on the sulfur atom displacing the adenosine-3',5'-diphosphate group.

As noted previously, glucuronyl transferases also react with phenols and aliphatic alcohols to form glucuronides. Because of the limited availability of PAPS as compared with UDPGA in most animal species, the glucuronidation of these alcohols and phenols usually predominates.

It is readily apparent that conjugation of an alcohol or a phenol with sulfate will increase its water solubility. However, because of the generally greater activity of the glucuronyl transferase reactions in most animal species, sulfate conjugation is considered to be of lesser

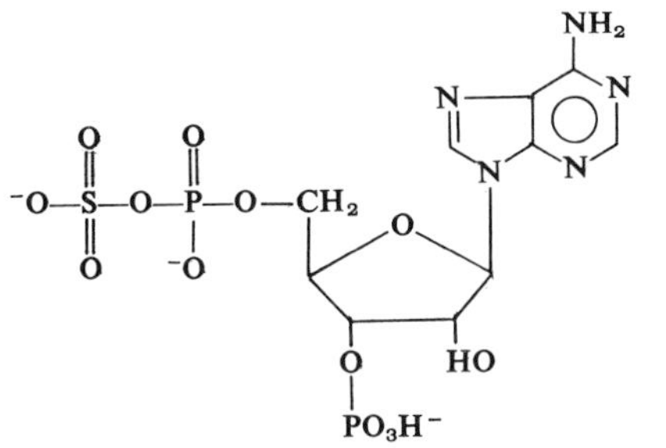

Figure 4–7. 3'-Phosphoadenosine-5'-phosphosulfate.

importance relative to facilitating the excretion of hydrophobic alcohols and phenols.

Amino Acid Conjugases

Aromatic carboxylic acids, arylacetic acids, and aryl-substituted acrylic acids undergo phase II (conjugation) reactions with α-amino acids. Although the most important reaction involves glycine, conjugation with glutamine is also seen in man and certain monkeys and conjugation with ornithine is seen in birds.

The sequence of reactions in the conjugation of benzoic acid with glycine is shown in Figure 4–8. The enzyme or enzymes that carry out the reaction of benzoic acid and other aromatic acids with coenzyme A (CoASH) appear to be located mainly in the mitochondria of hepatocytes. The enzymes that carry out this "activation reaction" appear to have a broad specificity for the types of aromatic acids that are substrates. This formation of the CoA derivatives of the

aromatic acid renders the carbonyl carbon of these acids more susceptible to nucleophilic attack by the α-amino nitrogen of glycine or glutamine in the subsequent step leading to the formation of the glycine or glutamine conjugate. The glycine or glutamine N-acyl transferase enzymes catalyzing the transfer of the benzoyl CoA group or other aromatic acyl CoA groups to glycine or glutamine are located in both the mitochondria and cytosol. These transferases appear to have a specificity for the α-amino acid, catalyzing the transfer of the acyl CoA group to glycine in the case of one enzyme and to glutamine in the case of another.

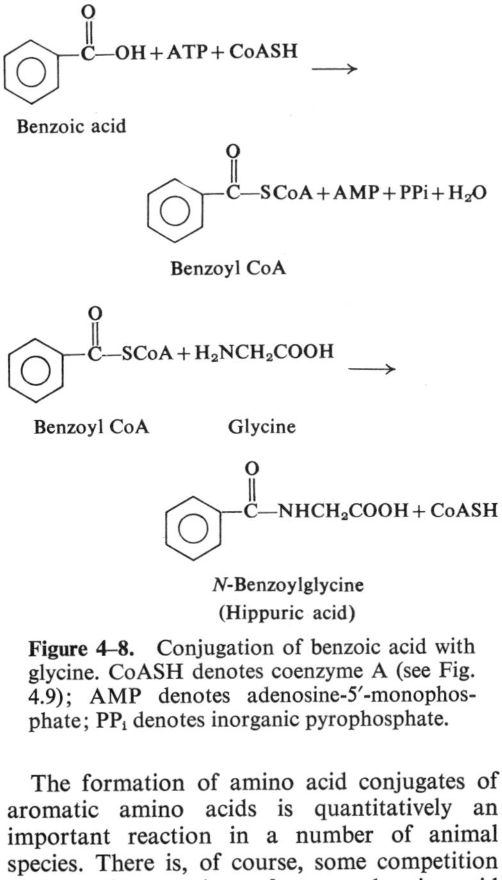

Figure 4–8. Conjugation of benzoic acid with glycine. CoASH denotes coenzyme A (see Fig. 4.9); AMP denotes adenosine-5'-monophosphate; PP$_i$ denotes inorganic pyrophosphate.

The formation of amino acid conjugates of aromatic amino acids is quantitatively an important reaction in a number of animal species. There is, of course, some competition between glucuronyl transferases and amino acid conjugases relative to metabolism of these aromatic acids. The degree to which glucuronide formation or amino acid conjugation predominates depends on both the animal species and structure of the acid.

Methyl Transferases

Methylation is not a quantitatively important pathway for metabolism of foreign compounds. In addition, methylation does not generally increase the water solubility of the product relative to the parent compound. Nevertheless, methylation is still generally considered to be a phase II reaction. The functional groups involved in methylation reactions are aliphatic and aromatic amines, N-heterocyclics, mono- and polyhydric phenols, and sulfhydryl-containing compounds.

The coenzyme for methylation reactions is S-adenosylmethionine (SAM) (Fig. 4–9). The methyl group bound to the sulfonium ion in SAM has considerable carbonium ion character and is transferred by nucleophilic attack of the alcohol oxygen, the amine nitrogen, and the sulfhydryl group on the methyl group giving S-adenosylhomocysteine and the methylated substrate as products. Examples of the products formed in methylation reactions involving foreign compounds are shown in Table 4–5. A number of enzymes are present in various animal tissues and particulate fractions of these tissues that are capable of carrying out methylation reactions using SAM as a cofactor. Some of these enzymes

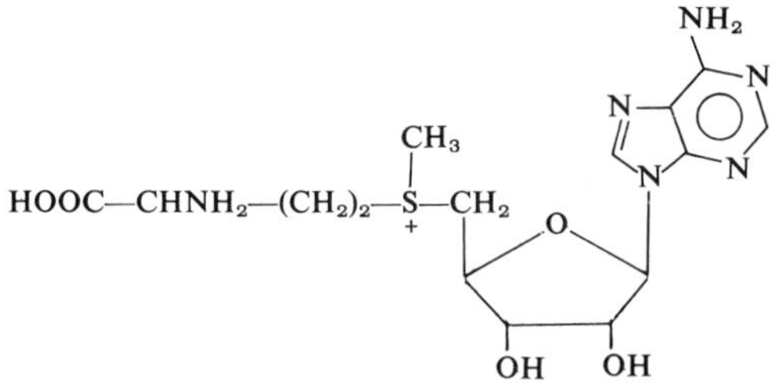

Figure 4–9. S-Adenosylmethionine.

are quite specific. For example, the enzyme catechol-O-methyl transferase carries out methylation reactions on the important endogenous amines dopamine and norepinephrine. However, the enzyme is also capable of methylating foreign compounds with two adjacent hydroxyl groups such as catechol (reaction 2, Table 4–5). Other methyl transfer enzymes are less specific, for example, the system found in the hepatic endoplasmic reticulum that can methylate various sulfhydryl compounds. In general, the enzymes carrying out methylation reactions with foreign compounds have not been characterized to any significant extent.

N-Acetyl Transferases

Acetylation is a common reaction of aromatic primary amines, hydrazines, hydrazides, sulfonamides, and certain primary aliphatic amines. Although the acetyl transferase enzymes can also transfer an acetyl group to alcohol and sulfhydryl groups, this reaction only appears to occur with endogenous substrates. No transfer of an acetyl

Table 4–5. EXAMPLES OF PRODUCTS OF METHYLATION REACTIONS

SUBSTRATE	PRODUCT
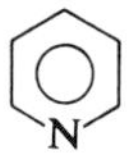 1. Pyridine	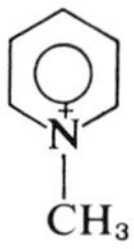
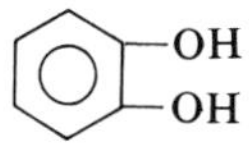 2. Catechol	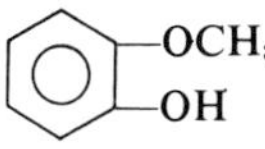
3. $(C_2H_5)_2N-\overset{\overset{\textstyle S}{\|}}{C}-SH$ Diethyldithiocarbamate	$(C_2H_5)_2N-\overset{\overset{\textstyle S}{\|}}{C}-S-CH_3$

group to an alcohol or sulfhydryl moiety of a foreign compound has yet been reported.

The enzymes carrying out acetyl transfer reactions are designated as acetyl coenzyme A: amine N-acetyl transferases. The cofactor for these reactions is acetyl coenzyme A. The structure of acetyl coenzyme A is shown in Figure 4–10. These enzymes, which are located in the soluble fraction of cell of various tissues, catalyze the transfer of the acetyl group from acetyl coenzyme A to the amine function of the foreign compound. Examples of the products formed in N-acetyl transferase–catalyzed reactions are shown in Table 4–6. In each case an acetyl group is added to a primary amine group to form an amide.

There appear to be multiple forms of N-acetyl transferase enzymes in animal tissues. There are also enzymes in animal tissues that carry out the deacetylation of amines. The degree to which a particular animal species excretes foreign amines as acetyl conjugates depends on the relative rates of acetylation and deacetylation of these compounds. Man appears to be relatively deficient in deacetylation enzymes.

Acetylation occasionally results in a decrease in the water solubility of an amine and increased toxicity. This is particularly true of some sulfonamides used therapeutically. Thus, like methylation reactions, N-acetyl transferase–catalyzed reactions have a variable effect on the toxicity of amines but are still considered to be phase II reactions.

Miscellaneous Reactions

An important reaction in the detoxication of cyanide is catalyzed by the enzyme rhodanese. The reaction catalyzed by rhodanese is shown in Figure 4–11. Although thiosulfate can act as a

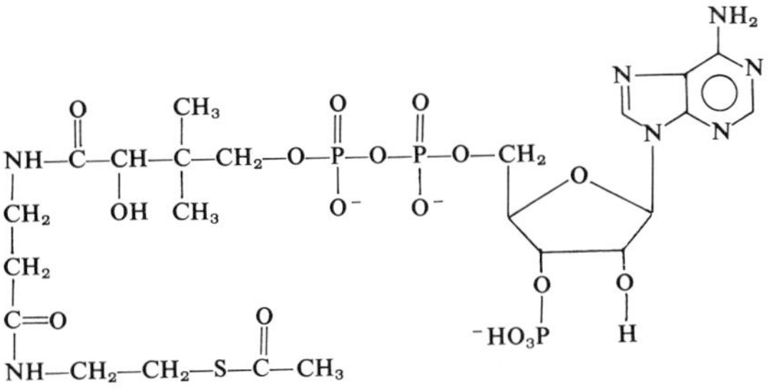

Figure 4-10. Acetyl coenzyme A.

donor of sulfur both *in vitro* and *in vivo* for formation of thiocyanate, it does not appear to be the endogenous donor of sulfur for this reaction. The nature of the endogenous sulfur

Table 4-6. EXAMPLES OF PRODUCTS OF *N*-ACETYL TRANSFERASE REACTIONS

SUBSTRATE	PRODUCT
1.	
2. R—NH—NH₂ substituted hydrazine	R—NH—NH—C(=O)—CH₃
3. R—SO—NH₂ aryl-substituted sulfonamide	R—SO—NH—C(=O)—CH₃

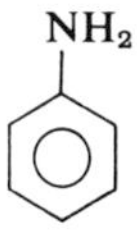

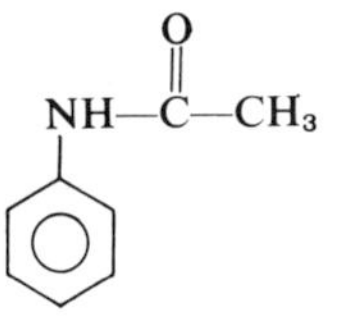

donor is unknown at this time. Thiocyanate is much less toxic than cyanide. Thus the reaction catalyzed by rhodanese is a true detoxication reaction.

Insects carry out conjugation reactions in which glucose replaces the glucuronide conjugation seen in other animal species. Ester and ether glucosides are formed using UDP-glucose as the cofactor.

Oxygen (O_2) is reduced by both enzymatic and nonenzymatic processes to the superoxide radical (O_2^-). This radical species of oxygen is postulated to be formed *in vivo* in animals through the activity of some iron-sulfur oxidation-reduction enzymes and certain flavoproteins (i.e., xanthine oxidase). The superoxide radical is a highly reactive species of oxygen and would likely cause

$$CN^- + S_2O_3^{2-} \longrightarrow SCN^- + SO_3^{2-}$$

cyanide thiosulfate thiocyanate sulfite

Figure 4-11. Detoxification reaction of cyanide catalyzed by rhodanese.

irreversible damage to cells in which it is produced if some means were not available to metabolize it. There is present in respiring plant and animal tissues enzymes given the name superoxide dismutase. Superoxide dismutase catalyzes the reaction $O_2^- + O_2^- + 2H^+ \rightarrow H_2O_2 + O_2$. Thus, the enzyme catalyzes the transformation of two molecules of superoxide radical to a molecule each of hydrogen peroxide and oxygen. Hydrogen peroxide is less reactive than superoxide radical. In addition, there are enzymes in plant and animal tissues capable of metabolizing hydrogen peroxide to less reactive products (O_2, H_2O). These include catalase, peroxidase, and glutathione peroxidase.

Heretofore we have referred to the individual reactions catalyzed by various phase I and phase II enzyme systems. It is often the case that a number of these enzyme systems will act consecutively or concurrently on a substrate or metabolites of that substrate. Shown in Figure 4-12 is an example, using benzene as a model, of the action of a number of phase I and phase II enzyme systems on a single substrate. In reaction (1) the benzene is oxidized by the cytochrome P-450–containing monooxygenase system to benzene oxide. The benzene oxide may spontaneously rearrange (2) or be converted to the

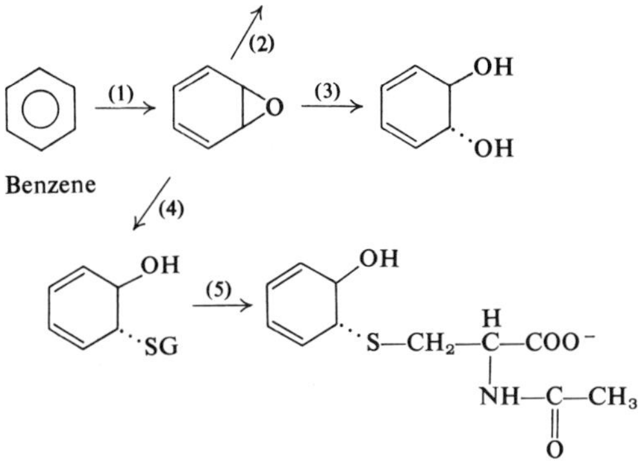

Figure 4-12. Metabolism of benzene by phase I and phase II enzyme systems. ⋯SG denotes a glutathione derivative.

corresponding dihydrodiol by the action of epoxide hydratase (3). The benzene oxide may also be subject to reaction with glutathione in a reaction catalyzed by glutathione-transferase (4) forming a glutathione derivative that may undergo further reaction to form the mercapturic acid derivative (5). Phenol formed on spontaneous rearrangement of benzene oxide (2) may undergo conjugation reactions with either sulfate, catalyzed by sulfate transferase (6), or glucuronic acid, catalyzed by glucuronyl transferase.

FACTORS THAT AFFECT THE RATES OF METABOLISM OF FOREIGN COMPOUNDS

Foreign compounds can be toxic per se or be metabolized in animal organisms to products that cause toxic effects. The rate of metabolism of toxic compounds to less toxic products or less toxic compounds to more toxic products is of considerable importance concerning the overall toxicity observed on exposure of animals to these compounds. Therefore, it is important to discuss factors that affect the rates of metabolism of foreign compounds.

One of the important factors controlling the rate of metabolism of foreign compounds is the concentration of the compound at the active center of enzymes involved in the metabolism of the compound in question. The concentration at the active centers of these enzymes depends on a number of properties of the compound. These properties are discussed below.

Rate of Absorption

The rate of absorption of a compound from the intestine, lung, or skin (depending on the route of exposure) is an important factor controlling the concentration of a compound at the active centers of enzymes involved in its metabolism. In general water-soluble compounds are less rapidly absorbed than lipid-soluble compounds.

Transfer Across Cell Membranes

The ease with which a compound crosses cell membranes is also important relative to its concentration at the active sites of enzymes involved in its metabolism. Most of the enzymes involved in the metabolism of foreign compounds are located intracellularly as opposed to being found in the blood or in the lumen of the gastrointestinal tract. Therefore, any compound must cross one or more membranes in order to reach the active site of enzymes involved in its metabolism. A simplistic but useful model of cell membranes is that they consist of a lipid bilayer, which is penetrated at intervals by protein molecules. In addition, there appear to be small pores in the membrane through which small-molecular-weight water-soluble compounds can pass (inorganic ions, urea, etc.). Because of the lipid-like nature of cell membranes those foreign compounds which are less water soluble generally gain access to the interior of cells more readily than those which are more water soluble. An important factor controlling the water solubility of foreign compounds is whether they contain ionizable groups in the molecule. Thus compounds containing amine, carboxyl, phosphate, sulfate, phenolic hydroxyl and other groups that are ionized at physiologic pH values are generally more water soluble and are less readily transferred across cell membranes than compounds not containing these groups.

Protein Binding

Intra- and extracellular proteins have the capacity to bind foreign compounds and reduce the concentrations of these compounds at the active sites of enzymes involved in their metabolism. This capacity to bind foreign compounds results from the presence in proteins of hydrophobic regions that will bind lipid-soluble (water-insoluble) compounds and hydrophilic regions that contain polar side chains of amino acids capable of forming hydrogen and electrostatic bonds with polar groups in water-soluble foreign compounds. For example, the ratio of protein bound to unbound dieldrin in rat blood is 440:1 (Hayes, 1975). Thus, proteins and in particular serum proteins have a capacity for nonspecific binding of foreign compounds. This binding reduces the availability of these compounds for metabolism.

Excretion

The more rapid the excretion of a toxic foreign compound or its toxic product by an animal organism, the less is the opportunity for interaction of the toxic compound or product with critical target molecules in the organism. The excretion of absorbed foreign compounds or their metabolites may occur by way of the urine, feces, expired air, milk, and sweat. Factors that increase the rate of excretion of foreign compounds and/or their metabolites by these routes generally decrease the toxicity of these compounds and/or their metabolites. There are exceptions, however. For example, the urinary excretion of mercury facilitated by administration of water-soluble chelating agents sometimes leads to kidney damage.

There are also various physiologic factors that control the rate of metabolism of foreign compounds. Included among these factors are the species, strain, sex, and age of the animal. Other factors controlling rates of metabolism are the time of day (circadian rhythms), temperature, pregnancy, disease states, and the nutritional status of the animal.

Species Differences

There are many examples of marked species differences in the rate of metabolism of a given dose of a foreign compound by a particular enzyme or group of enzymes. These differences are most generally related to differences in the activity of a particular enzyme or enzymes among those species. For example, there are large species differences in the rates of hydroxylation of biphenyl at the 2 position. Whereas the mouse has a high activity for 2-hydroxylation of biphenyl, the rat does not appear to possess a cytochrome P-450–containing monooxygenase capable of carrying out 2-hydroxylation of this compound. In man arylacetic acids are conjugated predominantly with glutamine whereas in the rat conjugation with glycine is the major reaction. Very little conjugation of foreign compounds with glucuronic acid is seen in the cat. Similarly, little or no conjugation with sulfate is seen in the pig.

Strain Differences

Strain differences in the metabolism of foreign compounds are also seen. Thus, various mouse strains vary in their ability to metabolize the drug hexobarbital and the environmental contaminant benzo(a)pyrene. Large interstrain differences in the ability of rats to metabolize various drugs have also been observed. These strain differences result from genetically determined differences in the activity of the various enzymes involved in the metabolism of foreign compounds.

Sex Differences

A marked difference in the response of female as compared to male rats to a number of toxic foreign compounds has been noted. For example, the widely used organophosphate insecticide parathion is approximately twice as toxic to female as compared to male rats. This decreased susceptibility of the male rat to parathion is related to a greater activity of the hepatic cytochrome P-450 monooxygenase enzyme system, which metabolizes parathion to nontoxic metabolites. This greater activity of the cytochrome P-450 monooxygenase enzyme system in male rats appears to be androgen related since castration or estrogen treatment of male rats or testosterone treatment of female rats tends to decrease the sex differences seen in rats in response to foreign compounds. Although there are sex-dependent differences in metabolism and physiologic response to foreign compounds in other species, these appear to be infrequent in comparison to those in the rat.

Effect of Age on Metabolism of Foreign Compounds

The oxidative metabolism of foreign compounds is markedly reduced in fetal and newborn mice, rats, guinea pigs, and rabbits. It has not been possible to consistently attribute this decreased activity of the cytochrome P-450 monooxygenase system to a reduced level of component enzymes (cytochrome P-450, NADPH-cytochrome c reductase). However, a decreased level of some enzyme is suggested by the ability of inducers of this enzyme system to increase its activity in newborn animals.

Enzymes involved in conjugation reactions are also decreased in activity in fetal and newborn guinea pigs, rats, and mice. In these animal species the ability to carry out oxidative and conjugation reactions increases rapidly after birth reaching adult levels in 30 to 45 days.

In contrast to the animal species noted above, the human fetus has the ability to metabolize foreign compounds although, in general, at a rate that is less than that seen in adults. A major exception is the ability of the human fetus to form glucuronides. The inability to form a glucuronide conjugate with bilirubin is a cause of jaundice in premature human infants. The decreased ability or lack of ability to form glucuronides is a result of a decreased activity or absence of the enzyme glucuronyl transferase.

Circadian Rhythms

An influence of the time of day on the rate of metabolism of foreign compounds is often seen within a given animal species. This variation in the rate of metabolism is often correlated with variations in endocrine functions as influenced by the light-dark cycle to which the animal is exposed. Thus, the in vitro metabolism of compounds such as aminopyrine and hexobarbital by the hepatic cytochrome P-450 monooxygenase system of rats is variable depending on the time of day of sacrifice of the animals. This variation in enzyme activity is thought to be largely the result of a variation in the levels of the enzymes of the P-450 monooxygenase system.

Nutritional Status

The activity of the enzymes and enzyme systems involved in the metabolism of foreign compounds is markedly affected by the nutritional state of experimental animals. Thus, in animals suffering from calcium, copper, selenium, vitamin C, or protein deficiency there is a decreased ability of enzymes from these animals to catalyze the *in vitro* oxidative metabolisms of a variety of substrates. It is likely that the decreased rate of metabolism of these substrates is the result of alteration in the levels of the enzymes involved in the metabolism of these compounds. However, a decreased availability of cofactors for these reactions may also be implicated.

Enzyme Induction

The activity of the hepatic cytochrome P-450–containing monooxygenase systems in various animal species including man can be markedly increased by exposure to a large number of drugs, pesticides, and industrial chemicals. This process of increased activity of these enzyme systems on exposure to chemicals is referred to as enzyme induction. As a result of induction of these enzyme systems an increase is seen in the *in vivo* and *in vitro* rate of metabolism of substrates for the cytochrome P-450–containing monooxygenase enzyme systems. The number of compounds known to induce the activity of these enzyme systems is large (> 300). There is no consistent structural relationship between the compounds capable of bringing about induction. The major features these compounds have in common is that they are lipid soluble and generally have a relatively long half-life in the animal species in which they act as an inducer.

The induction of the cytochrome P-450–containing monooxygenases enzyme systems seen after treatment with these compounds is accompanied by an increase in the amount of smooth endoplasmic reticulum in the liver. Also accompanying the increase in monooxygenase enzyme activity is an increase in the levels of the enzymes cytochrome P-450, and, in most cases, NADPH–cytochrome *c* reductase. An increase in UDP–glucuronyl transferase activity is also seen on exposure to a number of these inducers. However, no increase in other enzymes involved in conjugation reactions is seen. The levels of two or more distinctly different species of cytochrome P-450 appear to be increased on exposure of animals to the various inducers. The inducers have been roughly divided into two categories depending on the enzymatic and spectral properties of the cytochrome P-450 species they induce. One of these groups contains those compounds which are "phenobarbital-like" in their induction. These compounds induce species of cytochrome P-450 in which the spectral maximum of the reduced cytochrome P-450-carbon monoxide complex is at 450 nm. The other group contains those compounds which are

"3-methylcholanthrene-like" in their induction. These compounds induce species of cytochrome P-450 in which the spectral maximum of the reduced cytochrome P-450-carbon monoxide complex is at 448 nm. These different species of cytochrome P-450 also show some differences in substrate specificity. For example, the species induced by 3-methylcholanthrene and similar inducers show greater specificity for hydroxylation of polycyclic aromatic hydrocarbons than the species induced by phenobarbital.

The induction of the activity of the cytochrome P-450–containing monooxygenases by phenobarbital and 3-methylcholanthrene is inhibited by prior treatment of rats with protein synthesis inhibitors such as ethionine, dactinomycin, or puromycin. These and other data indicate that the induction of cytochrome P-450 monooxygenase activity is the result of increased synthesis of cytochrome P-450 and, in the case of "phenobarbital-like" induction, NADPH–cytochrome *c* reductase.

A large number of foreign compounds have also been shown to inhibit the cytochrome P-450 monoxyogenase–catalyzed metabolism of other foreign compounds *in vivo* and *in vitro*. Foremost among these compounds are SKF 525-A, piperonyl butoxide, disulfiram, propylthiouracil, pyrazole, and 3-aminotriazole. The evidence currently available suggests that these compounds inhibit the metabolism of other substrates by acting as alternate substrates for the cytochrome P-450–containing monooxygenase systems.

Whether the induction or inhibition of the cytochrome P-450–containing monooxygenase enzyme systems leads to an increase or a decrease in the toxicity of a particular compound is dependent on the toxic properties of the compound in question. If the monooxygenase-catalyzed metabolism of the compound leads to the formation of less toxic products, then induction of the monooxygenase system will generally result in a decrease in the toxicity of the compound to induced as compared to noninduced animals. On the other hand, inhibition of the monooxygenase enzyme system may lead to an increased toxicity due to increased half-life of the parent compound and an increased concentration of the more toxic parent compound at the site of critical target molecules. The opposite argument would generally apply to compounds whose monooxygenase-catalyzed products are more toxic than the parent compounds.

CONCLUSIONS

There are present in animal tissues a number of enzymes and enzyme systems that catalyze metabolic reactions involving foreign compounds. A unique feature of these enzymes is that they generally possess broad substrate specificity. That is, they possess the ability to carry out reactions on compounds of widely varied structure. In general, these reactions render foreign compounds more water soluble and more easily excreted. Thus, the toxicity of these compounds is generally decreased. However, there are a number of documented instances in which metabolism renders some of these compounds more toxic. There are also wide species and strain differences in the rates of metabolism of foreign compounds that contribute to species differences in response to toxic compounds. These differences are largely the result of differences in the activities of the enzymes involved in the metabolism of these compounds. Thus, the ability of a particular animal species to metabolize a foreign compound is subject to a host of variables, which makes predictions of the qualitative and quantitative aspects of the metabolism of a foreign compound difficult. However, an understanding of the metabolic disposition of a foreign chemical in any animal species may often offer a logical explanation for the toxic effect(s) of that chemical in that species.

REFERENCES

Gillette, J. R.: Significance of mixed oxygenases and nitroreductase in drug metabolism. *Ann. N.Y. Acad. Sci.*, **160**:558–70, 1969.

Gorrod, J. W.: Differentiation of various types of biological oxidation of nitrogen in organic compounds. *Chem. Biol. Interact.*, **7**:289–303, 1973.

Gram, T. E., and Gillette, J. R.: Biotransformation of drugs. In Bacq, Z. M. (ed.): *Fundamentals of Biochemical Pharmacology.* Pergamon Press Ltd., New York, 1971, pp. 571–609.

Hayes, W. J.: *Toxicology of Pesticides.* Williams & Wilkins Co., Baltimore, 1975.

Jakoby, W. B., and Keen, J. H.: A triple-threat in detoxification: the glutathione *S*-transferases. *Trends Biochem. Sci.*, **2**(10):229–31, 1977.

Jakoby, W. B.; Habig, W. H.; Keen, J. H.; Ketley, J. N.; and Pabst, M. J.: Glutathione S-transferases: catalytic aspects. In Arias, I. M., and Jakoby, W. B. (eds.): *Glutathione: Metabolism and Function.* Raven Press, New York, 1976, pp. 189–211.

La Du, B. N.; Mandel, H. G.; and Way, E. L.: *Fundamentals of Drug Metabolism and Drug Disposition.* Williams & Wilkins Co., Baltimore, 1971.

Testa, B., and Jenner, P.: *Drug Metabolism: Chemical and Biochemical Aspects.* Marcel Dekker Inc., New York, 1976.

Williams, R. T.: *Detoxication Mechanisms*, 2nd ed. Chapman and Hall, Ltd., London, 1959.

Ziegler, D. M., and Mitchell, C. H.: Microsomal oxidase. IV: Properties of a mixed-function amine oxidase isolated from pig liver microsomes. *Arch. Biochem. Biophys.*, **150**:116–25, 1972.

Chapter 5

FACTORS INFLUENCING TOXICOLOGY

John Doull

INTRODUCTION

It has been pointed out in previous chapters of this book that, in order for a toxic effect to occur in a biologic system, it is necessary for the toxic agent or its metabolites or conversion products to reach an appropriate receptor in the biologic system and to do so at a sufficiently high concentration and for a long enough time to initiate the toxic manifestation. With this requirement as a background, it is easy to understand how changes in the dose, route, and duration of exposure can influence the biologic response to a single toxic agent. However, even when these factors are rigidly controlled, there is still likely to be a great deal of variation in the response of individual members of a population to a specific toxic agent. Some of this variation can be attributed to factors that influence the absorption, distribution, metabolism, or excretion of the toxic agent, and it is the purpose of this chapter to consider these and other factors that have been shown to affect the toxic response.

It is convenient to divide the factors that influence toxicity into those that are related to (1) the poison or toxic agent, (2) the exposure situation, and (3) the subject. The factors that are related to the subject can be further divided on the basis of whether they are internal (inherent in the subject) or external to the subject (environmental). This general classification has been used in preparing the listing of toxicity-influencing factors shown in Table 5–1.

Much of the controversy that is associated with the interpretation of the results of supposedly comparable toxicologic investigations is the result of a failure to recognize the importance of these factors and the ability of even slight changes in the experimental protocol to alter markedly the response of the test system. Toxicologists need to keep these factors in mind in carrying out their predictive responsibilities (safety evaluation) and also in their activities related to detection (forensic toxicology) and to the diagnosis and treatment of poisoning (clinical toxicology).

Table 5–1. A CLASSIFICATION OF TOXICITY-INFLUENCING FACTORS

1. *Factors Related to the Toxic Agent*

   Chemical composition (pH, choice of anion, etc.)
   Physical characteristics (particle size, method of formulation, etc.)
   Presence of impurities or contaminants
   Stability and storage characteristics of the toxic agent
   Solubility of the toxic agent in biologic fluids
   Choice of the vehicle
   Presence of excipients: adjuvants, emulsifiers, surfactants, binding agents, coating agents, coloring agents, flavoring agents, preservatives, antioxidants, and other intentional and nonintentional additives

2. *Factors Related to the Exposure Situation*

   Dose, concentration, and volume of administration
   Route, rate, and site of administration
   Duration and frequency of exposure
   Time of administration (time of day, season of the year, etc.)

3. *Inherent Factors Related to the Subject*

   Species and strain (taxonomic classification)
   Genetic status (littermate, siblings, multigeneration effects, etc.)
   Immunologic status
   Nutritional status (diet factors, state of hydration, etc.)
   Hormonal status (pregnancy, etc.)
   Age, sex, body weight, and maturity
   Central nervous system status (activity, crowding, handling, presence of other species, etc.)
   Presence of disease or specific organ pathology

4. *Environmental Factors Related to the Subject*

   Temperature and humidity
   Barometric pressure (hyper- and hypobaric effects)
   Ambient atmospheric composition
   Light and other forms of radiation
   Housing and caging effects
   Noise and other geographic influences
   Social factors
   Chemical factors

FACTORS RELATED TO THE TOXIC AGENT

Composition of Sample

It is evident that the toxicity of a specific agent can be influenced by the composition of the particular sample used for the studies. Impurities or contaminants may be present that are considerably more or less toxic than the test agent or that can actually modify the response of the biologic system to the test agent. In the testing of agents for carcinogenic activity, for example, it is frequently necessary to consider whether the tumors were produced by an impurity rather than the test agent or whether the impurity could have functioned as an activator or cocarcinogen under the experimental conditions of the test. A related problem with impurities is that they may vary from batch to batch so that the results obtained with a particular sample of the test agent are not reproducible. Because of these problems, it is not surprising that adequate specifications for identity and purity are considered to be prerequisites for sound toxicologic assessment. It must be kept in mind, however, that the results of toxicologic studies that are carried out using such highly purified samples of the test agent may not accurately predict the hazard associated with exposure to that agent when it is prepared in pilot plant or large-scale production facilities. This problem can only be solved by carrying out additional studies to verify the toxicity of the agent in the "real-world" situation and by monitoring the hazard associated with continued use of the agent. Other toxicity-influencing factors that are directly related to the toxic agent include its stability, pH, and the selection of the anion or chelate or other binding group for the test agent.

Formulation Factors

The formulation process provides another group of factors that are associated with the toxic agent and are capable of markedly altering its toxicity. Formulation factors can increase or decrease toxicity directly by altering the chemical nature of the agent or by affecting the solubility, which influences the absorption of the toxic agent into the biologic system. Substances used in formulation of a product may also alter toxicity indirectly by changing the susceptibility of the biologic system to the toxic agent.

Vehicle. One of the most important of the formulation factors is the vehicle, which is defined as a substance (usually a liquid) used as a medium for suspending or dissolving the active ingredient. In practice, an attempt is made to select vehicles that have little or no toxic or pharmacologic activity of their own and that exert a relatively minor effect, if any, on the toxicity of the active ingredient. Common examples of vehicles used for laboratory toxicity investigations include water, saline, polyethylene glycols, vegetable oils, dimethylsulfoxide, and various organic solvents. Insoluble materials are often administered as suspensions in natural gums (acacia, tragacanth, etc.) or synthetic colloids (methyl cellulose, carboxymethyl cellulose, etc.). Since the toxicity of the active ingredient is likely to be quite different if it is given as a suspension rather than as a solution, the selection of the vehicle becomes a crucial part of the experimental protocol for any type of toxicity study.

Adjuvants. Adjuvants are formulation factors that are used to enhance the pharmacologic or toxic effect of the active ingredient. They are said to be additive when the adjuvant produces its effect by acting on the same biologic receptor as the active ingredient and synergistic when the adjuvant acts through a different biologic mechanism than the active ingredient. Examples of adjuvants used in toxicologic formulations include the addition of piperonyl butoxide to enhance the insecticidal activity of the pyrethrins and the use of mercaptobenzothiazole to enhance the fungicidal activity of the dithiocarbamates.

Binding Agents. Formulation ingredients such as petrolatum and kaolin may be added to provide a more agreeable or convenient preparation for administering the active ingredient. Such agents generally tend to delay absorption and thus to reduce toxicity.

Enteric Coating, Sustained-Release Preparations, etc. Other formulation factors that influence absorption of the active ingredient and consequently its toxicity are tablet size and hardness, and the use of specialized techniques to delay absorption (enteric coating, sustained-release preparations, etc.). Micronizing is a technique that is used to enhance the absorption of drugs, pesticides, and other agents by reducing the particle size (air milling) of the active ingredient. The effect of particle size on absorption and retention is particularly important when the exposure occurs by inhalation. Much of the information concerning the effects of these and other formulation factors on absorption has been obtained by measuring the level and disappearance of the active ingredient from the plasma or other body fluid of the test species. This approach, which is called pharmacokinetics, has been of great value in characterizing the bioavailability of drug formulations. Concepts derived from this type of investigation (apparent volume of distribution, half-life, single versus steady-state kinetics, etc.) are obviously equally important in other types of toxicologic investigations (see Chap. 3).

Miscellaneous Formulation Factors. Other agents that may be important in toxicologic studies with drugs or foods include coloring and flavoring agents, antioxidants, stabilizers, preservatives, and emulsifiers or surfactants. Some of the chemical agents that are used for these purposes (intentional additives) are listed in Table 5–2. Inadvertent or unintentional additives such as pesticides, reaction products, or lubricants may also be present in samples of foods, drugs, or other chemicals.

By using a pure sample of the test agent and by applying it to the test object (the experimental animal or other biologic system) in an undiluted

Table 5–2. CHEMICAL AGENTS USED AS FORMULATION INGREDIENTS

1. *Suspending Agents:* acacia, cellulose gum, carboxymethyl cellulose, etc.
2. *Preservatives:* sodium benzoate, emthyl *p*-hydroxybenzoate, propyl *p*-hydroxybenzoate chlorobutanol, phenylmercuric nitrate
3. *Surfactants:* polysorbate 80, Span 20, Span 60, Myrj 52
4. *Lubricants:* calcium stearate, cornstarch, magnesium stearate, talc, lycopodium
5. *Binders:* starch, gelatin, sugars, natural and synthetic gums, waxes
6. *Coating agents:* shellac, gelatin, carnauba wax
7. *Disintegrators*; corn and potato starch, cellulose derivatives (Solkafloc, Amvicel, etc.)
8. *Diluents:* sucrose, lactose, mannitol, milk solids, starch, kaolin, calcium carbonate, dicalcium phosphate
9. *Stabilizers:* sodium bisulfite, sodium sulfite
10. *Solvents:* ethanol, glycerine, propylene glycol, benzyl alcohol, isopropyl alcohol
11. *Excipients:* magnesium oxide, beeswax, Carbowaxes, mineral oil, petrolatum, silic acid, titanium dioxide, zein

form it is possible for the toxicologist to avoid the complicating influence of all of these formulation factors. However, most agents are not suitable for this type of exposure because of their toxicity or physical form, and even in those situations where such studies are feasible the results may be questioned on the basis that the laboratory experiments do not accurately predict the hazard associated with the conditions of general usage of the agent.

FACTORS RELATED TO THE EXPOSURE SITUATION

The major toxicity-influencing factors relating to the exposure situation are the dose and concentration of the toxic agent, the duration and frequency of the exposure, and the route, site, and rate at which the toxic agent is administered. The effect of variations in the dose, route, duration, and frequency of exposure has been considered in Chapter 2, and there is additional information on the effect of the route of administration on the toxic response in Chapter 3. The discussion here will be restricted, therefore, to selected additional factors, the effects of which on toxicity tend to be somewhat more variable and which are generally less well recognized in the design and interpretation of toxicologic investigations.

Volume and Concentration Factors

It is customary to use several concentrations of the test agent for parenteral and oral toxicity tests so that the total volume administered for each dosage level will remain relatively constant and to keep the volume of solution administered small in relation to the size of the biologic test system. A common recommendation for oral dosing, for example, is that the volume of material administered should not exceed 2 to 3 percent of the body weight, and many toxicology protocols specify an upper limit of 0.5 ml for intravenous dosing in rodents and 2 ml for larger laboratory animals. Although recommendations such as these tend to minimize the effects of volume and concentration on toxicity, other considerations (such as solubility) may require the use of very dilute solutions. As one might anticipate, the toxicity of drugs given by the oral route tends to be increased when they are given in more dilute solutions but the reverse situation can occur with agents whose toxic effects are due mainly to local irritation (Balazs, 1970). A common problem associated with the administration of the toxic agent in large volumes is vehicle toxicity. Since the intravenous LD50 of distilled water in the mouse is 44 ml/kg and that of isotonic saline is 68 ml/kg, the intravenous injection of less than 1 ml of a hypotonic solution could be lethal for this species (Balazs, 1970). Other problems associated with the administration of large volumes in toxicity studies include the possibility of excessive hydration and impaired renal clearance of the toxic agent, a laxative effect when large volumes of vegetable oils are used as a vehicle, and changes in the rate of gastric passage and subsequent intestinal absorption. When large volumes are administered, these effects can be partially minimized by the use of dose fractionation and a moderate extension of the exposure period. In some cases it may also be possible to use different sites of administration (subcutaneous or intramuscular administration). A number of other practical suggestions for handling the problems associated with the bulk administration of toxic agents can be found in a text on predictive toxicometrics (Boyd, 1972).

Volume effects also need to be considered in chronic toxicity testing. In most studies of this type, the toxic agent is added to the food. With test agents having a low toxicity, the percent of toxic agent in the diet may have to be increased to the point where the bulk of the agent interferes with nutrition. By failing to recognize this possibility, the investigator may erroneously attribute growth retardation and its subsequent physiologic effects to the toxic agent rather than to the dietary restriction imposed by the experimental protocol. One approach to this situation is to use equivalent amounts of an inert material in formulating the diet for the control groups, so that all exposure groups (including the controls) experience the same dietary restriction. Another approach is to use pair feeding of the control groups, in which the paired controls are allowed only the amount of food consumed by the experimental animals.

Site and Rate of Administration

Most of the evidence concerning the toxicity-influencing effects of the administration site have been obtained with the parenteral route, although regional effects have been detected for dermal absorption and data on the comparative toxicity of oral versus rectal administration are available (Boyd, 1972). Differences in the toxicity of strychnine and ammonium chloride have been shown in mice following subcutaneous injection into dorsal or ventral sites, and there are numerous examples of differences in intravenous toxicity when different veins are used to administer the test agent (Balazs, 1970). Some of these effects can be attributed to the metabolic or excretory role of the liver or kidneys and the ability of the investigator to minimize the initial effects of these organs on the toxic agent by judicious selection of the administration site. In those situations where administration site differences in toxicity have been detected, it may be possible to use the data as a basis for preliminary predictions regarding the translocation, deposition, inactivation, or site of excretion of the toxic agent. One can, of course, obtain the same type of information by comparing the toxic effects of an agent given intravenously or subcutaneously with those obtained when the agent is given orally or intraperitoneally or in some other manner that ensures passage through the portal circulation to the liver.

With few exceptions, fractionation of the dose of a toxic agent reduces toxicity (see Chapter 2 for a discussion of duration-frequency relationships) and this is particularly striking for agents

that are rapidly metabolized or excreted. An obvious explanation for this reduced toxic response is that the dose fractionation simply provides the biologic test system with more time to carry out the detoxification processes (metabolism, excretion, binding, etc.) that are available for the biotransformation of the toxic agent in that system. On this basis, one would expect the effects of dose fractionation to be less marked in toxicity studies with highly cumulative agents. The reduction in toxicity that occurs when toxic agents are given by slow infusion rather than as a single intravenous administration can also be attributed to increased metabolism or excretion or other detoxication processes. It is understandable that compounds in which the toxic effects are due to a metabolite rather than the parent compound would not be expected to conform to the above generalization. There are other experimental situations in which fractionation of the dose has produced an increase rather than the expected decrease in the toxic response. In one such study, it was found that the increased toxicity of a phenothiazine derivative (Dixyrazine) when fed in the diet over that resulting from single daily gavaging was due to the interaction of the agent and a constituent of the diet to form a more toxic product (Boyd, 1972). Similar paradoxic results have been reported for administration rate change studies with cardiac glycosides, pentylenetetrazol, and sodium cyanide (Balazs, 1970). It is evident, therefore, that changes in the rate of administration of a toxic agent can be expected to produce changes in the toxic response to that agent but that the magnitude and even the direction of these effects may be somewhat unpredictable.

Even in those situations where the toxic agent is administered as a single dose, the toxic response may be influenced by the rate at which the agent is administered. Intravenous injections given in a few seconds can produce transient concentrations in nearby organs that are several hundred times greater than those that are produced by giving the toxic agent over the period of a minute, a rate that approximates a complete circulation of the blood in man (Goldstein et al., 1974).

Diurnal and Seasonal Factors

Changes in the susceptibility of biologic systems to toxic agents may be related to the time of day at which they are administered, the season of the year, or even a longer period (years, decades, etc.). Most of the diurnal variations have been shown to be related to the eating and sleeping habits of the test species. In a nocturnal animal such as a rat, there is almost certain to be more food in the stomach in the morning than in the late afternoon and it is not surprising, therefore, that there is a diurnal variation in the toxicity of such drugs as caffeine, which has been shown to be more toxic in fasted rats. Similarly, agents that affect activity would be expected to produce somewhat different results when given during the day while the animals are normally sleeping than when given at night, which is a more active period for rats and many other species. It is of interest that Boyd (1972) has been able to increase diurnal activity in rats by starvation so that the effects of toxic agents on locomotor activity could be measured throughout the day. Continuous lighting may also be used to increase activity of nocturnal animals during normal daylight hours. As will be discussed elsewhere in this chapter, hormonal changes in the test species can produce day-to-day variations in the susceptibility of animals to toxic agents and such changes may also be responsible for some of the seasonal variations that have been reported for different species of animals to standard doses of toxic agents. Another possibility for seasonal and also yearly changes in susceptibility is the variability in the weather or local atmospheric conditions. These and other environmental conditions that can influence toxicity will also be discussed in the subsequent sections of this chapter.

FACTORS RELATED TO THE INTERNAL ENVIRONMENT OF THE SUBJECT

Taxonomic Classification

Before considering the various factors that are inherent in the biologic system and that may produce differences in susceptibility between individuals or groups of similar animals, it is appropriate to consider the kind of differences that can exist between animals from different taxonomic levels. This consideration is of great importance in toxicology since it is the basis for almost all toxicologic predictions, particularly those in which an attempt is made to establish the safety of an agent for use in man on the basis of tests in other species. Although there is growing recognition of the fact that a completely accurate evaluation of the toxicity of an agent in a particular species can only be obtained by carrying out the toxicologic studies in the desired species, the situations where such information can be obtained directly from man (poisoning cases and industrial exposure associated with the manufacture of the agent, etc.) rarely provide the type of dose-response and mechanism information that can be obtained by planned experiments in other species. Thus, even if it were possible to avoid the ethical considera-

tions associated with the deliberate exposure of man to potentially toxic agents, animal tests would still be needed to characterize the environmental hazard of the agent and probably to elucidate its mechanism of action.

Attempts to establish safety for man on the basis of tests in other species are complicated primarily by the increasing divergence that is encountered as one ascends through the different taxonomic levels. Using the classification shown in Table 5–3, for example, it is not surprising that comparisons made between animals or groups of animals that are closely related taxonomically are more likely to be predictive than those involving different taxonomic levels and consequently greater taxonomic diversity. Since comparisons between animals or groups of animals at different taxonomic levels can be influenced simultaneously by all of the inherited differences associated with evolutionary changes responsible for each of the classification levels,

Table 5–3. SAMPLE COMPARISONS IN COMPARATIVE TOXICITY EXPERIMENTS

Kingdom	Animals versus plants
Branch	Mesozoa versus Parazoa
Phylum	Chordata versus Invertebrata
Class	Mammalia versus Aves
Order	Rodentia versus Primates
Family	Muridae versus Sciuridae
Genus	*Rattus* versus *Mus*
Species	*R. rattus* versus *R. norvegicus*
Strain	Wistar versus Sprague-Dawley rat
Litter	Litter versus litter
Individual	Littermate versus littermate

it is not surprising that species and strain differences in susceptibility to a toxic agent are generally greater than sibling and littermate differences.

This biologic diversity that interferes with the ability of the toxicologist to make reliable predictions for different taxonomic levels is, on the other hand, a great advantage to the toxicologist who is seeking to discover new pesticides or chemotherapeutic agents. By taking advantage of some aspect of this biologic diversity (such as the ability of the host to detoxify a compound by a metabolic process that does not exist in the pest or parasite) it may be possible to develop an agent that is lethal for the undesirable species and harmless for all other species. In order to fully utilize both the uniformity and diversity of different taxonomic levels, it is evident that the toxicologist needs both qualitative and quantitative information about these intertaxonomic relationships. Studies of this type have been given the name "comparative pharmacology and toxicology" and interest in this area has markedly increased in the last few years (Cafruny, 1967). However, it should be pointed out that the same general ideas and basic principles were identified earlier as "selective toxicity" in a book by Adrian Albert (1960).

Attempts to define the mechanisms responsible for variation in species susceptibility to toxic agents have been particularly informative. It is now evident that many of the species differences in susceptibility to toxic agents can be explained by differences in the rate and pattern of the metabolism of the toxic agent. Examples of such differences in metabolism include (1) the failure of dogs to acetylate arylamines and the consequent differences in the metabolism of such agents as p-aminobenzoic acid in dogs from that seen in man and rabbits, (2) the inability of the guinea pig to acetylate S-aryl cystein, and (3) the deficiency of glucuronyl transferase in the cat when compared to man, who is able to form conjugated glucuronides to acetylate aromatic amines and to acetylate S-aryl cystein to mercapturic acid (Koppanyi and Avery, 1966).

In addition to differences in the rate and pattern of metabolism as the basis for species difference in susceptibility to toxic agents, differences in renal and biliary excretion, plasma protein binding, tissue distribution, and response of the "receptor site" have been postulated (Burns, 1970) and experimentally verified for some toxic agents. The effect of species differences in biliary excretion on toxicity and the possible role of enterohepatic circulation in producing similar effects have been discussed in Chapter 3 and additional information can be found in a review by Smith (1970).

The importance of plasma protein binding on toxicity can be illustrated by the occurrence of kernicterus (entry of bilirubin into the brain) as an unexpected toxic effect of the sulfonamides in premature and newborn infants. In this situation, the sulfonamides (and other drugs such as vitamin K) were found to be producing the toxic effect (kernicterus) by displacing bilirubin from its plasma-binding sites. The premature infant is unusually susceptible in this situation since it is deficient in the conjugating system responsible for coupling bilirubin with glucuronic acid. Another example of a difference in susceptibility to the effects of a drug that may be related to protein binding is provided by the clinical variations that occur in response to "standardized" doses of digitoxin in man.

If the difference in susceptibility to the toxic effects of a specific agent in two different species are due to differences in the rate and pattern of metabolism or plasma binding of the toxic agent in these species, then it should be possible in some cases at least to eliminate these differences by using experimental procedures that would ensure that the free plasma concentration of the toxic agent was identical in the two species. Experiments of this type have been carried out with carisoprodol (a muscle relaxant), with a variety of barbiturates, and with phenylbutazone and several related derivatives (Burns, 1970). Despite the marked differences that some of these agents exhibited in metabolism, there was a good correlation between the plasma level and the measured pharmacologic effect. This type of study supports the concept that quantitative species differences are most likely to occur as a result of metabolic differences between the species. Metabolic differences are less likely to provide a satisfactory explanation for qualitative differences in toxicity between species. For example, it has long been recognized that the rodenticidal activity of squill is dependent on the fact that the rat does not vomit and thereby retains the toxic agent whereas man and many other species eliminate this poison by emesis.

Genetic Status

It has long been recognized that strain differences in susceptibility to toxic agents may be explained by comparing the genetic status of the susceptible and nonsusceptible strains. The ability of genetic factors to explain the variation in susceptibility of individual members of a particular strain or group of individuals is a more recent development. Although studies in this area have been given the name "pharmacogenetics," most of the examples of genetic effects on drug response have been discovered as the result of differences in toxicity rather than in the desired drug response.

One of the first demonstrations of the role of inheritance in biologic response was the observations that the variation in the susceptibility of some rabbits to the toxic effects of atropine could be explained by the presence of an enzyme, atropine esterase, in the blood of the resistant animals. These observations not only explained why some rabbits were resistant to the toxic effects of atropine but they also provided a reasonable explanation for a species difference in susceptibility to atropine since atropine esterase has not been found in other species examined, including man.

A similar genetic explanation has been demonstrated for the prolonged apnea that is produced in some individuals with the administration of standard doses of succinylcholine. Individuals who have an atypical or low serum cholinesterase (pseudocholinesterase) level may exhibit prolongation of the muscular relaxation and apnea-producing effects of succinylcholine since this enzyme is responsible for the hydrolysis and consequent termination of the pharmacologic effect of succinylcholine. Studies by Kalow (1962) and others have demonstrated the existence of three distinct genotypes of cholinesterase in human serum (atypical, fluoride resistant, and silent gene), and a fourth variant has subsequently been detected on the basis of its electrophoretic bands.

Other genetically controlled drug toxicity relationships include the production of polyneuritis in individuals who exhibit an impaired ability to acetylate isoniazid and the acute hemolytic anemia that develops in individuals having a deficiency in the enzyme glucose-6-phosphate dehydrogenase (G6PD) when such individuals are treated with the antimalarial primaquine. Individuals with the G6PD deficiency have also been found to be more susceptible to the hemolytic effects of other drugs (sulfonamides, aspirin, vitamin K, etc.) and toxic agents (benzene, naphthalene, methylene blue, acetanilide, phenylhydrazine, etc.). A decreased response to the administered agent resulting from genetic factors has been demonstrated with coumarin in man, and a similar explanation has been suggested for the development of resistance to the coumarin rodenticide warfarin in rat populations in Scotland and Denmark. High insulin tolerance has been observed in an inbred strain of mice, and geneticists have used the inability of various individuals to detect a bitter taste with phenylthiourea to demonstrate the bimodality of response of groups of individuals due to this inherited trait. Other examples of genetically controlled differences in response to toxic agents can be found in the appropriate chapters of the books by Kalow (1962), Goldstein and associates (1974), and Loomis (1974) and in various review articles and monographs (Beutler, 1969; Kalow, 1965; LaDu, 1965).

Since most toxic agents must ultimately combine with their target receptors in order to produce their toxic manifestations, it is reasonable to expect that the toxic effect will be greatly influenced by the genetically determined structure of the protein receptor. If the specificity of the protein receptor and even the presence or absence of the receptor are primarily inherited characteristics, then it is likely that the "biologic variation" that exists between individuals, strains, and even species is more dependent on genetic factors responsible for specific receptors than on commonly suggested explanations involving environmental changes such as enzyme induction, immunologic responses, and so forth. Support for this hypothesis is provided by the demonstration that the variation in the amino acid sequence of homologous proteins

that occurs between species and even within individuals of the same species is genetically determined. The recommendation that the term "idiosyncrasy" be redefined to mean a genetically determined abnormal reactivity to a drug or toxic agent (Goldstein et al., 1974) is indicative of the growing importance of the genetic status as a toxicity-influencing factor.

Nutritional Status and Dietary Factors

Dietary factors can influence toxicity in several ways. As mentioned previously in this chapter, the formulation of the toxic agent into the diet may result in inactivation of the toxic agent (chelation, hydrolysis, etc.) or the formation of a more toxic product. Dietary factors also enter into the variability associated with the exposure situation (palatability, rate, and volume effects, etc.). In addition to these effects, dietary factors can produce changes in the body composition, physiologic and biochemical functions, and nutritional status of the subject and thereby influence toxicity.

Because of the possible effect of dietary composition and time of feeding on the absorption of the toxic agent, it is customary to use fasted animals for toxicity studies. One problem here is that the catabolic effects of starvation influence toxicity. Fasting for periods as short as two hours has been shown to decrease liver glycogen in rats and mice, and fasting for eight hours will also reduce blood glucose and produce changes in the activity of several of the drug-metabolizing enzymes. As one might expect, the stresses of starvation (body weight and organ hydration changes, pyloric ulcers, adrenal and thymus effects, etc.) have been shown to influence the toxic response to a variety of drugs and other agents. Murasmugenic diets (reduced total caloric intake) increased the toxicity of caffeine and DDT in rats, and low-protein diets (kwashiorkorigenic diets) have been shown to increase the toxicity of a variety of pesticides and other agents (Boyd, 1972). On the other hand, low-protein diets have been found to protect rats against the hepatotoxicity and lethality of carbon tetrachloride and dimethylnitrosamine exposure but not against the effects of chloroform and aflatoxin on the liver. It has been suggested (McLean and McLean, 1969) that the differences in the effect of low dietary protein on the toxicity of aflatoxin and dimethylnitrosamine can be explained by the decreased availability of the microsomal enzyme system in the protein-deficient animal. In this regard, it is of interest that the toxicity of chloroform can be enhanced by high-fat diets or by the addition of a microsomal stimulator such as DDT to the diet. The ability of dietary DDT or other microsomal stimulators to influence the toxicity of a specific agent is generally dependent on whether the microsomal conversion of the specific toxic agent results in a metabolite that is more or less toxic than the parent compound.

High-protein diets have also been shown to influence toxicity (decreased thioacetamide effects on the liver) and have been used clinically in combination with high-carbohydrate diets in patients whose livers have been damaged by toxic agents and some types of disease states. Vitamin deficiency is another dietary-related effect that may influence toxicity, and vitamin C deficiency has been shown to affect the rate of drug metabolism in guinea pigs. Diets that contain a high tyramine content (some types of aged cheeses, wine, beer, chicken liver, etc.) enhance effects of monoamine oxidase inhibitors, and similar toxic reactions can be produced by adding the MAO inhibitor to the diet and administering catecholamine-releasing drugs. Although foods are generally considered to be nontoxic unless adulterated or contaminated with specific toxic agents, Boyd (1972) has produced a variety of toxic manifestations by administering large doses of specific proteins (casein, lactalbumin, soy protein), fats (cottonseed oil, corn oil), and carbohydrates (glucose, sucrose, starch).

These examples illustrate the complex relationships that may exist between the diet, feeding patterns, nutritional status, and the toxic agent in conducting studies to demonstrate the existence of a food-related hazard and characterizing its mechanism of action.

Sex and Hormonal Status

Male and female animals of the same strain and species usually exhibit only slight differences in susceptibility to toxic agents. There are, however, some notable exceptions, and because of this possibility the experimental protocol for both acute and chronic toxicity tests generally specifies that the tests include both sexes. Since most of the examples of male-female differences in toxicity have been shown to be under direct endocrine control, a typical follow-up protocol for toxic agents that exhibit a sex effect is to determine whether the effect can be reduced or eliminated by castration or the administration of hormones and whether it is present in immature animals.

One of the most striking examples of a male-female difference in toxicity is the nephrotoxic effect of chloroform in male mice of certain strains. Female mice of the same strains show virtually no effect from chloroform exposures that are lethal for the males. Castration or the administration of estrogens reduces the effect in the male, and treatment with androgens induces

susceptibility to chloroform in the female. Sex differences in toxicity have been observed with some of the organophosphate insecticides. Female rats are more susceptible to the toxic effects of Di-Syston, Guthion, EPN, and parathion (thionate organophosphate derivatives) than are male rats, but the reverse situation occurs with methyl parathion. Sex-related effects in the organic phosphate insecticides are most likely to occur in those compounds that require metabolic activation to produce cholinesterase inhibition. Direct-acting cholinesterase inhibitors such as trichlorfon (Dipterex) exhibit little or no sex difference in susceptibility. Castration and hormone treatment reverse the sex-related effects of Guthion and parathion, and weanling male and female rats are equally susceptible to these agents.

Many of the barbiturates exhibit a sex-related difference in toxicity, which is most commonly manifested by a longer sleep time in female rats than in male rats. With hexobarbital, these effects can be correlated with metabolism of the parent compound by the liver microsomal enzymes and the rapid metabolic rate in the male can be reduced by estrogen pretreatment.

Other examples of agents that are more toxic in the female than in the male are phenacetin (rat), acetylsalicylic acid (rat), benzene (rabbit, man), dinitrophenol (cat), ethionine (rat), ethyl-o-ethylphenyl urea (rat), folic acid (mouse), nicotine (rat), picrotoxin (rat), squill (rat), warfarin (rat), and strychnine (rat). Examples of agents that are more toxic to the male than to the female include epinephrine (rat), alcohol (rat), digoxin (dog), ergot (rat), monocrotaline (rat), nicotine (mouse), ouabain (rat), and lead (rat). In many of these examples, the sex effect occurs in a single species and often only in a particular strain of that species. Hormonal treatment affects many of these sex differences, but the response is not always in the expected direction (toward the condition of resistance or susceptibility exhibited by the opposite sex). In some cases the sex effect can only be demonstrated when the animals are fed a protein-deficient diet (monocrotaline response) (Hurst, 1958).

From the above discussion, it is evident that the most likely explanation for sex-related differences in toxicity is that the enzymatic biotransformation of the agent is influenced by sex hormones. Experimental support for this hypothesis has been obtained for several of the examples listed. The sex effect observed with strychnine, for example, is not evident when the agent is given intravenously, and liver microsomal preparations from male rats metabolize strychnine to its metabolites at a faster rate than similar preparations from female rats.

Conversely, parathion (which is also more toxic to female rats) is metabolized more rapidly by liver microsome preparations from female than from male rats, but with this agent the metabolite (paraoxon) is more toxic than the parent compound. As one would anticipate, there is no evidence for a sex effect with paraoxon in rats. Sex hormones are also capable of producing a protein-sparing effect, and it has been suggested that this action or the fact that females have a lower fat-free body weight may explain some of the sex-related differences in toxicity that do not appear to be directly related to alterations in metabolism of the parent agent.

In addition to the toxicity differences that may occur between male and female animals, there are a number of other hormonally dependent situations that may influence the toxicity of various agents. Pregnancy has been shown to increase markedly the susceptibility of mice to some types of pesticides, and similar effects have been reported for lactating animals exposed to heavy metals. Hyperthyroidism and hyperinsulinism may alter the susceptibility of animals, including man, to toxic agents, and Boyd (1972) has suggested that many of these effects are due to stress-mediated hormonal mechanisms. Adrenalectomized rats are generally more susceptible to toxic agents, and stimulation of the pituitary adrenal axis increases the activity of drug-metabolizing enzymes.

Age, Maturity, and Body Weight

Although it has long been recognized that the immature animal or neonate is not simply a miniature of the mature or adult, it is only relatively recently that the mechanisms responsible for these age-dependent variations in toxicity have been investigated. An examination of the comparative toxicity of various agents in neonates and adults (Done, 1964) indicates that the toxicity ratio can vary from 0.002- to 16-fold but that there does appear to be some general consistency within pharmacologic classes. Newborn animals appear, for example, to be less susceptible to central nervous system (CNS) stimulants and more susceptible to CNS depressants. Many of these differences can be explained by the qualitative and quantitative differences in detoxification processes in newborn and adult animals. In rabbits, for example, the liver microsomal enzyme system starts to develop at about the first week after birth, and newborn animals from other species exhibit a similar lack of drug-metabolizing enzymes. Increased membrane permeability in the newborn (particularly at the blood-brain barrier) has been suggested as another possible mechanism for age-related differences in toxicity. Differences in the hepatic

and renal clearance of toxic agents between newborn and adult animals have been shown to occur and may also be involved in age-dependent toxicity effects (Balazs, 1970). In this respect, it is of interest that differences in the rate of drug metabolism have been shown in senescent animals and thus metabolic and excretion patterns may be contributing to toxicity variation at both extremes of the life-span rather than simply in the newborn.

The necessity for dose adjustment is well recognized in pediatrics and in certain other clinical conditions (administration of antibiotics to patients with renal impairment, etc.). In toxicologic studies it is customary to adjust the dose on the basis of the body weight in anticipation that this will tend to minimize variation between animals and species. With animals having a large body weight, there is often a disproportionate increase in drug toxicity, and many investigators have suggested other approaches such as the use of the body surface area or the factor of two-thirds of the body weight (which approximates the metabolically active weight). None of these experimental approaches is satisfactory for all experimental situations, and it is evident that the investigator will be required to make some compromise between convenience and precision in administrating toxic agents to biologic systems.

Emotional Status

Prior to the demonstration that the toxicity of amphetamine and other CNS stimulants can be increased by crowding, little attention was given to the possibility of emotional or other CNS factors influencing toxicity. It is now recognized that such studies can be affected not only by the number of animals per cage but also by the size of the cage, the type of bedding, the material used to construct the cage, and particularly by the manner and frequency of handling that the animal receives during the toxicity test. Efforts are also being made to demonstrate that emotional factors influence the susceptibility of man to toxic agents in his environment, and epidemiologists increasingly include consideration of such effects as urbanization, noise, adaptive response to change, and other social and economic pressure in the etiology of disease states associated with air and water pollution.

Miscellaneous Internal or Inherent Factors

Traditionally the toxicity of a specific toxic agent has been evaluated on the basis of tests carried out in healthy adult animals. The predictions that derive from such studies, since they are applied to the total population, cover not only the healthy animals in that population but those subjects in all stages of poor health, those with various disease conditions, and a host of subjects having various degrees of organ pathology. Since these deviations from the normal state of health are likely to influence the toxic response in the exposed individual, toxicologists are becoming increasingly concerned about the need to include diseased animals in the experimental population and to evaluate the effects of specific types of organ pathology on the toxicity response. It would be logical, for example, to include tests on hypertensive animals as part of the toxicologic investigation of a new diuretic agent and to investigate the effects of various types of kidney disease on the pharmacologic and toxicologic effects of the diuretic. It is possible, however, that the toxicologic evaluation would be of greater clinical value if it included, in addition, an investigation of the toxic effects of this diuretic in individuals with myocardial damage, or with diabetes, or any of a host of other disease states in which the drug might be used. The possibilities of this type of testing are of course virtually limitless and therefore beyond the realm of practical possibility. A compromise approach to this problem is to use normal healthy animals to identify the tissues or organs where the toxic effects predominate and then to carry out additional studies in animals that have various types of preexisting damage or disease in only these organs. Although relatively few studies of this type have been carried out, it is evident that preexisting pathologic damage can alter the toxic response of a particular organ and that greater cognizance will have to be taken of this fact in the toxicologic testing programs of the future.

A closely related aspect of this problem is the use of diseased animals to demonstrate toxic effects that are too subtle or of insufficient severity to be detectable in normal, healthy animals. The use of animals with various types of precancerous lesions as test objects for carcinogens has been partially successful, and it has been possible to demonstrate toxic effects with subthreshold dosage of pulmonary irritants by using animals with preexisting emphysema. In addition to the value of this approach in detecting toxic effects that might otherwise be missed, such test methods may provide the additional advantage of shortening the time required for the induction of the toxic manifestation (e.g., in carcinogenic testing).

Another example of an inherent factor that could influence the response to a toxic agent is the bacterial composition of the gastrointestinal tract. Possible effects here might include the actual composition of the toxic agent, changes in the rate and amount of absorbed toxic agent, and variation in the rate in which the toxic agent is eliminated in the feces.

Individuals who are exposed to a long-lasting cholinesterase inhibitor are more likely to show cholinergic signs of toxicity when given a second exposure to the same or to a different cholinesterase inhibitor. A similar situation occurs in lead workers who have a substantial body burden of lead. In this situation, the exposed individual may show no symptoms of toxicity prior to the second exposure (which may be at a subtoxic level). It would be of value to be able to evaluate the available reserve capacity in a tissue or organ to resist the effects of the toxic exposure and to include this evaluation as one of the toxicity-influencing factors that are inherent in the subject.

EXTERNAL ENVIRONMENTAL FACTORS

In the introduction to this chapter it was pointed out that there are basically only three kinds of factors that influence biologic response—those related to the poison, those related to the exposure situation, and those related to the subject—and that for convenience, the subject-related factors would be further divided into those that are inherent, or a part of the subject, and those that are external to the subject but are a part of his environment. Since we have referred to the inherent factors as internal environmental factors, it is appropriate to refer to the latter group of factors as external environmental factors. The external environmental factors can be further subdivided in terms of whether they derive from the subject's chemical environment, physical environment, or social environment. It is evident that these external environmental factors are only capable of influencing toxic response insofar as they are able to produce some type of internal modification in the biologic test object and that elucidation of the mechanism whereby such effects are produced will, in fact, enable many of the external environmental factors to be reclassified in terms of the internal environmental system that they affect. However, since this kind of mechanistic information is not available for most of the external environmental factors, it is necessary for the present to consider these factors as a separate group.

Physical Environmental Factors

The three physical environmental factors whose effects have been investigated most extensively are temperature, pressure, and radiation. However, there are accumulating experimental data that indicate that other less-studied modalities such as magnetism, acceleration, vibration, gravity, etc., are also capable of influencing biologic response in both experimental animals and man.

Temperature. As mentioned previously, the concentration of a specific toxic agent or its metabolites at the biologic receptor is influenced by the processes of absorption, storage, metabolism, and elimination. Each of these processes is to some extent temperature-dependent, and it is not surprising that both increased and decreased environmental temperatures have been demonstrated to influence toxic responses in animals and in man. Furthermore, in most cases the biologic receptor consists of an enzyme or an enzyme system that can be predicted to exhibit variations that are dependent upon the surrounding temperature. The situation is often complicated, however, by the fact that many toxic agents directly affect the temperature-regulation processes and in so doing alter the response of the biologic system to either heat or cold. It is evident, therefore, that any investigation of the interrelationship between temperature and toxic response should include the study of the effects of the toxic agent on temperature regulation as well as the study of the effect of environmental temperature on drug response.

On the basis of the above observations, one might anticipate that in general the response of a biologic system to a toxic agent would be decreased with a decrease in environmental temperature, but that the duration of the response would be more likely to be prolonged as a result of cold exposure. There are many toxic agents whose affects are consistent with this hypothesis (temperature is directly correlated with the magnitude and inversely correlated with the duration of drug response), but there are also exceptions to both parts of this hypothesis. In one of the earliest attempts to relate drug response to body temperature it was observed that colchicine is more toxic to rats than to frogs. Since this difference in toxicity could be eliminated by increasing the temperature of the frogs, it was concluded that the toxic effects of colchicine resulted from a metabolite rather than from a direct result of the agent itself. The cardiac glycosides represent another class of drugs whose toxicity has long been recognized to be dependent upon environmental temperature. Digitalis, like colchicine, is more toxic to the rat than the frog. Here again, however, the difference in toxicity can be abolished by increasing the environmental temperature of the poikilotherm. In both of these situations the duration of the response is prolonged by cold exposure. In contrast to this situation, cold exposure potentiates the toxicity of strychnine, nicotine, atropine, and malathion. Although pentylenetetrazol (Metrazol) is frequently listed as a drug that is

relatively unaffected by hypothermia, other types of CNS stimulants have been found to be significantly more toxic in the hibernating ground squirrel. Even within a single category of drugs such as the organic phosphate insecticides, there are marked differences in the effect of cold exposure on toxicity. With parathion, a directly acting cholinesterase inhibitor, hyperthermia increases toxicity. However, the toxicity of sarin, another direct-acting cholinesterase inhibitor, is increased by hypothermia. Additional information on these and other effects of temperature can be found in reviews by Cremer and Bligh (1969), Doull (1972), and Weihe (1973).

Pressure Effects. Most of the current interest in the effects of increased and decreased barometric pressure on the toxicity of drugs and other chemical agents is related to the clinical uses of hyperbaric oxygen and to concerns about the efficacy and toxicity of drugs and other chemical agents in space medicine. It has long been recognized, however, that the effects of such agents as digitalis and ethanol are influenced by the altitude in which the tests are carried out. There is also a fairly extensive literature on the effect of increased environmental pressure on the response of divers and caisson workers to drugs and toxic agents. In virtually all of these studies the effects of the increased or decreased barometric pressure on the pharmacologic and toxic effects of the specific agent have been attributed to changes in the environmental oxygen tension, rather than to a direct pressure effect. However, it has recently been reported that morphine is less toxic to rats kept in an altitude chamber at reduced pressure but with an oxygen tension equivalent to that at ground level, and similar results have been obtained with chlorpromazine, amphetamine, and meperidine (Doull, 1972). Of particular interest in this respect are the experiments of Kylstra and associates (1967) in which abnormal muscular activity has been observed in mice with liquid-filled airspaces (animals breathing oxygenated saline or fluorocarbons), for which these workers have suggested a CNS origin. At the very least, severe pressure changes are likely to produce variable degrees of stress, which in turn can influence the toxic response. It is evident, therefore, that the investigation of the potential toxicity of a possible contaminant in a aerospace life-support system or in saturation diving or in some other undersea activity may require considerations of the interactions of pressure, the total gaseous environment, and the toxic agent under test.

It frequently becomes difficult to separate the effects of the physical environment on the toxic response from the effects of the toxic agent on the response of the biologic system to the physical factor. It has long been recognized, for example, that one can at least partially counteract both the pulmonary and some of the CNS toxicity of acute hyperbaric oxygen exposure by the administration of anesthetics or other CNS depressants. However, hyperbaric oxygen exposure has been shown to significantly shorten the sleeping time of barbiturate-treated mice, although these effects do not seem to be due to changes in the biotransformation of the drugs. One might anticipate from such studies that physicians would need to make some adjustment in drug dosage level when using intravenous barbiturates under conditions of either increased or decreased environmental oxygen tension, but such considerations have not proven to be a serious problem in most clinical hyperbaric oxygen facilities. It has, in fact, been possible to use almost all classes of drug with little or no modification of the usual dosage routines.

Hyperbaric oxygen exposure has also been used in the treatment of poisoning by carbon monoxide, cyanide, and barbiturates and has been recommended for use in the management of other types of acute poisoning. It has also proven to be a useful tool for enhancing the tumoricidal activity of radiation. Although the mechanisms responsible for these types of interactions are largely unknown at the present time, there is experimental data that support the hypothesis that free radical formation may provide a linkage between oxygen and radiation effects at the molecular level. Regardless of the mechanism involved there is no doubt that changes in barometric pressure and the associated changes in oxygen tension can influence the response of the biologic test system to toxic agents and that these effects need to be considered as a part of the total environmental influence on biologic response. For further information and references on oxygen toxicity, the reader may wish to consult the reviews by Bean (1965), Clark and Lambertsen (1971), and Doull (1972).

Radiation. Most of the experimental data that relate to interactions between radiation and toxic effects in the biologic test object have been obtained from programs designed to find chemical protectants against radiation injury or radiation sensitizers. There has been relatively little attempt to investigate the possible effects of ionizing radiations on the response of biologic systems to toxic agents and only a modest amount of research on the effect of ultraviolet and visible light on either the pharmacologic or toxic effects of drugs and chemical agents. However, since radiation exposure is known to affect blood tissue barriers, to modify enzyme systems, and to produce disturbances in the normal ex-cretory patterns of numerous species, including man, it is reasonable to expect that such exposure would be capable of influencing the distribution, metabolism, and excretion of at least some of the drug and toxic agent. It is also reasonable to assume that these effects by and large must be of relatively small magnitude since the radiation therapist is able to use most drugs and therapeutic agents at dosage levels and in treatment schedule that are identical to those employed in non-irradiated patients.

Most of the current interest in the effects of radiation on the pharmacologic and therapeutic response of biologic systems to drugs and chemical agents is related to the experimental mechanisms involved rather than to the practical clinical situation.

Whole-body radiation exposure has been shown to produce a dose-dependent decrease in the pseudocholinesterase activity of the ilia of both rats and mice, and there are some changes in the response of the irradiated rat intestine to drugs such as acetylcholine and physostigmine. However, there is no significant change in the acute toxicity of the cholinergic carbamate or organophosphate insecticides in animals given lethal exposures of whole-body ionizing radiation and there is also no apparent change in the antidotal efficacy of atropine in such animals (Doull, 1972).

During the period when released histamine was considered to be responsible for some of the toxic effects of radiation exposure, attempts were made to demonstrate changes in the response of irradiated animals to injected histamine; and it appeared, at least in certain strains of mice, that such differences could be demonstrated and that these changes could be antagonized by the use of antihistamines.

Another group of drugs where radiation exposure appears to produce a significant change in response is the CNS stimulants. The toxicity of both amphetamine and pentylenetetrazol is increased in irradiated animals, whereas that of pentobarbital, chloralose, and other CNS depressants is decreased. This decrease in toxicity can be produced by irradiation of the head only which suggests that the mechanism responsible for this effect is a faster entry into the brain and a region-specific sensitization phenomenon. There is, however, no change in the analgesic effect of agents such as morphine, codeine, methadon, or meperidine, and there is little significant change in either the toxicity or the analgesia produced by the antipyretic analgesics such as aspirin, aniline, aminopyrine, and antipyrine. Radiation exposure has been reported to potentiate the emetic effect of apomorphine, and it is of interest that this effect persists for several weeks after single whole-body x-ray exposure (Doull, 1972).

One explanation for the change in the response of irradiated animals to drugs is provided by the studies of DuBois (1967) and associates, who have demonstrated a dose-dependent, reversible inhibition of the microsomal enzyme system in the liver of young, irradiated animals. It is evident, therefore, that, in spite of the fact that the clinical experience relating to the use of drugs in irradiated patients is generally reassuring, there may well be some drugs and toxic agents that need to be used with caution.

Many of the effects that have been demonstrated with ionizing radiation could also be produced under the proper experimental conditions by ultraviolet radiation, although there is even less experimental data here than exists for the effects of ionizing radiation. A somewhat different type of response is that of erythema and liver necrosis produced with 8-methoxypsoralin in mice exposed to ultraviolet light. Diurnal variations have been detected in the acute toxicity of several compounds and, although most of these are probably related to hormonal factors, it is possible to alter some of these responses by changing the light-dark exposure cycles. Variations in the length of day have also been suggested as a cause of some of the seasonal variations that have been observed in the toxicity of some drugs and chemical agents (Paget, 1970).

Chemical Environmental Factors

Environmental chemicals are capable of influencing toxic response in a variety of ways. Some of those that are related to the formulation and administration of the specific toxic agent have been considered in earlier sections of this chapter. Reference has also been made previously to the ability of chemical agents in the environment to influence the biologic test system in such a way that its susceptibility to toxic agents is altered. Mention has been made, for example, of the ability of chemical agents to produce changes in the metabolism of a toxic agent by means of induction of the liver microsomal enzyme systems, and to this should be added the possibility that environmental chemical agents may alter the receptor for the toxic agent in the biologic test system or the absorption, distribution, and excretion of the toxic agent. Since this subject has been covered previously in Chapters 3 and 4, it will not be considered further here.

Social Environmental Factors

The manner in which an animal or biologic specimen responds to a toxic agent is influenced not only by the immediate exposure situation but also by certain historic considerations. The handling of the animal prior to the exposure situation, for example, can produce CNS effects in the animal that influence its response to toxic agents. In experiments with laboratory animals sensory input to brain, which can modify hormonal and peripheral nervous system output, is clearly altered by the way in which the animal is housed, that is, whether it is caged singly or in groups, the number of animals per group, the nature of the cage itself, solid versus mesh, the type of litter material in the cage, the manner in which food and water are provided, the noise level, and the activity pattern within the animal room. All of these are recognized as factors that can influence the outcome of toxicity testing procedures. (See Chapter 6 for additional information on the relationship between behavior and toxicity.)

REFERENCES

Albert, A.: *Selective Toxicity.* John Wiley & Sons, Inc., New York, 1960.

Balazs, T.: Measurement of acute toxicity. In Paget, G. E. (ed.): *Methods in Toxicology.* F. A. Davis Co., Philadelphia, 1970.

Bean, J. W.: Factors influencing clinical oxygen toxicity. *Ann. N. Y. Acad. Sci.,* **117**:145–55, 1965.

Beutler, E.: Drug induced hemolytic anemia. *Pharmacol. Rev.,* **21**:73–103, 1969.

Boyd, E. M.: *Predictive Toxicometrics.* Sci. Tech., Ltd., Bristol, 1972.

Burns, J. J.: Species differences in drug metabolism and toxicological implications. *Proc. Eur. Soc. Study Drug Tox.,* **11**:9–13, 1970.

Cafruny, E. J. (symposium chairman): Proceedings of an international symposium on comparative pharmacology. *Fed. Proc.,* **26**:963–1265, 1967.

Clark, J. M., and Lambertsen, C. J.: Pulmonary oxygen toxicity: a review. *Pharmacol. Rev.,* **23**:37–133, 1971.

Cremer, J. E., and Bligh, J.: Body-temperature and responses to drugs. *Br. Med. Bull.,* **25**:299–306, 1969.

Done, A. K.: Developmental pharmacology. *Clin. Pharmacol. Ther.,* **5**:432–79, 1964.

Doull, J.: The effect of physical environmental factors on drug response. Hayes, W. I. (ed.): *Essays in Toxicology.* Academic Press, Inc., New York, 1972.

DuBois, K. P.: Inhibition by radiation of the development of drug-detoxification enzymes. *Radiat. Res.,* **30**:342–50, 1967.

Goldstein, A.; Aronow, L.; and Kalman, S. M.: The time course of drug action. In *Principles of Drug Action,* 2nd ed. John Wiley & Sons, Inc., New York, 1974.

Hurst, E. W.: Sexual differences in the toxicity and therapeutic action of chemical substances. In Walpole, A. L., and Spinks, A. (eds.): *The Evaluation of Drug Toxicity.* Little, Brown & Co., Boston, 1958.

Kalow, W.: Heredity and the response to drugs. In *Pharmacogenetics.* W. B. Saunders Co., Philadelphia, 1962.

——: Dose-response relationships and genetic variation. *Ann. N. Y. Acad. Sci.,* **123**:212–18, 1965.

Koppanyi, T., and Avery, M. A.: Species differences and the clinical trial of new drugs: a review. *Clin. Pharmacol. Ther.,* **7**:250–70, 1966.

Kylstra, J. A.; Nantz, R.; Crowe, J.; Wagner, W.; and Saltzman, H. A.: Hydraulic compression of mice to 166 atmospheres. *Science*, **158**:793–94, 1967.

LaDu, B. N.: Altered drug response in hereditary disease. *Fed. Proc.*, **24**:1287–92, 1965.

Loomis, T. A.: *Essentials of Toxicology*, 2nd ed. Lea & Febiger, Philadelphia, 1974.

McLean, A. E. M., and McLean, E. K.: Diet and toxicity. *Br. Med. Bull.*, **25**:278–81, 1969.

Paget, G. E.: The design and interpretation of toxicity tests. In Paget, G. E. (ed.): *Methods in Toxicology*. F. A. Davis Co., Philadelphia, 1970.

Smith, R. L.: Species differences in the biliary excretion of drugs. *Proc. Eur. Soc. Study Drug Tox.*, **11**:19–32, 1970.

Weihe, W. H.: The effect of temperature on the action of drugs. *Annu. Rev. Pharmacol.*, **13**:409–25, 1973.

Chapter 6

CHEMICAL CARCINOGENS*

John H. Weisburger and Gary M. Williams

INTRODUCTION

Toxicology is the science that deals with the adverse effects and mechanism of action of chemical agents in animals and man. The production of cancer by chemicals is a very special aspect of an adverse toxicologic reaction. In many respects, carcinogenic agents are similar to other toxicologic and pharmacologic agents. For example, chemical carcinogens in a given experimental setting show dose-response relationships. Chemical carcinogens undergo biotransformation, as would any similarly structured pharmacologic agents. In addition, the response to chemical carcinogens varies with the species, strain, and sex of the experimental animal, as is the case with other pharmacologic agents. Chemical carcinogens interact with other environmental agents; their effect is sometimes enhanced and sometimes decreased, as occurs with other pharmacologic agents. Yet, there are some very important differences that make chemical carcinogenesis a specialized field of toxicology. Chemical carcinogens of the kind that we will describe as genotoxic differ from most other kinds of toxins in that (1) their biologic effect is persistent and delayed; (2) divided doses are in some cases more effective than an individual large dose; and (3) the underlying mechanisms, particularly in respect to interaction with host genetic elements and other macromolecules, are distinct.

Early Discoveries in Chemical Carcinogenesis

Historically, several types of chemicals were discovered to have carcinogenic potential in experimental systems after having first been suspected of causing cancer in man (Shimkin, in Schottenfeld, 1975; Sontag, 1979). Soot and coal tars were first suspected to be carcinogenic in the late eighteenth

* We are indebted to Ms. B. Meyer, Ms. N. Harris, Ms. T. Gelchie, Ms. G. Friedenberg, and Ms. I. Hoffmann for excellent assistance in preparing this chapter. The authors are supported through a Cancer Center Support (Core) Grant and a Biomedical Research Support Grant, CA-17613 and PR-05775, from the U.S. Public Health Service, DHEW.

century when Sir Percivall Pott observed that many of his patients who had cancer of the scrotum were chimney sweeps. In Great Britain where soft coal has been used for many centuries, it was customary to train young boys as chimney sweeps. Men of small stature were preferred to mechanically dislodge soot from the narrow chimneys. Exposure to soots, therefore, began at a young age. Subsequent research has indicated that individuals are more sensitive to carcinogens when exposure first occurs early in life. The first experimental documentation that coal tar could cause cancer in animals was produced by Yamagiwa and Ichikawa, who reported in 1916 that coal tar applied to the ear of rabbits yielded cancer at the point of application. In the 1920s the English school, directed by Kennaway, fractionated coal tar and discovered the carcinogenic potency of pure polynuclear aromatic hydrocarbons, such as dibenz(a,h)anthracene and benzo(a)pyrene.

The aromatic amines are another type of chemical carcinogen whose investigation also stems from the discovery of cancer, in humans exposed to them. In this instance, the German physician Rehn noted a cluster of cases of cancer of the urinary bladder among workers in the dye industry. The experimental evidence that the amines to which these workers were exposed could be carcinogenic did not appear until 1937 when Hueper and associates found that 2-naphthylamine could cause bladder cancer in dogs, reproducing the lesions seen in humans.

A third type, the carcinogenic azo dyes, has not been implicated in human cancer. The illustrious pharmacologist Ehrlich discovered that exposure to scarlet red led to a reversible proliferation of liver cells. It was not until 25 years later (1932–1934) that Kinosita and Yoshida independently discovered the carcinogenic effect of some azo dyes in rodents.

In the intervening years many other classes and types of chemicals were found to be carcinogenic (National Cancer Institute, 1975; International Agency for Research on Cancer, 1978). Some, such as vinyl chloride, were discovered after they were suspected of being involved in the development of cancer in man. Others, such as the polycyclic aromatic hydrocarbons, were discovered as a result of studies relating structure and activity in certain types of compounds. Some chemicals were found to be carcinogenic in the course of routine bioassays for the detection of adverse effects in chronic toxicity studies. This was the case with N-2-fluorenylacetamide and dimethylnitrosamine. Some chemicals were also discovered to be carcinogenic during investigations that attempted to reproduce in laboratory animals adverse effects that had been observed in man or domestic animals. A study dealing with the possible causative factors of amyotrophic lateral sclerosis prevalent on Pacific islands led to the finding that the plant product cycasin was a potent carcinogen. Other tests delving into the factor responsible for turkey x-disease, which accounted for extensive losses of livestock, pinpointed aflatoxin B_1 and, later, other mycotoxins as effective hepatotoxins and potent carcinogens. The powerful carcinogenicity of bis(chloromethyl)ether was observed first in the laboratory, and a few years later the effect was noted in individuals exposed occupationally.

DEFINITION OF CHEMICAL CARCINOGENS

Chemical carcinogens are defined operationally by their ability to induce tumors. Four types of response have generally been accepted as evidence of tumorigenicity: (1) an increased incidence of the tumor types occurring in controls; (2) the occurrence of tumors earlier than in controls; (3) the development of types of tumor not seen in controls; and (4) an increased multiplicity of tumors in individual animals. Although the term "carcinogen" literally means giving rise to carcinomas, i.e., epithelial malignancies, in general usage it also includes agents producing sarcomas of mesenchymal origin. Furthermore, even benign tumors are included as evidence of carcinogenicity, a practice justified by the fact that no real carcinogen producing exclusively benign tumors has yet been identified. Chemicals capable of eliciting one of these tumorigenic responses, and which are thereby classified as carcinogens, comprise a highly diverse collection of chemicals, including organic and inorganic chemicals, solid-state materials, hormones, and immunosuppressants. For some of these chemicals, such as tumor enhancers or promoters, the designation "carcinogen" is perhaps unfortunate, but inescapable, since these chemicals in specific situations do increase the yield of spontaneously occurring cancers. In order to draw attention to the differences in properties of the diverse agents that can be considered as carcinogens, we have developed a classification based on the mode of action of carcinogens. This classification is important not only for theoretic, fundamental reasons, but also because different types and classes of carcinogens require distinct regulatory actions to ensure safety.

MODE OF ACTION OF CHEMICAL CARCINOGENS

Attempts to elucidate the mechanism of action of chemical carcinogens have focused on their interactions with cellular macromolecules. Details on the nature of these interactions are covered in the section on Reactions of Carcinogens; so here only our current understanding of the significance of the different actions of carcinogens will be considered. Carcinogens interact with numerous tissue constituents and produce a number of effects. The paramount concern in this field is to identify the actions essential to the production of neoplasms.

The neoplastic state is heritable at the cellular level (i.e., the progency of the division of a neoplastic cell inherit the neoplastic potential), and thus theories on the mechanisms by which chemicals convert normal cells to malignant ones must ultimately explain how the effect becomes permanent. Investigators concerned with the interactions of carcinogens with proteins and RNA have postulated that effects on these macromolecules can eventually be rendered permanent

Table 6–1. CONSIDERATIONS INDICATING THAT DNA IS A CRITICAL TARGET FOR CARCINOGENS

1. Many carcinogens are or can be metabolized to electrophiles that react covalently with DNA. In these cases, this reaction can usually be detected by induction of DNA repair.
2. Many carcinogens are also mutagens.
3. Defects in DNA repair such as in xeroderma pigmentosum predispose to cancer development.
4. Several heritable or chromosomal abnormalities predispose to cancer development.
5. Initiated dormant tumor cells are persistent, consistent with a change in DNA.
6. Cancer is heritable at the cellular level and, therefore, may result from an alteration of DNA.
7. Most, if not all, cancers display chromosomal abnormalities.
8. Many cancers display aberrant gene expression.

through epigenetic mechanisms on gene expression creating a new stable state of differentiation (see Hiatt et al., 1977).

The important discovery that carcinogens interact with DNA provided a basis on which the permanent neoplastic state could be explained by a direct alteration in the genotype. A number of considerations support the view that DNA is a critical target of carcinogens (Table 6–1). At present, the mechanisms by which the direct interaction of a carcinogen with DNA could lead to malignant conversion are much better understood than those postulating a role for an indirect protein or RNA interaction (see Reactions of Chemical Carcinogens).

Theories on the mechanisms of action of chemical carcinogens have usually sought to provide a unifying account. The pioneering studies of the

Millers (in Hiatt *et al.*, 1977) that revealed that many classes of carcinogens could give rise to electrophilic reactants that interacted with cellular macromolecules have been developed into a major generalization that states that the ultimate carcinogenic forms of chemical carcinogens "usually, if not always, are electrophilic reactants" (Miller and Miller, in Searle, 1976). Those who favor epigenetic mechanisms of carcinogenesis visualize that such electrophilic reactants would react with protein or RNA to produce the changes involved, by quite indirect mechanisms, such as faulty differentiation. On the other hand, those who subscribe to genetic mechanisms of carcinogenesis regard the ability of carcinogens to interact with DNA as critical and have developed a further generalization that carcinogens are mutagens (Ames, in Hiatt *et al.*, 1977; Ames, in Asher and Zervos, 1978). These generalizations on the action of carcinogens, however, have not been demonstrated to apply to all chemical carcinogens.

As noted above, chemical carcinogens comprise an extremely diverse group of agents, and thus it would be truly remarkable if they all acted on cells in the same manner. In fact, there are a number of carcinogenic chemicals such as plastics, asbestos, and hormones that have not been documented to alter DNA or to be mutagenic and whose structure does not suggest an obvious reactive form (i.e., electrophilic reactant). Thus, it seems likely that more than one mode of action is involved in the overall carcinogenic effects of different chemicals. To facilitate consideration of this possibility, we have proposed a mechanistic classification of carcinogens that separates them into two major categories, genotoxic and epigenetic (Williams, 1979; in Butterworth, 1979).

Carcinogens that interact with and alter DNA would be classified as genotoxic. This category contains the "classic" organic carcinogens that are electrophilic reactants either in their parent form or after metabolism. As will be developed more fully in the section on Bioassay, carcinogens in this category can be identified by their genotoxic effects through *in vitro* short-term tests. It seems highly likely that DNA alteration is the basis for the carcinogenicity of these compounds.

The category of epigenetic carcinogens contains all classes of carcinogens for which no evidence of genotoxicity has been found. If further study confirms the lack of a DNA interaction for these chemicals, then obviously this would be excluded as their mechanism of action. Other possible mechanisms may involve chronic tissue injury, hormonal imbalance, immunologic effects, or promotional activity on cells that are either genetically altered or have been independently altered by genotoxic carcinogens. Less likely but also deserving consideration are epigenetic effects mediated through covalent interactions with protein or RNA, as discussed above, leading to faulty differentiation (Griffin and Shaw, 1979).

It is important to note that this proposal does not preclude that genotoxic carcinogens could also have epigenetic effects. Indeed, the potency of some carcinogens may reside in their genotoxic as well as promoting actions.

CLASSES OF CHEMICAL CARCINOGENS

The proposed mechanistic classification of "carcinogens" separates them into eight classes (Weisburger and Williams, 1980). These in turn can be divided into the two general categories genotoxic and epigenetic (Table 6–2).

The genotoxic category would contain the agents that function as electrophilic reactants, as originally postulated by the Millers (in Searle, 1976; Hiatt *et al.*, 1977). Also, because some inorganic chemicals have displayed such effects, we have tentatively placed them in this category. However, the studies of Loeb and colleagues (in Schrauzer, 1978) on effects of inorganic chemicals on the fidelity of DNA polymerases suggest that these might yield abnormal DNA by a mechanism distinct from the electrophilic genotoxic compounds.

The second broad category, designated as epigenetic carcinogens, would comprise those carcinogens for which no evidence of direct interaction with genetic material exists. This category contains solid-state carcinogens, hormones, immunosuppressants, cocarcinogens, and promoters.

This classification, if ultimately validated, has major implications for risk extrapolation to humans of data on experimental carcinogenesis. Genotoxic carcinogens, because of their effects on genetic material, pose a clear qualitative hazard to humans. These carcinogens are occasionally effective after a single exposure, act in a cumulative manner, and act together with other genotoxic carcinogens having the same organotropism. Thus, the level of human exposure acceptable for "no risk" to ensue needs to be evaluated most stringently in the light of existing data and relevant mechanisms. Often, with powerful carcinogens, zero exposure is the goal.

On the other hand, with some classes of epigenetic carcinogens, it is known that their carcinogenic effects occur only with high and sustained levels of exposure that lead to prolonged physiologic abnormalities, hormonal imbalances, or tissue injury. Consequently, the risk from exposure may be of a quantitative nature. This is almost certainly the case with estrogens,

Table 6–2. CLASSES OF CARCINOGENIC CHEMICALS

TYPE	MODE OF ACTION	EXAMPLE
A. Genotoxic		
1. Direct-acting or primary carcinogen	Electrophile, organic compound, genotoxic, interacts with DNA	Ethylene imine, bis(chloromethyl)ether
2. Procarcinogen or secondary carcinogen .	Requires conversion through metabolic activation by host or *in vitro* to type 1	Vinyl chloride, benzo(a)pyrene, 2-naphthylamine dimethylnitrosamine
3. Inorganic carcinogen	Not directly genotoxic, leads to changes in DNA by selective alteration in fidelity of DNA replication	Nickel, chromium
B. Epigenetic		
4. Solid-state carcinogen	Exact mechanism unknown; usually affects only mesenchymal cells and tissues; physical form vital	Polymer or metal foils, asbestos
5. Hormone	Usually not genotoxic; mainly alters endocrine system balance and differentiation; often acts as promoter	Estradiol, diethylstilbestrol
6. Immunosuppressor	Usually not genotoxic; mainly stimulates "virally induced," transplanted, or metastic neoplasms	Azathioprine, antilymphocytic serum
7. Cocarcinogen	Not genotoxic or carcinogenic, but enhances effect of type 1 or type 2 agent when given at the same time. May modify conversion of type 2 to type 1	Phorbol esters, pyrene, catechol, ethanol, *n*-dodecane, SO_2
8. Promoter	Not genotoxic or carcinogenic, but enhances effect of type 1 or type 2 agent when given subsequently	Phorbol esters, phenol, anthralin, bile acids, tryptophan metabolites, saccharin

which are carcinogenic at high, chronic exposure levels in animal studies, or otherwise every individual would develop cancer. Thus, with epigenetic carcinogens, it may be possible to establish a "safe" threshold of exposure, once their mechanism of action is elucidated.

The types of chemicals found in each of the eight major classes are reviewed in the following discussion.

1. Direct-Acting or Primary Carcinogens

Table 6–3 lists the classes of agents that are direct acting and gives a few typical examples for each type. It will be noted that inherent in the chemical structure of such agents is the property of chemical reactivity. Chemically such materials can be considered electrophilic reactants that can interact with nucleophilic reagents. The direct-acting carcinogens include strained lactones, like β-propriolactone, propane sulfone, and α,β-unsaturated larger-ring lactones, epoxides, imines,

nitrogen mustard derivatives, alkyl and other sulfate esters, and some active halogen derivatives, like bis(chloromethyl)ether (Van Duuren, in Homburger, 1976; Searle 1976; Hiatt *et al.*, 1977). Although one would expect such reactive chemicals to be carcinogenic under a variety of conditions, some agents like methyl methanesulfonate are not highly carcinogenic in animals, mainly because they undergo secondary hydrolytic decomposition, or their reactive groupings provide ready targets to more specific detoxification reactions. These reagents need to be further evaluated because some of them are more than idle laboratory curiosities and, as with dimethyl sulfate, have been reported to induce cancer in man when they were handled without adequate precautions (Druckrey *et al.*, 1966).

Halo Ethers and Other Active Halogen Compounds. Chemicals in which the halogen-carbon bond is chemically activated through electron transfer such

Table 6–3. EXAMPLES OF DIRECT-ACTING OR PRIMARY CARCINOGENS

Alkyl Imines Ethylene imine	H_2C—CH—R $\diagdown$ $\diagup$ N H
Alkylene Epoxides 1,2,3,4-Butadiene epoxide	H_2C—CH—CH—CH_2 $\diagdown O \diagup$ $\diagdown O \diagup$
Aryl Epoxides (+)-7β-8α-Dihydroxy-9^d,10a-epoxy- 7,8,9,10-tetrahydrobenzo(a)pyrene	
Small-Ring Lactones β-Propiolactone	H_2C—CH_2 $\mid$ $\mid$ O—C=O
Propane sulfone	CH_2—CH_2 $\mid$ $\diagdown$ CH_2—SO_2 O
Sulfate Esters Dimethyl sulfate Methyl methanesulfonate 1,4-Butanediol dimethanesulfonate (Myleran)	$CH_3OSO_2OCH_3$ $CH_3SO_2OCH_3$ $CH_3SO_2O(CH_2)_4OSO_2CH_3$
Mustards Bis(2-Chloroethyl)sulfide (mustard gas, Yperite)	$ClCH_2CH_2$ $\diagdown$ $\quad$ S $\diagup$ $ClCH_2CH_2$
Bis(2-Chloroethyl)amine (nor-nitrogen mustard; $R = H$ $\quad$ nitrogen mustard; $R = CH_3$)	$ClCH_2CH_2$ $\diagdown$ $\quad$ N—R $\diagup$ $ClCH_2CH_2$
Cytoxan (Endoxan)	$ClCH_2CH_2$ $\quad$ O $\quad$ N—CH_2 $\diagdown$ $\quad\parallel$ $\quad\quad\quad CH_2$ $\quad$ N—P $\diagup$ $\quad\quad\quad$ O—CH_2 $ClCH_2CH_2$
2-Naphthylamine mustard (Chlornaphazine)	$ClCH_2CH_2$ $\diagdown$ $\quad$ N $\diagup$ $ClCH_2CH_2$
Triethylenemelamine	H_2C—CH_2 $\diagdown$ $\diagup$ N H_2C $\diagdown$ $\quad$ $\diagup CH_2$ $\quad$ N $\quad$ N H_2C $\diagup$ $\quad$ $\diagdown CH_2$
Active Halogen Compounds Bis(chloromethyl)ether Ethylene bromide (or dibromide) Benzyl chloride Methyl iodide Dimethylcarbamyl chloride	$ClCH_2OCH_2Cl$ $BrCH_2CH_2Br$ $C_6H_5CH_2Cl$ CH_3I $(CH_3)_2NCOCl$

Table 6–3 *(continued)*

Nitrosamides and Nitrosoureas

N-Methylnitrosourea

$$CH_3\overset{\displaystyle |}{\underset{\displaystyle NO}{N}}\!-\!CONH_2 \longrightarrow CH_3^+$$

N-Methylnitrosourethan

$$CH_3\!-\!\overset{\displaystyle |}{\underset{\displaystyle NO}{N}}\!-\!COOC_2H_5 \longrightarrow CH_3^+$$

N-Methyl-N'-nitro-N-nitrosoguanidine

$$CH_3\!-\!\overset{\displaystyle |}{\underset{\displaystyle NO}{N}}\!-\!\overset{\displaystyle \parallel}{\underset{\displaystyle NH}{C}}NHNO_2 \longrightarrow CH_3^+$$

N-Methyl-N'-acetyl-N-nitrosourea

$$CH_3\!-\!\overset{\displaystyle |}{\underset{\displaystyle NO}{N}}\!-\!CONHCOCH_3 \longrightarrow CH_3^+$$

---

as certain halo ethers are extremely powerful alkylating agents and carcinogens. The most important example is bis(chloromethyl)ether, discovered first to be carcinogenic by Van Duuren, Laskin, and their associates in laboratory experiments (Van Duuren et al., in Homburger, 1976). It was subsequently found that this highly reactive alkylating agent, an important chemical intermediate in industry, has led to cancer of the upper respiratory tract in humans exposed to apparently low levels of this chemical (Pasternack et al., 1977). In animal models inhalation in as little as 0.1 ppm was carcinogenic (Nelson, in Saffiotti and Wagoner, 1976; Nelson, in Hiatt et al., 1977).

The higher homologs appear to be less active. Bis(chlorethyl)ether induces tumors of the liver and other organs in mice but appears to be inactive in the rat. Additional data need to be generated with these types of chemical carcinogens. Knowledge of the relevant mechanisms would be important, to distinguish halohydrocarbons which are not genotoxic and may operate via a mechanism of promotion and those which are genotoxic.

Halogenated benzopyranes and benzofurans are also suspected to be carcinogenic. The carcinogenicity of polychlorinated biphenyls (PCB) may stem, in part, from such contaminants (Allen and Norback, in Hiatt et al., 1977). A powerful carcinogen, considering the low dosages used, was 2,3,7,8-tetrachlorodibenzo-p-dioxin. Ingestion by rats of 2,200 parts per trillion or 0.1 μg/kg/day induced squamous cancer in the respiratory tract and in the oral cavity and liver cancer, the latter in females only (Kociba et al., 1978). More research in this area is required to secure solid data. The relevant mechanisms may depend on the formation of a carbonium ion stemming from the loss of chlorine from an activated carbon atom vicinal to the ether group as in bis(chloromethyl)ether. Those compounds are listed as direct acting, but more research is needed; there are some indications that they may be procarcinogens.

Ethylene dibromide and dibromochloro-propane are endowed with the properties typical of genotoxic direct-acting carcinogens by virtue of their activity as mutagens and also their property of inducing mainly forestomach cancers in mice or rats after oral administration (Olson et al., 1973). Tris or tris(2,3-dibromo-propane)phosphate, a textile flame retardant, is mutagenic and carcinogenic, likewise by mechanisms

to be established (McCann and Ames, in Hiatt et al., 1977; Van Duuren et al., 1978a). These chemicals, utilized extensively in chemical industry and in agricultural practice, can be classified as powerful carcinogens since they induce tumors quickly and in high yield. They also have systemic effects. Dibromo-chloro-propane led to atrophy in Leydig cells and sterility in the animal models, and through inadvertent exposure also in men.

Nitrosamides and Nitrosoureas. Agents such as N-methylnitrosourea, N-methylnitrosourethan, and N-methyl-N'-nitro-N-nitrosoguanidine (Table 6–3), unlike sulfate esters or mustards, for example, are chemically stable in the anhydrous state. However, under aqueous conditions they undergo hydrolytic decomposition, possibly modified by specific enzymes, to liberate an alkylating moiety. The carcinogenicity of these compounds is further discussed together with the nitrosamines to which they are structurally related.

2. Procarcinogens or Secondary Carcinogens

Direct-acting ultimate carcinogens also result from the biochemical metabolic activation of precursor compounds, often called parent, pre- or procarcinogens (Table 6–4). Most of the chemical carcinogens known fall into this type (Searle, 1976; Hiatt et al., 1977; Miller, 1978; Weisburger and Williams, 1979). Until about 1968 the large family of polycyclic aromatic hydrocarbons was thought to be direct acting, for this type includes very potent carcinogens, acting almost universally at the site of application in minute amounts (Searle, 1976; Arcos, 1978; Jones and Freudenthal, 1978). On the basis of studies to be described, however, it now seems that this class must undergo biochemical activation (Conney, Heidelberger, and Jerina, in Ts'o and DiPaolo, 1974; Sims and Grover, 1974). From the fact that the polycyclic aromatic hydrocarbons have such a broad spectrum of activity it can be deduced that the enzymic component provided by the host is fairly widely distributed in many species and target tissues.

The majority of other types of procarcinogens,

Table 6-4. EXAMPLES OF PROCARCINOGENS, OR SECONDARY CARCINOGENS

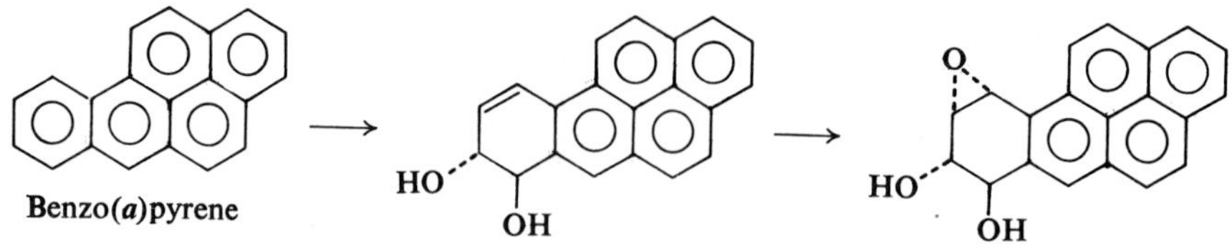

Benzo(*a*)pyrene

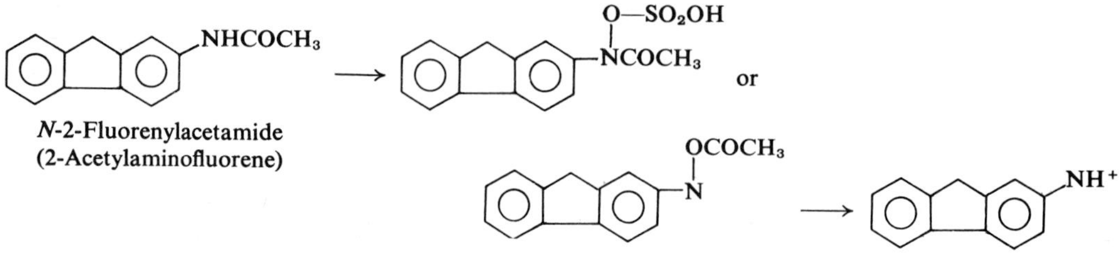

HO OH

HO OH

$NHCOCH_3$

O—SO_2OH
$NCOCH_3$ or

N-2-Fluorenylacetamide
(2-Acetylaminofluorene)

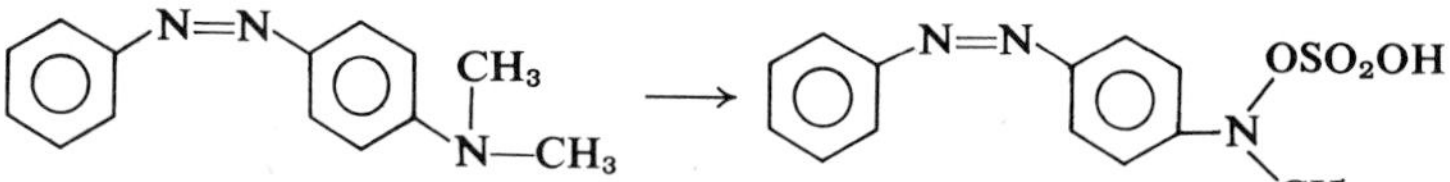

$OCOCH_3$
N

NH^+

N=N

CH_3
N—CH_3

4-Dimethylaminoazobenzene

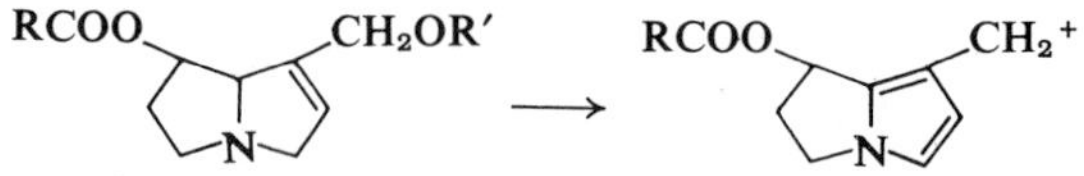

N=N

OSO_2OH
N
CH_3

$RCOO$ CH_2OR'

N

Senecio (or pyrrolizidine)
alkaloids

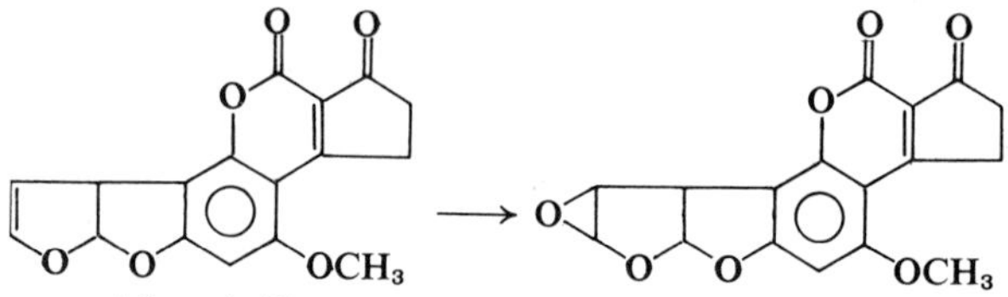

$RCOO$ CH_2^+

N

Aflatoxin B$_1$

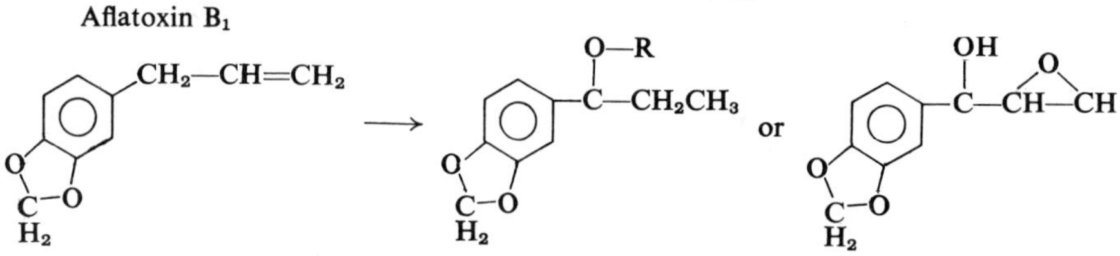

OCH_3

OCH_3

CH_2—CH=CH_2

O—R
C—CH_2CH_3 or

OH O
C—CH—CH

C
H_2

C
H_2

C
H_2

Safrole

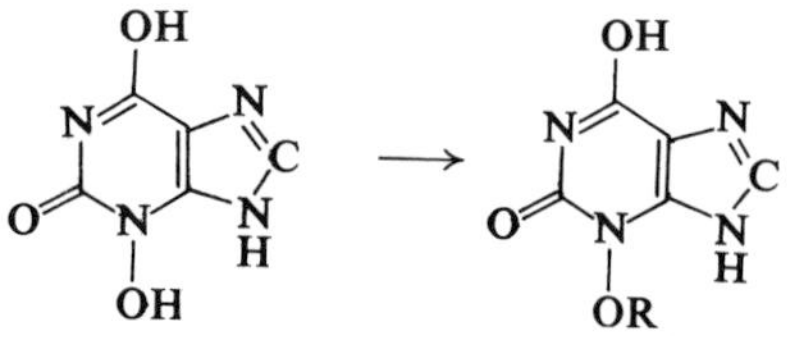

OH

N N
C
O N N
H
OH

3-Hydroxyxanthine

OH

N N
C
O N N
H
OR

CH_3NCH_3 $\longrightarrow$ $\left[CH_3NCH_2OH \right]$ $\longrightarrow$ CH_3^+
$|$ $|$
NO NO

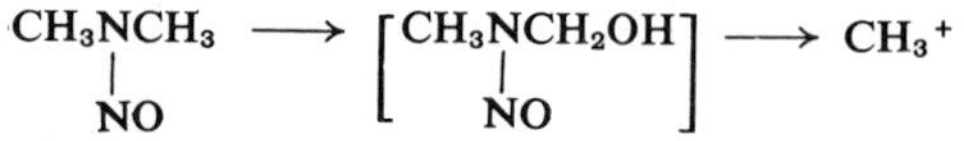

Dimethyl-
nitrosamine

Table 6–4   (*continued*)

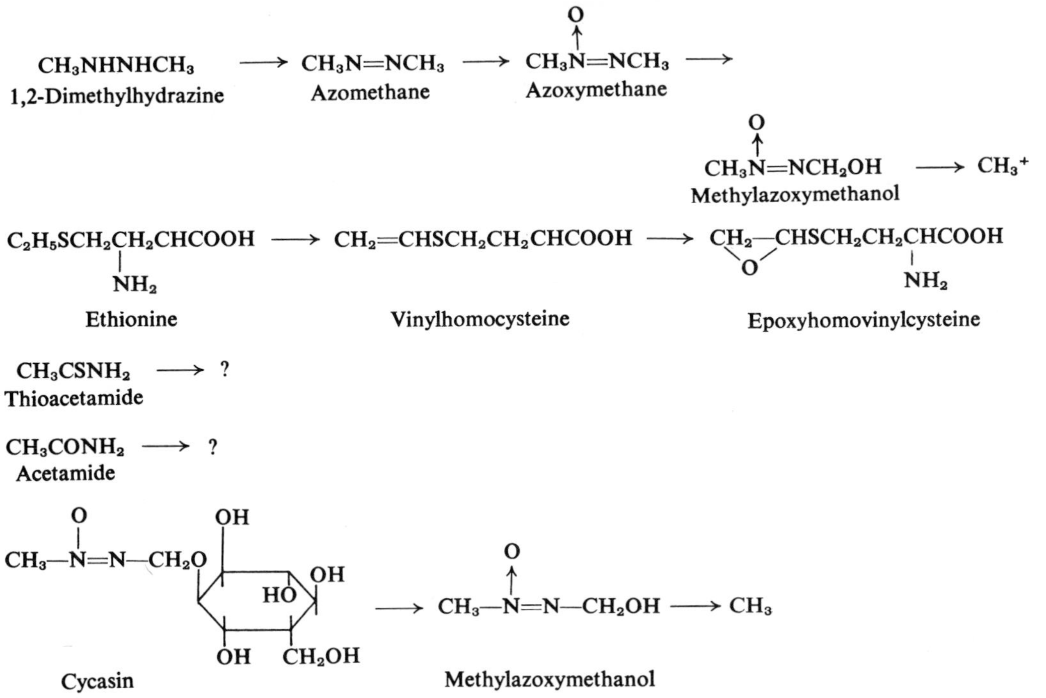

$$CH_3NHNHCH_3 \longrightarrow CH_3N{=}NCH_3 \longrightarrow CH_3\overset{\overset{O}{\uparrow}}{N}{=}NCH_3 \longrightarrow$$

1,2-Dimethylhydrazine   Azomethane   Azoxymethane

$$CH_3\overset{\overset{O}{\uparrow}}{N}{=}NCH_2OH \longrightarrow CH_3{}^+$$

Methylazoxymethanol

$$C_2H_5SCH_2CH_2\underset{\underset{NH_2}{|}}{C}HCOOH \longrightarrow CH_2{=}CHSCH_2CH_2CHCOOH \longrightarrow CH_2\underset{\diagdown O\diagup}{-}CHSCH_2CH_2\underset{\underset{NH_2}{|}}{C}HCOOH$$

Ethionine   Vinylhomocysteine   Epoxyhomovinylcysteine

$$CH_3CSNH_2 \longrightarrow \ ?$$

Thioacetamide

$$CH_3CONH_2 \longrightarrow \ ?$$

Acetamide

$$CH_3\overset{\overset{O}{|}}{-}N{=}N{-}CH_2O \ \ \longrightarrow CH_3\overset{\overset{O}{\uparrow}}{-}N{=}N{-}CH_2OH \longrightarrow CH_3$$

Cycasin   Methylazoxymethanol

---

however, were obviously in need of metabolic activation, for they produced tumors only under certain conditions at specific sites, and never at the point of application. Eventually, it was found that carcinogenesis in specific organs can be related in many instances either to specific enzymic activation processes in some types of cells or to the release of active intermediates from transport forms of the activated intermediate. Thus, the large class of procarcinogens includes types of chemicals such as the polynuclear aromatic hydrocarbons, certain aromatic amines, alkylnitrosamines and related compounds, mycotoxins such as aflatoxin B_1, pyrrolizidine alkaloids, plant toxins such as safrole, or cycasin, thioamides, and the antimetabolite ethionine.

Polycyclic or Heterocyclic Aromatic Hydrocarbons. This type contains some of the most extensively studied chemical carcinogens (Table 6–5). As noted above, there are historic reasons for such an emphasis. While a number of environmental products such as soot, coal, tar, tobacco smoke, petroleum, and cutting oils contain hydrocarbons, there is not yet any clear evidence that these products are carcinogenic to man and experimental animals because of their polycyclic aromatic hydrocarbon content. However, there is also no sound reason not to involve those carcinogens, for example, in lung cancer seen in cigarette smokers or tar-roofing workers (Wynder and Hecht, 1976). The initial investigators who applied hydrocarbon

to their own skin saw that local reaction and inflammation, such as are also seen in rodents, occurred rapidly. For this reason, the test was discontinued. Many rodent species are exquisitely sensitive to chemical carcinogens of this type (Arcos, 1978; Jones and Freudenthal, 1978). In mice, skin application of the more powerful agents such as 3-methylcholanthrene, 7,12-dimethylbenz(a)anthracene, and benzo(a)pyrene leads rather quickly to carcinoma formation. Subcutaneous injection produces sarcomas in rats or mice. Oral administration in sesame oil to 50-day-old female Sprague-Dawley rats results in the rapid induction of breast cancer, a model influenced by endocrine control as is the case in human females (Weisburger and Williams, 1979). However, administration of polycyclic aromatic hydrocarbons to rhesus monkeys and other primates has so far not been highly successful in yielding tumors. On the other hand, application of a crude petroleum oil to monkeys has induced cancer (Adamson *et al.*, 1972).

Within the large class of polycyclic hydrocarbons there have been many structure-activity studies. Data so generated have led to theoretic developments relating electronic structure of the chemical to carcinogenic activity. For detailed discussions of these aspects the reader is referred to reviews by Arcos (1978) and in Searle (1976). Suffice it to say that many of the results obtained can be interpreted in the light of contemporary concepts in terms of chemical structure and susceptibility to biochemical activation and detoxification.

Briefly, the situation can be summarized as follows. Many of the polycyclic aromatic hydrocarbons that

Table 6–5. EXAMPLES OF CARCINOGENIC POLYCYCLIC OR HETEROCYCLIC AROMATIC HYDROCARBONS

Bay region

L region

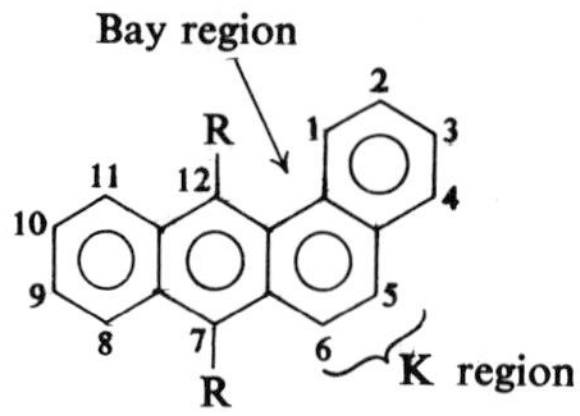

Benz[a]anthracene; R = H
7,12-Dimethylbenz[a]anthracene;
R = CH₃

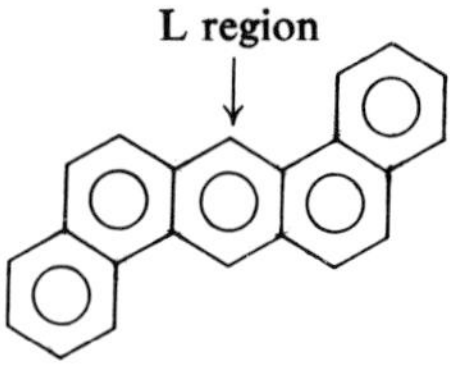

Dibenz[a,h]anthracene

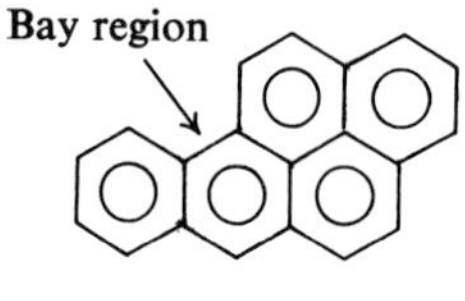

Bay region

H₃C—

Benzo[a]pyrene

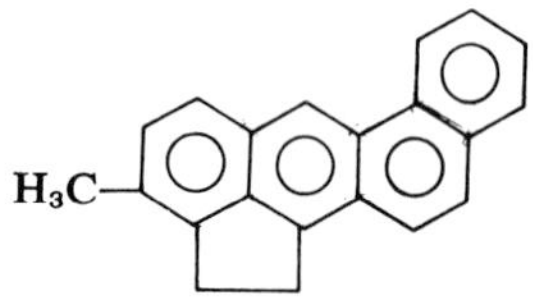

3-Methylcholanthrene

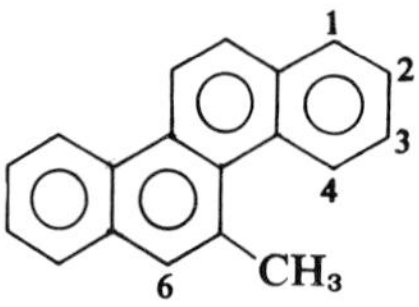

CH₃

5-Methylchrysene

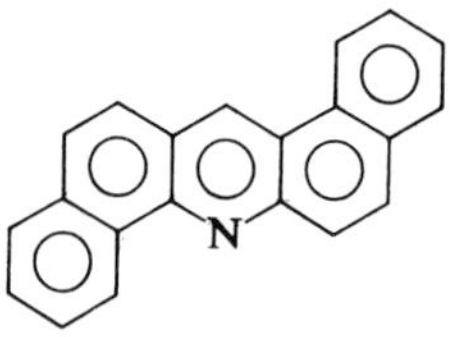

Dibenz[a,h]acridine

are carcinogenic are derived from a benz(a)anthracene skeleton. Anthracene itself is not carcinogenic, but benz(a)anthracene appears to have weak carcinogenicity. Addition of another benzene ring in select positions results in agents with powerful carcinogenicity such as dibenz(a,h)anthracene or benzo(a)pyrene, which are "natural" products resulting from incomplete combustion processes of carbonaceous materials. In addition, substitution of methyl groups on specific carbons of the ring also enhances carcinogenicity. Thus, 7,12-dimethylbenz(a)anthracene (DMBA) is one of the most powerful synthetic polycyclic aromatic hydrocarbon carcinogens known. Historically, on the basis of theoretic developments related to the electronic structure of these hydrocarbons, a certain area of the molecule, called the K region, was related specifically to the carcinogenic potential of a given compound (Pullman, in Ts'o and DiPaolo, 1974). On the other hand, substitution of another portion of the molecule, the L region such as the 7 and 12 carbons in benz(a)anthracene, increased carcinogenic potency; if these parts were free, there was a decrease. This simple scheme was a strong stimulus to research in structure-activity relationships for over 20 years. However, exceptions appeared with polycyclic aromatic hydrocarbons composed with fewer than or more than five rings and failed when chemicals with alkyl and in particular methyl substitution were involved. As noted above, because the

polycyclic hydrocarbons were powerful local carcinogens it was thought that they were direct acting. This was so, even though Boyland proposed as early as 1950 that an epoxide might be an active metabolite (Sims and Grover, 1974). In 1968, based on the fact that Gelboin, and also Sims, noted that DNA binding of isotope from a labeled polycyclic hydrocarbon was higher in the presence of a microsome fraction of liver, the view of investigators changed and extensive research on the reactive metabolites from polycyclic hydrocarbons began. It was already known with several other classes of carcinogens, especially the carcinogenic arylamines and nitrosamines, that metabolism led to reactive intermediates. It was Sims who first proposed the now prevalent and documented view that activation of polycyclic hydrocarbons was not likely to be on the K region, but rather stems from a two-step oxidation, with the eventual formation of a dihydrodiol epoxide. Several groups in Europe and North America have rounded out this picture. The organic chemist Jerina (1977) and the pharmacologist Conney developed the sequence of steps for several polycyclic hydrocarbons and called the reactive sites the Bay region. It would appear that thus far this activation process is broadly applicable to many polycyclic hydrocarbons, including methyl-substituted chemicals like 11-methylcyclopentenophenanthrene, 5-methylchrysene, and 7,12-dimethylbenz(a)anthracene (Jones and Freudenthal, 1978; Gelboin and Ts'o, 1978). It is possible that the metabolic conversion to other epoxides may also play a role and that there may be multiple active forms, especially with respect to distinct target organs. Nonetheless, the main active ultimate carcinogen most likely is in the form of a diol epoxide, and in fact in the form of one of the several possible stereoisomers (Buening et al., 1978; Gelboin and Ts'o, 1978; Griffin and Shaw, 1979; Coon et al., 1980).

This fact documents once more most strikingly that not all chemicals can cause cancer, that we do not live in a sea of nonspecific chemical carcinogens, but that the property of causing cancer is highly stereospecific and depends very strongly on the structure of the chemical and on the metabolic capability of the host to produce activated metabolites, counteracted by the ability to make protective detoxified metabolites.

As a result of the efforts of Lacassagne, Buu-Hoi, and others who synthesized and tested a number of polynuclear heterocyclic compounds, it has been found that some of them are quite carcinogenic, usually at the point of injection (Arcos, in Ts'o and DiPaolo, 1974; Schmeltz and Hoffmann, 1977; Sellakumar et al., 1977). Thus, despite the presence of hetero atoms in the molecules, they probably react by mechanisms similar to those of their homocyclic polynuclear aromatic hydrocarbons. Some of these materials have been found in natural products, in pyrolyzed proteins, and in tobacco smoke (Sugimura, in Hiatt et al., 1977) so that their study assumes increasing importance in understanding their mechanism of action and in attempting to reduce their effectiveness.

Aromatic Amines. The first reports relating the occurrence of bladder cancer in man exposed to aromatic amines labeled these cancers "aniline" cancers, for the workmen were exposed to a variety of aniline derivatives as intermediates in dyestuff manufacture (Eckardt, 1959; Scott, 1962; Schimkin, in Schottenfeld, 1975). In the intervening years, however, it has been found that 2,4,6-trimethylaniline produces liver tumors in rats (Table 6–6). Also, toluene-2,4-diamine was a carcinogen in rats.

Currently, tests suggest that a number of substituted anilines, particularly where the substitution is by an ortho-methyl group, may be carcinogenic. In a high-dose-level, long-term feeding test, even aniline itself has produced a low yield of subcutaneous sarcomas. The relevant mechanism has not yet been clarified, and at this time a statement of human risk is difficult to make on the basis of these results. The main reason for this qualification is that the monocyclic arylamines were carcinogenic only upon continuous intake of high dose levels, and at least with aniline, the type of lesion produces, namely subcutaneous sarcoma, is unusual and unexpected. On the other hand, ortho-toluidine and more so ortho-anisidine and para-cresidine also induced cancer in the urinary bladder, though only at high dose levels (National Cancer Institute bioassays, 1978; 1979). The significance of these results in relation to possible human exposure to these relatively simple compounds requires further research efforts.

It is noteworthy, however, that arylamines, when substituted in an *ortho* position by an electron donating methyl or certain halogens, appear to be more powerful than the unsubstituted compounds. As will be discussed below, certain polycyclic arylamines in which the amino group is in an alpha position to the adjoining ring are not usually carcinogenic because

Table 6–6. EXAMPLES OF CARCINOGENIC AROMATIC AMINES

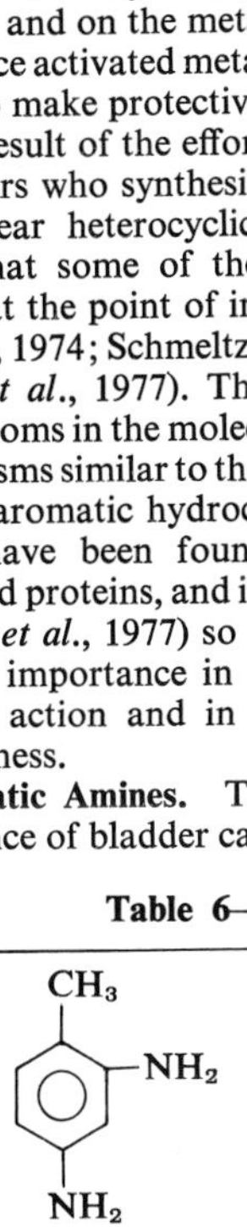

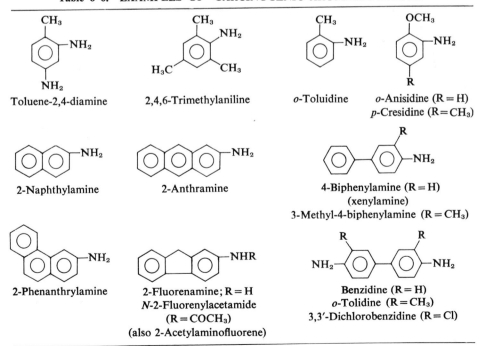

Toluene-2,4-diamine

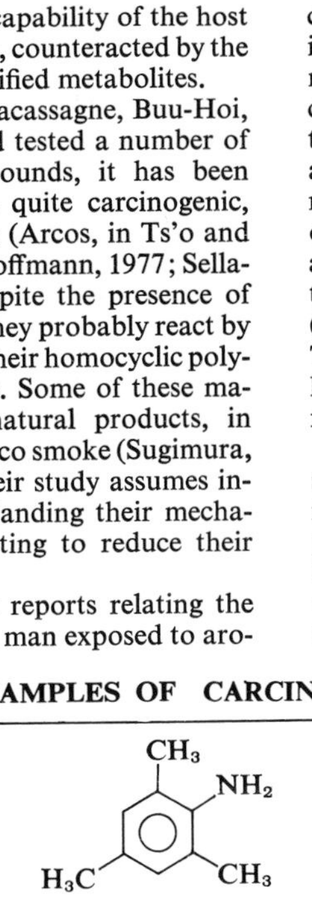

2,4,6-Trimethylaniline

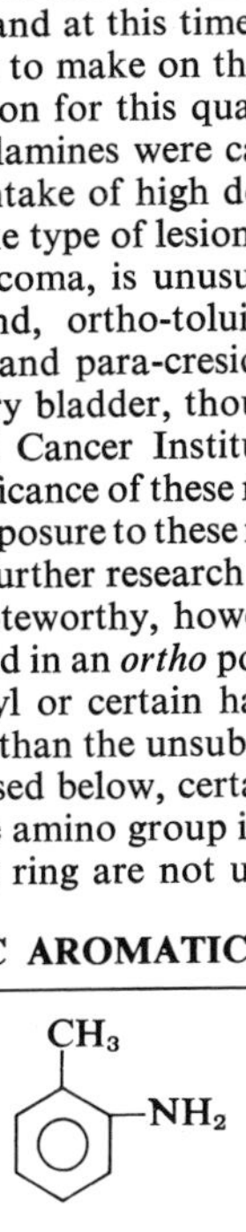

o-Toluidine

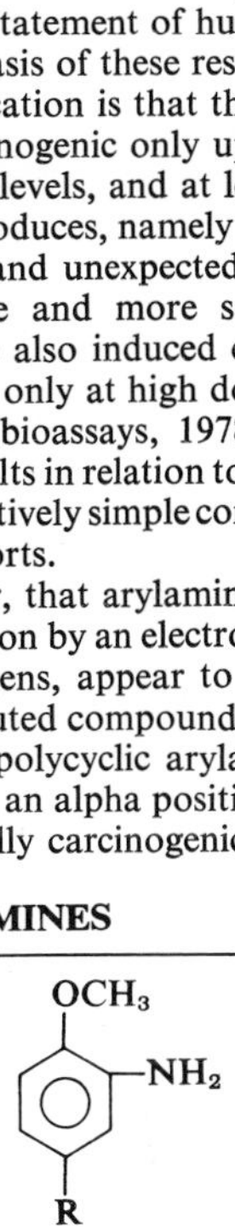

o-Anisidine (R = H)
p-Cresidine (R = CH₃)

2-Naphthylamine

2-Anthramine

4-Biphenylamine (R = H)
(xenylamine)
3-Methyl-4-biphenylamine (R = CH₃)

2-Phenanthrylamine

2-Fluorenamine; R = H
N-2-Fluorenylacetamide
(R = COCH₃)
(also 2-Acetylaminofluorene)

Benzidine (R = H)
o-Tolidine (R = CH₃)
3,3'-Dichlorobenzidine (R = Cl)

such compounds undergo the required N-hydroxylation only with difficulty, in contrast to arylamines with an amino group in other parts of the ring. However, it would appear that such inactive arylamines become weakly but definitively active if an orthomethyl group is inserted as, for example, 1-amino-2-methylanthraquinone. The reason is not yet understood, but may hinge on this substitution with methyl groups directing metabolic activation in a manner similar to that for larger polycyclic aromatic hydrocarbons. Thus, the active forms of such chemicals might be in the form of an epoxide, or a dihydrodiol epoxide. Current research will no doubt elucidate this question.

2-Naphthylamine has demonstrated carcinogenicity in several species, including man, rhesus monkey, dog, mouse, and hamster, but curiously not in rat (Clayson, 1962; Searle, 1976; Arcos, 1978). 1-Naphthylamine, an important industrial intermediate, has been thought to cause cancer in man, but animal experimentation has not substantiated the assertion that it is carcinogenic. Industries manufacturing 1-naphthylamine should make every effort to avoid the simultaneous presence of 2-naphthylamine as an impurity. Such manufacturing facilities also produce other possibly carcinogenic aromatic amines. Thus, it would seem that the suspected carcinogenicity of 1-naphthylamine in man may not in fact be due to this particular pure chemical entity but relate to carcinogenic impurities.

4-Aminobiphenyl (4-biphenylamine or xenylamine) is carcinogenic in man and in a number of laboratory animals. It is no longer manufactured in most countries because of this hazard. On the other hand, experimentation indicates that 2-biphenylamine is not carcinogenic. Among the higher homologs 4-aminoterphenyl is also carcinogenic, as would be expected.

Benzidine, an important industrial chemical intermediate, is carcinogenic in several animal species under a variety of conditions, as are substitute benzidines like o-tolidine, the ortho-dimethyl derivative, and also the 3,3'-dichloro compound. In the same class is methylenedianiline (or 4,4'-diaminodiphenylmethane) and derivatives (Stula et al., 1978).

Among the tricyclic arylamine derivatives a number of interesting structure-activity relationships have been found. 2-Aminofluorene (or 2-fluorenamine), a good but never-used experimental insecticide, and its acetyl derivative were discovered to be carcinogenic in most species in chronic toxicity studies (Weisburger, 1978).

Exceptions are the guinea pig and the steppe lemming. Tests in rhesus monkey are negative so far, but have perhaps been underway for an insufficient period (Adamson, 1972). There are no human data because extensive exposure of man has not occurred. The 1- and 3-isomers of fluoreneamine compounds are weakly if at all carcinogenic, and the 4-isomer does not seem to be carcinogenic in rodents.

In the anthracene and phenanthrene series similar observations are recorded. Thus, 1-anthramine and 1-phenanthrylamine are not carcinogenic, whereas the 2-isomers are highly active. 2-Anthramine, in addition to causing a variety of tumor types distant from the point of application, also induces skin cancers in rats on cutaneous application. Also, 2-phenanthreneamine is a good leukemogen and leads to a variety of other tumors in rats.

There have not been many tests of higher homologs. However, 6-aminochrysene, an α-substituted arylamine, appears to be carcinogenic to the liver when administered to newborn mice. Recent data show that it also induces skin tumors in mice after cutaneous application. This compound has been used in chemotherapy of splenomegaly secondary to malaria and also in chemotherapy of cancer in man, particularly breast cancer. Chronic feeding exposure in the rat gave no evidence of carcinogenicity. The reason for the activity of 6-aminochrysene in mice may be due to the fact that it behaves like a polycyclic hydrocarbon activated in the ring by the substituent amino group, rather than to the fact that it is an aromatic amine.

Many but not all carcinogenic aromatic amines administered to rodents cause cancer of the liver, or the urinary bladder especially in male animals. In females, breast cancer is often the usual result. Depending on the specific structure of the aryl moiety, lesions at a number of other target sites are seen (Clayson, in Searle, 1976; Arcos, 1978). For example, 4-aminostilbene usually leads to cancer of the external ear duct and 3-methyl-2-naphthylamine and 3-methyl-4-aminobiphenyl derivatives frequently cause intestinal, particularly colon, cancer (Weisburger, 1979). In the dog, and even in the hamster, these agents produce cancer in the urinary bladder (Deichmann and Lampe, 1967). The evidence thus far is that the urinary bladder is the site also affected in man exposed occupationally to certain of the carcinogenic aromatic amines.

Nitro derivatives of carcinogenic aromatic amines have also been found to lead to tumor formation. More information in this area is essential because certain of these nitro derivatives are still used extensively as industrial chemical intermediates. As will be discussed below, nitro compounds can be reduced fairly readily to hydroxylamino derivatives and thence to the amines. The enzymatic systems performing such reductions are less stereospecific than those for the biochemical hydroxylation of amines. Hence it may be that nitro derivatives would exhibit less stringent structure-activity relationships than the amines. In the few instances where this hypothesis was tested, arylhydroxylamines, except phenylhydroxylamine, have been found uniformly carcinogenic. For example, whereas 1-naphthylamine is inactive, 1-naphthylhydroxylamine is carcinogenic, in fact more so than the 2-isomer. Interestingly 1-nitronaphthalene has not been found active. Likewise in the fluorene series, N-acetyl-1-hydroxylamino- and 3-hydroxylaminofluorene are carcinogenic, whereas the corresponding amines are not.

One interesting carcinogen is 4-nitroquinoline N-oxide (Nagao and Sugimura, 1976) (Table 6–7). Investigation of the mechanism of action of this compound has proved most fruitful. Whereas early developments seemed to suggest that the nitro group was lost or could react with sulfhydryl groups, it now appears fairly certain that the required activation reaction is reduction to the corresponding 4-hydroxylaminoquinoline N-oxide. This latter compound can

Table 6–7. EXAMPLES OF CARCINOGENIC NITRO
AND OTHER HETEROCYCLIC COMPOUNDS

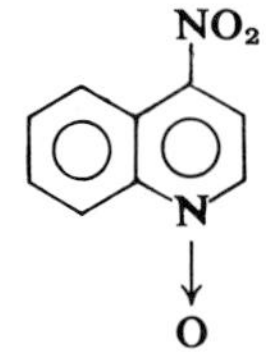

4-Nitroquinoline N-oxide

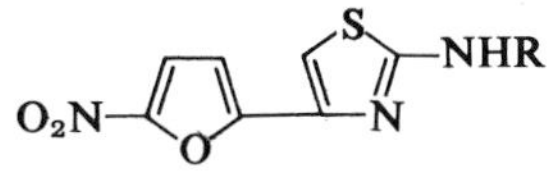

N-[4-(5-Nitro-2-furyl)-2-thiazolyl]-

formamide (R = —$\overset{\text{O}}{\overset{\|}{\text{CH}}}$)

N-[4-(5-Nitro-2-furyl)-2-thiazolyl]-
acetamide (R = —$\text{CH}_3\text{C}=\text{O}$)

N-[4-(5-Nitro-2-furyl)-2-thiazolyl]-
hydrazide (R = —$\text{NH}\overset{\text{}}{\underset{\|}{\text{CH}}}$)
$\overset{}{\underset{\text{O}}{}}$

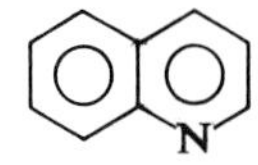

Quinoline

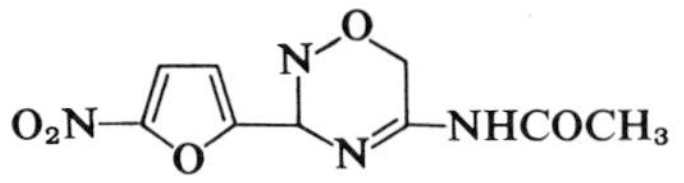

5-Acetamido-3-(5-nitro-2-furyl)-
6-H-1,2-4-oxadiazine

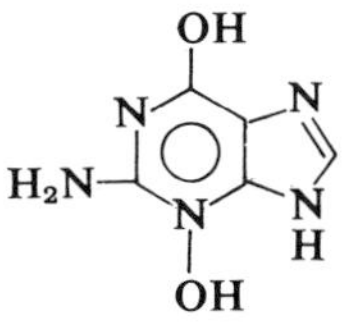

Guanine-3-oxide

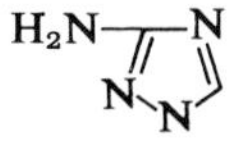

3-Amino-1,2,4-triazole

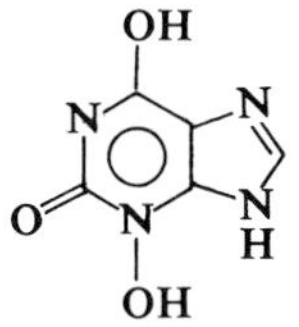

3-Hydroxyxanthine

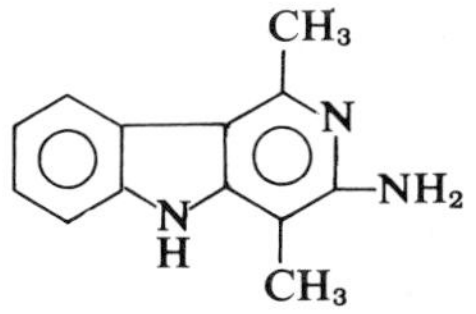

3-Amino-1,4-dimethyl-5H-
pyridol(4,3b)indole

induce pancreatic cancer, especially with azaserine. The corresponding amino derivative, or a compound lacking the N-oxide function, is not carcinogenic. 4-Nitroquinoline N-oxide is carcinogenic under many different conditions. It yields papillomas and carcinomas when painted on the skin of mice, especially if followed by a promoting agent like croton oil. When the compound is injected subcutaneously in rodents, sarcomas result. When it is given parenterally by intraperitoneal or intravenous injection, tumors are seen at a variety of sites, testifying to the potency of this agent and to the capability of many tissues to convert it to the active intermediate. The corresponding 4-nitropyridine-N-oxides require 3-alkyl substitution to be carcinogenic, implying a stabilized quinoid structure of an intermediate hydroxylamino compound as key reactant for neoplastic potential.

While 4-aminoquinoline-N-oxide appears not carcinogenic, it was recently found that quinoline itself does have carcinogenic properties, leading to hepatocellular cancer and hemangioendotheliomas in rats and mice, but not in hamsters and guinea pigs (Shinohara et al., 1977). Quinoline is not only an industrial product but is found in tobacco smoke. The relevance of the basic fraction of tobacco smoke, including quinoline, to cancer in man remains to be established (Schmeltz and Hoffmann, 1977).

Combustion products of gasoline-type hydrocarbons contain nitroolefins with some carcinogenic potential (Lampe and Deichmann, 1964). Further exploration of this area would seem rewarding.

Many nitrofuran derivatives have been synthesized since this particular structure has demonstrated practical use as drugs, particularly compounds with exquisite antibacterial activities used in agricultural practices as well as in medical applications such as against urinary tract infections.

A number of such compounds are very potent carcinogens for several distinct target organs, depending on the structure of the chemical and the test system (for general review, see Bryan, 1978). For example, nitrofuran derivatives are known to quickly induce cancer of the breast in rats, or cancer of the urinary bladder in several species. AF-2 or furylfur-amide was used as a food additive mainly in Japan until it was found to be highly mutagenic and carcinogenic (Sugimura and Matsushima, in Magee, 1976). As a rule, many 2-nitrofuran compounds are carcinogenic. Any such chemical requires detailed testing prior to widespread public use (Arcos, 1978). It seems probable that these chemicals are converted biochemically to the corresponding reactive hydroxyl-amino derivatives as carcinogenic intermediates.

Whereas the field of cancer research has led to many studies of structure-activity relationships among aromatic homocyclic compounds, there have been relatively few such investigations with the heterocyclic analogs even though these latter represent fundamental structures on which many important drugs are based. Very recently it has been found that such heterocyclic chemicals are found in "nature," as a result of the combustion or pyrolysis of protein-containing materials. The current status of this field indicates that many such chemicals are mutagenic. However, there is only preliminary information as to their carcinogenicity (Kawachi et al., 1979). Yet, this is a potentially important area, since the production of such chemicals as α- and β-carboline derivatives may account for the incidence of important cancers in man as a function of mode of cooking of foods, of pyrolysis during smoking of tobacco, and in general in relation to life-style (Weisburger, 1979).

One agent proposed for drug use in the United States and actually so used in Europe, 3-phenyl-5β-diethylaminoethyl-1,2,4-oxadiazole, was carcinogenic (Barron, 1963). Likewise, 3-aminotriazole, still used under some conditions in agriculture, definitely induces thyroid tumors in rodents. The mechanism appears to be due to interference with the synthesis of thyroxine and thus alteration in the pituitary-thyroid feedback system. There are additional reports, however, that 3-aminonitriazole can also cause liver tumors in mice and rats (Napalkov, in Truhaut, 1967). Certainly additional studies need to be conducted on the carcinogenicity of other heterocyclic amines, with emphasis on those to which man may be exposed.

Brown and associates discovered that 3-hydroxy-xanthine and N-oxide are oncogenic (in Nieburgs, 1978). When injected they yield sarcomas at the point of administration as well as effects at remote tissues. It appears that these materials are carcinogenic not because their incorporation into nucleic acids produces fraudulent macromolecules because antimetabolites that are incorporated into DNA have not been found to be carcinogenic so far. Instead, 3-hydroxy-xanthine and similar oncogenes are biochemically activated by mechanisms similar to those operating on the carcinogenic aromatic amines.

Azo Dyes. Just after the British school, led by

Kennaway, reported on the first successful induction of cancer in animals with pure polynuclear aromatic hydrocarbons, Yoshida (see Odashima et al., 1975) and Kinosita, working in separate laboratories, discovered in the early 1930s the carcinogenicity of some azo dye derivatives (Shimkin, in Schottenfield, 1975). Of interest was the fact that these compounds, 4-dimethylaminoazobenzene (formerly commonly called butter yellow because it was used in some countries to color butter and margarine) and o-aminoazotoluene, induced liver and bladder cancer after feeding (Table 6–8). In other words, the cancers were produced at a point remote from the site of introduction. Their action was quite different from that of the then-known carcinogenic hydrocarbons that induced cancer at the point of application. As a result of these discoveries many additional azo dyes were synthesized and examined for carcinogenic activity for the purpose of establishing structure-activity relationships, paralleling similar efforts with the polycyclic hydrocarbons. It was hoped that such studies would give insight into the specific mechanism of action, and indeed these pioneering studies did clarify a number of important points. One of the salient conclusions drawn from such studies was that not all agents belonging to a given class of chemicals were carcinogenic. In fact, very delicate alterations in structure modified the carcinogenic potential considerably. For instance, 4'-methyl-4-dimethylamino-azobenzene is carcinogenic but the 4'-ethyl analog is not. 4-Dimethylaminoazobenzene is the highly active standard carcinogen, but the 4-diethyl derivative is not. The reader is referred to specialized reviews for a detailed discussion of these structure-activity relationships (Searle, 1976; Arcos, 1978). It can be said, however, that some of the variations in activity as a function of structure stem from the susceptibility of the specific molecule to detoxification enzyme systems or, in reverse, to biochemical activation systems. However, not all of the data can be interpreted in terms of enzyme-mediated alterations of these molecules.

Most of the azo dyes studied are materials with one azo link. All other things being equal, they are usually not carcinogenic if they contain polar substituents like sulfonic acid residues. Thus, pure amaranth, with such a structure, is not carcinogenic. Of current use in commerce are some dyestuffs that have not yet been evaluated for chronic toxicity and possible carcinogenicity. These molecules contain polar groups and several azo links. Metabolic splitting of such compounds by reduction of the azo bonds has been shown to release the corresponding aromatic amines such as benzidine that are mutagenic and known carcinogens in animals and in man (see Hiatt et al., 1977). Since such dyestuffs can be metabolized not only by mammalian enzymes, but also even better by bacterial enzymes in the gut, exposure to them is potentially harmful. Thus, direct blue 6, black 38, and brown 95 have been active as rat liver carcinogens (NCI Bioassay Program, 1978; Thomas et al., 1978). With few exceptions, the carcinogenic azo dyes do not cause tumors at the point of injection. In rats, the usual end point is liver cancer, in mice, liver or urinary bladder tumors. A few of these agents studied in the hamster

Table 6-8. AZO DYES

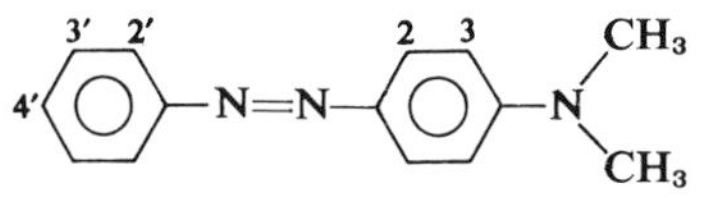

4-Dimethylaminoazobenzene
(N,N-Dimethylphenylazoaniline)
(many halogen, methyl, methoxy,
etc. derivatives)

Carcinogenic

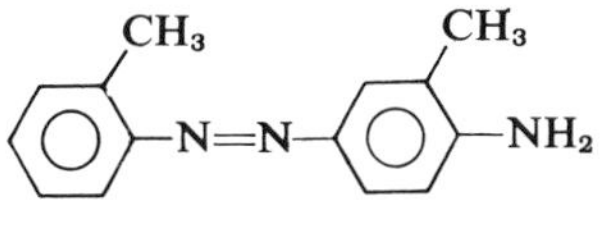

o-Aminoazotoluene

Carcinogenic

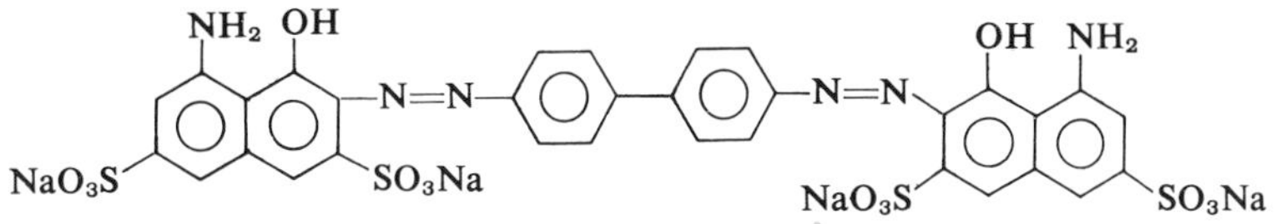

Direct blue 6

Carcinogenic

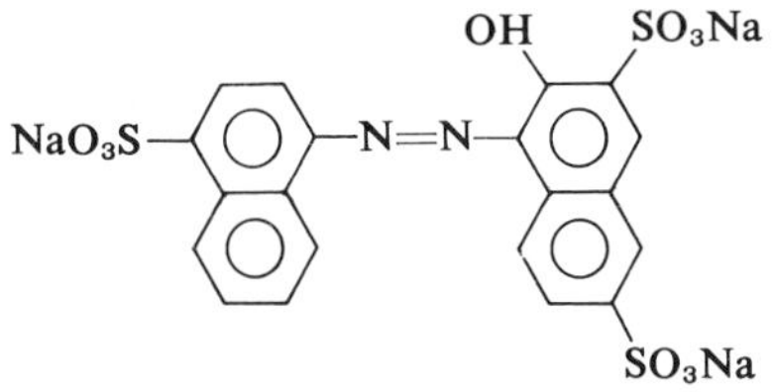

Amaranth
(FD + C Red No. 2)

Not carcinogenic

induced bladder tumors, an effect also seen in the dog (Saffiotti, in Deichman and Lampe, 1967). The carcinogenic azo dyes are valuable tools for the investigation of the mechanisms of carcinogenesis in model systems. Thus far, there is no known case of cancer in man that can be traced to exposure to such dyes.

Nitrosamines and Nitrosamides. This major class of important chemical carcinogens was discovered only in the last 25 years. While attempting to discover the cause of jaundice and liver damage seen in workmen exposed to a number of products, including dimethylnitrosamine, Barnes and Magee (see Magee *et al.*, in Searle, 1976) found that this agent was highly hepatotoxic in rodents and that it reproduced the lesions seen in man. Subsequently, they discovered that this agent was among the most carcinogenic materials then known. As was the case with other types of chemical carcinogens, this discovery led to an intensive effort to establish structure-activity relationships. The group headed by Druckrey (see Preussmann, 1977; Magee *et al.*, in Searle, 1976; Eisenbrand *et al.*, in Odashima *et al.*, 1975) studied over 100 alkyl or alkylarylnitrosamines, amides, and ureas (Table 6-9). Whereas with the carcinogens discussed thus far there were rather severe structure-related limitations, i.e., relatively few in a given class of agents were actually carcinogenic, in the nitrosamine series just the opposite appeared to be the case.

Many alkyl or alkylarylnitrosamines are carcinogenic. In rodents, the symmetric dialkyl compounds under some conditions exhibit delicate and yet specific organotropism; i.e., they preferentially cause cancer in a given organ. For example, dimethyl- and diethylnitrosamine usually cause liver cancer in rats while the dibutyl derivative causes cancer of the urinary bladder, and the diamyl compound causes cancer of the lung in rats. The dose rate also plays a role. Dimethylnitrosamine administered to rats in relatively low doses for a long time leads to cancer of the liver whereas a few or indeed a single large dose results in renal carcinomas. Asymmetric nitrosamines, especially those with at least one methyl group, often result in cancer of the esophagus, as do some nitrosamines based on cyclic secondary amines. In hamsters, on the other hand, diethylnitrosamine also causes cancer in the respiratory tract, and diketopropylnitrosamine or 2,6-dimethylnitrosomorpholine in the ductal pancreas.

The antibiotic streptozotocin, a drug used mainly in cancer chemotherapy, has the structure of an N-methylnitrosamine. As expected, this drug is carcinogenic, interestingly to the pancreas islet cells. It is also diabetogenic, unless nicotinamide is administered at the same time.

Similar in structure and probable mechanism of action are the alkyl and dialkylaryltriazeno deriva-

Table 6–9. CARCINOGENIC NITROSAMINES AND KEY ORGANS AFFECTED IN RODENTS

Compound	Structure	Organs affected
Dimethylnitrosamine	CH_3 / CH_3 $>$N—NO	Liver, kidneys, lungs
Diethylnitrosamine	CH_3CH_2 / CH_3CH_2 $>$N—NO	Liver, lungs, esophagus
Dibutylnitrosamine	$CH_3CH_2CH_2CH_2$ / $CH_3CH_2CH_2CH_2$ $>$N—NO	Bladder, liver, lungs
Diketopropylnitrosamine	CH_3COCH_2 / CH_3COCH_2 $>$N—NO	Ductal pancreas (hamster) Liver, lung, (rat, mouse)
Methylamylnitrosamine	CH_3 / $CH_3CH_2CH_2CH_2CH_2$ $>$N—NO	Esophagus, liver
Methylphenylnitrosamine (Methylnitrosoaniline)	CH_3 / C_6H_5 $>$N—NO	Esophagus
Nitrosopiperidine	CH_2 $\begin{smallmatrix}CH_2CH_2\\ CH_2CH_2\end{smallmatrix}$ N—NO	Esophagus, liver, nasal sinuses
N'-Nitrosonornicotine	(structure) N—NO	Esophagus, respiratory tract
Streptozotocin [2-Deoxy-2-(3-methyl-3-nitrosoureido)D-glucopyranose	CH_2OH ... $HNCONCH_3$, NO	Pancreas islet cells

tives. These materials, some of which are industrial products, have interesting carcinogenic properties.

Hoffmann *et al.* (see Schmeltz and Hoffmann, 1977; Hecht *et al.*, 1979) discovered that several nitrosamines derived from alkaloids like nicotine, in particular nitrosonornicotine, are found in tobacco. The mechanism of their formation seems to rest on a possibly bacterially mediated nitrosation of nicotine during the curing process. These and related nitrosamines are found also in tobacco smoke. In rats they cause mainly cancer of the esophagus, in hamsters cancer of the upper respiratory tract. The contribution of these chemicals to carcinogenesis in man smoking cigarettes or chewing tobacco products is not yet known. Individuals who smoke and drink alcoholic beverages have a high risk of cancer of the oral cavity and esophagus (Wynder and Gori, 1975). The relevant mechanism may be an induction by alcohol of enzymes capable of metabolizing nitrosamines like nitrosonornicotine, or polycyclic aromatic hydrocarbons found in smoke, in the target tissues.

Nitrosamines as a class are converted to active electrophilic reactants through oxidation (Magee *et al.*, in Searle, 1976; Preussmann, 1975; Arcos *et al.*, in Gelboin and Ts'o, 1978; Egan, 1978; Walker *et al.*, 1978). With the prototype dimethylnitrosamine, an active intermediate has been thought to be the unstable hydroxymethyl compound, which is converted to a methyl carbonium ion. The effect of hexamethylphosphoramide may be based on similar properties (Ashby *et al.*, 1978). Cyclic nitrosamines can conceptually be metabolized by hydroxylation alpha or beta to the N-nitroso function. Recent developments demonstrate that the key activation reaction appears to be alpha-hydroxylation (Hecht *et al.*, 1979).

Because biochemical activation of these compounds appears to take place in all species so far studied, these compounds are among the most dangerous carcinogens known. Whereas even the highly potent polycyclic hydrocarbons, like 3-methylcholanthrene, have so far failed to reliably cause cancer in monkeys, it was found that a number of nitrosamine derivatives led to cancer relatively rapidly in rhesus monkeys. For example, diethylnitrosamine has induced liver cancer in less than two years and in more recent experiments in less than one year (Adamson, 1972). There are species differences in relation to the tissue primarily affected. Diethylnitrosamine leads chiefly to liver cancer in rats or mice, but in the hamster, lung cancer is the main lesion although liver tumors also result.

Diphenylnitrosamine itself is not carcinogenic. The structural requirement for carcinogenicity is that at least one alkyl group capable of metabolism be attached to the nitrosamine. If the alkyl group is bulky, for example, a tertiary butyl group, and oxidizes metabolically with difficulty, the nitrosamine is unlikely to be carcinogenic.

The question now arises as to whether these versatile carcinogens contribute to the occurrence of cancer in man. The medical literature includes several case reports of individuals with acute intoxication by certain nitrosamines, mostly dimethylnitrosamine, an industrial intermediate to the point of overt hepatotoxicity. Yet, even though certain of these cases date to 1937, there is no reliable information that any of these individuals ever developed cancer due to this exposure. Nonetheless, as we have discussed, the properties especially of the smaller dialkylnitrosamines like dimethyl- or diethylnitrosamine categorize them as very powerful, versatile carcinogens in animals. Thus, it is important to minimize human exposure. However, in the last 20 years the chemical analytic technology has progressed enormously. Highly sensitive and specific techniques such as those utilizing the termal electron analyzer permit the reliable determination in the environment of nitrosamines at the parts-per-billion and even parts-per-trillion level (Egan, 1978). On the other hand, it requires continuing exposure to alkylnitrosamines at the level of parts per million or infrequent exposure to amounts of parts per thousand to induce cancer in animals. For this reason the biologic significance of concentrations of parts per billion or lower is obscure, yet these are the amounts present, for example, in certain foodstuffs, like bacon (Tinbergen and Krol, 1977). In fact, it is quite likely that larger amounts of such carcinogens were present in the food chain in previous years or decades, before the potential hazards due to such chemicals were known. It is sound policy to exert every responsible effort to lower exposure of people to these chemicals without, however, unnecessary alarming the public at large to cancer risks that may in reality be quite minimal, compared to other much larger risks.

Nitrosation of alkylureas, alkylamides, and esters produces some of the most remarkable carcinogens known (Table 6–10). Because many of these agents, chemically quite stable in the anhydrous state, do not require specific enzymic activation but spontaneously release an active intermediate in the presence of aqueous, preferably alkaline, systems, such materials are carcinogenic in virtually all living systems, even under *in vitro* conditions (Druckrey, in Odashima *et al.*, 1975; Preussmann, 1975; Magee *et al.*, in Searle, 1976). Certain of these materials were actually used commercially in industry and in chemical laboratories because of their ability to be hydrolyzed by alkali and yield reactive intermediates. For example, methylnitrosourea was the classic reagent for the laboratory preparation of diazomethane, itself utilized to esterify carboxylic acids, phenols, and the like. Since their potential hazard was demonstrated, these chemicals have not been used for this purpose. Instead methylnitrosotoluenesulfonamide, which is not carcinogenic, is utilized. However, diazomethane itself is a highly carcinogenic chemical, yielding tumors in the respiratory tract, especially the lung, in rats and mice. Thus, where this and similar chemicals are em-

Table 6–10. CARCINOGENIC NITROSAMIDES
AND UREAS, AND ARYL TRIAZENO
COMPOUNDS

N-Methylnitrosourea (R = O; R' = H; N'-acetyl, R' = COCH₃) N-Methyl-N'-nitro-N-nitrosoguanidine (MNNG) (R = NH; R' = NO₂)	$CH_3-N-CRNHR'$ $\quad\quad\; |$ $\quad\quad\; NO$
N-Methylnitrosourethan	$CH_3-N-COOC_2H_5$ $\quad\quad\; |$ $\quad\quad\; NO$
1-Phenyl-3,3-dimethyltriazene	
4-(3,3-Dimethyl-1-triazeno) imidazole-5-carboxamide	

ployed, extreme care and adequate facilities (hoods) are a must.

Given by oral administration, alkylnitrosoureas, alkylnitrosourethan, and the closely related N-methyl-N'-nitro-N'-nitrosoguanidine, nitrosobiuret, and N-methyl-N-nitroso-N'-acetylurea produced tumors in the gasrointestinal tract (Druckrey, in Odashima *et al.*, 1975; Sugimura, in Busch, Vol. 8, 1973). In fact, the latter three compounds are the chemicals of choice to induce cancer of the glandular stomach, a frequent lesion in humans in countries such as Japan, parts of Latin America, Iceland, Scandinavia, and certain other countries of Europe (Weisburger, 1979). Until these reagents were discovered, it was very difficult to induce cancer of the glandular stomach for model studies mimicking accurately the lesion seen in man.

It has been demonstrated that the treatment of certain foods, especially fish or beans frequently eaten in areas where stomach cancer is high, with nitrite, yields mutagenic activity, which recently has been shown to induce also cancer of the glandular stomach in rats. In addition, similar interaction between nitrite and primary amines like spermidine also yielded reactive intermediates, as assayed by mutagenic properties. While some of these interactions do correspond to the epidemiologic data on the incidence of gastric cancer, this association requires further research. Other foods eaten in areas such as China, at high risk for cancer in the upper respiratory and the upper gastrointestinal tract, also have been shown to contain specific nitrosamines (Higginson, 1977; Kraybill and Mehlman, 1977; Walker *et al.*, 1978). This association is also suggestive, but more specific relevant data need to be established. This entire area deserves more intense exploration, since, if validated, a relationship between nitrite, nitrosamines, nitrosamides, and specific human cancers prevelant in diverse parts of the world will have been demonstrated (Leonard, 1978).

It is important to note that these nitrosation reactions can be inhibited by preferential competitive neutralization of nitrite with naturally occurring and synthetic materials like vitamin C, vitamin E, sulfamate, and certain antioxidants like BHT, BHA, gallic acid, and the like. These reactions have been put to practical use. Thus, certain meats preserved with nitrite are at the same time treated with ascorbate or erythrobate, which has served to lower appreciably the amount of detectable dimethylnitrosamine, nitrosopyrrolidine, and other nitrosamines in the treated meats (Tinbergen and Krol, 1977). In addition, this interaction has been noted to bear on the considerable lowering of the incidence of stomach cancer in the United States during the last 40 years, and in the reduced risk of stomach cancer in migrant populations from countries where this type of cancer is still high to the United States (Weisburger, 1979). This neutralization of nitrite by vitamin C is being used also in certain pharmaceutic preparations with a potential nitrosatable substituent, by formulating such drugs with vitamin C or vitamin E.

Upon parenteral, especially intravenous, injection, some of the alkylnitrosoureas, particularly the ethyl derivative, yield tumors of the brain (Druckrey, in

Odashima *et al.*, 1975). Related alkylnitrosoureas provide unique means of specifically inducing neurogenic tumors and related lesions. Again, such tumors were difficult to produce, and indeed there was no really reliable means of doing so until these agents were discovered. Some are also active transplacentally yielding a high incidence of cancer in the offspring after a single dose to a pregnant female given at the proper time (Rajewsky, in Hiatt *et al.*, 1977). The question can be asked whether the relatively rare cancers of the brain and nervous system stem from a similar transplacental effect with as-yet-unknown intermediates.

The specific organotropic effect of this class of powerful carcinogens is as yet poorly understood. For example, Odashima *et al.* (1975) discovered that N-butylnitrosourea causes leukemia in several species, mainly of the granulocytic type as seen in humans.

As was discussed, many types of nitrosamines, symmetric and asymmetric, dialkyl and alkylarylnitrosamines, and the related nitrosoureas, nitroso esters, and triazene derivatives are highly potent, versatile chemical carcinogens. Because of their ease of transformation to the active ultimate carcinogen in many species, such materials are among the most potentially dangerous. Since the discovery of the carcinogenicity of the prototype dimethylnitrosamine consequent to an adverse effect in man, there have been numerous studies of diverse nitrosamines synthesized in the laboratory. The determination of their possible carcinogenicity has led to considerable advances in finding tools for the induction of specific types of cancer in high yield in animal model systems.

Nitrosamines and related materials can be synthesized very readily in the laboratory by reaction of nitrous acid with the corresponding secondary amine. The question arose as to whether such a synthesis could also take place in biologic systems, including man. The first attempt along these lines involving diethylamine and nitrite administered to rats gave no indication that such a combination took place *in vivo*. However, Sander (in Odashima *et al.*, 1975) made the important discovery that the less strongly basic amines were readily converted to nitrosamines under physiologic conditions prevailing in the stomach of experimental animals, and subsequently others not only provided sound evidence that nitrosamines, nitrosoureas, and similar hazardous materials were formed by chemical synthesis, but, more important, demonstrated that the administration of nitrite and the appropriate amine yielded almost the same toxic and carcinogenic effect as the corresponding nitrosamine derivative. Thus, it was discovered by combined chemical and bioassay techniques that the less basic amines, ureas, or esters are subject to nitrosation and gave rise to cancer in experimental systems.

In most areas, nitrite is utilized as a deliberate or an adventitious food additive. Nitrate is ubiquitous in the environment and is also used as a component of food preservatives. Under some conditions, nitrate is reduced to nitrite, particularly by microbiologic systems. This reduction is likely to occur in leftover food stored at room temperature, a relatively common occurrence in less-advanced countries where household refrigerators are uncommon (Weisburger,

1979). The reduction also occurs readily mediated by oral bacterial flora, in the mouth of individuals having eaten foods, especially plants, high in nitrate (Tannenbaum, in Hiatt et al., 1977). Secondary amines and similar nitrosatable substrates likewise are widespread in the environment and they also arise by digestive processes. Sander (loc. cit.) noted that nitrosation of specific secondary amines occurred most readily within the human stomach at a pH of 3 to 5.

More recent developments indicate that tertiary and quaternary amines, and in particular dimethylamino derivatives, can react with nitrite under similar conditions releasing dimethylnitrosamine (Lijinsky, in Tinbergen and Krol, 1977). Many drugs have a structure such that they could undergo such reactions, and this remains to be explored in regard to the etiology of human cancer. In such an evaluation, the organotropism of dimethylnitrosamine needs to be kept in mind; in every animal species so far tested it has yielded either liver or kidney cancer after oral intake.

Symmetric Dialkylhydrazines. Laqueur (in Odashima et al., 1975; in Kraybill and Mehlman, 1977), while studying the possible relationship of flour made from the cycad nut to a neurotoxic syndrome seen on some Pacific islands, discovered that this flour led to a variety of cancers in the liver, kidney, and digestive tract of rats (Table 6–11). Laqueur, Matsumoto, and others subsequently established that the active principle was cycasin, the β-glucoside of methylazoxymethanol. The pure compound failed to elicit cancer both in germ-free rats and, after intraperitoneal injection, in conventional animals. It was concluded that this material (1) was not secreted to a great extent in the bile, (2) was not hydrolyzed by mammalian tissues because of the absence of the required enzyme β-glucosidase in adult animals, and (3) was hydrolyzed by the gut microflora with the subsequent release of

the active principle, presumed to be methylazoxymethanol. Numerous studies have since documented these facts. The interesting discovery was made that subcutaneous injection of cycasin in newborn, but not adult, animals did lead to cancer, implying that the required β-glucosidase was present in the subcutaneous tissue of newborn rats.

Methylazoxymethanol itself leads to cancer in various species of conventional and germ-free animals, irrespective of the mode of administration. Interestingly, in rodents, the main type of cancer induced is in the colon, although duodenal, liver, kidney, and ear duct cancer is also found. In addition, the compound under some conditions induces hepatomegalocytosis; so while this compound is not entirely stable at physiologic pH, its organospecificity suggested the need to search for enzymatically mediated activation mechanisms. Zedeck, and Fiala (in Copeland and Rawson, 1977) have evidence that the enzyme may be related to alcohol dehydrogenase, which yields eventually, via several steps, methylcarbonium ions, presumed to be the active ultimate carcinogen, formed in the cell from precursor material. Thus, the natural product cycasin yields the same ultimate carcinogen as does dimethylnitrosamine after biochemical oxidation by host systems. Yet, dimethylnitrosamine does not yield colon cancer, albeit a stabilized synthetic derivative of the unstable putative metabolite of dimethylnitrosamine, namely methylhydroxymethylnitrosamine, in the form of its acetoxy derivative, can induce colon cancer, and thus has a close structural and biologic similarity to methylazoxymethanol.

Because of his interest in Laqueur's findings with cycasin, Druckrey (in Odashima et al., 1975) examined the carcinogenic properties of 1,2-dimethylhydrazine, which was postulated to be oxidized to methylazoxymethanol. 1,2-Dimethylhydrazine was, in fact, found to be highly carcinogenic in many

Table 6–11. DIALKYLHYDRAZINES AND RELATED CARCINOGENS

$$CH_3NHNHCH_3$$

1,2-Dimethylhydrazine

$$CH_3N=NCH_3$$
$$\downarrow$$
$$O$$

Azoxymethane

$$CH_3N=N-CH_2O\text{---glucose}$$
$$\downarrow$$
$$O$$

Methylazoxymethanol-glucoside (cycasin)

$$CH_3N=N-CH_2OH$$
$$\downarrow$$
$$O$$

Methylazoxymethanol

$$R-\langle\text{benzene}\rangle-CH_2NHNHCH_3$$

Natulan (procarbazine)
$R=CONHCH(CH_3)_2$
Benzylmethylhydrazine
$R = H$

species, yielding the same type of tumors as methyl-azoxymethanol. Azoxymethane, a metabolite chemically related to 1,2-dimethylhydrazine, produces the same pattern of response. Of considerable interest is the fact that in rodents these compounds cause a high incidence of cancer of the lower intestinal tract, colon, and rectum. These materials thus provide new tools to induce and study types of cancers that are prevalent in man in the United States and Western Europe (Magee *et al.*, 1976; Farber *et al.*, 1977; Weisburger *et al.*, in Hiatt *et al.*, 1977).

Curiously, the very closely related 1,2-diethylhydrazine has an entirely different target organ. Administration of this material yields primarily cancer of the lung and liver (Preussman, 1975). More information is required to understand the specific localization of the effect of this series of compounds.

Among substituted methylhydrazine derivatives, the antitumor agent Natulan (procarbazine hydrochloride) has been found to be highly carcinogenic in several test systems. While the exact mechanism is not known, it is presumed to depend on the metabolic liberation of methyl carbonium ions, as is true for symmetric 1,2-dimethylhydrazine. The parent compound, 1-methyl-2-benzylhydrazine, has a similar pattern of carcinogenicity.

1,2-Dimethylhydrazine is metabolized to the gas azomethane, which is exhaled in part in the breath of animals given 1,2-dimethylhydrazine. A next step further yields azoxymethane, and thence methylazoxymethanol (Zedeck, and Fiala, in Copeland and Rawson, 1977). Under some conditions, such as administration of low levels of 1,2-dimethylhydrazine in the drinking water, the tumor distribution seen, namely vascular tumors, particularly in the liver, is different from that when high doses are given orally or subcutaneously, i.e., intestinal cancer. In hamsters, oral administration of symmetric dimethylhydrazine leads also to blood vessel tumors, mainly in the liver (Toth, in Copeland and Rawson, 1977). It is presumed that the metabolic activation is different and proceeds via monomethylhydrazine, a chemical that induces mostly such vascular tumors, although under some circumstances tumors in the cecum but not in other parts of the intestinal tract are noted. The metabolic activation of methylhydrazine may be akin to that of hydrazine itself, namely the series of steps acetylation, N'-oxidation, and release of an active acylonium ion. This sequence has not yet been demonstrated for this particular series of compounds, but Nelson *et al.* (in Jerina, 1977; see also Gillette *et al.*, in Gelboin and Ts'o, 1978) have shown this to obtain for several hydrazine drugs. A highly carcinogenic natural product found in some types of mushrooms is N-methyl-N-formylhydrazine (Toth and Nagel, 1978).

When administered at high dose levels, hydrazine itself has been shown to reliably induce pulmonary tumors in mice, although the effect in rats is very much less pronounced, resulting in a low incidence of liver tumors and possibly, in one experimental series, lung tumors. It is interesting to note that in the C3H strain of mouse, a strain prone to develop spontaneous mammary tumors, hydrazine inhibits the occurrence of mammary tumors while simultaneously inducing lung tumors. The mechanism of this effect is not understood. It was found that the closely related hydroxylamine also inhibited mammary tumor formation in C3H mice. This chemical, however, is not carcinogenic (Weisburger and Williams, 1979).

Some substituted hydrazines, including the important drug isoniazid, also lead to pulmonary tumors in specific strains of mice (Swiss or strain A), perhaps because of metabolic release of hydrazine. Tests of isoniazid in other strains of mice or in other rodent species have afforded dubious evidence of carcinogenicity. However, a number of other drugs and chemicals that possess this type of structure, potentially giving rise to hydrazine during metabolism, have induced pulmonary tumors in susceptible strains of mice (Shimkin and Stoner, 1975).

Dioxane. This important commercial solvent was first found to be carcinogenic when administered at sizable dosages, 1 percent in drinking water to rats. In early experimentation this was found to induce carcinomas. In later tests it was also noted that some animals had nasopharyngeal cancers. It would appear, therefore, that the administration of the compound in drinking water leads to the nasal lesion, possibly by the introduction of the solution or the vapors from the solution into the air passages. The mechanism of action has not been completely clarified, but would depend, however, on an alpha-hydroxylation with formation of an active electrophile (Woo *et al.*, 1978; Young *et al.*, 1978). There is evidence for a dose dependency of the metabolic change.

Benzene. Occupational exposure under quantitatively ill-defined conditions to benzene has led to a number of cases of leukemia (Laskin and Goldstein, 1977). The historic prevailing hygienic conditions lead to the suspicion that the then-existing air concentrations were high. However, there are no real data. Recently, the threshold limit value was set at 1 ppm.

Despite several attempts to induce the disease in animal models, there are no published reports of a successful induction of leukemia. Inasmuch as leukemias in animals can be readily induced by viruses, or by immunosuppressive drugs in animals and man (see comment in this chapter), the question as to the mode of action of benzene in inducing leukemia in specific occupational groups remains open, but may also involve an indirect immunosuppressive action by a benzene metabolite. Benzene is not known to be genotoxic, although the putative metabolite arene oxide should be. If benzene in man acts by virtue of a general, or more likely specific, immunosuppressive effect, it will be important to develop methods to screen people for the presence of occult leukemia viruses, an important goal in any case.

Thioamides. In connection with the determination of the safety of certain food additives, it was discovered that thiourea, thioacetamide, and similar thioamides were carcinogenic (Table 6–12) (Searle, 1976). The main target organs are the thyroid and in some instances the liver. The action on the thyroid is thought to be due to an interference with the synthesis of thyroxine leading to an imbalance of the pituitary–thyroid gland relationships. Thus, an increased flow of thyrotropic hormone is generated by the pituitary, stimulating thyroid growth and contri-

Table 6–12. CARCINOGENIC THIOAMIDES AND MISCELLANEOUS CARCINOGENS

$$CH_3\overset{\displaystyle S}{\overset{\displaystyle \|}{C}}NH_2$$

Thioacetamide

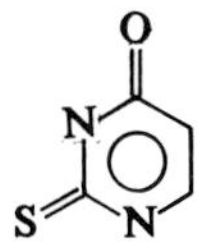

$$NH_2\overset{\displaystyle S}{\overset{\displaystyle \|}{C}}NH_2$$

Thiourea

$$CH_3CH_2SCH_2CH_2\underset{\displaystyle NH_2}{CHCOOH}$$

Ethionine

Thiouracil

$$CH_2{=}CH{-}S{-}CH_2{-}CH_2{-}\underset{\displaystyle NH_2}{CH}{-}COOH$$

Vinylhomocysteine

H_2NCOOR
Urethan (ethyl carbamate) R = —CH₂—CH₃)
Vinyl carbamate (R = —CH=CH₂)

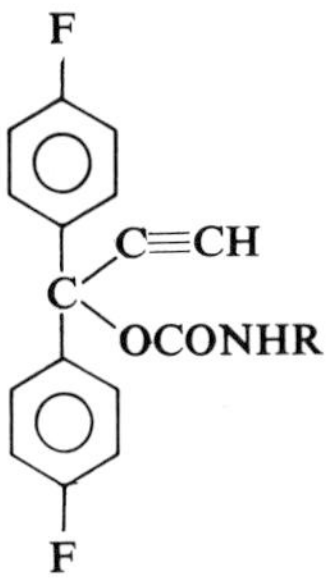

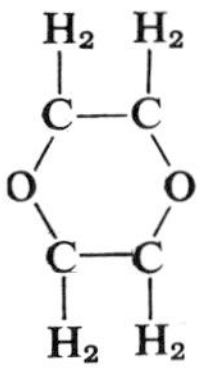

1,1(4,4′-difluoro)-diaryl-2-propynyl-N-cycloalkylcarbamate
(R = cycloheptyl or cyclooctyl)

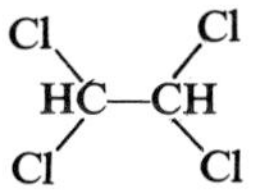

Dioxane

CCl_4
Carbon tetrachloride

Tetrachloroethane

$BrCH_2CH_2Br$
Ethylene bromide

$CH_2{=}CHCN$
Acrylonitrile

$CH_2{=}CH_2Cl$
Vinyl chloride

buting to tumor formation. In addition, a direct, local effect of the carcinogen or a metabolite in the thyroid appears necessary. The action on the liver by agents like thiouracil and thioacetamide has not yet received a sound fundamental explanation.

Acetamide, a related chemical, when given to rats in doses as large as 1 to 5 percent in the diet, elicits hepatocellular carcinomas in approximately one year. The mechanism of action of this chemical on the liver is quite different from that of the corresponding thioacetamide, the latter being effective in much lower dosages in a shorter span of time. Also, the effect of acetamide can be counteracted by the simultaneous administration of arginine glutamate suggesting, but certainly not proving, that abnormal metabolism of ammonia is somehow related to the carcinogenic effect.

Urethan. The carcinogenicity of urethan, ethyl carbamate, was discovered while it was used as an anesthetic agent during investigations in radiobiology (Searle, 1976). Since that time, numerous studies have been done with urethan. In mice, this agent readily induces pulmonary tumors, even with a single large dose. Different strains of mice exhibit variable responsiveness (Shimkin and Stoner, 1975). Most sensitive are strain A mice, whereas C57BL mice are among the strains responding less readily. Cutaneous application or oral administration followed by a promoting skin treatment (see below) with croton oil or pure phorbol esters leads to skin tumors. In rats, urethan is only weakly carcinogenic, but in the hamster this agent has produced melanotic lesions on the skin. In mice, urethan is active by the transplacental route and is passed to offspring in the milk. Thus administered, it leads to a variety of neoplasms in different organs.

In a series of related carbamates, the methyl ester is not carcinogenic and fails to inhibit the effect of the active ethyl ester. The propyl, isopropyl, and butyl esters are weakly active while the higher homologs are inactive. N-Hydroxyurethane exhibits the same degree of carcinogenicity as does urethan. The structure-activity relationships and the inactivity of the methyl derivative may relate to the fact that the metabolic pathway involves a dehydrogenation of the ethyl group, with formation of vinyl carbamate, which can then further undergo epoxidation (Table 6–12; Dahl et al., 1978).

Ethionine. This agent was synthesized as an antimetabolite to L-methionine and used in the study of transmethylation reactions in relation to the biochemistry of this essential amino acid. The hepatoxic and carcinogenic effect of ethionine was discovered many years later by Farber. Under acute conditions, ethionine interferes with the cellular energy supplying mechanisms centering around ATP and is incorporated into RNA (Kuchino et al., 1978), and the hepatoxic effect may stem in part from this effect. The mechanism underlying the more chronic action of ethionine leading to liver tumors in rats has not yet been explained. Weisburger et al. (unpublished) observed that whereas ethionine is not mutagenic, the vinyl analog is highly mutagenic. Thus, the activation pathway of ethionine may procede via vinylhomocysteine, further converted to an epoxide, in a manner similar to the documented example of urethane converted to vinyl carbamate and of aflatoxin B$_2$ metabolized to aflatoxin B$_1$ (Table 6–12; see above; Roebuck et al., 1978). It is not known whether the fairly polar homocysteine part of the molecule is further degraded as well, as part of the metabolic activation. Many known carcinogens are relatively nonpolar, facilitating absorption and passage across lipid membranes without active transport.

Carbon Tetrachloride and Related Halohydrocarbons. Carbon tetrachloride is a classic hepatoxic agent, affecting virtually all species, including man (see Chapters 10 and 18). That this chemical can also induce liver tumors has been reported in a number of strains of mice under several experimental conditions. Rats seemed curiously resistant, until it was found that most strains of rats used succumbed early to pronounced hepatoxic effects. With strains less prone to these effects, it was noted that hepatocellular carcinoma could be induced with proper scheduling of carbon tetrachloride intake. Most sensitive were the Japanese or Yoshida strain, followed by the Osborne-Mendel rat. In one test, carbon tetrachloride also induced hepatocellular carcinoma in the Syrian golden hamster, but this study apparently requires confirmation, for in one more recent set of tests no liver tumors were obtained.

In mice, particularly in females, chloroform is also hepatoxic and carcinogenic, but considerably less so than carbon tetrachloride. In the Osborne-Mendel strain rat, a small yield of kidney cancers were also noted. Many chlorinated hydrocarbons are not only hepatoxic, but quite nephrotoxic. There have been cases of human hepatoxicity with carbon tetrachloride and with chloroform. The latter had been used in medical practice as an anesthetic agent, until the hepatotoxicity was noted, and this application was discontinued. Nonetheless, there are no records of any human cancers stemming from such documented toxic exposures to these chemicals.

A comprehensive carcinogen test program by the U.S. National Cancer Institute on diverse chlorohydrocarbons, both fully saturated or with an ethylenic bond, uniformly induced liver tumors in male and female mice, gave evidence of severe nephrotoxicity, and in several instances had a low-yield carcinogenic effect on the kidney of Osborne-Mendel strain rats (Weisburger, E. K., in Falk, 1977). The findings have been attributed to the possible but not demonstrated formation of epoxide derivatives in the ethylene compounds. However, inasmuch as the saturated ethane derivative had similar tumorigenic properties, it would seem that the formation of an electrophilic epoxide may not be responsible for the demonstrated tumor formation. In fact, in the usual test for mutagenicity, providing indirect evidence for the formation of an electrophilic reactant, these compounds were generally negative. Even DDT and related chemicals, which also induce only mouse liver tumors, are negative in the hamster, and only weakly active in the rat, and are furthermore not mutagenic, can be classified with this group of halohydrocarbons. There is no evidence at all that human exposure under the more intense conditions during the industrial production of such chemicals or during their use, for example, in agricultural practice has demonstrated any carcinogenic risk to man (Deichman, 1974). How then account for the unquestionable demonstration of liver tumor formation in mice? Weisburger and Williams (in Asher and Zervos, 1978) have suggested that the induction of liver tumors in mice may be due to promotion of an as-yet-unknown, possibly endogenous gene change in mouse liver. Peraino et al. (in Slaga et al., 1978) have actually demonstrated such a phenomenon of promotion by DDT and related materials that are enzyme inducers in rat liver. Validation of this concept of a promoting rather than genotoxic action of chlorinated hydrocarbons is not only an important distinction from a theoretic point of view, but is even more relevant in terms of regulatory actions indicated to prevent chronic disease.

On the other hand, bromohydrocarbons are genotoxic, and in addition to causing liver tumors in mice also induce forestomach tumors in rats and mice rather quickly in high yield. They are clearly carcinogens and have distinct properties from the chloro compounds above. *Tris*, or tris (2,3-dibromopropyl)-phosphate, is also genotoxic and carcinogenic (Van Duuren et al., 1978a).

Microbiologic Carcinogens. A number of carcinogens are formed in nature by microorganisms or plants (Tables 6–13, 6–14). The mechanism of action of a number of these agents, particularly the antibiotics, is unknown. However, most of these naturally occurring carcinogens clearly require metabolic activation.

Mycotoxins. Investigations of the cause of an enormous loss of turkey poults with fulminating liver necrosis in Great Britain early in 1960 led to the discovery of a mold toxin produced on feeds contaminated with a strain of *Aspergillus flavus*. The toxin accounted for the pronounced hepatotoxicity of such contaminated meals (Wogan, in Homburger, 1976; in Kraybill and Mehlman, 1977). Further tests showed that the agent responsible, named aflatoxin B$_1$, not only was highly hepatoxic but was one of the most powerful carcinogens known, inducing liver tumors in several species after dietary intake of very low levels, of the order of ppb. The mold usually pro-

Table 6–13. CARCINOGENS FOUND IN MICROORGANISMS AND PLANTS

MICROORGANISMS	PLANTS
Aflatoxins	Tobacco, snuff
Sterigmatocystin	Betel nut
Luteoskyrin	Cycasin
Islanditoxin	Pyrrolizidine (Senecio)
Griseofulvin	alkaloids
Actinomycins	Coltsfoot
Mitomycin C	Bracken fern
Adriamycin	Mushroom toxins
Daunomycin	Safrole
Elaiomycin	β-Asarone (calamus oil)
Ethionine	Thiourea, goitrogens
Azserine	Phorbol esters*
Nitrosonornicotine	
Streptozotocin	

* Cocarcinogen and promoter.

duces four types of aflatoxin: B_1, B_2, G_1, and G_2. Because these agents exhibit characteristic fluorescence patterns, they were isolated and their structure established in record time, a significant achievement in the area of toxicologic studies.

Among the four isomers found, aflatoxin B_1 is much more toxic and carcinogenic than the G_1 analog. The G_2 derivative is virtually not carcinogenic. Aflatoxin B_2, on the other hand, is definitely but slightly carcinogenic, probably because there is an enzyme that converts aflatoxin B_2 to B_1 to a small extent (Roebuck et al., 1978). All of the structural elements draw attention to the double bond in the furan portion of the molecule (Lin et al., 1978). There is evidence that the ultimate carcinogen of the various aflatoxins involves an epoxide. Inasmuch as there are many other competing metabolic steps, including the production of ring-hydroxylated metabolites and of the demethylated phenol, it would seem that the epoxide is indeed a highly active carcinogen. The

other parts of the molecule, including the potentially reactive lactone ring, are not concerned directly with the carcinogenic activity but apparently provide bulk. Smaller parts like the difuran rings alone, for example, are not active.

Aflatoxin B_1 is highly hepatocarcinogenic in rats and in trout and is also appreciably carcinogenic in a number of other experimental species, including nonhuman primates. The major target organ is the liver, but under some conditions kidney and colon tumors have been seen in rodents. Interestingly, strains of mice treated thus far do not seem to show an effect on the liver, except with newborn mice. Adult mice develop lung tumors.

Even though in highly sensitive species like the rat, or the trout, aflatoxin exhibits carcinogenicity when fed in the diet at levels as low as 1 ppb, it is current FDA policy not to condemn foods with less than 15 ppb aflatoxin B_1. This is probably a judicious compromise since many foods would have to be banned were a strict "zero tolerance" required. It is also likely that such small amounts appear innocuous in man, since primary liver cancer in the U.S. has a relatively low incidence and in fact has decreased over the last 50 years (Linsell and Peers; Weisburger et al., in Hiatt et al., 1977; American Cancer Society, 1978), perhaps because our foods now are monitored for this and other hepatocarcinogens like dimethylnitrosamine or nitrosopyrrolidine. On the other hand, in countries like certain African nations, where staple foods have demonstrated high aflatoxin B_1 contamination of the order of ppm, primary liver cancer is one of the main, important neoplastic diseases (Schottenfeld, 1975; Higginson, 1977; Newburgs, 1978). This is an association that is probably but not necessarily causal. In this region, hepatitis B antigen is also endemic, and it has been thought that there might be a potentiating effect between this antigen and mycotoxicosis (Gyorkey et al., 1977; Trichopoulos et al., 1978). Currently, the International Agency for Research in Cancer is conducting a pilot experiment in Swaziland to remove the mycotoxins from foods and

Table 6–14. NATURAL PRODUCT CARCINOGENS

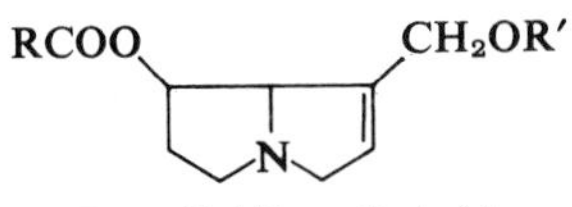

Pyrrolizidine alkaloids

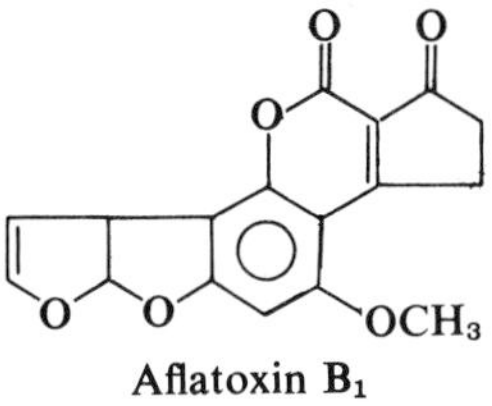

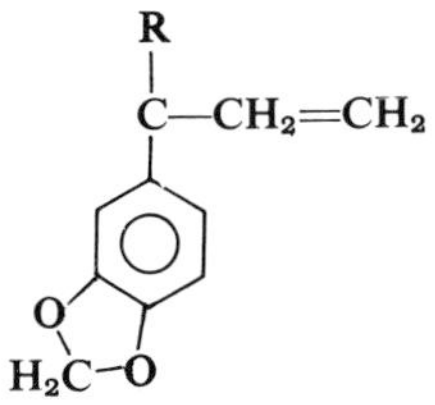

Safrole (R = H)
1'-Hydroxysafrole (R = —OH)

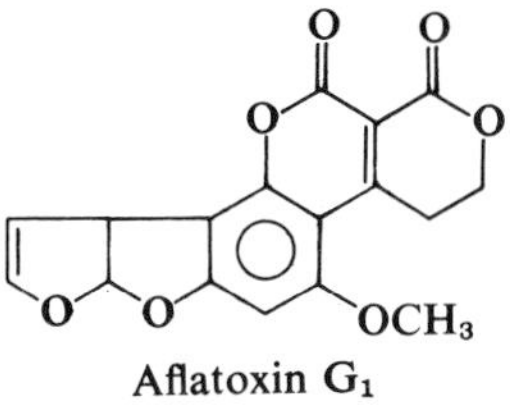

Aflatoxin B_1

Aflatoxin G_1

determine whether this will result in a decreased incidence of primary liver cancer, which is now high, as is the dietary level of aflatoxin B_1.

Sterigmatocystin is a related mycotoxin that is also carcinogenic and is likewise found in mold-contaminated food crops and may also play a role in human liver cancer.

Antibiotics. These natural products enter the human environment for a variety of uses, mainly as drugs. Data are beginning to accumulate that suggest that several of these agents such as daunomycin, dactinomycin, and streptozotocin may be carcinogenic (Schmähl et al., 1977; Uraguchi and Yamazaki, 1978). Except for streptozotocin, which has a nitrosamine type of structure (see above) and thus may be expected to have carcinogenic potency, the mechanism of carcinogenic action is not clear. Such molecular structures have been shown in part to bind strongly, but often reversibly, to DNA, perhaps by intercalation. Additional experiments in search of minor, more permanent, bonding would be interesting.

Azerine. Azerine, which is produced by *Streptomyces*, has been of interest as an antitumor agent. It inhibits purine biosynthesis through inhibition of the enzyme 2-formamido-N-ribosylacetamide 5'-phosphate: L-glutamine amido-ligase. Azaserine was shown to produce primarily pancreas and kidney cancer in rats. This organotropism correlates with localization of the agent (Longnecker and Curphey, 1975). The mechanism of action is not clear, but the enzyme inhibition has been shown to be due to alkylation of the sulfhydryl group of a cysteine residue in the enzyme, and azaserine is mutagenic without metabolic activation. Thus, a genotoxic action seems probable. The effect of azaserine on the pancreas is potentiated by 4-hydroxylaminoquinoline-N-oxide.

Plant Carcinogens. *Tobacco.* The best known of all plant carcinogens with a major impact as a cause of human cancer is the group of agents in the tobacco plant (Wynder and Gori, 1977). It contains certain carcinogens such as nitrosonornicotine and related agents even before burning and pyrolysis. Tobacco smoke is most complex and contains diverse classes of carcinogens, cocarcinogens, accelerators, and promoters. The carcinogens include polycyclic aromatic hydrocarbons, heterocyclic compounds, phenolic derivatives, etc. The reader is referred to specialized reviews for details (Hiatt et al., 1977; Schmeltz and Hoffmann, 1977; Hoffmann et al., in Gelboin and Ts'o, 1978). The total increase in human cancer in men since 1930 and in women since 1960 is accounted for by the smoking of manufactured cigarettes, by men, since about 1915, and by women since about 1940. Newer low-tar products now on the market seem to have a lower, but not zero risk. The reader is again referred to specialized reviews for this important area of toxicology.

Betel chewing (see Newburgs, 1978) likewise leads to cancer in humans with this habit, which can be easily prevented by reeducation, especially of the young generation.

Safrole. This chemical is typical of a number of related methylenedioxyalkyl or allylbenzenes, which are natural and synthetic flavoring agents. Thus far,

only safrole has been studied in some detail. Rather appreciable amounts, 0.5 percent in the diet, are needed in order to demonstrate carcinogenicity. This may be because the biochemical activation reactions, involving 1'-hydroxylation and probably also epoxidation on the exocyclic double bond, occur to a small extent only. In addition, there are further as-yet-unspecified metabolic reactions on the 1'-hydroxy derivative, yielding the ultimate carcinogenic form (Miller, 1978).

A derivative, dihydrosafrole, yielded tumors in the esophagus of rats, through unknown mechanisms.

Senecio Alkaloids. These interesting natural products, used extensively as teas or as drugs in some civilizations, have a distinct effect on the liver (Wogan, in Homburger, 1976; in Kraybill and Mehlman, 1977). There is no question that continuing administration of these agents leads to hepatomegalocytosis, mainly because they exert a pronounced antimitotic effect.

Certain of these alkaloids have an unquestioned carcinogenic effect in rats, the only species so far used in these tests. It is thought that the intake of such alkaloids in some areas of the world, perhaps together with mycotoxins and in the presence of viral agents such as hepatitis B, may contribute to liver cancer prevalent in these areas. These chemicals require metabolic activation, possibly to specific pyrrole derivatives in which, upon biochemical oxidation of the ring, the exocyclic ester as a leaving group splits to yield an electrophilic compound (Miller and Miller, in Searle, 1976; Miller, 1978).

Bracken Fern. In investigating the causes of hematuria and bladder cancers in cattle in Turkey and other regions, it was found that the consumption of bracken fern was etiologically related to the development of these lesions (Jarrett et al., 1978). In rats, administration of bracken fern has an effect not only on the urinary bladder but also on the upper intestinal tract (Hirono et al., 1978).

There is possible human exposure to the carcinogen in bracken fern since it has been demonstrated in the milk of cows consuming this plant (Pamukcu et al., 1978). The specific carcinogens are not yet known. It will be important to determine the structure since in several species, urinary bladder cancer seems to be the main lesion. Even when man is not exposed to occupational bladder carcinogens or carcinogens affecting the bladder in tobacco smoke, there are cases of bladder cancer, usually late in life. Could they be due to agents from bracken fern, perhaps ingested with cow's milk?

Miscellaneous Plant Carcinogens. In a search for agents associated with the high incidence of cancer of the esophagus in certain parts of the Caribbean, extracts of specific plants appeared to have carcinogenic activity. The relationship of such activity to cancer of the esophagus is, however, obscure, inasmuch as this disease is also seen in people who smoke cigarettes and consume alcoholic beverages in large amounts (Fraumeni, 1975). These customs appear prevalent in the same regions. An extract of mycelia of *Candida parapsilosis* produced sarcomas when injected into mice. The active principle has not yet been identified. Injection of an extract of the plant *Kra-*

meria ixina caused a high incidence of subcutaneous sarcomas in rats.

3. Inorganic Carcinogens

Relatively few investigators have concerned themselves with the possible carcinogenicity of inorganic chemicals (Hernberg, in Hiatt *et al.*, 1977; Sunderman, 1978; Schrauzer, 1978). There have been no systematic studies dealing with derivatives of the various elements. Compounds of uranium, polonium, and radium have demonstrated carcinogenicity attributed chiefly to their radioactive properties. Uranium, radium, and the derived radon gas have been implicated in the development of lung cancer in individuals engaged in mining ores. Miners who smoke cigarettes are at higher risk, indicating a possible synergistic effect between ore dust, radiation, and cigarette smoking (Lee and Kotin, 1972; Hiatt *et al.*, 1977).

In man, small-molecule inorganic compounds have been shown definitely carcinogenic only in the case of certain nickel derivatives by a process that was abandoned in the mid-1930s (Doll *et al.*, 1977). Workmen on the job since that time appear not to have appreciable risk, an impressive demonstration of prevention of occupational cancer by altering exposure conditions without detracting from commercial production.

In addition, human exposure to certain complex ores like chromates apparently has a high risk, particularly of cancer in the respiratory tract. It is not certain whether the disease process is due to a direct carcinogen reaction by chromate or whether the neoplastic change is due more to a type of solid-state carcinogenesis, akin to that of asbestos discussed below.

Connections have been established with deliberate or inadvertent intake of radioactive elements or their compounds that concentrate in certain organs or tissues. Thus, intake of labeled iodine and derivatives, concentrating in thyroid gland, has been known to give rise to cancer in that organ. Chemicals that concentrate in bone, like strontium derivatives, in their labeled forms can induce osteosarcomas. Parenthetically, a number of these elements are the main contributors to the cancer hazard associated with radioactive fallout, consequent to the aboveground use of nuclear weapons. Medical use of thorotrast is known to induce liver cancer (Truhaut, 1967; Schmähl *et al.*, 1977).

Among the inorganic chemicals titanium, nickel, chromium, cobalt, lead, manganese, and beryllium, and certain of their derivatives have been found to be carcinogenic under specific experimental conditions. Among these, salts of nickel and titanium appear to be most powerful. In most instances, these chemicals lead to cancer formation at the point of application, as for example the rapid formation of sarcoma after subcutaneous injection of nickel sulfide in rats; on the other hand, oral lead acetate induces kidney cancer in rats, and inhalation of beryllium salts or ores has induced pulmonary carcinoma in rats and rhesus monkeys. Manganese, however, antagonizes the effect of the nickel salts (Sunderman, 1978).

Selenium derivatives have had a controversial history in relation to carcinogenicity (see Schrauzer, 1978). There have been suggestions years ago that such compounds may be hepatocarcinogenic. Inorganic selenium derivatives are extremely hepatotoxic but do not appear to be carcinogenic. In fact, it seems that selenium is an essential element that controls the function of gluthathione peroxidase, among other key enzymes. Also, selenium derivatives inhibited carcinogenicity in several experimental systems and interfered with the mutagenicity of other carcinogens. There have been suggestions that soil geochemistry, especially in relation to a deficiency of selenium, coincides with a higher incidence of several important cancers, an obvious subject for more research.

Arsenic likewise has been called carcinogenic. There seems to be an association between trivalent inorganic arsenic exposure of humans through drinking water or certain occupations and the development of lung and skin cancer and lymphomas. However, the exposure situation may not be to arsenic alone, but simply to a complex environment containing excess arsenic, together with other materials. There are other regions where water contains arsenic with no apparent excess of cancer. Also, so far animal tests of arsenic derivatives have not yielded firm evidence that inorganic arsenic compounds can cause cancer, a truly exceptional situation (Frost, in Schrauzer, 1978). Roesman *et al.* (1977) have noted that arsenic can affect DNA repair.

Magnesium deficiency seems to be able to induce lymphomas by as-yet-unknown mechanisms, perhaps involving immunodeficiency.

Little is known about the mechanism of the oncogenic action of inorganic chemicals. They do not seem to operate directly as electrophiles, like the corresponding ultimate organic molecule carcinogens. There are certain indications that they are active in rapid bioassay systems (Casto *et al.*, 1979) and thus may be genotoxic. However, a potentially important conceptual advance stems from the research of Loeb (in Schrauzer, 1978) indicating that certain metal ions affect the fidelity of the polymerases involved in the biosynthesis of DNA, thus yielding abnormal DNA through this mechanism. Further research is required to fully define the relevance of these observations to the carcinogenicity of inorganics.

4. Solid-State Carcinogens

The discovery that plastics implanted subcutaneously in rodents could lead to sarcoma formation was made by accident. The Oppenheimers attempted to produce hypertension in rats by inserting plastic foils around the kidneys. They noted abnormal cellular formations, followed by granuloma development and eventually neoplastic tissue in the area of implantation.

This initial finding was explored by a number of investigators. The salient conclusion was that the chemical composition of the implanted material was relatively unimportant. Indeed, thin disks or sheets of metal like gold were as effective as a variety of polymers. The important factors were the size and shape of the insert. Smooth materials were more effective than rough, perforated disks and sheets were less effective than solid ones. The latent period was often quite long, more than one year in mice or rats (Brand *et al.*, 1977). No mechanism of action has emerged from these combined studies (Grasso, 1971). Because it was difficult to develop additional experimental approaches to this problem, investigators in the field have turned away from this area in recent years, especially since there appeared to be no human counterpart to solid-state carcinogenesis. However, the literature has provided a number of case reports in which a sarcoma was found around vascular grafts in humans. A few of these cases have in common the fact that the individuals involved were young at the time of implant, which may provide a clue to further epidemiologic investigations as well as laboratory studies (Schmähl *et al.*, 1977).

Asbestos. The data on the carcinogenic risk due to the inorganic polymer asbestos came from both clinical and laboratory observations (Fraumeni, 1975; Saffiotti and Wagoner, 1976; Selikoff, in Hiatt *et al.*, 1977). In view of the extensive use of asbestos and asbestos products in commerce, these observations assume key importance. There appear to be some differences in effect depending on the origin, physical structure, and minor chemical components with the broad class of asbestos-containing materials.

The mechanism of action of asbestos is unknown. Asbestos alone, in the pleural cavity in animal models and in man, leads to mesotheliomas. The latent period is usually long. Importantly, other fibers, such as fine fibrous glass, will also produce a high incidence of tumors under the same conditions (Stanton, in Bogovski *et al.*, 1973). Thus, the mechanism is remindful of solid-state carcinogenesis, especially since the lesion obtained is not epithelial, but mesenchymal. In support of this conclusion, no evidence for genotoxicity of asbestos has been developed from *in vitro* tests.

Asbestos is different from organic molecule chemical carcinogens insofar as it is not metabolized and excreted but remains permanently in the body. Thus, even limited exposure to high levels, as used to be the case in occupational situations, leads to a continuing presence of inhaled asbestos. Men exposed to asbestos in the large-scale ship-building effort in the early 1940s are currently at high risk for this disease. The latent period in man is 25 years or more, in general. Cases of disease have been seen even in relatives of workmen, who, through indirect exposures such as laundering work clothing, inhaled this material. Thus, this type of carcinogen can be considered more dangerous even than organic carcinogens, although the latter are genotoxic, because of the fact that asbestos remains permanently in the body.

In addition, of great importance is the fact that, as is true for certain other solid surfaces that remain permanently in tissues such as the lung, asbestos particles and other minerals and ores, such as in uranium mining, hematite mining, and the like, potentiate the action of other carcinogens, such as cigarette smoke, reaching the same organ (Selikoff, in Hiatt *et al.*, 1977). While asbestos by itself does not usually yield lung cancer, there is solid evidence that asbestos dust and smoking cigarettes contributes not additively but synergistically to the development of lung cancer in humans. It is important, therefore, to control exposure to asbestos and other mineral dust. For those individuals who were unfortunately exposed to asbestos years or decades ago, their risk for disease, particularly lung cancer, can and should be minimized by instituting smoking withdrawal programs immediately.

There is some information that asbestos fibers ingested during high-level occupation exposure also contribute to cancer in the gastrointestinal tract. Although more information in this area is required, animal studies so far have not demonstrated any effects in these target organs.

Iron-Carbohydrate Complexes. Iron supplementation has been achieved by subcutaneous administration of drugs such as iron dextran or iron dextrin. Subcutaneous injection in rodents of such drugs yielded local sarcomas (Golberg *et al.*, 1961). A high proportion of injected compound remains at the site of administration in some species. Thus, a physical mechanism of oncogenesis requires consideration (Roe, in Truhaut, 1967; Grasso, 1976). Schmähl *et al.* (1977) have recorded a few reports of subcutaneous tumors which may have been associated with iron dextran injection, but noted that no direct association has been established between drug injection and oncogenesis in millions of patients treated.

5. Hormones

Hormones, especially of the estrogen type have been shown to cause cancer over 40 years ago (Shimkin, in Schottenfeld, 1975; Searle, 1976). Current concepts show that estrogens, such as the naturally occurring hormone estradiol or the synthetic estrogen diethylstilbestrol (Table 6–15), can cause cancer in animals and in man when they are administered chronically at high level or when they are present through disturbances of normal endocrine balances in unphysiologic amounts for long periods of time (Herbst, in Hiatt *et al.*, 1977; Weisburger and Williams, 1979). This is probably even true in the case of young women, offspring of mothers treated with large amounts of diethylstilbestrol during pregnancy. The relevant mechanism, to be established in detail, may hinge on the faulty differentiation of the complex endocrine apparatus in the fetus, exposed to abnormally high levels of natural or

Table 6–15. TYPICAL COCARCINOGENS (CC) AND PROMOTERS (P)

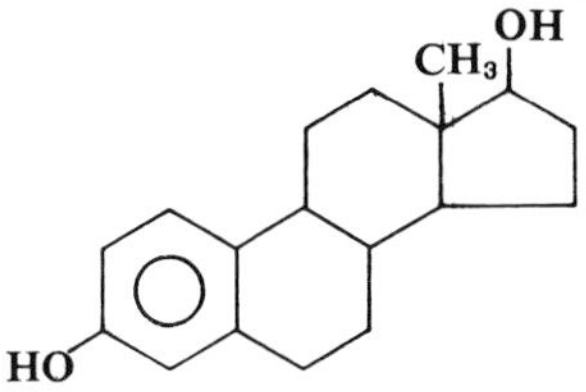

Estradiol (P)

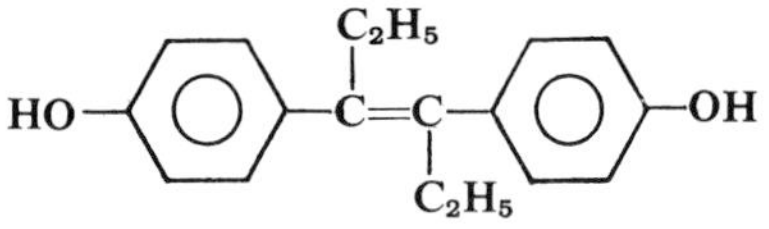

Diethylstilbestrol (P)

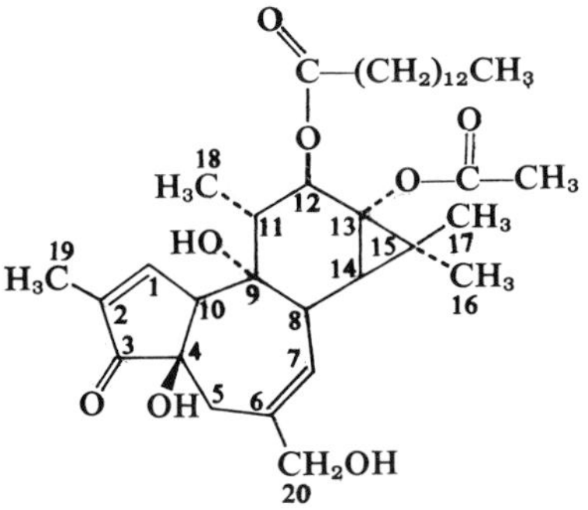

Phorbol esters (CC,P)

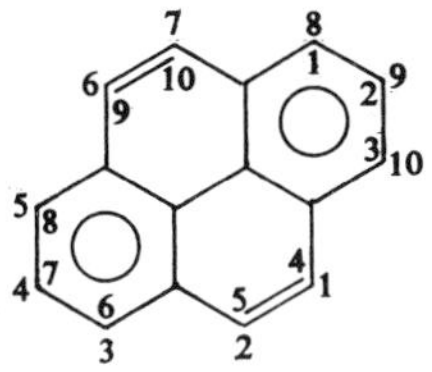

Pyrene (CC)

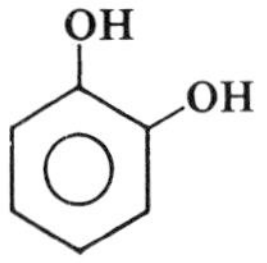

Catechol (CC)

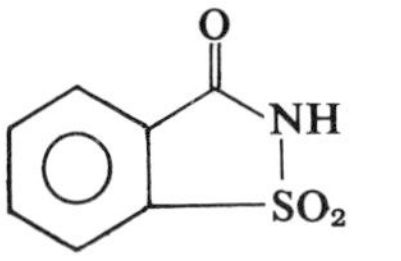

Saccharin (P)

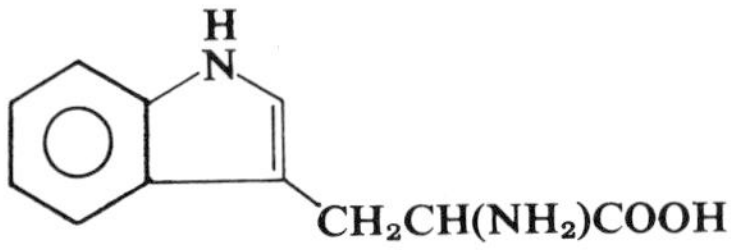

Tryptophan (P)

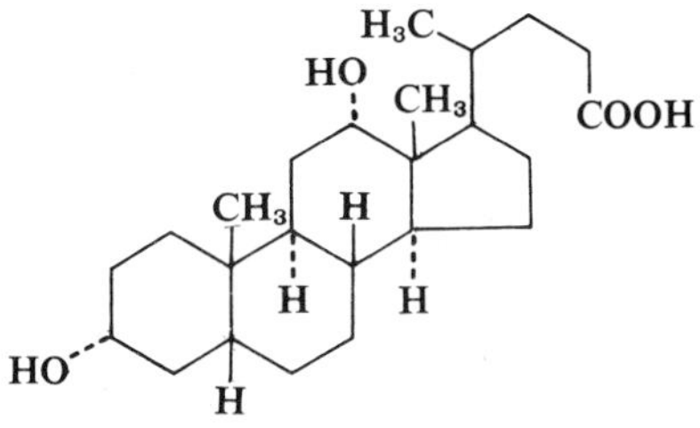

Deoxycholic acid (P)

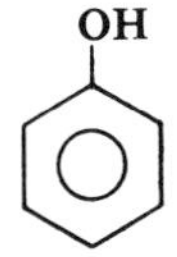

Phenol (P)

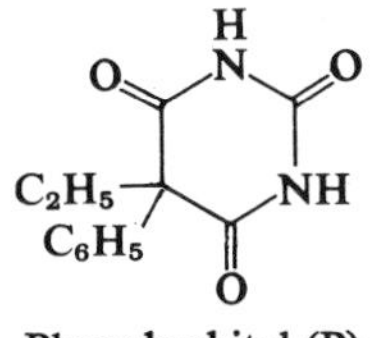

Phenobarbital (P)

synthetic estrogens, which becomes apparent in the offspring at the time of sexual maturation. In animals and in man cancer development is most likely due to promoting action and not due to a direct modification of the genetic apparatus. Thus, hormones and hormonal balances act through epigenetic mechanisms. The initiating agent leading to an altered DNA in man and in certain instances of animal neoplasms "induced" by excess estrogen is not known. In certain animal models, for example, breast cancer in mice, a viral element is associated with carcinogenesis (Becker, 1975; Hiatt et al., 1977). In postmenopausal women maintained on estrogen, there is a high risk of endometrial cancer, where again the actual inducer is not known. In some relatively rare instances, considering the widespread use of oral contraceptives, liver tumors were seen. In all of these cases, the hormones can be considered to have promoted the lesions, actually caused by unknown inducers, which in the case of liver tumors may be akin to the hepatitis B antigen (Weisburger and Williams, 1979).

The actual mechanism of promotion by estrogen is no doubt complex and may involve systemic general hormonal imbalances, including pituitary hormones like prolactin as well as also possibly adrenal and thyroid hormones (Hiatt et al., 1977). Androgen has rarely caused cancer. There are a few case reports of liver cancer in males taking large amounts of androgen as anabolic agents or muscle builders in athletes. As a rule, hormones need to be considered as powerful physiologic effectors, which when present in abnormal amounts for a long time are likely to lead to neoplasia.

6. Immunosuppressive Drugs

With the development of surgical techniques allowing organ transplantation, it has become necessary to prevent rejection by giving maintenance doses over long periods of time of immunosuppressive drugs or sera. It was found that a number of patients so treated developed tumors, usually leukemias or sarcomas but rarely solid cancers (Hoover, in Hiatt et al. 1977; Penn, 1978). Similar findings have been made in animal models given immunosuppressive sera or drugs like azathioprine, 6-mercaptopurine, and the like. The involvement of immune processes in primary carcinogenesis has not been well documented and is a controversial area (Prehn, 1974). Immunosuppressive treatment, whether sera or drugs, induced mainly leukemias, lymphomas, or reticulum cell sarcomas in mice or rats (Weisburger and Williams, 1979). In these animal models the primary inciting agent is often an oncogenic virus, and the same may be true in humans. Thus, it is thought that neoplasia stems from an epigenetic phenomenon, by which immunosuppression allows development of tumors initiated by a distinct genotoxic event.

7. Cocarcinogens

Cocarcinogens are agents that increase the overall carcinogenic process caused by a genotoxic carcinogen when administered together with the carcinogen (Table 6–15). The relevant mechanisms can be one or more of several possibilities: (1) The cocarcinogen intervenes in the metabolism of a genotoxic carcinogen by increasing the level of the active ultimate carcinogenic metabolite or by decreasing the detoxification process. (2) A cocarcinogen may increase non-

specifically or specifically the growth of cells with an altered genotype reflecting neoplastic change. This mechanism is identical to that applying to promoters to be discussed below.

The demonstration of cocarcinogenesis was made in the laboratories of Shear and, especially, of Berenblum and Shubik (see Berenblum, 1974; Slaga et al., 1977; Scribner and Süss, 1978). The latter group noted that application of a carcinogenic polycyclic aromatic hydrocarbon to mouse skin together with croton oil, the seed oil of the euphorbiacea Croton tiglium L., gave a much higher incidence of skin cancer than in controls given the carcinogen alone. The cocarcinogenic action of croton oil was found to be species specific, not being demonstrable in the rabbit, rat, or guinea pig.

The active principles in croton oil eventually isolated and identified by Hecker (in Slaga et al., 1978) were in the form of phorbol esters. These materials act also as promoters. It is not known whether they affect the metabolism of the carcinogen.

Tobacco smoke, as described, contains relatively small amounts of genotoxic carcinogens such as polycyclic aromatic hydrocarbons, certain nitrosamines, and possibly certain pyrolysis products of proteins in the form of α- or β-carbolines and related materials (Wynder and Hecht, 1976; Hiatt et al., 1977). However, tobacco smoke also includes cocarcinogens typified by catechol and other phenolic compounds mainly in the acidic fraction. Here also the mechanism of carcinogenicity is not known. In fact, active research in this field is important, including the development of methods to detect reliably such cocarcinogens.

The cocarcinogenic factors in tobacco smoke are thought to play an important role in the overall effect of the smoke in leading to cancer in man (Wynder et al., in Slaga et al., 1978). Thus, cocarcinogenicity represents not only a theoretic concept, valuable to dissect the complex sequence of events concerned with cancer causation, but also has practical importance in human disease risk.

8. Promoters

Promoters are agents that increase the tumorigenic response to a genotoxic carcinogen when applied after the carcinogen (Table 6–15). The demonstration of this phenomenon in the laboratories of Rous and Berenblum and Shubik (see Berenblum, 1974) gave rise to the "two-stage" concept of carcinogenesis, initiation and promotion.

Croton oil, studied by Berenblum and Shubik, has a highly specific and exquisite promoting activity on mouse skin as with its cocarcinogenic action. In an impressive series of experiments it has been shown that the genotoxic event, application of a polycyclic aromatic hydrocarbon, can be followed by months and in fact one year later by a promoting stimulus such as application of the phorbol esters from croton oil and still result in production of skin tumors (Van Duuren et al., 1978b).

Not all promoters are cocarcinogenic and not all cocarcinogens are promoters. Thus, phenol, for example, in tobacco tar, is a promoter, but not cocarcinogenic.

Although, phorbol esters remain a popular experimental model, a number of other promoters for different organ systems have been discovered. Bile acids have been shown to be promoters in colon carcinogenesis (Reddy et al., in Slaga et al., 1978). Hormones increase carcinogenicity through a mechanism of promotion when present in abnormal amounts. Peraino (in Slaga et al., 1978) observed that certain inducers of liver metabolic enzyme systems, such as phenobarbital, DDT, and BHT, when administered after minimal doses of primary hepatocarcinogens exerted a powerful promoting effect. In most instances, these same chemicals when administered together with hepatocarcinogens decreased carcinogenicity, most likely by increasing detoxification reactions especially those concerned with conjugation.

The mechanism of the promoting effect of chemicals when administered after a primary carcinogen is not yet known. A substantial portion of the effects of phorbal esters on various cell types can be accounted for by their activity on cellular membranes (Sivac in Slaga et al., 1978). Recent findings with phorbol esters indicate an ability to produce gene derepression and repression (see Slaga et al., 1978). In addition, phenobarbital has been shown to enhance the development of preneoplastic liver lesions (Pitot et al., 1978; Williams, in Slaga et al., 1978; Kitagawa et al., 1979). Many, if not all, of these chemicals, like DDT and other chlorinated hydrocarbons and phenobarbital, increase the incidence of mouse liver tumors and very rarely cause cancer in the rat liver. It can be postulated that this occurs by a mechanism of promotion of the preexisting abnormal liver cells that eventually give rise to the "spontaneously" occurring liver lesions and neoplasms in old mice and rats. The nature of the "inducing" agent yielding the abnormal cells is obscure. It could be genetic in these inbred strains, but variations in incidence between different colonies raise the possibility of an exogenous factor. In the mouse this may be an agent akin to the hepatitis virus prevalent in mice. The few liver cancers occasionally seen in rats given phenobarbital or DDT may result from an intake of diets contaminated with mycotoxins or some nitrosamines.

Tryptophan Metabolites. The role of the metabolites of this important essential amino acid in producing cancer was discovered in connection with studies on the effect of such agents on the urinary bladder (Clayson, 1962). Implantation of pellets containing hydroxyanthranilic acid, 3-hyroxykynurenine, and related aminohydroxy derivatives led to the induction of bladder tumors in mice and rats. Even though considerable research has been done in this area, it is not yet certain whether the specific chemicals incriminated are actually carcinogenic. One of the reasons for exerting prudence in drawing conclusions is that these metabolites of tryptophan are quite unstable and may have decomposed in the course of formulation prior to administration to the experimental animals.

Tryptophan was not carcinogenic when fed at a level of 5 percent in the diet to mice and rats (NCI Bioassay, 1978). On the other hand, Radomski et al. demonstrated that large amounts of tryptophan fed to dogs induced hyperplasia of the urinary bladder but no cancer was seen. Pretreatment of the dogs with small amounts of 2-naphthylamine followed by tryptophan yielded cancer of the bladder but the animals on carcinogen alone had none. Cohen et al. with a similar approach pretreated rats with amounts of a nitrofuran, FANFT, yielding only a small incidence of urinary bladder cancer in rats. Addition to the diet of 2 percent tryptophan, or of 5 percent saccharin, gave a sizable yield of bladder cancer suggesting that tryptophan or certain tryptophan metabolites have a promoting effect (see Friedell, 1977). Perhaps further support for this view comes from an experiment of Ross and Brass feeding diets containing 10, 20, and 40 percent casein to groups of 600 rats each in an aging study; a dose-related incidence of urinary bladder cancer was noted with an incidence of 1.8, 3.6, and 6.4 percent, respectively (see Weisburger and Williams, 1979).

Since promotion, an epigenetic phenomenon, is highly dose dependent, requires the presence of the agent for a long time, and importantly is reversible, such agents, while believed to be involved in human cancer causation (Weisburger and Williams, 1979), necessarily require different risk evaluation considerations than genotoxic carcinogens.

METABOLISM OF CHEMICAL CARCINOGENS

With few exceptions, endogenous as well as exogenous chemicals can and do undergo metabolic reactions (Weisburger and Williams, in

Becker, 1975; Searle, 1976; Hathaway, 1977; Hiatt *et al.*, 1977; and Miller, 1978). In the special case of chemical carcinogens such reactions lead only to loss of activity in the case of the primary direct-acting electrophilic carcinogens. In view of their reactive nature, such reactions can be straightforward chemical processes, involving an SN_1 or an SN_2 type of chemical interaction with cellular nucleophiles. Other reactions, which differ as a function of the structure of the carcinogen, can be enzyme mediated. The relative effectiveness of agents depends in part on the relative rates of interaction between the chemical representing genetic material, DNA, versus competing reactions with other cellular nucleophiles. Thus, the relative activity in a given series of chemicals hinges principally on such competing interactions and also metabolic detoxification reactions. Stability during transport, permeability across membranes, and similar factors also play a role.

The detoxification of compounds, as is true for drugs and other chemicals, depends on the chemical structure, species, strain, and environmental conditions. Alkylating agents such as methyl methanesulfonate are detoxified via an SN_2-type reaction by nucleophiles such as proteins, by water itself, and by esterases (Van Duuren, in Homburger, 1976). Oxidative reactions on the alkyl group are also possible. Aromatic rings are likely to undergo a hydroxylation reaction yielding phenolic compounds that are conjugated with glucuronic or sulfuric acid, and then excreted. In addition, the metabolic introduction of hydroxy groups on the phenyl ring may increase or decrease hydrolysis of the alkyl or arylalkyl esters and decrease carcinogenic potency.

Similar considerations with respect to the detoxification reactions and mechanisms apply to the nitrogen mustard type of compound. It has been found that, in general, a mustard derived from an aromatic or heterocyclic ring system has somewhat longer half-time *in vivo* as compared to an aliphatic mustard. For this reason, the former has more systemic effects.

Reactivity toward nucleophilic reactants also controls hydrolytic destruction of lactone and similar structures built on strained ring systems. Thus, β-propiolactone is more carcinogenic than higher homologs because of its reactivity (Van Duuren, in Homburger, 1976).

In general, the rate of hydrolytic attack of these direct-acting chemicals either by water in the host or mediated, in the case of esters, by enzymes relates to carcinogenicity. Such agents are also "detoxified" readily by sulfur amino acids and peptides such as glutathione, yielding eventually the corresponding mercapturic acids. Reactions such as these produce compounds that are more toxic because of their reaction with specific life-supporting enzymes and of lower carcinogenicity than might be expected from the reactive nature of these types of carcinogens.

By definition, all direct-acting carcinogens should also be active in mutagenic assays, transformation tests, DNA repair tests, and similar rapid bioassay systems (Ames, in Hiatt *et al.*, 1977; Hollaender, 1971–1979; Williams, 1979). There is no known exception at this time. In fact, because the cell systems, especially bacterial, used for the rapid bioassays are often less likely to provide competing nucleophiles to the same extent as occurs *in vivo*, this type of agent is detected more readily in such rapid bioassay tests than *in vivo*. In other words, considering their high reactivity and electrophilic character, they are often much less carcinogenic than might be expected.

Certain chemicals which can intercalate into the DNA strands are mutagenic to phage and bacteria (Lerman, 1964). However, it seems that this is seen mainly with activated metabolites that can interact covalently with DNA. There is very weak evidence that mutagenicity stems from intercalation only, and there is no documentation that carcinogenicity in mammalian systems arises from pure intercalation without covalent binding (Van Duuren *et al.*, 1969; McCann and Ames, in Hiatt *et al.*, 1977; W. T. Speck and H. S. Rosenkranz, unpublished data).

Carcinogens Requiring Biochemical Activation: Procarcinogens

Most of the chemical carcinogens in the environment belong to this class. In contrast to direct-acting carcinogens, which are chemically reactive and therefore do not persist in the environment, procarcinogens are often chemically stable entities. They are subject to a great variety of metabolic reactions by mammalian as well as bacterial systems. In the past, biochemical reactions were considered detoxification reactions (Searle, 1976; Parke and Smith, 1977; Gorrod and Beckett, 1978). It was the search for active carcinogenic biochemical derivatives of procarcinogens that gave new insight into metabolic reactions that were not detoxification, but instead toxication or activation reactions (Weisburger and Williams, in Becker, 1975; Jerina, 1977, and Miller, 1978). Liver is the organ with the greatest capacity for metabolizing chemical carcinogens (Weisburger and Williams, 1975). Most metabolism is toward detoxified metabolites, and thus, activated metabolites often account for only a small portion of a dose of a procarcinogen. Therefore, in order to detect such active metabolites, it is necessary to account, as quantitatively as possible, for all of the metabolites of a given agent. A determination of only the main metabolites, as is often performed in studies of drug, food additive, or pesticide metabolism, would probably fail to identify the key active metabolites.

A combination of the techniques of biochemical pharmacology through *in vivo* and *in vitro* studies with the techniques of mutagenicity or DNA repair testing constitutes a most useful new technique to assess whether a given chemical is converted even in small yield to a potentially harmful electrophile by measuring whether there is any reactive product formed, detected through the techniques mentioned during *in vivo* or *in vitro* metabolism (Asher and Zervos, 1978). As such a reactive product is detected, separation techniques can be directed to isolating the reactive metabolite for the purpose of structural identification. It would appear that these procedures would be useful not only for academic purposes but in general to assess whether or not under certain circumstances a potentially harmful product is present or generated through metabolism. Since, as we noted above, the major metabolites of chemicals are often of little toxicologic consequence, it would seem that this approach would permit a decision to be made as to possible adverse effects stemming from a given material. As we will discuss, not all such indications of electrophile characteristics necessarily imply hazard, and thus, no immediate regulatory decision should be taken with materials that have apparent electrophile character. On the other hand, the presence of this property cannot be ignored and must be investigated in detail.

The metabolic fate of several carcinogens is dependent on or influenced by action of the bacterial flora in the gut (Kraybill and Mehlman, 1977; Weisburger, 1978). Cycasin, the β-glucoside of methylazoxymethanol, is split in adult animals only by the mediation of bacterial enzymes. With other agents, the bacterial flora may assume mainly a detoxifying role, by virtue of its hydrolytic and reducing capability (Copeland and Rawson, 1977). Inasmuch as diet and other conditions modify the gut microflora, the metabolism of carcinogens, drugs, and chemicals affected by the flora could thus be indirectly modulated (Wynder *et al.*, 1975; Parke and Smith, 1977).

It is outside the scope of this chapter to elaborate on all the known metabolic activation reactions for chemical carcinogens. Instead, the general principles of these activation reactions will be discussed. Most of these reactions consist of biochemical oxidation or hydroxylation, performed by endoplasmic reticulum enzyme systems (see Chap. 4 of this volume). The endoplasmic reticulum studied very extensively in liver that is rich in this component exists in virtually all tissues in all species, but in differing amounts and often with a specificity for certain substrates. It is this feature that accounts in great part for the organ-specific localization of the action of individual chemical carcinogens. Carcinogens are active at certain sites under specific conditions because of the presence of the necessary activation enzyme system.

In some cases reductive enzymes yield activated intermediates as, for example, the conversion of nitroaryl or nitroheterocyclic compounds to the corresponding hydroxylamino derivatives. Thus, the active intermediate of 4-nitroquinoline N-oxide is the corresponding 4-hydroxylamino derivative. In other cases, the active intermediate from such a transport form by enzymic systems in certain target organs, as for example the urinary bladder. In others yet, enzymes such as an alcohol dehydrogenase appear involved.

Some carcinogens require a series of activation steps. For example, the aromatic amine N-2-fluorenylacetamide first undergoes N-hydroxylation (Weisburger and Williams, in Becker, 1975; Miller, 1978). The N-hydroxy metabolite is carcinogenic under conditions where the parent compound is not, as for example in guinea pigs. However, the N-hydroxy derivative itself is not chemically highly reactive as such and thus needs additional metabolic activation, which is provided by esterification of the N-hydroxy group by sulfate or acetate, or a peroxidase reaction, thus yielding a chemical with alkylating (or more accurately arylamidating) properties (Irving, in Griffin and Shaw, 1979).

When organic chemicals can be transformed to electrophilic reagents within cells, they are almost certain to act as genotoxic carcinogens. However, administration of the same chemicals in their reactive form may be innocuous, for they can react with competing nucleophilic substrates such as water or select protein or peptide end groups such as glutathione. Thus, the above-mentioned sulfate ester of N-hydroxy-N-2-fluorenylacetamide is not carcinogenic when administered to animals, simply because it undergoes rapid side reactions prior to reaching targets where it could be carcinogenic. Certain alkylating agents undergo similar reactions and are less carcinogenic than might be surmised on the basis of their structure. On the other hand, agents like alkylnitrosoureas or alkylnitrosourethan, which, because of their chemical configuration, can readily penetrate organ and cellular membranes and release the active alkyl carbonium ions inside cells by spontaneous hydrolytic mechanisms, are among the most dangerous carcinogenic chemicals. Thus, intracellular activation is a major factor in the carcinogenicity of many chemicals.

Metabolism and Mode of Action of Promoters

The most studied of promoters, which, however, thus far have a limited target, namely epithelial cells of mouse skin and subcutaneous mesenchymal tissue of rodents, belong to the class of phorbol esters. These chemicals are subject to esterases that hydrolyze the side-chain ester groups, reactions that seem associated with loss of promoting activity (Hecker, in Slaga *et al.*, 1978). Thus, the active principle may be the parent compound, although it contains reactive groupings possibly subject to biochemical change in the target tissue. The mode of action of phorbol ester in regard to the specificity of its promoting effect is not yet understood. Certain enzymes like ornithine decarboxylase are characteristically increased concomitant with the effect (Boutwell, in Slaga *et al.*, 1977). Phenols and catechols are promoters and cocarcinogens in certain tissues. Bile acids, especially secondary bile acids produced by bacterial metabolism from primary bile acids, are promoters in the large bowel. The mechanism of those effects is not understood (see Slaga *et al.*, 1977).

REACTIONS OF CHEMICAL CARCINOGENS

Historically because of the color produced in the tissue, it was noted that carcinogens of the azo dye type reacted with liver proteins in a sensitive species. The hues of the dyes bound to tissue proteins were pH dependent. As sensitive and specific techniques, mainly the use of carcinogens tagged with isotope, were established and as new knowledge on the function, isolation, and purification of other key cellular macromolecules such as various types of RNA and DNA became available, it was discovered that many chemical carcinogens could combine with these cellular entities (Ts'o and DiPaolo, 1974; Searle, 1976: Hiatt *et al.*, 1977; Miller, 1978; Weisburger, 1978).

This statement applies only to genotoxic carcinogens, which can be considered the primary causes of neoplastic disease. Nonetheless, chemicals operating through an epigenetic mechanism such as cocarcinogens and promoters do appear to play important roles in the context of several of the products associated with human cancer risks such as fractions of tobacco smoke, or promoters such as hormones or bile acids stemming from dietary conditions.

In proteins, the main reactive sites appear to be tryptophan, tyrosine, methionine, and perhaps histidine, all of which are nucleophilic reactants. In one instance reaction with glycogen has been documented. It would seem that the active carcinogenic electrophilic reactants derived from parent procarcinogens can and do interact with a variety of nucleophilic macromolecules in the cell. Additional information is needed to relate these documented chemical interactions to the carcinogenic process.

As with protein, RNA is also a target for electrophilic reactants. Interactions have been demonstrated with transfer RNA, messenger RNA, and ribosomal RNA. Such interactions are very likely involved in the inhibition of protein synthesis that occurs with toxic doses of carcinogens.

The ability of carcinogens to interact with DNA was disputed in the early years when protein interactions were of principal interest. However, the demonstration of the interaction of polycyclic aromatic hydrocarbons with DNA by Brookes, Lawley, Heidelberger, Sims, and Gelboin (see Ts'o and DiPaolo, 1974) opened this area of investigation. Subsequently numerous carcinogens of the electrophilic reactant type have been found to bind to DNA. Current interest has turned to examination of the bases to which carcinogens bind and the nature of the adducts. The overall chemistry of some of these interactions has been established (Pegg, 1977). For example, methyl carbonium ions from several sources, like the direct-acting alkylating agent methyl methanesulfonate, from the nitrosourea methylnitrosourea, from the procarcinogen nitrosamine dimethylnitrosamine, or from the hydrazine 1,2-dimethylhydrazine, all alkylate guanylic acid in DNA at several positions (Pegg and Hui, 1978). According to current views, the interaction at the 0-6 position appears associated with carcinogenicity. However, alkylation at N-7 occurs often to a greater extent with the methyl carbonium ions but does not seem to relate to carcinogenesis (Magee *et al.*, in Searle, 1976). With aflatoxin B_1 through the metabolically produced epoxide, reaction at N-7 seems relevant. With the metabolite derived from *N*-2-fluorenylacetamide, interaction is at C-8. With the polycyclic aromatic hydrocarbon benzo(a)pyrene, through its activated form, the 7,8-dihydrodiol-9,10-epoxide, the reaction is through the 10 carbon of the benzo(a)pyrene metabolite to the 2-amino position in guanylic acid (Gelboin and Ts'o, 1978). In addition, there are minor interactions with the other purines and pyrimidines in DNA.

Thus, considerable knowledge has accrued on the interaction with DNA of those carcinogens that we have termed genotoxic.

However, the altered steric and chemical properties of DNA with covalently bound carcinogen adducts in relation to transcription of the genetic code into phenotypic characteristics as well as the duplication of this DNA are not known. Nonetheless, it seems fairly certain that it is these covalently bound carcinogen products that result in mutagenicity and carcinogenicity.

MODIFYING FACTORS IN CHEMICAL CARCINOGENESIS

A number of studies involving mixtures of chemical carcinogens have indicated that when these agents act on the same target organ, the effects are additive and sometime synergistic (Lee and Kotin, 1972; Odashima et al., 1975; Preussmann, 1975, Schmähl, et al., 1977). For example, administration of a carcinogenic azo dye and diethylnitrosamine, both of which affect the liver, results in an increased incidence of liver tumors. On the other hand, agents that have distinct organ specificity often exert their carcinogenic effect independently. The tumor incidence in the various target organs is the same as it is in when the two agents are administered separately. The latent period, too, is the same provided it is similar for both agents. For example, a carcinogenic azo dye that affects the liver and 4-dimethylaminostilbene, which affects the ear duct, do not interact. When given jointly, both types of tumors are seen. In some cases of human cancer, multiple primary neoplasms coexist, suggesting that the patients may have been exposed to effective dosages of distinct carcinogens with separate organotropic effect.

More detailed and realistic studies of such interactions between carcinogens are needed in order to complement our knowledge and to relate experimental findings to the complexity of the environment with potential carcinogenic implications for man.

There are also noncarcinogenic chemicals that augment, sometimes very appreciably, the effect of a primary carcinogen. Best studied along these lines are the cocarcinogens (see above). Some 30 years ago, it was found by Shear and by Berenblum and Shubik that a number of irritant substances, for example, croton oil applied to the skin of mice, when administered subsequent to a small dose of a carcinogenic polycyclic aromatic hydrocarbon, quickly led to extensive tumor formation. Conditions could be devised whereby minimal tumor induction was seen, within the confines of the experiment, when either the polycyclic hydrocarbon alone or the croton oil treatment alone was applied—hence, the name cocarcinogenesis or two-stage carcinogenesis. Application of the polycyclic aromatic hydrocarbon was referred to as initiation and the subsequent treatment with croton oil was called promotion. Initiation was visualized as the interaction of a primary carcinogen, like benzo(a)-pyrene or 3-methylcholanthrene, with specific receptors of the cells, leading to largely irreversible changes. The promotion step was thought to consist of an enhanced growth and development of such abnormal cells. The main reason for the concept that initiation was irreversible was that weeks, months, even a year could elapse between the application of the primary carcinogen and the subsequent treatment with the cocarcinogen leading to tumor formation (Homburger, 1976; Van Duuren et al., 1978b; Berenblum, in Griffin and Shaw, 1979).

Promotion, on the other hand, involves chiefly the growth and development of so-called dormant or latent tumor cells, resulting from the interaction of the primary carcinogen and specific receptors in susceptible cells, the initiation step (Slaga et al., 1977). Promotion could be described as any situation yielding an increased growth rate of dormant cells, especially if this condition singled out preferentially the development of the tumor cells. The active principle of croton oil, in the form of phorbol esters, may act as such a promoter with respect to mouse skin, although normal cells are not completely immune to their effect. Sulfur, sulfur dioxide, aldehydes, phenols, sulfur compounds, and, above all, dodecane represent other examples of stimulators of the effect of polycyclic aromatic hydrocarbons and other carcinogens for mouse skin (Slaga et al., 1977). In some of these instances it is not certain whether the dramatic increase in carcinogenicity results from a typical promoting effect or from a more effective action of the primary carcinogen given simultaneously, rather than sequentially. Such sizable enhancing effects may account for the carcinogenicity of petroleum products, cutting oils, and the like, which may be much greater than might be suspected from their content of carcinogenic polycyclic aromatic hydrocarbons.

The initiation-promotion scheme has been most fruitful in mechanistic studies and has permitted investigators to follow a primary carcinogenic event including the early transformed tumor cells or latent tumor cells, and the subsequent steps during which such cells are stimulated to grow. Obviously, the underlying mechanisms are different.

By definition, cocarcinogens modify the effectiveness of a carcinogen present at the same time whereas promotion occurs subsequent to the exposure to a carcinogen. Current views are that promotion selectively or generally increases duplication of transformed cells. Cocarcinogens can act likewise. However, they can also modify the metabolism of a carcinogen either by increasing the production of the active ultimate carcinogen, or by decreasing the effectiveness of detoxification reactions, or by inhibiting DNA repair.

In the last few years, these theoretic models for cocarcinogenesis and promotion have assumed practical importance.

Alcohol is an excellent promoting agent or cocarcinogen (see Fraumeni, 1975). Whereas individuals who smoke cigarettes rarely develop cancer in the upper GI tract or the oral cavity, people who both smoke cigarettes and drink alcoholic beverages have a seriously increased risk in those sites. The mechanism in part stems from increased production in the oral cavity or in the esophagus of ultimate carcinogens from procarcinogens present in tobacco. In addition, alcohol may serve as an indirect promoting stimulus through mechanisms, possibly dietary deficiencies, that remain to be clarified (Wynder et al., 1975).

There seems to be good reason for the theory that lung cancer induction in man, due to excessive exposure to cigarette smoke, may be due to the presence of relatively small amounts of primary carcinogens and higher amounts of promoting agents (Wynder and Hecht, 1976; Schmeltz and Hoffman, 1977; Hoffmann et al., in Slaga et al., 1978; Van Duuren et al., 1978b). Two lines of evidence are available: (1) the known primary carcinogens present in a condensate (or tar) of cigarette smoke do not account for the potent carcinogenic effect of such condensates on mouse skin, and (2) the risk of lung cancer decreases relatively rapidly and appreciably in individuals who stop smoking. Promotion is a reversible effect, requiring the continuing presence of the promoting agent, whereas initiation by primary carcinogens does not, or at least much less so. If the effect of tobacco smoke were due only to primary carcinogens, the risk should not decrease so appreciably upon cessation of the habit.

There have been new data indicating that cancer of the large bowel, breast, prostate, ovary, and endometrium may depend to a very considerable extent not only on a carcinogenic but also on a promoting phenomenon (Slaga et al., 1978; Hiatt et al., 1977; Weisburger and Williams, 1979). The evidence stems from a consideration of the diverse incidence of these diseases in various parts of the world, as well as a study of the relevant mechanism in animal models (Magee et al., 1976; Farber et al., 1977; Copeland and Rawson, 1977). A high-risk region, like the United States, for the types of neoplasms enumerated above is typified by an intake of diets high in fat. On the other hand, the population of a country where the incidence is low usually consumes diets low in fat. Simulation of such conditions in animal models showed that animals on a high-fat diet developed, for example, colon or breast cancer in higher yield after similar doses of the appropriate carcinogens. In the case of colon cancer, it was demonstrated that the high-fat diet led to a high flow of bile acids through the gut, and it was shown independently that bile acids were good promoters in colon carcinogenesis. Humans with a high-fat diet also had higher intestinal levels of bile acids. Further evidence supporting this phenomenon came from an explanation for the lower risk of Finnish people for colon cancer, through their simultaneous intake of a high-fiber bran diet while consuming high levels of fat, in which the fiber acted as a nonspecific diluent and possibly specific absorbent of bile acids. With the endocrine-related cancers like breast or prostate, current data show that dietary fat modulates hormonal balances, which in turn act as promoters.

Thus, a better understanding of the phenomenon of promotion may provide an additional tool to reduce cancer risk, complementing procedures to lower exposure to carcinogens. This may be a fruitful approach insofar as animal experiments have indicated that with the same level of carcinogens, the incidence of cancer induced can be influenced very powerfully by changing the promotional stimulus.

Inasmuch as promotion is an epigenetic phenomenon that is highly dose dependent and also reversible, it is a system that can be utilized to reduce the risk of cancer development, even though exposure to a carcinogen may have taken place years before and hence is beyond control. Thus, a reduction of dietary fat, reducing the promoting stimulus for large bowel cancer by lowering the amount of bile acids in the gut or by increasing fiber intake, which would lower the concentration of bile acids, would be a conceptually effective means to reduce large-bowel cancer risk. Similarly, reducing the fat intake would serve to adjust the hormonal balances to that typical of a low-risk region and consequently be potentially useful in minimizing cancer development in the endocrine-sensitive target organs, such as breast or prostate.

Of further practical importance are the new findings that the essential amino acid L-tryptophan can act as a promoter, presumably through metabolites, of urinary bladder cancer (see Friedell, 1977). It would seem that saccharin and possibly cyclamate are also promoters. Therefore, these chemicals do not act as largely irreversible genotoxic carcinogens, but operate in a reversible manner and their effect is highly dose dependent. More efforts are needed to delineate the precise mode of action of these chemicals and establish no-effect levels in comparison to other promoting stimuli.

On the other hand, it is known from studies of migrants from Japan to the United States that the early events leading to gastric cancer are largely irreversible (Weisburger, 1979). Animal models involving carcinogens like methylnitrosourea or methylnitronitrosoguanidine indicate that gastric carcinogenesis is the result of interaction between carcinogen and target tissue, which is not highly subject to promoting effects although high levels of sodium chloride and of certain detergents have potentiated the effect of gastric carcinogens in animal models. The conclusion is that each type of cancer in man and each class of carcinogen have specific operational characteristics, which need to be understood as a rational basis for preventive efforts.

Another newly developed series of interactions deal with the presence in various tissues of rather complex enzyme systems concerned with DNA repair (Hiatt *et al.*, 1977; Van Lancker, 1977). One specific characteristic of carcinogens is that they react with DNA at specific sites. This reaction sets in motion the events leading to cancer unless the tissue concerned under the conditions of the exposure can repair this lesion. This series of reactions has been utilized to detect chemical carcinogens through rapid bioassay tests (Stich *et al.*, in Odashima *et al.*, 1975; Williams, 1978). In addition, DNA repair has been useful to account in part for the organospecificity of certain chemical carcinogens. For example, methylnitrosourea reacts readily with DNA of the kidney, liver, and brain. However, the liver can repair the lesion readily, the kidney somewhat less readily, but the brain does so with difficulty. This is why under certain experimental conditions methylnitrosourea induces brain cancer in rodents (Rajewsky *et al.*, in Hiatt *et al.*, 1977). More research hopefully will delineate the relevance of DNA repair in carcinogenesis and pinpoint further means of controlling cancer.

Experimental situations have also been documented where the effect of chemical carcinogens was decreased by antagonistic influences (Homburger, 1976; Wattenberg, 1978). The joint administration of a chemical carcinogen and a structurally analogous noncarcinogenic chemical has sometimes resulted in inhibitory effects, especially if the noncarcinogenic analog was present in large excess. For example, non- or weakly carcinogenic, partially hydrogenated polycyclic hydrocarbons have reduced the carcinogenicity of the fully aromatic structure. A 30 molar excess of acetanilide reduced the carcinogenicity of N-2-fluorenylacetamide on the liver and several other target organs in several species. The underlying mechanisms may be different in these cases.

The mechanism accounting for such antagonistic effects could involve (1) competitive displacement at the level of the target, (2) variation in the effectiveness of an activating enzyme system, or (3) a more general systemic effect leading to altered detoxification mechanisms or changed receptor ratios.

The carcinogenic effect of a given chemical is dependent on the rate of metabolism of the chemical. This metabolic rate can be influenced by environmental or host-controlled factors, other carcinogens, or noncarcinogenic agents (Gelboin and Ts'o, 1978).

A variation of these factors will alter the ratio of activated metabolite over detoxified metabolites. Obviously an increase in this ratio is likely to yield a picture of increased or synergistic effect; a decrease, one of reduced or antagonistic action. Most such studies have dealt with an evaluation of effects at the level of liver microsomal enzymes, but some dealt with effects on organs such as skin, lung, breast, and intestinal tract, whereas others experimented with carcinogens in tissue culture.

In the last few years our understanding of the operation of microsomal enzymes has increased considerably, in connection with the study not only of the metabolism of chemical carcinogens, but of drugs and exogenous chemicals generally. A number of recent reviews deal with these complex reaction systems (Hathaway, 1977; Hiatt *et al.*, 1977; Jerina, 1977; Parke and Smith, 1977; Gelboin and Ts'o, 1978; Gorrod and Becker, 1978). In general, agents that augment the effectiveness of microsomal enzymes lead to increased detoxification reactions and thus often, but not always, decrease carcinogenicity.

The pioneering experiment of Conney, Miller, and Miller (see Miller, 1978) demonstrated that dietary 3-methylcholanthrene increased the level of an enzyme system concerned with reduction of the azo link in the carcinogenic dyestuff 4-dimethylaminoazobenzene giving noncarcinogenic split products and thus explained the inhibition of the carcinogenicity of the dye by the hydrocarbon. Indeed, it is this experiment that gave insight into the relationship between chemicals capable of increasing the levels of such enzyme systems and the subsequent physiologic effects. It was this experiment in which one carcinogen, 3-methylcholanthrene, was found to inhibit the effect of another carcinogen, 4-dimethylaminoazobenzene, which laid the foundation for the entire field of enzyme induction in relation to drug metabolism.

Since that time numerous other chemicals such as DDT, BHT, phenobarbital, and benzoflavones were found to induce enzymes and thus reduce the carcinogenicity of these azo dyes and similar carcinogens (Wattenberg, 1978). Unfortunately, many of these studies have been performed only in rats; experimentation with other species is needed since species differences have already been reported. For example, it was found that administration of 3-methylcholanthrene decreased the ratio of N-hydroxy-N-2-fluorenylacetamide, an activated carcinogenic intermediate derived from N-2-fluorenylacetamide, to detoxification metabolites in the rat, but increased the ratio in the hamster. Parallel to these findings are the biologic and toxicologic findings that in the rat 3-methylcholanthrene reduces the carcinogenicity of N-2-fluorenylacetamide, but increases it in the hamster (Weisburger, 1978).

A major element for the reduced carcinogenicity is the increased detoxification through conjugation reactions with formation of glucuronides, sulfates, or glutathione conjugates. Peraino (*loc. cit.*) made the important observation that if DDT, phenobarbital, or compounds with similar properties are administered not at the same time as a carcinogen, but subsequently, there is not a decreased carcinogenic effect but an increase. These chemicals and drugs thus act as promoters. The exact mechanism is not yet understood, but it may depend on an increased duplication of transformed cells.

Man, in all probability, reacts to carcinogens in a manner not too different from either the rat or the hamster. In connection with observations on differences in drug reactions, the noted pharmacologist Brodie in 1964 raised the question "which man?" when discussing man's response to drugs. Man is genetically heterogeneous and lives under varied environmental conditions. Thus, a certain level of carcinogenic and indeed also toxic hazards will affect some men some of the time, depending on a large number of variables (Weisburger and Williams, 1979).

Chemical-Viral Interactions

Although sufficient human data have not yet been accumulated, there is excellent experimental evidence that some types of tumors in animals have a viral origin, e.g., certain leukemias, lymphomas, and mammary tumors in mice (Becker, 1975; Hiatt *et al.*, 1977). An antecedent viral hepatitis had been postulated to account for the occurrence of liver cancer in man in tropical countries (Higginson, 1977). With the development of alternatives such as consumption of foodstuffs contaminated with mycotoxins or Senecio alkaloids, the viral hypothesis as single factor has diminished in importance. However, studies still underway have recently reintroduced the concept of a possible viral-chemical interaction in connection with studies on the Australia or hepatitis B antigen, which is often found associated with patients with liver cancer (see Trichopoulos *et al.*, 1978).

Some experiments have permitted the conclusion that an antecedent or existing viral infection with specific nononcogenic viruses may potentiate the effect of chemical carcinogens (Nieburgs, 1978). There are a number of possible explanations for such interactions. One concept is that cells or tissues containing viruses may have greater sensitivity, perhaps because their rate of cell multiplication is altered or their cellular receptors are more exposed. Another possible explanation is that cells containing viruses have an altered metabolic capability and hence different metabolic activation potential as far as the carcinogen is concerned. Another theory is that chemical carcinogens act by derepressing latent viral elements in cells. Still another concept is that cancer is the result of derepressing of elements of ceullular genetic information characteristic of neoplasia. From the pragmatic point of view of evaluating the possible carcinogenic risk attached to environmental chemicals, the possible augmenting action of viral elements in animal and even in man (benzene?) needs to be considered.

In animal models, specific viruses have been demonstrated to induce leukemias, lymphomas, or sarcomas, but in humans the participation of viruses in these types of cancers has not yet been made (Becker, 1975; Hiatt *et al.*, 1977). Another question is whether chemicals that under some conditions can induce leukemia in animals or in man operate by activating through unknown mechanisms a viral carcinogen. This is a serious possibility. Indeed, drugs with immunosuppressive properties induce in animals and in man mainly these kinds of neoplasms, namely, leukemias, lymphomas, or sarcomas. In an animal model, spontaneous and chemically induced leukemias have been inhibited through a form of vaccination, an interesting and possibly fruitful lead (Pottathil *et al.*, 1978).

Environmental Factors

Diet. Developments in the field of azo dye carcinogenesis drew attention many years ago to the fact that diet can modify the effectiveness of chemical carcinogens. Rats fed a rice diet, low in protein and riboflavin, were highly sensitive to liver tumor formation when treated with 4-dimethylaminoazobenzene, but a diet containing adequate amounts of protein and vitamin B_2 reduced and in some cases prevented the carcinogenic effect. Miller and Mueller (see Searle, 1976; Miller, 1978) found that this diet-mediated change in carcinogenicity stemmed from an alteration in the level of azo dye reductase, which in turn altered the effective dosage of the carcinogen.

There are other more recent examples in which diet exerted an effect on the outcome of the carcinogenic process by controlling the effectiveness of enzymes concerned with the activation versus detoxification of the chemical carcinogens (Newberne, 1976). For example, administration of the potent liver carcinogen dimethylnitrosamine to rats on a protein-free diet has virtually no effect on the liver, mainly because of a severe decrease of microsomal enzymes in this organ (Magee *et al.*, in Searle, 1976). However, rats so treated exhibit tumors in the kidneys after a fairly long latent period. The acute toxicity of the mycotoxin aflatoxin B_1 is considerably reduced when rats are on a low-lipotrope diet, but the carcinogenicity to the liver is enhanced (Newberne, 1976).

Tumor induction in the mammary gland of rats is decreased when the animals are fed fat-restricted diets, but augmented on high-fat diets (see Wynder *et al.*, 1975). Skin tumor formation in mice likewise is decreased when the food intake is low. In this instance, it has been demonstrated that the degree of tumor formation was dependent on the amount of food intake during the promoting phase. When the animals were placed on a restricted food intake during the application of the primary carcinogen, but were fed *ad libitum* during the promotion phase, the tumor incidence was identical to that seen in well-fed control animals. On the other hand, normal food intake during initiation by carcinogen, followed by diet restriction during the promotion phase, reduced tumor incidence, pointing clearly to the fact that in this instance the developmental phases of cancer cells are inhibted by lower food intake.

There are similar data from human populations with apparently lower cancer incidence, when on restricted diets. Environmental factors must also be taken into account, however.

Specific Dietary Elements. *Protein.* Most rodent diets contain 18 to 25 percent protein. As the protein content increases above 50 percent, there appears to be a voluntary reduction in the number of total calories consumed. Thus, in situations where caloric intake influences tumor induction, animals fed diets with elevated protein levels have been found to have fewer tumors. A diet restricted in protein, on the other hand, has a lesser effect. In fact, in the case of the carcinogenic azo dyes mentioned earlier, a protein-restricted diet appears to increase the relative efficiency of the carcinogen. Diets completely devoid of protein, which can be administered only for limited periods of time, may decrease the effectiveness of certain carcinogens in specific target organs. Protein-restricted diets may result in a significant decrease in the number of enzymes bound to the endoplasmic reticulum and a subsequent decrease in the biochemical activation of carcinogens.

Fats. With several types of chemical carcinogens, in particular those affecting the endocrine-sensitive organs like the breast or the colon, the effectiveness of the carcinogen can be increased appreciably by a high-fat diet. As discussed previously, these considerations also appear to hold in man (Weisburger and Williams, 1979). The relevant mechanisms appear identical; namely, they depend on increased promotion (see Promoters). This factor appears quite important in providing rational approaches to the prevention of important types of human cancer.

Carbohydrates and Starches. The starches contained in most commercial experimental diets exert relatively little influence on tumor induction. Semipurified diets, on the other hand, containing highly soluble carbohydrates such as glucose and sucrose,

may enhance absorption of a carcinogen fed in the diet, thus enhancing toxicity. In humans, the risk of colon cancer has been related to low-residue, highly digestible foods, in contrast to diets high in roughage and residues (Burkitt and Trowell, 1975; Weisburger, 1979).

Animal experiments have confirmed that certain fibers like bran or pectin reduce the carcinogenicity of certain colon carcinogens. With many other types of carcinogens a difference is seen when animals are placed on a low-residue semipurified diet, compared to a diet composed of natural foodstuffs. In most instances, the carcinogen is somewhat less effective on the latter diets, although there are exceptions, for reasons that are not clear.

Micronutrients. A number of micronutrients, such as specific vitamins and minerals, are essential cofactors for the effective operation of many key enzymes (Schrauzer, 1978). Thus, a deficiency in specific micronutrients would obviously have an effect on the physiology of the host, and on the pharmacologic and toxicologic responses to exogenous agents, including carcinogens. The effect of riboflavin on the carcinogenicity of azo dyes in the rat liver has already been discussed. In addition, riboflavin appears to be involved in tumor induction processes at other sites by a mechanism that has not yet been determined.

Vitamin A has been implicated in the differentiation of epithelial tissues. Saffiotti and coworkers, DeLuca and associates, Bjelke, and Cone and Nettesheim (see Newberne, 1976) have reported that vitamin A levels may affect the induction of pulmonary tumors in rodent systems or in man. The mycotoxin aflatoxin B_1, which usually induces liver cancer in rats, has also caused colon cancer when animals were fed a diet low in vitamin A. Under other conditions of low intake of aflatoxin B_1, colon cancer was seen even with chow diets. Borderline vitamin A deficiency appears to have a potentiating effect in smokers with respect to lung cancer. There are additional data that other types of human cancer such as cancer of the cervix and of the lung arise somewhat more frequently in people with limited vitamin A levels. Recently, vitamin A analogs, namely retinoic acid derivatives, have been shown to inhibit carcinogenesis in several target organs (Sporn, 1976).

Low-lipotrope diets, also high in fat, exhibit a potentiating effect in carcinogenesis with certain liver carcinogens through mechanisms not entirely worked out but that would appear to be related to a deficiency of specific essential nutrients rather than the effect of the high fat level. Clearly more data are necessary in order to assess the involvement of particular cofactors in tumor induction in epithelial tissues.

Vitamin E and other synthetic antioxidants, such as butylated hydroxytoluene, propyl gallate, and ethoxyquin, have modified the tumor induction with certain carcinogens in a number of target organs (Wattenberg, 1978). In some cases, the effect was noted at low levels of these agents, where it can be assumed that the action hinged on their antioxidant properties. Selenium derivatives, together with α-tocopherol, also appeared to decrease tumor incidence (Jannsson *et al.*, in Schrauzer, 1978). In some other cases when high levels of the antioxidants were administered, the effect was traced directly to modification of enzyme levels, mainly in the liver, which led to changes in the activation and detoxification of metabolites of carcinogens.

Most semipurified diets and foods composed of natural ingredients contain adequate amounts of minerals. There is a paucity of information concerning the specific involvement of mineral elements in tumor induction processes. Magnesium-free diets have been reported to lead to leukemia in certain strains of rats. Iodine-deficient diets have led to thyroid tumors as a result of the disturbance of homeostatic equilibrium between pituitary and thyroid.

Dietary elements, particularly micronutrients such as vitamins A, E, and B, may provide some degree of protection against carcinogenic materials. As was discussed above, vitamin C and E prevent the formation of nitrosamines and nitrosamides and thus reduce or eliminate cancer risk at various target organs like the liver and upper gastrointestinal and respiratory tract (Weisburger, 1979). Further study of the mechanism of action of dietary factors may suggest means of lowering the prevalence of certain types of cancers in man.

Host-Controlled Factors

Species and Strains. Studies of chemical carcinogens can be carried out only in model animal systems although a few pioneers did some self-experimentation. The question has often been asked as to how animal carcinogenicity data can be extrapolated to man. *Homo sapiens*, unlike most experimental species, is genetically heterogeneous. In addition, there are wide variations in environment, diet, and life-style. Thus, one would not expect a uniform response to exogenous agents such as carcinogens. In pharmacology and medicine, it is a well-accepted fact that patients need to be considered as individuals when prescribing dosages of drugs. Animal systems, on the other hand, can be controlled much more effectively. Indeed, highly inbred strains of genetically uniform rodents, mice, rats, and hamsters are available. Animals can be housed under standard conditions, fed uniform purified diets, and, in essence, treated identically. Thus, it can be expected that response to carcinogens would be more uniform in experimental animals than in man. Nonetheless, cancer induction processes are very complex (Weisburger and Williams, 1979). Many chemical carcinogens need biochemical activation and undergo biochemical detoxification and metabolism. The active form attacks specific molecular and cellular receptors in some cells at a given stage of the mitotic cycle. Repair processes operate to limit key alterations. Latent tumor cells must reproduce, a function that can be affected considerably by host factors. All of these steps are, of course, strain and species dependent, and thus, it can be expected that the response to a given chemical carcinogen is a function of strain and species. Men are not uniform, and it is probably true that some men will respond some of the time to a given carcinogenic challenge. One of the key elements in the response of any species, including man, would appear to be the biochemical potential in activating or deactivating exogenous carcinogens. Promoting stimuli, stemming from elements such as the biosynthesis of cholesterol and bile acids or hormonal balances, of immune competence, and of endogenous viral flora, also are distinct as a function of species and strains.

Age. This is an important variable in studies on carcinogenesis (Homburger, 1976). This fact may well be true also in man. Currently existing data on lung cancer incidence as a function of number of cigarettes smoked per day indicate that the incidence is lower in Japan than in the United States; the habit of chronic smoking begins later in Japan than in the United States. Conversely, in occupational or other pursuits where exposure to chemical carcinogens is possible, or even unavoidable, selection of older personnel would serve to minimize the risk. There are actually two reasons for this policy. One, as noted, is that older individuals are probably less sensitive, and second, in view of the sometimes long latent period required for tumor development, their age would preclude that eventuality from occurring.

Some carcinogens cross the placental barrier. In certain cases, the enzyme system necessary to produce activated metabolites is sufficiently developed in the fetus to give adequate level of the required intermediates. In others, the mother may generate the active intermediate in a transportable form, which is released in the fetus by select enzyme systems. Certain types of carcinogens that do not require enzymes to develop the reactive ultimate carcinogen, like alkylnitrosoureas, are sometimes extremely effective transplacentally. However, for reasons that are not yet clear, methylnitrosourea is much less effective than the ethyl homolog as a transplacental carcinogen.

The method of experimental transplacental carcinogenesis has been developed by several investigators, including Shabad, DiPaolo, and Pienta, as a means of detecting possible environmental carcinogens in a simplified procedure (Mehlman *et al.*, 1976, 1977). The agent is given to a pregnant female and the fetuses are explanted into tissue culture. With some carcinogens abnormal transformed tumor cells are visualized after a short period of time. This interesting technique has broad potential usefulness and needs further exploration.

It is quite probable that cancers occurring in childhood are the result of transplacental exposure. An important series of cases were discovered where young prepubertal girls exhibited a rare form of vaginal cancer that was traced to the fact that their mothers had been treated with sizable doses of the hormone diethylstilbestrol in order to maintain a successful pregnancy (Herbst, in Hiatt, 1977).

Newborn animals also exhibit higher sensitivity to certain carcinogens than older animals. Thus, injection of newborn mice with any one of a number of chemical carcinogens results in tumors, primarily of the liver and lung, approximately a year after the administration of the carcinogen. Carcinogens may be effective when administered to young animals but ineffective when administered to older animals. For example, the polycyclic aromatic hydrocarbons do not usually induce liver cancer when administered to young adult mice or rats, but do so when given to newborn animals. Likewise, aflatoxin B_1 fails to induce liver tumors in mice when administered after weaning, but does induce tumors when given at birth. Hamsters, too, appear to be more sensitive to aflatoxin B_1 at birth than after weaning but the difference in sensitivity is not as great as that in rats (Homburger *et al.*, 1978; see Homburger, 1976).

Many investigators utilize weanling animals in experiments with chemical carcinogens. Such animals are quite sensitive, and with agents of low carcinogenicity requiring a long latent period for tumor development, it is useful to begin with animals as young as possible. However, in some instances weanling animals are considerably more sensitive to the toxic effect of an agent. Hence, failure to adjust dosages upward as the animal develops the capability of tolerating higher levels may result in fewer tumors and a longer experimental period.

Sex and Endocrine Balance. Epidemiologic data on human cancer incidence show that some types of cancer occur more frequently in males than in females, and vice versa (Fraumeni, 1975; American Cancer Society, 1979). In experimental animals, likewise, some chemical carcinogens affecting specific target organs appear to induce cancer more frequently in one than the other sex, even when a nonendocrine organ is involved. For example, N-2-fluorenylacetamide induces liver cancer primarily in male rats although females of certain strains are not entirely resistant (Miller, 1978; Weisburger, 1978). On the other hand, o-aminoazotoluene is somewhat more active in female mice than in males in leading to liver cancer. Dimethyl- or diethylnitrosamine produces liver cancer often, but not always, with similar efficiency in males and females; a variety of carcinogens cause pulmonary tumors in male and female mice with equal frequency (Shimkin

and Stoner, 1975). In nonendocrine target organs the sex-linked effectiveness of a given carcinogen stems mostly from a sex-dependent activity of enzyme systems necessary for the conversion of a procarcinogen to the active ultimate carcinogen. For example, in the case of N-2-fluorenylacetamide-induced liver cancer in males, the key difference resides in the levels of the enzyme sulfotransferase giving rise to the active sulfate ester of N-hydroxide-N-2-fluorenylacetamide (Miller, 1978). Levels of enzyme are six to eight times higher in male than in female rats. Alternatively, a sex difference in carcinogenic susceptibility may stem from varying ratios of detoxification enzymes. For example, for some substrates glucosiduronic acid formation is higher in females than in males (Parke and Smith, 1977).

The endocrine system is important in relation to tumor growth in endocrine-sensitive tissues such as the gonads, adrenals, prostate, and breast (Homburger, 1976; Hiatt *et al.*, 1977; Weisburger and Williams, 1979). Also, alteration in the hormonal balance, e.g., by gonadectomy or hypophysectomy, may affect the carcinogenic process even in nonendocrine organs if endocrine-sensitive enzyme systems are required for activation or detoxification of the carcinogen or for the growth and development of the tumor, as noted above. In any case, the situation is quite complex, for endocrine glands and their target organs are interconnected by delicately balanced feedback pathways. Alteration in one hormone level usually leads to repercussions in the entire system, yielding a new equilibrium point. In most species, and particularly in females, regular and periodic oscillations occur, corresponding to the normal estrus cycle. Age, in turn, plays a role in the endocrine responsiveness. Thus, superimposition of an exogenous toxicant with an affinity for any of the endocrine-susceptible organs may also indirectly affect other organs in the body. Addition of a hormone may have an even more complex action. The long-term effect of chemicals on the endocrine balance and the periodicity of the system must also be considered. Hormones such as those contained in the oral contraceptives may have an entirely different action in animals like rodents or dogs with an estrus cycle quite unlike that of the human female. It has been shown that continuous administration of hormonally active preparations to rodents results often in the development of tumors, especially in the breast. This may not necessarily constitute a carcinogenic risk for sexually mature human females receiving the same preparation in low dosages on a rhythmic basis tailored to the normal menstrual cycle. In fact, such treatment may serve to maintain the individual in hormonal balance and reduce the risk of cancer development in endocrine-responsive organs. On the other hand, exposure of newborn or immature animals, humans, or fetuses to an exogenous agent may permanently affect the differentiation of endocrine organs and thus lead to cancer later in life due to either hormonal imbalance or aberrant tissue receptor response to existing hormones (Weisburger and Williams, 1979). Such may have been the case of young, pubertal girls, children of mothers given large doses of the estrogenic drug diethylstilbestrol during pregnancy, and thus affecting the fetus.

Pharmacologic and Toxicologic Implications of Carcinogenesis: Dose-Response and Zero Tolerance

Extensive experimentation with a variety of chemical carcinogens, including polycyclic aromatic hydrocarbons, aromatic amine derivatives, alkylating drugs, and alkylnitrosamines, has established the fact that, as is the case with other pharmacologic agents, the response to chemical carcinogens is dose dependent (Eckhardt, 1959; Druckrey, in Truhaut, 1967; International Symposium, 1976; Mehlman et al., 1976; Mehlman et al., 1977; Cederlöf et al., 1978; Cranmer et al., 1978; Hoel and Rall, 1978; Leonard, 1978; Whittemore, 1978; Weisburger and Williams, 1979).

There is, however, one way in which chemical carcinogens are quite distinct from ordinary pharmacologic agents. Drugs and indeed toxic chemicals exert their action rapidly, almost instantaneously. As the drug ingested is metabolized and excreted, the effect diminishes to the vanishing point, and in virtually all instances there is no residual action, with the possible exception of agents affecting the immune system or causing allergies. In general, subsequent exposures act anew in the same manner without any long-lasting effects. In contrast, while the onset of the interaction between a chemical carcinogen and specific tissues is fundamentally similar, in that the agent undergoes metabolism as do other drugs, the key, often biochemically activated, ultimate carcinogen reacts with specific tissue receptors and leaves a long-lasting imprint in such receptors. Thus, with chemical carcinogens, a given dose results in a permanent alteration of a certain number of cells in specific tissues. Subsequent dosages add to such a change. After a sufficient number of such altered cell systems have been produced, their subsequent multiplication results in a visible neoplastic area. Because the metabolic capability varies with the carcinogen and the tissue in which it exerts its action, the time required to produce a detectable tumor will vary. Thus, time as well as dose is a factor in

assessing properties of chemical carcinogens as compared to drugs. It is in this way that carcinogens differ from ordinary toxic agents. A number of small doses give no overt signal of their presence and in due time can yield tumors within the life-span of a host. With noncarcinogens such low dosages of a toxic agent would be completely innocuous.

In contrast, therefore, to the effect of pharmacologic agents generally, carcinogens are distinct insofar as a same total dose when administered as smaller doses over a longer period of time can actually be more effective in leading to cancer than when given as fewer individual larger doses in a short time. In the extreme, several chemicals that are potent carcinogens when administered chronically are not active at all when given acutely as a single large dose. There are, however, carcinogens that can induce cancer with a single dose.

These concepts have been established with several of the well-known classes of powerful, highly active carcinogens. There have been relatively few studies on the effect of dose rate or even dose-response with weaker carcinogens such as safrole, acetamide, or o-toluidine. Shimkin et al. (1966, see Shimkin and Stoner, 1975) examined the potential of inducing pulmonary tumors in mice with alkylating drugs of diverse structures. It was found that the strongly carcinogenic drugs were active over a broad dose range. However, there were some that gave evidence of some carcinogenicity only at the highest but not lower dose levels. Current studies, involving larger numbers of animals, on the dose-responses to several carcinogens will obviously assist in yielding more information on the shape of the dose-response curve at low levels of carcinogens (Cornfield, 1977; Hiatt et al., 1977; Cranmer et al., 1978; Scherer and Emmelot, in Griffin and Shaw, 1979; Littlefield et al., 1979).

Nonetheless, the capability of analytic chemists to measure accurately at the parts-per-billion and even the parts-per-trillion level has led to the detection in our food chain of amounts of this order of magnitude of several types of powerful carcinogens. Questions have been raised as to the biologic significance of these analytic findings. Several of the chemicals like nitrosopyrrolidine, found in bacon, can induce liver cancer in several species with appropriate higher dosages, of the order of ppm to parts per thousand (Preussmann, 1975; Leonard, 1978). Primary liver cancer is rarely seen in populations that consume fried bacon. Is this evidence for a no-effect level? Similar questions can be raised for the trace amounts of the hormone diethylstilbestrol, of select pesticides, and even, as discussed above, of mycotoxins. It is a controversial subject, where opinions abound and facts are few, and probably, as Weinberg (1972) has aptly stated, this socially important question is currently beyond the reach of exact science. It is transscience. It requires logical deductive reasoning, not emotional extrapolation without scientific, meaningful justification.

Animal bioassays for carcinogenicity often record only the incidence in treated groups compared to the control group. More sensitivity is obtained if the parameters for evaluation include the latent period, often considered to be the time when the experimental group has reached 50 percent tumor incidence, or the total time required for all animals to show tumors. Other relevant parameters include the dose, the dose rate, the type of tumor, and the multiplicity of tumors, which, when considered in relationship to dosage, yields a finer estimation of dose-response in comparative studies.

In a given experimental setting such dose-response relationships have been demonstrated. Two sets of data are usually obtained. With increasing dose (1) the percent tumor yield increases and (2) time required for tumor development decreases. In most cases the overall tumor yield in any specific organ is proportional to the total dose, but the speed or rate of tumor appearance is related to the amount in an individual dose (Druckrey, in Truhaut, 1967).

Reports of cancer resulting from occupational exposure to specific carcinogens have rarely yielded quantitative data, for the extent, amount, and length of exposure were rarely conducive to accurate measurement. Nonetheless, adequate data do exist in several areas to show that human cancer incidence is also proportional to dose. For example, Nelson (in Saffiotti and Wagoner, 1976; see Pasternack et al., 1977) tabulated cancer incidence in workmen exposed to vinyl chloride or to bis(chloromethyl)ether and noted a gross relationship between dose and effect. Workmen engaged in uranium or asbestos mining exhibited a risk of cancer broadly related to the length of time an individual was engaged in these particular occupations. We have recently completed a critical examination with a number of chemicals and generally found appropriate dose-response relationships. In particular, with the drug chlornaphazine, where intake was reasonably well established, there appeared to be proportionality between the percent of people with bladder cancer and the amount of drug consumed. Many of these dose-response relationships were observed in limited populations of people exposed occupationally or iatrogenically (Schmähl et al., 1977). There is sound evidence with large population groups that there is a dose dependency, for example in users of cigarettes where the risk is proportional to the number of cigarettes smoked per day, all other things being equal (Wynder and Hecht, 1976; Hoffmann et al., in Gelboin and Ts'o, 1978). In fact, the curve is concave upward, showing that higher doses are considerably more effective than smaller doses. It cannot be said that a smoker of, for example, three cigarettes per day would have zero risk, but it can be said that such a smoker has a very small risk indeed, compared to someone smoking 30 cigarettes per day, a dose range factor of only 10.

The question can then be asked whether a dose would be found with chemical carcinogens that would correspond to a no-effect level. Since, as we discussed above, the methods of chemical analysis have become ultrasensitive, this question has been the subject of much discussion.

A number of classic papers have attempted to deal with this area (Wynder, 1973). It is scientifically difficult to approach and arrive at conclusions that can be applied pragmatically to the real world in which we live. Thus far, experimental studies with carcinogens have involved relatively small groups of animals. With smaller doses, the number of animals with induced tumor decreased and the latent period lengthened to the point where spontaneous tumors were seen also in untreated control animals. A mathematical impossibility was at hand. The question is whether such data obtained in lifetime studies on groups of 50 or even 100 animals can be extrapolated to assure "safety," i.e., absence of carcinogenic risk with a given material in several hundred million people. Investigators have tried to obtain more statistically valid results by increasing the number of animals, especially at low dose levels. While such studies would have an unquestionable theoretic benefit, it seems that such a refinement still may not contribute a broader base for an assurance of safety with respect to the possible presence of low levels of chemical carcinogens in the environment. The main reason for this stems from considerations, to be discussed in more detail below, that there are additive and even synergistic effects between chemical carcinogens, or even between non-carcinogenic environmental chemicals or conditions, and a single chemical carcinogen. Man does not live in a pure environment exposed to a single agent at a time (Lee and Kotin, 1972). Different types of cancers occur in various parts of the world, induced for the most part by naturally occurring "environmental" chemicals. Hence, every effort should be made to avoid adding effective levels of synthetic chemicals to the carcinogenic burden already upon us.

Nonetheless, current views show that we do not "live in a sea of carcinogens." Specific cancers in man have specific single or multifactorial, yet defined or definable risk factors (Wynder and Gori, 1977; Weisburger and Williams, 1979). In the general public, cancer of the lung has a number of such known risk factors, whereas cancer of the breast or cancer of the colon has an entirely different set of such risk factors. It should be the aim of toxicology and oncology to define broadly these very specific risk factors so as to provide a sound, scientific basis for rational disease prevention. The pessimistic, almost hopeless statement that we live in a sea of carcinogens does not seem to be conducive, on the other hand, to such rational approaches to prevention.

Immunologic Factors

Immunologic factors have been found in some instances to alter the rate and extent of tumor development. Recent views concerning an alteration of surface antigens during transformation of normal to tumor cells would support the theory that immunologic mechanisms could have an effect on tumor cell growth rate (Baldwin, in Homburger, 1976; Stutman, in Hiatt et al., 1977). Immunologic mechanisms have been thought to play a role in the greater sensitivity of newborn animals to chemical carcinogens, for in some species and strains the immunologic competence in the newborn is either totally lacking or considerably less than that present in the adult animal. Thus, the immature immunologic system may fail to recognize a transformed tumor cell as being abnormal. There are, however, cases in which damages in immunologic competence failed to alter the latent period of tumor production.

Immunologic status appears to be more important with respect to the question whether or not metastases occur than in relation to the early effects in the carcinogenic process. Since diet under some conditions affects the immune system, this is one additional pathway whereby diet may influence cancer induction.

BIOASSAY OF CHEMICAL CARCINOGENS

The evaluation of the carcinogenicity of chemicals cannot be based exclusively on chronic testing in animals. This is because there are various modes of action of chemical carcinogens (see above and Table 6–2), which are not necessarily revealed by chronic bioassay. Of prime importance, evidence of genotoxic versus epigenetic effects (see section on Mode of Action) is not obtained in such chronic tests. Since such information is crucial to proper risk extrapolation to humans, we have proposed a *"decision point approach"* to carcinogenicity evaluation (Weis-

burger and Williams, in Asher and Zervos, 1978). In addition to establishing a framework within which the information required for risk extrapolation can be obtained, this approach also provides a guide to the elimination of unnecessary procedures in chemical and toxicologic evaluation. The decision point approach is outlined in Table 6–16.

Table 6–16. DECISION POINT APPROACH TO CARCINOGEN EVALUATION

A. Structure of chemical
B. *In vitro* short-term tests
   1. Bacterial mutagenesis
   2. DNA repair
   3. Mammalian mutagenesis
   4. Sister chromatid exchange
   5. Cell transformation
B′. Decision point: tests under A and B
C. Limited *in vivo* bioassays
   1. Skin tumor induction in mice
   2. Pulmonary tumor induction in mice
   3. Breast cancer induction in female Sprague-Dawley rats
   4. Altered foci induction in rodent liver
C′. Decision point: tests under A, B, and C
D. Chronic bioassay
E. Final evaluation: all tests

A. Structure of Chemical

For a number of reasons, the evaluation begins with a consideration of structure. Of principal importance is the fact that predictions as to whether or not a given chemical might be carcinogenic can be made with fair success within certain types of chemicals (Arcos, 1978; Ashby, 1978; Asher and Zervos, 1978; Cramer et al., 1978; Hoel and Rall, 1978; Van Duuren, in Nieburgs, 1978). This is particularly true in the case of chemicals of a type that includes known carcinogens. For example, within the large series of azo dyes, Miller and Miller, as well as Yoshida, Kinosita, Druckrey, and Schmähl, have provided data on carcinogenicity versus structure. Carcinogens of this type are usually substituted with amino groups in a para position, whereas inclusion of relatively polar substituents like sulfonic acid abolishes carcinogenicity. On the basis of this knowledge alone, for example, it is not likely that pure FD and C Red #2 or FD and C Red #40, which bear such deactivation substituents on both sides of the azo bond (Table 6–8), would be carcinogenic. On the other hand, more complex tetrazo dyes that include a potentially carcinogenic benzidine residue, available on reduction, are carcinogenic. Within the arylamine type of chemicals, ortho-substituted (next to the vicinal ring) polynuclear arylamines like 1-naphthyl-amine or 1-fluorenylamine are not carcinogenic whereas the 2-isomers are powerfully active in rodents, and 2-naphthylamine also in man. This is because the 1-isomers do not undergo to a significant extent a required metabolic activation reaction, namely, N-hydroxylation. Also, the guinea pig, in contrast to rodents or man, does not have the necessary enzymes to carry out this key step, N-hydroxylation, even with the 2-isomers, and therefore the arylamines so far tested are not carcinogenic in this species. Thus, potential metabolites must also be given con-sideration.

Information on structure and metabolism pro-vides a guide to the selection among limited bio-assays at stage C and, as more information accrues, may eventually contribute to selection of specific short-term tests at stage B.

B. In Vitro *Short-Term Tests*

The status of *in vitro* assays is that no indi-vidual test that has been studied adequately has detected all carcinogens tested. Thus, from this practical consideration alone a battery of tests is desirable. However, the importance of a battery becomes obvious upon consideration of the com-plexity of metabolism and mechanism of action of chemical carcinogens. As indicated earlier, carcinogens can be classified as genotoxic or epigenetic. Most *in vitro* tests identify genetic effects and thus would detect only genotoxic carcinogens. If epigenetic carcinogens are to be detected, additional tests will have to be de-veloped. Known species differences in response to carcinogens can be related to a large extent (but not exclusively) to metabolism, and thus, tests with different metabolic capabilities are important.

A detailed review of aspects of short-term tests has appeared recently (Hollstein *et al.*, 1979).

A screening battery must include microbial mutagenesis tests, developed mainly by Ames, Bridges and Green, deSerres, Malling Rosen-kranz, Matsushima, and Sugimura (see Brusik in Butterworth, 1979; Hollaender, 1971–1979; Mehlman *et al.*, 1976, 1977; Montesano *et al.*, 1976), because they have been the most sensitive, effective, and readily performed screening tests thus far. In deciding what other tests to include, it is important to consider the contribution of the proposed test in terms of metabolic capability, re-liability, and biologic significance of the end point (Williams, 1979a). The bacterial mutagenesis tests require a mammalian enzyme preparation to provide for metabolism of procarcinogens, and hence, any test that is dependent on an enzyme preparation does not expand the metabolic capability of the battery since this factor is the

limiting part of a test series. Among proposed short-term tests employing enzyme preparations are those measuring as indicators DNA fragmen-tation, inhibition of DNA synthesis, and DNA repair.

DNA repair is a specific response to DNA damage and, unlike DNA fragmentation and inhibition, cannot be attributed to toxicity (Hiatt *et al.*, 1977; Van Lancker, 1977; Williams, 1979b). Therefore, DNA repair tests offer an end point of greater biologic significance and are recommended in preference to these other tests. Similarly, mutagenesis of mammalian cells is a definitive end point like bacterial mutagenesis and therefore is also recommended. Sister chromatid exchange is included because of its sensitivity and ease and objectivity of measure-ment, even though its significance is not yet fully understood. Cell transformation is included because this alteration is potentially the most relevant to carcinogenesis. However, much more needs to be done to clarify the significance of this end point. Other *in vitro* tests that appear not to enhance the sensitivity of a battery include degranulation of rat liver rough endoplasmic reticulum, and tetrazolium reduction (Purchase *et al.*, 1978).

1. Bacterial Mutagenesis. Valuable bacterial screening tests have been developed in the labora-tories of Ames and Rosenkranz (see Hiatt *et al.*, 1977). The Ames test measures back mutation to histidine independence of histidine mutants of *Salmonella typhimurium* and can be conducted with strains that are also repair deficient, possess abnormalities in the cell wall to make them per-meable to carcinogens, and carry an R factor-enhancing mutagenesis. Hence, these organisms are highly susceptible to mutagenesis making them sensitive indicators. The test developed by Rosenkranz and associates utilizes DNA repair-deficient *Escherichia coli* and measures their enhanced susceptibility to cell killing by carcino-gens. In this system, a chemical that interacts with DNA is more toxic to the repair-deficient strain than to wild type *E. coli* because the mutant strain cannot repair the damage. Thus, by mea-surement of relative toxicity an indication of DNA interaction is obtained. These tests are de-pendent upon mammalian enzyme preparations for metabolism of carcinogens. The capability of the Ames test to detect certain carcinogens has been enhanced by application of preincubation of the compound and the activation system with the test organism (Sugimura *et al.*, in Montesano *et al.*, 1976).

2. DNA Repair. The covalent interaction of chemicals with DNA provokes an enzymatic re-pair of the damaged regions of DNA known as excision repair. In this process an incision is made in the strand of DNA near the point of damage and an endonuclease removes the damaged region. The gap is filled by resynthesis of a patch using the opposite strand as a template and then the patch is closed by a ligase. Several of these steps could be measured as an indication of repair, but the resynthesis of the patch is most widely used to monitor repair in screening systems. Repair synthesis can be measured in a variety of ways (Williams, 1979b). Several of the definitive procedures are technically sufficiently demanding so that they have not received much attention for screening purposes. Of the two procedures that have, autoradiographic measurement of repair synthesis has the advantage over liquid scintillation counting in that it excludes cells in replicative synthesis, whereas these are part of the background with liquid scintillation counting. In addition, with liquid scintillation counting, increases in incorporation can result from changes in uptake or the pool size of thymidine without any repair occurring. Furthermore, autoradiography affords a determination of the percentage of cells in the affected population that responds. Two additional complications with most repair assays are that they require suppression of replicative DNA synthesis if continuously dividing lines are being used, and that they are dependent upon enzyme preparations for metabolic activation. Both these complications are overcome in the hepatocyte primary culture/ DNA repair assay, which uses freshly isolated, nondividing liver cells that can metabolize carcinogens and respond with DNA repair synthesis measured autoradiographically (Williams, 1979, 1980). This assay has demonstrated substantial sensitivity and reliability with activation-dependent procarcinogens. It also offers the advantages of expanded metabolic capability and biologic significance of the end point. Thus, it is a valuable addition to bacterial mutagenesis assays in a screening battery.

3. **Mammalian Mutagenesis.** The three mutational assays in mammalian cells that have been used for carcinogen screening are resistance to purine analogs, bromodeoxyuridine, and ouabain. Of these, purine analog resistance is the most widely used. In this assay, mutants lacking the purine salvage pathway enzyme hypoxanthine-guanine phosphoribosyl transferase are identified by their resistance to toxic purine analogs such as 8-azaguanine or 6-thioguanine that kill cells that utilize the analogs. This assay has the advantage over ouabain resistance in that it involves a nonessential function, unlike the membrane ATPase system involved in ouabain resistance, and thus there are no lethal mutants. Its advantage over the measurement of thymidine kinase-deficient mutants by resistance to bromodeoxy-

uridine is that the gene for hypoxanthine-guanine phosphoribosyl transferase is on the X chromosome rather than a somatic chromosome, as with thymidine kinase, and consequently the gene is more mutable because there is only one functional copy in each cell. The target cells used in purine analog resistance assays have almost all been fibroblast-like, such as the V79 line, and have displayed little ability to activate carcinogens. This deficiency has been overcome by providing exogenous metabolism mediated by either cocultivated cells (Huberman, in Montesano *et al.*, 1976) or enzyme preparations (Hsie, in Butterworth, 1979). The latter again offers no extension in metabolic capability over that used for bacterial systems. However, the use of freshly isolated hepatocytes as a feeder system (Williams, 1979a) offers additional possibilities since the metabolism of hepatocytes has been shown to be different from that of liver enzyme preparations as regards the presence of conjugating capability in the hepatocytes. Another interesting development is the finding that liver epithelial cultures can be mutated by activation-dependent carcinogens (Williams, 1979a) and may therefore provide another system with additional self-contained metabolic potential.

4. **Sister Chromatid Exchange.** Sister chromatid exchange is an exchange at one locus between the sister chromatids of a chromosome, which does not result in an alteration of overall chromosome morphology. Exchanges between sister chromatids were first demonstrated by Taylor (Wolff, 1977) using radiographic techniques to label one chromatid of each chromosome, and leave the other unlabeled. New methods for detecting exchanges have been developed from the discovery by Zakharov and Egolina (Wolff, 1977) that two rounds of DNA replication in the presence of bromodeoxyuridine resulted in the unifilar substitution of one chromatid and the bifilar substitution of its sister chromatid such that the two stained differentially with Giemsa. An extension of this approach, which is perhaps the most widely used method for differentiating sister chromatids, is the FPG or harlequin method that combines staining with a fluorescent dye plus Giemsa (Wolff, 1977). Using this technique, the observation of sister chromatid exchanges induced by chemicals is one of the quickest, easiest, and most sensitive tests for genetic damage. Sister chromatid exchanges are suspected to be due to a recombination event which may occur at the DNA replication fork, but at present, the lesions responsible for exchanges are unknown (Wolff, 1977). Therefore, in the application of this test, the possibility of a positive result with noncarcinogens must always be kept in mind. Thus far, this response has not

been validated with a very extensive array of chemicals. Kinsella and Radman (1978) have reported the interesting observation that the promoter, 12-0-tetradecanoylphorbol 13-acetate, induced exchanges and postulated that this could be a mechanism for promotion. Other possibilities exist (see Promoters), but, regardless, this finding indicates that agents which are not genotoxic, as we have defined the concept in terms of damage to DNA, may, nevertheless, ultimately produce positive effects in this system. More research on the limitations of SCE is obviously required.

5. Cell Transformation. The first reliable system for transformation of cultured mammalian cells was introduced by Sachs and associates (see Ts'o and DiPaolo, 1974; Odashima *et al.*, 1975; Hiatt *et al.*, 1977). This system utilizing hamster fibroblasts was subsequently developed into a colony assay for quantitative studies by DiPaolo and has been adapted as screening test by Pienta *et al.* In addition, a quantitative focus assay for transformation using mouse cells has been devised in the laboratory of Heidelberger. The correlation between transformation and malignancy appears to be good in these systems, but a subject of concern is frequency of induced transformation. Nevertheless, they provide an indication of the activity of chemicals which could be due to either genotoxic or epigenetic mechanisms. Also, because human cancers usually involve epithelial tissues, transformation in epithelial systems is actively being pursued (Williams, 1976; Grisham *et al.*, 1978). However, these systems have not yet been perfected for routine test approaches, since the end-point transformation is currently difficult to quantify. Another approach under development is the use of cell systems carrying oncogenic viruses as a more sensitive means of detecting transforming chemicals.

Summary of Rapid *In Vitro* Tests. The six steps (A and B, 1–5) recommended thus far provide a basis for preliminary decision making.

If clear-cut evidence of genotoxicity in more than one test has been obtained, the chemical is highly suspect. Confirmation of carcinogenicity may be sought in the limited *in vivo* bioassays without the necessity of resorting to the more costly and time-consuming chronic bioassay.

Evidence of genotoxicity in only one test must be evaluated with caution. In particular, several types of chemicals such as intercalating agents are mutagenic to bacteria, but not reliably carcinogenic. Also positive results have been obtained with synthetic phenolic compounds or natural products with phenolic structures like flavones. *In vivo*, such compounds are likely to be conjugated and excreted readily and hence not likely carcinogenic risks to man. Therefore,

evidence of only bacterial mutagenesis must be evaluated with regard to the chemical structure and metabolism.

If all the preceding test systems yield no indication of genotoxicity, the chemical may be given a low priority for further testing depending on two criteria: (1) the structure of the material and (2) the potential human exposure. If substantial human exposure is likely, careful consideration should be given to undertaking the standard chronic bioassay. The chemical structure and the properties of the material provide direct obvious guidance on the proper relevant course of action. The basis for this statement is that epigenetic carcinogens such as solid-state materials, hormones, possibly some metal ions, and promoters that are negative in tests for genotoxicity operate by complex and as-yet-poorly-understood mechanisms. Thus, it is not certain that the limited *in vivo* bioassays would yield any results with such materials. Therefore, the chronic standard bioassay is, at this time, necessary to reveal any potential activity with these agents. It is indeed urgent to develop reliable means to detect such materials readily without requiring the large investment associated with a chronic bioassay.

The testing of metal ions in rapid bioassay tests may take advantage of the recently proposed concept that such ions affect the fidelity of enzymes concerned with DNA synthesis (Loeb, in Schrauzer, 1978). Obviously, the nature of the metal ion, of which there are only a limited number, would provide the necessary insight as to the need for testing such a material further and what kind of assay would most likely reveal adverse effects.

Compounds with hormone-like properties do exist outside of the strict androgen and estrogen type of material. As noted, such chemicals are potential cancer risks mainly because they interfere with the normal, physiologic endocrine balance. More research on ways and means to test for such properties quickly is required. It is known, for example, that certain drugs lead to release of prolactin from the pituitary gland. Chronic intake of such drugs causing a permanently higher prolactinemia would in turn alter the relative ratio of other hormones. At this time, any material with such properties needs to undergo a chronic bioassay to evaluate whether endocrine-sensitive tissues would be at higher risk. The interpretation of data needs to take into account the normal diurnal, monthly, and even seasonal cycles of the endocrine system and whether the test would have led to interference in this balanced, rhythmic system (Weisburger and Williams, 1979).

The implications of a positive response in specific chronic bioassays coupled with convincing data of the absence of genotoxicity are discussed under the final evaluation.

C. Limited In Vivo Bioassays

This stage of evaluation employs tests that will provide further evidence of potential hazard of chemicals positive for genotoxicity without the necessity of undertaking chronic bioassay.

A number of tests for *in vivo* genotoxicity have been developed; these include the dominant lethal test, host-mediated mutagenicity, chromosomal damage, testicular DNA synthesis inhibition and repair, sebaceous gland suppression, and DNA fragmentation all in various organs. A chemical that is negative in all the *in vitro* genotoxicity test is unlikely to be positive in any one of these *in vivo* tests, and so, at present, there is no basis for recommending one of these. Furthermore, a positive result in one of these *in vivo* tests would serve only as a further indication of the need for chronic bioassay, which, as discussed, is already the only recourse for suspect chemicals that are negative and the *in vitro* tests. Such *in vivo* tests therefore would serve only to establish priorities for chronic bioassay of chemicals negative in *in vitro* tests.

Thus, at this stage, the *in vivo* tests recommended are those that will provide evidence of carcinogenicity, including cocarcinogenicity and promotion in a relatively short period (i.e., 30 weeks or less). Unlike the *in vitro* tests, these are not applied as a battery, but rather used selectively according to the information available on the chemical.

1. Skin Tumor Induction in Mice. The carcinogenicity of a limited number of chemicals and crude products can be revealed readily upon continuous application to the skin of mice, producing papillomas or carcinomas, or upon subcutaneous injection, yielding sarcomas (Van Duuren, in Searle, 1975; in Homburger, 1976; Hoffmann *et al.*, in Gelboin and Ts'o, 1978). Also, activity as initiating agents can be rapidly determined by the concurrent or sequential application of a promoter, such as one of the phorbol esters (see Slaga *et al.*, 1977). Tars from coal, petroleum, or tobaccos are active in such systems, as are the pure polycyclic aromatic hydrocarbons and congeners contained in such products. Mouse skin responds positively because it appears to have the necessary enzymes to yield the active intermediates resulting in initiation, especially in the presence of cocarcinogens or promoters in the crude products. On the other hand, such mixtures rarely yield visceral tumors such as those in the liver, mainly because the liver can detoxify these chemicals quickly. However, lung and lymphoid tumors in sensitive mouse strains can be a secondary tumor site.

Mouse skin is useful primarily, therefore, for chemicals such as polycyclic hydrocarbons, also direct-acting chemical carcinogens such as sulfur or nitrogen mustard, bis(chloromethyl)ether, propiolactone, also alkylnitrosoureas. Arylamines and related carcinogens by themselves usually do not provide a positive response on mouse skin, although some exceptions are 2-anthramine and 3-methyl-2-naphthylamine, which are active in this system perhaps because these chemicals are converted to active epoxy intermediates, in the same manner as the polycyclic aromatic hydrocarbons. On the other hand, mouse skin does not appear to yield a positive result with a basic fraction of tobacco tar, even though this fraction is mutagenic and leads to cell transformation. Some arylamines and urethane, however, provide a positive indication but only upon promotion with phorbol ester.

2. Pulmonary Tumor Induction in Mice. Andervont and Shimkin pioneered with the model involving the development of lung tumors in specific sensitive strains of mice, especially the strain A/Heston and related strains like A/J. As Shimkin and Stoner (1975) point out, a singular advantage of the assay system is that, in addition to an end point measuring the percent of animals with tumor compared to controls, the multiplicity of tumors is an additional parameter expressing the "strength" of any carcinogenic action. Most chemicals that are active in this system are also carcinogenic in other longer, chronic animal tests. Another useful aspect of this assay is that significant results are obtained in as short a time as 30 to 35 weeks, and sometimes faster. Extension of the test for a longer period is not desirable since the incidence of pulmonary tumors in control animals increases rapidly after 35 weeks, and thus the test loses sensitivity. A negative result in this test system, however, does not signify safety, inasmuch as not all classes of chemical carcinogens induce lung tumors.

3. Breast Cancer Induction in Female Sprague-Dawley Rats. Shay discovered and Huggins elegantly extended the finding that polycyclic hydrocarbons rapidly induced cancer in the mammary gland of young female random-bred Wistar rats and better in Sprague-Dawley rats. With powerful carcinogens, especially select polycyclic hydrocarbons, arylamines, or nitrosoureas, a positive result is obtained rapidly, in less than nine months. As in the case of lung tumor induction in mice, the multiplicity of mammary tumors provides an additional quantitative criterion to denote relative strength of the carcinogenic stimulus. As is true with lung tumors in mice, a positive response in this system has usually been demonstrated to occur in other animal bioassay models. A negative response does not mean safety (Weisburger, in Searle, 1975).

4. Altered Foci Induction in Rodent Liver. Research in a number of laboratories has established that during liver carcinogenesis several distinct liver cell lesions precede the development of carcinomas (Farber and Sporn, 1976). The earliest of these, the altered focus, when sufficiently developed can be demonstrated in routine histologic tissue sections. However, altered foci are abnormal in a number of properties that permit their reliable and objective identification at early stages by more sensitive techniques. Altered foci in rat liver display abnormalities in the enzymes γ-glutamyl transpeptidase, glucose-6-phosphatase, and adenosine triphosphatase, which have been used for their histochemical detection (Kitagawa, Scherer and Emmelot, in Farber and Sporn, 1976; Solt et al., 1977; Pitot et al., 1978). Another important marker for foci that permits histochemical identification is their resistance to iron accumulation (Williams, in Farber and Sporn, 1976). This latter property is more sensitive than the enzyme abnormalities and also, unlike the enzyme abnormalities, characterizes rat and mouse liver lesions. Therefore, induction of iron-resistant altered foci in mouse or rat liver can be used as a limited bioassay. With known carcinogens, foci have been detected within three weeks of carcinogen exposure and in high numbers by 12 to 16 weeks of exposure (Williams and Watanabe, 1978). Therefore, the recommended approach is that of 12 weeks' exposure to the test chemical with injection of subcutaneous iron during the last two weeks to produce the iron load that delineates the foci resistant to iron accumulation. Few carcinogens have yet been submitted to this regimen, but based upon current knowledge of the pathogenesis of liver cancer, this is anticipated to be a highly reliable test for liver carcinogens. Since the liver is the target for so many carcinogens because of its metabolic capability (Weisburger and Williams, in Becker, 1975), this test should possess substantial sensitivity.

Another approach to detecting altered foci employs their resistance to the cytotoxic effect of carcinogens (Tatematsu et al., 1977). In this approach administration of the test chemical is followed by exposure to N-2-fluorenylacetamide and partial hepatectomy (Solt et al., 1977). The N-2-fluorenylacetamide is metabolized by normal liver cells and affects them so that they cannot proliferate in response to the partial hepatectomy. In contrast, the cells in altered foci proliferate and become extremely conspicuous. The current complexity of this approach, involving administration of a known carcinogen and surgical manipulation, would appear to be a disadvantage compared to the demonstration of foci by resistance to iron accumulation. However, a sufficient data base is not available to recommend one approach over the other, and future developments in this active field may lead to significant improvements in these approaches.

Summary of Limited *In Vivo* Bioassays. The presence of two positive results, (1) in a battery of rapid *in vitro* bioassay tests indicating reliably genotoxicity and (2) in the limited *in vivo* bioassays, namely, skin painting, pulmonary tumor induction in mice, breast cancer induction in rats, or induction of liver altered foci, would make a product highly suspect as a potential carcinogenic risk to man. This is true especially if these results were obtained with moderate dosages and more so if there was evidence of a good dose response, particularly as regards the multiplicity of the lung or mammary gland tumors.

In the absence of genotoxicity, it is possible to test for promoting activity on mouse skin initiated with small doses of, for example, benzo(a)pyrene or 7,12-dimethylbenzo(a)anthracene. A material exhibiting endocrine properties likewise may show an effect in modifying breast cancer induction in animals given limited amounts of methylnitrosourea as an initiating dose. Similarly, promoters of urinary bladder cancer may be visualized by pretreatment with limited amounts of bladder carcinogen (Friedell, 1977).

Proven activity in more than one of the limited *in vivo* bioassays may be considered unequivocal qualitative evidence of carcinogenicity.

D. Chronic Bioassay

Current bioassay systems involve primarily rats, mice, and for some specific purposes hamsters (Grice, 1975; Weisburger, in Searle, 1975; Page, in Kraybill and Mehlman, 1977; Homburger, et al., 1978; Sontag, 1979). Because younger animals are often more sensitive, exposure begins at weaning or shortly thereafter. Newborn mice, and in some cases newborn rats and hamsters, have been recommended because they appear to show even higher sensitivity to carcinogens.

Certain bioassays have involved exposure of males and females of a parent generation that are mated during treatment, thus providing for possible transplacental exposure. The exposure is then continued during infancy. Recommendations to consider this procedure were made by a distinguished advisory group to the U.S. Food and Drug Administration led by Dr. P. Shubik, under the chairmanship of Dr. N. Nelson (Food and Drug Administration Advisory Committee, 1971). Its advantages and limitations require definition (Shubik, in Griffin and Shaw, 1979).

The induction of tumors by chemicals is quite

specific and structure-related. Within the field of polycyclic aromatic hydrocarbon carcinogenesis, where literally hundreds of chemicals have been studied after skin application or subcutaneous injection, many structure-activity correlations have resulted, as described in this paper. These demonstrate very clearly that structures that are closely related chemically, and even stereoisomers, may show quite divergent carcinogenic properties under otherwise identical conditions (Buening et al., 1978; Gelboin and Ts'o, 1978). Similar observations have been made with other types of chemical carcinogens (Searle, 1975; Hiatt et al., 1977).

Many types of chemical carcinogens show dose-response effects, as do other pharmacologic agents. However, with carcinogens, the time factor needs to be considered because cancer induction under a variety of conditions, even with powerful carcinogens, requires a certain minimum period of time. This is because the entire process is very complicated, from the biochemical activation of the agent leading to transformation of cells in specific tissues, to the growth and development of abnormal cells to a visible neoplasm. This entire process has been thought to take at least one-eighth of the life-span of a species. Thus, mice, rats, and hamsters, with an average life of two to three years, usually develop detectable cancer in no less than three months after treatment with most carcinogens. With longer-lived species, including primates, the process may be expected to take much longer. For example, diethylnitrosamine induces malignant liver cancer in rats in as little as three to five months, whereas in the rhesus monkey the same point was reached in one to three years (Adamson, 1972). 2-Naphthylamine induces cancer in the urinary bladder of a hamster in about a year (Saffiotti et al., in Deichmann and Lampe, 1967), whereas under most conditions, two or more years are required in the dog or the monkey. Hence, the trend has been to use even shorter-lived species as a means to decrease the time required for bioassays (Weisburger, in Searle, 1975).

A high dose is expected to induce a certain yield of cancers in a given target organ more rapidly than a lower dose, even though the latter, given sufficient time, may eventually induce the same yield of tumors. In addition, varying the dosage may lead to shifts in target organs, mainly because of alterations in metabolic pathways, and possibly also tissue-related factors such as cell turnover times and repair mechanisms. For example, a few large doses of dimethylnitrosamine induced cancer of the kidneys after a fairly long latent period, whereas continuous low dosing with the same agent consistently resulted in a high incidence of liver cancer with a shorter latent period (Magee et al., in Searle, 1975). The underlying mechanism is largely understood in terms of DNA repair capability.

Cancer resulting from potent carcinogens such as those with demonstrated activity in man can be detected in mice or rats rather quickly, often in less than one year. Weaker agents take longer, even at high dose levels, and it may be necessary to observe the animals for their entire lifetime. Similar relationships can be demonstrated to hold for man. For example, it has been shown that the development of pulmonary carcinoma in man as a result of smoking of cigarettes is proportional to the number of cigarettes smoked per day, and the age of appearance is inversely related to cigarette consumption (Wynder and Hecht, 1976).

During studies of pathogenesis of certain cancers it was found that with some specific chemicals, antecedent precancerous lesions could be detected in some organs, sometimes long before a definitive tumor could be diagnosed. If this were true for all chemical carcinogens, their early detection by rapid examination of tissues for such specific adverse effects would be greatly facilitated, and, indeed, the reliable detection of such lesions in the liver is the basis for a proposed limited in vivo bioassay (see above). However, in some tests in rats, autopsies performed one year after the beginning of treatment have given no diagnostic sign although neoplasms were present after 18 months (Weisburger, in Searle, 1975). When tissues were found to be normal in a study lasting less than a lifetime, the conclusion would not necessarily be justified that an agent was not carcinogenic. However, with older animals, complications arise that hinder the interpretation of the tests unless specific precautions are taken. The difficulties hinge on a number of facts. As animals age, they (1) die from causes unrelated to carcinogen treatment and are thus lost to the experiment without necessarily exhibiting cancer and (2) exhibit spontaneous tumors, most often in the endocrine-sensitive organs, again not related to the treatment. Sufficiently large numbers of animals in the study permit statistical evaluation of the significance of the results despite these handicaps.

Some investigators recommend lifetime studies, which, when animal colonies are carefully maintained, permit some strains of rats to live as long as three years and mice to live as long as two and one-half years. Most current procedures, however, involve exposure of groups of male and female rats, mice, or hamsters in experiments that terminate after two years for rats and 21 to 24 months for mice and hamsters, depending on strain, thus allowing optimum survival time for nonexposed controls. An advantage of this scheme is that 70 to 90 percent of the experimental animals live to the end of the test. Thus, fresh tissues are secured for subsequent microscopic study. In lifetime studies it is sometimes difficult to avoid losses of valuable material due to autolysis when the animals die spontaneously.

Furthermore, the question of the length of administration of the test compound requires consideration. With food additives and related materials, where humans are conceivably exposed during their life-span, it would seem useful to administer the compound throughout the test series, or even through a partial two-generation study, discussed above. With industrial chemicals and other materials where the potential exposure may be intermittent, a period of 18 months might be more useful. This seems sufficiently long, since even with a weak carcinogen it is logical to assume that the processes leading toward tumor induction have been initiated, although no accurate comparative study to ascertain this point experimentally has been performed. Thus, discontinuing administration of the compound after 18 months and maintaining the animals for three to six additional months may be useful to support the development of any tumor produced and lead to regression of any abnormal, yet noncancerous lesion. At the same time, the toxic stress of compound administration is removed, and thus a beneficial, more prolonged survival of the animals might actually be facilitated.

Another consideration is the dosage and mode of compound administration. Contemporary procedures call for the determination of the maximally tolerated dose (MTD) in preliminary assays, under the same conditions selected for the test series. Acute LD50 determinations, while valuable by themselves, do not necessarily contribute information that will be useful in determining doses tolerated under chronic conditions. If a chemical leads to changes in the processing enzymes, the chronically tolerated dose could be higher or lower than an acute toxic dosage, depending on how the balance of activation or toxication over detoxification metabolites is altered.

With active carcinogens, the induction of tumors may be seen at several dose levels. Such studies have shown that even with powerful carcinogens there are doses at which no effect is obtained within the allotted life-span of the animals (see Druckrey, in Truhaut, 1967; in Searle; Hoel and Rall, 1978). More studies in the low-dosage ranges would be desirable with larger numbers of animals than have been used heretofore, to establish whether a significant number of tumors would thus be seen. The entire problem of very small doses is still open and may be difficult to resolve satisfactorily. Analytic chemistry has advanced impressively, permitting accurate determinations of chemicals at parts per-billion and even parts-per-trillion levels. Even with powerful carcinogens and with consideration of possibly synergistic interactions, the question remains whether levels in this range have any biologic significance, especially in defining human risk. In the absence of data and facts, this area is bound to be controversial.

Even in simplified test series it is advisable to utilize at least two dose levels. The main reason is to ensure adequate survival of at least one of the groups of animals for the planned experimental period. If the preliminary toxicology leads to the selection of a high dose level that is tolerated for six to nine months but then results in death of the experimental group without cancer or adverse effects, the entire study will have to be repeated. Thus, to save time, a similar group of animals is started simultaneously at a lower dose level; one-half or one-third of the MTD generally is adequate and usually permits survival of the animals for the necessary length of time. An active carcinogen would show a response, proportional to dose, at both dosages. If the MTD shortens life-span, animals at that level might exhibit a lower cancer incidence than those on the reduced dosage, living longer.

With weaker carcinogens, active when given at the MTD, it has been found that the second dose level fails to induce significant cancer in a chronic test with the usual number of animals at risk. Hence, careful selection of dosages is mandatory in order to detect relatively low degrees of carcinogenicity, unless, of course, larger numbers of animals are used.

Modes of Administration and Selection of Animal Type. The primary direct-acting carcinogens will amost always cause cancer in any tissue to which they are directly applied. On the other hand, procarcinogens, which require metabolic or chemical conversion, rarely do so and in contrast exhibit sometimes quite specific organotropic affinity, depending on the biochemical potential of a given tissue. Even so, the mode of administration can influence the tumor yield at a given site, since it dictates pathways of internal distribution and metabolism and hence the concentration in a tissue. For example, dibutylnitrosamine given subcutaneously to rats leads almost exclusively to tumors in the urinary bladder (Druckrey, in Odashima et al., 1975). After subcutaneous injection, absorption leads to direct passage via the blood into renal pathways. On the other hand, oral administration produces tumors in the liver, lung, and urinary bladder because these additional organs receive a sufficient concentration of the agent. Tryptophan suppresses the response of the liver, without altering the high carcinogenicity to the bladder, a phenomenon already seen with another carcinogen, N-2-fluorenylacetamide (see various authors, in Deichmann and Lampe, 1967).

In general, the mode of administration should logically mimic potential exposure of humans. Thus, food additives would normally be fed or given by gavage. Cosmetics would be applied to the skin. Drugs given by parental injection would be thus tested.

However, if the only question asked is whether a given chemical structure has carcinogenic potential that, as discussed previously, is a highly specific, nonrandom property, then the mode of administration may depend more on such mechanistic aspects. The mode is used that would be most likely to reveal a carcinogenic effect based on the chemical structure of the agent. In any case, with many chemical carcinogens, particularly the more powerful agents, an effect is observed, irrespective of the mode of intake. This statement does not imply, however, that there is not an optimum procedure for each chemical.

A note of caution is in order, though, with respect to the interpretation of tumors in rodents seen at the site of single or repeated subcutaneous injection. This technique offers a number of advantages. With direct-acting carcinogens, the site of injection is the area where tumors are formed, often quickly and with small amounts of chemical. Where a chemical also has systemic effects, such can be observed, provided complete autopsies are performed, as is essential anyhow in studies of this type. Nonetheless, certain products induce local sarcomas, which has been taken as definitive evidence of oncogenic potential. In fact, such materials may not be realistically active in terms of hazards to the public, who are exposed to such materials by some way other than the parenteral route, or as adult individuals. An example is the induction of sarcoma upon subcutaneous injection or implantation of polymers or certain chemicals into rats or mice. This would normally not reflect an oncogenic risk to man (see Schmähl et al., 1977). Other chemicals leading to sarcoma at the site of injection, but that are probably innocuous, are generally characterized by polar structures, as in detergents, soaps, emulsifiers, or organic salts. Grasso (1971) and others have proposed examination of early lesions as a means of discriminating between agents that are true local-acting carcinogens, such as the polycyclic hydrocarbons, and those that may induce tumors as artefacts, such as detergents, where the latter give rise to early lesions.

Within the numerous strains and substrains of rodents species, mice, rats, and hamsters, it would

be of paramount importance to select a strain that is readily available; has good breeding performance; is a generally healthy animal, with disease-free, extended survival; and at the same time exhibits moderate or good sensitivity to carcinogens. Some investigators prefer to use random-bred animals, mainly for the reason that the data obtained need to be extrapolated to the heterozygous human population. This point is not necessarily valid, for even inbred animals would respond, by and large, to a given carcinogenic challenge in a manner similar to that of some humans. All known human carcinogens with the possible exceptions of arsenic and benzene have also led to tumors in one or more animal systems. There is no reason to believe that the reverse would not be true; that is, an agent that reliably and unambiguously induces tumors in an animal species, even inbred strains, would constitute a certain risk for at least a portion of the human species. However, as we will discuss, there are select exceptions to this rule, based on an understanding of the underlying mechanisms. Because the variability and the reproducibility of tests are somewhat better in inbred animals, and also because certain transplantation experiments and related immunologic considerations are performed more readily or possibly exclusively in inbred animals or F_1 hybrid descendants of two distinct inbred strains, the trend has been toward the use of such inbred animals. However, even with random-bred animals, properly conducted tests can be executed reproducibly.

The number of animals to be used in a test series is dependent on several factors, including the reliable statistical evaluation of results. If the agent studied is a known carcinogen giving a high incidence of tumors in less than one year, the loss of animals due to treatment-unrelated causes may be minimal, and groups of 20 to 30 suffice. On the other hand, with an unknown agent or where the effect is weak, and therefore may be expected to be detectable only after a lengthy experimental period, a larger number of animals is required to compensate for deaths unrelated to treatment. If, for various reasons, the experimenter plans to kill some of the animals prior to the termination of the main tests, the initial number would have to be increased, so as to take into account this reduction in the group size of the animals at risk in any set.

With weak carcinogens, where the tumor incidence in any given tissue may be as low as 20 percent, it is necessary to have available at least 20 animals for final evaluation (four animals with a specific lesion). Assuming a low two-year survival of only 50 percent, it follows that 40 animals would be needed at the beginning of the test, in the example cited. Even then the significance would only be borderline. Current practice is to use 50, 100, or, for specific tests, even more animals per group. It is best to plan such tests with the advice and continuing consultation of professional statisticians.

Once an animal has been in any test series longer than a year, it is a valuable specimen. Every effort should be made not to lose it because of poor husbandry practices or inadequate professional supervision. Animals must be inspected every day and, toward the end of an experiment, twice a day. Animals in poor health should be examined to establish whether survival is possible. If unlikely, proper autopsy procedures should be instituted immediately. In long-term tests little is gained by maintaining an animal that is already in poor health for a few more days or weeks.

Autopsies should be performed by highly trained personnel, capable of detecting even minor grossly visible lesions. A complete autopsy includes opening of the skull and examination of the tissues of the nervous system, the brain, and the pituitary gland, as well as the other viscera. Proper fixation of tissues in suitable fluids, trimming of select tissues for histologic processing, and finally the microscopic study of stained sections should be supervised or performed by trained professionals. The entire assay hinges on the accurate execution of the total test series, but in particular it depends on the correct diagnosis and interpretation of the significance of any lesions noted. Again, individuals trained in experimental pathology should be part of the team designing and monitoring a test series. A responsible pathologist using correct diagnostic procedures will be in the best position to successfully conclude the study.

Control groups are as important as experimental groups. In smaller studies evaluating the carcinogenicity of only one or two compounds, the control group must be of the same size as each experimental group. Some effort can be saved if a number of chemicals or drugs are studied simultaneously, for then one control group can serve as reference point for a number of contemporary experimental groups. The control group should involve $A \times \sqrt{n}$, where A is the size of each group and n is the number of simultaneous experimental groups. If a vehicle is used, control groups treated with the vehicle alone, in addition to untreated control groups, are required in order to assess the possible influence of the treatment with the vehicle. In addition, it is desirable, if not mandatory, to include a positive control group of animals treated with a known, carefully selected carcinogen. If possible, this should have a structure similar to that of the unknown chemicals tested and/or perhaps have similar organ specificity. Often it is desirable to give this positive

control at two dose levels, one known to be effective quickly, as a means of assessing the responsiveness of the specific type of animals used. The other could be a lower dosage to mimic a weaker effect possible with the unknown compounds.

E. Final Evaluation

If the decision point approach has led to chronic bioassays, then fairly definitive data on carcinogenicity would be obtained. However, the results of the *in vitro* short-term tests *must* be considered for evaluation of possible mechanisms of action and risk extrapolation to humans. Convincing positive results in the *in vitro* tests coupled with documented *in vivo* carcinogenicity permit classification of the chemical as a genotoxic carcinogen. It would, therefore, be anticipated that the chemical could display the properties characteristic of such carcinogens, which include the ability under some circumstance to be effective as a single dose, cumulative effects, and synergism or at least additive effects with other genotoxic carcinogens. Genotoxic carcinogens, therefore, represent clear qualitative hazards to humans, and the level of exposure permitted must be rigorously evaluated and controlled. Along those lines, no distinction should be made between naturally occurring and synthetic carcinogens. In fact, there is growing evidence that the majority of human cancers stem from exposure to the former types of agents (Weisburger and Williams, 1980).

If, on the other hand, no convincing evidence for genotoxicity is obtained, but the chemical is carcinogenic in animal bioassays, then the possibility exists that the chemical is an epigenetic carcinogen. The strength of this conclusion depends on the relevance of the *in vitro* tests. For example, the finding that certain stable organochlorine pesticides do not display genotoxic effects in liver cell systems, which are identical to the *in vivo* target cell for these carcinogens, strongly supports the interpretation that these carcinogens may act by epigenetic mechanisms. The nature of these mechanisms is poorly understood at present and is probably quite different for different classes of carcinogens, as discussed in this chapter. They may involve chronic tissue injury, immunosuppressive effects, hormonal imbalances, blocks in differentiation, promotion of preexisting altered cells, or processes not yet known. Regardless, most types of epigenetic carcinogens share the characteristic of being active only at high, sustained doses, and up to a certain point, the lesion induced may be reversible. Thus, these types of carcinogens may represent only quantitative hazards to humans, and safe levels of exposure may be established by carrying out proper pharmacologic dose-response studies.

Kroes (1979) has recently suggested a similar approach.

EPILOGUE

During the last decade, sizable progress has been made in the basic sciences underlying toxicology with specific reference to chronic effects, including carcinogenesis. Thus, we have come to realize that the great diversity of chemical structures capable of causing cancer eventually depended on the specific property of such structures to be either electrophilic reactants as such, or after metabolic activation. At the same time, there has been further insight into the molecular target of such carcinogens as electrophilic reactants, namely, the genetic material in the cell, DNA. It has also been discovered that carcinogens covalently bound to DNA can be repaired and that some of the observed biologic effects, including that of organotropism, depended as much on such repair processes, or lack thereof, as on the metabolic activation and interaction with DNA.

The recognized interaction with DNA has provided the necessary scientific background to relate mutagenicity to carcinogenicity. In turn, this connection has provided a sound basis for utilizing the property of mutagenicity of chemicals as such or after metabolic activation as an assessment of potential carcinogenicity. In this review, we provide for the first time a classification of chemical carcinogens into genotoxic agents, as defined above, and of other agents capable of increasing cancer risk through mechanisms other than genotoxicity, namely, through epigenetic mechanisms. Inasmuch as current evidence shows that most classes of agents operating through such an epigenetic mode of action do so in a reversible, highly dose-dependent fashion, there are theoretic as well as regulatory implications in treating such agents in an entirely distinct manner. It is expected that further research utilizing this classification will provide better control of potentially harmful substances without a blind, blanket indictment of all agents that can cause cancer by whatever mechanism. This is important inasmuch as there are sound data with respect to the causes of the main human cancers, including that of cancer of the lung due to smoking of cigarettes, and cancer of the colon, breast, prostate, and perhaps pancreas due to certain dietary habits, to the effect that they depend as much on the presence of agents operating via epigenetic mechanisms as on genotoxic carcinogens. Thus, there is hope that these important types of cancer can be controlled by modifying not only the environment with respect to genotoxic carcinogens but also that of epigenetic carcinogens, and thus, human cancer risk can be reduced.

During the last decade the public has become much more aware of environmental cancer risks. This, in turn, has led to legislation and regulation at the state and federal level, and indeed in international forums, and to development of policies to control environmental cancer. The same public involvement has provided increased resources in toxicology from private and public funds, which have contributed to our base of knowledge. At the same time, however, the public, while aware of this field, is not well informed, insofar as matters that come to public attention via the public press and media are not necessarily those that would be most likely to protect the majority of the public. It is hoped that the principles and facts developed in this chapter will not only assist professionals concerned with toxicology and carcinogenesis, but can be translated to activities such that the public will be better informed and protected against avoidable cancer hazards.

REFERENCES

The references have been confined in the main to reviews or monographs so as to comply with editorial policy to limit the number of citations. Detailed references to the research literature can be found in the reports quoted. The reader is referred also to the continuing serials below as source material.

Advances in Cancer Research
Methods in Cancer Research.
Progress in Experimental Tumor Research.
International Agency for Research on Cancer: Monograph series and scientific publications.
Monographs, *Journal of the National Cancer Institute.*
Proceedings, Symposium of the Princess Takamatsu Cancer Research Fund, Tokyo (University Park Press, Baltimore).
Recent Results in Cancer Research (Springer-Verlag, Berlin).
Annual Review of Pharmacology and Toxicology.
Occasional reviews and symposia, *Cancer Research.*

Adamson, R. H.: Long-term administration of carcinogenic agents to primates. In Goldsmith, E. I., and Moor, J. (eds.): *Medical Primatology 1972.* Proceedings of Third Conference on Experimental Medicine and Surgery in Primates, Lyon, 1972, part 3. Basel, Karger, 1972, pp. 216–25.
American Cancer Society: *1979 Facts and Figures.* American Cancer Society, Inc., New York, 1978, p. 31.
Arcos, J. C.: Criteria for selecting chemical compounds for carcinogenicity testing: An essay. *J. Environ. Pathol. Toxicol.,* 1:433–58, 1978.
Ashby, J.; Styles, J. A.; and Paton, D.: Potentially carcinogenic analogues of the carcinogen hexamethylphosphoramide: Evaluation *in vitro. Br. J. Cancer,* 38:418–27, 1978.
Ashby, J.: Structural analysis as a means of predicting carcinogenic potential. *Br. J. Cancer,* 37(6):904–23, 1978.
Asher, I. M., and Zervos, C. (eds.): *Symposium on Structural Correlates of Carcinogenesis and Mutagenesis.* Office of Science, FDA, Rockville, Md., 1978.
Barron, C. N.: Observations on the chronic toxicity of 3-phenyl-5 beta diethylaminoethyl-1,2,4-oxadiazole in the rat and dog. *Exp. Mol. Pathol.,* Suppl. 2:1–27, 1963.
Becker, F. F. (ed.): *Cancer 1. A Comprehensive Treatise.* Plenum Press, New York and London, 1975.

Berenblum, I.: *Carcinogenesis as a Biological Problem.* Frontiers of Biology, Vol. 34. North-Holland Publishing Co., Amsterdam, 1974.

Bogovski, P.; Gilson, J. C.; Timbrell, V.; and Wagner, J. C. (eds.): *Biological Effects of Asbestos.* International Agency for Research on Cancer, Lyon, 1973.

Brand, I.; Buoen, L. C.; and Brand, K. G.: Foreign-body tumors of mice: Strain and sex differences in latency and incidence. *J. Natl. Cancer Inst.*, **58**:1443–47, 1977.

Bryan, G. T. (ed.): *Nitrofurans.* Raven Press, New York, 1978.

Buening, M. K.; Wislocki, P. G.; Levin, W.; Yagi, H.; Thakker, D. R.; Akagi, H.; Koreeda, M.; Jerina, D. M.; and Conney, A. H.: Tumorigenicity of the optical enantiomers of the diastereomeric benzo(a)-pyrene 7,8-diol-9,10-epoxides in newborn mice: Exceptional activity of (+)-7β,8α-dihydroxy-9α,10α-epoxy-7,8,9,10-tetrahydrobenzo(a)pyrene. *Proc. Natl. Acad. Sci. U.S.A.*, **75**:5358–61, 1978.

Burkitt, D. P., and Trowell, H. C. (eds.): *Refined Carbohydrate Foods and Disease.* Academic Press, Inc., New York, 1975.

Busch, H. (ed.): *Methods in Cancer Research.* Academic Press, Inc., New York, 1967–1980.

Butterworth, B. E. (ed.): *Strategies For Short-Term Testing For Mutagens/Carcinogens.* CRC Press, Inc., West Palm Beach, 1979.

Casto, B. N.; Meyers, J.; and DiPaolo, J. A.: Enhancement of viral transformation for evaluation of the carcinogenic or mutagenic potential of inorganic metal salts. *Cancer Res.*, **39**:193–98, 1979.

Cederlöf, R.; Doll, R.; Fowler, B.; Friberg, L.; Nelson, N.; and Vouk, V.: Air pollution and cancer: risk assessment methodology and epidemiological evidence. *Environ. Health Prespect.*, **22**:1–123, 1978.

Clayson, D. B.: *Chemical Carcinogenesis.* Little-Brown & Co., Boston, 1962.

Coon, J. M.; Conney, A. H.; Estabrook, R. W.; Gelboin, J. R.; Gillette, J. R.; O'Brien, P. J.: *Microsomes and Drug Oxidation.* Academic Press, New York, 1980.

Copeland, M. M., and Rawson, R. W.: Proceedings of the 1977 Workshop on Large Bowel Cancer, Houston, Texas. *Cancer*, **40**:2405–2763, 1977.

Cornfield, J.: Carcinogenic risk assessment. *Science*, **198**:693–99, 1977.

Cramer, G. M.; Ford, R. A.; and Hall, R. L.: Estimation of toxic hazard—a decision tree approach. *Food Cosmet. Toxicol.*, **16**:255–76, 1978.

Cranmer, M. F.; Lawrence, L. R.; Konvicka, A. J.; and Herrick, S. S.: NCTR computer systems designed for toxicologic experimentation. *J. Environ. Pathol. Toxicol.*, **1**:701–709, 1978.

Dant, B. A.; Miller, J. A.; and Miller, E. C.: Vinyl carbamate as a promutagen and a more carcinogenic analog of ethyl carbamate. *Cancer Res.*, **38**:3793–3804, 1978.

Deichmann, W. B.: The chronic toxicity of organochlorine pesticides in man. In McKee, William D. (ed.): *Environmental Problems in Medicine.* Charles C Thomas Publisher, Springfield, Ill., 1974, pp. 568–642.

Deichmann, W. B., and Lampe, K. F. (eds.): *Bladder Cancer. A Symposium.* Aesculapios Publishing Co., Birmingham, Ala., 1967.

Doll, R.; Mathews, J. D.; and Morgan, L. G.: Cancers of the lung and nasal sinuses in nickel workers: A reassessment of the period of risk. *Br. J. Ind. Med.*, **34**:102–105, 1977.

Druckrey, H.; Preussmann, R.; Nashed, N.; and Ivankovic, S.: Carcinogene alkylierende substanzen. I. Dimethyl sulfate, carcinogene Wirkung an Ratten und wahrscheinliche Ursache von Berufskrebs. *Z. Krebsforsch.*, **68**:103–11, 1966.

Eckardt, R. E.: *Industrial Carcinogens.* Grune & Stratton, Inc., New York, 1959.

Egan, H. (ed.): *Environmental Carcinogens, Selected Methods of Analysis.* IARC Scientific Publications, Vol. 1. International Agency for Research on Cancer, Lyon, 1978.

Falk, H. F. (ed.): Conference on comparative metabolism and toxicity of vinyl chloride related compounds. *Environ. Health Perspect.*, **21**:1–328, 1977.

Farber, E.; Kawachi, T.; Nagayo, T.; Sugano, H.; Sugimura, T.; and Weisburger, J. H. (eds.): *Pathophysiology of Carcinogenesis in Digestive Organs.* University of Tokyo Press and University Park Press, Baltimore, 1977.

Farber, E., and Sporn, M. B.: Symposium. Early lesions and the development of epithelial cancer. *Cancer Res.*, **36**:2476–2706, 1976.

Food and Drug Administration Advisory Committee on Protocols for Safety Evaluation: Panel on carcinogenesis report on cancer testing in the safety evaluation of food additives and pesticides. *Toxicol. Appl. Pharmacol.*, **20**:419–38, 1971.

Fraumeni, J. F., Jr. (ed.): *Persons at High Risk of Cancer.* Academic Press, Inc., New York, 1975.

Friedell, G. H. (ed.): National Bladder Cancer Conference. *Cancer Res.*, **37**:2734–2973, 1977.

Gelboin, H. V., and Ts'o, P. O. P. (eds.): *Polycyclic Hydrocarbons and Cancer*, Vol. 1. Academic Press, Inc., New York, 1978.

Golberg, L.; Smith, J. P.; and Baker, S. B., de C.: The significance of sarcomas induced in rats and mice by iron-dextran. *Biochem. Pharmacol.*, **8**:233, 1961.

Gorrod, J. W., and Beckett, A. H. (eds.): *Drug Metabolism in Man.* Taylor & Francis Ltd, London, 1978.

Grasso, P.: Physiochemical and other factors determining local sarcoma production by food additives. *Food Cosmet. Toxicol.*, **9**:463–78, 1971.

Grasso, P.: Review of tests for carcinogenicity and their significance to man. *Clin. Toxicol.*, **9**:745–60, 1976.

Grice, H. C.: *The Testing of Chemicals for Carcinogenicity, Mutagenicity, and Teratogenicity.* Canadian Department of Health and Welfare, Ottawa, 1975.

Griffin, A. C., and Shaw, C. R. (eds.): *Carcinogens: Identification and Mechanisms of Action.* Raven Press, New York, 1979.

Grisham, J. W.; Charlton, R. K.; and Kaufman, D. G.: *In vitro* assay of cytotoxicity with cultured liver: Accomplishments and possibilities. *Environ. Health Perspect.*, **25**:161–71, 1978.

Gyorkey, F.; Melnick, J. L.; Mirkovic, R.; Cabral, G. A.; Gyorkey, P.; and Hollinger, F. B.: Experimental carcinoma of liver in Macaque monkeys exposed to diethylnitrosamine and hepatitis B virus. *J. Natl. Cancer Inst.*, **59**:1451–57, 1977.

Hathaway, D. E. (ed.): *Foreign Compound Metabolism in Mammals.* The Chemical Society, London, 1977.

Hecht, S. S.; Chen, C. B.; and Hoffmann, D.: Tobacco specific nitrosamines: Occurrence, formation, carcinogenicity, and metabolism. *Accounts Chem. Res.*, **12**:92–98, 1979.

Hiatt, H. H.; Watson, J. D.; and Winsten, J. A. (eds.): *Origins of Human Cancer. Proliferation*, Vol. 4. Cold Spring Harbor Laboratory, New York, 1977.

Higginson, J.: The role of the pathologist in environmental medicine and public health. *Am. J. Pathol.*, **86**:459–84, 1977.

Hirono, I.; Ushimaru, Y.; Kato, K.; Mori, H.; and Sasaoka, I.: Carcinogenicity of boiling water extract of bracken, *Pteridium aquilicum. Gann*, **69**:383–88, 1978.

Hoel, D. G., and Rall, D. P.: NIEHS Extrapolation II Conference, Pinehurst, Calif., March 10–12, 1976. *Environ. Health Perspect.*, **22**:125–85, 1978.

Hollaender, A. (ed.): *Chemical Mutagens, Principles and*

Methods for Their Detection. Plenum Press, New York, 1970–1980.

Hollstein, M.; McCann, J.; Angelosanto, F.; and Nichols, W.: Short-term tests for carcinogens and mutagens. *Mutat. Res.*, **65**:133–226, 1979.

Homburger, F. (ed.): *The Physiopathology of Cancer.* S. Karger, Basel, New York, London, 1976.

Homburger, F.; Adams, R. A.; Soto, E.; and Van Dongen, C. G.: Chemical carcinogenesis in Syrian hamsters. *Fed. Proc.*, **37**:2090–91, 1978.

International Agency for Research on Cancer: *Monograph Series, Evaluation of the Carcinogenic Risk of Chemicals to Humans.* IARC, Lyon, France, 1972–1978.

International Symposium, Threshold doses in chemical carcinogenesis, Heidelberg. *Oncology*, **33**:50–100, 1976.

Ito, N.; Tatematsu, M.; Hirose, M.; Nakanishi, K.; and Murasaki, G.: Enhancing effect of chemicals on production of hyperplastic liver nodules induced by *N*-2-fluorenylacetamide in hepatectomized rats. *Gann*, **69**:143–44, 1978.

Jarrett, W. F. H.; McNeil, P. E.; Grimshaw, W. T. R.; Selman, T. E.; and McIntyre, W. I. M.: High incidence area of cattle cancer with a possible interaction between an environmental carcinogen and a papilloma virus. *Nature*, **274**:215–17, 1978.

Jerina, D. M.: *Drug Metabolism Concepts.* ACS Symposium Series. 44. American Chemical Society, Washington, D.C., 1977.

Jones, P. W., and Freudenthal, R. I. (eds.): *Polynuclear Aromatic Hydrocarbons.* Raven Press, New York, 1978.

Kawachi, T.; Nagao, M.; Yahagi, T.; Takahashi, Y.; Mori, Y.; Sugimura, T.; and Takayama, S.: Mutagens and carcinogens in food. International Cancer Conference, Buenos Aires. Plenum Press, New York, 1979.

Kinsella, A. R., and Radman, M.: Tumor promoter induces sister chromatid exchanges: Relevance to mechanisms of carcinogenesis. *Proc. Natl. Acad. Sci. U.S.A.*, **75**:6149–53, 1978.

Kitagawa, H.; Pitot, H. C.; Miller, E. C.; and Miller, J. A.: Promotion by dietary phenobarbital of hepatocarcinogenesis by 2-methyl-*N*,*N*-dimethyl-4-aminoazobenzene in the rat. *Cancer Res.*, **39**:112–15, 1979.

Kociba, R. J.; Keyes, D. G.; Beyer, J. E.; Carreon, R. M.; Wade, C. E.; Dittenber, D. A.; Kalnins, R. P.; Frauson, L. E.; Park, C. N.; Barnard, S. D.; Hummel, R. A.; and Humiston, C. G.: Results of a two-year chronic toxicity and oncogenicity study of 2,3,7,8-tetrachlorodibenzo-p-dioxin in rats. *Toxicol. Appl. Pharmacol.*, **46**:279–303, 1978.

Kraybill, H. F., and Mehlman, M. A. (eds.): *Environmental Cancer,* Vol. 3. Halsted Press, New York, 1977.

Kroes, R.: Animal Data: Interpretation and Consequences. In Kriek, E., and Emmelot, P. (eds.): *Proceedings of the Symposium on Environmental Carcinogenesis: Occurrence, Risk Evaluation and Mechanisms of Action of Chemical Carcinogens,* Elsevier/No. Holland Biomedical Press, Amsterdam, 1979.

Kuchino, Y., Sharma, O. K., and Borek, E.: Lysine transfer RNA$_2$ is the major target for L-ethionine in the rat. *Biochemistry*, **17**:144–47, 1978.

Laskin, S., and Goldstein, B. D. (eds.): *J. Toxicol. Environ. Health,* Suppl. 2, 1977.

Lee, D. H. K., and Kotin, P. (eds.): *Multiple Factors in the Causation of Environmentally Induced Disease.* Academic Press, Inc., New York, 1972.

Leonard, B. J. (ed.): Toxicologic aspects of food safety. *Arch. Toxicol.*, Suppl. 1, Springer-Verlag, Berlin, Heidelberg, New York, 1978.

Lerman, L. S.: Acridine mutagens and DNA structure. *J. Cell. Physiol.*, **64** (Suppl. 1):1–18, 1964.

Lin, J. K.; Kennan, K. A.; Miller, E. C.; and Miller, J. A.: Reduced nicotinamide adenine dinucleotide phosphate-dependent formation of 2,3-dihycro-2,3-dihydroxyaflatoxin B$_1$ from aflatoxin B$_1$ by hepatic microsomes. *Cancer Res.*, **38**:2424–28, 1978.

Littlefield, N. A.; Farmer, J. H.; Sheldon, W. G.; and Gaylor, D. W.: Effects of dose and time in a long-term, low-dose carcinogenic study. *J. Environ. Pathol. Toxicol.*, **33**:17, 1979.

Longnecker, D. S., and Curphey, T. J.: Adenocarcinoma of the pancreas in azaserine-treated rats. *Cancer Res.*, **35**:2249–58, 1975.

Magee, P. N.; Takayama, S.; Sugimura, T.; and Matsushima, T. (eds.): *Fundamentals in Cancer Prevention.* University of Tokyo Press and University Park Press, Baltimore, 1976.

Mehlman, M. A.; Shapiro, R. E.; and Blumenthal, H. (eds.): *New Concepts in Safety Evaluation.* Halsted Press, New York, 1976.

Mehlman, M. A.; Cranmer, M. F.; and Shapiro, R. F.: The status of predictive tools in application to safety evaluation: Present and future. Carcinogenesis and mutagenesis, *J. Environ. Pathol. Toxicol.*, **1**:1–352, 1977.

Miller, E. C.: Some current perspectives on chemical carcinogenesis in humans and experimental animals: Presidential address. *Cancer Res.*, **38**:1479–96, 1978.

Montesano, R.; Bartsch, H.; and Tomatis, L. (eds.): *Screening Tests in Chemical Carcinogenesis.* International Agency for Research on Cancer, Lyon, 1976.

Nagao, M., and Sugimura, T.: Molecular biology of the carcinogen, 4-nitroquinoline 1-oxide. *Adv. Cancer Res.*, **23**:132–69, 1976.

National Cancer Institute: *Survey of Compounds Which Have Been Tested for Carcinogenic Activity.* Public Health Publication No. 149. U.S. Government Printing Office, Washington, D.C., 1951–1975.

Newberne, P. M.: Environmental modifiers of susceptibility to carcinogenesis. *Cancer Detect. Prev.*, **1**:129–73, 1976.

Nieburgs, H. E. (ed.): *Prevention and Detection of Cancer.* Marcel Dekker, Inc., New York, 1978.

Odashima, S.; Takayama, S.; and Sato, H. (eds.): *Recent Topics in Chemical Carcinogenesis. Gann Monograph,* No. 17. University Park Press, Baltimore and Tokyo, 1975.

Olson, W.; Haberman, R.; Weisburger, E.; Ward, J.; and Weisburger, J.: Induction of stomach cancer in rats and mice with halogenated aliphatic fumigants. *J. Natl. Cancer Inst.*, **51**:1993–95, 1973.

Pamukcu, A. M.; Erturk, E.; Yalciner, S.; Milli, U.; and Bryan, G. T.: Carcinogenic and mutagenic activities of milk from cows fed bracken fern (*Pteridium aquilicum*). *Cancer Res.*, **38**:1556–60, 1978.

Parke, D. V., and Smith, R. L. (eds.): *Drug Metabolism—from Microbe to Man.* Taylor & Francis Ltd., London, 1977.

Pasternack, B. S.; Shore, R. E.; Albert, R. E.: Occupational exposure to chloromethyl ethers. *J. Occupat. Med.*, **19**:741–46, 1977.

Pegg, A. E.: Formation and metabolism of alkylated nucleosides: Possible role in carcinogenesis by nitroso compounds and alkylation agents. *Adv. Cancer Res.*, **25**:195–259, 1977.

Pegg, A. E., and Hui, G.: Formation and subsequent removal of O^6-methylguanine from deoxyribonucleic acid in rat liver and kidney after small doses of dimethylnitrosamine. *Biochem. J.*, **173**:739–48, 1978.

Penn, I.: Tumors arising in organ transplant recipients. *Adv. Cancer Res.*, **28**:31–36, 1978

Pitot, H. C.; Barsness, L.; Goldsworthy, T.; and Kitagawa, T.: Biochemical characterization of stages of hepatocarcinogenesis after a single dose of diethylnitrosamine. *Nature*, **271**:456–58, 1978.

Pottathil, R.; Huebner, R. J.; and Meier, H.: Suppression of chemical (DEN) carcinogenesis in SWR/J mice by goat antibodies agains endogenous murine leukemia viruses. *Proc. Soc. Exp. Biol. Med.*, **159**:65–68, 1978.

Prehn, R. T.: Immunomodulation of tumor growth. *Am. J. Pathol.*, 77:119–22, 1974.

Preussmann, R.: Chemische Carcinogene in der menchlichen Umwelt. In *Handbuch der allgemeinen Pathologie*, Vol. VI/6, Part 2. Springer, Berlin, Heidelberg, New York, 1975, pp. 421–594.

Purchase, I. F. H.; Longstaff, E.; Ashby, J.; Styles, J. A.; Anderson, D.; Lefevre, P. A.; and Westwood, F. R.: An evaluation of 6 short-term tests for detecting organic chemical carcinogens. *Br. J. Cancer*, 37:873–959, 1978.

Roebuck B. D.; Siegel, W. G.; and Wogan, G. N.: *In vitro* metabolism of aflatoxin B$_2$ by animal and human liver. *Cancer Res.*, 38:999–1002, 1978.

Rossman, T. G.; Meyn, M. S.; and Troll, W.: Effects of arsenite on DNA repair in *Escherichia coli. Environ. Health Perspect.*, 19:229–33, 1977.

Saffiotti, U., and Wagoner, J. K. (eds.): Occupational carcinogenesis. *Ann. N.Y. Acad. Sci.*, 271:1–516, 1976.

Schmähl, D.; Thomas, C.; and Auer, R.: *Iatrogenic Carcinogenesis.* Springer-Verlag, Berlin, Heidelberg, 1977.

Schmeltz, I., and Hoffmann, D.: Nitrogen containing compounds in tobacco and tobacco smoke. *Chem. Rev.*, 77:295–311, 1977.

Schottenfeld, D. (ed.): *Cancer Epidemiology and Prevention.* Charles C Thomas Publisher, Springfield, Ill., 1975.

Schrauzer, G. N. (ed.): *Inorganic and Nutritional Aspects of Cancer.* Plenum Press, New York, 1978.

Scott, T. S.: *Carcinogenic and Chronic Toxic Hazards of Aromatic Amines.* Elsevier Publishing Co., Amsterdam, New York, 1962.

Scribner, J. D., and Süss, R.: Tumor initiation and promotion. *Int. Rev. Exp. Pathol.*, 18:137–98, 1978.

Searle, C. E. (ed.): *Chemical Carcinogens.* ACS Monograph 173, American Chemical Society, Washington, D.C., 1976.

Sellakumar, A.; Stenback, F.; Rowland, J.; and Shubik, P.: Tumor induction by 7H-dibenzo(c,g) carbazole in the respiratory tract of Syrian hamsters. *J. Toxicol. Environ. Health*, 3:935–39, 1977.

Shimkin, M. B., and Stoner, G. D.: Lung tumors in mice: Application to carcinogenesis bioassay. *Adv. Cancer Res.*, 21:2–58, 1975.

Shinohara, Y.; Ogiso, T.; Hananouchi, M.; Nakanishi, K.; Yoshimura, T.; and Ito, N.: Effect of various factors on the induction of liver tumors in animals by quinoline. *Gann*, 68:785–96, 1977.

Sims, P., and Grover, P. L.: Epoxides in polycyclic aromatic hydrocarbon metabolism and carcinogenesis. *Adv. Cancer Res.*, 20:166–274, 1974.

Slaga, T. J.; Sivak, A.; and Boutwell, R. K. (eds.): *Mechanisms of Tumor Promotion and Cocarcinogens.* Raven Press, New York, 1978.

Solt, D. B.; Medline, A.; and Farber, E.: Rapid emergence of carcinogen-induced hyperplastic lesions in a new model for the sequential analysis of liver carcinogenesis. *Am. J. Pathol.*, 88:595–610, 1977.

Sontag, J. (ed.): *Carcinogens in Industry and Environment.* Marcel Dekker, Inc., New York, 1979.

Sporn, M. B.; Dunlop, N. M.; Newton, D. L.; and Smith, J. M.: Prevention of chemical carcinogenesis by vitamin A and its synthetic analogs(retinoids). *Fed. Proc.*, 35:1332–38, 1976.

Stula, E. F.; Barnes, J. R.; Sherman, H.; Reinhardt, C. F.; and Zapp, J. A., Jr.: Liver and urinary bladder tumors in dogs from 3,3'-dichlorobenzidine. *J. Environ. Pathol. Toxicol.*, 1:475–90, 1978.

Sunderman, F. W., Jr.: Carcinogenic effects of metals. *Fed. Proc.*, 37:40, 1978.

Tatematsu, M.; Shirai, T.; Tsuda, H.; Miyata, Y.; Shinohara, Y.; and Ito, N.: Rapid production of hyperplastic liver nodules in rats treated with carcinogenic chemicals: A new approach for an in vivo short-term screening test for hepatocarcinogens. *Gann*, 68:499–507, 1977.

Thomas, A. W.; Boeniger, M. F.; Weber, M. G.; Stein, H. P.; Upton, A. C.; and Millar, J. D.: Direct black 38, direct blue 6, direct brown 95, benzidine derived dyes. *Am. Ind. Hyg. Assoc. J.*, 39(8):A18–A24, 1978.

Tinbergen, B. J., and Krol, F.: *Nitrite in Meat Products.* Centre for Agriculture Publ. and Documentation, Wageningen, Zeist, The Netherlands, 1977.

Toth, B., and Nagel, D.: Tumors induced in mice by N-methyl-N-formylhydrazine of the false morel *Gyromitra esculenta. J. Natl. Cancer Inst.*, 60:201–204, 1978.

Ts'o, P. O. P., and DiPaolo, J. A. (eds.): *Chemical Carcinogenesis.* Marcel Dekker, Inc., New York, 1974.

Trichopoulos, D.; Gerety, R. J.; Sparros, L.; Tabor, E.; Xirouchaki, E.; Munoz, N.; and Linsell, C. A.: Hepatitis B and primary hepatocellular carcinoma in a European population. *Lancet*, 2:1217–19, 1978.

Truhaut, R. (ed.): *Potential Carcinogenic Hazards from Drugs.* UICC Monograph Series, Vol. 7. Springer-Verlag, Berlin, 1967.

Uraguchi, K., and Yamazaki, M. (eds.): *Toxicology, Biochemistry and Pathology of Mycotoxins.* Halsted Press, New York, 1978.

Van Duuren, B. L.; Lowengart, G.; Seidman, I.; Smith, A. C.; and Melchionne, S.: Mouse skin carcinogenicity tests of the flame retardants tris(2,3-dibromopropyl)phosphate, tetrakis (hydroxymethyl)phosphonium chloride, and polyvinyl bromide. *Cancer Res.*, 38:3236–40, 1978a.

Van Duuren, B. L.; Sivak, A.; Katz, C.; and Melchionne, S.: Tumorigenicity of acridine orange. *Br. J. Cancer*, 23:587–90, 1969.

Van Duuren, B. L.; Smith, A. C.; and Melchionne, S. M.: Effect of aging in two-stage carcinogenesis on mouse skin with phorbol myristate acetate as promoting agent. *Cancer Res.*, 38:865–66, 1978b.

Van Lancker, J. L.: DNA injuries, their repair, and carcinogenesis. In Grundmann, E., and Kirsten, W. H. (eds.): *Current Topics in Pathology*, Vol. 64. Springer-Verlag, Berlin, Heidelberg, 1977.

Walker, E. A.; Castegnaro, M.; Griciute, L.; and Lyle, R. E. (eds.): *Environmental Aspects of N-Nitroso Compounds.* IARC Scientific Publications No. 19, International Agency for Research on Cancer, Lyon, 1978.

Wattenberg, L. W.: Inhibitors of chemical carcinogenesis. *Adv. Cancer Res.*, 26:197–226, 1978.

Weinberg, A. M.: Science and trans-science. *Science*, 177:211, 1972.

Weisburger, E. K.: Mechanisms of chemical carcinogenesis. *Ann. Rev. Pharmacol. Toxicol.*, 18:395–415, 1978.

Weisburger, J. H.: Mechanism of action of diet as a carcinogen. *Cancer*, 43:1987–95, 1979.

Weisburger, J. H., and Williams, G. M.: Chemical carcinogenesis. In Holland, J. F., and Frei, E., III (eds.): *Cancer Medicine*, 2nd ed. Lea & Febiger, Philadelphia, 1980.

Whittemore, A. S.: Quantitative theories of oncogenesis. *Adv. Cancer Res.*, 27:55–88, 1978.

Williams, G. M.: The use of liver epithelial cultures for the study of chemical carcinogenesis. *Am. J. Pathol.*, 85:739–53, 1976.

Williams, G. M.: The status of *in vitro* test systems utilizing DNA damage and repair for the screening of chemical carcinogens. *J. Assoc. Official Anal. Chem.*, 63:857–63, 1979.

Williams, G. M.: The detection of chemical mutagens/carcinogens by DNA repair and mutagenesis in liver cultures. In DeSerres, F. J., and Hollander, A. (eds.): *Chemical Mutagens*, Vol. VI. Plenum Press, New York, 1980.

Williams, G. M., and Watanabe, K.: Quantitative kinetics of development of N-2-fluorenylacetamide-induced, altered (hyperplastic)hepatocellular foci resistant to iron accumulation and of their reversion or persistence following removal of carcinogen. *J. Natl. Cancer Inst.*, **61**:113–21, 1978.

Wolff, S.: Sister chromatid exchange. *Annu. Rev. Genet.*, **11**:183–201, 1977.

Woo, Y.-T.; Argus, M. F.; and Arcos, J. C.: Effect of mixed-function oxidase modifiers on metabolism and toxicity of the oncogen dioxane. *Cancer Res.*, **38**:1621–25, 1978.

Wynder, E. L.: The Delaney clause controversy. *Prev. Med.*, **2**:123–70, 1973.

Wynder, E. L., and Gori, G. B.: Contribution of the environment to cancer incidence: An epidemiologic exercise. *J. Natl. Cancer Inst.*, **58**:825–32, 1977.

Wynder, E. L., and Hecht, S.: *Lung Cancer*. UICC Technical Report Series, Vol. 25, Geneva, 1976.

Wynder, E. L.; Peters, J. A.; and Vivona, S. (eds.): Symposium: Nutrition in the causation of cancer. *Cancer Res.*, **35**:3231–3550, 1975.

Young, J. D.; Braun, W. H.; and Gehring, P. J.: Dose-dependent fate of 1,4-dioxane in rats. *J. Toxicol. Environ. Health*, **4**:709–26, 1978.

Chapter 7

GENETIC TOXICOLOGY

William G. Thilly and *Howard L. Liber*

INTRODUCTION

Genetic toxicology is the study of the inter-action of chemical and physical agents with the process of heredity. One of the practical results of research in this field has been the development of a series of microbial (prokaryotic and eukaryotic) assays for the various kinds of genetic damage caused by environmental chemicals. These "short-term tests" are, without question, the reason for today's general interest in the field. Students should understand, however, that these assays are the products of scientific research based on a broad foundation of genetic and molecular knowledge. The use of these genetic assays obliges the user to acquire the knowledge and understand the assumptions, which predicate their design and define their limits, in determining the level of hazard associated with a test substance.

As an area of basic research, genetic toxicology has its own molecular problems to unravel, but even the most molecularly oriented researchers are simultaneously responsible for participating in the evaluation of the sources of risk and for ultimately reducing the incidence of serious and widespread human diseases. Many of the heritable diseases of humans already have been shown to arise as a result of change in DNA structure, chromosomal structure, or chromosome number. It is assumed that other heritable diseases arise via these kinds of genetic errors despite the absence of rigorous demonstrations for each case. Less clear is the relationship between genetic change and cancer. This relationship rests (1) on the demonstration that nearly all chemicals that induce genetic change in any of a variety of biologic systems are also capable of inducing tumors in experimental animals; and, vice versa (2) on the apparent monoclonal constitution of tumors; and (3) on the heritable nature of the cancer cell's phenotype. Monoclonal constitution of atherosclerotic plaques has led to the suggestion that this important disease state also has an origin in genetic damage. However, it must be clearly understood that the causal relationships have not

yet been established in these examples, and that the testing of these possibilities is an important area of present intellecutal activity. This chapter will consider only the heritable human diseases as having an etiology of genetic damage, *res ipsa loquitur*. Were other diseases to arise via errors in genetic mechanisms, the discussions presented here might apply to their etiology as well.

Genetic toxicology, as a field of research, combines the powerful tools of genetic and molecular biology with an important goal (the reduction of genetic disease) directly related to the well-being of society. To introduce the scientific substance of this field, we first define in the best structural terms available the nature of the genetic lesions of humans. We then review the association of these lesions with specific human diseases, consider the incidence of these diseases individually and as a class, and consider our reasons for believing that there are separate kinds of genetic disease possible having separate environmental etiologies.

Returning to the structural genetic lesions, we discuss illustrative methods by which their induction by chemicals can be studied and identify those chemicals and chemical classes that have been shown to be genetically active. Finally, we turn to the central assumption of today's thinking in applied genetic toxicology: that reliable identification and regulation of substances genetically active in microbial (prokaryotes and eukaryotes) genetic assay systems will reduce the incidence of genetic disease.

CLASSIFICATION OF GENETIC LESIONS BASED ON THE MOLECULAR LEVEL OF ERROR IN TRANSMISSION

Human genetic diseases arise from *at least* three separate modes of failure to transmit genetic information accurately and quantitatively.

Gene-locus mutations or "point mutations" are changes in the DNA sequence within a gene. Either substitution of an incorrect base pair or addition or deletion of a small number of base pairs constitutes the nature of this kind of lesion. The process of forming gene-locus mutations is called *mutagenesis* by microbiologists, although many mammalian workers use this term to refer to all genetic changes. In this discussion, "*mutagenesis*" is used *solely* to designate the production of gene-locus or point mutations.

This use of the term "mutagenesis" to designate gene-locus mutation is complemented by the use of the term "clastogenesis" (break production) to designate the process of genetic change, which appears as microscopically observable addition, deletion, or rearrangement of parts of the chromosomes in eukaryotic species. Students are warned, however, that some authors include the processes resulting in the gain or loss of whole chromosomes in their use of the term "clastogenesis" (or mutagenesis for that matter). The gain or loss of whole chromosomes might better be separated in our thinking from chromosomal breakage, since its molecular mechanism and sensitivity to chemical or physical agents is probably quite different. Unfortunately, a single term for the gain or loss of whole chromosomes has not yet gained wide use among genetic toxicologists. We will use the somewhat cumbersome word "*aneuploidization*" for our discussions. (See Table 7–1.)

Table 7–1.   DEFINITIONS

Mutagenesis:	Occurrence of "point" or "gene-locus" mutation (base-pair substitutions and small additions or deletions)
Clastogenesis:	Occurrence of chromosomal breaks resulting in gain, loss, or rearrangement of pieces of chromosomes
Aneuploidization:	Gain or loss of one or more intact chromosomes

The terms "mutagenesis," "clastogenesis," and "aneuploidization" thus define specific structural changes in the cellular genetic complement. Each definition should be used in its most general sense, and when a particular mechanism is found to produce one of these structural changes, one should continue to consider other molecular mechanisms and to assess the fraction of actual lesions of the particular class that are produced by the newly demonstrated process.

Mutagenesis involves one of the six possible base-pair substitutions (i.e., two transitions $AT \rightarrow GC$, $GC \rightarrow AT$; and four transversions $AT \rightarrow TA$ or CG, $GC \rightarrow CG$ or TA;) or the addition or deletion of any number of base pairs in an existing sequence (e.g., $\dfrac{-AAAAAA-}{-TTTTT-} \rightarrow$

$\dfrac{AAAXXAAA}{TTTYYTTT}$, an addition of two base pairs). Base-pair mutation at the DNA or genotypic level would be expected, on the basis of molecular biology, to be observed only under one of two conditions: (1) a triplet codon is changed to the codon for a new amino acid, and then only when the amino acid substitution changes some important property of the protein such as its catalytic activity or resistance to protease attack; (2) a protein synthesis termination sequence is generated in the mRNA $\left(\text{DNA sequences } \dfrac{TAG}{ATC}, \right.$ $\left. \dfrac{TGA}{ACT}, \dfrac{TGG}{ACC} \right)$ instead of a triplet codon for an amino acid. Naturally, the premature termination must also modify biologic activity of the protein to be observed. Most students are certain they are adept in handling these simple concepts. It is a good idea to calculate the probability of any single base substitution changing the *charge* at a particular amino acid site, inserting a proline, for example, or generating a chain-terminating or "nonsense" codon, to test one's own adeptness. What is the probability, for instance, of generating a nonsense codon via an $AT \rightarrow GC$ transition?

Addition or deletion of base pairs, when the number of base-pair changes is not a multiple of three, will drastically change the amino acid sequence of the protein coded after the mutation and will probably have an effect on protein function similar to a chain-terminating mutation. These are called *frameshift mutations*. Additions or deletions of three base pairs (or multiples of three) would have the effect of adding or deleting one (or more) amino acid(s) from the coded protein. Thus the effect of an addition or deletion of three base pairs would probably mimic base-pair substitution, because only changes in protein structure affecting catalysis, protease resistance, etc., would be observed as a phenotypic change. There is some imprecision in our definition of addition or deletion mutations, in that it is (1) usually applied to a small number of base pairs, and (2) possible that such mutations arise from several independent molecular mechanisms. Events involving, for example, ten or more bases are usually termed "large additions" or "large deletions" and, if large enough (greater than 10^4 base pairs, for instance), enter the undefined area between point mutation and chromosomal breakage in eukaryotic cells.

Error in the nondamaging, but as-yet-undefined, processes of recombination involving double-stranded DNA exchanges between chromosomes could result in genetic addition or deletion, which would not necessarily be morphologically detectable in chromosomes.

The phenotypic effects of clastogenesis or aneuploidization may, in large part, be anticipated to reflect the gain or loss of multiple genes, except in cases where rearrangements following clastogenesis might change the nature of the control systems under which some or all of the involved genes operate. It is not only for this reason however, that clastogenesis and aneuploidization have been distinguished in this chapter, but because the processes may have differing modes of induction and spectra of chemical sensitivity.

EXAMPLES AND FREQUENCIES OF HUMAN GENETIC DISEASES

It is one thing to define the different genetic lesions in terms of the structural changes in the DNA or the chromosomes and quite another to consistently use these definitions in discussions of both human genetic diseases and of the mechanisms by which the lesions are produced. In the matter of human genetic diseases, distinction between aneuploidization and clastogenesis is not often made, but sufficient data are now available to make reasonable estimates of their respective frequencies in liveborn infants. Accurate division of the thousands of recorded heritable syndromes between those of mutagenic and submicroscopic clastogenic origin, however, is not at present possible. Even in cases where altered protein sequences have been demonstrated, it would seem doctrinaire to the point of imprudence to insist that such lesions, involving only a few base pairs, could not arise as the result of unequal crossing over or of other aberration of recombination. We shall attempt to present the available information in a manner linking possible genetic mechanism to human disease as closely as possible.

Errors of Chromosomal Number and Structure

Hook and Hamerton (1977) have recently summarized the results of seven studies of chromosomal abnormalities in newborns. Of some 56,952 infants examined, 353 were found to have a microscopically detectable lesion (0.62 percent). We may class 189 of the abnormalities as aneuploidization, of which 107 were found in the sex chromosomes and 82 were found among the remaining autosomal chromosomes. Table 7–2 summarizes these data. This total frequency of 0.33 percent for abnormalities of chromosome number in newborns should be contrasted to the report of Boué et al. (1975) in which a total chromosomal abnormality frequency of 6.15 percent was found in spontaneously aborted fetuses less than 12 weeks of age, and the finding of Creasy and Alberman reported by Carr and Gedeon (1977) that the total chromosomal abnormality frequency in spontaneous abortuses up

to 27 weeks of age was 30.5 percent. Of these, the errors of chromosomal number comprised a major fraction (93 percent). These data suggest that the various trisomies are selected against *in utero*, probably from fertilization onward, so that the observed frequency among newborns is a gross underestimate of the frequency of occurrence of aneuploidization in human gametogenesis. Such a conclusion is consistent with *in vitro* observations that chromosomal anomalies induced by physical or chemical agents are generally associated with cell reproductive death.

Carr and Gedeon (1977) also summarized data showing that triploidy and tetraploidy account for some 23 percent of the chromosomal anomalies in spontaneous abortions, but reference to Hook and Hamerton (1977) shows only one case of triploidy in the 56,952 newborns examined, suggesting extreme selective pressure against polyploidy during gestation.

Table 7–2. FREQUENCY OF ANEUPLOIDY IN HUMAN NEWBORN*

	TOTAL OBSERVED	PERCENT
Sex Chromosomes		
47,XYY	35	0.061
47,XXY	35	0.061
47,XXX	28	0.049
45,XO	2	0.004
Other	7	0.012
Autosomes		
+D	3	0.005
+E	7	0.012
+G	71	0.125
Other	1	0.002
Total examined = 56,952		

* Summarized from Hook and Hamerton (1977).

When the trisomies were examined for each of the 22 autosomes, an extra chromosome 16 accounted for 116/368 of all trisomies encountered, while no examples of extra chromosomes 1 or 5 were found (Carr and Gedeon, 1977). This contrasts with the predominance of an extra chromosome 21 among trisomies in newborns, again emphasizing the intrauterine selection processes in determining the frequency of particular chromosomal number abnormalities in liveborn infants.

Of the many etiologic factors examined in an attempt to find the cause of aneuploidization in humans, only maternal age has been found to yield a positive correlation that is statistically significant. This does not mean that the events of aneuploidization occur only in female gametogenesis. In an analysis of the origin of the extra chromosome 21 in Down's syndrome, some 7 of

31 were found to be of paternal origin. However, the frequency of trisomies does not significantly increase with paternal age as it does in the case of maternal age. Redrawn in Figure 7–1 is the summary of Vogel (1970) of the maternal age dependence of trisomies 13 (Patau's syndrome), 18 (Edward's syndrome), and a deletion of the short arm of chromosome 18. The continuous interaction of the parent with the chemical and physical environment might be expected to yield a monotonic increase in total genetic insults, and, thus, these age dependence data are particularly important in considering possible approaches to human genetic toxicology.

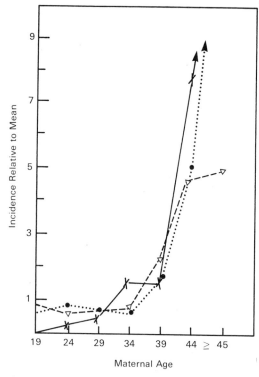

Figure 7–1. Chromosomal abnormalities and maternal age; (∇) D_1 trisomy (Patau's syndrome, 172 cases); ($\bullet$) trisomy 18 (Edward's syndrome, 153 cases); (X) $E_{18}p$ (35 cases). (Redrawn from Vogel, F.: Spontaneous mutation in man. In Vogel, F., and Rohrborn, G. [eds.]: *Chemical Mutagenesis in Mammals and Man.* Springer Verlag, New York, 1970.)

When the data regarding microscopically detectable chromosomal breaks in newborns are summarized (Table 7–3), the total number of balanced (total chromosomal material is apparently unchanged) and unbalanced (some loss or gain of chromosomal material is evident) rearrangements is 144 in the six studies of 56,952 infants, for a frequency of 0.25 percent (Hook

Table 7–3. FREQUENCIES OF ABNORMALITIES OF CHROMOSOME STRUCTURE*

	TOTAL OBSERVED	PERCENT
Balanced rearrangements	110	0.2
(Translocations and inversions)	0	0
Unbalanced rearrangements	34	0.06
(Translocations)	11	0.019
(Inversions)	1	0.002
(Deletions)	5	0.009
(Supernumerary)	10	0.018
(Other)	7	0.012
Total examined = 56,952		

* Summarized from Hook and Hamerton (1977).

and Hamerton, 1977). Carr and Gedeon (1977) summarize a number of studies involving spontaneous abortuses and report a range of 1.3 to 3.8 percent of detectable translocations. As was the case with trisomy, an intrauterine selective pressure seems to be operative. However, a conservative estimate that the intrauterine selective pressure permits only 0.0033/0.605 = 0.54 percent of chromosomal number errors arising in gametogenesis should be compared to the apparently smaller intrauterine selective pressure against the live, full-term birth of a fetus carrying a recognizable chromosomal break 0.0025/0.038 = 6.6 percent. A simple model of the probability of coming to term being an inverse function of the amount of DNA involved in the particular lesion is not incompatible with these calculations. As was the case with chromosomal number abnormalities, a higher probability of occurrence is found in infants of older mothers for some categories of chromosomal breaks. A good example is the occurrence of the syndrome associated with a deletion of the long arm of chromosome 18, which was found by Cenani and Pfeiffer and reported by Vogel (1970) to increase markedly with maternal age. No demonstration of dependence of chromosomal breaks on paternal age has been found. As recently as 1978, D. S. Borgaonkar has catalogued the several hundred chromosomal variants and anomalies observed in man, but specific anomalies continue to be added to the literature.

Errors Apparently at the Gene Level

Human genetic diseases that are not detectable on the basis of chromosomal abnormalities include, but are not limited to, diseases for which a change in the structure or the function of a protein, such as an enzyme, has been ascertained. Because this subclass of diseases is so readily identifiable with the well-studied microbiologic examples of point or gene-locus mutants, it is assumed sometimes that such genetic changes result from similar mutagenic processes. However, we must emphasize that such molecular evidence pointing to a gene-locus mutational origin is available for only a small portion of the diseases known to behave in a mendelian manner without any microscopically evident chromosomal malformation. Despite this problem we will base our estimate of the total genetic damage suffered via the etiologic route of mutagenesis on the data available for this kind of disease. Error arising from this mode of estimate would be an overestimate of the relative importance of mutagenesis in causing human genetic disease.

Carter (1977) estimated that some 7/1,000 newborns in European populations suffered from diseases that behaved as autosomal dominants, 2.5/1,000 from autosomal recessive diseases, and 0.4/1,000 from X-linked disease, for a total incidence of diseases of putative mutagenic origin of about 1 percent. McKusick (1975) has catalogued the human disease syndromes that behave as mendelian traits and lists a total of 2,336. New syndromes continue to be reported. Of these, 141 are identified as relating to enzyme deficiencies, and 34 others are associated with a nonenzymic protein such as in hemophilia A (factor VIII deficiency). Frequencies of occurrence for individual syndromes among the autosomal dominants and X-linked recessives range from a high of about 10^{-4} for the X-linked Duchenne-type muscular dystrophy to about 10^{-5} for achondroplasia (autosomal dominant) and to less than 10^{-6} as a best estimate for a large fraction of all known syndromes, for which only one or two cases have ever been identified. Vogel and Rathenberg (1975), in particular, have tried to take into account the various factors influencing the measurement of incidence of mutagenic disease and the calculation from these measurements of an average mutation rate in man. They also summarize the data that permit the conclusion that many of the diseases associated with mutagenesis do *not* display any increasing frequency with increasing maternal age, but, in contrast to the syndromes associated with chromosomal number and size abnormalities, display a strong positive correlation with paternal age. Several of Vogel's examples are redrawn for summary in Figure 7–2. No data are available regarding the frequency of gene-locus mutations in human abortuses; so calculations of selective pressure *in utero* are therefore impossible. A further point is that many genetic defects may not be evident until a considerable time after birth. Thus, the total incidence among infants represents, somewhat, an underestimate of the frequency of genetic disease (see also Chap. 8).

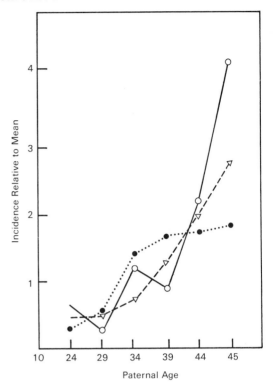

Figure 7–2. Gene locus mutation and paternal age: (∇) achondroplasia ($n = 77$); ($\bullet$) myositis ossificans ($n = 40$). (Redrawn from Vogel, F.: Spontaneous mutation in man. In Vogel, F., and Rohrborn, G. [eds.]: *Chemical Mutagenesis in Mammals and Man.* Springer Verlag, New York, 1970.)

At the biochemical level, Harris (1975) has summarized the amino acid sequences associated with the hemoglobin variants in man and pointed out that all of the possible transitions and transversions of base-pair substitution mutation may be deduced to have occurred in causing these abnormalities. Harris's treatment of the biochemical effects of genetic disease is a necessary part of a student's education in this area.

This brief summary of human genetic disease is meant to give a quantitative understanding of the incidence of disease putatively arising from aneuploidization (0.4 percent), from clastogenesis (0.3 percent), and from mutagenesis (1 percent). Also, it is useful to remember that maternal age affects the frequency of chromosomal number errors and chromosomal breakage frequencies for some, but apparently not all, specific lesions, and that paternal age affects the frequency of putative point mutations for some, but apparently not all, of the genetic lesions of that class. These data are sufficient to direct attention to genetic diseases as a major health problem, the amelioration of which deserves a high priority in the minds of those capable of understanding the problem and contributing to solutions.

TOXICOLOGIC PARADIGM

Other chapters of this text discuss many facets of man's interaction with the chemical environment. It is important to remember that genetic damage is not simply a question of classic genetics or molecular biology of the gene. As diagrammed in Figure 7–3, a series of processes separate

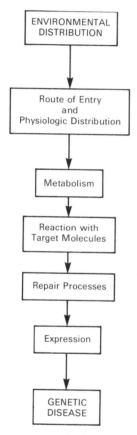

Figure 7–3. Toxicologic paradigm.

the chemical in the environment from the appearance of a genetically afflicted individual. Affecting the probability that a molecule of a particular chemical will cause a genetic error are its concentration in the environment; its physical/chemical characteristics, which affect the probability that it will enter the body and be distributed to the possible target tissues; the nature of the distribution system in man; the nature of the metabolic systems in the tissues to which the compound is distributed and the properties of the resulting metabolic products; the ability of

the compound or its metabolites to react with cellular target molecules, especially DNA; the ability of the cells to remove the products of such reactions and restore the prior biologic state through such processes as DNA repair; the ability of the tissue to recognize and suppress the multiplication of cells with aberrant properties; and the opportunity of whatever potential genetic change has been caused to be expressed. In the remaining sections of this chapter we discuss experimental models in terms which, for reasons of brevity, do not always give proper emphasis to the processes preceding the reaction of a chemical with the genetic material. However, it is the responsibility of genetic toxicology to continue to retest assumptions and to create experimental systems that mimic, in as many quantitative and qualitative conditions as possible, the processes of chemical-biologic interactions as they occur in humans.

Since human subjects cannot be exposed to test substances for the purpose of determining mutagenic potential, approximations must be devised that will yield a reliable differentiation between hazardous and nonhazardous substances. In order to faithfully mimic the exposure and response of humans, all of the pharmacokinetic, metabolic, genetic, and intercellular organizational characteristics of humans should be taken into account. Unfortunately, many important facts about humans are, for all practical purposes, unknown. Thus, in choosing an organism such as *S. typhimurium*, *D. melanogaster*, or *M. mus*, biochemical differences between these species and man may well be anticipated, and, indeed, many are already known in the processes of metabolism of xenobiotics and DNA repair. Within the many cell types in the human, however, there are many differences in metabolic activity toward mutagenic chemicals, and the possibility has not been eliminated that there can be important differences in the way that cells in different tissues excise chemical adducts in DNA and replace the missing sequences.

Additionally, there are important differences between the way that people seem to be exposed to chemical mutagens and the way that most determinations of mutagenic potential are performed. It would seem that people are exposed to a great variety of chemicals in amounts that rarely raise concentrations in body fluids above the nanomolar range for any one chemical. These low-concentration exposures of cells *in vivo* continue for essentially the preparental lifetime of the individual and the whole lifetime of the individual in models in which cancer and aging are regarded as diseases of mutational origin. This mode of exposure, low concentration, and long time is not the way that experiments have been performed to date. Nearly all experiments expose test animals or cells to effective concentrations in the micromolar-to-millimolar range for periods rarely in excess of one day. This is a constraint placed by the economic need to keep exposures short and the biologic requirement resulting from the fact that low-concentration exposures simply do not induce sufficient mutation to be statistically significant. Thus, it is incumbent upon the genetic toxicology community to develop experimental systems to test directly the relationship between time and concentration of exposure and the induction of genetic error.

CYTOGENETICS AND TOXICOLOGY

The Normal Human Genome

The normal human chromosomal complement or "karyotype" contains 46 chromosomes: 22 pairs of autosomes designated 1, 2, 3 . . . 22; and two sex chromosomes, XX in females and XY in males. Morphologically, the chromosomes are best characterized at mitosis, when they assume an extremely condensed conformation and, thus, become visible in the light microscope. They can be described as X-shaped objects consisting of two biarmed-shaped chromatids in which the two pairs of arms join at the region called the centromere (Fig. 7–4). The length (both relative

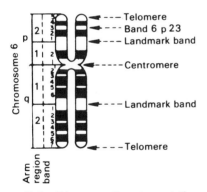

Figure 7–4. Diagrammatic representation of chromosome 6 in metaphase. (From Sanchez, O., and Yunis, J. J.: New chromosomal techniques and their medical applications. In Yunis, J. J. [ed.]: *New Chromosomal Syndromes.* Academic Press, Inc., New York, 1977.)

and absolute) of each chromatid arm is constant for each chromosome, but varies among chromosomes. This variation in size is the basis for the first discrimination among chromosomes, in which seven groups (A to G) are described.

More recently, however, several staining techniques have been developed that reveal each

chromosome to have a distinctive series of light and dark bands, by which it may be readily identified (Fig. 7–5). For example, Q bands refer to the banding patterns seen with quinacrine and G bands with giemsa. Other banding techniques exist as well (Sanchez and Yunis, 1977), and the patterns change during mitosis. The short arm of a chromosome is called p (for petite), while the long arm is q (measured from the centromere). Each arm is broken into regions, which are further subdivided into bands.

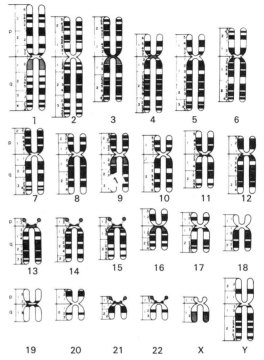

Figure 7–5. Diagrammatic representation of metaphase chromosome bands as observed with the Q- and G-staining methods; centromere representative of Q-banding method only. (From *Paris Conference [1971]: Standardization in Human Cytogenetics.* Birth Defects: Original Article Series, **VIII**: 7, 1972.)

As techniques for describing normal chromosomal morphology become more refined, it becomes possible to recognize chromosomal damage at a finer level. For example, the exchange of chromosomal regions of equal length between two different chromosomes (balanced translocations) can be identified by noting the characteristic banding patterns of the regions exchanged. The example shown in Figure 7–6 represents the changes that can be observed when chromosomes 2 and 6 exchange chromosomal material in a balanced fashion; i.e., none is lost to the cell; it has, however, been rearranged such that genes

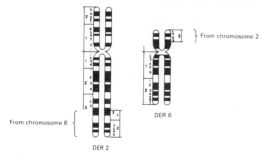

Figure 7–6. Schematic representation of a balanced translocation 2/6. (From Sanchez, O., and Yunis, J. J.: New chromosomal techniques and their medical applications. In Yunis, J. J. [ed.]: *New Chromosomal Syndromes*. Academic Press, Inc., New York, 1977.)

that were on chromosome 2 are now on chromosome 6, and vice versa.* Translocations need not be balanced and may or may not affect the size of the chromosomes enough to be detectable by nonbanding techniques.

Abnormal Genomes

Abnormal karyotypes are designated by giving the total number of chromosomes observed, followed by the number of the chromosome involved, if known. For instance, Down's syndrome is associated with an additional chromosome 21, and the karyotype is designated (47, 21 +), while Turner's syndrome, in which only one X chromosome is found, is designated (45,XO). If an addition or deletion is noted in part of a chromosome, the shorthand designation is to indicate the chromosomes involved and, if possible, whether it is the long or short arm of the chromosome(s), as in 18q⁻ syndrome (46, 18q⁻), where there occurs a deletion of part of the long arm of chromosome 18. Computer classification of structural abnormalities leads to a simple six-digit designation, giving the chromosome involved first, then the arm designation (p or q), then the region, band, and subbands according to the Paris Conference (1971). 05p140 would indicate an aberration in the *short* arm (p) of chromosome 5 in region *1* (there is only one) in the 4th band, but without any designation of subband position *0*.

Aneuploidization. Aneuploidy is responsible for several of the most common genetic diseases. Klinefelter's (47, XXY) and Down's (47, 21 +) syndromes are generally due to trisomies, while

Turner's (45, XO) is due to a monosomy. The mechanism by which such aberrant cells arise is thought to be via nondisjunction, in which a dividing cell does not distribute the chromosomes equally to its daughters. Thus, a sperm or egg could contain two sex chromosomes or two chromosomes 21. The actual molecular/physical reason that the cell fails to divide properly is unknown. Studies with mice (Szemere and Chandley, 1975) have shown that x-rays can induce nondisjunction in males. In this study, 23/1,000 meiotic cells from irradiated animals were trisomic, as compared to 0/200 in controls. Studies in *Drosophila* have revealed that x-rays (Mavor, 1924) and heat (Grell, 1971) increase the apparent frequency of nondisjunction.

Assay systems have been developed in diploid yeasts that detect nondisjunction by the emergence of a recessive characteristic after loss of a sister chromosome containing the dominant variant (Parry and Zimmerman, 1976). Heat, UV light, and x-irradiation were shown to cause nondisjunction.

Higher orders of aneuploidy are occasionally seen in humans, especially in the sex chromosomes. Genotypes containing up to five sex chromosomes have been reported. These cases are thought to be the result of successive nondisjunctions during the two meiotic divisions (Hamerton, 1971). Triploid and tetraploid (containing 69 or 92 chromosomes, respectively) babies are very rare, although they form a significant fraction of aborted fetuses. Triploidy may be the result of fertilization by two sperm, while tetraploidy is most likely due to failure of cytokinesis at the first cleavage division. Almost all of these aneuploid situations can also exist in mosaic form, with normal 46-chromosome karyotypes, generally due to mitotic nondisjunctions at some point after the first division of the fertilized ovum.

In conclusion, although there is no evidence indicating that chemicals cause aneuploidy in humans, these kinds of defects should be considered as *potential* toxicologic problems until further information is available.

Clastogenesis. There is a large literature dealing with cytogenic observations of individual chromosomal structural aberrations in many species of eukaryotic cells. The method is straightforward: the desired cells are collected, and their growth halted in metaphase by colcemid or colchicine. They are then fixed, stained, and examined under the microscope (see Cohen and Hirschhorn, 1971). The types of abnormalities scored include single chromatid gap, an unstained region on a single chromatid without a definite boundary whose dimensions are no more than the width of the chromatid; single chromatid

---

* This kind of exchange often has no effect on the functionality of the cell in which it occurs, because no genetic material has been lost. However, were this cell to undergo *meiosis*, it could produce gametes, which are partially trisomic and monosomic, depending on how the chromosomes segregated.

break, a clean, unstained region with a definite boundary whose space between boundaries is greater than the width of the chromatid; isochromatid gap, an unstained region on *both* chromatids without a definite boundary whose dimensions are no more than the width of the chromatids; isochromatid break, a clean, unstained region on *both* chromatids with a definite boundary whose space between boundaries is greater than the width of the chromatids; dicentric chromosome, the rejoining of two chromosomes by either short or long arms, resulting in a new chromosome with *two centromeres*; translocations, the exchange of material between two chromosomes (e.g., Kihlman, 1971).

Numerous studies have been performed in which cells were exposed to a chemical or physical agent and then examined for increased frequency of chromosomal aberrations. Several different types of systems have been used, and these are summarized and exemplified below.

1. *In vivo* studies: animals (generally mice) are treated with a chemical, and chromosomal aberrations are scored in their bone marrow cells, peripheral lymphocytes, and spermatogonia (e.g., Tates and Natarajan, 1976).

2. *In vivo* F_1 studies: animals are treated with a chemical, and their offspring are examined for abnormalities. As an example, Sotomayor and Cumming (1975) observed an increase in translocations in the male offspring of mice treated with cyclophosphamide.

3. Human studies: human peripheral lymphocytes can easily be examined for chromosome damage. Groups examined usually include industrial workers exposed to chemicals (e.g., Bauchinger *et al.*, 1976; Meretoja *et al.*, 1977) and patients undergoing treatment with various drugs (Watson *et al.*, 1976).

4. *In vitro* studies: many different cell types have been used for *in vitro* clastogenesis work. *In vitro* use of human cells allows the researcher to treat with any chemical desired, which of course cannot be done with humans.

By means of illustration, a recent publication typical of this genre, remarkable for its clarity, is summarized here. Dr. J. R. Honeycombe of the Institute of Cancer Research, London, investigated the clastogenic effects of 1,4-dimethane sulphonoxybutane (BUS, busulfan) on lymphocyte cultures freshly derived from normal males and females. The test compound was coincubated for three days with whole blood samples diluted with culture medium, which were treated with phytohemagglutinin to stimulate the division of a subpopulation of the blood lymphocytes. At the end of three days, when most cells had completed at least two mitoses after growth stimulation, colcemid, which blocks formation of the

mitotic spindle and thus prevents completion of mitosis after chromosome condensation, was added to the culture to increase the number of cells in metaphase. The cells were collected, fixed, spread on a microscope slide, treated with trypsin, and subsequently stained to produce the G-banding pattern. The appearance of chromosomal anomalies could be (1) counted and (2) assigned to specific regions in the banding pattern. Figure 7–7 summarizes her principal ob-

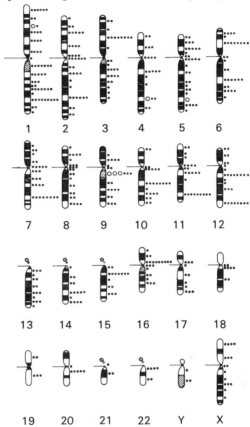

Figure 7–7. Distribution of breakpoints on a G-band karyogram of the human chromosome complement. The dark spots (●) represent one breakpoint and the clear circles (○) represent ten breakpoints. (From *Paris Conference [1971]: Standardization in Human Cytogenetics*, Birth Defects: Original Article Series, **VIII**: 7, 1972.)

servations and illustrates the concept of chromosome banding and its use in seeking clues to the mechanisms of chemical clastogenesis. The data demonstrate a nonrandom distribution of breaks among chromosomes and among regions of the same chromosome. (Nonrandom distributions have also been observed after treatment of human cells with mitomycin C [Cohen and Shaw, 1964; Morad *et al.*, 1973] and chlorambucil

[Reeves and Margoles, 1974].) Particularly interesting is the apparent occurrence of breaks in the unstained areas of the G banding. Finding the molecular explanation for this kind of specificity is one of the principal challenges to genetic toxicology today.

Figure 7–8 summarizes the data relating the concentration of test agent to the number of aberrations observed. Quantitative data of this kind are necessary in comparing the relative potency of different chemicals, or in studying the mechanisms of clastogenesis by comparing results with the same compound performed under different experimental conditions.

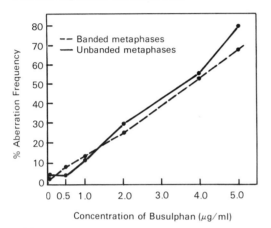

Figure 7–8. The relationship between percent aberration frequencies (i.e., total number of aberrations in 100 cells) for banded and unbanded chromosomes and BUS concentration in μg/ml for one individual (male, age range 20 to 30). (From Honeycombe, J. R.: The effects of busulphan on the chromosomes of normal human lymphocytes. *Mutat. Res.*, **57**:35–49, 1978.)

5. The micronucleus test: this is a proposed bioassay system for chromosome damage based on the production of "micronuclei," which are presumably composed of chromosome fragments resulting from breakage (Countryman and Heddle, 1976). Agents that cause other types of chromosome damage often induce increases in micronuclei frequency (e.g., Wild, 1978). The major advantage of this system of identification and enumeration of specific chromosome aberrations is its apparent simplicity of scoring. At this writing, this approach is still being evaluated as a possibly more efficient means of assessing clastogenic potential of chemicals.

EXPERIMENTAL MUTAGENESIS

Basic Principles

Independent of species, mutagenesis is defined as a change in the linear structure of DNA. Un-

like aneuploidy or clastogenesis, this change in sequence is not detectable by microscopy. These genotypic changes must be expressed in a way that they can be identified through recognizable "phenotypic" changes. A commonly used phenotypic change is the loss of the function of a particular enzyme (forward mutation, i.e., away from the wild phenotype) or the regaining of the function of an enzyme (reversion, i.e., toward the wild phenotype). In a growing number of experimental systems, the genetic basis of the observed phenotypic changes has been demonstrated by sequencing the affected protein or the DNA itself and showing the molecular nature of the change in one or several examples. However, there are any number of assays in which only the loss of enzyme activity or acquisition of a trait (e.g., drug resistance) closely associated with the function of an enzyme has been demonstrated. The existence of mutations in the associated DNA sequences for the structure of the enzyme or the molecules that control its synthesis or degradation is, in such cases, assumed or inferred from the behavior of the assay; i.e., frequency is affected by mutagenic stimuli; occurrence is shown to be a spontaneous event independent of selective conditions, etc. Still other assays are based on observations of morphologic changes in phenotype, such as colony size, shape, or color in microbiologic systems; wing shape, the presence of distinctive wing veination, or absence of bristles in *Drosophila*; or coat color or marking in mice. The enzyme or functional protein associated with these phenotypic changes is, in most cases, unknown. Their genetic origin is demonstrated by classic genetic techniques of mating and back crossing. Hollaender (1971a, 1971b, 1973, 1976) has edited a series of volumes, each containing detailed descriptions of a wide variety of genetic assays involving species from bacteria and fungi through insects and rodents to humans. While most of the mutagenesis literature involves the measurement of change in one or a small number of genetic loci by detecting an associated phenotypic change, it is also possible to examine the products of hundreds of soluble proteins, and noting the appearance or disappearance of electrophoretic bands, indicating a mutation. This approach has been discussed by Harris (1975) and applied broadly to the study of genetic diversity in human populations.

Mathematical Modeling of Induced Mutation.
When a noxious agent is introduced into a large population of people, fruit flies, or cells, depending on the agent and its effective concentration, some individuals are mutated at individual genetic loci and some individuals die. Death, however, has very little to do with mutation at the genetic loci used in most investigations, because those

loci are chosen by the investigator as sites where mutations confer no selective disadvantage. Thus, death, which probably occurs because of some nongenetic effect of the agent, can be modeled as an event independent of the mutation caused by the test agent. This is important in that the assumption of independence makes modeling a lot easier, but more importantly, it emphasizes that there are two distinct biologic processes occurring, death and mutation.

Given independence of death and mutation, there are four kinds of individuals in a population following treatment with a test agent:

Fraction A, dead and mutated;
Fraction B, not dead and mutated;
Fraction C, dead and not mutated;
Fraction D, not dead and not mutated.

The fraction of cells that are dead is simply A + C, and the fraction that are mutant for the selected phenotype is A + B. The alert will reason that individuals that are dead are going to be difficult to identify as mutant or not mutant, since in most assays, growth under selective conditions or growth to maturity is required for such identification. Here, again, the independence of death and mutation is found to be a fundamental assumption, because the number we wish to determine $A + B/(A + B + C + D)$ is equal to $B/(B + D)$; i.e., the fraction of all cells mutated is equal to the fraction of mutant cells among surviving cells.

Both mutation and death can be modeled as occurring from one or more chemical reactions in one or more cellular target molecules of fixed size. For this discussion, we will use the simplest example, that of a single fixed target requiring one reaction (hit) to cause death and another fixed target, usually smaller, which requires only one hit to cause mutation. This kind of modeling is known as "target theory" and has been used in radiation biology for decades. A good general treatment can be found in Elkind and Whitmore (1967).

The fraction of all cells that are mutated by treatment can be designated M and the fraction killed designated T. Another way of saying this is that the probability of any individual in the population suffering death is T and of sustaining a particular mutation is M. Now, it is possible that any cell might be hit in the death target 0, 1, 2, 3, . . . times, and this is equally true for hits in the mutation target. Thus, the requirements of a discrete variable, having an infinite number of possible integral values, independence of events, and statistical equilibrium, are fulfilled, which permits description of the situation in terms of the Poisson distribution (Wadsworth and Bryan, 1960). Using the Poisson distribution allows us to derive the result that the probability of surviving,

$S = 1 - T$, is the probability of not having any lethal hits. Expressing the average number of lethal hits in any lethal target, in terms of a second-order chemical reaction between the treatment parameter D and the target parameter α, permits us to write the relationship between survival and treatment as

$$S = e^{-\alpha D}$$

which is applicable even as T approaches 1. Another way to look at this is to note that for small T, $T = \alpha D$; i.e., killing is proportional to target size and the treatment parameter. Mutation can be modeled in the same way as killing. The only adjustment is that an independent mutational target parameter β must be chosen so that $M = \beta D$.

α and β then represent "inverse target sizes" and D is a parameter that depends on the concentration and duration of exposure of the target to the test agent. Another term for D is dose. In our cozy world of arithmetic models, then, experiments would give results as in Figure 7–9, in

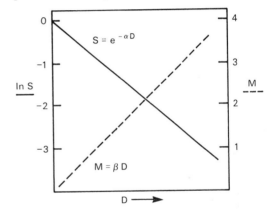

Figure 7–9. Survival and mutation as a function of dose when killing and mutation are modeled as simple first-order reactions between a cellular target and the dosing agent.

which the surviving fraction S decreases as an exponential function of D, and the mutant fraction increases linearly with D. In experimental practice, it should be obvious that mutant fraction, M, is actually calculated by first determining the surviving fraction, S, and dividing that number into the fraction of individuals treated that are mutant. This is because the mutants counted are, of course, both mutant *and* alive and represent the fraction $M \times S$ of the treated population. Since we want to know M, we simply divide $M \times S$ by S.

More often than not, however, experimental results do not reasonably approximate Figure 7–9. Often, results indicate that at low values of

D, very little change, if any, appears to occur in survival or mutant fractions, as shown in Figure 7–10. Curves of this shape are often described as

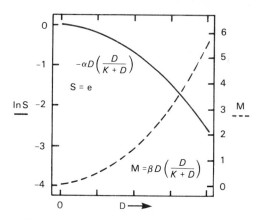

Figure 7–10. Survival and mutation as functions of dose under the assumption that chemical hits are linear with dose (αD or βD) and that the probability of nonrepair is approximated by $\dfrac{K}{K + D}$.

"threshold" responses because significant change is not observed at D below some low value. Some workers have suggested that these curves arise from the removal of potentially toxic and mutagenic lesions by a repair system which is saturated at high D. Thus for D greater than some minimal level, all additional damage could kill or mutate, as in Figure 7–9. In distinction to this "saturable repair" model, one should also consider an "unsaturated repair" model, as in Figure 7–10, in which the probability of a chemical event is just αD for a lethal target and the probability of *nonrepair* is approximated by $\dfrac{D}{K + D}$. K is a function related to the ability of the cell to repair itself by an unsaturated enzyme system; i.e., K is much bigger than D.

Other mechanisms should be considered. Any saturable function such as a rate-limiting cellular uptake step could yield the threshold response. A chemical could preferentially react with a cellular component (e.g., glutathione) so that other, slower reactions would be relatively insignificant until the pool of reactant component was exhausted. The important thing to remember is that the existence of a shoulder in a survival or mutation curve is not sufficient to prove the existence of a DNA repair or any other kind of cellular recovery system.

There are, no doubt, other mechanistic models that would lead, predictably, to threshold responses. This simplification of the subject for the purpose of introduction should not obscure the fact that actual experimental results are nearly always more complicated than hypothetic models. Students may wish to devise means to explain mutation response curves such as in Figure 7–11 in which the compound ICR-191 was reported to induce mutation linearly with concentrations from 0 to 1.5 μM, and then plateaued in both human and hamster cell mutation assays at the hgprt locus (DeLuca *et al.*, 1977; O'Neill *et al.*, 1978).

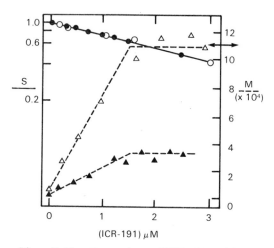

Figure 7–11. Comparison of ICR-191 toxicity ($\bigcirc$) and mutagenicity ($\triangle$) to hamster cells (O'Neill *et al.*, 1978) and to human cells ($\bullet$, $\blacktriangle$) (DeLuca *et al.*, 1977) in 16- and 24-hour exposures, respectively. Can you explain the apparent plateau at 1.5 μM?

Examples

Ames Assays.   Bruce Ames and his colleagues at the University of California at Berkeley carefully selected, from a group of hundreds of different point mutations in the *his* operon of *Salmonella typhimurium*, a set of three point mutations that demonstrated a low frequency of spontaneous reverse mutation and could be readily reverted to the wild phenotype by exposure to known chemical mutagens (Ames *et al.*, 1975).

It was known from the pioneering work of Benzer (1961) that some chemicals, such as methylnitronitrosoguanidine (MNNG), were active in causing base-pair substitution mutations, but not addition or deletion mutations, while other compounds, such as 9-aminoacridine, exhibited an opposite mutational activity. Ames, thus, chose a strain sensitive to the "base-pair mutagens" and two strains sensitive to addition or deletion mutagens. The term"frameshift" mutagen has been applied to addition or deletion mutagens, even though frameshifts result only when addition or deletion of base pairs not evenly divisible by three occurs. The base-pair mutation carrying strain TA1535 (*S. typhimurium*, Ames, strain number) was mutant in the hisG gene coding for the enzyme phosphoribosyl ATP synthetase, which is required for histidine synthesis. The mutation itself was designated his G46. The actual nature of the base substitution (whether transition or transversion) has not yet been determined. The mutation his G46 made the carrier strain auxotrophic for histidine. Thus, reverse mutation to the wild phenotype could be detected by the appearance of bacterial colonies growing in the absence of exogenous histidine. Similarly, reversion of strain TA1538 indicated ability of a test compound to delete two base pairs, $\frac{G-C}{C-G}$, from the sequence $\frac{GCGCGC}{CGCGCG}$ in the structural gene for histidine dehydrogenase. This mutation is designated his D3052. Reversion of strain TA1537 indicated that a $\frac{C}{G}$ base-pair addition occurred in a sequence $\frac{GG}{CC}$ in the gene for histidine aminotransferase, the mutation being designated his C3076. This set of mutants each contained an additional deletion mutation, designated uvrB, that eliminated a DNA repair system that normally protects *Salmonella* from mutation by ultraviolet light. The effect of choosing strains carrying the uvrB defect was to increase the sensitivity of the strains to most chemical mutagens. Yet another mutation, rfa, was also incorporated, which changed the nature of the lipopolysaccharide bacterial cell wall, such that it became more permeable to chemicals like the polycyclic and heterocyclic hydrocarbons and, thus, more sensitive to the mutagenic activity of such compounds.

Still greater sensitivity to mutagenesis by some chemicals, e.g., aflatoxin B_1, was conferred to the tester strains by inserting a plasmid, pKm101, which presumably carried an error-prone DNA repair system. An increase in sensitivity did not occur with pKm101 addition for all compounds, and some diminution resulted for alkylating agents. Addition of the plasmid to strain TA1535 resulted in strain TA100 and addition to strain TA1538 resulted in strain TA98.

Studies using the Ames strains have confirmed the earlier observations that the kind of genetic lesion predominantly induced is related to chemical structure of the test agent. However, while the nature of the chemical lesion may often determine the pathway of genetic change, this is not always the case, since errors apparently can arise from inaccurate resynthesis of DNA strands after removal of the chemical lesion by cellular enzymes. Using the Ames strains' response to 0.32 μM aflatoxin B_1, after being in a one-hour liquid incubation in the presence of rat liver microsomes, illustrates this point. Of the strains not carrying the error-prone repair associated plasmid (TA1535, TA1537, TA1538), only the base-pair substitution carrying strain TA1535 mutation is reverted. But, when pKm101 is added to strains TA1535 or TA1538, creating strains TA100 and TA98, both the base substitution and the addition mutation are reverted under the same conditions. The implication is that, as a result of the action of the putative error-prone repair system, errors of the addition and deletion variety can now occur during the process of repairing the damage caused by aflatoxin B_1 treatment.

As this chapter is being written, techniques for the use of Ames' doubly repair-deficient and permeable strains are in a state of reexamination and improvement. The original studies of several hundred compounds were performed with standard bacterial plating techniques, but the requirement for performance of tens of thousands of assays yearly in testing laboratories has led to the suggestion that serial dilution approaches be substituted. Our own experience with the Ames *S. typhimurium* strains in assays of forward mutation to drug (8-azaguanine) resistance (presumably via mutation inactivating one of the several enzymes necessary for metabolizing the base analog to a form incorporable into RNA) has led us to suggest that the single forward assay can effectively replace the set of reversion assays without compromising the sensitivity of the Ames assay in detecting the activity of a broad spectrum of chemical mutagens for *S. typhimurium* (Skopek *et al.*, 1978a, 1978b). The economics of large-scale testing dictate that simple machines must be designed and constructed that will permit automation of the bacterial mutation assay. Aside from variation from Ames' original specific protocols regarding determination of mutant fraction, important changes with regard to the incorporation of metabolic elements may confidently be anticipated. At this time, most assayists incorporate a postmitochondrial supernatant fraction, prepared from rat liver after the method of deDuve *et al.* (1962), into the growth medium during the time of coincubation of the bacteria and the test agent. This subcellular fraction contains the mixed-function oxygenation system responsible for the metabolism of many chemically unreactive chemicals to chemically reactive derivatives, which can, in turn, damage DNA. Evidence is accumulating, however, that this use of the rat liver postmitochondrial supernatant is not a realistic approximation of the metabolic behavior of the intact liver. Efforts are progressing to permit facile use of whole rat liver cells, in which the organization of the endoplasmic reticulum is not disrupted, thus permitting (presumably) a fair semblance of *in vivo* metabolic dynamics. Looking to the future, one can envisage the need, development, and use of freeze-stored aliquots of human tissues as the source of the metabolic element in microbiologic mutation assays.

Rodent and Human Cell Mutation Assays. The development by the Szybalskis of selection conditions for the presence or absence of the activity of the X-linked enzyme, hypoxanthine-guanine phosphoribosyltransferase (Szybalski, 1964), has permitted the development of mammalian cell mutation assays and their use in studying the process of mutagenesis. Credit must also be given to the developers of the techniques for growing mammalian cells as clones, particularly to Puck and his colleagues (Puck and Marcus, 1955). Without their contributions, mammalian cell mutation assays would have been impossible. The principles underlying the assays are the same as for bacterial cell mutation assays. One must obtain an independent estimate of the fraction of cells that both have survived treatment and have been mutated. For quantitative assay of mutation at the hgprt locus in mammalian cells, some specific knowledge is needed of the behavior of cell interactions in culture and the nature of the phenotype of the hgprt⁻ state relative to drug (6-thioguanine) resistance.

When mammalian cells are cultured while adhering to glass or plastic petri dishes, cells will approach each other and form an intercellular junction through which small molecules may pass. The junction of an hgprt⁺ cell and an hgprt⁻ cell would create a two-cell unit, which behaves as if it were hgprt⁺, because the enzymic product of the wild type cell would be readily distributed to the mutant cell. Thus, observation of cell cultures at densities permitting intercolony contact leads to underestimation of the number of hgprt⁻ cells, i.e., the number of cells capable of forming colonies in the presence of 6-thioguanine (Fujimoto *et al.*, 1971).

The development of phenotypic resistance to 6-thioguanine is delayed many generations after treatment with mutagenic agents. This places a requirement on the assay that cells be cultured for some time (as many as 14 generations) to permit phenotypic expression. We have hypothesized that this long phenotypic lag arises from a trivial requirement for loss by protein degradation and dilution via cell division of all or nearly all of the HGPRT molecules existing prior to the mutagenic event (Thilly *et al.*, 1978). The fact

that some 2×10^6 molecules of HGPRT appear in a mammalian cell in culture and that degradation half-lives are on the order of 24 to 48 hours in culture will permit students to calculate the number of days or generations to be expected for the duration of phenotypic lag for mutation at hgprt. Data for this locus in mouse, hamster, and human cell mutation experiments are now available for a wide variety of chemical mutagens. No particular differences have so far been observed between hamster cell and human cell response to a number of mutagens. Other selection systems have been introduced and applied with varying degrees of success to quantitative studies of chemically induced mutation. The selection system of resistance to bromodeoxyuridine via loss of the activity of thymidine kinase is particularly noteworthy, since the period of phenotypic lag is demonstrably shorter than is the case for 6-thioguanine resistance. This system has been evaluated in a heteroploid line of mouse lymphoma cells by Clive and his associates. The possibility of using this selection system in human diploid cells is well worth considering. However, the tk gene is located on autosome 17 in humans, so the assay requires isolation of heterozygotes for thymidine kinase activity. Clive *et al.* (1973) achieved this in the mouse line by mutation to the homozygous-deficient state, and then selected thymidine kinase–positive cells, which were found to behave as heterozygotes, from the homozygous population. This selection process has now been successfully completed for a diploid human lymphoblast line (Skopek *et al.*, 1978c).

If students detect that this business of measuring mutant fractions in mammalian cell populations has a few unexpected problems, then this discussion has served a useful purpose. However, the force of logic indicates that the development of assays for mutagenesis (as well as aneuploidization and clastogenesis) in apparently genetically normal human cells can yield better approximations of potential human genetic hazard than estimates derived from the response of cells derived from nonhuman species. In fairness to those who presently espouse the use of nonhuman mammalian assays, there are no known examples of a chemical causing significantly different amounts of mutation in rodent cells than in man. The observations of Rauth (1967) and others that caffeine is able to potentiate the lethal effects of ultraviolet irradiation (which is, presumably, damaging DNA almost exclusively in the cell) in rodent cell lines, but not in human cell lines, points to a sound basis for suspicion that the postirradiation recovery processes can be substantially different. This idea is given greater weight by the demonstration of Roberts and his associates (1973) that the kinetics of DNA synthesis following treatment with methylnitrosourea differed qualitatively between the human HeLa cell line and the hamster cell line, V79.

SPECTRA OF GENETIC DAMAGE CAUSED BY PHYSICAL AND CHEMICAL AGENTS

Review of the vast literature on genetic damage, caused by all physical and chemical agents, will convince a student that, while an agent can be effective in causing one of the several kinds of genetic damage, it will not necessarily cause all kinds. Barthelmess (1970) reviewed the available data regarding environmental chemicals' ability to cause gene mutations in viruses and bacteria and their ability to cause chromosomal defects of structure and/or number in plants, insects, and mammals at the cellular or organismal level. Examples of the point that some chemicals are fairly specific in their antigenetic potential can readily be obtained from this tabular survey. For instance, 2-aminopurine is an active mutagen in bacteria but causes no chromosomal defects in insects, an action spectrum that seems to be true of base analogs incorporated into DNA in general, Colchicine has been examined in a number of cell types, and it causes errors of chromosome number but relatively few errors of chromosome structure. This action can reasonably be ascribed to effects of colchicine on mitotic spindle formation. Benzoic acid, reported to be a bacterial mutagen, was reported negative as a clastogen in human cells. However, very few quantitative studies simultaneously comparing mutagenic and clastogenic effects have been reported. Table 7–4 reduces the data of Kao and Puck (1969) to a comparison of the relative ability of several agents to cause chromatid exchanges or gene-locus mutation in cultured Chinese hamster ovary cells. Relative to ethyl methane sulfonate, methylnitronitrosoguanindine was found to be about four times *less* mutagenic but seven times *more* clastogenic. Caffeine, a potent clastogen, was found to be nonmutagenic. On the other hand, ICR-191, a half-mustard substituted acridine, had substantial mutagenic activity but little clastogenic potency.

The differences cited here are only a sample of the diversity of action spectra available through literature study. Summary reviews have, however, not yet appeared.

APPROACHES TO MECHANISM

We have now reviewed the facts that humans suffer from genetic error at the level of DNA sequence, from genetic error in the arrangement of DNA sequences within a chromatid, from gain or loss of sequences within a chromatid, and from the gain or loss of a whole chromatid(s).

We have reviewed the data showing that among the gene-locus chemical mutagens, some are predominantly active by inducing base substitution, while others predominantly induce addition or deletion mutation. We have noted that the potency of a substance as a gene-locus mutagen is not related to its potency in inducing higher rates of recombination (sister chromatid exchange), inducing clastogenesis, or inducing aneuploidy. Indeed, we have noted that a strong case can be made for the independence of these phenomena of genetic error at the level of human epidemiology, structural/molecular change involved in the error detected in humans, and in the kinds of chemicals that produce the errors in experimental systems.

These phenomena of gene-locus mutation, recombination, clastogenesis, and aneuploidy are all increased in experimental systems by one class of chemicals or another, and we do not yet

Table 7–4. RELATIVE CLASTOGENIC vs. MUTAGENIC ACTIVITY AMONG CHEMICAL AND PHYSICAL AGENTS*†

AGENT	RELATIVE MUTAGENIC ACTIVITY (GLY LOCUS)	RELATIVE CLASTOGENIC ACTIVITY (CHROMATID EXCHANGES)
Ethyl methone sulfonate	100	100
Methyl nitronitrosoguanidine	27	710
Ultraviolet light	12	350
ICR-191	3	< 13
Caffeine	0	340
Hydroxylamine	0	88

* Summarized from Kao and Puck (1969).
† All compared at a survival of approximately 14 percent.

understand how the chemicals cause the error in the orderly hereditary process. This process, highly schematized, is presented in Figure 7–12 to serve as a basis for discussion.

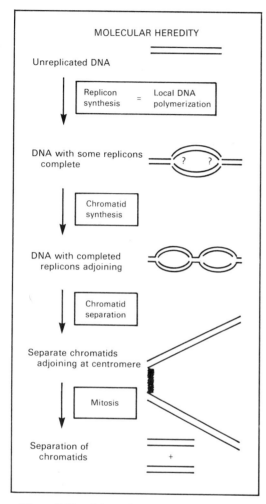

MOLECULAR HEREDITY

Unreplicated DNA

Replicon synthesis = Local DNA polymerization

DNA with some replicons complete

Chromatid synthesis

DNA with completed replicons adjoining

Chromatid separation

Separate chromatids adjoining at centromere

Mitosis

Separation of chromatids

Figure 7–12. Schematized DNA and chromosome replication shown in terms of DNA strands.

At the simplest level, replicative DNA synthesis is a polymerization on a DNA template catalyzed by enzymes under a narrow range of solvent/solute conditions. The fidelity of synthesis relative to the template may well be expected to be changed by anything affecting either the template or the catalysis. Much present research (Essigmann et al., 1977; Weinstein and Grunberger, 1974) is centered on a model in which chemicals react covalently with DNA, and the processes that follow result in an altered DNA sequence. A number of reasonable suggestions

have been advanced as to the nature of these processes. Individual base-pairing affinities could be altered allowing base substitutions to occur with detectable frequencies (see Drake, 1970). Distortion of the DNA helix could lead to single-strand breaks and excision of the locally altered sequence. Synthesis using the unchanged single strand as template, followed by joining to the unaltered sequence, would accomplish a "repair" of the damaged DNA. If this repair synthesis were, for reasons of catalysis, less faithful in replicating from a template than normal replicative synthesis, then mutation could result through repair itself. In phage it is known (Howard-Flanders et al., 1968) that repair of some damage by ultraviolet light occurs after replicative DNA synthesis reaches or passes the point of chemical reaction in the DNA. This process in phage involves genetic recombination, and it is suggested that such mechanisms could operate in higher animals as well. Postreplication repair in rodent and/or human cells may be regarded justly as an area in which our collective ignorance exceeds our collective knowledge.

However, many mutagens do not covalently link to DNA and do not induce any DNA repair activity (e.g., proflavin), and their mode of action is receiving less attention than those compounds which do form chemical bonds to DNA. It is possible that some compounds stabilize irregular DNA replicative intermediates, leading to synthesis with addition or deletion of one or several nucleotides.

Some chemicals, such as beryllium (Be^{2+}), apparently lead to base-substitution mutation by replacing Mg^{2+}, a normal enzymatic cofactor involved in the catalytic steps of polymerization (Sirover and Loeb, 1976). Mutator genes coding for altered polymerases of decreased fidelity are known in microbial systems. There is no shortage of mechanistic possibilities by which a chemical could befoul this fairly intricate process of template-guided polymerization, in which one error in 10^9 base-pair additions represents about a tenfold increase in gene-locus mutation over that observed in normal, untreated human cells in culture.

DNA synthesis leading to synthesis of an entire chromatid is, of course, not a simple polymerization. As the replicon sequences within a chromatid are synthesized, they should have, for an appreciable time, structures where two-stranded DNA adjoins four-stranded DNA. It is unknown if these structures are sites of recombination or chromatid breakage, but they would seem prime candidates in terms of explaining such phenomena as specificity of sites for sister chromatid exchange or clastogenesis. Finally, the two sister chromatids must separate at mitosis, a process that must involve a molecular dissociation within the centromere and a successful process of mechanical separation involving the mitotic spindle apparatus. At this level, a chemical might be active in aneuploidization and cause genetic damage without ever reacting in any way with DNA or any of the constituents of chromatin.

CENTRAL PREMISE

The goal of reducing genetic disease in humans may be reached by a number of technologic paths; one would be gene or enzyme replacement therapy for afflicted individuals. It is not beyond present technical ability to develop viral transport vectors, which might carry specific genetic information to a sufficient fraction of tissue cells, to eliminate or ameliorate the symptoms of a deficiency disease. Another approach, of demonstrated use in reducing genetic disease in newborns is to augment the already active intra-uterine surveillance system through cytogenetic and biochemical analysis of fetal cells collected by amniocentesis. This approach places the decision of whether or not a fetus with demonstrable genetic error will be brought to term upon the parents. A variation on this approach is genetic counseling, for older potential parents or known heterozygous carriers of harmful mutations, to voluntarily forego parenthood. These approaches have in common the advantage that they deal with genetic error independent of the cause of error.

The central premise of the present legal and regulatory approach to environmental mutagens is that they are causing genetic error in humans, and that the human exposure to these chemicals can be reduced by timely and conscientious effort. As scientists, we should recognize that two important, and as-yet-untested, assumptions, underlie the central premise:

1. Environmental mutagens cause aneuploidy, chromosome breaks, gene-locus mutations, or other genetic damage in humans.

2. The environmental mutagens that can be controlled by conscientious effort represent an important source of human mutagens.

Actually, much of the present interest in environmental mutagens is related to the widespread belief that cancer is caused by a mutagenic event. If this is the case, then the central premise is supported by the clear association between many occupational chemical exposures and cancer incidence in man, not to mention the causation of lung cancer by smoke inhalation.

Finally, we should emphasize that, even if the central premise is correct, existing genetic errors in the human population include a large portion

of autosomal recessive traits (e.g., cystic fibrosis is carried, perhaps, by one person in 70 in the heterozygous state). Such errors, if not increased by new mutations, will take many centuries to reduce in frequency of diseased infants. Aneuploidies and many autosomal dominant and X-linked diseases would be significantly reduced in a human generation, however, if the rate of new error were decreased to zero.

REFERENCES

Ames, B. N.; McCann, J.; and Yamasaki, E.: Methods for detecting carcinogens and mutagens with the *Salmonella*/mammalian-microsome mutagenicity test. *Mutat. Res.*, 31:347–64, 1975.

Barthelmess, A.: Mutagenic substances in the human environment. In Vogel, F., and Röhrborn, G. (eds.): *Chemical Mutagenesis in Mammals and Man.* Springer-Verlag, New York, 1970, pp. 69–147.

Bauchinger, M.; Schmid, E.; Einbrodt, H. J.; and Dresp, J.: Chromosome aberrations in lymphocytes after occupational exposure to lead and cadmium. *Mutat. Res.*, 40:57–62, 1976.

Benzer, S.: On the topography of the genetic fine structure. *Proc. Natl. Acad. Sci. (USA)*, 47:403–15, 1961.

Borgaonkar, D. S.: *Chromosomal Variation in Man, A Catalog of Chromosomal Variants and Anomalies*, 2nd ed. The Johns Hopkins University Press, Baltimore, 1978.

Boué, J.; Boué, A.; and Lazar, P.: Retrospective and prospective epidemiological studies of 1500 karyotyped spontaneous human abortions. *Teratology*, 12:11–26, 1975.

Carr, D. H., and Gedeon, M.: Population cytogenetics of human abortuses. In Hook, E. B. and Porter, I. H. (eds.): *Population Cytogenetics. Studies in Humans.* Academic Press, Inc., New York, 1977, pp. 1–10.

Carter, C. O.: Monogenic disorders. *J. Med. Genet.*, 14:316–20, 1977.

Clive, D.; Flamm, W. G.; and Patterson, J. B.: Specific-locus mutational assay systems for mouse lymphoma cells. In Hollaender, A. (ed.): *Chemical Mutagens: Principles and Methods for their Detection*, Vol. 3. Plenum Press, New York 1973, pp. 79–104.

Cohen, M. M., and Hirschhorn, K.: Cytogenetic studies in animals. In Hollaender, A. (ed.): *Chemical Mutagens: Principles and Methods for their Detection*, Vol. 2, Plenum Press, New York, 1971, pp. 515–34.

Cohen, M. M., and Shaw, M. W.: Effects of mytomycin C on human chromosomes. *J. Cell. Biol.*, 23:386–95, 1964.

Countryman, P. I., and Heddle, J. A.: The production of micronuclei from chromosome aberrations in irradiated cultures of human lymphocytes *Mutat. Res.*, 41:321–32, 1976.

deDuve, C.; Wattiaux, R.; and Baudhuin, P.: Distribution of enzymes between subcellular fractions in animal tissues. *Adv. Enzymol. Relat. Subj. Biochem.*, 24:291–358, 1962.

DeLuca, J. G.; Kaden, D. A.; Krolewski, J.; Skopek, T. R.; and Thilly, W. G.: Comparative mutagenicity of ICR-191 to *S. typhimurium* and diploid human lymphoblasts. *Mutat Res.*, 46:11–18, 1977.

Drake, J. W.: *The Molecular Basis of Mutation.* Holden Day, San Francisco, 1970, chap. 10.

Elkind, M. M., and Whitmore, G. F.: *The Radiobiology of Cultured Mammalian Cells.* Gordon and Breach, New York, 1967.

Essigmann, J. M.; Croy, R. G.; Nadzan, A. M.; Busby, W. F., Jr.; Reinhold, V. N.; Büchi, G.; and Wogan, G. N.: Structural identification of the major DNA adduct formed by aflatoxin B_1 in vitro. *Proc. Natl. Acad. Sci. (USA)*, 74:1870–74, 1977.

Fujimoto, W. Y.; Subak-Sharpe, J. H.; and Seegmiller, J. E.: Hypoxanthene-guanine phosphoribosyltransferase deficiency: chemical agents selective for mutants or normal cultured fibroblasts in mixed and heterozygote cultures. *Proc. Natl. Acad. Sci. (USA)*, 68:1516–19, 1971.

Grell, R. F.: Induction of sex chromosome nondisjunction by elevated temperature. *Mutat Res.*, 11:347–49, 1971.

Hamerton, J. L.: Klinefelter's syndrome. In *Human Cytogenics*, Vol. II. Academic Press, Inc., New York, 1971, chap. 1.

Harris, H.: *The Principles of Human Biochemical Genetics*, 2nd ed. North Holland/American Elsevier, New York, 1975.

Hollaender, A. (ed.): *Chemical Mutagens: Principles and Methods for Their Detection*, Vol. 1. Plenum Press, New York, 1971a.

Hollaender, A. (ed.): *Chemical Mutagens: Principles and Methods for Their Detection*, Vol. 2. Plenum Press, New York, 1971b.

Hollaender, A. (ed.): *Chemical Mutagens: Principles and Methods for Their Detection*, Vol. 3. Plenum Press, New York, 1973.

Hollaender, A. (ed.): *Chemical Mutagens: Principles and Methods for Their Detection*, Vol. 4. Plenum Press, New York, 1976.

Honeycombe, J. R.: The effects of busulphan on the chromosomes of normal human lymphocytes. *Mutat. Res.*, 57:35–49, 1978.

Hook, E. B., and Hamerton, J. L.: The frequency of chromosome abnormalities detected in consecutive newborn studies—differences between studies—results by sex and severity of phenotypic involvement. In Hook, E. B., and Porter, I. H. (eds.): *Population Cytogenetics: Studies in Humans*. Academic Press, Inc., New York, 1977, pp. 63–80.

Howard-Flanders, P.; Rupp, W. D.; Wilkins, B. M.; and Cole, R. S.: DNA replication and recombination after UV irradiation. *Cold Spring Harbor Symp. Quant. Biol.*, 33:195–208, 1968.

Kao, F. T., and Puck, T. T.: Genetics of somatic mammalian cells IX. Quantitation of mutagenesis by physical and chemical agents. *J. Cell. Physiol.*, 74(3):245–58, 1969.

Kihlman, B. A.: Root tips for studying the effects of chemicals on chromosomes. In Hollaender, A. (ed.): *Chemical Mutagens: Principles and Methods for Their Detection*, Vol. 2. Plenum Press, New York, 1971, pp. 489–514.

Mavor, J. W.: The production of non-disjunction by x-rays. *J. Exp. Zool.*, 39:381–432, 1924.

McKusick, V. A.: *Mendelian Inheritance in Man, Catalogs of Autosomal Dominants, Autosomal Recessive, and X-linked Phenotypes*, 4th ed. The Johns Hopkins University Press, Baltimore, 1975.

Meretoja, T.; Vainio, H.; Sorsa, M.; and Härkönen, H.: Occupational styrene exposure and chromosomal aberrations. *Mutat. Res.*, 56:193–97, 1977.

Morad, M.; Jonasson, J.; and Lindsten, J.: Distribution of mitomycin C induced breaks on human chromosomes. *Hereditas*, 74:273–82, 1973.

O'Neill, J. P.; Fuscoe, J. C.; and Hsie, A. W.: Mutagenicity of heterocyclic nitrogen mustards (ICR compounds) in cultured mammalian cells. *Cancer Res.*, 38:506–509, 1978.

Paris Conference (1971): Standardization in human cytogenetics. In Bergsma, D. (ed.): *Birth Defects.*

Original Article Series, Vol. 8, No. 7. The National Foundation, New York, 1972.

Parry, J. M., and Zimmerman, F. K.: The detection of monosomic colonies produced by mitotic chromosome non-disjunction in the yeast *Saccharomyces cerevisiae*. *Mutat. Res.*, 36:49–66, 1976.

Puck, T. T., and Marcus, P. I.: A rapid method for viable cell titration and clone production with HeLa cells in tissue culture: the use of x-irradiated cells to supply conditioning factors. *Proc. Natl. Acad. Sci. (USA)*, 41:432–37, 1955.

Rauth, A. M.: Evidence for dark-reactivation of ultraviolet light damage in mouse L cells. *Radiat. Res.*, 31:121–38, 1967.

Reeves, B. R., and Margoles, C.: Preferential location of chlorambucil-induced breakage in the chromosomes of normal human lymphocytes. *Mutat. Res.*, 26:205–208, 1974.

Roberts, J. J., and Ward, K. N.: Inhibition of postreplication repair of alkylated DNA by caffeine in Chinese hamster cells but not HeLa cells. *Chem. Biol. Interact.*, 7:241–64, 1973.

Sanchez, O., and Yunis, J. J.: New chromosomal techniques and their medical applications. In Yunis, J. J. (ed.): *New Chromosomal Syndromes*. Academic Press, Inc., New York, 1977, pp. 1–54.

Sirover, M. A., and Loeb, L. A.: Metal-induced infidelity during DNA synthesis. *Procl. Natl. Acad. Sci. (USA)*, 73:2331–35, 1976.

Skopek, T. R.; Liber, H. L.; Krolewski, J. J.; and Thilly, W. G.: Quantitative forward mutation assay in *Salmonella typhimurium* using 8-azaguanine resistance as a genetic marker. *Proc. Natl. Acad. Sci. (USA)*, 75:410–14, 1978a.

Skopek, T. R.; Liber, H. L.; Kaden, D. A.; and Thilly, W. G.: Relative sensitivities of forward and reverse mutation assays in *Salmonella typhimurium*. *Proc. Natl. Acad. Sci. (USA)*, 75:4465–69, 1978b.

Skopek, T. R.; Liber, H. L.; Penman, B. W.; and Thilly, W. G.: Isolation of a human lymphoblastoid line heterozygous at the thymidine kinase locus: Possibility for a rapid human cell mutation assay. *Biochem. Biophys. Res. Commun.*, 84:411–16, 1978c.

Sotomayor, R. E., and Cumming, R. B.: Induction translocations by cyclophosphamide in different germ cell stages of male mice: Cytological characterization and transmission. *Mutat. Res.*, 27:375–88, 1975.

Szemere, G., and Chandley, A. C.: Trisomy and triploidy induced by x-irradiation of mouse spermatocytes. *Mutat. Res.*, 33:229–38, 1975.

Szybalski, W.: Chemical reactivity of chromosomal DNA as related to mutagenicity: Studies with human cell lines. *Cold Spring Harbor Symp. Quant. Biol.*, 29:151–60, 1964.

Tates, A. D., and Natarajan, A. T.: A correlative study on the genetic damage induced by chemical mutagens in bone marrow and spermatogonia of mice. I. CNU-ethanol. *Mutat. Res.*, 37:267–78, 1976.

Thilly, W. G.; DeLuca, J. G.; Hoppe, H., IV; and Penman, B. W.: Phenotypic lag and mutation to 6-thioguanine resistance in diploid human lymphoblasts. *Mutat. Res.*, 50:137–44, 1978.

Vogel, F.: Spontaneous mutation in man. In Vogel, F., and Röhrborn, G. (eds.): *Chemical Mutagenesis in Mammals and Man*. Springer Verlag, New York, 1970, pp. 16–68.

Vogel, F., and Rathenberg, R.: Spontaneous mutation in man. *Adv. Hum. Genet.* 5:223–318, 1975.

Wadsworth, G. P., and Bryan, J. G.: *Introduction to Probability and Random Variables*. McGraw-Hill Book Company, Inc., New York, 1960.

Watson, W. A. F.; Petrie, J. C.; Galloway, D. B.; Bullock, I.; and Gilbert, J. C.: *In vivo* cytogenic activity of sulphonylurea drugs in man. *Mutat. Res.*, **38**:71–80, 1976.

Weinstein, I. B., and Grunberger, D.: Structural and functional changes in nucleic acids modified by chemical carcinogens. In Ts'o, P. O. P., and DiPaolo, J. A. (eds.): *Chemical Carcinogenesis*, Part A. Marcel Dekker, Inc., New York, 1974, pp. 217–35.

Wild, D.: Cytogenic effects in the mouse of 17 chemical mutagens and carcinogens evaluated by the micronucleus test. *Mutat. Res.*, **56**:319–27, 1978.

Chapter 8

TERATOGENS

Raymond D. Harbison

INTRODUCTION

The biologic functions that make up the processes of reproduction and organogenesis are varied in nature and in their susceptibility to adverse influences in the environment. Since 1941, when Gregg first drew attention to the association of death, blindness, and deafness among offspring of women exposed to rubella (German measles) during pregnancy, the scientific community has recognized that exogenous environmental agents contribute to fetal death and congenital malformation in the human. Some 20 years later, the occurrence of 10,000 malformed infants born of mothers who had taken thalidomide during pregnancy (McBride, 1961) and the birth of nearly 20,000 defective children following an epidemic of rubella (Warkany, 1971) confirmed the association of environmental factors and congenital defects.

Whereas many disorders of early childhood can be either prevented or effectively treated, very little progress has been made in the prevention of congenital defects. Consequently, these defects have become one of the leading causes of death during late intrauterine life and account for one of the largest groups of patients in pediatric wards. In the United States no less than one-third of the capacity of these wards is devoted to treatment of children with congenital defects and their sequelae.

The term "congenital defect" refers to all morphologic, biochemical, and functional abnormalities produced before or at birth. Congenital malformations or anomalies refer merely to structural aberration. Congenital defects may not be detected at birth, but if detected later are definitely attributable to antenatal developmental disorders or defects. A wide variety of abnormal conditions and diseases are detectable during neonatal life or adolescent development for which a congenital background may be suggested. The final manifestation may be as a readily detected abnormal morphologic development or as a subtle behavioral, learning, biochemical, or

functional defect with less readily recognized effects.

In the United States some 200,000 birth defects are recorded each year, accounting for about 7 percent of all live births (National Foundation, 1975). More than 560,000 infant deaths, spontaneous abortions, stillbirths, and miscarriages are recorded due to defective fetal development.

Chemical agents can affect embryo development in such a way that defects in one or another organ system are produced. If only embryonic somatic cells are affected and germ cells escape damage, that individual only will be affected. Since this is usually the case, most congenital defects are not hereditary. Substances that cause defects of fetal development are called teratogens. Estimates are that from 1 to 5 percent of congenital defects in the human are drug or chemical related (Wilson, 1973).

The number of drugs taken during pregnancy averages about nine. Women of childbearing age are also exposed occupationally to industrial chemicals. About 125,000 women work in environments containing potential teratogens: solvents, chemical reagents, etc. The incidence of birth defects in offspring of these women could be two to three times higher than the expected rate. The contribution of environmental chemical contamination to the incidence of birth defects is at present unknown.

Incidence figures for congenital defects are often underestimated because a great variety of congenital defects and disorders are not detectable during early postnatal life. Among these disorders may be mental retardation, defects of the sense organs, abnormal sexual development, and certain enzyme defects. The lower defect detection rate at birth can be seen where the results of reexaminations of series of children studied soon after birth are compared (Table 8–1). In all cases, fewer defects were noted during the first few days of life when compared to follow-up studies.

In view of the multiple etiology of malformations, discussed below, the detection rate or over-

Table 8–1. INCIDENCE (%) OF CONGENITAL DEFECTS*

FREQUENCY AT BIRTH	FOLLOW-UP OBSERVATION TIME	FINAL FREQUENCY
1.5	4 years	10.1
2.4	3–6 years	16.0
1.7	5 years	2.3
3.5	1 year	6.9
1.1	9 months	3.1

* From Saxén, H., and Rapola, J.: *Congenital Defects.* Holt, Rinehart & Winston, Inc., New York, 1969.

all incidence of congenital defects may not be useful in detecting specific causative factors. Where a teratogen results in a variety of malformations, the overall incidence is the only point of reference, but slight increases in some malformations will be masked by the permanent "background" caused by many teratogens. The effect of thalidomide would never have been recognized as an increase in the overall incidence of congenital defects; however, using phocomelia, a marker defect of low incidence, a causal relationship between drug ingestion and defect could easily be made. Epidemiologic studies of human populations have revealed a great number of marked differences and changes in the incidence of various malformations in different populations and at different periods. For example, incidence of central nervous system abnormalities is higher in Scotland when compared

to the United States (Saxén and Rapola, 1969). Seasonal variations as well as environmental influences can also alter the incidence of defects. Using specific marker defects, the increased incidence of rubella can be correlated with the increased incidence of congenital deafness. The increased sales of the drug thalidomide can be correlated with the increased incidence of phocomelia.

EMBRYOLOGY

The complex and remarkable process of embryogenesis is a precisely programmed sequence of cell proliferation, differentiation, migration, and, finally, organogenesis. Embryogenesis involves complex cellular interaction in both time and space. A graphic display of the developmental sequence of embryonic and fetal growth is shown in Figure 8–1. The critical periods during human development can be divided into an embryonic period and a fetal development period with most organogenesis complete during the first trimester. During the earliest stages, the first two weeks, rapid cell proliferation takes place. The numerous products of these early cell divisions have different potentialities, depending on their relative positions in the embryonic mass. This sequence of events is not generally disturbed by teratogens except that any damage may result in early death of the embryo. During the embryonic period, most major morphologic abnormalities may be produced, while physiologic defects and minor

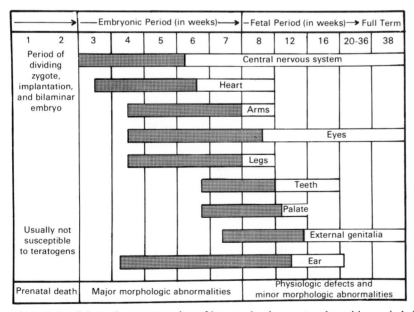

Figure 8–1. Schematic representation of human development and sensitive periods for production of maldevelopment. Cross-hatching represents highly sensitive periods; clear area represents stages that are less sensitive to teratogens.

Table 8–2.   COMPARATIVE GESTATIONAL DEVELOPMENT*

	MAN	RAT	MOUSE	RABBIT	HAMSTER
Implantation period	6½ da	8 da	5 da	9 da	7 da
13 to 20 somite	27 da	11 da	9 da	10 da	9 da
End of embryonic period	12–14 wk	14 da	13 da	11 da	10 da
End of metamorphosis	20 wk	17 da	17 da	15 da	14 da
Fetal development	20–34 wk	18–22 da	18–20 da	16–32 da	15–16 da
Parturition	36–40 wk	21 da	19 da	32 da	15 da

* Data derived from Witschi (1956) and Rugh (1968).

morphologic abnormalities may be produced during the period of fetal development. Final morphologic and functional development occurs at various times in different organs and is sometimes completed only after birth.

A comparative development chart is shown in Table 8–2. This table sequences several developmental stages of man, mouse, rat, hamster, and rabbit.

Although it is widely known that under certain conditions some aspects of reproduction are vulnerable to physical and chemical factors in the environment, for example, both the germ cells and the early embryo may be damaged by relatively small doses of ionizing radiation or chemicals, it is generally assumed that a placental barrier protects the embryo and/or fetus against most levels of chemical exposure. On the contrary, the placenta, which performs admirably in maintaining the growing embryo, does not selectively protect the intrauterine organism from harmful agents administered during pregnancy. The placental barrier has been found to act like a sieve. Except for compounds of large molecular weight, and those with strong electronegative or electropositive charges (heparin and most neuromuscular blocking agents), almost all pharmacologic substances and other chemicals can and do pass from the maternal to fetal bloodstream. Generally, substances with a molecular weight of less than 600 pass the placental barrier. Placental transfer of chemicals varies greatly during the stages of gestation and among species (Harbison *et al.*, 1975; Stevens and Harbison, 1974).

CRITICAL PERIODS

Human experience and animal experiments have taught us that susceptibility to teratogenic agents varies with the developmental stage at the time of exposure. The most prominent example of a specific chemical-induced alteration during a specific time of gestational development is thalidomide. Thalidomide was teratogenic when taken during gestational days 34 through 50 (McBride, 1961). Generally, ear anomalies were associated with intake between the thirty-fourth and thirty-eighth days, arm anomalies were seen

between the fortieth and forty-fourth days, and aplasia of the femur or tibia between the forty-fourth and forty-eighth days. A variety of malformations of internal organs, such as intestinal atresia, imperforate anus, and aplasia of the gallbladder and appendix, also occurred, either associated with skeletal defects or occasionally alone. A teratogenic response is determined by the developmental stage at the time of exposure as well as the inherent toxicity of the agent. There are special times during fetal development when defects can be induced and sharply limited critical periods for various specific defects.

Considering fertilization as the beginning of development, the first subdivision is that beginning with cleavage of blastomeres and continuing through completion of the blastocyst. Fabro and Sieber (1969) have found that many chemicals and drugs accumulate in the blastocyst and the fluids bathing the blastocyst. Cleavage involves little morphologic differentiation of cells except that as numbers increase, relationships to the surface change. During the early phase of cell proliferation, malformations are not produced. At this time, the embryo may be killed, or if it survives, it develops normally. It is also difficult to produce abnormalities very late in fetal development since the process of organogenesis has been completed.

In each species there is therefore a relatively short critical period of sensitivity to teratogens, when early organogenesis is in progress. This period extends from the time of implantation to the end of the embryonic period (Table 8–2). In the rat and mouse, the sensitive period extends from about the fifth to the fourteenth day of the approximately 20-day gestation period. In the human the critical embryologic development period extends from the third week through the third month of pregnancy.

Time of drug administration dramatically affects the incidence of malformations (Fig. 8–2). The embryocidal and embryopathic effects produced by exposure of pregnant rats to rubratoxin are seen primarily following treatment on gestational days 8 through 13. Dactinomycin, which disrupts organogenesis by blocking synthesis of RNA, caused death

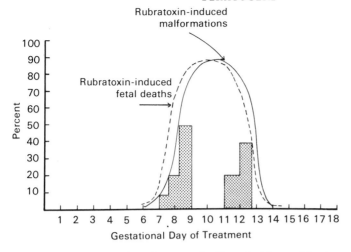

Figure 8–2. Critical timing of teratogenic effects. Incidence of death or malformation is shown on the ordinate and day of treatment is shown on the abscissa. Rubratoxin (0.8 to 1.0 mg/kg) was administered to pregnant rats on gestational days 7 through 15 (Evans and Harbison, 1977). Fetal death and malformations were induced with greatest frequency following treatment on gestational days 9 through 11. Actinomycin-induced malformations are shown as stippled bars. Actinomycin, 0.3 mg/kg, was administered to pregnant rats (Tuchmann-Duplessis and Mercier-Parot, 1960). The peak incidence of malformations was seen following treatment on gestational days 7 through 9. Tetrahydrocannabinol-induced malformations are shown as cross-hatched bars. Tetrahydro-cannabinol, 50 mg/kg, was administered to pregnant mice (Harbison *et al.*, 1977). The peak incidence of malformations was seen following treatment on gestational days 11 and 12.

of nearly all fetuses when administered to pregnant rats during the first few days of pregnancy. The embryocidal effects fell to about 10 percent when the drug was given as late as the thirteenth day. The incidence of malformations among surviving fetuses showed an extremely sharp peak when the drug was given between the seventh and ninth days (Fig. 8–2). Similarly, tetrahydrocannabinol produced 65 percent incidence of fetal death when administered to pregnant mice during days 8 and 9, but only 28 percent when administered on days 12 and 13. Orofacial anomalies were seen, however, only after tetrahydrocannabinol treatment of pregnant mice on gestational days 10–13. Parathion was embryocidal when administered to pregnant mice on gestational days 12,

13, and 14 (Harbison, 1975), while administration of parathion during early gestation was only one-third as toxic.

Specific critical periods for various malformations in the mouse, caused by a single teratogen, diphenylhydantoin, are shown in Table 8–3. The sensitive periods correlate well with the known sequence of organogenesis in this species. If the time in gestation when a particular organ completes its differentiation is known, then a congenital defect of that organ could only be caused by a teratogen that acted prior to that time. This rule often enables discrimination between a suspected teratogen and an unusual occurrence as the cause of a human malformation because the timing is not compatible with the observed effect.

Table 8–3. CRITICAL TIMING OF TERATOGENIC EFFECTS OF DIPHENYLHYDANTOIN IN THE MOUSE

Gestational Treatment Days	DAY OF PREGNANCY					
	6–8	9–10	11–12	13–14	15–16	17–19
Orofacial	0	24	63	57	4	0
Eye defects	0	19	0	0	0	0
Limb defects	0	12	0	0	0	0
CNS defects	0	28	0	0	0	0
Skeletal defects	0	44	52	57	3	0
Kidney defects	0	25	17	7	4	0

* Diphenylhydantoin, 150 mg/kg, was administered to pregnant mice at the designated gestational days. Figures are percentages of all surviving fetuses displaying the malformation.

† From Harbison, R. D., and Becker, B. A.: Relation of dosage and time of administration of diphenylhydantoin to its teratogenic effect in mice. *Teratology*, **2**:305–12, 1969.

EXPERIMENTAL TERATOGENESIS

Since recognition of chemical-induced teratogenesis in man, suitable laboratory animal models to determine prenatal safety of drugs have been sought. Various types of adverse effects on the human fetus have been reported for about 200 different drugs. Of the almost 2,000 chemicals tested in mammals, about one-third have demonstrated teratogenicity in various experimental designs. The teratogenic potential of drugs and chemicals has been primarily tested in mice, rabbits, and rats, although primates have occasionally been used. All these animals, like humans, have a placenta, so chemicals are exposed to maternal tissues and subjected to maternal metabolism before entering the embryo or fetus. Gestation in the animal model is short (three weeks in rat or mouse), multiple births are normal (so each treated female yields a large amount of experimental data), and housing and maintenance of large numbers of animals are practical because of their small size and low cost. The most serious limitation in the use of rodents is the different structure, and possibly different function as well, of their placenta as compared with that of the human. In contrast, the placental structure and function, as well as the pattern of embryologic development, in the nonhuman primates are similar to those in the human. The primates respond to known teratogens that affect humans, such as thalidomide, rubella virus, and androgenic steroids.

Chick embryos are useful to study the action of a proximate teratogen, one that acts directly, without the necessity of prior metabolic transformation. The teratogen can be placed in direct contact with the developing embryo. A good correlation was found for the teratogenic effects of diverse compounds in chick embryos and in rodents. The presence of a yolk sac in both species may explain why some agents that are teratogenic in chicks and rodents are less active in primates, as is the case with trypan blue.

Prior to 1960, the only governmental recommendations for testing drugs during the reproductive cycle of animals were conventional six-week chronic-toxicity tests in male and female rodents; these were followed during two pregnancies. Fetal survival was the main parameter measured in the "litter test." Since this time, and in response to the thalidomide episode, guidelines for reproduction studies for safety evaluation of drugs for human use have been issued (FDA, 1966). Similar protocols have been issued for evaluation of food additives, pesticides, and household products (FDA, 1970; CPSC, 1977). These tests are more comprehensive and include testing during the teratogen-susceptible period of reproduction. Current guidelines may be divided into three phases.

Phase I, which addresses general reproduction, requires treatment or exposure of male rodents, usually rats, for 60 days and female rodents for 14 days followed by mating at the end of this period. Treatment of inseminated females is continued during gestation and weaning. Half of the pregnancies are terminated midgestation and the embryos are examined. The other half are allowed to deliver and wean their offspring. Weanlings are killed and subjected to gross and visceral examination for abnormalities. This study phase determines effects on reproduction, early stages of gestation, late stages of gestation, parturition, and lactation.

Phase II requires treatment of two species of pregnant animals during only the period of organogenesis of gestation. Fetuses are delivered by cesarean section one day prior to parturition. Fetuses are subsequently examined for gross, visceral, and skeletal abnormalities. This study phase determines embryotoxic and teratogenic potential.

Phase III emphasizes effects on postnatal development and late gestation. Pregnant female rodents are treated or exposed during the last third of gestation and through weaning. The purpose of this study is to determine effects on late fetal development, labor and delivery, lactation, neonatal viability, and growth and development of the newborn.

The recommended phases of study are just guidelines, and interpretation of results may be open to criticism because of poor choice of animal models, chronicity of administration or exposure, absence of data on chemical metabolism and placental transfer, and lack of knowledge regarding mechanisms of teratogenesis.

DOSE

Chemical-induced teratogenic effects are dose related. A suitable dosage of teratogen will produce some defective offspring, some normal offspring, and some fetal deaths. Dose-response curves for teratogens may have steep or shallow slopes. Correspondingly, the dosage of a chemical that is teratogenic lies within a zone between that which will kill the fetus and that which has no effect. Teratogens have a threshold below which teratogenic effects are not produced. The dose-response relationship for diphenylhydantoin is shown in Figure 8–3. At dosages below 50 mg/kg, no cleft palates were produced. At dosages of 50 mg/kg and above, a dose-response relationship was observed. At dosages above 75 mg/kg, greater than 60 percent of the fetuses were killed *in utero*. At dosages of 75 mg/kg and

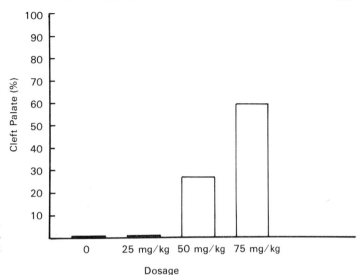

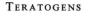

Figure 8–3. Dose-response relationship for diphenylhydantoin. Pregnant mice were treated with diphenylhydantoin on gestational days 11, 12, and 13. (Data from Harbison, R. D., and Becker, B. A.: Relation of dosage and time of administration of diphenylhydantoin to its teratogenic effect in mice. *Teratology*, **2**:305–12, 1969.)

below, no significant increase in *in utero* deaths was recorded. Embryolethal effects can often be distinguished from teratogenic effects (Gebhardt, 1970).

CLASSES OF CYTOTOXIC TERATOGENS

The term "cytotoxic chemical" was initially used to describe a number of chemically unrelated agents that had in common the ability to inhibit the growth of tumors. They act specifically on cells in cycle. The embryo and fetus are highly susceptible to cytotoxic agents, because they constantly have groups of cells in the growth phase. Acutely toxic doses may cause cellular death and result in fetal death. Survivors may show symptoms of damage to systems that contain cells in cycle and with a short cycle time. Chronic administration of low doses may produce cellular abnormalities in several systems.

The mechanism by which chemicals cause cell death is not clear, but effects have been ascribed to some form of unbalanced growth, RNA and protein synthesis being out of phase with DNA synthesis. The phenomenon of unbalanced growth has been described in detail for a number of cytotoxic agents. Cytotoxins may be grouped together according to their mechanisms of action.

Alkylating agents are very reactive toward molecules that have negative charges (nucleophiles), such as ionized carboxylic and phosphoric acids and thiols, or that have negative areas due to presence of amine groups. These agents react with many biologic constituents, including nucleic acids, proteins, nucleotides, and amino acids. Some alkylating agents have cytotoxic properties as parent compounds. These include nitrogen mustards, sulphonoxyalkanes, aziridines (ethylenamines), and oxiranes (epoxides). Their chemical reactivity depends on the positively charged form, which reacts with negatively charged nucleophiles. Bifunctional alkylating agents that are teratogenic include busulfan, chlorambucil, cyclophosphamide, METEPA, nitrogen mustard, thio-TEPA, triethylenemelamine, and uracil mustard. The mechanism of teratogenic activity of bifunctional alkylating agents is inter- or intrastrand cross-linking of DNA as well as alkylation of other essential macromolecules.

Chemical teratogens that require metabolism or bioactivation to *electrophilic reactants* include acetylaminofluorene, aflatoxin, alkyltriazenes, aminoazobenzene, benzanthracenes, benzpyrenes, carbon tetrachloride, cycasin, 1,2-diethylhydrazine, ethionine, methylcholanthrene, nitrosourea, pyrrollizidine alkaloids, diphenylhydantoin, and thalidomide. Most frequently it is the liver that produces a variety of electrophilic reactants that, like the alkylating agents, covalently bind to macromolecules. Metabolism or bioactivation may also be extramicrosomal or be carried out by fetoplacental tissue or gut bacteria.

A number of organic chemicals have been identified as either inherently electrophilic or able to be converted *in vivo* to electrophilic reactants. If the appropriate level of reaction takes place with essential macromolecules, then a cellular transformation will occur. The degree and nature of the cellular lesion will depend on a number of variables, the most important of which are

1. Stage of embryo or fetal development when chemical is administered.

2. Dosage of chemical, route of administration, and exposure schedule.

3. Ability of chemical to pass placenta and penetrate embryonic tissue.

4. Ability of maternal tissues (especially liver) to detoxify or to bioactivate chemical.

5. Biologic and chemical half-life of the material or its metabolite.

6. Stage of the cell cycle when the chemical is present at a cytotoxic concentration.

7. Capacity of embryonic tissues to detoxify or bioactivate chemical.

8. Ability of the damaged cells to repair or recover from the cytotoxic lesion.

These variables explain why an agent may be found to be highly teratogenic under one set of experimental conditions and inactive in another.

Antimetabolites inhibit pathways of purine or pyrimidine biosynthesis and formation of thymidylic acid. These compounds include aminopterin, azaguanine, azathioprine, azauracils, cytosine arabinoside, diaminopurine, halogenated pyrimidines, mercaptopurine, methotrexate, primethamine, and thioguanine. The mechanism for inhibition of nucleic acid replication is the incorporation into nucleic acids of the antimetabolites as base analogs and the subsequent inhibition of replication.

Intercalating agents insert between base pairs of DNA and interfere with transcription and replication. These compounds are teratogenic and include acriflavine, dactinomycin, chloroquine, daunomycin, quinacrine, and mithramycin.

Amino acid antagonists inhibit protein and nucleic acid synthesis by interfering with incorporation of specific amino acids required for protein or nucleic acid synthesis. These compounds include asparaginase, azaserine, DON, *p*-fluorophenylalanine, hadacidin, and mimosine. Specific interference with asparagine, aspartic acid, glutamine, methionine, phenylalanine, and tyrosine utilization has been reported.

Spindle poisons condense with microtubular protein and interfere with formation of cellular organelles and the spindle apparatus. These teratogenic compounds include colchicine, griseofulvin, podophyllotoxin, vinblastine, and vincristine.

Many teratogenic chemicals are bioactivated *in vivo*. Without exception, it has been found that the active metabolite is an electrophilic reactant. A compound known to be an electrophilic reactant (for example, an alkylating agent) or bioactivated to an electrophilic reactant must therefore be considered a potential teratogen. The chemical half-life of the reactant determines whether it can travel from the site of formation, usually maternal liver, to sensitive embryonic tissues. Very reactive intermediates, such as the $CCl_3 \cdot$ radical formed from carbon tetrachloride, will be unstable and react at the site of formation instead of traveling to the embryonic or fetal tissue. Carbon tetrachloride is very toxic to adult liver where it is bioactivated, but not very toxic in newborn rats whose metabolic enzymes are not fully developed (Reynolds, 1967). This is in agreement with the weak teratogenic action of carbon tetrachloride. A short half-life does not exclude a compound from being teratogenic, however. For example, aflatoxins are metabolized by the liver to epoxides that have very short half-lives and act mainly on the liver (Garner, 1974). Despite the short half-lives of the metabolites, the aflatoxins are teratogenic (Elis and DiPaolo, 1967). This may be explained by a chemical equilibrium between the epoxide and a more stable oxipen or bioactivation *in situ* by fetal tissue.

Nitrosamines are similarly activated in the liver to reactive electrophilic carbonium ions that are hepatotoxic. Nitrosamines are not powerful inducers of transplacental cancer because the active metabolite is too unstable to reach the fetus and the fetus is unable to activate the nitrosamines until shortly before birth. Chemically related nitrosoureas can be detected in the embryo and are teratogenic because they are stable enough to cross the placenta. Monoalkyltriazenes, which are formed from dialkyltriazenes by metabolic demethylation, are chemically stable, having chemical half-lives of the order of ten minutes. The chemical stability of the monoalkyltriazenes allows time for diffusion from maternal liver and penetration of embryonic tissue resulting in teratogenicity. Removal of the sugar residue from cycasin *in vivo* produces an electrophilic reactant that is stable enough to be teratogenic. Metabolic activation of the cycasin is dependent on species, age, and condition of the test species; thus teratogenicity of the compound is widely variable. Ethionine is bioactivated in the liver to S-adenosyl-L-ethionine, which can ethylate macromolecules causing cell abnormalities. Adenosylethionine is chemically stable and can penetrate to embryonic tissues and cause teratogenic effects. Aminoazobenzenes are teratogenic (Sugiyama *et al.*, 1960). These chemicals are bioactivated by *N*-hydroxylation and subsequently esterified, forming unstable intermediates that rearrange to electrophilic amidonium ions. Polycyclic hydrocarbons may be metabolically converted to epoxides that are very reactive electrophiles. This class of chemicals is highly teratogenic. Not all the polycyclic hydrocarbons are metabolically converted to epoxides, however, and not all the hydrocarbons are alike in their teratogenic properties. Benzpyrene is not an effective teratogen, while 7,12-dimethylbenzanthracene produces a high incidence of defects. Pyrrollizidine alkaloids have a structure similar to that of mitomycin C, and both are probably active only after conversion to a pyrrole analog.

PATHOGENESIS

Many teratogenic agents are selectively toxic for the fetus. There is often a wide range between the dose that induces fetal malformation and the dose that causes maternal toxicity. The most dangerous teratogens are those tolerated by the mother at a dose that is selectively damaging to fetal organogenesis. That fetal defects are so easily produced without significant harm to the mother is consistent with the effects of rubella and of thalidomide in humans. By contrast, maternal disorders, such as hemorrhagic anemia and liver damage, are not teratogenic. This emphasizes the risk that drugs and other environmental agents, otherwise innocuous, might be responsible for unexplained human malformations.

Teratogens can induce *in utero* death followed by abortion or resorption. Fetal death and the incidence of malformations among survivors generally run a parallel course. There is an association between intrauterine death, spontaneous abortion, stillbirth, and congenital defects. These facts indicate a close relationship between teratogenesis and the more general problem of reproductive wastage.

Teratogenic agents act selectively on developing cells and tissues to initiate abnormal embryogenesis. The mechanisms of selectivity of teratogens are varied and many of the early changes induced in developing systems are at a molecular or subcellular level. Proposed mechanisms for direct actions of cytotoxic agents have been discussed. In addition, other mechanisms of teratogenicity are alterations in precursor and substrate availability, which alter energy sources, change membrane characteristics, produce osmolar imbalance or enzyme inhibition, or alter chromosomes. These teratogenic effects may not result in cellular death, but may produce changes in developing cells to alter their subsequent course of development. The pathogenic effects of these indirect mechanisms, as well as the direct cytotoxic effects to produce abnormal embryogenesis, are altered cellular death, failure of cell interactions, reduced biosynthesis, impeded morphogenetic movement, or mechanical disruption of cells and tissues. Finally, too few cells or cell products may be produced to effect localized morphogenesis or functional maturation, and the results are imbalances in growth and differentiation. Teratogens may initiate one or more mechanisms and any one mechanism may be the result of different types of teratogens.

Most developmental defects involve deficiencies of tissue elements or of their biochemical products. Even final defects that do not overtly involve tissue deficiency may involve cell death during early pathogenesis (Scott *et al.*, 1975). Certain cytotoxic agents, by killing cells and initially causing localized cellular depletion, may ultimately result in a tissue-excess abnormality such as polydactyly. This paradoxic situation is produced because cellular depletion was greater in limb bud mesoderm than in ectoderm, resulting in an imbalance in the inductive influence thought to be exerted by the apical ectodermal ridge in determining the number of digital rays in the mesoderm. Localized deficiencies of cells result in imbalances between interacting groups of cells but may also be followed by a rebound in proliferative rate. General cell necrosis less than

the critical amount causing death of the embryo slows the rate of growth, and the resulting effect will be growth retardation. Functional deficits can also occur following damage inflicted during organogenesis. This can be explained as being the result of unreplenished cellular depletion or other tissue derangements critical to later functions. Growth retardation, at first considered simply slowed proliferation, may be an alteration of complex metabolic and transport activities essential to support normal growth, and failure to grow may reflect a variety of functional deficits. This is best exemplified by the fetal alcohol syndrome (Jones, 1975) and small-for-gestational-date babies produced as a result of *in utero* heroin addiction (Finnegan *et al.*, 1975). Dependence of normal function on gross as well as minute structural integrity has been emphasized, but physiologic functions are interdependent and failure of one may result in breakdown of another.

The differences and interrelationships among death, malformations, growth retardation, and functional deficits are poorly understood. Recently, in evaluating adverse influences on development, it has become apparent that growth retardation and functional deficits result in as great a morbidity among offspring as do morphologic abnormalities. Although structural defects are more conspicuous, functional defects are as incapacitating. No estimation of adverse effects on development can be considered complete unless it includes all manifestations of abnormal development. Evaluation of postnatal development is suggested in routine teratologic studies (CPSC, 1977).

TERATOGENIC MECHANISMS— A CATALOG

Mutation is a mechanism of teratogenesis. This defect is heritable and results from changes in sequence of nucleotides of DNA. Information encoded in DNA will be erroneously transcribed into RNA and ultimately into proteins. Some 20 to 30 percent of human developmental errors can be attributed primarily to mutation in a prior germ line. If the effect is in a germinal cell, the mutation will be hereditary. If the effect is in a somatic cell, it will be transmitted to all descendants of that cell, but will not be hereditary. Somatic mutations in the early embryo may affect enough progeny cells to produce a demonstrable structural or functional defect. Mutations are caused by ionizing radiation, chemical mutagens such as nitrous acid, alkylating agents, many carcinogens, and other factors leading to chromosomal breaks or crossovers (Freese, 1971). They may also result from interference with the normal processes of DNA repair.

Chromosomal nondisjunction and breaks give rise to excesses, deficiencies, or rearrangements of chromosomes or chromatids. These abnormalities are the cause of about 3 percent of human developmental defects but are not hereditary. Whole-chromosomal aneuploidy occurs during meiotic division in maturation of germ cells or during ordinary mitosis when newly divided chromosomes fail to separate, resulting in nondisjunction, which has no counterpart in mutagenesis. Nondisjunction occurs with greater frequency in germ cells of aged parents and also after aging of germ cells in the genital tract before fertilization. Chromosomal aberrations result from viral infections, irradiation, and chemical agents.

Chromosome deficiency is poorly tolerated and is usually lethal to the cell or organism, although the absence of one sex chromosome in Turner's syndrome is tolerated with only slight effect on development. Chromosome excess is usually detrimental. Trisomies of smaller autosomes are compatible with survival beyond birth, but are associated with moderate to severe developmental disorders (mongolism and chondrodystrophy) except in the case of excess sex chromosomes, which results in only mild defects.

Mitotic interference is produced by cytotoxic agents inhibiting synthesis of DNA, thereby slowing or arresting mitosis. The mitotic spindle can be prevented from forming or be dissolved after formation, by chemical agents that interfere with polymerization of tubulin into the microtubules of the spindle (Malawista *et al.*, 1968). Without a spindle, chromosomes do not separate at anaphase. Also, even when spindles are formed, chromosomes may not be able to separate because of apparent stickiness or physical continuity known as bridges. These conditions are produced by high-dosage radiation and radiomimetic chemicals (Hicks and D'Amato, 1966).

Altered nucleic acid integrity or function is the mechanism by which many antibiotics and antineoplastic drugs are teratogenic. The effects are biochemical changes interfering with nucleic acid replication, transcription, natural base incorporation, or RNA translation (protein synthesis), without producing heritable changes in DNA of germ cells. The agents altering nucleic acid integrity or function have been previously described and defined. Some of the agents interfere with replication or integrity of DNA. Antipurines, -pyrimidines, and -folates are teratogenic by producing erroneous incorporations into DNA or RNA. Interference with RNA translation and protein synthesis is a mechanism for the teratogenic action of cytotoxic agents. Agents that interfere with protein synthesis are generally embryocidal but can be teratogenic.

Lack of precursors and substrates needed for biosynthesis is a mechanism of teratogenesis. Biosynthesis can be altered by specific dietary deficiencies of vitamins and minerals. These deficiencies can be teratogenic, embryocidal, and growth inhibiting to offspring of pregnant mammals. The embryo may often manifest deficiency by death or by abnormal development before the mother shows serious signs of deprivation.

Deficiencies of other essential materials can occur in spite of adequate supplies of such materials in the maternal diet. Presence of analogs or antagonists to vitamins, essential amino acids, purines, pyrimidines, etc., may result in utilization of abnormal metabolites in biosynthesis instead of normal precursors. Incorporation of these analogs or antagonists causes abnormal development or death of early embryos (Seegmiller and Runner, 1974).

Adequate supplies of normal precursors and substrates in the maternal diet may not be absorbed from the maternal digestive tract or transported across the placenta. There are examples of absorption failures as a mechanism of teratogenesis (Volpintesta, 1974). Failure of absorption from maternal gut resulting in teratogenicity has been reported for copper due to excess zinc or sulfate (swayback lambs) and iodine in presence of high calcium (cretinism).

Azo dyes and tissue antisera inhibit placental transport of essential metabolites and are teratogenic (Lloyd *et al.*, 1968; Brent, 1971). The mechanism of these teratogens is to interfere with transfer of metabolites essential for normal embryonic growth, creating a nutritional deficiency. This effect is known only in rodents and rabbits, which are unique among mammals in being dependent for early placental transport on the inverted yolk sac placenta. No instance of failed placental transport has been demonstrated in higher mammals.

Energy supplies can be altered and result in abnormal fetal development (Bowman, 1967; Cox and Gunberg, 1972; Shepard, 1970). Inadequate glucose sources produced by dietary deficiencies or induced hypoglycemia reduce energy (ATP) generation and cause abnormal fetal development. Interference with glycolysis by 6-aminonicotinamide and iodoacetate also reduces energy generation and results in fetal defects. Interference with the citric acid cycle by 6-aminonicotinamide or riboflavin deficiency reduces energy generation and is teratogenic. Finally, impairment of terminal electron transport by hypoxia, dinitrophenol, or cyanide also reduces ATP generation and utilization and results in defective offspring.

Enzymatic function is essential for differentiation and growth. Some teratogens act specifically on enzymes to alter development (Jaffe, 1974; Johnson, 1974; Runner, 1974). Teratogenic folic acid antagonists inhibit dihydrofolate reductase. 5-Fluorouracil inhibits thymidylate synthetase and is teratogenic. Hydroxyurea produces aberrant development by inhibiting ribonucleoside diphosphate reductase. Acetazolamide inhibits carbonic anhydrase and alters fetal development. Cytosine arabinoside inhibits DNA polymerase. 6-Aminonicotinamide inhibits glucose-6-P dehydrogenase. These teratogens are enzyme inhibitors and subsequently alter fetal growth and development.

Osmolar imbalance is another mechanism of teratogenesis. Hypoxia produces early fluid osmolyte changes resulting in edema, hematomas, and blisters. These in turn lead to pathogenetic effects such as mechanical distortion and tissue ischemia, which reaches extremities and surface structures of the head, where abnormal embryogenesis ultimately occurs. Similar pathogenetic effects follow osmolyte imbalances resulting from trypan blue, hypertonic solutions, and adrenal cortical hormones. Tail and extremity malformations induced by injecting pregnant mice with hypertonic saline solutions result from damage following edema, blisters, and hemorrhages (Tanaka *et al.*, 1968). Benzhydryl piperazine-induced orofacial malformations have been attributed to edema known to occur in embryos after treatment (Posner, 1972) Fluid accumulations, hemorrhages, and blisters have been reported in rodent embryos after trypan blue treatment. Abnormal fluid accumulations can cause tissue distortions sufficient to lead to malformations.

Alterations of membrane characteristics can lead to osmolar imbalances, as described above. Solvents such as dimethyl sulfoxide (DMSO) produce swellings and blisters associated with ionic shifts between compartments in chick embryos by altering permeability of cell membranes and other membranes (Browne, 1968). Teratogenic doses of vitamin A, leading to hypervitaminosis A, produce ultrastructural damage to cellular membranes in rodent embryos (Morriss, 1973; Nakamura *et al.*, 1974).

GENETIC FACTORS INFLUENCING TERATOGENESIS

The distinction between genetic and purely phenotypic abnormalities is not easily made. Most congenital malformations are not associated with any obvious abnormality of the chromosomes and are not heritable. The nonheritable nature of the abnormalities has been demonstrated by brother-sister matings of malformed animals and also on a large scale in humans. However, genetic factors play an important part

in determining sensitivity to teratogens as well as in the probability of spontaneous malformation. An indication of the role of genetic factors is the observed difference in sensitivity between species and between strains of the same species. The azo dye trypan blue produced exencephalic offspring in three rat strains at frequencies of 17, 50, and 97 percent, respectively. Cortisone produced cleft palate in 100 percent of strain A mice but only 20 percent in strain C57BL. This difference is the result of earlier midline fusion of the palate in the more resistant strain. Cortisone produced cleft palate in rabbits but no malformations in rats. Yet cortisone strongly potentiated the actions of another teratogen, vitamin A, in rats. That these genetically determined differences are not necessarily due to differences in metabolism or transplacental passage of teratogens may be seen from similar findings in chick embryo. Injection of teratogens into the yolk sac of various strains on the fourth day produced micromelia (short upper extremities) at frequencies varying from 5 to 100 percent.

Among multiparous animals, some fetuses escape defects while others in the same litter suffer severe and even multiple malformations. For example, trypan blue administered to 200 pregnant rats on the seventh, eighth, and ninth days of gestation produced death and resorption of nearly one-half of the fetuses, numerous malformations in one-half the survivors, and no effect in the remaining one-quarter (Wilson, 1955). Response differences could not be ascribed to differences between mothers, as dead, malformed, and normal fetuses appeared to be randomly distributed among individual rats and even in the same uterine horn (Wilson, 1959). Vitamin A deficiency produced retinal defects, ectopic ureters, and diaphragmatic hernia. Riboflavin deficiency produced shortened long bones and mandible, fused ribs and toes, and cleft palate. Folic acid deficiency affected virtually every organ and system in the body. Irradiation produced anophthalmia, encephalocele, and renal agenesis. Teratogen-specific effects were also obtained in the chick, where maternal and placental factors are excluded. Active forms of all vitamins are required by all growing cells. Quantitative differences in these requirements at critical stages of development of each organ must underlie the differential effects of teratogenic treatments, so that at any given time one organ is more sensitive to riboflavin deficiency, another to vitamin A deficiency, etc.

TYPES OF TERATOGENS

A variety of agents have been studied and are teratogenic in animal models (Table 8–4). Fetal malformation produced by nutritional deficiency

Table 8–4. TERATOGENS IN ANIMAL MODELS*

Dietary deficiency: vitamins A, D, and E, ascorbic acid, riboflavin, thiamine, nicotinamide, folic acid, pantothenic acid, trace metals (Zn, Mn, Mg, Co), protein

Hormone deficiency: pituitary, thyroid, insulin (alloxan diabetes)

Vitamin antagonists: antifolic drugs, 6-aminonicotinamide, 3-acetylpyridine

Hormone antagonists: thiouracil derivatives

Vitamin excess: vitamin A, nicotinic acid

Hormone excess: cortisone, hydrocortisone, thyroxine, vasopressin, insulin, androgens, estrogens, epinephrine

Carbohydrates: galactose, 2-deoxyglucose, bacterial lipopolysaccharides

Antibiotics: dactinomycin, penicillin, tetracyclines, streptomycin

Sulfonamides: hypoglycemic sulfonamides, sulfanilamide

Heavy metals: methyl mercury, phenylmercuric acetate, inorganic mercury salts, lead, thallium, strontium, selenium, chelating agents (EDTA)

Azo dyes: trypan blue, Evans blue, Niagara sky blue 6B

Agents producing hypoxia: carbon monoxide, carbon dioxide, etc.

Drugs and chemicals: nicotine, eserine, quinine, pilocarpine, ricin, saponin, chlorpromazine and derivatives, thiadiazole, triazene, boric acid, salicylate, hydroxyurea, acetazolamide, chlorcyclizine, meclizine, thalidomide, rauwolfia, vinca, veratrum alkaloids, triparanol (MER-29), serotonin, imipramine, 2,3,4,8-tetrachlorodibenzo-*p*-dioxin, nitrosamines, caffeine, barbital, carbutamide, diphenylhydantoin, amphetamine, glutethimide, morphine (Schardein, 1976; Shepard, 1976)

Insecticides, herbicides, fungicides (Wilson, 1977b)

Solvents: dimethyl sulfoxide, chloroform, 1,1-dichloroethane, carbon tetrachloride, benzene, xylene, cyclohexanone, propylene glycol, alkane, sulfonates, acetamides, formamides

Natural substances: rubratoxin B, aflatoxin B_1, ochratoxin A, ergotamine, locoweed, jimson weed

Physical agents: hypo- and hyperthermia, hypoxia, radiation

Infections: 10 viruses known, including rubella and cytomegalovirus, syphilis, gonorrhea

---

* Data derived from Schardein, 1976; Cahen, 1964; Carter, 1971; Kalter, 1968; Warkany, 1959; Woollam, 1965.

is of interest because of its possible relationship to human congenital malformations. The first published data on chemical teratogenesis dealt with vitamin A deficiency in pigs (Hale, 1935). A vitamin A–deficient diet throughout pregnancy produced abnormal offspring with a variety of malformations. Subsequent matings of the same sow yielded normal offspring as did brother-sister matings between malformed animals. Since

this time, the teratogenic effects of other vitamin deficiencies have been established.

Hormone deficiencies and excesses are teratogenic either by the hormone acting alone or in concert with another chemical. For example, cortisone can increase the incidence of malformations caused by vitamin A, whereas insulin antagonizes the effects. Thyroxine antagonizes the teratogenic action of vitamin A while the antithyroid compound methylthiouracil increases that teratogenic effect. Moreover, thyroxine can reduce the incidence of a spontaneous genetically determined anomaly, cleft lip, in mice. Thus, disturbances of hormonal balance may play a role in the etiology of malformations in the human. Concealed endocrinopathies may account for some fetal wastage.

Trace element deficiencies can be teratogenic as well. This has been demonstrated for zinc, manganese, and cobalt (DiPaolo and Kotin, 1966). The effect of zinc deficiency was demonstrated by feeding the chelating agent EDTA to pregnant rats from day 6 to day 21. Malformations were prevented by simultaneous feeding of zinc carbonate (Swenerton and Hurley, 1971).

Administration of the azo dye trypan blue to rats at a dose of 10 mg between gestational days 7 and 10 produces malformations of brain (hydrocephalus), eyes, vertebral column, and cardiovascular system (Wilson, 1955). Similar malformations are produced in rabbits and chicks. Trypan blue never reaches the rat embryo, but accumulates in maternal reticuloendothelial system and in the placenta. The dye is excluded by the yolk sac that encloses the rat embryo at about the ninth day of gestation. When injected into the yolk sac of embryo explants, the dye is teratogenic even on the eleventh day (Gilbert and Gillman, 1954). Trypan blue gains access to the embryonic blastocyst throughout the gestation period. The dye is localized in lysosomes of the yolk sac and inhibits several lysomal enzymes, which interferes with the hydrolytic digestion of the yolk, thus impairing fetal nutrition. Yolk sac function is of little importance in primates; thus trypan blue is more teratogenic in chick embryo and rodents than in primates (Beck *et al.*, 1967). There are structural requirements for teratogenic activity among azo dyes. Shifting sulfonate substitutions or substitution of methyl groups greatly reduces the teratogenic activity of the dyes.

HUMAN TERATOGENESIS

From the time man has been capable of leaving any records, monsters resulting from biologic malformations have been of considerable interest. Mothers tend to attribute the birth of a defective child to some unusual event during pregnancy. This prejudices objective retrospective investigations into causative factors that may have operated some nine months prior to the birth. The mother of the defective child is either unlikely to remember this period or likely to exaggerate or imagine events during pregnancy.

It has only rarely been possible to observe an experiment on teratogenesis in the human. Cases have been reported in which acute hypoxia produced by carbon monoxide or morphine overdose was followed by birth of a malformed child; however, cause-and-effect relationships in such episodes are uncertain. Aminopterin, an antifolic drug, is an abortifacient occasionally used for this purpose. Surviving fetuses of such abortion attempts were grossly malformed (Warkany and Kalter, 1961). Progestational steroids, used for treatment of habitual abortion, have produced masculinization of the female fetus (Jackson, 1959). For this reason, progesterone-containing oral contraceptives are contraindicated during suspected pregnancy. Toxoplasmosis and syphilis during pregnancy produce fetal malformations by direct invasion and destruction of fetal tissue (Warkany and Kalter, 1961). Methyl mercury ingestion by pregnant women produced cerebral palsy in offspring, even though the mothers were symptom free (Matsumoto et al., 1965).

Rubella infection during pregnancy produces cataracts and other eye abnormalities, deafness, cardiac defects, and mental retardation. Heart and eye defects occurred predominantly during first- or second-month infection. Rubella contracted after the third month of gestation was without effects. Approximately 20 percent of women who contract rubella during the first trimester will give birth to a defective child.

Thalidomide, a sedative-hypnotic, was introduced in the late 1950s in West Germany, England, and other countries. This drug was nontoxic and the therapeutic dose was about 100 mg, but patients have recovered from ingestion of as much as 14 g taken with suicidal intent.

Shortly after introduction of thalidomide, there was an increase in the number of infants born with phocomelia, shortening or complete absence of the limbs. Not a single case of phocomelia was seen in the decade 1949–1959 at the University Pediatric Clinic in Hamburg. A single case was reported in 1959, 30 cases in 1960, and 154 cases in 1961. Occurrence of phocomelia increased in many parts of the world when thalidomide was in use. In 1961, a pediatrician reported a suspected association between phocomelia and ingestion of thalidomide during pregnancy. In virtually every case, thalidomide was ingested between the third and eighth weeks of pregnancy. Thalidomide was withdrawn from the market in 1961. The drug was never approved by the Food and Drug Administration, and therefore never in general use in the United States. Ultimately, 10,000 infants were deformed by thalidomide.

Thalidomide produces a characteristic pattern of malformation, including malformations of the extremities (phocomelia), ears, and face. Upper extremities were involved in about 80 percent of the cases. Defects ranged from complete absence of all the bones of an extremity to hypoplasia of the thenar eminence. There was a predilection for abnormalities of the radius and thumb. Involvement of the lower extremities with hypoplasia or absence of the tibia and femur was less commonly encountered. Ear anomalies ranging from hypoplasia to anotia were seen in approximately 20 percent of the cases. Capillary hemangiomas extending from the upper lip over the nose to the glabella were frequently seen. A variety of malformations of internal organs, such as intestinal atresia, imperforate anus, and aplasia of the gallbladder and appendix, also occurred either associated with skeletal defects or occasionally as the only abnormality.

Routine teratogenicity testing of new drugs resulted from the thalidomide experience. Thalidomide, as well as other teratogens, displays a strong species specificity. At first congenital abnormalities could not be produced in rats, but in certain strains of white rabbits, thalidomide administered between the eighth and sixteenth days of pregnancy led to limb malformations (Larsen, 1963). Subsequently, work with rats showed that this species was sensitive, but only on the twelfth day of gestation (Bignami et al., 1962). Finally, a thalidomide-induced syndrome, which resembled that seen in humans, was produced in monkeys.

Species differences in thalidomide-induced teratogenicity may be explained by variations in metabolic pathways. Thalidomide is extensively metabolized and the proximate teratogen is a metabolite rather than the parent compound. Recently, Fabro et al. (1976) have proposed a chemically reactive metabolite as the ultimate teratogen.

Following the thalidomide episode, investigation of the teratogenicity of drugs and chemicals intensified, both for established drugs as well as for new ones. However, at present, only a few drugs have been identified as teratogens in man.

All cytotoxic anticancer drugs, such as alkylating agents, antimetabolites, plant alkaloids, antibiotics, and those cytotoxic agents previously discussed, depend on their ability to block biosynthetic processes necessary for cellular replication, to act directly on DNA, or to inhibit cell division. They may be expected to cause fetal death or a wide variety of developmental abnormalities if administered during the critical period of organogenesis. The folic acid antagonist 4-aminopteroylglutamic acid (aminopterin) is of special clinical interest. The drug has been used as an abortifacient. Fetuses that survive aminopterin exposure during the first trimester present a typical malformation syndrome, which includes hydrocephalus, absent or partially ossified skull bones, micrognathia, palate defects, low-set ears, hypertelorism, and anomalies of the extremities.

Courrier and Jost (1942) produced fetal masculinization in pregnant rabbits with ethinyltestosterone. Wilkins (1960), some 18 years later, reported 70 cases of masculinization of the human female fetus following prenatal use of various progestational compounds used to maintain pregnancy in habitual aborters or to control bleeding during pregnancy. An additional 30 cases of masculinized infants were reported after the use of norethindrone. The genital deformity ranged between varying degrees of clitoral enlargement and labioscrotal fusion. Labial fusion occurred if progestin was given before the thirteenth week of gestation, and clitoral enlargement could be produced during the second and even third trimesters. The expression of masculinization depended on the relative androgenicity and dose of the preparation used. Of the available steroid esters, 17-alpha-hydroxyprogesterone is least androgenic. There are no clinical data to suggest that the small amount of progestins contained in oral contraceptives have a similar masculinizing effect in escaped pregnancies. Estrogen-induced masculinization has also been documented following the use of diethylstilbestrol during the first trimester. Diethylstilbestrol may stimulate the fetal adrenal to increase its androgenic output or cause abnormal estrogen metabolism in some mothers. Administration of testosterone or its analogs during the susceptible period of gestation has also been shown to cause virilization of the female fetus.

Studies in the last decade have suggested that ethanol is a teratogen (Lemoine *et al.*, 1968; Jones *et al.*, 1973, 1974). Some children born to alcoholic mothers have pre- and postnatal growth failure, microcephaly, developmental delay, and other anomalies termed the "fetal alcohol syndrome." Craniofacial anomalies include small eyelid folds and other defects (myopia, ptosis, and strabismus), maxillary hypoplasia, and anomalies of the ears. Skeletal anomalies, cardiac defects, abnormal palmar creases and, in girls, hypoplasia of the labia majora are also found. Teratogenic anomalies are probably due to the ethanol rather than malnutrition because linear growth is curtailed more than weight growth; in case of generalized maternal malnutrition fetal weight is curtailed more. The growth rate appears to be irreversibly reduced: infants with fetal alcohol syndrome have remained small and mentally defective when placed in foster homes. The percentage of fetuses at risk to the teratogenic effects of ethanol is not known, but, as with all drugs and chemicals, the pregnant woman should be advised to minimize her exposure to ethanol.

Thyroxine is teratogenic in laboratory animals, but its clinical use for treatment of maternal hypothyroidism does not affect fetal thyroid development. Maternal thyrotropic hormone (TSH) does not readily cross the placenta. All antithyroid agents affect function and development of the fetal thyroid-pituitary axis. Administration of thiouracils for treatment of maternal hyperthyroidism pose a threat of congenital goiter in the fetus. Promiscuous use of iodides during pregnancy also poses a threat to fetal development. Congenital goiter, resulting in tracheal compression and neonatal respiratory death, has occurred after prolonged administration of iodide-containing cough and antiasthma preparations. Transplacental passage of excessive amounts of iodide depresses hormone synthesis in the fetal thyroid. The compensatory increase in fetal TSH is responsible for the goitrous enlargement.

A number of other drugs and chemicals are suspected teratogens in humans because of animal studies or clinical suspicion. Drugs include anticonvulsants, anorexogenics, oral hypoglycemics, and alkylating agents (Wilson, 1973). Included in this list of possible teratogens are aspirin, antibiotics, antituberculous drugs, quinine, imipramine, and insulin. Catz and Abuelo (1974) further classified trimethoprim-sulfisoxazole, barbiturates, diphenylhydantoin, dextroamphetamine, antacids, nicotinamide, iron, and antihistamines as suspected teratogens. Forfar (1974) added alcohol, dicoumarol, excess vitamins A and D, smoking, chloroquine, LSD, lithium, quinacrine, phenylbutazone, meprobamate, promethazine, pyrimethamine, and others to the list. Tuchmann-Duplessis (1965) suspected antitumor drugs, busulfan, mercaptopurine, cyclophosphamide, and chlorambucil. Meclizine, sulfonamides, trifluoperazine, phenmetrazine, cortisone, podophyllotoxin, serotonin, and tetracycline have also been frequently mentioned as possible human teratogens. Insecticides, herbicides, fungicides, metals, and solvents are considered candidate teratogens (Wilson, 1977b). However, the human risk at current usage conditions is generally not known.

In addition to teratogenic effects resulting from drug and chemical exposure, overt chemical and drug toxicity may also result from drug and chemical administration in late gestation or at

Table 8–5. DRUG AND CHEMICAL TOXICITY IN THE HUMAN FETUS

Alcohol	Muscular hypotonia, withdrawal
Antibacterials	
Streptomycin	8th nerve damage
Tetracyclines	Deposition in bone, discoloration of teeth, inhibition of bone growth
Sulfonamides	Kernicterus, anemia
Novobiocin	Hyperbilirubinemia
Chloramphenicol	Death (gray syndrome)
Erythromycin	Liver damage
Nitrofurantoin	Hemolysis
Anticoagulants	
Coumarin	Hemorrhage, death
Sodium warfarin	
Antidiabetics	
Tolbutamide	Thrombocytopenia
Chlorpropamide	Prolonged hypoglycemia
Phenformin	Lactic acidosis
Insulin (shock)	Fetal loss
Ammonium chloride	Acidosis
Adrenocortical hormones	Adrenocortical suppression
Prednisolone	Acute fetal distress, fetal death
Antihistamines	Infertility
Antithyroid drugs	Hypothyroidism
Barbiturates, diphenylhydantoin	Coagulation defects, withdrawal syndrome (barbiturates only)
Phenobarbital excess	Neonatal bleeding, death
Chlordiazepoxide	Withdrawal syndrome
Diazepam	Hypothermia
Meprobamate	Retarded development
Sedatives	Behavioral changes
Meperidine	Neonatal depression
Primidone	Withdrawal syndrome
Heroin, morphine, methadone	Withdrawal syndrome, neonatal death
Mepivacaine	Fetal brachycardia and depression
Reserpine	Nasal congestion, lethargy, respiratory depression, brachycardia
Phenothiazines	Hyperbilirubinemia, depression, hypothermia
Hexamethonium bromide	Neonatal ileus
Cholinesterase inhibitors (pesticides)	Transient muscle weakness
Magnesium sulfate	Central depression and neuromuscular block
Quinine	Thrombocytopenia
Iophenoxic acid	Elevation of serum PBI
Chloroquine	Death
Alphaprodine	Platelet dysfunction
Thiazide diuretics	Thrombocytopenia, salt and water depletion, neonatal death
Lithium	Cyanosis and flaccidity
Primaquine, pentaquine	Hemolysis
Vitamin K analogs, excess	Hyperbilirubinemia
Intravenous fluids, excess	Fluid and electrolyte abnormalities
Smoking	Premature birth, small babies, perinatal loss
Vaccinations	Fetal vaccinia
Polio vaccine, live	Fetal loss
Oral progestins, androgens, estrogens	Advanced bone age
Salicylates, large amounts	Bleeding
Anesthetics (general anesthetics)	Newborn depression
Solvents	Newborn depression

birth (Table 8–5). Drugs ingested during late pregnancy or during labor and delivery are excreted by the newborn during the first seven to eight days of neonatal life (Hill, 1974). However, some may take longer and effects may become manifest very late. Estrogen treatment produced a delayed effect. Daughters of women treated during pregnancy some 14 to 22 years earlier with diethylstilbestrol or dienestrol diacetate to maintain pregnancy developed vaginal alterations, including rare neoplasms (Greenwald et al., 1971; Herbst et al., 1971). The toxicity induced by drugs and chemicals in the adult can also be produced in the fetus during late gestational development or during parturition.

Cortisone is a suspect teratogen but there is not yet enough evidence to incriminate it. Cortisone produces 100 percent cleft palate in certain genetic strains of white mice. A review of 260 pregnancies during which cortisone or its analogs were used at pharmacologic doses for a variety of indications showed that 90 percent of pregnancies terminated with normal infants at birth. Of the remaining 10 percent, there were seven stillborn infants, one abortion, 15 premature infants, and two infants with cleft palate. Another study of a steroid used during pregnancy for treatment of rheumatic fever showed an overall low probability of teratogenicity. On the basis of available evidence, cortisone is probably safe to use in cases of grave maternal illness in which glucocorticoid therapy is indicated and its use should not be made a source of added maternal apprehension. Administration of steroids during pregnancy for minor indications such as eczema or mild asthma, however, is an unjustified risk.

Insulin is an endocrine agent that is widely used during pregnancy. There is no clinical evidence that controlled insulin therapy for treatment of maternal diabetes has teratogenic effects in humans. Insulin shock, however, may lead to fetal death and congenital malformation.

Oral sulfonylurea hypoglycemia agents, tolbutamide and chlorpropamide, have been incriminated as possible human teratogens. These produce malformations, primarily eye defects, in animal models. Several isolated cases of multiple congenital anomalies have been reported following their use. However, maternal diabetes itself is associated with an increased incidence of malformation; therefore, more data are needed to evaluate the real danger of sulfonylurea-induced defects.

Antihistamine antiemetics, such as meclizine and cyclizine, used in treatment of nausea and vomiting of early pregnancy, have also been incriminated as suspect teratogens. Large doses of meclizine produce a high incidence of cleft palate in rats. The evidence, although scanty, circumstantial, and mostly retrospective, prompted one European country to remove the drug from the market. Subsequently, other studies emerged, some incriminating the drug as teratogenic and others declaring it innocent. Retrospective studies have been inconclusive and prospective data available do not show any cause-and-effect relationship.

The most recent drugs creating teratogenic concern are the hallucinogens. Lysergic acid diethylamide (LSD), mescaline, and 2-bromo-d-lysergic acid have been reported to produce severe malformations in the hamster. There are conflicting reports on the teratogenic effect of LSD in the rat. In the human adult, LSD has been associated with breaks and other structural abnormalities of chromosomes. Chromosomal breaks have also been reported in the offspring of mothers who ingested LSD during pregnancy, and there have been isolated reports of the association of LSD taken early in pregnancy with the birth of malformed infants. However, chromosomal breakage that occurs for other reasons, such as in measles, has not been associated with congenital malformations, and the instances of human LSD-congenital malformation are too few for statistical evaluation. Prospective experiments involving deliberate administration of LSD are obviously not permissible. Retrospective studies with users of illicit LSD are virtually impossible to evaluate because of multiple drug use, uncertain purity of LSD, unknown dosage and timing, inadequate nutritional status of abusers, and biases associated with all retrospective studies. There is no convincing evidence to implicate LSD as a teratogen in humans, yet the possibility cannot be excluded (Long, 1972; Emerit et al., 1972).

Some contaminants to which people may be exposed in the general environment or through occupational contact are teratogenic in animal models. Dioxin (2,3,7,8-tetrachlorodibenzo-p-dioxin), a potent mutagen, carcinogen, and teratogen, is a contaminant of the herbicide 2,4,5-trichlorophenoxyacetic acid (2,4,5-T), widely used in agriculture and as a defoliant for military purposes (Jackson, 1972; Sparschu et al., 1971). The fungicide captan (N-trichloromethylthio-4-cyclohexene-1,2-dicarboximide) is also teratogenic (Verrett et al., 1969). The CNS of the fetus appears to be especially sensitive to toxic effects of methylmercury. Pregnant women who have been exposed to doses of methylmercury without incurring typical poisoning symptoms have borne children who developed cerebral palsy. Other neurologic symptoms included chorea, ataxia, tremors, seizures, and mental retardation (Koos and Longo, 1976). Lead, another major environmental pollutant, may also be teratogenic (Matsumoto et al., 1965; Scanlon, 1972).

SUMMARY

Experimental teratology and clinical observations have provided evidence for several principles of teratology. The susceptible period for production of congenital malformations is the first trimester of pregnancy, the stage of organogenesis. Subtle congenital defects can also be produced by drugs and chemicals during the second and third trimester. These defects are generally functional or biochemical aberrations. A simple teratogen can produce a variety of malformations. For example, rubella virus interferes with normal development of the eye (cataracts), the ear (deafness), the heart (patent ductus), and the brain (mental retardation). The same malformation can be produced by a variety of teratogens. Trypan blue and hypervitaminosis A produce spina bifida in the rat. Genetic and environmentally induced malformations may be phenocopies and clinically indistinguishable. Masculinization of the female fetus, genetically induced by the adrenogenital syndrome, may be indistinguishable from the ambiguous genitalia of the fetus masculinized by the androgenic effect of progestational compounds administered early in pregnancy. Teratogenic effects vary in different species and in different strains of the same species. This genetic difference is the major stumbling block in preclinical testing of drugs. Thalidomide, the most potent human teratogen known, produces little, if any, effect in the rat and mouse. The smallest teratogenic dose in man was 0.5 to 1.0 mg/kg. The largest dose producing no effect in mouse and rate was 4,000 mg/kg. Only moderate embryopathy was produced in the rabbit at a dosage of 2.5 mg/kg. Acetylsalicylic acid, with a long history of safe use in human pregnancy, is responsible for a high incidence of malformation in the rat. Cortisone, which produced 100 percent cleft palate in the offspring of certain strains of white mice, has no known effect on the development of other strains. Most human malformations are due to an interaction between genetic and environmental factors.

Pregnant women should obviously not be exposed to drugs and chemicals known to be teratogenic, but these same agents may be harmless and useful in men, in women beyond menopause, and in children; therefore, these agents cannot practically be eliminated from our environment. A critical question is whether pregnancy can be recognized soon enough to avoid exposure to these teratogens. A schematic presentation of the problem is shown in Figure 8–1. The sensitive period for teratogenesis is the phase of organ differentiation. The period of organogenesis in the human embryo begins at about the twentieth day of gestation (first somite stage) and continues through the first trimester (Hamilton *et al.*, 1962). Subtle morphologic and biochemical differentiation continues throughout the second and third trimesters. Women with regular menses ovulate 14 days (12 to 16 days) prior to the onset of the next menstrual period. Fertilization takes place within a day or two following ovulation (Fluhmann, 1956). At fetal age 20 days, the missed period is about one week overdue and pregnancy tests are positive. The length of the menstrual cycle varies between women and among individual women. About 30 percent of all women have a range of 15 days between their shortest and longest cycles. Thus, most women will be unaware they are pregnant during the critical period of organogenesis. Safeguards for exposure during this period are negligible. Whenever a woman of childbearing age is treated with drugs or exposed to chemicals in the environment, the possibility of pregnancy should be kept in mind. This includes agents that are considered harmless, e.g., caffeine, nicotine, and alcohol. These agents as yet have not been shown harmless. Even aspirin is capable of causing blood-clotting disorders in the neonate when administered to mothers during the week prior to birth. The risk of chemical teratogenesis is accentuated during the first trimester.

Congenital malformations occur spontaneously and can also be produced by external physical or chemical treatments. The causes of the spontaneous events are unknown. Experimentation is confined to laboratory animals, while human data are statistically derived. Requirements for animal testing have slowed the development of new drugs. An effective human data collection system is needed (Ingalls and Klingberg, 1965) Prospective statistical investigations in humans may provide associations between as-yet-unsuspected chemicals and drugs and the subsequent birth of a defective child.

On the whole, it would seem wise to avoid exposure to drugs, chemicals, viruses, bacteria, and physical forces during pregnancy. Since this seems impractical, there is little choice other than to continue to emphasize major areas of responsibility. The physician's responsibility is to be continuously aware of teratogenic potential when prescribing drugs and biologicals during the reproductive years. The mother's responsibility is to avoid promiscuous self-medication and exposure to industrial chemicals. Benefits and risks should be carefully weighed before exposure of a pregnant woman to drugs and chemicals, particularly during the first trimester.

Chemical teratogenesis is a challenging new area of toxicology. We have little understanding of the mechanisms of chemical-induced teratogenesis. Also, we do not know whether chemical teratogens are responsible for spontaneous human malformations. Increasing experimentation and knowledge of biochemical events of normal embryogenesis will permit a better understanding of teratogenesis. Practical means may be developed for diagnosis and prevention of congenital defects.

REFERENCES

Beck, F.; Lloyd, J. B.; and Griffiths, A.: Lysosomal enzyme inhibition by trypan blue: a theory of teratogenesis. *Science,* **157**:1180–82, 1967.

Bignami, G.; Bovet, D.; Bovet-Nitti, F.; and Rosnati, V.: Drugs and congenital abnormalities. *Lancet,* 2:1332–33, 1962.

Borisy, G. G., and Taylor, E. W.: The mechanism of action of colchicine. I. Binding of colchicine-^{3}H to cellular protein. *J. Cell Biol.,* **34**:525–34, 1967.

Bowman, P.: The effect of 2,4-dinitrophenol on the development of early chick embryos. *J. Embryol. Exp. Morphol.,* **17**:425–31, 1967.

Brent, R. L.: Antibodies and malformations. In Tuchmann-Duplessis, H. (ed.): *Malformations Congenitales des Mammiferes.* Mason et Cie, Paris, 1971, pp. 187–220.

Browne, J. M.: Physiological effects of dimethylsulfoxide (DMSO) on the chick embryo. *Teratology,* **1**:212, 1968.

Cahen, R. L.: Evaluation of the teratogenicity of drugs. *Clin. Pharmacol. Ther.,* **5**:480–514, 1964.

Carter, C. O.: Incidence and aetiology. In Norman, A. P. (ed.): *Congenital Abnormalities in Infancy,* 2nd ed. Blackwell Scientific Publications, Oxford and Edinburgh, 1971.

Catz, C. S., and Abuelo, D.: Drugs and Pregnancy. *Drug Ther.,* **4**(4):79–91, 1974.

Commission on Drug Safety, Report. *Conference on Prenatal Effects of Drugs.* Chicago, 1963.

Courrier, R., and Jost, A.: Intersexualité foetale provoquée par la prégnéninolone au cours de la grossesse. *C. R. Séances Soc. Biol. Ses Filiales,* **136**:395–96, 1942.

Cox, S. J., and Gunberg, D. L.: Energy metabolism in isolated rat embryo hearts: Effect of metabolic inhibitors. *J. Embryol. Exp. Morphol.,* **28**:591–99, 1972.

CPSC, Consumer Product Safety Commission: *Toxicity Testing of Household Products.* Document 1138. Washington, DC, 1977.

DiPaolo, J. A., and Kotin, P.: Teratogenesis-oncogenesis: a study of possible relationships. *Arch. Pathol.*, **81**:3–23, 1966.

Elis, J., and DiPaolo, J. A.: Aflatoxin B1. Induction of malformations. *Arch. Pathol.*, **83**:53–57, 1967.

Emerit, I.; Roux, C.; and Feingold, J.: LSD: No chromosomal breakage in mother and embryos during rat pregnancy. *Teratology*, **6**:71–74, 1972.

Evans, M. A., and Harbison, R. D.: Prenatal toxicity of rubratoxin B and its hydrogenated analog. *Toxicol. Appl. Pharmacol.*, **39**:13–33, 1977.

Fabro, S., and Sieber, S. M.: Penetration of drugs into the rabbit blastocyst before implantation. In Pecile, A., and Finzi, C. (eds.): *International Symposium on the Foeto-Placental Unit, Milan, 1968.* Excerpta Medica International Congress Series, No. 183. Amsterdam, 1969, pp. 313–20.

Fabro, S.; Shull, G.; and Dixon, R.: Further studies on the mechanism of teratogenic action of thalidomide. *Pharmacologist*, **18**:231, 1976.

FDA, Food and Drug Administration: *Guidelines for Reproduction Studies for Safety Evaluation of Drugs for Human Use.* Washington, DC, 1966.

FDA, Food and Drug Administration, Advisory Committee on Protocols for Safety Evaluations, Panel on Reproduction: Report on reproduction studies in the safety evaluation of food additives and pesticide residues. *Toxicol. Appl. Pharmacol.*, **16**:264–96, 1970.

Feehan, E. B.: More on mollies (and tetracycline). *N. Engl. J. Med.*, **282**:1048, 1970.

Finnegan, L. P.; Kron, R. E.; Connaughton, J. F., Jr.; and Emich, J. P.: Neonatal abstinence syndrome: Assessment and management. In Harbison, R. D. (ed.): *Perinatal Addiction.* Spectrum Publications, New York, 1975, pp. 141–58.

Fluhmann, C. F.: *The Management of Menstrual Disorders.* W. B. Saunders, Philadelphia, 1956.

Forfar, J. O.: Epidemiology of drug-induced malformations. *Biochem. Soc. Trans.*, **2**:690–95, 1974.

Freese, E.: Molecular mechanisms of mutations. In Hollaender, A. (ed.): *Chemical Mutagens. Principles and Methods for Their Detection*, Vol. I. Plenum Press, New York, 1971, pp. 1–56.

Garner, C.: Moulds, bacteria and cancer. *New Scientist*, **63**:325–27, 1974.

Gebhardt, D. O. E.: The embryolethal and teratogenic effects of cyclophosphamide on mouse embryos. *Teratology*, **3**:273–78, 1970.

Gilbert, C., and Gillman, J.: The morphogenesis of trypan blue induced defects of the eye. *S. African J. Med. Sci.*, **19**:147–54, 1954.

Gregg, N. M.: Congenital cataract following German measles in the mother. *Trans. Ophthalmol. Soc. Aust.*, **3**:35–46, 1941.

Greenwald, P.; Barlow, J. J.; Nasca, P. C.; and Burnett, W. S.: Vaginal cancer after maternal treatment with synthetic estrogens. *N. Engl. J. Med.*, **285**(7):390–92, 1971.

Hale, F.: Relation of vitamin A to anophthalmos in pigs. *Am. J. Ophthalmol.*, **18**:1087–92, 1935.

Hamilton, W. J.; Boyd, J. D.; and Mossman, H. W.: *Human Embryology*, 3rd ed. Williams & Wilkins Co., Baltimore, 1962.

Harbison, R. D.: Parathion-induced toxicity and phenobarbital-induced protection against parathion during prenatal development. *Toxicol. Appl. Pharmacol.*, **32**:482–93, 1975.

Harbison, R. D., and Becker, B. A.: Relation of dosage and time of administration of diphenylhydantoin to its teratogenic effect in mice. *Teratology*, **2**:305–12, 1969.

———: Effect of phenobarbital and SKF 525A pretreatment on diphenylhydantoin teratogenicity in mice. *J. Pharmacol. Exp. Ther.*, **175**:283–88, 1970.

Harbison, R. D.; MacDonald, J. S.; Sweetman, B. J.; and Taber, D.: Proposed mechanism for diphenylhydantoin-induced teratogenesis. *Pharmacologist*, **19**:179, 1977.

Harbison, R. D.; Mantilla-Plata, B.; and Lubin, D. J.: Alteration of Δ^9-tetrahydrocannabinol-induced teratogenicity by stimulation and inhibition of its metabolism. *J. Pharmacol. Exp. Ther.*, **202**:455–65, 1977.

Harbison, R. D.; Olubadewo, J.; Dwivedi, C.; and Sastry, B. V. R.: Proposed role of the placental cholinergic system in the regulation of fetal growth and development. In Morselli, P. L.; Garattini, S.; and Sereni, F. (eds.): *Basic and Therapeutic Aspects of Perinatal Pharmacology.* Raven Press, New York, 1975, pp. 107–20.

Health and Welfare of Canada: *The Testing of Chemicals for Carcinogenicity, Mutagenicity, and Teratogenicity.* 1973.

Herbst, A. L.; Ulfelder, H.; and Poskanzer, D. C.: Adenocarcinoma of the vagina. Association of maternal stilbestrol therapy with tumor appearance in young women. *N. Engl. J. Med.*, **384**(16):878–81, 1971.

Hicks, S. P., and D'Amato, C. J.: Radiosensitivity at various stages of the mitotic cycle and cellular differentiation. In Woollam, D. H. W. (ed.): *Advances in Teratology*, Vol. I. Logos Press, London, 1966, pp. 215–27.

Hill, R. M.: Will this drug harm the unborn infant? The doctor's dilemma. *South. Med. J.*, **67**:1476–80, 1974.

Ingalls, T. H., and Klinberg, M. A.: Implications of epidemic embryopathy for public health. *Am. J. Public Health*, **55**:200–208, 1965.

Jackson, H.: Antifertility substances. *Pharmacol. Rev.*, **11**:135–72, 1959.

Jackson, W. T.: Regulation of mitosis. III. Cytological effects of 2,4,5-trichlorophenozyacetic acid and of dioxin contaminants in 2,4,5-T formulations. *J. Cell Sci.*, **10**:15–25, 1972.

Jaffe, N. R.: Specific activity and localization of enzymes associated with osteochondrodysplasia in the developing rat. *Teratology*, **9**(3):A–22, 1974.

Johnson, E. M.: Organ specific patterns of abnormal molecular differentiation. *Teratology*, **9**(3):A–23–24, 1974.

Jones, K. L.: The fetal alcohol syndrome. In Harbison, R. D. (ed.): *Perinatal Addiction.* Spectrum Publications, New York, 1975, pp. 79–88.

Jones, K. L.; Smith, D. W.; Streissguth, A. P.; and Myrianthropoulos, N. C.: Outcome in offspring of chronic alcoholic women. *Lancet*, **1**:1076–78, 1974.

Jones, K. L.; Ulleland, C. N.; and Streissguth, A. P.: Pattern of malformation in offspring of chronic alcoholic mothers. *Lancet*, **1**:1267–71, 1973.

Kalter, H. *Teratology of the Central Nervous System.* University of Chicago Press, Chicago, 1968.

———: Correlation between teratogenic and mutagenic effects of chemicals in mammals. In Hollaender, A. (ed.): *Chemical Mutagens: Principles and Methods for Their Detection*, Vol. I. Plenum Press, New York, 1971, pp. 57–82.

Koos, B. J., and Longo, L.: Mercury toxicity in pregnant women, fetus and newborn infant. *Am. J. Obstet. Gynecol.*, **126**:390–409, 1976.

Landauer, W.: On the chemical production of developmental abnormalities and of phenocopies in chicken embryos. *J. Cell Comp. Physiol.*, **43**(Suppl. 1):261–305, 1954.

———: Gene and phenocopy: Selection experiments and tests with 6-aminonicotinamide. *J. Exp. Zool.*, **160**:345–54, 1965.

Landauer, W., and Clark, E. M.: On the role of riboflavin in the teratogenic activity of boric acid. *J. Exp. Zool.*, **156**:307–12, 1964.

Larsen, V.: The teratogenic effects of thalidomide,

imipramine HCl and imipramine-N-oxide HCl on white Danish rabbits. *Acta Pharmacol. Toxicol.*, 20:186–200, 1963.

Lemoine, P.; Harousseau, H.; Borteyru, J. P.; Menuet, J. C.: Les enfants des parents alcooliques: anomalies observées. A propos de 127 cas. *Quest. Medicale*, 21: 476–82, 1968.

Lloyd, J. B.; Beck, F.; Griffiths, A.; and Parry, L. M.: The mechanism of action of acid bisazo dyes. In Campbell, P. N. (ed.): *The Interaction of Drugs and Subcellular Components in Animal Cells.* Churchill, London, 1968, pp. 171–202

Long, S. Y.: Does LSD induce chromosomal damage and malformations? A review of the literature. *Teratology*, 6:75–90, 1972.

Malawista, S. E.; Sato, H.; and Bensch, K. G.: Vinblastine and griseofulvin reversibly disrupt the living mitotic spindle. *Science*, 160:770–71, 1968.

Matsumoto, H.; Koya, G; and Takeuchi, T.: Fetal minamata disease. A neuropathological study of two cases of intrauterine intoxication by a methyl mercury compound. *J. Neuropath. Exp. Neurol.*, 24:563–74, 1965.

McBride, W. G.: Thalidomide and congenital abnormalities. *Lancet*, 2:1358, 1961.

Miller, E. C., and Miller, J. A.: Studies on the mechanism of activation of aromatic amine and amide carcinogens to ultimate carcinogenic electrophilic reactants. *Ann. N. Y. Acad. Sci.*, 163:731–50, 1969.

Morriss, G. M.: The ultrastructural effects of excess maternal vitamin A on the primitive streak stage rat embryo. *J. Embryol. Exp. Morphol.*, 30:219–42, 1973.

Nakamura, H.; Yamawaki, H.; Fujisawa, H.; and Yasuda, M.: Effects of maternal hypervitaminosis A upon developing mouse limb buds. II. Electron microscopic investigation. *Congenital Anomalies*, 14:271–83, 1974.

National Foundation/March of Dimes: *Facts.* National Foundation, New York, 1975.

Persaud, T. V. N.: Teratogenic effect of hypoglycin-A. *Adv. Teratol.*, 5:77–95, 1972.

Posner, H. S.: Significance of cleft palate induced by chemicals in the rat and mouse. *Food Cosmet. Toxicol.*, 10:839–55, 1972.

Reynolds, E. S.: Liver parenchymal cell injury. IV. Pattern of incorporation of carbon and chlorine from carbon tetrachloride into chemical constituents of liver in vivo. *J. Pharmacol. Exp. Ther.*, 155:117–24, 1967.

Rugh, R.: *The Mouse. Its Reproduction and Development.* Burgess Publishing Corp., Minneapolis, 1968.

Runner, M. N.: A specific developmental defect related to an ubiquitous enzyme. Induced micromelia in the chick embryo traceable to defects in dehydrogenase and molecular assembly. In Janerich, D. T.; Skalko, R. G.; and Porter, I. H. (eds.): *Congenital Defects. New Directions in Research.* Academic Press, Inc., New York, 1974, pp. 275–81.

Saxén, L., and Rapola, J.: *Congenital Defects.* Holt, Rinehart & Winston, Inc., New York, 1969.

Scanlon, J.: Fetal effects of lead exposure. *Pediatrics*, 49:145–46, 1972.

Schardein, J. L.: *Drugs as Teratogens.* CRC Press, Cleveland, 1976.

Scott, W. J.; Ritter, E. J.; and Wilson, J. G.: Studies on induction of polydactyly in rats with cytosine arabinoside. *Dev. Biol.*, 45:103–11, 1975.

Seegmiller, R. E., and Runner, M. N.: Normal incorporation rates for precursors of collagen and mucopolysaccharide during expression of micromelia induced by 6-aminonicotinamide. *J. Embryol. Exp. Morphol.*, 31:305–12, 1974.

Shepard, T. H.: *A Catalog of Teratogenic Agents*, 2nd ed. John Hopkins University Press, Baltimore, 1976.

Shepard, T. H.; Tanimura, T.; and Robkin, M. A.:

Energy metabolism in early mammalian embryos. *Dev. Biol.*, 4:42–58, 1970.

Sieber, S. M., and Fabro, S.: Identification of drugs in the preimplantation blastocyst and in the plasma, uterine secretion and urine of the pregnant rabbit. *J. Pharmacol. Exp. Ther.*, 176:65–75, 1971.

Sparschu, G. L.; Dunn, F. L.; and Rowe, V. K.: Study of the teratogenicity of 2,3,7,8-tetrachlorodibenzo-*p* dioxin in the rat. *Food Cosmet. Toxicol.*, 9:405–12-1971.

Stevens, M. W., and Harbison, R. D.: Placental transfer of diphenylhydantoin: Effects of species, gestational age, and route of administration. *Teratology*, 9:317–26, 1974.

Stevenson, A. C.: Frequency of congenital and hereditary disease, with special reference to mutation. *Br. Med. Bull.*, 17:254–59, 1961.

Sugiyama, T.; Nishimura, H.; and Fukui, K.: Abnormalities in mouse embryos induced by several aminoazobenzene derivatives. *Okajimas Folia Anat.*, 36:195–201, 1960.

Swenerton, H., and Hurley, L. S.: Teratogenic effects of a chelating agent and their prevention by zinc. *Science*, 173:62–63, 1971.

Tanaka, S.; Ihara, T.; and Mizutani, M.: Apical defects in rat fetuses observed after intraperitoneal injection of high concentration of sodium chloride. *Congenital Anomalies*, 8:197–209, 1968.

Tuchmann-Duplessis, H.: Design and interpretation of teratogenic tests. In Robson, J. M.; Sullivan, F. M.; and Smith, R. L. (eds.): *Embryopathic Activity of Drugs.* Little, Brown & Co., Boston, 1965, pp. 56–93.

Tuchmann-Duplessis, H., and Mercier-Parot, L: The teratogenic action of the antibiotic actinomycin D. In Wolstenholme, G. E. W., and O'Connor, C. M. (eds.): *CIBA Foundation Symposium on Congenital Malformations.* Little, Brown & Co., Boston, 1960, pp. 115–28.

Verrett, M. J.; Mutchler, M. K.; Scott, W. F.; Reynaldo, E. F.; and McLaughlin, J.: Teratogenic effects of captan and related compounds in the developing chicken embryo. *Ann. N. Y. Acad. Sci.*, 160(Art 1.):334–43, 1969.

Volpintesta, E. J.: Menkes kinky hair syndrome in a black infant. *Am. J. Dis. Child.*, 128:244–46, 1974.

Warkany, J.: Congenital malformations in the past. *J. Chronic Dis.*, 10:84–96, 1959.

————: *Congenital Malformations—Notes and Comments.* Year Book Medical Publishers, Chicago, 1971.

Warkany, J., and Kalter, H.: Congenital malformations. *N. Engl. J. Med.*, 265(20):993–1001, 1961.

Wilkins, L.: Masculinization of female fetus due to use of orally given progestins. *J.A.M.A.*, 172:1028–32, 1960.

Wilson, J. G.: Teratogenic activity of several azo dyes chemically related to trypan blue. *Anat. Rec.*, 123:313–34, 1955.

————: Experimental studies on congenital malformations. *J. Chronic Dis.*, 10:111–30, 1959.

————: Teratogenic interaction of chemical agents in the rat. *J. Pharmacol. Exp. Ther.*, 144:429–36, 1964.

————: Present status of drugs as teratogens in man. *Teratology*, 7:3–16, 1973.

————: Current status of teratology—general principles and mechanisms derived from animal studies. In Wilson, J. G., and Fraser, F. C. (eds.): *Handbook of Teratology*, Vol. I. Plenum Press, New York, 1977a, pp. 47–74.

————. Environmental chemicals. In Wilson, J. G., and Fraser, F. C. (eds.): *Handbook of Teratology*, Vol. I. Plenum Press, New York, 1977b, pp. 357–85.

Witischi, E.: *Development of Vertebrates.* Saunders, Philadelphia, 1956.

Woollam, D. H. M.: Principles of teratogenesis: Mode of action of thalidomide. *Proc. R. Soc. Med.*, 58:497–501, 1965.

UNIT II
SYSTEMIC TOXICOLOGY

Chapter 9

TOXIC RESPONSES OF THE CENTRAL NERVOUS SYSTEM

Stata Norton

INTRODUCTION

The central nervous system (CNS) is protected from toxicants by the blood-brain barrier. The "barrier" is a functional concept based on observations that some substances that enter and affect many of the soft tissues of the body, such as liver, kidney, and muscle, are excluded from the brain. Not all substances are preferentially excluded from the brain; for example, most anesthetics, analgesics, and tranquilizers penetrate readily. Nonpolar, lipid-soluble compounds usually penetrate the blood-brain barrier, while highly polar compounds tend to be excluded. In the immature brain, the barrier is generally not as effective, and toxic doses of some compounds, such as inorganic lead salts, may accumulate in the CNS of children, while the adult develops marked effects on the peripheral nervous system instead. Because of specificity of this kind in regard to uptake of substances in the brain, there is a considerable amount of research and speculation regarding the anatomic features that relate to the functional barrier.

Three concepts have received major consideration (Bondareff, 1965; Kuhlenbeck, 1970). One theory is that the blood-brain barrier may be due to the presence of glial cells. Much of the brain capillary endothelium is invested with astrocytic processes, and these present a barrier to free access of substances to the neurons in many places. In some brain areas, such as the median eminence of the hypothalamus and the area postrema of the fourth ventricle, the capillaries are not wrapped with glial processes and substances can reach the neurons more readily. Another theory is that unique properties of brain endothelial cells may constitute a barrier. Zonulae occludentes are structures joining blood capillary endothelial cells together to form tight junctions that are impermeable to many large molecules. However, small molecules may penetrate to the neuron through the junctions and through the cytoplasm of the endothelial cells and glia. In addition to the barrier presented by tight junctions, the endothelial cells in the CNS have other special properties. Normal endothelial cells lack pinocytotic vesicles in their cytoplasm and pores in the luminal endothelial membrane, which are present in capillaries in other tissues (Hirano *et al.*, 1978). These pinocytotic vesicles may appear in the endothelial cells of the CNS in various pathologic conditions in which the permeability of the blood-brain barrier is increased. The vesicles may transport some chemicals across the endothelial lining of small blood vessels in the CNS. When blood-brain barrier permeability is increased, some proteins (e.g., horseradish peroxidase) or chemicals combined with protein (e.g., Evans blue dye bound to albumin) may be observed in these intracellular vesicles (Westergaard *et al.*, 1977). Conditions that are known to increase vesicles are postirradiation brain edema (Cervós-Navarro and Rozas, 1978), ischemia (Welsh and O'Connor, 1978), and hypertension (Hazama, *et al.*, 1978).

The concept that the extracellular space may act as a barrier is also worthy of consideration. The extracellular basement membrane between the endothelial cells of the capillary and the glia and neurons is an ordered fibrillar mucoprotein structure and may have unique properties, as it does in the kidney, allowing it to serve as a "sieve" to transport molecules needed for cell nutrition and to regulate electro-osmotic flow of water while excluding other substances.

In the peripheral nervous system (PNS) the blood-neural barrier is present in some places and absent in others. The details of areas of the nervous system in which a barrier is absent are given in Table 9–1. In both the central and peripheral nervous system fenestrated epithelial cells have been found in areas that are permeable to large molecules such as horseradish peroxidase. The susceptibility of these barrier-free areas to some toxic substances compared with the greater resistance of other areas of the central nervous system has been proposed to be due to differences in ease of penetration of the toxicant through the spaces between the epithelial cells (Jacobs *et al.*, 1976; Jacobs, 1977; Olney *et al.*, 1977).

Even those toxic substances which can penetrate brain tissue do not affect equally all of the cell types in the brain. Different brain areas usually have different sensitivities to toxicants, reflecting unique biochemistry of the cells as well as differences in degree of vascularization of brain areas. The three kinds of glial cells in the brain differ in their roles in the CNS and in their sensitivities to toxic agents. Astrocytes are closely associated with neurons in gray matter and have been called the nurse cells of neurons because they are thought to be essential in maintaining the stable microenvironment needed for neuronal function. The oligodendrocyte in the CNS has a

Table 9–1. REGIONS OF THE NERVOUS SYSTEM THAT HAVE A DEFICIENT BARRIER AS MEASURED BY PENETRATION OF MACROMOLECULES

AREA	REFERENCES
Central Nervous System	
Median eminence with arcuate nucleus	Reese and Brightman, 1968
Median preoptic region	Brightman and Reese, 1969
Choroid plexus Area postrema	Olsson and Hossman, 1970
Peripheral Nervous System	
Dorsal root ganglia Autonomic ganglia	Brierley, 1955 Olsson, 1968 Jacobs *et al.*, 1976 Jacobs, 1977

role similar to that of the peripheral Schwann cell and invests neuronal axons with spiral wrappings of myelin. Microglia are phagocytic cells with primary functions resembling peripheral leukocytes. The role of the microglia in response to toxicants has not been widely investigated.

Although the brain is a highly vascularized organ, not all portions are equally supplied with blood. The variation in degree of vascularization accounts for some of the variation in sensitivity of brain areas to hypoxia. For example, the globus pallidus is more poorly vascularized than the cerebral cortex (hence the name, pallidus) but has about the same density of cell bodies in the tissue. In the adult brain, white matter is generally less vascularized than gray matter (Friede, 1966), but the lower oxygen requirement of the myelinated axons, which make up much of the white matter, makes white matter generally less sensi-

tive than gray matter with its high cell body-to-neuropil ratio.

Apart from known differences in distribution of blood capillaries in the brain, there are other unique differences that account for variation in response of anatomic areas to toxicants. Some of these differences may be due to functional demands on cells. It has been proposed that excitatory amino acids may damage hypothalamic neurons by causing excessive stimulation and metabolic exhaustion of the cells (Olney, 1971). Quantitative differences in essential cell components may make one cell type more sensitive than another type. Small neurons, such as granule cells in the cerebellum and visual cortex, are preferentially killed when the whole brain is exposed to methyl mercury. The amount of cytoplasm and rough endoplasmic reticulum, which binds mercury, is less than in larger cells, and thus the small cells may be more likely to be overwhelmed by the effects of mercury (Jacobs *et al.*, 1977).

Studies of the microchemistry of the brain reinforce concepts of the diversity of structure of different areas. High concentrations of norepinephrine, serotonin, acetylcholine, and dopamine are found in various pathways of the phylogenetic "old brain," including the hypothalamus, reticular formation, basal ganglia, and limbic system. However, experimental techniques are not yet sophisticated enough to allow generalizations to be made regarding the role of brain structures and amine levels in specific functions.

Certain large cells in the central nervous system, such as cortical and hippocampal pyramidal cells, cerebellar Purkinje cells, and motor cells in the ventral horn of the spinal cord, have unusually large nuclei and the DNA is largely present as euchromatin, the form of chromatin most closely associated with transcription (Arrighi, 1974). These cells often have several nucleoli. All these structural differences point to high metabolic activity in these cells and thus increased susceptibility to anoxic damage. In fact, anoxia, in the presence of functional activity such as occurs in epileptic convulsions, is known to damage these cells (Chason, 1971).

The preceding considerations can be summarized to suggest the principle that governs responses of elements of the nervous system to toxicants: selective damage to one or more areas or components is achieved by selective exposure due to differences in ease of penetration to some cells through barriers, by selective anoxia via differences in blood flow and metabolic requirements of some elements, or by selective sensitivity resulting from qualitative or quantitative chemical differences in cell components. Identification of the selective nature of the damage from toxic agents is essential in determination of mechanism of action of toxicants but also has further value in analyzing the relation of brain structure to function.

STRUCTURAL TOXICITY

General Responses of Cells to Injury

When cells are damaged by exposure to toxic chemicals either by direct contact with the chemical or by secondary effects such as anoxia subsequent to diminished oxygen supply, some similar effects are observed. These effects are swelling of the cell and cytoplasmic organelles, dispersion of the rough endoplasmic reticulum (RER), and swelling of the nucleolus. The changes are accompanied by decreases in cytoplasmic pH, in activity of oxidative enzyme systems, and in synthesis of protein and other cell components. Differences in response relate more to quantitative differences in amount and rate of change in organelles of different cell types than to qualitative differences. Thus, it has been pointed out (Scarpelli and Trump, 1971) that cells with little capacity for anaerobic metabolism but with rapid ionic shifts through the external membrane, such as myocardial cells and neurons, are susceptible during anoxia to rapid edema from the loss of integrity of the cell membrane. On the other hand, liver cells, exposed to carbon tetrachloride, will first show changes in the endoplasmic reticulum, diminished protein synthesis, and lipid accumulation. However, both the electrically excitable cells and liver cells will show both types of injury responses over a period of hours.

The neuron is a cell that has little capability for anaerobic metabolism and a high metabolic rate. The oxygen consumption of neurons is ten times higher than the oxygen consumption of glia (Ruščák et al., 1968). This combination of metabolic conditions puts the neuron at more risk than glial cells from anoxia. Neuronal damage starts within a few minutes after cessation of blood flow to the brain, and death of some neurons occurs before complete cessation of oxygen or glucose transport. Certain cells are more sensitive to anoxia than others. The sequence of vulnerability can be described in order of decreasing sensitivity: neurons, oligodendrocytes, astrocytes, microglia, and cells of the capillary endothelium.

Three types of anoxia are generally recognized: anoxic, ischemic, and cytotoxic.

Anoxic Anoxia. Primary oxygen lack (also called anoxic anoxia, which is a rather awkward term) is a term applied to inadequate oxygen supply in the presence of adequate blood flow. Such a primary condition can result from direct interference with respiration by toxic substances. For example, neuromuscular blocking agents, such as d-tubocurarine chloride, can cause respiratory paralysis by interference with the action of acetylcholine, the chemical transmitter at the neuromuscular junction. Respiratory paralysis can cause death of some neurons because of failure of oxygenation of blood. Circulation of blood to the brain is not prevented in respiratory failure, except as the eventual result of cardiac failure from continued anoxia. If respiration is restored before cardiovascular failure occurs, neurons in the CNS that are sensitive to anoxia may be destroyed without death of the organism. However, inadequate oxygen supply can also result from interference with the oxygen-carrying capacity of blood. Examples are the production of carboxyhemoglobin by carbon monoxide and methemoglobin by nitrites.

Ischemic Anoxia. This results from a decrease in arterial blood pressure to a level below that which supplies the brain adequately with oxygen. Ischemic anoxia differs from anoxic anoxia in that stagnation of the blood in the brain leads to an inadequate supply of needed substances and an accumulation of metabolic products such as lactic acid, ammonia, and inorganic phosphate. Cardiac arrest from toxic substances is one obvious cause of inadequate blood flow. Increased venous pressure in cardiac failure is an additional complication. Reduced cerebral blood flow, is, of course, not limited to cardiac failure. Extreme hypotension from vasodilation, particularly if the head is elevated, can also cause brain ischemia. Hemorrhage or thrombosis of cerebral vessels causes local ischemic anoxia of the brain areas supplied by these vessels and may further complicate the consequences of toxicants.

Cytotoxic Anoxia. Cytotoxic anoxia is a consequence of interference with cell metabolism in the presence of an adequate supply of both blood and oxygen. Cytotoxic anoxia may result from hypoglycemia, produced, for example, by an excess of insulin, or it may result from metabolic inhibitors such as cyanide, azide, dinitrophenol, malononitrile, and methionine sulfoximine. In contrast to the great susceptibility of the neurons of the adult brain to ischemic and anoxic anoxia, it is the oligodendroglia that are more susceptible to injury from repeated episodes of hypoglycemia or repeated toxic doses of metabolic inhibitors. In addition to producing cytotoxic anoxia, some of these agents may also produce ischemic anoxia; these combined effects are discussed later in more detail.

Effects of Anoxia. When a cell is damaged by acutely developing anoxia, a rapid sequence of changes is observed. The following description is characteristic of ischemic anoxia or the condition in which an aerobic cell with an electrically excitable membrane is deprived of glucose and oxygen and removal of metabolic products via blood flow is prevented. It is presumed that lesser degrees of anoxia and greater energy reserves in the cell would be reflected in variations in the intensity and type of change.

Early ischemic changes are seen in mitochondria and the cytoplasmic sap. These are related to the loss of oxidative enzyme activity with decreased ATP, decreased ATP synthesis, increased glycolysis, and decreased glycogen. As a consequence, the activity of the energy-dependent sodium pump in the cell membrane decreases and the neuron starts to pick up water. As intracellular lactate increases, the pH of the cell drops, resulting in clumping of nuclear chromatin. Loss of mitochondrial granules and slight clumping of the nuclear chromatin can be seen by the electron microscope in the first five minutes of ischemia (Trump and Arstila, 1975). The diminished activity in oxidative and phosphate-releasing enzymes can be attributed also to changes in cytoplasmic pH and ionic strength (Robinson *et al.*, 1975). The continual increase in intracellular sodium ion and influx of water results in swelling of the cell body, lysosomes, and mitochondria and dilation of the rough endoplasmic reticulum (Trump and Arstila, 1975). All of these rapid changes are diagrammed in Figure 9–1.

The second-phase changes in anoxic neurons have been known in detail for many years and have been called Spielmeyer's triad of late ischemic neuronal changes: (1) shrinkage of cell cytoplasm, (2) disappearance of Nissl substance, and (3) nuclear pyknosis with loss of nucleolar detail. These changes occur both *in vivo* (Brierley *et al.*, 1971) and in cell cultures *in vitro*. Vanderhaeghen and Logan (1971), on the basis of *in vitro* studies, have proposed that Spielmeyer's late ischemic changes accompany the development of an alkaline intracellular pH during recovery from anoxia. That is, the shift in pH from acidic, during the early phases of anoxia, to alkaline reflects a recovery from anaerobic glycolysis with its accumulation of lactic acid and other intermediary metabolites in the early phase, to a phase characterized by a pH of approximately 7.4 associated with adequate aerobic metabolism. This shift in pH can explain the characteristic disappearance of Nissl substance in injured neurons. Nissl substance is composed of endoplasmic reticulum and fine granules containing ribonucleic acid (RNA) (Palay and Palade, 1955). Disappearance of RNA may be related to the activation of a poly-nucleotidase, alkaline ribonuclease type II, at the time of restoration of an alkaline pH, following an acidic pH phase during which some damage must have occurred.

There are two responses of cells in the CNS that result in brain edema. The acute, neuronal response to hypoxia has just been described. Although astrocytes are resistant cells, relative to neurons, cerebral edema resulting from swelling of astrocytes may occur as a response to brain hypoxia with accumulation of lactate, ammonia, and inorganic phosphate. The early hypoxic changes found in astrocytes have been proposed, as with neurons, to be a consequence of the acidosis resulting from anaerobic glycolysis. The astrocyte may respond in a manner similar to that of the extracellular space of other tissue (deRobertis, 1963). According to this theory, brain edema following hypoxia may be due to increased fluid accumulation inside the astrocytes rather than to accumulation of fluid in spaces between cells.

Although the changes described above refer to effects of anoxia, these changes have been dwelt on because the toxic responses of cells to chemical agents are often remarkably similar to responses to anoxia. This is not entirely unexpected since any toxic substance that interferes with glucose metabolism, ATP synthesis, or protein synthesis or that acts directly on cell membranes to affect permeability would be affecting cell metabolism at one or another place in the system that maintains the integrity of the cell.

Chronic Changes in Cell Organelles. Intracellular changes in response to toxic agents may be chronic rather than acute. For example, changes may slowly occur in the fibrous skeleton of the cell (the microtubules, about 240 Å in diameter, and neurofibrils, 40 to 100 Å in diameter). Both these structures are abundant in neurons and glia, and they may be functionally associated with transport of substances in axons and other cell processes (Schlaepfer, 1971). Toxic responses to some agents such as mitotic inhibitors result in development of intracellular neurofibrillar tangles. For example, intracisternal injection of vincristine or colchicine produces neurofibrillar tangles in neurons in experimental animals. Patients receiving the vinca alkaloids in leukemia therapy may also develop these changes (Shelanski and Wiśniewski, 1969). In some chronic disease states, such as Alzheimer's disease, the tangles consist primarily of double-stranded helices of 100-Å filaments (Crapper *et al.*, 1976). The relationship of these cell inclusions to altered function is not known. Weakness and paralysis can develop in animals and patients treated with mitotic inhibitors, and it has been suggested that damage to these

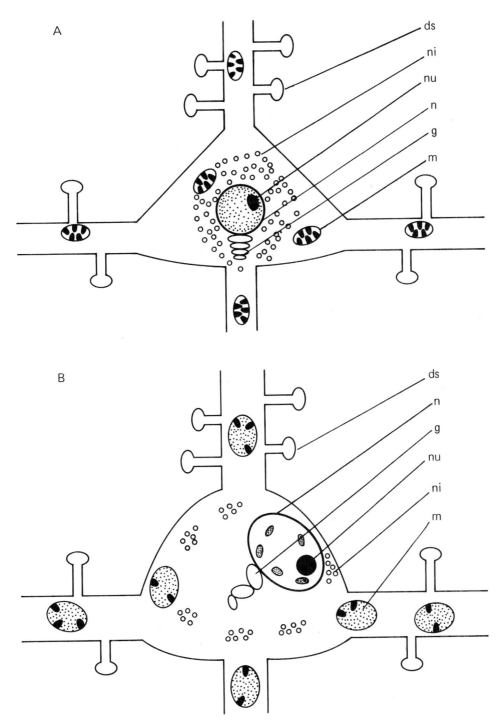

Figure 9–1. Anoxic changes in neurons. *A.* Normal neuron: *ds*, dendritic spine; *ni*, Nissl substance (RER); *nu*, nucleolus; *n*, nucleus; *g*, Golgi substance; *m*, mitochondrion. *B.* Anoxic neuron: swelling of dendritic spines, mitochondria, nucleus, nucleolus, and Golgi substance; clumping of chromatin in the nucleus (pyknosis) and dispersion of Nissl substance (chromatolysis). Lysosomes (not shown) also swell.

tubular cytoplasmic organelles may result in failure of protein synthesis or transport of essential substances to the terminals of cell axons in the peripheral nervous system (PNS).

Responses of the Immature and Mature Nervous System

In addition to the selective sensitivity of different cell types in the nervous system, certain anatomic areas are more prone to damage than other areas. Some of the sites that have been identified with damage from toxic substances are listed in Figures 9–2 and 9–3. Often when an anatomically delineated area is damaged, the location of the damage follows the anatomic boundaries so that it is appropriate to speak of damage to the globus pallidus, hippocampus, etc. For a description of the anatomic and functional relationship of defined areas in the brain, an extensive literature is available. General information can be found in reference texts such as the one by Crosby and coauthors (1962).

Two explanations have been suggested for the selective sensitivity of different brain areas to toxic substances. Spielmeyer in 1922 proposed that differences in vascular distribution are such that some areas of the brain are uniquely sensitive to altered blood flow. The Vogts, also in 1922,

contended that there exist differences in neuronal composition, metabolism, or function that do not depend on differences in vascular supply and that determine sensitivity to toxic states. Although it is apparent that both concepts are involved in toxic reactions of the nervous system, there is convincing evidence that the response to many substances must depend on unique neuronal biochemistry and function apart from regional vascular patterns. A distinction must also be made in regard to the degree of maturity of the nervous system at the time of exposure. In some animals, humans included, where the young are born with a relatively immature nervous system, the pattern of neonatal toxic damage may differ from that of the mature nervous system. Major differences in cell structure and sensitivity are related to the degree of development of the blood-brain barrier, the degree of myelination of tracts (oligodendroglial or Schwann cell investiture of axonal processes), the degree of arborization of dendritic and axonal processes, and the extent of development of blood capillaries.

Immature Nervous System. In the immature brain the pattern of lesions in anoxic anoxia differs from the lesions in metabolic disturbances (cytotoxic anoxia). The cerebral neocortex and the cerebellum are often unaffected in experimental neonatal anoxia under conditions when

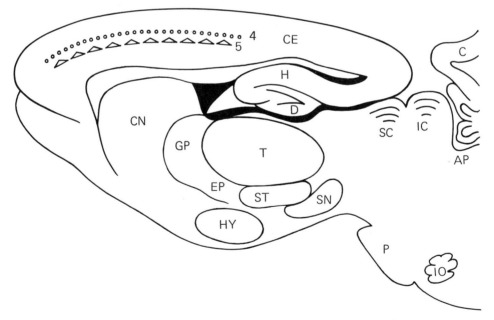

Figure 9–2.   Diagram of representative mammalian brain (rat brain) in longitudinal section showing areas referred to in text. *CE*, cerebral cortex with layer 4 granule cells and layer 5 pyramidal cells; *C*, cerebellum; *H*, hippocampus with *D*, fascia dentata (dentate gyrus); basal ganglia (*CN*, caudate nucleus; *GP*, globus pallidus; and *EP*, entopeduncular nucleus); *T*, thalamus; *SC*, superior colliculus; *IC*, inferior colliculus; *AP*, area postrema; *ST*, subthalamus; *SN*, substantia nigra; *HY*, hypothalamus; *P*, pons; *IO*, inferior olivary nucleus.

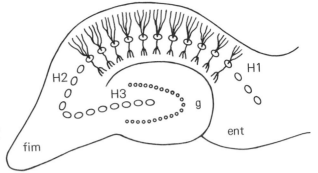

Figure 9–3. Diagram of representative mammalian hippocampus with pyramidal cell areas (*H1, H2, H3*) labeled with the terminology of Rose (1927) for human hippocampus. Comparable areas for the rodent brain are *H1* (*CA1*); *H2* (*CA3*); *H3* (*CA4*); *g*, granule cells; *fim*, fimbria; *ent*, entorhinal area.

the neonatal somatic afferents and many diencephalic areas are severely affected. In the immature brain, anoxic encephalopathy may result in extensive damage to the brainstem as well as to sensory relay nuclei (lateral thalamic atrophy) but with apparent sparing of the neocortex. The basal ganglia and hippocampus commonly show damage (Windle, 1963). However, the neocortex can be damaged under conditions of partial asphyxia where blood supply is maintained in the presence of low oxygen (Myers, 1973). Results from several lines of investigation have led to the concept that the maintenance of some blood flow and a supply of glucose but with lack of oxygen may result in a lower pH than lack of oxygen and glucose (Ljunggren *et al.*, 1974). Under these conditions both the immature neocortex and basal ganglia may be damaged, the latter particularly when an episode of total ischemia follows partial ischemia (Myers, 1975).

As in the adult, interference with glucose metabolism affects the cerebral cortex, cerebellar folia, and hippocampus (especially area H_1). Bilirubin encephalopathy (kernicterus) affects areas that are often resistant to anoxic anoxia: globus pallidus, fascia dentata, and area H_2 of the hippocampus (Malamud, 1963). The subthalamus is also affected, and the superior olivary nucleus is often involved. A complex progression of behavioral effects has been described, related to some of these types of damage. (For a discussion of prenatal toxicity, see Chapter 8.)

Mature Nervous System. The mature nervous system can be distinguished from the immature nervous system in that the cells most sensitive to oxygen lack are neurons in the cerebral cortex, cerebellar cortex, and hippocampus. In the cerebral cortex, neurons of the fourth layer, which has major afferent connections from the sensory systems, are the ones commonly damaged in severe anoxia (Scholz, 1953). These sensitive neurons are small granule cells. Small cells in layer 5 may also be lost following anoxia. Large motor pyramidal cells are more resistant. In the cerebellar cortex the decreasing order of sensitivity is Purkinje cells, granule cells, and then Golgi cells (Scholz, 1959). In the hippocampus the pyramidal cells of field H_1 are most sensitive, followed by H_3 and the granular layer of the fascia dentata. In general, cells that are rich in cell processes with small cell bodies are especially vulnerable to anoxia, whereas motor cells with long axons and fewer processes are less sensitive (Jacob, 1963). With prolonged anoxia the adult may show damage to the basal ganglia and the associated subthalamic nucleus and substantia nigra. Ischemia with rapid cessation of blood flow is likely to result in a brainstem pattern of damage involving the inferior colliculus and inferior and superior olivary nuclei. Repeated episodes of anoxia usually result in damage to white matter. (See Figures 9–2 and 9–3 for general localization of the anatomic areas in the brain affected by anoxia.)

Reversibility of Damage

The principal event in irreversible damage to the nervous system can be described simply as neuronal death, since these differentiated cells cannot divide and be replaced. However, normal function may be restored for an individual even after considerable damage from exposure of the nervous system to toxic substances. Redundancy of function in a population of neurons and plasticity of organization are the methods by which restoration of function is presumed to occur after the death of some neurons. When some neurons die, other cells already having the same function may be adequate to maintain normal activity, or, failing this, other neurons may acquire the needed function. In situations where neither course is possible, for example in extensive damage to a specialized population of neurons or brain nucleus, then some loss of function must result.

Some degree of recovery of function usually occurs after nonfatal neurotoxic reactions. When cell death is not involved, the neurotoxic reaction lasts only until the toxic agent is removed or metabolized or until cell constituents altered by the toxic event have regenerated. Reversible toxic reactions are often associated with toxicants but also occur after therapeutic administration of drugs. From this point of view, neurotoxicity could be considered to include all undesired nervous system effects of drugs or other chemicals. However, it is probable that many reversible toxic changes occurring in neurons or glial cells during therapeutic use of drugs may be closely related to the mechanisms of therapeutic activity. For example, the synaptic clefts between axons and dendrites of neurons are considered to be especially vulnerable to exogenous chemicals carried by the bloodstream, since the postsynaptic membrane is the site of receptors for chemical transmitters in the nervous system. Many psychoactive drugs are thought to cause psychic changes by altering neuronal transmission. This may involve blocking the access of normal chemical transmitters to postsynaptic receptors, acting as false transmitters, or affecting concentrations of transmitters through effects on synthesis, storage, release, reuptake, or enzymatic inactivation mechanisms. These effects are proposed to occur in areas of the CNS in which specific transmitter mechanisms are involved, that is, the anatomic areas in the brain that normally have high concentrations of some biogenic amines, particularly serotonin, norepinephrine, dopamine, acetylcholine, and gamma amino butyric acid. Examples of compounds presumed to act therapeutically by altering neurotransmitters are monoamine oxidase inhibitors, cholinesterase inhibitors, reserpine, phenothiazines, and L-DOPA. Other drugs, such as general anesthetics, appear to affect neurons generally, probably through a reversible effect on electrically excitable neuronal membranes.

The functional state of the CNS called "general depression" commonly results from overexposure to many solvents used in industrial operations. A state in which awareness or consciousness of workers is impaired is clearly a matter of concern, even though the effect may be completely reversible on removal of the worker from the exposure. Many fat solvents, like alcohol, either inhaled or ingested cause "general depression," characterized initially by drowsiness, difficulty in concentrating, and mood changes and progressing to slurred speech, ataxia, and disorientation followed by loss of consciousness. These effects mimic the effects of general anesthetics and may well have the same mechanism of action.

To the extent that reversible toxicity differs only quantitatively from therapeutic actions of drugs, these effects are appropriately discussed in numerous reviews and books on the subject of neuropharmacology.

FUNCTIONAL TOXICITY

The functioning of the nervous system in the presence of damage from toxic agents is obviously both of great importance and complexity. The nervous system possesses considerable redundancy of structure, which may mask functional change until the reserve capacity of the system is exceeded by the amount of damage. The nervous system is also capable of developing tolerance or adapting to some types of damage; hence function may return to normal during continuous exposure to a toxic substance. Thus damage may exist in the nervous system that can be detected by cytologic or neurochemical methods when functional damage is not detected. On the other hand, alterations in gait, visual-motor performance, emotional state, and many other behavioral parameters may, at times, be the earliest and most sensitive signs of nervous system toxicity. In the subsequent discussion the alterations in behavior that can occur as consequences of toxic damage to the nervous system are divided into alterations of the sensory, motor, and integrative functions of the nervous system.

Examples will be given in which motor functions are directly affected, such as peripheral neuropathies. Sensory functions, such as vision, may be damaged at various sites along the pathway from the sensory receptor to the cortex. Integrative processes, which are important and poorly understood functions of information processing by the brain, can be the functions primarily altered. Learning and memory are included in this group. Emotional components of behavior may be disturbed. It should be noted that when behavior is evaluated, it is difficult to examine the effects of toxicants on information processing apart from sensory and motor components since all behavioral tests must rely on evaluation of the output of the brain after information processing has taken place.

No analysis of the toxic effects of a chemical on the nervous system is complete without knowledge of effects on function. It might even be argued that without a functional change there is no toxicity to an organ. Such an argument ignores the equally valid concept that any irreversible change in an organ caused by an exogenous chemical is a toxic effect. The CNS differs from organs such as the liver in that neurons cannot divide once they have reached a mature state while hepatic cells retain the capacity to divide throughout the life of the organism. As an example, focal loss of a small number of granule cells in the cerebellum from a dose of

Peripheral Nervous System	Central Nervous System			Peripheral Nervous System
Anatomy	Function	Anatomy	Toxicity	Anatomy

	B. Symbol formation	Cerebral cortex Hippocampus	Impaired learning and memory	
		Mammillary bodies	Confusional states	
A. Sensory pathways	C. Sensory-motor integration			E. Motor pathways
	1. Life support systems	Hypothalamus Medulla	Impaired appetite reproduction, respiration	
	2. Voluntary and involuntary movement	Pyramidal motor system Basal ganglia system Cerebellum	Dyskinesias Activity changes Ataxias	
	D. Emotional overlay	Limbic lobe	Emotional instability Psychoses	

Figure 9–4. Types of functional changes resulting from effects on anatomic areas in the CNS.

methyl mercury will not be detected as locomotor changes or even as changes in fine movements. The nervous system not only has redundancy in this regard but also has the ability to compensate by adaptive mechanisms. Nevertheless, the loss of granule cells, in the above example, represents a reduction in the reserve capacity of the brain, which might well be detectable if additional demands were placed on the system.

As a generalization a distinction can be made between pharmacologic and toxicologic effects. Characteristically pharmacologic effects are short lasting and completely reversible while toxicologic effects often include irreversible damage. Because of this difference and the adaptability of the nervous system to damage, mentioned above, histopathologic studies have a place in toxicology that they do not have in pharmacology. In spite of the limitations on functional tests, they are also an integral part of the study of toxicology of the nervous system.

Five categories of nervous system function are shown in Figure 9–4. These categories are: sensory, motor, two integrative functions (symbol formation and sensory-motor integration), and emotional states associated with any of the other four functions. Symbol formation, including

language and visual symbols, incorporates learning and memory as the terms are commonly used in behavior studies. In a broader sense learning occurs in all integrative systems in Figure 9–4, perhaps to varying degrees. In this sense it could be said that the respiratory center "learns" tolerance to morphine-induced respiratory depression or that various complex visual-motor performances such as walking are "learned."

Sensory Functions

Damage to the senses of sight and hearing, alterations in the sensations of temperature, touch, and pain, and other paresthesias result from central demyelination and peripheral neuropathies. Neuronal atrophy in the cortical layers in specific sensory receiving areas can cause loss of sensation, such as cortical blindness, even though the remainder of the sensory pathway is intact. Lead encephalopathy and severe poisoning in children from organic mercury compounds may result in marked sensory damage, including blindness and hearing loss. Sensory neuropathies are commonly accompanied by numbness, tingling, and hypersensitivity to touch. The selective sensory fiber toxicity from organic mercury has already been mentioned. Inorganic lead salts and organophosphorus compounds, such as triorthocresyl phosphate, cause disturbances of both sensory and motor functions. Sensory damage alone can affect motor function since damage to muscle spindle afferents can be related to ataxia without direct damage to motor fibers.

Effective methods for detection of functional damage to senses, particularly vision and hearing, have been developed. Some of the most sensitive methods use operant conditioning techniques, which require discrimination of light intensity, tone intensity, or pitch. Examples of the use of these methods can be found in work of Stebbins and coworkers (Hawkins *et al.*, 1977) on damage to the cochlea of monkeys from dihydro-streptomycin and in the work of Luschei and coworkers (1977) on peripheral vision in monkeys intoxicated with methyl mercury. Generally these methods are time consuming and difficult to carry out successfully except in the hands of experienced investigators. Tests of motor function are used conjointly to establish the integrity of the motor system since the operant tests of sensory function rely on motor movements.

An interesting possibility for evaluation of sensory thresholds in humans as well as other animals is the startle response and comparable reflexes that involve the sensory and motor systems. Although the potential of these methods has been discussed (Reiter and Ison, 1977), very few data are available on the effects of toxic substances on reflex responses to stimuli.

Electrophysiologic methods have been used to monitor sensory pathways. For example, the visual-evoked potential, recorded from the surface of the cerebral cortex in the primary sensory receiving area, is a complex wave, and the components of this wave have been studied extensively. Damage to the visual pathway can be detected as alterations in the cortical wave form (Woolley, 1976).

Motor Functions

As with sensory systems, either demyelinating processes or neuronal damage can produce motor dysfunction. In addition to substances causing mixed motor and sensory neuropathy, motor fiber demyelination alone is the primary peripheral damage produced by compounds like isonicotinic hydrazide. The functional pathology seen with damage to motor nerve axons or terminals at skeletal muscle is weakness or paralysis of the involved muscles. Unsteadiness of gait may result from muscle weakness although ataxias may also result from damage to visual-motor integration without peripheral neuropathy. Several methods are available to monitor

motor function. Direct functional tests of nerve-muscle function rely on physiologic methods of recording conduction velocity or the compound action potential of peripheral nerves. Tests of conduction velocity have not proved very sensitive in detection of peripheral nerve damage because not all axons in a nerve are damaged simultaneously by a toxic chemical and the undamaged axons conduct normally. The compound action potential, which records the summed amplitudes of action potentials of all conducting fibers, is more sensitive since it will be reduced proportionately to the number of damaged fibers. However, it is a more difficult technique and is subject to more variation. Behavioral tests of complex motor movements are used and do detect muscle weakness although involvement of higher control centers is difficult to eliminate. Appropriate methods for laboratory animals are performance on a rotating rod (Kinnard and Carr, 1957; Watzman and Barry, 1968), measurement of gait (Mullenix *et al.*, 1975), or performance on a treadmill (Gibbins *et al.*, 1968).

Integrative Functions

In Figure 9–4, three categories of central nervous system function are listed: symbol formation, sensory-motor integration, and emotional state. Learning, using the term in the broad sense of adaptation, is a characteristic of all three. Therefore, functional tests related to these categories reflect damage only after the adaptive capability of the CNS has been exceeded.

Symbol Formation. Methods of measurement of memory and learning, in the restricted sense of symbolic integration of information, are of great importance in evaluation of toxic effects of chemicals on subtle behavioral parameters. When memory or learning is severely impaired, the type of functional damage may be called confusional states.

Various tests have been described that are intended to detect impairment of memory and learning ability in man, and these tests have counterparts in animal tests. Several tests of short-term memory in brain-damaged patients have been compared (Sterne, 1969). In clinical neurologic examinations a relation between lesion size and behavioral deficit has been reported (Boller *et al.*, 1970). Maze learning may also be compared in man and animals, and performance in visual maze learning has been shown to be altered by some kinds of organic brain damage in man (Milner, 1965) as well as by some brain lesions and toxic substances in experimental animals (Bullock *et al.*, 1966; Brown *et al.*, 1971).

One of the best localizations of cerebral

function known is in regard to memory. It has been shown that memory deficit is produced by bilateral hippocampal resection. This effect has been further specified by Barbizet (1969): "The syndrome of normal capacity of immediate memory and gradual forgetting indicates a change in the hippocampomammillary system regardless of the nature of the underlying lesion. It is not observed in cortical lesions." The coordinated pathway of memory involves: hippocampus–fornix–hypothalamus–mammillary body–mammillothalamic tract–thalamus–cortex. In this system the mammillary body is the integrating center. Lesions of the mammillary body can be produced by thiamine deficiency, both experimentally by pyrithiamine administration and in thiamine-deficiency diseases such as Wernicke's encephalopathy and Korsakoff's syndrome. Memory is impaired in these conditions.

Although there is a good correlation between experiments in animals and clinical observations regarding the anatomic substrate for memory, the general problem of correlation of behavioral effects of toxic substances in animals and man is difficult to resolve. Many studies on "memory" and "learning" have involved tests of function that have not been related to any anatomic damage. In animal tests, in particular, the failure of animals to perform a task may be related to many phenomena other than "memory" or "learning." Investigations in animals, including man, must test comparable functions if meaningful correlations are to be made, and this may be experimentally hard to achieve.

Sensory-Motor Integration. There are obvious difficulties in comparisons of toxic brain damage in man and other animals since the elaboration of language and the high level of concept formation and integration in man tend to obscure whatever exist as generalizations of these functions in the mammalian brain. However, these fundamental difficulties in the study of toxic effects are compounded by the failure to consider that brain function in man can be included in generalization of functions of other mammals. A start has been made in setting up tests for quantitative assessment of brain damage in various mammals, including man. These tests need to be compared for their predictive value in different kinds of brain damage. Some of the Halstead battery of tests, the Porteus maze, the Wisconsin card-sorting test, and reaction time tests appear to be useful predictors of the amount of general cortical impairment (Sterne, 1969; Strain and Kinzie, 1969; Vega, 1969).

Some fairly simple tests can be performed that correlate anatomic damage with functional damage. For example, finger-tapping speed and pegboard speed are measures of motor impersistence (Joynt et al., 1962; Vega, 1969). Preservation has been measured using a card-sorting test (Milner, 1963). Careful studies using tests of reaction time in man have shown a correlation between the size of brain lesions and the degree of slowing of reactions (Boller et al., 1970). Not only localized lesions but also general cortical atrophy, measured by enlarged cerebral ventricles, correlates with impairment of function on tests requiring visual motor performance (Chapman and Wolff, 1959; Vega and Parsons, 1967). Tests intended to measure general intelligence in normal individuals (IQ tests such as the Wechsler Adult Intelligence Scale) show poorer correlations with size of cortical lesions or degree of cortical atrophy. Very little is known of the presumed quantitative relationship between the amount of toxic agent and degree of functional brain damage in man or animals.

Tests that measure sensory-motor performance can be studied in animals. Since results with tests of sensory-motor performance in humans appear to correlate well with some types of brain damage, such tests should be extensively employed in animals. A simple test is general activity, measured either in a home cage or in a special apparatus. Functional damage to the CNS from carbon monoxide has been demonstrated in this way (Culver et al., 1975), and the alteration in activity correlates with morphologic changes in neurons (Norton and Culver, 1977). General activity, particularly circadian activity, is a measure of sensory-motor integration although many factors may modify it. Some other tests that can be used are measures of reaction times, such as shuttle-box avoidance tests, and the measurement of performance on a rotating rod, mentioned previously under motor function. Animals can be trained to exert a constant force on a lever and alterations in performance can be measured (Falk, 1969). The latter test requires extensive equipment and training of animals. Perhaps the simplest test is measurement of body weight in a chronic experiment. It should not be forgotten that the success of an animal in maintaining general body function is dependent on adequate CNS function. In a study of chronic administration of methyl mercury, Berthoud and coworkers (1976) found that body weight was altered at low doses and proposed that "defects in food and energy regulation may provide early indications of an incipient overt intoxication." Such a finding could result from a primary effect on any one of several major organs, including the CNS.

Emotional Responses. The limbic system, specifically the hippocampus, has a low seizure threshold, and some convulsions from toxic substances may result from effects on this system.

coverings. In addition to TOCP two related esters, cresyldiphenyl phosphate and *o*-isopropylphenyldiphenyl phosphate, are neurotoxic (Johannsen *et al.*, 1977). Not all species of animal are equally affected. Like man, the chicken and cat are sensitive to these compounds (Beresford and Glees, 1963). Adult animals are more sensitive than young. A second major class of organophosphorus compounds, the anticholinesterase insecticides, contains a few compounds that cause an identical delayed neuropathy. Delayed neurotoxicity has been reliably shown to occur in poisoning from DFP (diisopropyl fluorophosphate), leptofos (Abou-Donia and Preissig, 1976), and mipafox (Aldridge *et al.*, 1969; Johnson, 1969). However, the action of the compounds causing delayed neuropathies is distinguished from the action on cholinesterase by the marked species dependency, relative insensitivity of young animals, delay in development of the lesion, and specificity of the type of neurologic damage. Many related organophosphate insecticides, such as parathion and malathion, have not been shown to cause neuropathies in any species nor have the carbamate anticholinesterase insecticides.

After a single exposure of adequate magnitude to the neurotoxic organophosphorus compounds, axonal damage can be demonstrated after a delay of eight to ten days. In low-level exposures damage may appear only after chronic exposures of weeks or months. Axons are the primary target in both peripheral nerves and the long ascending and descending tracts of the spinal cord. The neuropathy is not reversed or prevented by thiamine. Originally it was proposed that the neurotoxic effects of organophosphorus insecticides might be due to cholinesterase inhibition. However, no good correlation was obtained between the inhibition of pseudo or true cholinesterase and the neurotoxic effect. Johnson and coworkers in a series of papers have proposed that the nervous system contains a neurotoxic esterase distinct from true or pseudocholinesterase. Phosphorylation of 80 percent or more of the neurotoxic protein by neurotoxic organophosphorus compounds reliably correlates with clinical neuropathy (Johnson, 1975).

Type 4. Agents Causing Primary Damage to Perikarya of Peripheral Neurons

The perikaryon (cell body) of a neuron is the main site of synthesis of protein that is essential for the normal function of the entire neuron including its long axon and multiply branched dendrites, which together may contain much more cytoplasm than the perikaryon. From the perikaryon many proteins and other cell constituents are transported centrifugally along the axon and dendrites. An extensive literature surrounding the phenomenon of axonal transport has developed (see, for example, Ochs, 1977), but the role of transport from the cell body in the development of axonal damage has yet to be clarified. The giant swellings that develop in some neuropathies are often associated with nodes of Ranvier in the Schwann cell and may represent areas where normal axon flow has ceased, with ballooning of the axons above the dammed-up areas. No matter where damage to a neuron occurs it can be difficult to identify the primary site. For example, in experimental axotomy Lieberman (1971) has proposed that "the nucleolus is perhaps the most sensitive indicator of changes in the functional state of the cell, and an increase in nucleolar volume is one of the earliest events of the axon reaction." The response to axotomy involves a burst of synthesis of ribosomal RNA in the nucleolus followed by an increase in cytoplasmic ribosomes and synthesis of structural proteins. Thus damage to the axon from any cause is unlikely to exist in the absence of perikaryal response. However, in only a few instances does it appear probable that the primary damage to the neuron is at the cell body and proceeds centrifugally rather than in the reverse direction. One of the aspects of neurotoxicity of organophosphorus compounds that has been stressed is the delayed appearance of the toxicity, the "silent phase" of 8 to 12 days before the onset of axonal or functional changes. Although compounds like the organomercurials affect the perikaryon, there is also a delay before the appearance of morphologic or functional changes.

Organomercury Compounds. The sensory cell bodies in the dorsal root ganglion of the spinal cord are more readily affected by organomercurials than other neurons, perhaps because of the lack of a blood barrier such as exists over much of the brain capillaries (Cavanagh, 1977). The earliest signs in experimental intoxication are in the cell bodies in which dispersion of the rough endoplasmic reticulum is seen in the electron microscope (Jacobs *et al.*, 1975). This dispersion of ribosomal material is equivalent to chromatolysis of Nissl substance observed in light microscopy. It should be noted, however, that chromatolysis is an early change after axotomy (Lieberman, 1971); so the presence of early effects on the cell body does not exclude a primary effect on peripheral portions of axons. Another early change is the diminished protein synthesis in these same cells as measured by incorporation of ^{14}C glycine (Cavanagh and Chen, 1971b). It has been proposed that organomercury compounds affect the entire neuron so that the whole fiber from the distal ending to the spinal root fragments at the same time (Cavanagh and Chen, 1971a).

The effects of organomercury compounds on central neurons are described below.

Vinca Alkaloids. Vincristine and vinblastine have been used therapeutically in the treatment of leukemia. Polyneuropathy, with sensory disturbances and motor nerve and muscle atrophy, is associated with their use (Shelanski and Wiśniewski, 1969). Aggregates of argentophilic filaments (100 Å) are found in the neurons of the brainstem, spinal cord, and dorsal root ganglia. The aggregates are localized primarily in the cytoplasm of the perikaryon, while the axons are less involved. In this, the effects of vinca alkaloids differ from the toxicity of iminodipropionitrile, the latter being associated primarily with axonal filament aggregates. The filaments in both conditions are not identical to the neurofibrillary degeneration associated with diseases such as Alzheimer's dementia or postencephalitic parkinsonism in which tangles of neurofibrils consist of double-stranded helices. The relationship of experimental and naturally occurring tangles to cell transport is a subject of considerable investigation since it is proposed that the neurofibrils normally transport substances from the perikaryon down the axon (Prineas, 1969; Johnson and Blum, 1970).

Iminodipropionitrile. The behavioral effect of this compound in mice and rats is to produce excitement and a "waltzing syndrome" associated with damage to axons in the spinal cord and brainstem. Although an increase in axoplasmic protein concentration and protein synthesis has been noted, Slagel and associates (1966) were unable to show a change in amount of RNA or base ratio of RNA in ventral horn cells and other brain areas. The toxic effects of this compound on axons thus appear to be independent of changes in RNA metabolism in the cell body. Mechanism of action of this chemical deserves further study.

Type 5. *Neuromuscular Junction of Motor Nerve*

Synaptic clefts and the terminals of myelinated axons are uniquely vulnerable to toxic chemicals. Since this location in the nervous system is designed to respond to chemical transmitters, it is not surprising that various exogenous chemicals may affect pre- and postsynaptic binding sites. The myelin sheath ends above the nerve terminal, and this area and the cleft between the motor nerve and muscle end plate are open to substances that can diffuse through the capillaries of skeletal muscle.

The pharmacology of the neuromuscular junction has been investigated in great detail, and extensive discussions of drug actions at the neuromuscular junction are available (e.g., Goodman and Gilman, 1975).

The effects of some toxic substances on the terminals of motor neurons are of unusual theoretic interest as well as being responsible for severe poisoning in humans.

Botulinum Toxin. When the depolarizing nerve action potential reaches the end of the axon, acetylcholine is released to cause an end-plate potential on the muscle side of the synapse. The end-plate potential, if of sufficient magnitude, will initiate the self-propagating muscle action potential. Botulinum toxic interferes with this sequence by preventing the release of acetylcholine from the axon terminal (Ambache, 1949). The binding of botulinum toxin to the terminal is irreversible and the muscle behaves as if denervated. The neuron responds as if the axon had been severed distally. After an early period of chromatolysis and swelling, there is an increase in nucleolar RNA followed by an increase in ribosomal RNA (Watson, 1969). Recovery from botulinum toxin involves sprouting of the nerve terminal and eventually formation of new contacts with the muscle (Duchen and Strich, 1968).

Tetrodotoxin. Tetrodotoxin has been responsible for deaths in humans as a result of consumption of improperly prepared puffer fish. Preparation of these fish as food by experienced handlers is required to prevent contamination of the flesh with the toxin from the liver. Death from tetrodotoxin results from skeletal muscle paralysis. However, sensory nerves are equally affected (Evans, 1969). The mechanism of action has been examined by various investigators, and it has been concluded that tetrodotoxin selectively blocks the sodium channels along the axon, preventing the inward sodium current of the action potential while leaving unaffected the outward potassium current (Kao, 1966).

Saxitoxin. Saxitoxin is the toxin produced by the dinoflagellate, *Gonylaulax*. When the toxin-containing plankton organism is ingested by shellfish, the mollusk becomes poisonous to man. The action of saxitoxin on the sodium channel of the neuron resembles the effect of tetrodotoxin (Hille, 1968).

Batrachotoxin. Batrachotoxin is one of several related toxic steroidal compounds present in extracts of the skin of the South American frog *Phyllobates aurotaenia* and used as an arrow poison. The action of batrachotoxin is antagonistic to the effects on sodium flux of tetrodotoxin and saxitoxin. Batrachotoxin depolarizes the nerve membrane by increasing the permeability of the resting membrane to sodium ions. In the absence of sodium ions, batrachotoxin has no effect on the nerve. If tetrodotoxin is applied externally to an axon, the effect of batrachotoxin is blocked, showing the opposite effect these two toxins have on sodium channels (Narahashi *et al.*, 1971; Bartels-Bernal *et al.*, 1977).

Additional details of these toxins are to be found in Chapter 21 on toxins of animal origin.

DDT (Dichlorodiphenyltrichloroethane). Several insecticides cause repetitive firing of the motor end plate through repeated depolarizations of the presynaptic nerve terminal. Repetitive discharge occurs in sensory, central, and motor neurons in DDT-poisoned insects (Narahashi and Haas, 1968). The central effects of DDT are discussed below.

Allethrin. Pyrethrum is an insecticide extracted from species of *Chrysanthemum*. The toxic effects of the insecticide include various nervous system effects (see Chapter 16 on Pesticides and Chapter 4 on Metabolism of Toxic Substances). Allethrin, a synthetic insecticide chemically resembling the natural pyrethrins, has been studied for its mechanism of action. The effect of allethrin on the neuromuscular junction resembles that of DDT. Allethrin causes repetitive firing of the motor end plate. Wouters and coworkers (1977) propose that this may be due to prolongation of the transient increase in sodium permeability during an action potential. The prolonged permeability has been reported in both vertebrates and invertebrates (Wang *et al.*, 1972). Allethrin also shows a negative temperature coefficient at the neuromuscular junction, i.e., repetitive firing increases with lower temperature. The greater sensitivity of invertebrates over vertebrates to the pyrethroids may be due, in part, to this negative temperature coefficient and the higher body temperature of the vertebrate.

Lead. In addition to causing peripheral neuropathy, lead has been shown to have a direct synaptic action. Manalis and Cooper (1973) demonstrated that lead depresses the end-plate potential by presynaptic block. It is proposed that lead competitively inhibits calcium-mediated release of acetylcholine (Kober and Cooper, 1976). The possible relation of these findings to lead neuropathies is unknown.

Type 6. Neurotoxicants Causing Localized CNS Lesions

The compounds in this group cause lesions restricted in distribution, affecting primarily localized anatomic areas in the CNS. Selective toxicity in the CNS may occur for several reasons. First, some areas are more exposed to substances present in blood. This has been discussed previously in the concept of the blood-brain barrier. Examples relating to areas lacking a blood-brain barrier are glutamic and kainic acids described below. Second, some areas have unique biochemical specialization for which the toxic substance has an affinity, such as pyrithiamine or mercury. Third, some areas in the CNS are affected indirectly as a result of changes elsewhere in the organism. One example of the response of the CNS to damage elsewhere is the specific condition in severe liver disease resulting in hepatic encephalopathy.

Hepatotoxicity. The neurologic syndrome that may occur as a result of alcoholic liver cirrhosis consists of ataxia, rigidity, tremor, facial grimacing, and mental changes such as emotional instability or dementia (Victor *et al.*, 1965). The primary histologic finding is the presence of Alzheimer type II astrocytes in the basal ganglia, cerebral cortex, and cerebellum. These astrocytes have enlarged nuclei and perikarya. Some loss of neurons may occur in the areas where the large astrocytes are found. The condition has been reproduced experimentally in rats using a portocaval shunt and gavage with ammoniated cationic resin (Norenberg *et al.*, 1974). In severe liver disease the ammonia concentration in the plasma may be increased several times above normal. It appears likely that the enlarged astrocytes are responding metabolically to the excess blood ammonia. Comparable changes in the CNS can be produced by chronic administration of carbon tetrachloride, which is a well-known hepatoxic substance. After several weeks of dosing with carbon tetrachloride, astrocytes are enlarged and neurons are diminished in size in both the basal ganglia (Hasson and Leech, 1967; Diemer, 1976b) and cerebellum (Diemer, 1976a). This is particularly evident in the nuclei of these cells. The change in size of the nuclei may reflect altered metabolic activity in the cells (Diemer, 1976b).

Methione Sulfoximine. Although alterations in nuclear or perikaryal size may occur as an adaptive process during chronic treatment with a toxicant, there may be differences in acute and chronic changes with some toxic compounds. Prolonged administration of methionine sulfoximine may cause damage to myelin (see Nitrogen Trioxide). Methionine sulfoximine inhibits glutamine synthetase, which is a key enzyme for handling ammonia in the brain. Large doses of methionine sulfoximine cause convulsions in rats after a delay of several hours. Prior to the onset of seizures, astrocytes in the cerebral cortex and basal ganglia enlarge and resemble the Alzheimer type II astrocytes seen in chronic hepatic encephalopathy (Guieterrez and Norenberg, 1975).

Glutamate. Large doses of monosodium L-glutamate produce hypothalamic and retinal lesions in newborn mice (Potts *et al.*, 1960). The lateral geniculate nucleus also shows degeneration but this may be secondary to the retinal damage. The site of hypothalamic damage is the arcuate nucleus. The effect on this nucleus is probably not specific for monosodium glutamate since there is evidence that other acidic amino acids, such as aspartate and cysteine, produce the same changes, whereas neutral or basic amino acids do not (Olney, 1971). There is some controversy as to whether or not monosodium glutamate affects the hypothalamus in monkeys (Reynolds et al., 1971). The rat is affected like the mouse (Burde et al., 1971). Other areas that are damaged by large doses of the acidic amino acids are the areas in which the blood-brain barrier is deficient, including the area postrema (Olney et al., 1977). The mechanism of damage is proposed to be the sustained state of depolarization, energy depletion, and ionic imbalance produced by large doses of excitatory acidic amino acids. The neuronal sites sensitive to depolarization by these compunds are localized on the perikaryon and dendrites. Axons are unresponsive (Schwarcz and Coyle, 1977). Kainic acid is an analog of glutamic acid and, like glutamate, destroys the neurons it excites (Olney et al., 1974). Kainic acid has been used experimentally by injection as a tool to destroy neurons in selected brain areas while leaving axons from distant neurons intact (McGeer et al., 1976).

Gold Thioglucose. Neuropil dissolution in the ventromedial nucleus of the hypothalamus of mice has been reported following administration of gold thioglucose, but the lesion is not limited to this nucleus and may involve various brain areas in which the blood-brain barrier is normally reduced or absent (Perry and Liebelt, 1961). This lesion, like the lesion following monosodium glutamate, induces obesity in mice. Debons and coworkers (Debons et al., 1970) have shown that the gold localizes in oligodendroglia in the ventromedial nucleus. Presumably the heavy metal is toxic to cells and produces "scarring." This lesion does not occur in alloxandiabetic mice, implying that the presence of "glucoreceptors" in the hypothalamus is necessary for the deposition of gold in the ventromedial nucleus. No changes in the CNS of man have been reported during use of gold thioglucose in arthritis.

Acetylpyridine. This compound is not of commercial importance but is an analog of nicotinic acid and may act as an antimetabolite for niacin. It causes highly selective damage limited to certain cells of the hippocampus (areas H_2 and H_3) in the mouse and in the squirrel monkey. In the squirrel monkey the lateral geniculate and inferior olivary nuclei are also damaged (Coggeshall and MacLean, 1958). MacLean (1963) has pointed out the uniqueness of this damage and its correlation with the high zinc concentration of areas H_2 and H_3, presumably associated with the high succinic dehydrogenase levels. Area H_1 (Sommer's sector), which does not contain high concentrations of zinc, is damaged by anoxic conditions but is not altered by 3-acetylpyridine. This chemical has been used experimentally to destroy the inferior olivary nucleus in the rat in investigations of the role of climbing fibers from neurons of the inferior olive. The Purkinje cells of the cerebellum have no contacts from climbing fibers in these animals and locomotion is seriously impaired (Sotelo et al., 1975). It has been proposed that the acute toxic effects are the result of synthesis of abnormal nucleotides in which pyridine is replaced by 3-acetylpyridine (Desclin and Escubi, 1974).

Pyrithiamine. Thiamine deficiency can be induced by administration of pyrithiamine, and the CNS lesions that result experimentally in mice from this compound closely resemble the lesions of thiamine deficiency (Wernicke's encephalopathy) in man. Selective damage to the mammillary bodies from pyrithiamine has been shown to be associated with a decrease in transketolase activity (Collins et al., 1970). Other brain areas that are high in transketolase activity may also be damaged, for example, the tegmentum of the pons in the rat.

DDT (Dichlorodiphenyltrichloroethane). Repeated administration of DDT to animals results in tremor, incoordination, muscular twitching, and weakness. With chronic exposure these changes become irreversible. In dogs, changes are found in the anterior horn cells and in the cerebellum (loss of Purkinje cells) and neurons in the dentate nucleus (Haymaker et al., 1946). Glial changes have not been reported. In rabbits, the changes are confined to the anterior horn cells of the spinal cord (Cameron and Burgess, 1945). Single large doses of DDT produce convulsions in monkeys and rats (Woolley, 1970). These effects have not been reported for man. The mechanism of the acute action of DDT on axonal firing has been elucidated in a series of papers by Narahashi and others (Narahashi and Haas, 1968). (See under Type 5 Neurotoxins.) The relation of the chronic effects to the acute toxicity of DDT is not known. Several related pesticides cause convulsions in acute overdose that resemble the effects of DDT. Experimentally, chronic doses of chlordane cause hyperexcitability and tremors. Large doses cause convulsions (Hyde and Falkenberg, 1976). Endrin (Revzin, 1966) and lindane (Hanig et al., 1976) also cause convulsions. The latter compound is of interest in that this effect was produced by a single topical application of 1 percent lindane on weanling rabbits. Since topical lindane is used in treatment of scabies, the production of convulsions by this route of application is of significance.

Mercury. Chronic exposure to low levels of inorganic mercury or its compounds produces psychologic changes (erethismus mercurialis), presence of colored mercury compounds in the anterior lens capsule of the eye (mercurialentis), slight tremor, and signs of autonomic nervous system dysfunction (especially excess salivation). No CNS lesions have been found during "micromercurialism," the stage of mercury poisoning with increased central and autonomic nervous system excitability.

The toxic signs of alkyl mercury compounds, such as methyl mercury, show differences from inorganic mercurials. This may be due to greater penetration of organic mercury compounds into the brain. Localization of inorganic mercury in cerebellar Purkinje cells has been reported (Cassano et al., 1969), whereas methyl mercury causes necrosis of the granule cell layer of the cerebellum (Hunter and Russell, 1954). The toxic effect of methyl mercury on cerebellar granule cells is of interest since the granule cells are more resistant than Purkinje cells to anoxia but are vulnerable to disorders of kidney and carbohydrate metabolism (Olsen, 1959). Focal atrophy of the cortex with sensory disturbances, ataxia, and dysarthria is found after organic mercury intoxications. The emotional changes and autonomic nervous system involvement with inorganic mercury are not seen with organic mercury. Sensory nerve fibers are rather selectively damaged; motor fibers are much less involved (Miyakawa et al., 1970, 1971). The primary mode of action of both kinds of mercury compounds may be interference with membrane permeability and enzyme reactions by binding of mercuric ion to sulfhydryl groups, but distribution of the organic and inorganic forms may differ. It has been pointed out that small neurons in the CNS are more likely to be damaged than large neurons in the same area by methyl mercury. The greater sensitivity of small cells may be due to their greater amount of membrane for the amount of cytoplasm, and a greater ratio of membrane/cytoplasm may increase the likelihood of membrane damage from mercury (Jacobs et al., 1977).

In recent years mercury compounds, especially organic mercury compounds, have been studied in great detail. Several reviews and detailed studies are available (Murakami, 1972; Shaw et al., 1975; Jacobs et al., 1977; Luschei et al., 1977).

Manganese. The hazards of manganese have been known for a long time. Reports in the medical literature on manganese encephalopathy, in persons exposed to manganese dusts, date back to 1837. In monkeys injected with manganese compounds or exposed to manganese aerosols, neuronal degeneration has been found in the globus pallidus, subthalamic nuclei, caudate nucleus, putamen, and cerebellum. Some liver damage also occurs (Pentschew et al., 1963). The functional disability in monkeys and man closely resembles the extrapyramidal signs and symptoms of parkinsonism. Emotional changes may be present as an early symptom of toxicity. Cotzias (1958) has written an extensive review of the subject.

The description of toxic effects of the various agents listed above has been limited to the effects on the nervous system even when these compounds have distinct and sometimes dramatic effects on other organs in the body. For example, the interaction of compounds causing liver damage with CNS effects has been mentioned. The diverse somatic effects of substances such as isoniazid, lead, vincristine, and anticholinesterase compounds are also recognized, but are outside the scope of a general survey of nervous system toxicants.

REFERENCES

Abou-Donia, M. B., and Preissig, S. H.: Delayed neurotoxicity from continuous low dose and administration of leptofos to hens. *Toxicol. Appl. Pharmacol.*, 38:595–608, 1976.

Aldridge, W. N.; Barnes, J. M.; and Johnson, M. K.: Studies on delayed neurotoxicity produced by some organophosphorus compounds. *Ann. N.Y. Acad. Sci.*, 160:314–22, 1969.

Aleu, F. P.; Katzman, R.; and Terry, R. D.: Fine structure and electrolyte analysis of cerebral edema induced by alkyl tin intoxication. *J. Neuropathol. Exp. Neurol.*, 22:403–13, 1963.

Ambache, N.: The peripheral action of *Cl. botulinum* toxin. *J. Physiol.*, 108:127–41, 1949.

Arrighi, F. E.: Mammalian chromosomes. In Busch, H. (ed.): *The Cell Nucleus*, Vol. 2. Academic Press, Inc., New York, 1974, pp. 1–32.

Auld, R. B., and Bedwell, S. F.: Peripheral neuropathy with sympathetic over-activity from industrial contact with acrylamide. *Can. Med. Assoc. J.*, 96:652–54, 1967.

Bank, W. J.; Pleasure, D. E.; Suzuki, K.; Nigro, M.; and Katz, R.: Thallium poisoning. *Arch. Neurol.*, 26:456–64, 1972.

Barbizet, J.: Psychophysiological mechanisms of memory. In Vinken, P. J., and Bruyn, G. W. (eds.): *Handbook of Clinical Neurology*, Vol. 3. John Wiley & Sons, Inc., New York, 1969.

Bartels-Bernal, E.; Rosenberry, T. L.; and Daly, J. W.: Effect of batrachotoxin on the electroplax of electric eel: Evidence for voltage-dependent interaction with sodium channels. *Proc. Natl. Acad. Sci. USA*, 74:951–55, 1977.

Bass, N. H.: Pathogenesis of myelin lesions in experimental cyanide encephalopathy. *Neurology*, 18:167–77, 1968.

Beresford, W. A., and Glees, P.: Degeneration in the long tracts of the cords of the chicken and cat after triorthocresylphosphate poisoning. *Acta Neuropathol. (Berl.)*, 3:108–18, 1963.

Berthound, H. R.; Garman, R. H.; and Weiss, B.: Food intake, body weight, and brain histopathology in mice following chronic methyl mercury treatment. *Toxicol. Appl. Pharmacol.*, 36:19–30, 1976.

Boller, F.; Howes, D.; and Pattern, D. H.: A behavioral evaluation of brain-scan estimates of lesion size. *Neurology*, 20:852–59, 1970.

Bondareff, W.: The extracellular compartment of the cerebral cortex. *Anat. Rec.*, 152:119–27, 1965.

Bradley, W. G., and Asbury, A. K.: Radioautographic studies of Schwann cell behavior. I. Acrylamide neuropathy in the mouse. *J. Neuropathol. Exp. Neurol.*, 29:500–506, 1970.

Brierley, J. B.: The sensory ganglia—recent anatomical, physiological and pathological contributions. *Acta Psychiat. Neurol. Scand.*, 30:553–76, 1955.

Brierley, J. R.; Brown, A. W.; and Meldrum, B. S.: The nature and time course of the neuronal alterations resulting from oligaemia and hypoglycaemia in the brain of *Macaca mulatta*. *Brain Res.*, 25:483–99, 1971.

Brightman, M. W., and Reese, T. S.: Junctions between initimately apposed cell membranes in the vertebrate brain. *J. Cell Biol.*, 40:648–77, 1969.

Brown, S.; Dragann, N.; and Vogel, W. H.: Effects of lead acetate on learning and memory in rats. *Arch. Environ. Health*, 22:370–72, 1971.

Brucher, J. M.: Neuropathological problems posed by carbon monoxide poisoning and anoxia. *Prog. Brain Res.*, 24:75–100, 1967.

Bullock, J. D.; Wey, R. J.; Zaia, J. A.; Zarembook, I.; and Schroeder, H. A.: Effects of tetraethyl lead on learning and memory in the rat. *Arch. Environ. Health*, 13:21–22, 1966.

Burde, R. M.; Schainker, B.; and Kayes, J.: Acute effects of oral and subcutaneous administration of monosodium glutamate on the arcuate nucleus in mice and rats. *Nature*, 233:58–60, 1971.

Cameron, G. R., and Burgess, F.: The toxicity of 2,2-bis(*p*-chlorphenyl) 1,1,1-trichlorethane (D.D.T.). *Br. Med. J.*, 1:865–71, 1945.

Carlton, W. W., and Kreutzberg, G.: Isonicotinic acid hydrazide-induced spongy degeneration of the white matter in the brain of Pekin ducks. *Am. J. Pathol.*, 48:91–106, 1966.

Cassano, G. G.; Viola, P. L.; Ghetti, B.; and Amaducci, L.: The distribution of inhaled mercury (Hg[203]) vapors in the brain of rats and mice. *J. Neuropathol. Exp. Neurol.*, 28:308–20, 1969.

Cavanagh, J. B.: Metabolic mechanisms of neurotoxicity caused by mercury. In Roizin, L.; Shiraki, H.; and Grčević, N. (eds.): *Neurotoxicology*. Raven Press, New York, 1977, pp. 283–88.

Cavanagh, J. B., and Chen, F. C. K.: The effects of methyl-mercury-dicyandiamide on the peripheral nerves and spinal cord of rats. *Acta Neuropathol. (Berl.)*, 19:208–15, 1971a.

———: Amino acid incorporation of protein during the "silent phase" before organo-mercury and *p*-bromophenylacetylurea neuropathy in the rat. *Acta Neuropathol. (Berl.)*, 19:216–24, 1971b.

Cavanagh, J. B.; Chen, F. C. K.; Kyu, M. H.; and Ridley, A.: The experimental neuropathy in rats caused by *p*-bromophenylacetylurea. *J. Neurol. Neurosurg. Psychiat.*, 31:471–78, 1968.

Cavanagh, J. B.; Fuller, N. H.; Johnson, H. R. M.; and Rudge, P.: The effect of thallium salts, with particular reference to the nervous system changes. *Quart. J. Med.*, 43:293–319, 1974.

Cervós-Navarro, J., and Rozas, J. I.: The arteriole as a site of metabolic change. *Adv. Neurol.*, 20:17–24, 1978.

Chapman, L. F., and Wolff, H. G.: The cerebral hemispheres and the highest integrative functions of man. *Arch. Neurol.*, 1:357–424, 1959.

Chason, J. L.: Nervous system and skeletal muscle. In Anderson, W. A. D. (ed.): *Pathology*, Vol. 2, 6th ed. C. V. Mosby Co., St. Louis, 1971.

Coggeshall, R. L., and MacLean, P. D.: Hippocampal lesions following administration of 3-acetylpyridine. *Proc. Soc. Exp. Biol. Med.*, 98:687–89, 1958.

Collins, R. C.; Kirpatrick, J. B.; and McDougal, D. B., Jr.: Some regional pathologic and metabolic consequences in mouse brain of pyrithiamine-induced thiamine deficiency. *J. Neuropathol. Exp. Neurol.*, 29:57–69, 1970.

Cotzias, G. C.: Manganese in health and disease. *Physiol. Rev.*, 38:503–32, 1958.

Crapper, D. R.; Krishnan, S. S.; and Quittkat, S.: Aluminum, neurofibrillary degeneration and Alzheimer's disease. *Brain*, 99:67–80, 1976.

Crosby, E. C.; Humphrey, T.; and Lauer, E. W.: *Correlative Anatomy of the Nervous System*. Macmillan Publishing Co., Inc., New York, 1962.

Culver, B., and Norton, S.: Juvenile hyperactivity in rats after acute exposure to carbon monoxide. *Ex. Neurol.*, 50:80–98, 1976.

Curley, A.; Kimbrough, R. D.; Hawk, R. E.; Nathenson, G.; and Finberg, L.: Dermal absorption of hexachlorophene in infants. *Lancet*, 2:296–97, 1971.

Davenport, J. J.; Farrell, D. F.; and Sumi, S. M.: "Giant axonal neuropathy" caused by industrial chemicals. *Neurology*, 26:919–23, 1976.

Debons, A. F.; Krimsky, I; From, A.; and Cloutier, R. J.: Gold thioglucose induction of obesity: Significance of focal gold deposits in hypothalamus. *Am. J. Physiol.*, 219:1403–1408, 1970.

deRobertis, E.: Morphological aspects of water and ion shifts in the CNS. In Schadé, J. P., and McMenemey, W. H. (eds.): *Selective Vulnerability of the Brain in Hypoxaemia*. F. A. Davis Co., Philadelphia, 1963.

Desclin, J. C., and Escubi, J.: Effects of 3-acetylpyridine on the central nervous system of the rat, as demonstrated by silver methods. *Brain Res.*, 77:349–64, 1974.

Diemer, N. H.: Number of Purkinje cells and Bergmann astrocytes in rats with CCl$_4$-induced liver disease. *Acta Neurol. Scand.*, 55:1–15, 1976a.

———: Glial and neuronal alterations in the corpus striatum of rats with CCl$_4$-induced liver disease. *Acta Neurol. Scand.*, 55:16–32, 1976b.

DiVincenzo, G. D.; Kaplan, C. J.; and Dedinas, J.: Characterization of the metabolites of methyl n-butyl ketone, methyl iso-butyl ketone and methyl ethyl ketone in guinea pig serum and their clearance. *Toxicol. Appl. Pharmacol.*, 36:511–22, 1976.

Dru, D.; Agnew, W. F.; and Greene, E.: Effects of tellurium ingestion on learning capacity of the rat. *Psychopharmacologia*, 24:508–15, 1972.

Duchen, L. W., and Strich, S. J.: The effects of botulinum toxin on the pattern of innervation of skeletal muscle in the mouse. *Quart. J. Exp. Physiol.*, 53:84–89, 1968.

Duckett, S., and Scott, T.: The localization of tellurium in tellurium-induced hydrocephalus. *Experientia*, 27:432–34, 1971.

Evans, M. H.: Mechanism of saxitoxin and tetrodotoxin poisoning. *Br. Med. Bull.*, 25:263–67, 1969.

Falk, J. L.: Drug effect on discriminative motor control. *Physiol. Behav.*, 4:421–27, 1969.

Friede, R. L.: *Topographic Brain Chemistry*. Academic Press, Inc., New York, 1966.

Fullerton, P. M., and Barnes, J. M.: Peripheral neuropathy in rats produced by acrylamide. *Br. J. Ind. Med.*, 23:210–21, 1966.

Gibbins, R. J.; Kalant, H.; and LeBlanc, A. E.: A

technique for accurate measurement of moderate degrees of alcohol intoxication in small animals. *J. Pharmacol. Exp. Therap.*, 159:236–42, 1968.

Goodman, L., and Gilman, A.: *The Pharmacological Basis of Therapeutics*, 5th ed. Macmillan Publishing Co., Inc., New York, 1975.

Gutierrez, J. A., and Norenberg, M. D.: Alzheimer II astrocytosis following methionine sulfoximine. *Arch. Neurol.*, 32:123–26, 1975.

Hanig, J. P.; and Yoder, P. D.; and Krop, S.: Convulsions in weanling rabbits after a single topical application of 1% lindane. *Toxicol. Appl. Pharmacol.*, 38:463–69, 1976.

Hasson, J., and Leech, R. W.: Experimental hepatocerebral disease. *Arch. Pathol.*, 84:286–89, 1967.

Hawkins, J. E., Jr.; Stebbins, W. C.; Johnsson, L.-G., Moody, D. B.; and Muraski, A.: The patas monkey as a model for dihydrostreptomycin ototoxicity. *Acta Otolaryngol.*, 83:123–29, 1977.

Haymaker, W.; Ginzler, A. M.; and Ferguson, R. L.: The toxic effects of prolonged ingestion of DDT on dogs with special reference to lesions in the brain. *Am. J. Med. Sci.*, 212:423–31, 1946.

Hazama, F.; Amano, S.; and Ozaki, T.: Pathological changes of cerebral vessel endothelial cells in spontaneously hypertensive rats with special reference to the role of these cells in the development of hypertensive cerebrovascular lesions. *Adv. Neurol.*, 20:359–69, 1978.

Heydlauf, H.: Ferric-cyanoferrate (II): An effective antidote in thallium poisoning. *Eur. J. Pharmacol.*, 6:340–44, 1969.

Hicks, S. P.: Brain metabolism *in vivo*. I. The distribution of lesions caused by cyanide poisoning, insulin hypoglycemia, asphyxia in nitrogen and fluoroacetate poisoning in rats. *Arch. Pathol.*, 49:111–37, 1950.

Hille, B.: Pharmacological modifications of the sodium channels of frog nerve. *J. Gen. Physiol.*, 51:199–219, 1968.

Hirano, A.; Ohsugi, T.; and Matsumura, H.: Pores and tubule-containing vacuoles in altered blood vessels of the central nervous system. *Adv. Neurol.*, 20:461–69, 1978.

Hunter, D., and Russell, D. S.: Focal cerebral and cerebellar atrophy in a human subject due to organic mercury compounds. *J. Neurol. Neurosurg. Pyschiat.*, 17:235–41, 1954.

Hurst, E. W.: Experimental demyelination in relation to human and animal disease. *Ann. J. Med.*, 12:547–60, 1952.

Hyde, K. M., and Falkenberg, R. L.: Neuroelectric disturbance as indicator of chronic chlordane toxicity. *Toxicol. Appl. Pharmacol.*, 37:499–515, 1976.

Innes, J. R. M., and Saunders, L. Z.: *Comparative Neuropathology*. Academic Press, Inc., New York, 1962.

Inturrisi, C. E.: Thallium-induced dephosphorylation of a phosphorylated intermediate of the (sodium + thallium-activated) ATPase. *Biochim. Biophys. Acta*, 178:630–33, 1969.

Jacob, H.: CNS tissue and cellular pathology in hypoxaemic states. In Schadé, J. F., and McMenemey W. H. (eds.): *Selective Vulnerability of the Central Nervous System in Hypoxaemia*. F. A. Davis Co., Philadelphia, 1963.

Jacobs, J. M.: Penetration of systemically injected horseradish peroxidase into ganglia and nerves of the autonomic nervous system. *J. Neurocytol.*, 6:607–18, 1977.

Jacobs, J. M.; Carmichael, N.; and Cavanagh, J. B.: Ultrastructural changes in the dorsal root and trigeminal ganglia of rats poisoned with methyl mercury. *Neuropathol. Appl. Neurobiol.*, 1:1–19, 1975.

———: Ultrastructural changes in the nervous system of rabbits poisoned with methyl mercury. *Toxicol. Appl. Pharmacol.*, 39:249–61, 1977.

Jacobs, J. M.; MacFarlane, R. M.; and Cavanagh, J. B.: Vascular leakage in the dorsal root ganglia of the rat, studied with horseradish peroxidase. *J. Neurol. Sci.*, 29:95–107, 1976.

Johannsen, F. R.; Wright, P. L.; Gordon, D. E.; Levinskas, G. F.; Radue, R. W.; and Graham, P. R.: Evaluation of delayed neurotoxicity and dose-response relationships of phosphate esters in the adult hen. *Toxicol. Appl. Pharmacol.*, 41:291–304, 1977.

Johnson, A. B., and Blum, N. R.: Nucleoside phosphatase activities associated with the tangles and plaques of Alzheimer's disease. *J. Neuropathol. Exp. Neurol.*, 29:463–78, 1970.

Johnson, M. K.: Delayed neurotoxic action of some organophosphorus compounds. *Br. Med. Bull.*, 25:231–35, 1969.

———: The delayed neuropathy caused by some organophosphorus esters: mechanism and challenge. *CRC Crit. Rev. Toxicol.*, 3:289–316, 1975.

Joynt, R. J.; Benton, A. L.; and Fogel, M. L.: Behavioral and pathological correlates of motor impersistence. *Neurology*, 12:876–81, 1962.

Kao, C. Y.: Tetrodotoxin, saxitoxin and their significance in the study of excitation phenomena. *Pharmacol. Rev.*, 18:997–1049, 1966.

Kennedy, G. L.; Dressler, I. A.; and Keplinger, M. L.: The concentration of hexachlorphene in the blood of albino rats as a function of time postexposure, number of exposures, route of exposure, previous exposure and age. *Toxicol. Appl. Pharmacol.*, 37:425–31, 1976a.

Kennedy, G. L.; Dressler, I. A.; Richter, W. R.; Keplinger, M. L.; and Calandra, J. C.: Effects of hexachlorophene in the rat and their reversibility. *Toxicol. Appl. Pharmacol.*, 35:137–45, 1976b.

Kennedy, P., and Cavanagh, J. B.: Spinal changes in the neuropathy of thallium poisoning. *J. Neurol. Sci.*, 29:295–301, 1976.

Kesson, C. M.; Baird, A. W.; and Lawson, D. H.: Acrylamide poisoning. *Postgrad. Med. J.*, 53:16–17, 1977.

Kimbrough, R. D., and Gaines, T. B.: Hexachlorophene effects on the rat brain. *Arch. Environ. Health*, 23:114–18, 1971.

Kinnard, W. J., Jr., and Carr, C. J.: A preliminary procedure for the evaluation of central nervous system depressants. *J. Pharmacol. Exp. Therap.*, 121:354–61, 1957.

Kober, T. E., and Cooper, G. P.: Lead competitively inhibits calcium-dependent synaptic transmission in the bullfrog sympathetic ganglion. *Nature*, 262:704–705, 1976.

Krehbiel, D.; Davis, G. A.; LeRory, L. M.; and Bowman, R. E.: Absence of hyperactivity in lead-exposed developing rats. *Environ. Health Perspect.*, 18:147–57, 1976.

Kuhlenbeck, H.: *The Central Nervous System of Vertebrates*, Vol. 3, Part I. Academic Press, Inc., New York, 1970.

Lampert, P.; Garro, F.; and Pentshew, A.: Tellurium neuropathy. *Acta Neuropathol. (Berl.)*, 15:308–17, 1970.

Lampert, P. W., and Schochet, S. S.: Electron microscopic observations on experimental spongy degeneration of the cerebellar white matter. *J. Neuropathol. Exp. Neurol.*, 27:210–20, 1968a.

———: Demyelination and remyelination in lead neuropathy. *J. Neuropathol. Exp. Neurol.*, 27:527–45, 1968b.

Lapresle, J., and Fardeau, M.: The central nervous system and carbon monoxide poisoning. II. Anatomical study of brain lesions following intoxication with carbon monoxide (22 cases). *Prog. Brain Res.*, 24:31–74, 1967.

Levine, S.: Anoxic-ischemic encephalopathy in rats. *Am. J. Pathol.*, 36:1–18, 1960.

———: Experimental cyanide encephalopathy. *J. Neuropathol. Exp. Neurol.*, 26:214–22, 1967.

Lewey, F. H.: Neurological, medical and biochemical signs and symptoms indicating chronic industrial carbon disulfide absorption. *Ann. Intern. Med.*, 15:869–83, 1941a.

———: Experimental chronic carbon disulfide poisoning in dogs. *J. Ind. Hyg. Toxicol.*, 23:415–36, 1941b.

———: Neuropathological changes in nitrogen trichloride intoxication of dogs. *J. Neuropathol. Exp. Neurol.*, 9:396–405, 1950.

Lieberman, A. R.: The axon reaction: A review of the principal features of perikaryal responses to axon injury. *Int. Rev. Neurobiol.*, 14:49–124, 1971.

Ljunggren, B.; Norberg, K.; and Siesjö; B. K.: Influence of tissue acidosis upon restitution of brain energy metabolism following total ischemia. *Brain Res.*, 77:173–86, 1974.

Luschei, E.; Mottet, N. K.; and Shaw, C.-M.: Chronic methylmercury exposure in the monkey (*Macaca mulatta*): Behavioral tests of peripheral vision, signs of neurotoxicity, and blood concentration in relation to dose and time. *Arch. Environ. Health*, 32:126–31, 1977.

McGeer, E. G.; Innanen, V. T.; and McGeer, P. L.: Evidence on the cellular localization of adenylcylase in the neostriatum. *Brain Res.*, 118:356–58, 1976.

MacLean, P. D.: Comments on the selective vulnerability of the hippocampus. In Schadé, J. F., and McMenemey, W. H. (eds.): *Selective Vulnerability of the Central Nervous System in Hypoxaemia*. F. A. Davis Co., Philadelphia, 1963.

Malamud, N.: Patterns of CNS vulnerability in neonatal hyperemia. In Schadé, J. F., and McMenemey, W. H. (eds.): *Selective Vulnerability of the Central Nervous System in Hypoxaemia*. F. A. Davis Co., Philadelphia, 1963.

Manalis, R. S., and Cooper, G. P. : Presynaptic and postsynaptic effects of lead at the frog neuromuscular junction. *Nature* 243:354–55, 1973.

Mettler, F. A.: Choreo-athetosis and striopallidonigral necrosis due to sodium azide. *Exp. Neurol.*, 34:291–308, 1972.

Milner, B.: Effects of different brain lesions on card sorting. *Arch. Neurol.*, 9:90–100, 1963.

———: Visually-guided maze learning in man: Effects of bilateral hippocampal, bilateral frontal, and unilateral cerebral lesions. *Neuropsychologia*, 3:317–38, 1965.

Miyakawa, T.; Deshimaru, M.; Sumiyoshi, S.; Teraoka, A.; and Tatetsu, S.: Experimental organic mercury poisoning. Pathological changes in muscles. *Acta Neuropathol.* 17:80–83, 1971.

Miyakawa, T.; Deshimaru, M.; Sumiyoshi, S.; Teraoka, A.; Udo, N.; Hattori, E.; and Tatetsu, S.: Experimental organic mercury poisoning—pathological changes in peripheral nerves. *Acta Neuropathol.* (Berl.), 15:45–55, 1970.

Miyoshi, K.: Experimental striatal necrosis induced by sodium azide. A contribution to the problem of selective vulnerability and histochemical studies of enzymatic activity. *Acta Neuropathol.* (Berl.), 9:199–216, 1967.

Miyoshi, K.; Matsuoka, T.; and Mizushima, S.: Familial holotopistic striatal necrosis. *Acta Neuropathol.* (Berl.), 13:240–49, 1969.

Mullenix, P.; Norton, S.; and Culver, B.: Locomotor damage in rats after X-irradiation *in utero*. *Exp. Neurol.*, 48:310–24, 1975.

Murakami, U.: The effect of organic mercury on intrauterine life. In Klingberg, M. A.; Abramovici, A.;

and Chemke, J. (eds.): *Drugs and Fetal Development*, Advances in Experimented Medical Biology, Vol. 27. Plenum Press, New York, 1972, pp. 301–36.

Myers, R. E.: Two classes of dysergic brain abnormality and their conditions of occurrence. *Arch. Neurol.*, 29:394–99, 1973.

———: Fetal asphyxia due to umbilical cord compression. *Biol. Neonate*, 26:21–43, 1975.

Narahashi, T.; Albuquerque, E. X.; and Deguchi, T.: Effects of batrachotoxin on membrane potential and conductance of squid giant axon. *J. Gen. Physiol.*, 58:54–70, 1971.

Narahashi, T., and Haas, H. G.: Interaction of DDT with the components of lobster nerve membrane conductance. *J. Gen. Physiol.*, 51:177–98, 1968.

Norenberg, M. D.; Lapham, L. W.; Nichols, L. W.; and May, A. G.: An experimental model for the study of hepatic encephalopathy. *Arch. Neurol.*, 31:106–109, 1974.

Norton, S., and Culver, B.: A Golgi analysis of caudate neurons in rats exposed to carbon monoxide. *Brain Res.*, 132:455–65, 1977.

Ochs, S.: Axoplasmic transport in peripheral nerve and hypothalamoneurohypophyseal systems. *Adv. Exp. Med. Biol.*, 87:13–40, 1977.

Olney, J. W.: Glutamate-induced neuronal necrosis in the infant mouse hypothalamus. *J. Neuropathol. Exp. Neurol.*, 30:75–90, 1971.

Olney, J. W.; Rhee, V.; and de Gubareff, T.: Neurotoxic effects of glutamate on mouse area postrema. *Brain Res.*, 120:151–57, 1977.

Olney, J. W.; Rhee, V.; and Ho, O. L.: Kainic acid: A powerful neurotoxic analogue of glutamate. *Brain Res.*, 77:507–12, 1974.

Olsen, S.: Acute selective necrosis of the granular layer of the cerebellar cortex. *J. Neuropathol. Exp. Neurol.*, 18:609–19, 1959.

Olsson, Y.: Topographical differences in the vascular permeability of the peripheral nervous system. *Acta Neuropathol.* (Berl.), 10:26–33, 1968.

Olsson, Y., and Hossman, K.-A.: Fine structural localization of exudated protein tracers in the brain. *Acta Neuropathol.* (Berl.), 16:103–16, 1970.

Overmann, S. R.: Behavioral effects of asymptomatic lead exposure during neonatal development in rats. *Toxicol. Appl. Pharmacol.*, 41:459–71, 1977.

Palay, S. L., and Palade, G. E.: The fine structure of neurons. *J. Biophys. Biochem. Cytol.*, 1:69–88, 1955.

Papez, J. W.: A proposed mechanism of emotion. *Arch. Neurol. Psychiat.*, 38:725–43, 1937.

Paterson, P. Y.: The demyelinating diseases: Clinical and experimental correlates. In Samter, M. (ed.): *Immunological Disease*, Vol. 2. Little, Brown & Co., Boston, 1971.

Pentschew, A.; Ebner, F. F.; and Kovatch, R. M.: Experimental manganese encephalopathy in monkeys. *J. Neuropathol. Exp. Neurol.*, 22:488–99, 1963.

Perry, J. H., and Liebelt, R. A.: Extra-hypothalamic lesions associated with gold-thioglucose induced obesity. *Proc. Soc. Exp. Biol. Med.*, 106:55–57, 1961.

Pleasure, D.; Towfighi, J.; Silberg, D.; and Parris, J.: The pathogenesis of hexachlorophene neuropathy: In vivo and in vitro studies. *Neurology*, 24:1068–75, 1974.

Pleasure, D. E.; Mishler, K. C.; and Engel, W. K.: Axonal transport of protein in experimental neuropathies. *Science*, 166:524–25, 1969.

Plum, F.; Posner, J. B.; and Hain, R. F.: Delayed neurological deterioration after anoxia. *Arch. Intern. Med.*, 110:18–25, 1962.

Potts, A. M.; Modrell, K. W.; and Kingsbury, C.: Permanent fractionation of the electroretinogram by sodium glutamate. *Am. J. Ophthalmol.*, 50:900–907, 1960.

Preziosi, T. J.; Lindenberg, R.; Levy, D.; and Christenson, M.: An experimental investigation in animals of the functional and morphologic effects of single and repeated exposures to high and low concentrations of carbon monoxide. *Ann. N. Y. Acad. Sci.*, 174:369–84, 1970.

Prineas, J.: The pathogenesis of dying-back polyneuropathies. I. An ultrastructural study of experimental tri-ortho-cresyl phosphate intoxication in the cat. *J. Neuropathol. Exp. Neurol.*, 28:571–97, 1969.

Reese, T. S., and Brightman, M. W.: Similarity in structure and permeability to peroxidase of epithelia overlying fenestrated cerebral capillaries. *Anat. Rec.*, 160:414, 1968.

Reiter, L. A., and Ison, J. R.: Inhibition of the human eyeblink reflex: an evaluation of the sensitivity of the Wendt-Yerkes method for threshold detection. *J. Exp. Psychol. Human Percept. Perform.*, 3:325–36, 1977.

Revzin, A. M.: Effects of endrin on telencephalic function in the pigeon. *Toxicol. Appl. Pharmacol.*, 9:75–83, 1966.

Reynolds, W. A.; Lemkey-Johnson, N.; Filer, L. J., Jr.; and Pitkin, R. M.: Monosodium glutamate: Absence of hypothalamic lesions after ingestion by newborn primates. *Science*, 172:1342–44, 1971.

Robinson, N.; Duncan, P.; Gehrt, M.; Sances, A.; and Evans, J.: Histochemistry of trauma after electrode implantation and stimulation in the hippocampus. *Arch. Neurol.*, 32:98–102, 1975.

Ruščák, M.; Ruščáková, D.; and Hager, H.: The role of the neuronal cell in the metabolism of the rat cerebral cortex. *Physiol. Bohemoslov.*, 17:113–21, 1968.

Saida, K.; Mendell, J. R.; and Weiss, H. S.: Peripheral nerve changes induced by methyl n-butyl ketone (MBk) and methyl ethyl ketone (MEK). *J. Neuropathol. Exp. Neurol.*, 35:113, 1976a.

———: Peripheral nerve changes induced by methyl n-butyl ketone and potentiation by methyl ethyl ketone. *J. Neuropathol. Exp. Neurol.*, 35:207–25, 1976b.

Sauer, R. M.; Zook, B. C.; and Garner, F. M.: Demyelinating encephalomyelopathy associated with lead poisoning in nonhuman primates. *Science*, 169:1091–93, 1970.

Sauerhoff, M. W., and Michaelson, I. A.: Hyperactivity and brain catecholamines in lead-exposed developing rats. *Science*, 182:1023–24, 1973.

Savolainen, H.; Lehtonen, E.; and Vaino, H.: CS₂ binding to rat spinal neurofilaments. *Acta Neuropathol.* (*Berl.*), 37:219–23, 1977.

Scarpelli, G. G., and Trump, B. F.: *Cell Injury*. University Association, Research in Educational Pathology. Upjohn Co., Kalamazoo, 1971.

Schlaepfer, W. W.: Experimental lead neuropathy: A disease of the supporting cells in the peripheral nervous system. *J. Neuropathol. Exp. Neurol.*, 28:401–18, 1969.

———: Vincristine-induced axonal alterations in rat peripheral nerve. *J. Neuropathol. Exp. Neurol.*, 30:488–505, 1971.

Scholz, W.: Selective neuronal necrosis and its topistic patterns in hypoxemia and oligenia. *J. Neuropathol. Exp. Neurol.*, 12:249–61, 1953.

———: The contribution of pathoanatomical research to the problem of epilepsy. *Epilepsia*, 1:36–55, 1959.

Schwarcz, R., and Coyle, J. T.: Striatal lesions with kainic acid: neurochemical characteristics. *Brain Res.*, 127:235–49, 1977.

Schwedenberg, T. H.: Leukoencephalopathy following carbon monoxide asphyxia. *J. Neuropathol. Exp. Neurol.*, 18:597–608, 1959.

Shaw, C.-M.; Mottet, N. K.; Body, R. L.; and Luschei, E. S.: Variability of neuropathologic lesions in experimental methyl mercurial encephalopathy in primates. *Am. J. Pathol.*, 80:451–70, 1975.

Shelanski, M. L., and Wiśniewski, H.: Neurofibrillary degeneration induced by vincristine therapy. *Arch. Neurol.*, 20:199–206, 1969.

Slagel, D. E.; Hartmann, H. A.; and Edstrom, J. E.: The effect of iminodipropionitrile on the ribonucleic acid content and composition of mesencephalic V cells, anterior horn cells, glial cells, and axonal balloons. *J. Neuropathol. Exp. Neurol.*, 25:244–53, 1966.

Slager, U. T.; Reilly, E. B.; and Brandt, R. A.: The neuropathology of barbiturate intoxication. *J. Neuropathol. Exp. Neurol.*, 25:237–43, 1966.

Sotelo, C.; Hillman, D. E.; Zamora, A. J.; and Llinás, R.: Climbing fiber deafferentation: its action on Purkinje cell dendritic spines. *Brain Res.*, 98:574–81, 1975.

Spencer, P. S., and Schaumburg, H. H.: Experimental neuropathy produced by 2,5-hexanedione—a major metabolite of the neurotoxic industrial solvent methyl n-butyl ketone. *J. Neurol. Neurosurg. Psychiat.*, 38:771–75, 1975.

———: Feline nervous system response to chronic intoxication with commercial grades of methyl n-butyl ketone, methyl i-butyl ketone and methyl ethyl ketone. *Toxicol. Appl. Pharmacol.*, 37:301–11, 1976.

Spielmeyer, W.: *Histopathologie des Nervensystems*. Julius Springer, Berlin, 1922.

Sterne, D. M.: The Benton, Porteus and WAIS digit span tests with normal and brain-injured subjects. *J. Clin. Psychol.*, 25:173–77, 1969.

Strain, G. S., and Kinzie, W. B.: Reducing misdiagnosis of schizophrenic patients on a test for brain damage. *J. Clin. Psychol.*, 25:262–69, 1969.

Tiller, J. R.; Schilling, R. S. F.; and Morris, J. N.: Occupational toxic factor in mortality from coronary heart disease. *Br. Med. J.*, 4:407–11, 1968.

Torack, R. M.: The relationship between adenosine triphosphatase activity and triethyltin toxicity in the production of cerebral edema of the rat. *Am. J. Pathol.*, 46:245–62, 1965.

Trump, B. F., and Arstila, A. U.: Cell membranes and disease processes. In Trump, B. F., and Arstila, A. U. (eds.): *Pathobiology of Cell Membranes*. Academic Press, Inc., New York, 1975.

Vanderhaeghen, J. J., and Logan, W. J.: The effect of the pH on the *in vitro* development of Spielmeyer's ischemic neuronal changes. *J. Neuropathol. Exp. Neurol.*, 30:99–104, 1971.

Vega, A.: Use of Purdue Pegboard and finger tapping performance as a rapid screening test for brain damage. *J. Clin. Psychol.*, 25:255–58, 1969.

Vega, A., and Parsons, O. A.: Cross-validation of the Halstead-Reitan tests for brain damage. *J. Consult. Clin. Psychol.*, 31:619–25, 1967.

Victor, M.; Adams, R. D.; and Cole, M.: The acquired (non-Wilsonian) type of chronic hepatocerebral degeneration. *Medicine*, 44:345–96, 1965.

Vigliani, E. C.: Clinical observations on carbon disulfide intoxication in Italy. *Industr. Med. Surg.*, 19:240–42, 1950.

Vogt, C., and Vogt, O. (J. Psychol. Neurol., Lpz. 28, 1922), quoted by A. Meyer. Blackwood, W.; Meyer, A.; McMenemey, W. H.; Norman, R. M.; and Russell, D. S. (eds.): *Greenfields' Neuropathology*, 2nd ed. Edward Arnold, Ltd., London, 1963.

Walsh, J. C., and McLeod, J. J.: Alcoholic neuropathy. An electrophysiological and histological study. *J. Neurol. Sci.*, 10:457–65, 1970.

Wang, C. M.; Narahashi, T.; and Scuka, M.: Mechanism of negative temperature coefficient of nerve blocking action of allethrin. *J. Pharmacol. Exp. Therap.*, 182:442–53, 1972.

Watson, W. E.: The response of motor neurons to intramuscular injection of botulinum toxin. *J. Physiol.*, 202:611–30, 1969.

Watzman, N., and Barry, H., III: Drug effects on motor coordination. *Psychopharmacologia*, **12**:414–23, 1968.

Welsh, F. A., and O'Connor.: Patterns of micro-circulatory failure during incomplete cerebral ischemia. *Adv. Neurol.*, **20**:133–149, 1978.

Westergaard, E.; van Deurs, B.; and Brondsted, H. E.: Increased vesicular transfer of horseradish peroxidase across cerebral endothelium evoked by acute hypertension. *Acta Neuropathol. (Berl.).*, **37**:141–52, 1977.

Windle, W. F.: Selective vulnerability of the central nervous system of rhesus monkeys to asphyxia during birth. In Schadé, J. F., and McMenemy, W. H. (eds.): *Selective Vulnerability of the Central Nervous System in Hypoxaemia.* F. A. Davis Co., Philadelphia, 1963.

Woolley, D. E.: Effects of DDT and of drug-DDT interactions of electroshock seizures in the rat. *Toxicol. Appl. Pharmacol.*, **16**:521–32, 1970.

————: Evaluation of behavioral and other neurological endpoints for assessing toxicity. In *Workshop on Behavioral Toxicology.* DHEW Publication No. NIH 76–1189, 1976, pp. 11–48.

Worden, A. N.; Palmer, A. C.; Noel, P. R. B.; and Mawdesley-Thomas, L. E.: Lesions in the brain of the dog induced by prolonged administration of monoamine oxidase inhibitors and isoniazid. *Proc. Eur. Soc. Study Drug Toxicol.*, **8**:149–61, 1967.

Wouters, W.; Van Den Bercken, J.; and Van Ginneken, A.: Presynaptic action of the pyrethroid insecticide allethrin in the frog motor end plate. *Eur. J. Pharmacol.*, **43**:163–71, 1977.

Chapter 10

TOXIC RESPONSES OF THE LIVER

Gabriel L. Plaa

INTRODUCTION

Liver injury induced by chemicals has been recognized as a toxicologic problem for close to 100 years (Sollmann, 1957; Zimmerman, 1976). Around 1880 scientists were concerned about the mechanisms involved in the hepatic deposition of lipids following exposure to yellow phosphorus. Hepatic lesions produced by arsphenamine, carbon tetrachloride, and chloroform were also studied in laboratory animals in the first 40 years of the twentieth century. During the same period the correlation between hepatic cirrhosis and excessive ethanol consumption became recognized.

It was recognized early that "liver injury" is not a single entity, that the lesion observed depends not only on the chemical agent involved but on the period of exposure. After acute exposure one usually finds lipid accumulation in the hepatocytes, cellular necrosis, or hepatobiliary dysfunction, whereas cirrhotic or neoplastic changes are usually considered to be the result of chronic exposures. Different biochemical alterations may lead to the same end point: no single mechanism seems to govern the appearance of degenerative changes in the hepatocytes or alterations in its function. Some forms of liver injury have been found to be reversible while others result in a permanently deranged organ. The mortality associated with various forms of liver injury varies. The incidence of injury differs among species, and the presence of a dose-response relationship may not always be apparent. It is no wonder that today the phrase "produces liver injury" has little meaning to the toxicologist; the form of injury requires precision before its consequences can be assessed.

MORPHOLOGIC AND FUNCTIONAL CONSIDERATIONS

The classic manner of presenting the relationships between the hepatic cell, its vascular supply, and the biliary system has been the configuration of the hexagonal lobule (Fig. 10–1). Rappaport (1969) reports that this concept was introduced by Kiernan in 1833. This configuration is still presented in some textbooks as the functional unit of the liver. In the center of this lobule, one finds the terminal hepatic venule (central vein) and at the periphery the portal space, containing a branch of the portal vein, an hepatic arteriole, and a bile duct. Based on this configuration, pathologic lesions of the hepatic parenchyma have been classified as centrilobular, midzonal, or periportal.

There is a growing body of evidence that indicates that the hexagonal lobule configuration does not correspond to the functional unit of the liver. The hexagonal lobule is not conspicuous under microscopic examination. Injection of colored gelatin mixtures into the portal vein or the hepatic artery has shown that terminal afferent vessels supply blood to only sectors of adjacent hepatic lobules. These sectors are found to be situated around terminal portal branches and extend from the central vein of one hexagon to the central vein of an adjacent hexagon. This had led Rappaport and coworkers to define the parenchymal mass in terms of functional units called the liver acini (Rappaport, 1969). The simple liver acinus consists of a small parenchymal mass that is irregular in size and shape and is arranged around an axis consisting of a terminal portal venule, an hepatic arteriole, a bile ductule, lymph vessels, and nerves (Fig. 10–2). This acinus lies between two or more terminal hepatic venules (central veins) with which its vascular and biliary axis interdigitates. There is no physical separation between two liver acini. The hepatic cells of the simple acini are in cellular and sinusoidal contact with the cells of adjacent or overlapping acini. Even with this extensive communication, the hepatic cells of one particular acinus are preferentially supplied by their parent vessels.

The simple acinus concept has also been developed to show that there are circulatory zones within each acinus. Rappaport (1969) has divided these into three, depending on their distance from the supplying terminal vascular

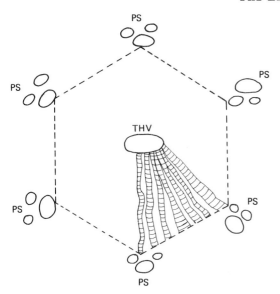

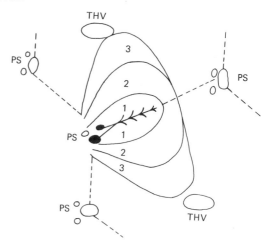

Figure 10–1. Schematic representation of the classic hexagonal lobule. *PS* is the portal space, consisting of a branch of the portal vein, a hepatic arteriole, and a bile duct; *THV* is the terminal hepatic venule (central vein).

Figure 10–2. Schematic representation of a simple hepatic acinus. *PS* is the portal space, consisting of a branch of the portal vein, a hepatic arteriole, and a bile duct; *THV* is the terminal hepatic venule (central vein); *1, 2,* and *3* represent the various zones draining off the terminal afferent vessel (in black). (Modified from Rappaport, A. M.: Anatomic considerations. In Schiff, L. [ed.]: *Diseases of the Liver*, 3rd ed. J. B. Lippincott Co., Philadelphia, 1969.)

branch (Fig. 10–2). It has also been demonstrated that three or more simple acini can constitute what is called a "complex acinus." This unit consists of the three simple units and a sleeve of parenchyma around the preterminal afferent vessels, the lymph vessels, and the nerves that eventually give origin to the terminal axial channels of the simple acini.

Although it has been assumed for quite some time that the various hepatic parenchymal cells within the liver lobule have the same kind of functional specificity, it is now becoming clear that there is a lack of uniformity; these differences have been brought into evidence by histochemical and electron microscopic techniques. Rappaport (1976) has reviewed the current knowledge and has superimposed the differing regions of metabolic activity upon his concept of zonal acinar circulation. In brief, the activity of respiratory enzymes has been found to be particularly high in the zone closest to the terminal afferent vessel (zone 1 in Figure 10–2), whereas the most distant zone (zone 3) has been found to be particularly rich in microsomal enzymes. Others (Wattenberg and Leong, 1962; Koudstall and Hardouk, 1969) have reported that centrilobular cells, as seen in the hexagonal lobular configuration, are relatively rich in some NADPH-dependent enzymes and that peripheral cells are relatively poor. Sweeney and coworkers

(1978a, 1978b) employed sedimentation velocity analysis as a means of studying hepatocytic heterogeneity in rats. They found significant heterogeneity among populations of hepatocytes and suggested that the larger cells were richer in mixed-function oxidase activity. Furthermore, enhancement of mixed-function oxidase by two different inducers (phenobarbital and 3-methylcholanthrene) resulted in quite different sedimentation-velocity patterns. The concept of heterogeneity in various hepatic cells and in various zones is only in a state of early development. However, one can already see that the concept may permit the rationalization of differing mechanisms of action in the development of hepatic lesions associated with hepatotoxic agents.

The classic descriptions of focal, midzonal periportal, and centrilobular lesions can be explained by Rappaport's zonal acinar configuration (Rappaport, 1969). It is possible to visualize that centrilobular necrosis, for instance, is located in a region that corresponds to the distal acinar zone of Rappaport (zone 3 in Fig. 10–2). It has also been said that regeneration occurs from cells located in the midzonal region of the classic representation; this would correspond to the acinar zone closest to the terminal afferent vessel (zone 1), a zone that has been shown to be particularly high in cytogenic enzyme activity. Therefore, it would appear that the acinar circulatory visualization of the hepatic lobule does not come in conflict with the earlier descriptions of pathologic lesions.

Morphologically, chemical-induced injury can manifest itself in different ways. The acute effects can consist of an accumulation of lipids (fatty liver) and the appearance of degenerative processes leading to death of the cell (necrosis). The necrotic process can affect small groups of isolated parenchymal cells ("focal necrosis"), groups of cells located in zones ("centrilobular, midzonal, or periportal necrosis"), or virtually all of the cells within an hepatic lobule ("massive necrosis"). The accumulation of lipids can also be zonal or more widespread. While the acute injury caused by the halogenated hydrocarbons, carbon tetrachloride and chloroform, usually consist of both necrosis and fat accumulation, it is not necessary that both features be present to constitute liver injury. For example, tannic acid, when administered acutely, produces centrilobular necrosis, but extensive fat accumulation does not seem to occur (Horvath et al., 1960). Thioacetamide also produces centrilobular necrosis without accumulation of lipids (Gupta, 1956). Ethionine, on the other hand, produces fatty livers upon acute administration with little or no necrosis (Rouiller, 1964).

Chemical-induced liver injury resulting from chronic exposure can produce marked alterations of the entire liver structure with degenerative and proliferative changes observed in the different forms of cirrhosis. Neoplastic changes may be another end point of chemical liver injury.

CLASSIFICATION OF CHEMICAL-INDUCED LIVER INJURY

There have been a variety of ways of classifying the hepatic lesions induced by various chemical substances. One has only to compare the review written by Drill in 1952 with another review written by Zimmerman in 1974 to appreciate the changes that have occurred in the thinking of investigators involved in this area. Before 1950, investigators were primarily interested in the injury produced by exposure to nontherapeutic agents likely to occur in an occupational environment. In 1974, one sees that the primary concern is about drug-induced injury. In addition to acute hepatic necrosis and lipid accumulation (Table 10–1), one sees growing interest in the cholestatic type of response (Table 10–2). This latter lesion results in diminution or cessation of bile flow, with the ensuing retention of bile salts and bilirubin. The retention of bilirubin leads to the production of jaundice. Industrial chemicals are not usually associated with this type of response, although a large number of drugs are (Table 10–2). In addition to the cholestatic lesion, one finds another one, a type of chemical-induced hepatitis that resembles closely that produced by viral infections. The drugs associated with this lesion are less numerous (Table 10–2). A number of drugs are also associated with a mixed type of lesion, that is, one that possesses both cholestatic viral-like hepatitic components (Perez et al., 1972; Zimmerman, 1974, 1978).

In 1959, Popper and Schaffner classified chemical-induced hepatic injury on the basis of the morphologic changes observed. Five groups of reactions were described. The first was called "zonal hepatocellular alterations without inflammatory reaction." The substances included in this category all produce zonal changes, either necrosis or fat accumulation (Table 10–1). These authors point out that because of its great reproducibility in several animal species, its dose dependence, and its predictable character, this type of lesion is probably the best-understood type of hepatic injury.

The second group described was called "intrahepatic cholestasis." This category contained drugs, without common chemical structural characteristics, that were capable of producing, in a very small percentage of the population, a jaundice resembling that produced by extrahepatic biliary obstruction (Table 10–2). The important histologic features associated with this response are the presence of bile stasis, dilation of the canaliculi with subsequent loss of the microvilli, and the occurrence of focal necrosis. There appeared to be no relationship between dose and response, and production of the lesion in animals was not possible with these substances.

The third category was called "hepatic necrosis with inflammatory reaction." The prominent feature here is the progression to a massive necrosis characteristic of viral hepatitis (Table 10–2). Again it was found that the incidence was extremely low, that dose dependency did not seem to exist, and that reproducibility of these lesions in animals was not possible.

The fourth group was called an "unclassified group." This category contained a variety of hepatic injuries that did not fit into any type of scheme. For a few of these, the lesions were associated with manifestations of pathology in several other organs.

The fifth group consisted of those producing "hepatic cancer." No drugs were contained in this last category. However, a number of chemicals are now recognized as being hepatocarcinogens in animals.

Zimmerman (1974) classified hepatotoxic substances in a somewhat different manner. He first classified them according to the supposed mechanism of action based on current knowledge. Second, he characterized them on the basis of the morphologic changes observed. Finally, he classified them according to the circumstances of exposure. On the basis of mechanism, he divided all of the agents into two broad categories: "intrinsic hepatotoxins" and those depending on "host idiosyncrasy" rather than on the intrinsic toxicity of the agent. For the "intrinsic

Table 10–1. EXAMPLES OF ACUTE HEPATOTOXIC CHEMICALS

CHEMICAL	PRODUCES NECROSIS	PRODUCES FATTY LIVER	REFERENCE*
Carbon tetrachloride	X	X	1
Chloroform	X	X	2
Trichloroethylene	X	X	3
Tetrachloroethane	X	X	3
Bromobenzene	X		4
Dimethylnitrosamine	X	X	5
Dimethylaminoazobenzene	X	X	3
Thioacetamide	X		6
Pyrrolizidine alkaloids	X	X	7
Aflatoxin	X	X	8
Penicillum islandicum	X	X	9
Amanita phalloides	X		10
Tannic acid	X		11
Phosphorus	X	X	2
Ethionine		X	3
Azaserine	X	X	12
Cycloheximide		X	13
Tetracycline		X	14
Cerium		X	15
Beryllium	X		16
Allyl alcohol	X		3
Allyl formate		X	17
Ethanol		X	18
Methotrexate		X	19
Mithramycin	X		19
Mitomycin C		X	19
Puromycin		X	19
Urethane	X		19
Galactosamine	X	X	20
Acetaminophen	X		21
Phenacetin	X		21
Furosemide	X		21
Emetine		X	22

* (1) Recknagel, 1967; (2) Drill, 1952; (3) Rouiller, 1964; (4) Koch-Weser et al., 1953; (5) Magee and Swann, 1969; (6) Gupta, 1956; (7) McLean, 1970; (8) Raisfeld, 1974; (9) Uraguchi et al., 1961; (10) Baccino et al., 1976; (11) Horvath et al., 1960; (12) Marchetti et al., 1970; (13) Jazcilevich and Villa-Trevino, 1970; (14) Hoyumba et al., 1975; (15) Lombardi and Recknagel, 1962; (16) Witschi and Aldridge, 1967; (17) Rees and Tarlow, 1967; (18) Middleton et al., 1975; (19) Zimmerman, 1974; (20) Decker and Keppler, 1974; (21) Mitchell et al., 1976a; (22) Dianzani, 1976.

agents," again a high incidence of toxicity in exposed individuals, dose dependency, and the ability to produce the lesion in experimental animals are found. For the "host idiosyncrasy" group, the opposite is found: very low frequency of injury, a lack of dose dependency, and a failure to produce the lesion in animals. When Zimmerman categorized morphologic changes, he divided them into three: cytotoxic, cholestatic, and mixed. From this, it is apparent that the classification of Popper and Schaffner (1959) is still the basis of the morphologic descriptions. However, it should be pointed out that according to Zimmerman's line of reasoning, it is possible to have either an intrinsic hepatotoxin or an idiosyncratic compound that manifests either of these morphologic changes. His final considerations concerned the circumstances of the exposure and were divided into two main categories: one he terms "toxicologic," which consists primarily of chemical overdosage, and the second, "iatrogenic," which consists of lesions produced during the course of therapeutic utilization of drugs.

On the basis of mechanism, hepatotoxic agents can be grouped in different ways. Although numerous attempts have been made to identify the biochemical lesion associated with a variety of compounds, the available knowledge is insufficient to allow for classification of agents by this manner. However, Zimmerman divided his "intrinsic hepatotoxins" into two broad categories. He called these the "direct" and the "indirect" hepatotoxins. According to his concept, a direct agent would be one that can injure

Table 10–2. EXAMPLES OF DRUG-ASSOCIATED LIVER INJURY

DRUG	REFERENCE*	DRUG	REFERENCE*
Intrahepatic Cholestasis			
Chlorpromazine	1	Ectylurea	1
Prochlorperazine	1	p-Aminosalicylic acid	1
Promazine	2	Chlorthiazide	1
Trifluoperazine	2	Thiouracil	1
Thioridazine	2	Methimazole	1
Mepazine	1	Carbimazole	3
Carbamazepine	2	Propylthiouracil	2
Amitriptyline	2	Metahexamide	5
Imipramine	3	Carbutamide	5
Iprindole	3	Acetohexamide	5
Chlordiazepoxide	4	Tolbutamide	3
Diazepam	5	Tolazamide	3
Methyltestosterone	3	Chlorpropamide	1
Norethandrolone	3	Sulfanilamide	1
Methandrolone	5	Sulfadiazine	1˙
Fluoxymestrone	3	Erythromycin estolate	3
Mestranol	5	Triacetyleandomycin	3
Norethyndrol	5	Sodium oxacillin	2
Estradiol	3	Nitrofurantoin	3
Arsphenamine	1	Oxyphenisatin	4
Carbarsone	1	Phenindione	5
Viral-like Hepatitis			
Iproniazid	1	Isoniazid	6
Phenylisopropylhydrazine	2	Pyrizinamide	4
Nialamide	2	Halothane	4
Phenelzine	2	Methoxyflurane	4
Tranylcypromine	4	p-Aminosalicylic acid	4
Imipramine	4	Ethionamide	4
Cinchophen	1	Zoxazolamine	1
6-Mercaptopurine	2	Acetohexamide	2
α-Methyldopa	4	Indomethacin	4
Carbamazepine	4	Trimethobenzamide	4
Ethacrynic acid	4	Phenindione	4
Phenylbutazone	4	Sulfamethoxazole	4
Colchicine	4	Sulfisoxazole	4
Oxyphenisatin	5	Papaverine	4
Dantrolene	7	Ibufenac	5

* (1) Popper and Schaffner, 1959; (2) Schaffner and Raisfeld, 1969; (3) Plaa and Priestly, 1976; (4) Perez *et al.*, 1972; (5) Zimmerman, 1974; (6) Mitchell *et al.*, 1976c; (7) Utili *et al.*, 1977.

many tissues, including the liver. As far as the hepatocyte is concerned, a direct agent should affect a number of organelles such as the endoplasmic reticulum, the mitochondria, and the lysosomes. Examples of this type of agent are carbon tetrachloride, phosphorus, and tannic acid. On the other hand, the indirect agents are thought to affect a particular metabolic pathway. This effect should lead to a crippling of the metabolic organization of the cell. Ethionine is an example; its interference with methionine for available ATP leads to the diminution of lipoprotein-transport molecules and the retention of fat. For the cholestatic lesions, one would find the anabolic steroids in the category of the indirect agents, although their precise mechanism of action is unknown. It appears that these substances interfere with bile formation. While these types of classifica-

tions assist in conceptionalizing what is occurring, it should be understood that, with additional knowledge of the events actually involved in the elaboration of the biochemical lesion, changes in the methods of classifying substances will certainly have to occur.

Agents that produce liver injury can be placed in two broad categories (Klatskin, 1969): those agents that produce toxic hepatitis and those agents that produce drug-induced hepatitis. Hepatotoxins can be defined as a heterogenous group of naturally occurring and synthetic chemical agents that produce a variety of hepatic lesions classified as forms of toxic hepatitis (Table 10–1). On the other hand, the drugs associated with liver injury in man appear to behave as sensitizing agents rather than as hepatotoxins (Table 10–2). The substances that produce toxic hepatitis have the following common characteristics: (1) they produce a distinctive lesion; (2) the severity of the lesion seems to be related to the dose administered; (3) while quantitative differences in potency can be found among individuals, generally the same type of lesion can be produced in all individuals; and (4) they usually appear after a predictable, usually brief, latent period. On the other hand, many of the drugs associated with liver injury in man do not fit these criteria for hepatotoxins because (1) the lesions cannot be produced in experimental animals; (2) the effects do not seem to be related to the dose; (3) there is an absence of a temporal relationship; (4) only a small fraction of the exposed population is susceptible; (5) the histologic pattern is more variable, and (6) often the lesions are accompanied by manifestations of hypersensitivity (allergic reactions).

From various classifications one can see that a variety of pathologic processes are involved in what is called, in general terms, "liver injury." Furthermore, many different kinds of substances can cause injury. The question that continually arises is whether the lesion is a manifestation of the hepatotoxic property of the substance in question or whether it is a manifestation of the host's response to the agent. When one considers host response, one must consider not only hypersensitivity (allergic) reactions but also exaggerated responses to minor alterations in hepatic function. With some anabolic steroids, jaundice develops only sporadically in man, yet diminished biliary excretory capacity is a regular occurrence. It is not known whether the jaundice seen on occasion is a result of an allergic response or whether it is an exaggerated manifestation of diminished biliary excretion. This leads one to reiterate the idea that classification schemes are extremely helpful, but they are only a means of sorting out the state of current views on liver function. As knowledge accumulates, conceptions can change and so must classifications.

CELLULAR SITES OF LIVER INJURY

For the last 50 years, many investigators have been interested in unraveling the hepatotoxic mechanisms involved in carbon tetrachloride–induced liver injury. The amount of information accumulated for this substance is much greater than that available for other substances. Also, in many studies with other agents, comparisons have been made with the effects obtained with carbon tetrachloride. In this sense, carbon tetrachloride has become a reference substance. The major interest in the early periods was devoted to the accumulation of fat associated with exposure to carbon tetrachloride. Consequently, early research efforts were oriented toward fat metabolism. The determination of biochemical mechanisms of action has been limited by the analytic techniques available at the time. Consequently, the efforts that were made to determine mechanisms of action centered around the evolution of biochemical approaches to the functioning of various organelles in the hepatocyte. The early work centered on the mitochondria since this was one of the first organelles whose biochemistry became well understood. As the elements of protein synthesis became better known, and with the discovery of the role of the endoplasmic reticulum in this event, investigations were carried out with this particular organelle. The various organelles that can be affected are summarized in Table 10–3.

Carbon tetrachloride can affect cellular membranes. Christie and Judah (1954) showed that carbon tetrachloride altered the permeability of the mitochondria; the activity of the enzymes involved in the Krebs cycle was found to be diminished in these preparations. These effects were shown to occur *in vivo* and *in vitro*. In addition, others (Dianzani, 1954; Dianzani and Bahr, 1954) demonstrated that there was an uncoupling of oxidative phosphorylation in mitochondria. Shifts of electrolytes, in particular calcium ion, were shown to occur early in the intoxication. The results of these observations led to the conclusion that the mitochondrial effects probably produced the fatty livers. This hypothesis no longer seems to be tenable (Recknagel, 1967; Judah, 1969) because the mitochondrial changes occur much later than does the appearance of fat accumulation. However, the eventual role of the mitochondrial changes in the development of necrosis has yet to be investigated fully.

Later experiments show that carbon tetrachloride can also affect the membranes of the endoplasmic reticulum. Recknagel and Lombardi in 1961 were the first to demonstrate that glucose-6-phosphatase, an enzyme associated with this structure, was markedly depressed very early after carbon tetrachloride administration. By electron microscopy, it was possible to show that the cisternae of the endoplasmic reticulum were dilated. It was further shown that protein synthesis associated with this structure was inhibited when one followed the incorporation of labeled amino acids into hepatic protein by liver microsomes (Smuckler *et al.*, 1961). Recknagel and Ghoshal (1966) demonstrated that carbon tetrachloride affects the lipid structure or microsomes derived from the endoplasmic reticulum and proposed that peroxidative decomposition of lipids in this organelle occurs early in the intoxication.

Table 10–3.　EXAMPLES OF HEPATOTOXINS AFFECTING
VARIOUS ORGANELLES

ORGANELLES AFFECTED	COMPOUND	REFERENCE[*]
Plasma membrane	*Amanita phalloides*	1
	Phalloidin	2
Endoplasmic reticulum	Carbon tetrachloride	3
	Thioacetamide	4
	Dimethylnitrosamine	5
	Phosphorus	6
	Ethionine	7
	Dimethylaminoazobenzene	8
	Allyl formate	8
	Pyrrolizidine alkaloids	9
	Galactosamine	10
	Tannic acid	11
Mitochondria	Carbon tetrachloride	3
	Pyrrolyzidine alkaloids	9
	Ethionine	7
	Allyl formate	8
	1,1-Dichloroethylene	12
	Phosphorus	8
	Hydrazine	13
	Dimethylnitrosamine	8
Lysosomes	Carbon tetrachloride	14
	Pyrrolizidine alkaloids	9
	Beryllium	15
	Amanita phalloides	16
	Ethionine	17
	Phosphorus	17
Nucleus	Pyrrolizidine alkaloids	9
	Dimethylnitrosamine	18
	Hydrazine	13
	Beryllium	19
	Aflatoxin	20
	Ethionine	17
	Tannic acid	11
	Galactosamine	10
	Thioacetamide	21

* (1) Baccino *et al.*, 1976; (2) Weiss *et al.*, 1973; (3) Recknagel, 1967; (4) Thoenes and Bannasch, 1962; (5) Magee and Swann, 1969; (6) Ghoshal *et al.*, 1969; (7) Anthony *et al.*, 1962; (8) Rouiller, 1964; (9) McLean, 1970; (10) Decker and Keppler, 1974; (11) Oler *et al.*, 1976; (12) Reynolds *et al.*, 1975; (13) Ganote and Rosenthal, 1968; (14) Dianzani, 1963; (15) Witschi and Aldridge, 1968; (16) Zuretti and Baccino, 1976; (17) Dianzani, 1976; (18) Emmelot and Benedetti, 1960; (19) Witschi, 1970; (20) Wogan, 1969; (21) Olason and Smuckler, 1976.

Another organelle that has been investigated is the lysosome. Dianzani (1963) showed that carbon tetrachloride and dimethylnitrosamine had little effect on lysosomes at a time when necrotic changes were already developing. In 1965, Baccino and coworkers demonstrated that, *in vitro*, carbon tetrachloride could cause lysosomal damage with the concomitant release of enzymes into the suspending medium. However, this effect could not be prevented by the administration of promethazine and diphenhydramine, two substances that exert protective effects against carbon tetrachloride *in vivo*. Alpers and Isselbacher

(1967) have also shown that release of lysosomal enzymes occurs at carbon tetrachloride concentrations that also inhibit leucine incorporation into protein. They found that lipid peroxidation seemed to be independent of this effect since carbon tetrachloride did not enhance peroxide formation in lysosomal fractions at a time when its effect on enzyme activity was maximal. Witschi and Aldridge (1967, 1968) have demonstrated that beryllium is taken up by rat lysosomes *in vivo* and that lysosomal enzymes are released. Since the release of enzymes is a late phenomenon, it is not known if this effect is the cause of the liver injury. For the moment, it appears that lysosomes play a relatively minor role in the development of necrosis.

Changes in membrane permeability have been demonstrated by a number of investigators. Calcium has been shown to accumulate in necrotic tissues. Work by Judah (1969) and others showed that treatment with promethazine or EDTA could remove the inhibition of enzymes due to a loss of semipermeable properties of the cells. Promethazine was also found to protect against carbon tetrachloride necrosis (Rees *et al.*, 1961). The interesting finding was that, while treatment with this substance protected against the necrosis, the fatty alterations were not affected. This important observation clearly showed that the two changes could be dissociated in the case of carbon tetrachloride. There is other evidence that suggests that altered permeability exists. Thiers and coworkers (1960) found striking increases in calcium in mitochondria from animals treated with carbon tetrachloride; these increases in calcium were paralleled by a decrease in potassium.

Altered membrane permeability of the hepatic cell can also lead to increased enzyme activity in the plasma. The activity of a number of hepatic cytoplasmic and mitochondrial enzymes has been found to increase in the plasma following carbon tetrachloride hepatotoxicity. The plasma activities of transaminases, lactic acid dehydrogenase, aldolase, and isocitric dehydrogenase, among others, have been used as diagnostic indicators of hepatic injury. Generally speaking, the plasma activities of cytoplasmic enzymes have been found to increase more rapidly than those of mitochondrial enzymes. Because of the time sequence involved, there is some doubt that the appearance of enzymes in the plasma results from necrosis; the early appearance of nonmitochondrial enzymes was thought to result from altered cell permeability (Dinman *et al.*, 1963). Most investigators have considered these increases in plasma enzyme activities to be the result of decreases of enzymes in hepatic tissue. However, Dinman and Bernstein (1968a, 1968b) have found that the activities of some liver enzymes are actually increased after exposure to carbon tetrachloride. Ideo and coworkers (1971) speculate that this result may be dependent upon the dose employed; they propose that low doses of carbon tetrachloride may increase hepatic enzyme synthesis and that this increase may overlap with the loss of activity due to cellular necrosis. On the other hand, with high doses of the substance, there may be a drop in protein synthesis that results in a net decrease of tissue enzyme activity. It should be pointed out that whether these increases are associated with changes in permeability or whether they reflect prenecrotic changes has little bearing on the empiric use of these enzymes for determining the presence of dysfunction.

MECHANISMS OF LIVER INJURY

Accumulation of Lipids

A number of agents that produce liver injury also cause the accumulation of abnormal amounts of fat in the parenchymal cells (Table 10–1). The lipid that accumulates is predominantly triglyceride. Triglyceride accumulation is the result of an imbalance between the rate of synthesis and the rate of release of triglyceride by the parenchymal cells into the systemic circulation. Lombardi (1966) has described four general mechanisms that can account for accumulation of triglycerides: (1) the rate of synthesis of hepatic triglyceride is normal, but the liver cell is unable to secrete the triglyceride into the plasma; (2) the secretion of hepatic triglyceride is normal, but the rate of synthesis is increased; (3) there is both an increase in the rate of synthesis and a block in the secretion of the synthesized triglyceride; and (4) the triglyceride synthesis takes place in a compartment of the cell other than the endoplasmic reticulum and thus this pool is not accessible to the normal secretory pathway.

In recent years, it has been shown by a number of investigators that a block of the secretion of hepatic triglyceride into the plasma is the basic mechanism underlying the fatty liver induced in the rat by carbon tetrachloride, ethionine, phosphorus, puromycin, or tetracycline, by feeding a choline-deficient diet, or by feeding orotic acid (Lombardi, 1966; Hoyumpa *et al.*, 1975). The accumulation of triglyceride in the hepatic cells is paralleled by a decrease in the concentration of plasma lipids and plasma lipoproteins. The plasma concentration of triglyceride in the fasted rat can be diminished to almost one-half its normal value within 30 minutes after exposure to carbon tetrachloride. By two hours, it is possible to show that liver triglycerides have begun to accumulate abnormally in the hepatic cell. The evidence demonstrating this type of action for carbon tetrachloride has been accumulated by pretreating animals with Triton WR-1339, a nonionic detergent that causes the secreted triglycerides to accumulate in the plasma by preventing the passage of plasma triglycerides into surrounding tissues (Recknagel *et al.*, 1960), by the use of the isolated perfused liver (Heimberg *et al.*, 1962), and by experiments following the incorporation of labeled fatty acids into liver and plasma triglycerides (Maling *et al.*, 1962; Schotz *et al.*, 1964). Tetracycline induces fatty livers in animals and man and interferes with triglyceride secretion (Seto and Lepper, 1954; Hoyumpa *et al.*, 1975).

This antibiotic also inhibits protein synthesis (Goldberg, 1965).

When hepatic triglyceride is released into the plasma, it is not released as such, but is combined with a lipoprotein. There is some evidence that indicates that carbon tetrachloride and ethionine can cause a fall in the level of circulating lipoprotein. It appears to be the very-low-density fraction of the lipoproteins that is principally affected. This fraction is considered to be the major portion involved in the transport of hepatic triglycerides to the extrahepatic tissues (Lombardi, 1966). It can be reasoned that a decrease in the amount of triglyceride combined with lipoprotein can occur if (1) synthesis of triglyceride and the other lipid moieties increases, (2) synthesis of the protein moiety is decreased, (3) the two moieties are formed but somehow do not associate, and (4) the formed lipoprotein is normal but somehow cannot be secreted by the cell. It has been possible to show that carbon tetrachloride, ethionine, phosphorus, and puromycin interfere with the synthesis of the protein moiety (Robinson and Seakins, 1962; Smuckler et al., 1962; Farber et al., 1964). Although there is evidence that all these substances can affect synthesis of lipoproteins, it is by no means clear that this is the only mechanism involved. With ethionine and phosphorus, it appears that this factor is most likely the key defect; however, with carbon tetrachloride, Recknagel (1967) has pointed out that on the basis of turnover rates of the apoprotein, it appears that the coupling phase of triglyceride secretion is probably affected by this agent. With tetracycline, impaired release of very-low-density lipoprotein occurs, but it is not known whether synthesis, conjugation, or secretion is the phase affected (Hoyumpa et al., 1975).

The function of the lipoproteins seems to be one of a vehicle, containing protein, phospholipid, and cholesterol; a defect could thus occur in the synthesis of the phospholipid or cholesterol moieties. In choline-deficient animals, a situation that results in the development of fatty liver, phospholipid synthesis is impaired. This effect of choline deficiency has been reported to result in impaired release of very-low-density lipoproteins (Lombardi and Oler, 1967). Orotic acid can produce fatty livers when fed to rats and also results in a block in the secretion of low-density lipoproteins (Windmueller and von Euler, 1971). Judah (1969) has reported that low levels of potassium ion bring about a reduction in the rate of transfer of lipoproteins across the liver cell membrane. The low potassium ion levels seen in ethionine intoxication may play a role in the triglyceride accumulation because of reduced lipoprotein secretion.

The important position of glycerophosphate in the regulation of synthesis of triglycerides is known, but there is little experimental evidence that suggests that this substrate is a key factor involved in the development of accumulation of triglycerides. The synthesis of triglyceride in cellular compartments other than the endoplasmic reticulum is also known. It is now thought that the triglycerides formed in the supernatant fraction are metabolically not as available as the triglycerides formed in endoplasmic reticulum (Schotz et al., 1964). However, very few studies have been done to assess the relative importance of this particular aspect in the eventual accumulation of hepatic triglycerides.

By electron microscopy, it has been possible to show that, in the endoplasmic reticulum, the accumulation of triglycerides causes the formation of droplets. Baglio and Farber (1965) have coined the term "liposomes" for these droplets. They have speculated that these liposomes may represent the morphologic expression of a block in the release of triglyceride; they postulate that a defective synthesis or secretion of lipoproteins may result in the accumulation of triglyceride in the cisternae of the endoplasmic reticulum. The major portion of the esterified fatty acids released by the liver appears as triglycerides in the very-low-density lipoprotein fraction. Hamilton and associates (1967) showed that when labeled free fatty acids are perfused through livers, osmiophilic particles appear within the Golgi vesicles within five minutes. They proposed that these particles represent the very-low-density lipoprotein formed from the free fatty acids. The investigators also reported a second type of osmiophilic particle resembling the liposomes found by Baglio and Farber in 1965. They attributed these to inadequate very-low-density lipoprotein transport with diversion of triglycerides to liposome formation. In later work, Mahley and coworkers (1969) showed that particles isolated from tubules and secretory vesicles of rat liver Golgi are similar to very-low-density lipoprotein on the basis of morphologic, flotational, chemical, and immunochemical properties. Recently microtubules have been suggested as playing a role in the secretion of very-low-density lipoprotein; a tubulin assembly-disassembly cycle exists in the liver, and interruption of the cycle by colchicine administration results in a blockade of very-low-density lipoprotein secretion (Jeanrenaud et al., 1977). Hepatotoxins have not been tried on this system.

It is possible that elevated triglyceride could result because of an increase in the rate of synthesis of this substance. Since there is evidence that the rate of synthesis is directly proportional to the concentration of the substrates present (fatty acids and glycerophosphate), it is theoretically possible that increased hepatic triglyceride synthesis could occur because of increased fatty acids or increased glycerophosphate. Increased fatty acids could result from a decreased oxidation of fatty acids, an increased synthesis of fatty acids, or an increased mobilization of fatty acids from peripheral stores. In the case of ethanol-induced fatty liver, impaired mitochondrial oxidation of fatty acids appears to be the primary abnormality seen in man (Hoyumpa et al., 1975), due to a shift in redox potential (increased NADH/NAD ratio). However, this may be accompanied by other abnormalities (Isselbacher, 1977). There is very little evidence to support the idea that fatty acid synthesis is involved in the development of fatty liver.

Increased mobilization of free fatty acids from adipose tissue has also been proposed as a possible mechanism for the development of fatty livers. However, after close scrutiny of the experimental evidence, it does not appear that such a mechanism could play a major role. For instance, in the case of ethionine, where it has been shown that the plasma concentration of fatty acids doubles, the net uptake by the liver is still normal (Lombardi, 1966). In the case of carbon tetrachloride, Recknagel (1967) has concluded that accelerated movement of fatty acids from peripheral stores is not a factor to be considered. It must be remembered that in the case of mobilization of fatty acids from adipose stores, the question is not whether this source of fat is needed for the accumulation of liver triglycerides, but whether an excessive amount of fatty acids is actually being released to the liver for uptake. Everyone agrees that fatty acids must be available from adipose tissue for the liver to synthesize triglycerides. In addition, the role of circulating free fatty acids has been amply demonstrated by interruption of the pituitary-adrenal axis with the resulting diminution of plasma free fatty acids. This leads to a block in the accumulation of triglycerides. However, in this situation, it appears that the peripheral stores plays a permissive role rather than a controlling role.

One can raise the question whether fat accumulation itself always represents an injurious response for the hepatocyte. As previously pointed out, a fatty liver does not necessarily lead to death of the hepatocytes; ethionine, puromycin, and cycloheximide all cause fat accumulation without producing necrosis. Promethazine protects rats against the necrogenic effects of carbon tetrachloride but does not abolish the fatty liver (Rees et al., 1961). Bucher and Malt (1971) have reviewed the biochemical and morphologic events associated with liver regeneration. Following partial hepatectomy in rats, there is a largely hormone-mediated mobilization of fat from adipose tissue. Neutral fat accumulates in the remainder of the liver

within 18 to 24 hours, reaching a value ten times that of normal livers and bringing about distortion of the normal lobular pattern. The capacity to secrete triglycerides increases, but liposomes begin to appear along with intracellular fat globules, indicating a relative delay in triglyceride secretion when compared with triglyceride accumulation. The hepatic cells, in the presence of this fat, still function as well as normal, if not more efficiently, while preparing for cell division at the same time. As Ingelfinger (1971) points out, in the face of this, can one say that excessive fat accumulation in itself is damaging?

Protein Synthesis

With many of the hepatotoxic substances that have been shown to produce necrosis, relatively similar morphologic changes have been reported to occur rapidly after the administration of the substance. Light microscopic examination reveals a loss of cytoplasmic basophilic material well before the appearance of necrosis in the hepatocyte. By electron microscopy, one sees vacuoles in the cytoplasm within one hour after the injection of carbon tetrachloride. At this time, the endoplasmic reticulum is also abnormal; the membranes are less well defined and dilated. Smuckler and coworkers (1962) observed dilatation of the cisternae of the endoplasmic reticulum and a loss of ribosome particles from the membrane surfaces. Similar observations have been reported to occur when rats have been treated with dimethylnitrosamine, carcinogenic azo dyes, ethionine, and thioacetamide (Magee, 1966).

Magee (1966) doubts that these changes actually represent early changes leading to necrosis. He feels that they are merely related to the inhibitory effects of these substances on protein synthesis. Ethionine, dimethylnitrosamine, carbon tetrachloride, thioacetamide, and galactosamine have all been shown to inhibit incorporation of amino acids into liver proteins. While a number of investigators have thought that inhibition of protein synthesis is the cause of liver necrosis, Magee (1966) points out that this cannot be considered to be entirely correct since, for at least ethionine, protein synthesis can be inhibited without inducing liver necrosis. Cycloheximide also inhibits protein synthesis for many hours, but does not result in liver necrosis (Farber, 1971). In fact, cycloheximide treatment has been shown to protect rats against hepatocytic necrosis induced by carbon tetrachloride and against acute necrosis of the biliary epithelium following α-naphthylisothiocyanate (Farber, 1975). Furthermore, Witschi and Aldridge (1967) showed that beryllium, a substance that produces midzonal necrosis, does not cause early inhibition of protein synthesis.

Extensive work has been carried out to determine how various agents affect protein synthesis (Dianzani, 1976). Ethionine inhibits amino acid incorporation into microsomal proteins. Ethionine replaces methionine and forms S-adenosyl-ethionine, which leads to a trapping of cellular adenine, a diminution in the rate of ATP synthesis, and inhibition of RNA synthesis. The ethionine, by its adenine-trapping effect, leads to accumulation of triglycerides in the liver within a few hours; this fatty liver appears to be a secondary consequence to the interference with protein metabolism (Farber, 1971).

Dimethylnitrosamine has also been shown to inhibit protein synthesis, and the effects are quite striking three hours after administration of the substance (Magee, 1966). The effects also occur in the microsomes rather than in the soluble supernatant fraction of liver homogenates. Mizrahi and Emmelot (1962) claim that dimethylnitrosamine probably affects protein synthesis by causing a loss of messenger RNA from the polyribosomes. They tentatively concluded that this loss of messenger RNA from the ribosomes may be due to methylation of the RNA. Mager and coworkers (1965) have reported results with dimethylnitrosamine that are consistent with the destruction of ribosome-bound messenger RNA.

Inhibition of protein synthesis in rat liver by carbon tetrachloride has been reported by Smuckler and coworkers (1961, 1962). A marked reduction of incorporation of amino acids into lipoproteins was observed as early as two hours after administration of carbon tetrachloride by Seakins and Robinson (1963). Decreased amino acid incorporation into hepatic proteins, albumin, and fibrinogen was found by Smuckler and coworkers (1962). Smuckler and Benditt (1965) found no evidence for inhibition of RNA synthesis after carbon tetrachloride; however, they did find that there were changes in the proportions of the various subunits found in ribosomal preparations.

More recently, Farber and coworkers (1971) have shown that pretreatment of rats with cycloheximide protects the liver against the ribosomal changes induced by carbon tetrachloride. This protection occurs during a time in which the changes induced by carbon tetrachloride on the endoplasmic reticulum still occur. These authors have interpreted their results to indicate that carbon tetrachloride exerts its effect on protein synthesis on single-unit ribosomes and not on the polysomes. It would thus appear that carbon tetrachloride can exert no effect when the ribosomes are aggregated in polysomes but only when they are present as monomers. In addition, these investigators have shown that damage to protein synthesis induced by carbon tetrachloride appears to be irreversible in contrast to the observations made with ethionine or puromycin. These observations may explain in part why carbon tetrachloride results in cell death whereas this does not occur with the other two substances.

Galactosamine also inhibits protein synthesis; reduced synthesis of RNA and plasma proteins, particularly coagulation factors, has been observed (Decker and Keppler, 1974). Uridine prevents or reverses the inhibition, which indicates that the depression is the result of the UTP deficiency induced by galactosamine. The galactosamine-1-phosphate formed in the liver leads to the accumulation of UDP-derivatives of galactosamine; in turn, this results in a depletion of hepatic UTP, UDP-hexoses, and a depression of uracil nucleotide–dependent biosynthesis of macromolecules. This is believed to result in injury to cellular organelles and necrosis of liver cells. Galactosamine-induced liver injury passes through several stages depending upon the dosage schedule (reversible acute hepatitis, chronic progressive hepatitis, cirrhosis, production of liver tumors), but is highly specific to this amino sugar. In addition, morphologic studies indicate that all hepatocytes are affected, to a varying degree, so that the result is an experimental model of diffuse liver cell injury (Medline et al., 1970).

Lipid Peroxidation

In 1966, Slater published a brief review concerning the necrogenic action of carbon tetrachloride. In this work, he speculated on a mechanism of action based on activation of the parent compound to a toxic metabolite. Slater pointed out that several of the observations concerning the nature of the hepatotoxic response to carbon tetrachloride led one to believe that it was not the parent compound that produced the toxic response. He proposed that homolytic cleavage of the carbon-chlorine bond occurred in the endoplasmic reticulum and that this resulted in the production of free radicals. He proposed that carbon tetrachloride is activated to a free radical and that the free radicals so formed then interact with neighboring lipid-rich material causing alterations in structure and function. Working independently, Recknagel arrived at the same conclusion (Recknagel and Ghoshal, 1966).

Butler (1961) demonstrated that carbon tetrachloride was metabolized to chloroform and concluded that this transformation was caused by homolytic cleavage, yielding free radicals that could alkylate sulfhydryl groups of enzymes. Wirtschafter and Cronyn (1964) proposed a general theory for solvent toxicity in which the reaction of the solvents with free radicals should be considered for the elaboration of toxic response. Furthermore, in 1948, Hove discovered that carbon tetrachloride lethality could be reduced by feeding vitamin E to rats maintained on semisynthetic, vitamin E–deficient diets. The protective effect of antioxidants was also investigated by Gallagher (1962), who showed that vitamin E, diphenyl-*p*-phenylenediamine (DPPD), and selenium all gave some measure of protection. The protective effect of DPPD was confirmed by DiLuzio and Costales (1965). Therefore, it was concluded that if lipid antioxidants protect the rat against carbon tetrachloride, it seemed reasonable to predict that destructive lipoperoxidation was involved in the toxic response.

Recknagel and Ghoshal (1966) hypothesized that free radicals arising from the homolytic cleavage of carbon tetrachloride attacked the methylene bridges of unsaturated fatty acid side chains of microsomal lipids, resulting in morphologic alteration of the endoplasmic reticulum, loss of activity of drug-metabolizing enzymes, loss of glucose-6-phosphatase activity, loss of protein synthesis, and loss of the capacity of the liver to form and excrete low-density lipoprotein. They were able to demonstrate that *in vitro* carbon tetrachloride could act as a prooxidant and that this effect of carbon tetrachloride was limited to the liver. As the lipid peroxidation occurred, the investigators were able to demonstrate the appearance of conjugated dienes, typical of peroxidized polyenoic fatty acids. In subsequent work, it was shown that, *in vivo*, the appearance of conjugated dienes occurred in animals and in man subjected to intoxicating doses of carbon tetrachloride. Phenobarbital treatment resulted in increased lipid peroxidation *in vivo* and SKF 525-A resulted in a diminution of the appearance of microsomal lipid peroxidation. The extensive investigative work carried out by Recknagel and his coworkers (Recknagel and Glende, 1973) has been the foundation of the lipid peroxidation theory as it concerns carbon tetrachloride liver injury.

Reynolds and Yee (1967) compared the patterns of incorporation of isotopic carbon from carbon tetrachloride, chloroform, dichloromethane, and methyl chloride into chemical constituents of liver organelles after oral administration of the substances. Of the four substances studied, only carbon tetrachloride and chloroform caused fatty liver and centrilobular necrosis. They found that only after carbon tetrachloride was glucose-6-phosphatase activity depressed in the liver; after chloroform, there was no indication that such a depression occurred. The doubling of RNA content in the cell sap has been considered to be a result of the degranulation of the

rat endoplasmic reticulum; of the four chloromethanes tested, only carbon tetrachloride had this property. In addition, this substance was the only one of the four that was found to cause transient influx of calcium into liver parenchymal cells. The shift in labeling patterns of cytoplasmic constituents of the liver, from cell sap to microsomes, from acid-soluble constituents to lipids, and from serine to methionine, with increasing chlorine content was consistent with the hypothesis that the hepatotoxicity of chloroform and carbon tetrachloride is due in part to homolytic cleavage of carbon tetrachloride and chloroform.

Comporti and coworkers (1965) have also provided evidence that carbon tetrachloride *in vitro* stimulates lipid peroxidation of rat liver microsomes. These authors were unable to find similar results with chloroform. Rat liver homogenates obtained from animals previously treated with carbon tetrachloride (one to two hours) were also reported to produce more lipid peroxides. DiLuzio and Hartman (1969) have demonstrated that animals treated with carbon tetrachloride had lower microsomal lipid-soluble antioxidant activity and concluded that this was consistent with enhanced lipid peroxidation.

Gordis (1969) has shown that five minutes after the intravenous injection of ^{14}C- or ^{36}Cl-carbon tetrachloride, liver lipids were labeled. Most of the radioactivity was found in the phospholipid fraction. His results were compatible with the formation of free radicals and offered an alternative to the lipid peroxidation theory of Recknagel (1967). Gordis visualized the possibility that free radicals derived from carbon tetrachloride would form chlorinated lipids that may be unsuitable as membrane components. Recently, Benedetti *et al.* (1977a, 1977b) have described the alterations induced by carbon tetrachloride in the lipids of the membranes of the hepatic endoplasmic reticulum one hour after treatment. The results indicate that both the simple addition of carbon tetrachloride free radicals to fatty acids and a chain termination addition reaction of carbon tetrachloride free radicals to fatty acid free radicals containing conjugated dienes occurred; the latter products were quite abnormal in physical chracteristics. In subsequent work, Benedetti *et al.* (1977c) were able to produce these alterations *in vitro* using liver microsomes incubated in the presence of carbon tetrachloride; in addition, they followed the production of malonic dialdehyde and monitored glucose-6-phosphatase activity under aerobic and anaerobic environments. The binding of carbon tetrachloride free radicals to microsomal lipids occurred in both environments. However, the lipids underwent peroxidation (production of malonic dialdehyde), and depression of glucose-6-phosphatase activity occurred only in the aerobic environment. These investigators concluded that peroxidative breakdown of unsaturated lipids, rather than covalent binding, was responsible for the inactivation of glucose-6-phosphatase. Glende *et al.* (1976) followed the conversion of carbon tetrachloride to chloroform *in vitro* using liver microsomes; lipid peroxidation, cytochrome P-450 content, glucose-6-phosphatase activity, and aminopyrine demethylase activity were also monitored. During the anaerobic conversion of carbon tetrachloride to chloroform no detectable diminution in cytochrome P-450 content was observed if lipid peroxidation was prevented; the activities of glucose-6-phosphatase and aminopyrine demethylase were also unaffected. When an aerobic environment was employed, loss of cytochrome P-450 accompanied the presence of lipid peroxidation (increased malonic dialdehyde production) and the activity of each enzyme decreased. Thus, the studies performed by both Benedetti *et al.* (1977c) and Glende *et al.* (1976) lead to the conclusion that the key event in carbon tetrachloride–induced alteration of microsomal enzyme activity is lipid peroxidation and not covalent binding of carbon tetrachloride–derived free radicals to microsomal lipids. However, although covalent binding of carbon tetrachloride free radicals, in itself, does not appear to be responsible for loss of enzyme activity, it appears to participate in the formation of a deranged species of microsomal lipid (Benedetti *et al.*, 1977a, 1977b, 1977c).

Alpers and coworkers (1968) studied the role of lipid peroxidation in the pathogenesis of carbon tetrachloride–induced inhibition of protein synthesis. They found that, *in vivo*, the administration of anti-oxidants did prevent the appearance of fatty livers and necrosis; however, protein synthesis, studied by the incorporation of leucine into hepatic proteins, was not altered by the administration of the antioxidant. These authors concluded that the demonstration of lipid peroxidation *in vitro* may not always imply functional damage to the subcellular component affected. They raised the possibility that *in vivo* inhibition of protein synthesis may not have a direct relationship to the degree of lipid peroxidation. There is still some controversy regarding the relative importance of carbon tetrachloride–induced lipid peroxidation in the subsequent pathologic changes and there are inconsistent results reported in the literature (Plaa and Witschi, 1976). Recknagel and Glende (1973) do recognize that there are a number of unknown factors that can contribute to cell death after lipid peroxidation has occurred; there is not a one-to-one correspondence between the initial lipid peroxidation and the eventual development of necrosis. More recently, it has been shown (Pesh-Imam *et al.*, 1978) that lipid peroxidation of microsomal lipids causes the production of diffusable and filterable toxic factors which are not free radicals, but which can lyse red blood cells or kill free-swimming protozoa. This observation opens a new way of explaining how a highly localized lipoperoxidative event could eventually alter membrane function of organelles distal from the original locus of peroxidation. The involvement of the additional factors in the pathogenesis of cellular necrosis has yet to be evaluated, but their discovery is extremely exciting.

Klaassen and Plaa (1969) studied the dose-response relationships involved in carbon tetrachloride and chloroform hepatotoxicity. They were able to confirm the presence of conjugated dienes *in vivo* after the administration of carbon tetrachloride, and also the depression of glucose-6-phosphatase activity as described previously. However, these authors were unable to show the presence of conjugated dienes after the administration of chloroform in doses that resulted in fatty livers and necrosis. Furthermore, they could find no depression of glucose-6-phosphate after administration of chloroform. Brown *et al.*, (1974) have reported that rats pretreated with phenobarbital, but not untreated rats, will produce conjugated dienes during chloroform anesthesia; depression of glucose-6-phosphatase activity also occurs after chloroform only in phenobarbital-pretreated rats (Lavigne and Marchand, 1974). Since chloroform-induced liver injury is more severe in phenobarbital-pretreated rats, the possibility exists that the initial lesion induced by chloroform in these animals is only aggravated by the appearance of lipid peroxidation. These findings cast doubt on the general applicability of lipid peroxidation as a mechanism for necrogenic halogenated hydrocarbons.

Lipid peroxidation has also been reported to occur after the administration of tetrachloroethane in mice (Tomokuni, 1970). This substance produces increases in liver triglycerides under these experimental conditions. Sell and Reynolds (1969) compared the lesion produced by iodoform to that produced by carbon tetrachloride. They found that, morphologically, the lesions were quite comparable. In addition, lipid peroxidation was found to occur within 30 minutes, being associated with a depression in glucose-6-phosphatase activity and calcium flux. There was also an increase in cell sap RNA. These findings are essentially identical to those observed after carbon tetrachloride intoxication. Lipoperoxidation has also been reported to occur after phosphorus poisoning in rats (Ghoshal *et al.*, 1969). Elevation of triglyceride levels was observed as well; however, the elevation of triglycerides was found to occur after the increases in lipid peroxidation.

Several other hepatotoxic substances have been shown to produce acute liver necrosis in the absence of *in vivo* demonstration of lipid peroxidation (Plaa and Witschi, 1976). 1,1-Dichloroethylene causes liver injury that is quite comparable to that produced by carbon tetrachloride; yet lipid peroxidation has not been observed. Dimethylnitrosamine and thioacetamide also do not seem to produce lipid peroxidation *in vivo*. There are also doubts about the importance of the phenomenon in ethylene dibromide–induced liver injury. With halothane the results obtained by Brown *et al.* (1974) are comparable to those observed with chloroform. DiLuzio (1973) proposed that lipid peroxidation also plays a role in acute ethanol-induced fatty liver. The subject is still controversial and the matter is yet to be resolved (Plaa and Witschi, 1976). While there is no doubt that lipid peroxidation does occur with some substances, it is evident that with others this factor is either absent or of doubtful significance.

Necrosis

Despite the great advances that have been made in understanding the morphologic and biochemical alterations associated with chemical-induced liver injury, it has to be realized that the knowledge acquired is still incapable of establishing which of the changes observed lead to cell death and which are secondary disturbances (Judah, 1969). This view has been shared by Farber (1971); current knowledge can inform the interested person as to what can be done to a cell and yet not destroy it. As stated by Judah (1969), "this advance in knowledge by attrition will continue."

This state of affairs has led Farber (1975) to suggest that perhaps our concepts of cell death are in error. Cell death has been considered for a long time to be a degenerative phenomenon, a "running down" of the metabolic activity of the cell. He suggests that under some conditions cell death may not be a passive event but may rather be the result of a more active process, like the overproduction of some enzyme or other protein ("cell suicide" instead of "cell homicide"). As support for this interesting concept Farber (1975) points out that cycloheximide, an inhibitor of protein synthesis, can protect certain cells against the necrogenic properties of carbon tetrachloride and α-naphthylisothiocyanate. Obviously, more work is needed to test the validity of this novel hypothesis.

Cholestasis

The mechanisms involved in drug-induced cholestasis are still very poorly understood. One of the major reasons for this deficiency lies in the fact that, with the possible exception of the steroids, it has been virtually impossible, or at least extremely difficult, to reproduce in animals the drug-induced cholestatic syndrome seen in man. However, it is possible to produce cholestatic responses in animals with certain chemicals that have no therapeutic utility. The induction of intrahepatic cholestasis in animals following the administration of certain bile salts, α-naphthylisothiocyanate (ANIT), certain steroids, and manganese has provided important contributions to the understanding of the characteristics, and perhaps the causes, of the cholestatic syndrome (Plaa and Priestly, 1976).

Lithocholic acid is a naturally occurring bile acid. In the liver, cholesterol is biotransformed to cholic and chenodeoxycholic acids. After entrance into the intestine, these bile acids can be deconjugated and converted to the so-called secondary bile acids by the intestinal flora. One of these products is lithocholic acid, a monohydroxy derivative. Javitt (1966) has demonstrated that the taurine conjugate of lithocholic acid (taurolithocholic acid) can produce acute changes in hepatic function when administered intravenously. The infusion of this substance in the rat results in a prompt diminution of bile flow and bile acid excretion. The cessation of bile flow is dose dependent and bile flow usually returns to normal within six hours. Javitt has shown that prolonged infusions of taurolithocholate result in hyperbilirubinemia. Schaffner and Javitt (1966) found that the canalicular microvilli were greatly reduced in size and number after administration of taurolithocholate; the Golgi apparatus was found to be dilated and vacuolated. Taurocholate can compete with taurolithocholate and can antagonize the cholestatic response induced by the later substance. The evidence suggests that taurolithocholate induction of cholestasis is due to its poor water solubility and precipitation of the substance in the biliary tract (Javitt and Emerman, 1968). However, recent studies (Boyer et al., 1977) indicate that this bile salt also modifies the structure and permeability of the membrane of the bile canaliculus by directly binding to components of the membrane; the role of this effect in cholestasis has not been clarified. In addition to the effects of this substance on biliary flow, taurolithocholate also causes a marked elevation in SGPT activity after its administration. This elevation in transaminase activity seems to be independent of the effect on bile flow, since it continues to appear even when cholestasis has been antagonized by the concomitant administration of taurocholate (Priestly et al., 1971). Others (Fisher et al., 1971; Miyai et al., 1971) have demonstrated cholestasis in isolated rat livers perfused with lithocholic, chenodeoxycholic, glycolithocholic, or taurolithocholic acid. The three α-sulfate esters of taurolithocholic acid and glycolithocholic acid were less cholestatic than the nonsulfated conjugates. Chenodeoxycholate causes hepatocellular necrosis in rats. Lithocholate and chenodeoxycholate differ in the mechanism by which they produce cholestasis (Plaa and Priestly, 1976). Chenodeoxycholate is cytotoxic and cholestasis seems to result from a generalized hepatocellular dysfunction, whereas lithocholate seems to interact directly with the bile secretory function of the canalicular membrane.

A single oral dose of ANIT produces both bile stasis and hyperbilirubinemia in the rat, and the cessation of bile flow occurs within 24 hours (Goldfarb et al., 1962). Electron microscopic studies carried out after acute ANIT administration have also indicated alterations of hepatocyte membrane (Rüttner *et al.*, 1964). ANIT has been found to affect several hepatocyte functions (Plaa and Priestly, 1976). In addition to the development of hyperbilirubinemia, sulfobromophthalein (BSP) retention and inhibition of microsomal drug-metabolizing activity have also been demonstrated.

The bilirubin retention induced by ANIT could be due to a number of defects in hepatic cell function (Plaa and Priestly, 1976). The maximal rate of biliary bilirubin excretion is diminished in ANIT-treated animals. ANIT can cause an increase in the synthesis of bilirubin from non-erythropoietic sources; this effect can be demonstrated two hours after the administration of ANIT. While all of these mechanisms could participate in the response, it is predominantly the decrease in biliary excretion of bilirubin that contributes to the hyperbilirubinemia observed.

There is a considerable amount of indirect evidence that indicates that the cholestatic properties of ANIT may be due to a metabolite (Plaa and Priestly, 1976). There is marked species variation; both the cholestatic and hyperbilirubinemic responses can be potentiated if the animals are pretreated with enzyme inducers; inhibitors of microsomal enzyme activity have been shown to diminish the ANIT response; temperature can also effect the response; inhibitors of protein synthesis have been shown to markedly reduce the cholestatic and hyperbilirubinemic responses to ANIT.

The cholestatic reaction associated with the clinical use of anabolic and contraceptive steroids has prompted experimental studies designed to characterize the response in animals. Although some canalicular dilatation has been observed in rats after administration of norethandrolone (Schaffner *et al.*, 1960), definite manifestations of intrahepatic cholestasis, such as hyperbilirubinemia and canalicular bile plugs, have not been established as norethandrolone effects in rats. Imai and Hayashi (1970) have reported that large doses of norethisterone produce jaundice consistently in mice. Canalicular bile plugs were observed after treatment with norethisterone, methyltestosterone, oxymetholone, mestranol, or norethandrolone. No plugs were observed when testosterone proprionate, progesterone, or 17β-estradiol was administered. Electron microscopy revealed dilatation of the bile canaliculi and a decrease in the appearance of microvilli. Various strains of male mice were shown to respond similarly; DS and C57BL strains were the most sensitive, whereas ICR mice were the least sensitive. Sprague-Dawley rats did not exhibit cholestasis, even when treated with larger doses of norethisterone. These observations indicate a species variation

and even a difference between strains. Anabolic steroids do cause BSP retention in rabbits (Lennon, 1966). With ethinyl estradiol, reduced bile flow was observed in rats (Gumucio and Valdivieso, 1971). Estrogens appear to be able to affect the permeability of the biliary tree, reduce bile salt–independent bile flow, and decrease the clearance of infused bile salts (Plaa and Priestly, 1976); it is not clear which parameter is of major importance in producing the cholestatic reaction. With various oral contraceptive steroids, decreased bile flow and a decrease in biliary excretory maximum for bilirubin have been reported (Heikel and Lathe, 1970), but the mechanism has not been elucidated.

Intrahepatic cholestasis can also be produced in rats by the administration of an intravenous load of manganese sulfate (Witzleben, 1972). This response is associated with the development of necrotic lesions, which varies from focal necrosis to subtotal midzonal necrosis. Widespread dilatation of bile canaliculi with loss of microvilli is observed 20 hours after treatment. The maximum biliary excretion of bilirubin is markedly diminished in the manganese-loaded rats; there is no correlation between the extent of necrosis and the cholestatic response. Manganese treatment followed by bilirubin infusion can cause a more severe cholestasis; recovery of bile flow is partial at 24 hours and essentially complete at 48 hours. Small doses of manganese produce cholestasis only if followed by an injection of bilirubin; a close relationship exists between manganese and bilirubin in order to elicit the fully developed cholestatic response (Klaassen, 1974; de Lamirande and Plaa, 1979).

In 1963, Keysser and coworkers reported that ethylphenylbutyramide could produce intrahepatic cholestasis in dogs. Bile plugs were observed in the bile canaliculi, but no significant changes were seen in the hepatic parenchymal cells. The dogs also demonstrated BSP retention. By electron microscopy it was possible to show that the canaliculus exhibited distended microvilli. Electron-dense material was also present in some canaliculi and in the Golgi apparatus. This substance also produces the same effect in rats; however, a much higher dose is required to produce cytochemical and electron microscopic changes in the liver (Williams *et al.*, 1964).

There is still considerable controversy as to whether phenothiazines and tricyclic antidepressants cause cholestasis in humans because of a direct toxic effect or because of a hypersensitivity reaction. These compounds have been the subject of extensive investigation in animals (Plaa and Priestly, 1976). There seems to be important species variation in chlorpromazine-induced hepatobiliary dysfunction. In the dog and rhesus monkey, a reduction in bile flow has been reported after its acute intravenous administration, whereas neither acute nor chronic administration has resulted in cholestasis in rats. The morphologic features of phenothiazine-induced cholestasis observed in humans have not been produced in laboratory animals. This lends credence to the hypersensitivity hypothesis.

With erythromycin estolate the data obtained with animals are very limited (Plaa and Priestly, 1976). Cytotoxicity, related to surfactant properties, was observed *in vitro* using preparations of isolated hepatocytes; reduced bile flow in the isolated perfused rat liver was also reported.

A number of mechanisms leading to cholestasis have been proposed based on various experimental results, but these are far from being definitive (Plaa and Priestly, 1976). These include impaired bile salt–independent canalicular bile flow (chlorpromazine, ethinylestradiol, ethacrynic acid), canalicular membrane function (ANIT, taurolithocholate, cytochalasin B), altered ductular cell permeability (ANIT), hypertrophic hypoactive smooth endoplasmic reticulum (bile salts, ANIT), and intracanalicular precipitation (taurolithocholate, chlorpromazine, erythromycin lactobionate).

Cirrhosis

Cirrhosis is a chronic morphologic alteration of the liver that has received a great amount of attention. No attempt will be made to cover the vast amount of literature pertaining to this liver lesion. Histologically cirrhosis is characterized by the presence of septae of collagen distributed throughout the major portion of the liver (Schinella and Becker, 1975). These appear to form fibrous sheaths in a three-dimensional network, which appear as bands in a two-dimensional histologic section; the circumscribed areas of aggregated liver cells appear as nodules. Invariably the pattern of hepatic blood flow is altered. In the majority of cases, single-cell necrosis appears as the major element in its pathogenesis. This necrotic process is associated with a deficiency in the repair mechanism of the residual cells; this deficiency leads to fibroblastic activity and scar formation. The pathogenesis of cirrhosis is not at all clearly understood. Other factors, such as intrahepatic vascular alterations, may play a contributory role in the development of cirrhosis.

Cirrhosis can be induced in animals by chronic administration of carbon tetrachloride, aflatoxin, or the administration of several chemical carcinogens. In humans, however, the single most important cause of cirrhosis is the chronic ingestion of alcoholic beverages (Lelbach, 1975; Rankin *et al.*, 1975). In the usual laboratory animal the production of cirrhosis, as seen in humans, is not possible by the chronic feeding of ethanol alone (Schinella and Becker, 1975). However, precirrhotic changes (increased hydroxyproline, increased proline incorporation into collagen, and increased collagen proline hydroxylase activity) have been observed after ethanol ingestion (Middleton *et al.*, 1975). Recently, Lieber and DeCarli (1976) reported the production of cirrhosis in baboons after long-term feeding of ethanol.

For a number of decades a controversy has existed whether ethanol itself causes cirrhosis in humans by a direct hepatotoxic effect or whether the nutritional deficiency, which is closely associated with alcoholism, is the primary cause (Hartroft, 1975; Lieber, 1975). In part, the major reason for evoking the element of nutritional deficiency has been the lack of success experienced when attempting to produce cirrhosis by feeding ethanol to animals maintained on an otherwise nutritionally adequate diet. The proponents of the nutrition theory (Hartroft, 1975) indicate that in dogs and rats the development of cirrhosis depends on the duration of the consumption of ethanol, the percentage of total calories provided by ethanol, and the composition of the accompanying diet; diets that are inadequate in choline, proteins, methionine, vitamin B_{12}, and folic acid favor the development of cirrhosis. Supplementation of the diets with these nutrients appears to abolish the effect of long-term feeding of ethanol. The proponents of the direct hepatotoxic theory (Lieber, 1975) emphasize the requirement of long-term ingestion of large quantities of ethanol by animals on nutritionally adequate diets, and the demonstrated effects of precirrhotic changes in the various animal models. Perhaps the usual laboratory species employed are more resistant to ethanol than are humans. The development of cirrhosis in the baboon (Lieber and DeCarli, 1976) maintained on an otherwise nutritionally adequate diet lends considerable weight in favor of the direct hepatotoxic theory. In any event, this new animal model may permit a better understanding of the pathogenesis of ethanol-induced cirrhosis.

Carcinogenesis

The problem of chemical carcinogenesis is covered elsewhere in detail (see Chapter 6). Consequently, only a cursory view of hepatocarcinogenesis will be described in this section.

A wide variety of chemicals have been shown to elicit carcinogenic changes in laboratory animals (Farber *et al.*, 1975; Wogan, 1976). In humans, however, apart from possibly vinyl chloride, no direct evidence exists that establishes any single chemical agent as the causative factor for liver cancer (Wogan, 1976). The evidence for humans appear to be largely indirect, the result of extrapolation or conclusions drawn on the basis of limited epidemiologic studies. Among naturally occurring substances that are liver carcinogens in animals one finds aflatoxin B_1 and other mycotoxins, some pyrrolizidine alkaloids, cycasin, and safrole. Among synthetic substances one finds some dialkylnitrosamines, some organochlorine pesticides, certain polychlorinated biphenyls, carbon tetrachloride, chloroform, vinyl chloride, dimethylaminoazobenzene, acetylaminofluorene, thioacetamide, urethane, ethionine, dimethylbenzanthracene, and galactosamine.

There is increasing evidence that chemical hepatocarcinogens do not induce cancer but rather initiate a chain of events that results in cancer (Farber, 1976). The initiating event may be a mutation, but perturbations in cell differentiation may also be involved. Many hepatocarcinogens interact with virtually all cell organelles; yet evidence is lacking that these changes play a major role as the precursor lesion. The acute inhibition of cell proliferation has been suggested to be of importance; perhaps this leads to an altered cell population that can grow in the presence of a cytotoxic environment (cell selection). The morphologic characteristics of hepatocellular carcinomas present a continuous spectrum from the highly differentiated to the anaplastic pattern. Organizationally, the hepatocytes are not arranged as in the normal adult liver, but assume a "pseudofetal" configuration; this organizational difference also expresses itself in biochemical patterns (emergence of fetal isozymes, production of α-fetoprotein and fetal antigens). Each individual neoplasm is unique (pattern of enzymes, antigenic composition, morphologic appearance), and this property is consistent with the hypothesis of an origin from a single clone of cells.

After initiation a long latent period (6 to 24 months in the rat) occurs before the liver cancer becomes evident. During this period ductular cell proliferation, hepatocytic changes, and hyperplastic nodules are observed. Farber (1976) proposes that the histogenesis of hepatocellular carcinoma involves a series of altered or new hepatocytic populations that evolve into malignant neoplasia; each population develops from its immediate precursor by a process of selection. At least four such populations appear as likely steps: enzyme-deficient foci, early hyperplastic nodules, late hyperplastic nodules, and hyperbasophilic foci. These could be pictured as proceeding in an ordered sequence from the target cell. However, an alternative scheme states that each new cell population is derived from the target cell, but is independent and unrelated to the others. The validity of either hypothesis is yet to be determined.

Little is known about the selection process that favors the development of malignant hepatocytes. Perhaps resistance to necrosis develops (selective cytotoxicity). Endogenous and exogenous modulating factors are known to affect the incidence and time of appearance of liver cancers; these include nutrients, hormones, drugs, and other chemicals. Their roles are very poorly understood as are immunologic factors and the presence of cirrhosis. The absence of such knowledge greatly limits extrapolation of results obtained in animals under controlled conditions to humans exposed in undefined conditions.

FACTORS INVOLVED IN LIVER INJURY

Biotransformation of Toxicants

The phenomenon of biotransformation to a more active metabolite is well known in pharmacology. It is now known to occur with hepatotoxic substances. There is considerable evidence that carbon tetrachloride is metabolized in the liver. McCollister and associates (1951) showed that a nonvolatile product could be detected in the urine of monkeys treated with carbon tetrachloride. They also demonstrated the formation of CO_2 from this substance. Butler (1961) showed that carbon tetrachloride was reduced to chloroform *in vivo*. It is now clear that the toxicity of carbon tetrachloride depends on cleavage of the carbon-chlorine bond. The work of a number of investigators (Recknagel and Glende, 1973) has led to the following observations: the cleavage occurs in the endoplasmic reticulum and is mediated by the mixed function oxidase system; carbon tetrachloride forms a type I binding spectrum with cytochrome P-450; NADPH-dependent flavoproteins do not appear to be involved; the products of the homolytic cleavage can become incorporated into microsomal lipids; free radical scavengers and lipid antioxidants protect against the liver injury; inducers of cytochrome P-450 can enhance liver injury. Stenger and Johnson (1971) showed that the enhancing effect of phenobarbital was due to an increase in the activity of hepatic drug–metabolizing enzymes and not only to the presence of proliferated hepatic smooth-surfaced endoplasmic reticulum. In rabbits, chloroform, hexachloroethane, and two other chlorinated metabolites have been found in various tissues 48 hours after the administration of carbon tetrachloride (Fowler, 1969).

The conversion of carbon tetrachloride to chloroform has also been measured in the liver of rats following inhalation of carbon tetrachloride (Dambrauskas and Cornish, 1970). These investigators were studying the development of tolerance of rats to subsequent doses of carbon tetrachloride. They found that animals preexposed to the halogenated hydrocarbons were resistant to the lethal and hepatotoxic effects of this substance. By whole-body and liver analyses, they were able to show that, in the tolerant rat, the amount of carbon tetrachloride converted to chloroform was significantly diminished. This delay in the conversion to chloroform was also demonstrated *in vitro* in livers from animals sacrificed after preexposure to carbon tetrachloride.

Chloroform has also been shown to be metabolized enzymatically by the liver (Paul and Rubinstein, 1963), and it was shown that glutathione activated the oxidation of chloroform (Rubinstein and Kanics, 1964). The hepatotoxicity of chloroform is augmented by phenobarbital pretreatment, and concomitantly chloroform markedly depletes hepatic glutathione in phenobarbital-treated rats, but not in normal animals (Docks and Krishna, 1976). Covalent binding of radiolabel derived from chloroform to microsomal proteins was shown *in vitro* and glutathione diminished the response. Free-radical intermediates have also been proposed to arise during chloroform activation (Brown *et al.*, 1974). Two groups of investigators (Mansuy *et al.*, 1977; Pohl *et al.*, 1977) demonstrated that *in vitro* microsomes derived from phenobarbital-treated rats were capable of converting chloroform to phosgene, a highly reactive electrophilic compound. They proposed that this activation proceeds through the hydroxylation of chloroform to trichloromethanol, which spontaneously dehydrochlorinates to produce phosgene. It has been concluded that the site of activation is cytochrome P-450 rather than NADPH cytochrome c reductase (Sipes *et al.*, 1977).

Biotransformation has also been shown to be important in the case of hepatic lesions produced by bromobenzene. In 1953, Koch-Weser and coworkers demonstrated that bromobenzene in rats produced centrilobular necrosis. The lesion could be prevented by the coadministration of cysteine and methionine, whereas the lesion was aggravated by prior fasting. When the animals were protected, urinary mercapturic acid rose. It was concluded that the liver injury produced by bromobenzene was due to a preferential depletion of cysteine and methionine caused by the conjugation of bromobenzene to mercapturic acid. Brodie and coworkers (1971) postulated that the necrosis was produced by an active metabolite of bromobenzene, presumably an epoxide, capable of reacting covalently with macromolecules in the liver cells. They showed that liver microsomes could convert bromobenzene into a compound that reacted covalently with glutathione. Furthermore, it was possible to show that inhibitors of microsomal drug-metabolizing enzymes, SKF 525-A or piperonyl butoxide, prevented the liver necrosis and that phenobarbital induction enhanced the liver injury

(Reid *et al.*, 1971). With phenobarbital, increased formation of mercapturic acids was seen. It was postulated that the epoxide formation is so great that normal amounts of glutathione cannot protect the tissue proteins from the alkylating agent. In this regard, diethyl maleate, which depletes hepatic glutathione, increases the incidence of hepatic lesions produced by low doses of bromobenzene. It appears that in bromobenzene necrosis, the toxic metabolite is bromobenzene epoxide; this metabolite is further degraded through the action of glutathione transferase and epoxide hydratase (Mitchell *et al.*, 1976a).

Acetaminophen-induced hepatotoxicity is also caused by a chemically reactive metabolite (Mitchell *et al.*, 1976a). The formation of this metabolite can be followed by the irreversible binding of radiolabel, derived from the acetaminophen, to liver protein. Little covalent binding occurs after subtoxic doses but it increases as the dose approaches the toxic range. Inducers of microsomal mixed-function oxidase enhance formation of the reactive metabolite and liver toxicity, whereas inhibitors reduce metabolite formation and toxicity. The reactive intermediate is further conjugated with glutathione and excreted as a mercapturic acid.

The experimental work carried out to unravel acetaminophen- and bromobenzene-induced liver injury has led to some very important observations. One is that hepatotoxicity need not be correlated with the pharmacokinetics of the parent substance or even its major metabolites, but may be correlated with the formation of quantitatively minor, highly reactive, intermediates. A second concept is that a threshold tissue concentration must be attained before liver injury is elicited; if it is not attained, injury does not occur. Third, endogenous substances like glutathione play an essential role in protecting hepatocytes from injury by chemically reactive intermediates; this provides the cell with a means of preventing the reactive metabolite from attaining a critical, effective concentration. Finally, other enzymic pathways, like glutathione transferase and epoxide hydratase, also play a role in protecting the hepatocyte by catalyzing the further degradation of the toxic reactive intermediates. Furthermore, these studies have provided investigators relatively simple biochemical procedures for uncovering the possible existence of potentially toxic chemically reactive metabolites or intermediates in new compounds. A better understanding of species variations in response to potential hepatotoxins is now possible using pharmacokinetics (Gillette, 1977).

The production of reactive metabolites that bind irreversibly to hepatic proteins has also been observed in animals with furosemide and acetyl-isoniazid (Mitchell *et al.*, 1976a). With furosemide a dose threshold exists for both necrosis and co-valent binding, but the threshold in mice is not due to depletion of hepatic glutathione. Apparently the threshold is caused by a change in the proportion of unchanged compound that is eliminated. At subthreshold doses most of the furosemide is highly bound to plasma proteins and eventually eliminated unchanged, whereas with high doses plasma binding becomes saturated and more furosemide becomes available for hepatic biotransformation. In the case of acetylisoniazid, the major metabolite of isoniazid, increased covalent binding to liver proteins and enhanced hepatotoxicity were observed in phenobarbital-pretreated rats; enhanced covalent binding was also observed with iproniazid. In both cases the reactive metabolites are thought to be free radicals arising from monoalkyl diazenes (Mitchell *et al.*, 1976b).

Other hepatotoxic responses have been shown to be due to the production of a toxic metabolite. The biotransformation of dimethylnitrosamine is linked to its hepatotoxic effect (Magee and Swann, 1969). The pyrrolizidine alkaloids in "bush teas" made from *Crotalaria fulva* result in venoocclusive hepatic disease. These substances are said to be converted to toxic metabolites in the liver (Mattocks, 1968). The cholestatic response produced by α-naphthylisothio-cyanate was enhanced by administering inducers of microsomal enzymes (Plaa and Priestly, 1976). Allyl alcohol and its precursor allyl formate produce periportal necrosis (Rouiller, 1964; Reid, 1972). Rees and Tarlow (1967) have shown that allyl formate is converted to a highly reactive aldehyde, acrolein, by alcohol dehydrogenase. Hepatotoxic reactive metabolites have been proposed (Hunter *et al.*, 1977) for thioacetamide and thioacetamide sulfite, the major metabolite of thioacetamide, to account for their acute necrogenic effects. Biotransformation has also been invoked to explain why halothane produces acute necrotic lesions only when this agent is given to animals pretreated with inducers of hepatic mixed-function oxidases (Brown *et al.*, 1974; Reynolds and Moslen, 1977). Reduced oxygen tensions enhance the hepatotoxicity and bioactivation of halothane (Brown and Sipes, 1977). The formation of a reactive epoxide has been proposed to account for the acute focal necrosis seen in rats given aflatoxin B_1; the biochemical characteristics of this epoxide are said to be similar to those described for bromobenzene epoxide (Mgbodile *et al.*, 1975).

Alteration of Hepatic Blood Flow

With some hepatotoxins it is possible to observe alterations in hepatic blood flow as a result of the injury. These alterations manifest themselves 24 hours or more after the injury. Hemorrhagic necrosis has been observed in rats after the administration of beryllium (Cheng,

1956). Dimethylnitrosamine produces hemorrhagic necrosis, where the center of the lobule becomes entirely occupied by blood (Barns and Magee, 1954). This "veno-occlusive" lesion can be observed ten days after administration of the substance (Magee and Swann, 1969). Similar lesions have been observed in animals and children ingesting *Crotalaria*, a pyrrolizidine alkaloid (Magee and Swann, 1969; McLean, 1970). This lesion seems to be a characteristic of those substances that produce hemorrhagic necrosis and are not typically found after administration of carbon tetrachloride. Butler and Hard (1971) attribute this to the fact that carbon tetrachloride induces a coagulative necrosis of the hepatocytes that does not affect the sinusoid lining cells, permitting the retention of an intact vascular pattern; however, dimethylnitrosamine affects both the parenchymal cells and the sinusoid lining cells, resulting in hemorrhage and a collapse of the trabecular reticulin framework around the central veins.

Himsworth (1954) postulated that carbon tetrachloride could act directly on hepatic cells and that this would cause swelling, resulting in a mechanical obstruction of sinusoidal blood flow. He felt that the cells distal to the swelling would become hypoxic and this would result in necrosis. However, Daniel and coworkers (1952), using radiographic techniques, could demonstrate no alteration in the blood flow of the liver. Stoner (1956), using the heated thermo-couple technique for indirectly measuring blood flow, was unable to show a diminution in hepatic blood flow after the administration of carbon tetrachloride or dimethylnitrosamine. In fact, an actual increase in flow was observed during the process of necrosis. In cats, the data indicate that diminished hepatic blood flow is not a causative factor in the initial phase of carbon tetrachloride liver injury and at a later time points an increased hepatic arterial blood flow was observed (Lautt and Plaa, 1974).

In 1960, Calvert and Brody put forth the idea that hepatic vasoconstriction, due to the elaboration of catecholamines, was the primary effect of carbon tetrachloride. The hypothesis was based on indirect evidence. High spinal cord transection at the level of C6 or C7 protected rats against the necrotic effects of carbon tetrachloride. Larson and Plaa (1965) showed that cordotomy resulted in hypothermia. They also showed that if cord-transected animals were placed in an incubator to maintain their body temperature, carbon tetrachloride was quite capable of producing its hepatic necrotic effects. Oxygen consumption of transected rats maintained at room temperature dropped markedly. It would thus appear that in hypothermic rats metabolic activity of the liver was diminished and this would explain the apparent protective effects of cervical cordotomy. Large infusions of norepinephrine, epinephrine, or mixtures of these substances did not result in lesions similar to those produced by carbon tetrachloride. Finally, in rats sympathectomized immunologically the hepatic lesion induced by carbon tetrachloride was still present (Larson *et al.*, 1965). Therefore, it appears that the vascular role attributed to carbon tetrachloride via release of catecholamines must be rejected as a primary cause of hepatic injury.

Potentiation of Hepatotoxicity

It is now well established that subjects exposed to several chemical agents simultaneously can exhibit altered pharmacologic or toxicologic responses. The effect of a second drug can have a marked influence on the response elicited by a previously administered drug and vice versa. In the field of therapeutics such drug interactions have been well described. With hepatotoxicity, interactions have been observed. Many of these have led to the discovery that biotransformation to a more active metabolite is involved in the hepatotoxic response.

In addition to these, other instances of potentiation of hepatotoxicity have been described. Individuals recovering from an acute ingestion of ethanol seem to be more susceptible to the liver-damaging properties of the halogenated hydrocarbons than do individuals not ingesting ethanol. Since the early investigators studying this phenomenon in animals used simultaneous administration of both agents, the explanation seemed to be that ethanol enhanced the absorption of the hydrocarbon (Stewart *et al.*, 1960). However, Guild and coworkers (1958) reported that ingestion of ethanol several hours before exposure to the hydrocarbons caused an enhanced toxic response. The latter phenomenon has been shown to be true in mice, rats, and dogs. The halogenated hydrocarbons that have been shown to exert an enhanced hepatotoxic response after ethanol pretreatment include carbon tetrachloride, chloroform, trichloroethylene, and 1,1,2-trichloroethane (Klaassen and Plaa, 1967).

Cornish and Adefuin (1967) showed that several aliphatic alcohols, such as methanol, ethanol, isopropanol, *n*-butanol, *sec*-butanol, and *tert*-butanol, also exert a similar potentiating effect on the acute inhalation toxicity of carbon tetrachloride. Several examples of potentiation

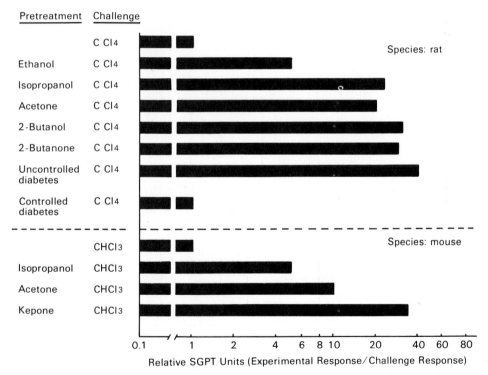

Figure 10–3. Potentiation of haloalkane-induced hepatotoxicity. Rats or mice were subjected to the specified various pretreatments before receiving a challenge dose of carbon tetrachloride or chloroform. Diabetes was produced by administering alloxan, either alone (*Uncontrolled*) or with insulin (*Controlled*). The severity of the liver injury was assessed 24 hours after the haloalkane challenge using serum glutamic pyruvic transaminase (SGPT) activity. Relative SGPT units were obtained by dividing the activity in the experimental group (Pretreatment plus Challenge) by the activity in the respective control group (Challenge alone). The details of each study can be found in the following references: Hewitt *et al.*, 1979; Traiger and Bruckner, 1976; Plaa *et al.*, 1975; Hanasono *et al.*, 1975a; Traiger and Plaa, 1974.

are depicted in Figure 10–3. The remarkable potentiating effect of isopropanol has been studied in detail (Plaa *et al.*, 1975), and it has been shown that the biotransformation of isopropanol to acetone plays a crucial role. Acetone itself can potentiate carbon tetrachloride hepatotoxicity. With ethanol the potentiation seems to be due to the presence of the unmetabolized alcohol; however, with isopropanol the effect seems to be caused by the presence of both unmetabolized alcohol and acetone. The results obtained with *n*-butanol resemble those of ethanol, whereas with 2-butanol they resemble those of isopropanol. It is interesting that 2-butanol is also metabolized to a ketone (2-butanone; methylethyl ketone) as is isopropanol (Traiger and Bruckner, 1976). The mechanisms underlying the potentiation observed are not known. However, it appears that somehow the interaction could be located within the enzyme systems associated with the endoplasmic reticulum. With isopropanol and acetone one could attempt to explain the potentiation on the basis of enhanced bioactivation of carbon tetrachloride (Sipes *et al.*, 1973). However, when one considers the quantitative aspects of the potentiation this explanation does not appear to be complete, and one wonders whether isopropanol and acetone alter the hepatic organelles in such a way that they become more susceptible to the injurious properties of carbon tetrachloride–derived free radicals (Côté *et al.*, 1974).

The interaction between isopropanol and carbon tetrachloride has been documented in an industrial accident in an isopropanol packaging plant, where workers exposed to both agents exhibited hepatotoxicity (Folland *et al.*, 1976). Isopropanol and acetone also cause enhanced hepatotoxicity in mice given chloroform, trichloroethylene, 1,1,2-trichloroethane, or 1,1,1-trichloroethane (Plaa *et al.*, 1975). So the interaction is not limited to carbon tetrachloride. A similar interaction has been observed in rats pretreated with 2-butanol or 2-butanone (Fig. 10–3) and challenged with carbon tetrachloride (Traiger and Bruckner, 1976). Recent results (Hewitt *et al.*, 1979) indicate that kepone can potentiate chloroform hepatotoxicity in mice (Fig. 10–3).

Experimentally, it was shown (Hanasono *et al.*, 1975a) that diabetes induced in rats by either alloxan or streptozotocin enhances the hepatotoxicity of carbon tetrachloride (Fig. 10–3). Reversal of the diabetic state by insulin treatment prevented the potentiated response. Alloxan-induced diabetes also enhanced the response to chloroform, 1,1,2-trichloroethane, and galactosamine (Hanasono *et al.*, 1975b). The mechanisms

underlying these potentiations have not been elucidated. However, one possible explanation would be that intrahepatic formation of ketone bodies, because of the uncontrolled diabetic state, enhances either the bioactivation process or alters the susceptibility of the organelles in a manner similar to what has been suggested to explain the enhanced response produced by acetone. Ketoacidosis occurs in alcoholism (Isselbacher, 1977) and perhaps this is involved in the enhancement of hepatotoxicity observed with ethanol. It is obvious that a considerable amount of work remains before these questions can be answered.

REFERENCES

Alpers, D. H., and Isselbacher, K. J.: The effect of carbon tetrachloride on rat-liver lysosomes. *Biochim. Biophys. Acta*, 137:33–42, 1967.

Alpers, D. H.; Solin, M.; and Isselbacher, K. J.: The role of lipid peroxidation in the pathogenesis of carbon tetrachloride-induced liver injury. *Mol. Pharmacol.*, 4:566–73, 1968.

Anthony, D. A.; Schaffner, F.; Popper, H.; and Hutterer, F.: Effect of cortisone on hepatic structure during subacute ethionine intoxication in the rat: An electron microscopic study. *Exp. Mol. Pathol.*, 1:113–21, 1962.

Baccino, F. M.; Cantino, D.; and Zuretti, M. F.: Studies on the hepatotoxicity of *Amanita phalloides* in the rat. I. Liver cell vacuolation. *Exp. Mol. Pathol.*, 24:159–75, 1976.

Baccino, F. M.; Rita, G. A.; and Dianzani, M. U.: Further experiments on the action of CCl₄ on lysosomes in vitro. *Enzymologia*, 29:169–84, 1965.

Baglio, C. M., and Farber, E.: Reversal by adenine of the induced lipid accumulation in the endoplasmic reticulum of the rat liver. *J. Cell Biol.*, 27:591–601, 1965.

Barnes, J. M., and Magee, P. N.: Some toxic properties of dimethylnitrosamine. *Br. J. Ind. Med.*, 11:167–74, 1954.

Benedetti, A.; Casini, A. F.; Ferrali, M.; and Comporti, M.: Early alterations induced by carbon tetrachloride in the lipids of the membranes of the endoplasmic reticulum of the liver cell. I. Separation and partial characterization of altered lipids. *Chem.-Biol. Interactions*, 17:151–66, 1977a.

Benedetti, A.; Casini, A. F.; Ferrali, M.; and Comporti, M.: Early alterations induced by carbon tetrachloride in the lipids of the membranes of the endoplasmic reticulum of the liver cell. II. Distribution of the alterations in the various lipid fractions. *Chem.-Biol. Interactions*, 17:167–83, 1977b.

———: Studies on the relationships between carbon tetrachloride-induced alterations of liver microsomal lipids and impairment of glucose-6-phosphatase activity. *Exp. Mol. Pathol.*, 27:309–23, 1977c.

Boyer, J. L.; Layden, T. J; and Hruban, Z.: Mechanisms of cholestasis—taurolithocholate alters canalicular membrane composition, structure and permeability. In Popper, H.; Biachi, L.; and Reutter, W. (eds.): *Membrane Alterations as Basis of Liver Injury*. MTP Press Ltd., Lancaster, 1977, pp. 353–69.

Brodie, B. B.; Reid, W. D.; Cho, A. K.; Sipes, G.; Krishan, G.; and Gillette, J. R.: Possible mechanism of liver necrosis caused by aromatic organic compounds. *Proc. Natl. Acad. Sci. U.S.A.*, 68:160–64, 1971.

Brown, B. R. and Sipes, I. G.: Biotransformation and hepatotoxicity of halothane. *Biochem. Pharmacol.* **26**:2091–94, 1977.

Brown, B. R., Jr.; Sipes, I. G.; and Sagalyn, A. M.: Mechanisms of acute hepatic toxicity: Chloroform, halothane, and glutathione. *Anesthesiology*, **41**:554–61, 1974.

Bucher, N. L. R., and Malt, R. A.: *Regeneration of Liver and Kidney.* Little, Brown & Co., Boston, 1971, pp. 135–37.

Butler, T. C.: Reduction of carbon tetrachloride in vivo and chloroform in vitro by tissues and tissue constituents. *J. Pharmacol. Exp. Ther.*, **134**:311–19, 1961.

Butler, W. H., and Hard, G. C.: Hepatotoxicity of dimethylnitrosamine in the rat with special reference to veno-occlusive disease. *Exp. Mol. Pathol.*, **15**:209–19, 1971.

Calvert, D. N., and Brody, T. N.: Role of the sympathetic nervous system in CCl₄ hepatotoxicity. *Am. J. Physiol.*, **198**:669–76, 1960.

Cheng, K. K.: Experimental studies on the mechanism of the zonal distribution of beryllium liver necrosis. *J. Pathol. Bacteriol.*, **71**:265–76, 1956.

Christie, G. S., and Judah, J. D.: Mechanism of action of carbon tetrachloride on liver cells. *Proc. Roy. Soc. Ser. B*, **142**:241–57, 1954.

Comporti, M.; Saccocci, C.; and Dianzani, M. U.: Effect of CCl₄ in vitro and in vivo on lipid peroxidation of rat liver homogenates and subcellular fractions. *Enzymologia*, **29**:185–204, 1965.

Cornish, H. H., and Adefuin, J.: Potentiation of carbon tetrachloride toxicity by aliphatic alcohols. *Arch. Environ. Health*, **14**:447–49, 1967.

Côté, M. G.; Traiger, G. J.; and Plaa, G. L.: Effect of isopropanol-induced potentiation of carbon tetrachloride on rat hepatic ultrastructure. *Toxicol. Appl. Pharmacol.*, **30**:14–25, 1974.

Dambrauskas, T., and Cornish, H. H.: Effect of pretreatment of rats with carbon tetrachloride on tolerance development. *Toxicol. Appl. Pharmacol.*, **17**:83–97, 1970.

Daniel, P. M.; Pritchard, M. M. L.; and Reynell, P. C.: The portal circulation in rats with liver-cells damage. *J. Pathol. Bacteriol.*, **64**:61–64, 1952.

Decker, K., and Keppler, D.: Galactosamine hepatitis: Key role of the nucleotide deficiency period in the pathogenesis of cell injury and cell death. *Pharmacol. Rev. Physiol. Biochem.*, **71**:77–106, 1974.

de Lamirande, E., and Plaa, G. L.: Dose and time relationships in manganese-biliriubin cholestasis. *Toxicol. Appl. Pharmacol.*, **49**:257–63, 1979.

Dianzani, M. U.: Toxic liver injury by protein synthesis inhibitors. In Popper, H., and Schaffner, F. (eds.): *Progress in Liver Diseases*, Vol. 5. Grune & Stratton, New York, 1976, pp. 232–45.

———: Uncoupling of oxidative phosphorylation in mitochondria from fatty livers. *Biochim. Biophys. Acta*, **14**:514–32, 1954.

———: Lysosome changes in liver injury. In de Reuck, A. V. S., and Cameron, M. P. (eds.): *Ciba Symposium on Lysosomes.* Little, Brown & Co., Boston, 1963, pp. 335–52.

Dianzani, M. U., and Bahr, G. F.: Electron microscope investigation of mitochondria isolated from normal and steatotic livers by differential centrifugation. *Acta Pathol. Microbiol. Scand.*, **35**:25–38, 1954.

DiLuzio, N. R.: Antioxidants, lipid peroxidation and chemical-induced liver injury. *Fed. Proc.*, **32**:1875–81, 1973.

DiLuzio, N. R., and Costales, F.: Inhibition of the ethanol and carbon tetrachloride induced fatty liver by antioxidants. *Exp. Mol. Pathol.*, **4**:141–54, 1965.

DiLuzio, N. R., and Hartman, A. D.: The effect of ethanol and carbon tetrachloride administration on hepatic lipid-soluble antioxidant activity. *Exp. Mol. Pathol.*, **11**:38–52, 1969.

Dinman, B. D., and Bernstein, I. A.: Acute carbon tetrachloride hepatotoxicity. IV. Liver and serum enzyme activity during the acute damage phase. *Arch. Environ. Health*, **16**:770–76, 1968a.

———: Acute carbon tetrachloride hepatotoxicity. V. Enzymatic and structural concomitants during the regenerative phase. *Arch. Environ. Health*, **16**:777–84, 1968b.

Dinman, B. D.; Hamdi, E. A.; Fox, C. F.; and Frajola, W. J.: CCl₄ toxicity. III. Hepatostructural and enzymatic change. *Arch. Environ. Health*, **7**:630–46, 1963.

Docks, E. L., and Krishna, G.: The role of glutathione in chloroform-induced hepatotoxicity. *Exp. Mol. Pathol.*, **24**:13–22, 1976.

Drill, V. A.: Hepatotoxic agents: Mechanism of action and dietary interrelationship. *Pharmacol. Rev.*, **4**:1–42, 1952.

Emmelot, P., and Benedetti, E. L.: Changes in the fine structure of rat liver brought about by dimethylnitrosamine. *J. Biophys. Biochem. Cytol.*, **7**:393–96, 1960.

Farber, E.: Biochemical pathology. *Annu. Rev. Pharmacol.*, **11**:71–96, 1971.

———: Some fundamental aspects of liver injury. In Khanna, J. M., Israel, Y., and Kalant, H. (eds.): *Alcoholic Liver Pathology.* Addiction Research Foundation, Toronto, 1975, pp. 289–303.

———: The pathology of experimental liver cell cancer. In Cameron, H. M.; Linsell, D. A.; and Warwick, G. P. (eds.): *Liver Cell Cancer.* Elsevier, Amsterdam, 1976, pp. 243–77.

Farber, E.; Liang, H.; and Shinozuka, H.: Dissociation of effects on protein synthesis and ribosomes from membrane changes induced by carbon tetrachloride. *Am. J. Pathol.*, **64**:601–22, 1971.

Farber, E.; Sarma, D. S. R.; Rajalakshmi, S.; and Shinozuka, H.: Liver carcinogenesis: A unifying hypothesis. In Becker, F. F. (ed.): *The Liver: Normal and Abnormal Functions*, Part B. Marcel Dekker, Inc., New York, 1975, pp. 755–71.

Farber, E.; Shull, K. H.; Villa-Trevino, S.; Lombardi, and Thomas, M.: Biochemical pathology of acute hepatic adenosinetriphosphate deficiency. *Nature* (*Lond.*), **203**:34–40, 1964.

Fisher, M. M.; Magnusson, R.; and Miyai, K.: Bile acid metabolism in mammals. I. Bile acid-induced intrahepatic cholestasis. *Lab. Invest.*, **21**:88–91, 1971.

Folland, D. S.; Schaffner, W.; Grinn, H. E.; Crofford, O. B.; and McMurray, D. R.: Carbon tetrachloride toxicity potentiated by isopropyl alcohol. *J.A.M.A.*, **236**:1853–56, 1976.

Fowler, J. S. L.: Carbon tetrachloride metabolism in the rabbit. *Br. J. Pharmacol.*, **37**:733–37, 1969.

Gallagher, C. H.: The effect of antioxidants on poisoning by carbon tetrachloride. *Aust. J. Exp. Biol. Med. Sci.*, **40**:241–54, 1962.

Ganote, C. E., and Rosenthal, A. S.: Characteristic lesions of methylazoxy-methanol-induced liver damage. *Lab. Invest.*, **19**:382–98, 1968.

Ghoshal, A. K.; Porta, E. A.; and Hartroft, W. S.: The role of lipoperoxidation in the pathogenesis of fatty livers induced by phosphorus poisoning in rats. *Am. J. Pathol.*, **54**:275–91, 1969.

Gillette, J. R.: Kinetics of reactive metabolites and covalent binding *in vivo* and *in vitro*. In Jollow, D. J.; Kocsis, J. J.; Snyder, R.; and Vainio, H. (eds.): *Biological Reactive Intermediates.* Pleunum Press, New York, 1977, pp. 25–41.

Glende, E. A., Jr.; Hruskewycz, A. M.; and Recknagel, R. O.: Critical role of lipid peroxidation in carbon tetrachloride-induced loss of aminopyrine demethylase, cytochrome P-450 and glucose-6-phosphatase. *Biochem. Pharmacol.*, 25:2163–70, 1976.

Goldberg, I. H.: Mode of action of antibiotics. II. Drugs affecting nucleic acid and protein synthesis. *Am. J. Med.*, 39:722–723, 1965.

Goldfarb, S.; Singer, E. J.; and Popper, H.: Experimental cholangitis due to α-naphthylisothiocyanate (ANIT). *Am. J. Pathol.*, 40:685–98, 1962.

Gordis, E.: Lipid metabolites of carbon tetrachloride. *J. Clin. Invest.*, 48:203–209, 1969.

Guild, W. R.; Young, J. V.; and Merrill, J. P.: Anuria due to carbon tetrachloride intoxication. *Ann. Intern. Med.*, 48:1221–27, 1958.

Gumucio, J. J., and Valdivieso, V. D.: Studies on the mechanism of the ethynylestradiol impairment of bile flow and bile salt excretion in the rat. *Gastroenterology*, 61:339–44, 1971.

Gupta, D. N.: Acute changes in the liver after administration of thioacetamide. *J. Pathol. Bacteriol.*, 72:183–92, 1956.

Hamilton, R. L.; Regen, D. M.; Gray, M. E.; and LeQuire, V. S.: Lipid transport in liver. I. Electron microscopic identification of very low density lipoproteins in perfused rat liver. *Lab. Invest.*, 16:305–19, 1967.

Hanasono, G. K.: Côté, M. G.; and Plaa, G. L.: Potentiation of carbon tetrachloride-induced hepatotoxicity in alloxan- or streptozotocin-diabetic rats. *J. Pharmacol. Exp. Ther.*, 192:592–604, 1975a.

Hanasono, G. K.; Witschi, H. P.; and Plaa, G. L.: Potentiation of the hepatotoxic responses to chemicals in alloxan-diabetic rats. *Proc. Soc. Exp. Biol. Med.*, 149:903–907, 1975b.

Hansen, C. H.; Pearson, L. H.; Schenker, S.; and Combes, B.: Impaired secretion of triglycerides by the liver; a cause of tetracycline-induced fatty liver. *Proc. Soc. Exp. Biol. Med.*, 128:143–46, 1968.

Hartroft, W. S.: On the etiology of alcoholic liver cirrhosis. In Khanna, J. M.; Israel, Y.; and Kalant, H. (eds.): *Alcoholic Liver Pathology*. Addiction Research Foundation, Toronto, 1975, pp. 189–97.

Heikel, T. A. J., and Lathe, G. H.: The effect of oral contraceptive steroids on bile secretion and bilirubin Tm in rats. *Br. J. Pharmacol.*, 38:593–601, 1970.

Heimberg, M.: Weinstein, I.; Dishmon, G.; and Dunkerley, A.: The action of carbon tetrachloride on the transport and metabolism of triglycerides and fatty acids by the isolated perfused rat liver and its relationship to the etiology of fatty liver. *J. Biol. Chem.*, 237:3623–27, 1962.

Hewitt, W. R.; Miyajima, H.; Côté, M.G.; and Plaa, G. L.: Acute alteration of chloroform-induced hepato- and nephrotoxicity by mirex and kepone. *Toxicol. Appl. Pharmacol.*, 48:509–27, 1979.

Himsworth, H. P.: *Liver and Its Diseases*, 2nd ed. Harvard University Press, Cambridge, Mass., 1954.

Horvath, E.; Solyom, A.; and Korpassy, B.: Histochemical and biochemical studies in acute poisoning with tannic acid. *Br. J. Exp. Pathol.*, 41:298–304, 1960.

Hove, E. L.: Interrelation between α-tocopherol and protein metabolism. III. The protective effect of vitamin E and certain nitrogenous compounds against CCl₄ poisoning in rats. *Arch. Biochem.*, 17:467–73, 1948.

Hoyumba, A. M., Jr.; Greene, H. L.; Dunn, G. D.; and Schenker, S.: Fatty liver: Biochemical and clinical considerations. *Digest. Dis.*, 20:1142–70, 1975.

Hunter, A. L.; Holscher, M. A.; and Neal, R. A.: Thioacetamide-induced hepatic necrosis. I. Involvement of the mixed-function oxidase enzyme system. *J. Pharmacol. Exp. Ther.*, 200:439–48, 1977.

Ideo, G.; DelNinno, E.; and de Franchis, R.: Behavior

of some enzymes and isoenzymes in plasma liver and bile of rats treated with carbon tetrachloride. *Enzyme*, 12:242–54, 1971.

Imai, K., and Hayashi, Y.: Steroid-induced intrahepatic cholestasis in mice. *Jap. J. Pharmacol.*, 20:473–81, 1970.

Ingelfinger, F. J.: Foreword. In Butcher, N. L. R., and Malt, R. A.: *Regeneration of Liver and Kidney*. Little, Brown & Co., Boston, 1971.

Isselbacher, K. J.: Metabolic and hepatic effects of alcohol. *N. Engl. J. Med.*, 296:612–16, 1977.

Javitt, N. B.: Cholestasis in rats induced by taurolithocholate. *Nature (Lond.)*, 210:1262–63, 1966.

Javitt, N. B., and Emerman, S.: Effect of sodium taurolithocholate on bile flow and bile acid excretion. *J. Clin. Invest.*, 47:1002–14, 1968.

Jazcilevich, S., and Villa-Trevino, S.: Induction of fatty liver in the rat after cycloheximide administration. *Lab. Invest.*, 23:590–94, 1970.

Jeanrenaud, B.; LeMarchand, Y.; and Patzelt, C.: Role of microtubules in hepatic secretory processes. In Popper, H.; Bianchi, L.; and Reutter, W. (eds.): *Membrane Alterations as Basis of Liver Injury*. MTP Press, Lancaster, 1977, pp. 247–55.

Judah, J. D.: Biochemical disturbances in liver injury. *Br. Med. Bull.*, 25:274–77, 1969.

Keysser, C. H.; Williams, J. A.; Van Petten, L. E.; and Coy, N.: Experimental production by 2-ethyl-2-phenyl butyramide of intrahepatic cholestasis. *Nature (Lond.)*, 199:498–99, 1963.

Klaassen, C. D.: Biliary excretion of manganese in rats, rabbits and dogs. *Topicol. Appl. Pharmacol.*, 29:458–68, 1974.

Klaassen, C. D., and Plaa, G. L.: Relative effects of various chlorinated hydrocarbons on liver and kidney function in dogs. *Toxicol. Appl. Pharmacol.*, 10:119–31, 1967.

————: Comparison of the biochemical alterations elicited in livers from rats treated with carbon tetrachloride, chloroform, 1,1,2-trichloroethane and 1,1,1-trichloroethane. *Biochem. Pharmacol.*, 18:2019–27, 1969.

Klatskin, G.: Toxic and drug-induced hepatitis. In Schiff, L. (ed.): *Diseases of the Liver*, 3rd ed. J. B. Lippincott Co., Philadelphia, 1969, pp. 498–601.

Koch-Weser, D.; de la Huerga, J.; Yesinick, C.; and Popper, H.: Hepatic necrosis due to bromobenzene as an example of conditioned amino acid deficiency. *Metabolism*, 11:248–60, 1953.

Koudstall, J., and Hardouk, M. J.: Histochemical demonstration of enzymes related to NADPH-dependent hydroxylating systems in rat liver after phenobarbital treatment. *Histochemie*, 20:68–77, 1969.

Larson, R. E., and Plaa, G. L.: A correlation of the effects of cervical cordotomy, hypothermia, and catecholamines on carbon tetrachloride-induced hepatic necrosis. *J. Pharmacol. Exp. Ther.*, 147:103–11, 1965.

Larson, R. E.; Plaa, G. L.; and Brody, M. J.: Immunological sympathectomy and CCl₄ hepatotoxicity. *Proc. Soc. Exp. Biol. Med.*, 116:557–60, 1965.

Lautt, W. W., and Plaa, G. L.: Hemodynamic effects of CCl₄ in the intact liver of the cat. *Can. J. Physiol. Pharmacol.*, 52:727–35, 1974.

Lavigne, J. G., and Marchand, C.: The role of metabolism in chloroform hepatotoxicity. *Toxicol. Appl. Pharmacol.*, 29:312–26, 1974.

Lelbach, W. K.: Quantitative aspects of drinking in alcoholic liver cirrhosis. In Khanna, J. M.; Israel, Y.; and Kalant, H. (eds.): *Alcoholic Liver Pathology*. Addiction Research Foundation, Toronto, 1975, pp. 1–18.

Lennon, H. D.: Relative effects of 17α-alkylated anabolic steroids on sulfobromophthalein (BSP) retention in rabbits. *J. Pharmacol. Exp. Ther*, **151**:143–50, 1966.

Lieber, C. S.: Alcohol and the liver: Transition from metabolic adaptation to tissue injury and cirrhosis. In Khanna, J. M.; Israel, Y.; and Kalant, H. (eds.): *Alcoholic Liver Pathology*. Addiction Research Foundation, Toronto, 1975, pp. 171–88.

Lieber, C. S., and DiCarli, L. M.: Animal models of ethanol dependence and liver injury in rats and baboons. *Fed. Proc.*, **35**:1232–36, 1976.

Lombardi, B.: Considerations on the pathogenesis of fatty liver. *Lab. Invest.*, **15**:1–20, 1966.

Lombardi, B., and Oler, A.: Choline deficiency fatty liver. Protein synthesis and release. *Lab. Invest.*, **17**:308–21, 1967.

Lombardi, B., and Recknagel, R. O.: Interference with secretion of triglycerides by the liver as a common factor in toxic liver injury. *Am. J. Pathol.*, **40**:571–86, 1962.

McCollister, D. D.; Beamer, W. H.; Atchison, G. J.; and Spencer, H. C.: Distribution and elimination of radioactive CCl$_4$ by monkeys upon exposure to low vapor concentration. *J. Pharmacol. Exp. Ther.*, **102**:112–24, 1951.

McLean, E. K.: The toxic actions of pyrrolizidine (senecio) alkaloids. *Pharmacol. Rev.*, **22**:429–83, 1970.

Magee, P. N.: Toxic liver necrosis. *Lab. Invest.*, **15**:111–31, 1966.

Magee, P. N., and Swann, P. F.: Nitroso compounds. *Br. Med. Bull.*, **25**:240–44, 1969.

Mager, J.; Bornstein, S.; and Halbreich, A.: Enhancement of the polyuridylic acid-directed phenylalamine polymerization in liver-microsome preparations from rats treated with carbon tetrachloride or dimethylnitrosamine. *Biochim. Biophys. Acta*, **95**:682–84, 1965.

Mahley, R. W.: Hamilton, R. L.; and LeQuire, V. S.: Characterization of lipo-protein particles isolated from the Golgi apparatus of rat liver. *J. Lipid Res.*, **10**:433–39, 1969.

Maling, H. M.; Frank, A.; and Horning, M. G.: Effect of carbon tetrachloride on hepatic synthesis and release of triglycerides. *Biochim. Biophys. Acta*, **64**:540–45, 1962.

Mansuy, D.; Beaune, P.; Cresteil, T.; Lange, M.; and Leroux, J.-P.: Evidence for phosgene formation during liver microsomal oxidation of chloroform. *Biochem. Biophys. Res. Comm.*, **79**:513–17, 1977.

Marchetti, M.; Ottani, V.; and Puddu, P.: Studies on azaserine-induced fatty liver in the rat. *Proc. Soc. Exp. Biol. Med.*, **133**:30–33, 1970.

Mattocks, A. R.: Toxicity of pyrrolizidine alkaloids. *Nature (Lond.)*, **217**:723–28, 1968.

Medline, A.; Schaffner, F.; and Popper, H.: Ultrastructural features in galactosamine-induced hepatitis. *Exp. Mol. Pathol.*, **12**:201–11, 1970.

Mgbodile, M. U. K.; Holscher, M.; and Neal, R. A.: A possible protective role for reduced glutathione in aflatoxin B$_1$ toxicity: Effect of pretreatment of rats with phenobarbital and 3-methylcholanthrene on aflatoxin toxicity. *Toxicol. Appl. Pharmacol.*, **34**:128–42, 1975.

Middleton III, H. M.; Dunn, G. D.; and Schenker, S.: Alcohol-induced liver injury: Pathogenetic considerations. In Becker, F. F. (ed.): *The Liver: Normal and Abnormal Functions*, Part B. Marcel Dekker, Inc., New York, 1975, pp. 647–77.

Mitchell, J. R.; Nelson, S. D.; Thorgeirsson, S. S.; McMurty, R. J.; and Dybing, E.: Metabolic activation: biochemical basis for many drug-induced liver injuries. In Popper, H., and Schaffner, F. (eds.): *Progress in Liver Diseases*, Vol. 5. Grune & Stratton, New York, 1976a, pp. 259–79.

Mitchell, J. R.; Snodgrass, W. R.; and Gillette, J. R.: The role of biotransformation in chemical-induced liver injury. *Environ. Health Perspect.*, **15**:27–38, 1976b.

Mitchell, J. R.; Zimmerman, H. J.; Ishak, K. G.; Thorgeirsson, U. P.; Timbrell, J. A.; Snodgrass, W. R.; and Nelson, S. D.: Isoniazid liver injury: Clinical spectrum, pathology, and probable pathogenesis. *Ann. Intern. Med.*, **84**:181–92, 1976c.

Miyai, K.; Price, V. M.; and Fisher, M. M.: Bile acid metabolism in mammals: Ultrastructural studies on the intrahepatic cholestasis induced by lithocholic and chenodeoxycholic acids in the rat. *Lab. Invest.*, **24**:292–302, 1971.

Mizrahi, I. J., and Emmelot, P.: The effect of cysteine on the metabolic changes produced by two carcinogenic n-nitrosodiakylamines in rat liver. *Cancer Res.*, **22**:339–51, 1962.

Oler, A.; Neal, M. W.; and Mitchell, E. K.: Tannic acid: Acute hepatotoxicity following administration by feeding tube. *Food Cosmet. Toxicol.*, **14**:565–69, 1976.

Olason, D., and Smuckler, E. A.: Changes in hepatic nuclei induced by acetamide and thioacetamide. *Arch. Pathol. Lab. Med.*, **100**:415–18, 1976.

Paul, B. B., and Rubinstein, D.: Metabolism of carbon tetrachloride and chloroform by the rat. *J. Pharmacol. Exp. Ther.*, **141**:141–48, 1963.

Perez, V.; Schaffner, F.; and Popper, H.: Hepatic drug reactions. In Popper, H., and Schaffner, F. (eds.): *Progress in Liver Disease*, Vol. 4. Grune & Stratton, New York, 1972, pp. 597–625.

Pesh-Imam, M.; Willis, R. J.; and Recknagel, R. O.: Red cell damage induced by peroxidized microsomes: The relationship between hemolytic activity and peroxide content. *J. Environ. Health Sci.*, **1**:81–95, 1978.

Plaa, G. L., and Priestly, B. G.: Intrahepatic cholestasis induced by drugs and chemicals. *Pharmacol. Rev.*, **28**:207–73, 1976.

Plaa, G. L.; Traiger, G. J.; Hanasono, G. K.; and Witschi, H. P.: Effect of alcohols on various forms of chemically induced liver injury. In Khanna, J. M.; Israel, Y.; and Kalant, H. (eds.): *Alcoholic Liver Pathology*. Addiction Research Foundation, Toronto, 1975, pp. 225–44.

Plaa, G. L., and Witschi, H. P.: Chemicals, drugs, and lipid peroxidation. *Ann. Rev. Pharmacol. Toxicol.*, **16**:125–41, 1976.

Pohl, L. R.; Bhooshan, B.; Whittaker, N. F.; and Krishna, G.: Phosgene: A metabolite of chloroform. *Biochem. Biophys. Res. Comm.*, **79**:684–91, 1977.

Popper, H., and Schaffner, F.: Drug-induced hepatic injury. *Ann. Intern. Med.*, **51**:1230–52, 1959.

Priestly, B. G.; Côté, M. G.; and Plaa, G. L.: Biochemical and morphological parameters of taurolithocholate cholestasis. *Can. J. Physiol. Pharmacol.*, **49**:1078–91, 1971.

Raisfeld, I. H.: Models of liver injury: The effect of toxins on the liver. In Becker, F. F. (ed.): *The Liver: Normal and Abnormal Functions*, Part A. Marcel Dekker, Inc., New York, 1974, pp. 203–23.

Rankin, J. G.; Schmidt, W.; Popham, R. E.; and de Lint, J.: Epidemiology of alcoholic liver disease—insights and problems. In Khanna, J. M.; Israel, Y.; and Kalant, H. (eds.): *Alcoholic Liver Pathology*. Addiction Research Foundation, Toronto, 1975, pp. 31–41.

Rappaport, A. M: Anatomic considerations. In Schiff, L. (ed.): *Diseases of the Liver*, 3rd ed. J. B. Lippincott Co., Philadelphia, 1969, pp. 1–49.

————: The microcirculatory acinar concept of normal and pathological hepatic structure. *Beitr. Path.*, **157**:215–43, 1976.

Recknagel, R. O.: Carbon tetrachloride hepatotoxicity. *Pharmacol. Rev.*, **19**:145–208, 1967.

Recknagel, R. O., and Ghoshal, A. K.: Lipoperoxidation as a vector in carbon tetrachloride hepatotoxicity *Lab. Invest.*, **15**:132–48, 1966.

Recknagel, R. O., and Glende, E. A., Jr.: Carbon tetrachloride hepatotoxicity: An example of lethal cleavage. *CRC Crit. Rev. Toxicol.*, **2**:263–97, 1973.

Recknagel, R. O., and Lombardi, B.: Studies of biochemical changes in subcellular particles of rat liver and their relationship to new hypothesis regarding pathogenesis of carbon tetrachloride fat accumulation. *J. Biol. Chem.*, **236**:564–69, 1961.

Recknagel, R. O.; Lombardi, B.; and Schotz, M. C.: A new insight into the pathogenesis of carbon tetrachloride fat infiltration. *Proc. Soc. Exp. Biol. Med.*, **104**:608–10, 1960.

Rees, K. R.; Sinha, P.; and Spector, W. G.: The pathogenesis of liver injury in carbon tetrachloride and thioacetamide poisoning. *J. Pathol. Bacteriol.*, **81**:107–18, 1961.

Rees, K. R., and Tarlow, M. J.: The hepatotoxic action of allyl formate. *Biochem. J.*, **104**:757–61, 1967.

Reid, W. D.: Mechanism of allyl alcohol-induced hepatic necrosis. *Experientia*, **28**:1058–61, 1972.

Reid, W. D.; Christie, B.; Krishna, G.; Mitchell, J. R.; Moskowitz, J.; and Brodie, B. B.: Bromobenzene metabolism and hepatic necrosis. *Pharmacology*, **6**:41–55, 1971.

Reynolds, E. S., and Moslen, M. T.: Halothane hepatotoxicity: Enhancement by polychlorinated biphenyl pretreatment. *Anesthesiology*, **47**:19–27, 1977.

Reynolds, E. S.; Moslen, M. T.; Szabo, S.; Jaeger, R. J.; and Murphy, S. D.: Hepatotoxicity of vinyl chloride and 1,1-dichloroethylene. *Am. J. Pathol.*, **81**:219–32, 1975.

Reynolds, E. S., and Yee, A. G.: Liver parenchymal cell injury. V. Relationships between patterns of chloromethane-C^{14} incorporation into constituents of liver *in vivo* and cellular injury. *Lab. Invest.*, **16**:591–603, 1967.

Robinson, D. S., and Seakins, A.: The development in the rat of fatty livers associated with reduced plasma-lipoprotein synthesis. *Biochim. Biophys. Acta*, **62**:163–65, 1962.

Rouiller, C.: Experimental toxic injury of the liver. In Rouiller, C. (ed.): *The Liver*, Vol. 2. Academic Press, Inc., New York, 1964, pp. 335–476.

Rubinstein, D., and Kanics, L.: The conversion of carbon tetrachloride and chloroform to carbon dioxide by rat liver homogenates. *Can. J. Biochem.*, **42**:1577–85, 1964.

Rüttner, J. R.; Spycher, M. A.; and Kuenzie, C.: Zur Pathologie des Ikterus: der ANIT-induzierte Ikterus der Ratte, ein Modell einer durch Zellmembran-schädigung bedingten toxichen Hepatose. *Pathol. Microbiol.*, **27**:403–409, 1964.

Schaffner, F., and Javitt, N. B.: Morphologic changes in hamster liver during intrahepatic cholestasis induced by taurolithocholate. *Lab. Invest.*, **15**:1783–92, 1966.

Schaffner, F.; Popper, H.; and Perez, V.: Changes in bile canaliculi produced by norethandrolone: Electron microscopic study of human and rat liver. *J. Lab. Clin. Med.*, **56**:623–28, 1960.

Schaffner, F., and Raisfeld, I. H.: Drugs and the liver: A review of metabolism and adverse reactions. *Adv. Intern. Med.*, **15**:221–51, 1969.

Schinella, R. A., and Becker, F. F.: Cirrhosis. In Becker, F. F. (ed.): *The Liver: Normal and Abnormal Functions*, Part B. Marcel Dekker, Inc., New York, 1975, pp. 711–23.

Schotz, M. C.; Baker, N; and Chavez, M. N.: Effect of carbon tetrachloride ingestion on liver and plasma triglyceride turnover rate. *J. Lipid Res.*, **5**:569–77, 1964.

Seakins, A., and Robinson, D. S.: The effect of the administration of carbon tetrachloride on the formation of plasma lipoproteins in the rat. *Biochem. J.*, **86**:401–407, 1963.

Sell, D. A., and Reynolds, E. S.: Liver parenchymal cell injury. VIII. Lesions of the membranous cellular components following iodoform. *J. Cell Biol.*, **41**:736–52, 1969.

Seto, J. T., and Lepper, M. H.: The effect of chlortetracycline, oxytetracycline, and tetracycline administered intravenously on hepatic fat content. *Antibiot. Chemother.*, **4**:666–72, 1954.

Sipes, I. G.; Krishna, G.; and Gillette, J. R.: Bioactivation of carbon tetrachloride, chloroform and bromotrichloromethane: Role of cytochrome P-450. *Life Sci.* **20**:1541–48, 1977.

Sipes, I. G.; Stripp, B.; Krishna, G.; Maling, H. M.; and Gillette, J. R.: Enhanced hepatic microsomal activity by pretreatment of rats with acetone or isopropanol. *Proc. Soc. Exp. Biol. Med.*, **142**:237–40, 1973.

Slater, T. F.: Necrogenic action of carbon tetrachloride in the rat: A speculative mechanism based on activation. *Nature (Lond.)*, **209**:36–40, 1966.

Smuckler, E. A., and Benditt, E. P.: Studies on carbon tetrachloride intoxication. III. A subcellular defect in protein synthesis. *Biochemistry*, **4**:671–79, 1965.

Smuckler, E. A.; Iseri, O. A.; and Benditt, E. P.: Studies on carbon tetrachloride intoxication. I. The effect of carbon tetrachloride on incorporation of labelled amino acids into plasma proteins. *Biochem. Biophys. Res. Commun.*, **5**:270–75, 1961.

―――: An intracellular defect in protein synthesis induced by carbon tetrachloride. *J. Exp. Med.*, **116**:55–72, 1962.

Sollmann, T.: *A Manual of Pharmacology*, 8th ed. W. B. Saunders Co., Philadelphia, 1957.

Stenger, R. J., and Johnson, E. A.: Further observations upon the effects of phenobarbital pretreatment on the hepatotoxicity of carbon tetrachloride. *Exp. Mol. Pathol.*, **14**:220–27, 1971.

Stewart, R. D.; Torkelson, T. R.; Hake, C. L.; and Erley, D. S.: Infrared analysis of carbon tetrachloride and ethanol in blood. *J. Lab. Clin. Med.*, **56**:148–56, 1960.

Stoner, H. B.: The mechanism of toxic hepatic necrosis. *Br. J. Exp. Pathol.*, **37**:176–98, 1956.

Sweeney, G. D.; Garfield, R. E.; Jones, K. G.; and Latham, A. N.: Studies using sedimentation velocity on heterogeneity of size and function of hepatocytes from mature male rats. *J. Lab. Clin. Med.*, **91**:432–43, 1978a.

Sweeney, G. D.; Jones, K. D.; and Krestynski, F.: Effects of phenobarbital and 3-methylcholanthrene pretreatment on size, sedimentation velocity, and mixed function oxygenase activity of rat hepatocytes. *J. Lab. Clin. Med.*, **91**:444–54, 1978b.

Thiers, R. E.; Reynolds, E. S.; and Vallee, B. L.: The effect of carbon tetrachloride poisoning on subcellular metal distribution in rat liver. *J. Biol. Chem.*, **235**:2130–33, 1960.

Thoenes, W., and Bannasch, P.: Elektronen- und lichtmikroskopische Untersuchungen am Cytoplasma der Leberzellen nach akuter und chronischer Thioacetamid Vergiftung. *Virchows Arch. (Pathol. Anat.)*, **335**:556–83, 1962.

Tomokuni, K.: Studies on hepatotoxicity induced by chlorinated hydrocarbons. II. Lipid metabolism and absorption spectrum of microsomal lipid in mice exposed to 1,1,2,2-tetrachloroethane. *Acta Med. Okayama*, **24**:315–22, 1970.

Traiger, G. J., and Bruckner, J. V.: The participation of 2-butanone in 2-butanol-induced potentiation of carbon tetrachloride hepatotoxicity. *J. Pharmacol. Exp. Ther.*, **196**:493–500, 1976.

Traiger, G. J., and Plaa, G. L.: Chlorinated hydrocarbon

toxicity—potentiation by isopropyl alcohol and acetone. *Arch. Environ. Health*, **28**:276–78, 1974.

Uraguchi, K.; Sakai, F.; Tsukioka, M.; Noguchi, Y.; and Tatsuno, M.: Acute and chronic toxicity in mice and rats of the fungus mat of *Penicillium islandicum* sopp added to the diet. *Jap. J. Exp. Med.*, **31**:435–61, 1961.

Utili, R.; Boitnott, J. K.; and Zimmerman, H. J.: Dantrolene-associated hepatic injury. *Gastroenterology*, **72**:610–16, 1977.

Wattenberg, L. W., and Leong, J. L.: Histochemical demonstration of reduced pyridinenucleotide dependent polycyclic hydrocarbon metabolizing systems. *J. Histochem. Cytochem.*, **10**:412–20, 1962.

Weiss, E.; Sterz, I.; Frimmer, M.; and Kroker, R.: Electron microscopy of isolated rat hepatocytes before and after treatment with phalloidin. *Beitr. Pathol.*, **150**:345–56, 1973.

Williams, J. A.; Salthouse, T. N.; and Keysser, C. H.: Fine structural and cytochemical changes in livers of rats dosed orally with 2-ethyl-2-phenyl butyramide. *Fed. Proc.*, **23**:297, 1964.

Windmueller, H. G., and von Euler, L. H.: Prevention of orotic acid-induced fatty liver with allopurinol. *Proc. Soc. Exp. Biol. Med.*, **136**:98–101, 1971.

Wirtschafter, Z. T., and Cronyn, M. W.: Free radical mechanism for solvent toxicity. *Arch. Environ. Health.*, **9**:186–91, 1964.

Witschi, H. P.: Effects of beryllium on deoxyribonucleic acid-synthesizing enzymes in regenerating rat liver. *Biochem. J.*, **120**:623–34, 1970.

Witschi, H. P., and Aldridge, W. N.: Biochemical changes in rat liver after acute beryllium poisoning. *Biochem. Pharmacol.*, **16**:263–78, 1967.

———: Uptake, distribution and binding of beryllium to organelles of the rat liver cell. *Biochem. J.*, **106**:811–20, 1968.

Witzleben, C. L.: Physiologic and morphologic natural history of a model of intrahepatic cholestasis (manganese-bilirubin overload). *Am. J. Pathol.*, **66**:577–82, 1972.

Wogan, G. N.: Metabolism and biochemical effects of aflatoxins. In Goldblatt, L. A. (ed.): *Aflatoxins*. Academic Press, Inc., New York, 1969, pp. 151–86.

———: The induction of liver cell cancer by chemicals. In Cameron, H. M.; Linsell, D. A.; and Warwick, G. P. (eds.): *Liver Cell Cancer*. Elsevier, Amsterdam, 1976, pp. 121–52.

Zimmerman, H. J.: Hepatic injury caused by therapeutic agents. In Becker, F. F. (ed.): *The Liver: Normal and Abnormal Functions*, Part A. Marcel Dekker, Inc., New York, 1974, pp. 225–302.

———: Experimental hepatotoxicity. In Eichler, O. (ed.): *Handbook of Experimental Pharmacology*, Vol. 16/5. Springer-Verlag, New York, 1976, pp. 1–120.

———: *Hepatotoxicity*. Appleton-Century - Crofts, New York, 1978.

Zuretti, M. F., and Baccino, F. M.: Studies on the hepatotoxicity of *Amanita phalloides* in the rat. II. Biochemical analysis of the lysosomal changes. *Exp. Mol. Pathol.*, **24**:176–92, 1976.

SUPPLEMENTAL READING

Becker, F. F.: *The Liver: Normal and Abnormal Functions*, Part A. Marcel Dekker, Inc., New York, 1974.

———: *The Liver: Normal and Abnormal Functions*, Part B. Marcel Dekker, Inc., New York, 1975.

Cameron, H. M.; Linsell, D. A.; and Warwick, G. P.: *Liver Cell Cancer*. Elsevier, Amsterdam, 1976.

Jollow, D. J.; Kocsis, J. J.; Snyder, R.; and Vaino, H.: *Biological Reactive Intermediates*. Plenum Press, New York, 1977.

Khanna, J. M.; Israel, Y.; and Kalant, H.: *Alcoholic Liver Pathology*. Addiction Research Foundation, Toronto, 1975.

Popper, H.; Bianchi, L.; and Reutter, W.: *Membrane Alterations as Basis of Liver Injury*. MTP Press Ltd., Lancaster, 1977.

Zimmerman, H. J.: *Hepatotoxicity*. Appleton-Century - Crofts, New York, 1978.

Chapter 11

TOXIC RESPONSES OF THE KIDNEY

Jerry B. Hook

INTRODUCTION

The mammalian kidney is an extremely complex organ, both anatomically and functionally. One primary renal function is excretion of wastes, but the kidney also plays a significant role in the regulation of total body homeostasis. The kidney is the predominant organ involved in regulation of extracellular volume and in control of electrolyte and acid-base balance. This organ is also the major site of formation of hormones that influence systemic metabolic functions: erythropoietin is a potent stimulus to erythrocyte formation; the relatively inactive 25-hydroxy-vitamin D_3 is metabolically activated to the active 1,25-dihydroxy-vitamin D_3; renin, the trigger to the formation of angiotensin and aldosterone, is formed in the kidney; and recent evidence indicates that the kidney produces several vasoactive prostaglandins and kinins. A toxicologic insult to the kidney could affect any or all of these functions. However, the effects usually reported following toxic insult reflect decreased elimination of wastes, i.e., an increase in blood urea nitrogen (BUN) or an increase in plasma creatinine. The frequency of reports of such changes associated with renal insult does not necessarily mean that excretory functions are primarily affected by nephrotoxins; rather, these are the renal functions that are traditionally measured. Thus, the use of BUN and plasma creatinine as clinical indices of nephrotoxicity reflects the state of technology but not necessarily the primary sites of nephrotoxicity.

RENAL PHYSIOLOGY AND PATHOPHYSIOLOGY

Functional Anatomy

Gross examination of a sagittal section of the kidney clearly demonstrates the demarcation between the two major anatomic areas, the cortex and the medulla (Fig. 11–1). The cortex constitutes the major portion of the kidney and consequently receives most of the total nutrient blood flow to the organ. Thus, when a blood-borne toxicant is delivered to the kidney, a high percentage of the material will reach sites in the cortex. In a single pass through the kidney most chemicals will have a greater propensity to influence cortical, rather than medullary, function. A smaller percentage of the total chemical delivered to the kidney would reach the medulla. However, because of the low blood flow to the medulla and because of the anatomic arrangement of the *vasa rectae* and loops of Henle (Fig. 11–1), the possibility of a chemical being trapped in the countercurrent mechanism is high. Thus, a foreign compound could remain in the medulla at relatively high concentrations.

A discussion of the functional anatomy of the kidney is most appropriately based on the functional unit of the kidney, the nephron (Fig. 11–1). The nephron may be considered in three portions: the vascular element including the afferent and efferent arterioles, the glomerulus, and the tubular element. All nephrons have their primary vascular elements and glomeruli in the cortex. The proximal convoluted tubule is localized in the cortex and sends the *pars recta* (straight portion) of the proximal tubule and loops of Henle deep into the substance of the kidney. Those glomeruli close to the medulla (juxtamedullary glomeruli) are associated with nephrons that send their loops of Henle deep into the medulla. Other glomeruli closer to the surface of the kidney often form nephrons whose loops of Henle are contained within the cortex (Fig. 11–1). The relative proportion of nephrons with long versus short loops varies with species.

Each element of the nephron unit has specific functions, all of which may be influenced by nephrotoxins. The vascular element serves to (1) deliver waste and other materials to the tubule for excretion; (2) return reabsorbed and synthesized materials to the systemic circulation; and (3) deliver oxygen and metabolic substrates to the nephron; it is within the vascular element of the afferent arteriole that renin is formed. The glomerulus is a specially developed capillary bed. It is unique in that it is the only capillary bed in

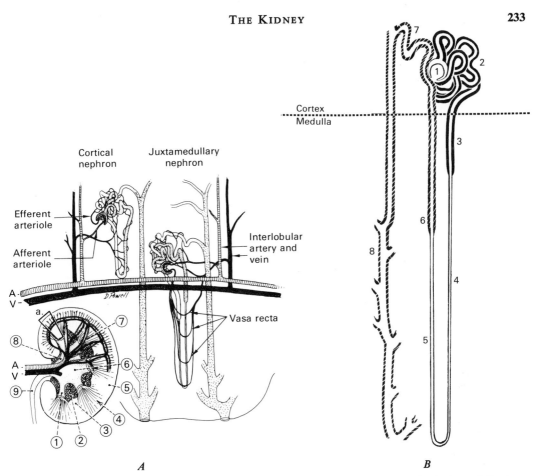

Figure 11–1. *A.* Sagittal section of a mammalian (human) kidney is illustrated in the lower left. *A* and *V* refer to renal artery and vein, respectively; (*1*) minor calix; (*2*) fat in sinus; (*3*) renal column of Bertin; (*4*) medullary ray; (*5*) cortex; (*6*) pelvis; (*7*) interlobar artery; (*8*) major calix; (*9*) ureter. Insert (*a*) from the upper pole of the kidney is enlarged to illustrate the relationships between the nephrons and the vasculature. (From Tisher, C. C.: Anatomy of the kidney. In Brenner, B. B., and Rector, F. C., Jr. [eds.]: *The Kidney.* W. B. Saunders Co., Philadelphia, 1976.)

B. Anatomy of a juxtamedullary nephron. Note the demarcation between cortex and medulla: (*1*) glomerulus; (*2*) proximal convoluted tubule; (*3*) proximal straight tubule (pars recta); (*4*) descending limb of the loop of Henle; (*5*) thin ascending limb of the loop of Henle; (*6*) thick ascending limb of the loop of Henle; (*7*) distal convoluted tubule; (*8*) collecting duct. (Modified from Gottschalk, C.W.: Osmotic concentration and dilution of the urine. *Am. J. Med.*, **36**:670–85, 1964.)

the body positioned between vasoactive arterioles. The glomerulus is a relatively porous capillary and acts as a selective filter of the plasma. Based on molecular size and net charge, certain materials will be filtered into the lumen of the tubule and others will be retained in the circulation (Fig. 11–2). The tubular element of the nephron selectively reabsorbs the bulk of the filtrate; approximately 98 to 99 percent of the salts and water are reabsorbed. There is virtually complete reabsorption of filtered sugars and amino acids and selective elimination of waste materials. Furthermore, the tubular element, particularly the proximal tubule, actively secretes

material into the urine. Secretory activity is responsible for most excretion of certain organic compounds and for the elimination of hydrogen and potassium ions. The tubular element is also actively involved in the synthesis of ammonia and glucose and the activation of vitamin D. (For a more detailed consideration of renal structure and function see Valtin [1973] or Brenner and Rector [1976].)

The cellular response to a toxic insult may vary from an imperceptible biochemical aberration to cell death with resulting necrosis. Functionally, toxicity may be reflected as a minor alteration in transport capability (e.g., transient glucosuria,

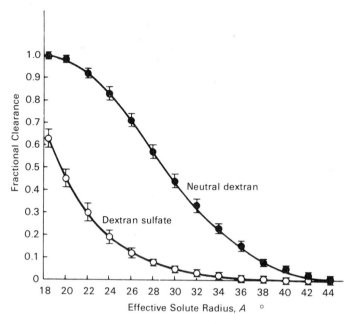

Figure 11–2. Fractional clearances (clearance compared to inulin clearance) of neutral dextran and dextran sulfate by rat kidney plotted as a function of effective molecular radius. As effective molecular radius increases, the fractional clearance, which reflects glomerular permeability, decreases. The permeability to neutral dextran is considerably greater than that of the charged dextran sulfate. (From Brenner, B. M., *et al.*: Determinants of glomerular permselectivity: Insights derived from observations *in vivo. Kidney Int.*, **12**:229–37, 1977. Reprinted with permission.)

aminoaciduria), as polyuria with decreased concentrating capacity, or as frank renal failure with anuria and elevated BUN. Depending on the magnitude of the insult, these changes may be reversible, permanent, or lethal. Theoretically, these effects may be brought about in one of several ways: (1) Vasoconstriction could decrease renal blood flow and glomerular filtration rate, reducing urine flow and eventually resulting in an increase in BUN. If prolonged, vasoconstriction would lead to tissue ischemia with resultant loss of function and eventually tissue destruction. (2) The nephrotoxin could directly affect the glomerular element, altering permeability such that filtration at the glomerulus is compromised. (3) Alternatively, or in combination with these other possibilities, the administration of a nephrotoxin could directly influence tubular function. Either specific reabsorptive or secretory mechanisms could be influenced by the toxicant, or the general permeability of the tubule could be influenced such that the normal ability of the tubule to act as a barrier to diffusion could be altered.

Reason for Susceptibility of the Kidney

The kidney is a highly dynamic organ. Renal blood flow is quite high; the two kidneys together receive about 25 percent of the cardiac ouput. Approximately one-third of the plasma water reaching the kidney is filtered, and from this material approximately 98 to 99 percent of the salt and water is reabsorbed. Maintenance of normal function requires delivery of large amounts of metabolic substrates and oxygen to the kidney. Because of the high blood flow, any

drug or chemical in the systemic circulation will be delivered in relatively high amounts to this organ. As salt and water are reabsorbed from the glomerular filtrate, the materials remaining (including the potential toxicant) in the urine may be concentrated in the tubule. Thus, a nontoxic concentration of a chemical in the plasma could become toxic in the kidney subsequent to concentration within the urine. Furthermore, a chemical reaching the kidney might be concentrated in the cells in one or both of the following ways. If the material is actively secreted into the tubular urine, it will first be accumulated within the cells of the proximal tubule in concentrations higher than in plasma. This process will expose these cells to very high concentrations of the agent, which could produce toxicity. Similarly, a material that is reabsorbed (even by passive means) from the urine into the blood will pass through the cells of the nephron in a relatively high concentration, potentially leading to intracellular toxicity.

As pointed out above, the renal medulla offers unique problems concerning nephrotoxicity. Because of the low blood flow to the medulla, relatively less potential toxicant might enter this region by the bloodstream than would enter the cortex. However, any materials in the tubular urine will by necessity pass through the loop of Henle and the collecting duct in the medulla. The countercurrent mechanisms within the medulla may trap the compound, leading to establishment of a high concentration within the lumen of the nephron.

The kidney is sensitive to extrarenal factors

that would decrease blood pressure or blood volume, as in shock or hemorrhage. Such changes may rapidly induce signs of ischemia and functional deficit in this highly active metabolic organ. The kidney is under the influence of the sympathetic nervous system, and changes in neural activity can markedly influence renal function. A direct effect of the renal sympathetic nerves on renal vascular resistance and on renin secretion has been documented many times. More recent evidence suggests that renal nerve activity might directly influence proximal tubular function as well. Therefore, any change in systemic homeostasis that would alter sympathetic nerve activity could also influence the kidney. Similarly, dehydration may occur due to decreased water intake, elevated body temperature, or a secondary effect of a chemical. This could lead to decreased plasma volume, which could decrease glomerular filtration. Probably of greater importance in this case is the fact that in the presence of antidiuretic hormone the urine would be maximally concentrated and the possibility of a chemical reaching excessively high concentrations in the urine would be maximized.

Assessment of Renal Function

Evaluation of the effect of a chemical on renal function can be accomplished by several methods. The methods used depend on the complexity of the question to be answered. For instance, to determine if there had been *an* effect on kidney function, unanesthetized intact animals could be used. More information can probably be gained by quantifying renal function in anesthetized animals, where renal function can be determined in a steady state. To learn about specific biochemical or functional lesions, studies are often done *in vitro*. Lastly, histopathologic studies can provide a great deal of information about renal integrity.

There are many advantages to determining the effect of a chemical agent in the intact, unanesthetized animal. These studies can be done serially during the course of a feeding program to monitor an alteration in renal function. The standard battery of tests includes measurement of urine volume, urinary pH, and excretion of sodium and potassium. The appearance of sugar and/or excess protein in the urine would indicate abnormalities in renal function as would changes in urine sediment. Abnormalities in urine osmolality might indicate a deficit in renal medullary function. Small blood samples can be drawn directly, taken from the tail or from the orbital sinus of the eye, and the BUN and plasma creatinine can be estimated. A relatively simple test is the ability of the animal to eliminate a load of a compound whose mechanism of renal

handling is known. The compound most commonly used is phenolsulfonphthalein (PSP). These are all relatively general tests and can provide information about abnormalities of total kidney function. More recently, attempts have been made to develop noninvasive tests that might provide more specific information. Several groups have attempted to utilize the appearance of enzymes in the urine as indices of renal function. Enzymuria in general can indicate abnormality of function, and the specific enzymes involved might provide information about selective sites of damage. The appearance in the urine of enzymes of renal origin (enzymes that are specific to the kidney, such as maltase or trehalase) could indicate specific destruction of the renal proximal tubules (Berndt, 1976), whereas alkaline phosphatase in the urine could arise from renal or prerenal (e.g., hepatic) damage.

The use of anesthetized animals provides more information concerning toxic insult to the kidney. The commonly used animals are dogs, rabbits, and rats. In anesthetized preparations, systemic blood pressure and glomerular filtration rate in the steady state can be monitored. Glomerular filtration rate is usually estimated from the clearance of inulin. The clearance of urea as estimated by BUN is not particularly definitive because urea is a by-product of protein metabolism and any toxic insult that would influence protein metabolism (poor nutrition, hepatotoxicity) could influence BUN. The polysaccharide inulin provides information about glomerular filtration rate regardless of the state of protein metabolism. Renal blood flow can be estimated from renal plasma flow using the renal clearance and/or renal extraction of para-aminohippuric acid (PAH). Alternatively, radio-labeled microspheres or an electromagnetic flowmeter may be used to specifically measure renal blood flow. The ability of the kidney to reabsorb or secrete electrolytes is estimated as the fractional excretion of sodium, potassium, bicarbonate, chloride, etc. Fractional excretion takes into account the filtered load, thus allowing comparisons of electrolyte transport between treated and control animals even if renal hemodynamics have changed. Another estimate of nephron function in terms of the ability to remove electrolyte and water from specific sites along the nephron is to quantify the clearance of free water (which reflects the ability of the kidney to remove almost all sodium from the urine). In addition, the concentrating capacity in the anesthetized animal can be used to estimate medullary function (Berndt, 1976).

Very elegant studies have been conducted in dogs and rats using micropuncture. Using this technique, individual nephron or vascular segments are punctured and fluid collected and pressures monitored. Thus, the technique can be used to distinguish between vascular, tubular, and glomerular changes following nephrotoxicity (Biber et al., 1968; Oken, 1976).

To more specifically quantify the effects of a nephrotoxin, a variety of in vitro techniques may be employed. In vivo techniques might demonstrate that the renal clearance of a particular compound is diminished, but it may be difficult to distinguish between effects directly on hemodynamics, metabolism, or transport if all are altered by a nephrotoxin. The toxic effects of chemicals may be evaluated in vitro by directly adding the agent to the preparation or following administration to the animal. This allows a distinction to be made between an effect on the kidney due to direct chemical insult and secondary effects, such as those subsequent to metabolism, for example. The renal cortical slice technique has been used extensively to evaluate the influence of nephrotoxins on the transport of organic anions such as PAH and organic cations such as N-methylnicotinamide (NMN) or tetraethylammonium (TEA). Attempts have been made to evaluate transport in a reabsorptive direction using the nonmetabolized amino acid analog α-aminoisobutyric acid and the nonmetabolized sugar α-methyl-d-glucoside. In addition, the ability of the kidney to produce ammonia and glucose from added substrates can be quantified in vitro and can provide more specific information about metabolic alterations produced by a nephrotoxin. Isolated tubular preparations may be employed to evaluate the influence of nephrotoxins on selected areas of the nephron. Micropuncture and microperfusion techniques have also been utilized in attempts to identify specific loci of action of nephrotoxins.

Histopathologic examination of tissue can demonstrate structural changes that have occurred in response to nephrotoxins and can often identify selected areas that have been affected. For instance, light microscopy can demonstrate the papillary necrosis produced by nonnarcotic analgesics and can isolate the proximal tubular damage induced by mercury, chromium, and other heavy metals. Histopathology will often show that an injury has occurred even in a situation in which function was not noticeably altered. The use of standard light microscopy can also provide information concerning the appearance in the tubule of protein casts, of sloughed brush border and crystals or stones in the kidney and urine. Very elegant experiments have been conducted using microdissection techniques. Following nephrotoxic insult, entire tubules have been carefully dissected and specific areas of damage have been identified by light

microscopy (Biber et al., 1968). Many histochemical techniques are also available to evaluate renal response to poisons. Electron microscopy provides information concerning subcellular localization of tubular injury. Changes in mitochondria can very easily be identified, as can alterations in other organelles. Electron microscopy has been extensively employed in efforts to understand the changes in glomerular structure that might account for changes in permeability following nephrotoxins.

Compensation for Renal Damage

The kidney has a remarkable ability to compensate following loss of renal mass. Within a short time after surgical removal of one kidney, the remaining kidney hypertrophies to such an extent that standard clinical signs of renal function provide no indication of tissue loss (Fig. 11-3). This ability to compensate becomes a problem when attempting to evaluate the effect of nephrotoxins and points out that distinctions must be made between acute and chronic renal injury. A single dose of a nephrotoxin may produce profound, acute changes in renal function, but if the injury is not lethal and if no other insult is forthcoming, the kidney may compensate and regain normal function in a short time (Fig. 11-4). Similarly, chronic administration of a low dose of a nephrotoxin may bring about significant changes in structure of the kidney, but during the course of administration, the kidney may compensate so that no marked changes are seen in the standard renal tests. The consequences of these effects are profound, for if kidney function is evaluated at a time far removed from single injury a classic function test might reveal no changes, even though there had been a great deal of tissue damage. Following chronic administration no change in kidney function may be seen until the ability of the kidney to compensate is exceeded. Then, within a short period of time the animal might develop life-threatening renal failure.

Sites of Action of Nephrotoxins

Few data are available that define specific cellular or subcellular sites of action of nephrotoxins. Only rarely have specific receptors (in the classic sense of the word) for specific nephrotoxins been identified. Rather, in many cases it appears that several tissue constituents may be influenced by a poison. There are two interrelated reasons for this apparent lack of specificity: (1) In contrast to a specific pharmacologic effect of a chemical that requires activation or inhibition of a specific endogenous receptor, cell damage may follow interruption of one or several of the many required cellular functions; (2) certain kidney

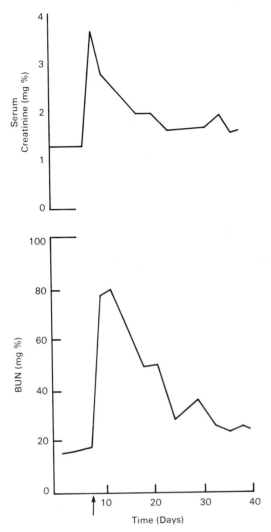

blood flow to the kidney is delivered to the cortex, which is predominantly proximal tubule. In addition, active secretion of compounds occurs in the proximal tubule, and changes brought about by concentrating a chemical within the tubular lumen would be expected to produce their effects first in the proximal nephron. There appear to be differences in sensitivity along various segments within the proximal nephron. The proximal convolution is the primary site of reabsorption of glucose and amino acids and seems to be more sensitive to certain metals like chromium. The *pars recta* (or straight portion) has a greater capacity to secrete organic compounds, and it is in this area where damage due to mercury, cephaloridine, and other organic compounds appears first.

This is not to say, however, that there are not specific receptors for certain nephrotoxins in the kidney. Localization of sites of nephrotoxins to areas of the tubule other than the proximal nephron strongly argues for specific biochemical receptors for some types of nephrotoxic agents. For instance, the loop of Henle appears to be the site of damage produced by analgesic mixtures (aspirin and phenacetin) and other materials that act in the medulla, such as fluoride ion. The distal convoluted tubule is a relatively small part of the total nephron and appears not be be selectively damaged by most nephrotoxins. However, compounds such as amphotericin have been shown to influence the ability of the kidney to acidify the urine, which is probably a distal tubular event. The collecting duct appears to be relatively insensitive to most nephrotoxins. For instance, following intoxication with analgesic mixtures, histologic evaluation of the medulla shows that most of the ascending limbs of the loop of Henle have been destroyed, whereas the collecting ducts appear to be unaffected. Damage due to outdated tetracyclines may occur in this area.

The glomerulus is a primary site of action of several chemicals and is also susceptible to immunologic injury. The evidence to date indicates that the primary barrier to filtration is the glomerular basement membrane. Following toxic insult, changes in glomerular permeability may occur, leading to loss of proteins in the urine. It had previously been suggested that nephrotoxins might change the diameter of pores in the glomerulus, allowing larger materials to pass through. However, by light microscopy the tissue does not appear to be more porous, but appears to be somewhat thicker after several nephrotoxins. More recent evidence has indicated that the net electrical charge on the glomerular membrane may be altered by toxicants, thereby changing the ability of the glomerular membrane to attract or repel charged molecules (Fig. 11–5).

Figure 11–3. The effect of a three-fourths nephrectomy on renal function tests in a dog. Serum creatinine and BUN were measured on alternate days for eight days. At the arrow the animal was anesthetized and one kidney removed. Approximately 50 percent of the branches of the renal artery entering the renal pelvis of the remaining kidney were ligated. The surgical wound was closed and the animal allowed to recover. In the immediate postoperative period there was a significant increase in serum creatinine and BUN, but within a short time these estimates of renal function returned to within normal limits.

cells may be more susceptible to damage merely because they are exposed to concentrations of chemicals many times higher than are other cells of the body, leading to nonspecific cellular damage. For instance, many nephrotoxins appear to have their primary site of action on (in) the proximal tubule. This is reasonable since most

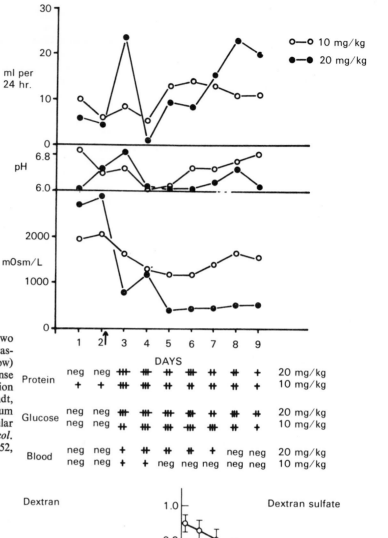

Figure 11–4. The effect of two doses of subcutaneous potassium dichromate (at the arrow) in rats. The rapidity of response and the quick return of function are illustrated. (From Berndt, W. O.: The effect of potassium dichromate on renal tubular transport processes. *Toxicol. Appl. Pharmacol.*, **32**:40–52, 1975.)

	1	2	3	4	5	6	7	8	9	
Protein	neg	neg	+++	+++	++	+++	++	++	+	20 mg/kg
	+	+	+++	+++	++	++	++	++	+	10 mg/kg
Glucose	neg	neg	+++	+++	+++	+++	++	+++	++	20 mg/kg
	neg	neg	++	+++	+++	+++	+++	++	+	10 mg/kg
Blood	neg	neg	+	++	++	++	+	neg	neg	20 mg/kg
	neg	neg	+	+	neg	neg	neg	neg	neg	10 mg/kg

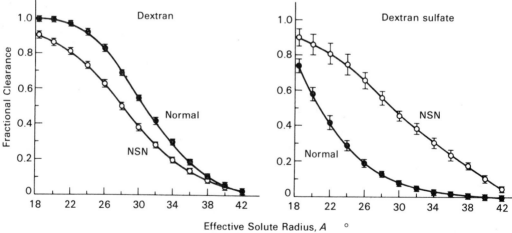

Figure 11–5. The effect of nephrotoxic serum nephritis (*NSN*) on glomerular permeability to neutral dextran and dextran sulfate. NSN, like puromycin aminonucleoside, appears to alter the charge on the glomerular membrane, thereby producing a net increase in permeability to dextran sulfate. (From Brenner, B. M., *et al.*: Determinants of glomerular permselectivity: Insights derived from observations *in vivo*. *Kidney Int.*, **12**:229–37, 1977. Reprinted with permission.)

SPECIFIC NEPHROTOXINS

Heavy Metals

Most heavy metals are potent nephrotoxins. Relatively low doses of a variety of metals produce a similar set of signs and symptoms characterized by glucosuria, aminoaciduria, and polyuria (Fig. 11–4). If the dose of the metal is increased, there will be renal necrosis, anuria, increased BUN, and death. Most metals probably produce their nephrotoxicity by a similar mechanism. Following a toxic metal insult the histologic picture is one of necrotic proximal tubules with lumens filled with proteinaceous material. It has been suggested that tissue destruction could lead to the sloughing of proximal tubular cells into the lumen resulting in tubular occlusion. Occlusion could be of sufficient magnitude to increase intratubular pressure, resulting in decreased glomerular filtration rate. However, this is probably an oversimplistic explanation. Oken (1976) has observed that when tubules are occluded after several nephrotoxins, intraluminal pressure is reduced, not elevated. The apparently low glomerular filtration rate may be partially explained by an increased permeability of the tubule to glomerular markers such as inulin, suggesting that filtration may occur and the tubule no longer is an effective barrier to reabsorption of inulin, producing an apparent decrease in glomerular filtration rate. Oken (1976) suggested that little leakage of inulin occurs, but since reabsorptive capacity of the tubule was reduced, the fall in glomerular filtration rate was due to decreased glomerular permeability or reduced glomerular blood flow. Indeed, there appears to be a significant vascular component of the nephrotoxicity of heavy metals. Protection against a great deal of nephrotoxicity to several heavy metals is offered by feeding animals a high-salt diet prior to challenge with the poison. Since the high salt would decrease renin release by the kidney, a renin-angiotensin mechanism has been proposed to explain vasoconstriction. This interpretation has not, however, been universally accepted. Several investigators have recently suggested an involvement of renal prostaglandins in this vasoconstriction. However, even in the absence of vasoconstriction, changes in renal function, particularly in the proximal tubule, occur following heavy metals. Probably the frank nephrotoxicity that occurs in response to heavy metals is due to a combination of ischemia secondary to vasoconstriction and direct cellular toxicity of these materials.

The kidney appears to possess several mechanisms that tend to protect the organ from heavy metal damage. Following low-dose exposure, significant concentrations of metal are found in renal tissue prior to development of physiologic signs of toxicity. Renal lysosomes appear to play an active role in such a protective mechanism (Fowler et al., 1975). This binding of metals by lysosomes may be stimulated by chronic low-level exposure, and the accumulation may be due to one of several mechanisms, including lysosomal endocytosis of a metal protein complex, autophagy of intoxicated organelles such as mitochondria, and/or binding of the metal to acidic lipoproteins within the lysosome. In addition, the smooth endoplasmic reticulum proliferates in the pars recta cells following exposure to mercury, and apical extrusion of endoplasmic reticulum packets may eliminate mercury from the kidney (Fowler, 1972). Exposure to very high concentrations of metals may inundate these mechanisms, resulting in the manifestations of cellular responses to injury.

Mercury. The toxicity of mercury has been recognized since antiquity. Mercury may be introduced into the body as elemental mercury, as inorganic mercury, or as organic mercury such as diuretics. More recently, organic mercury as an environmental pollutant, methylmercuric chloride, has produced renal damage in man and animals. A considerable amount of data has accumulated on the nephrotoxicity of mercury because it has been used extensively as a model compound to produce acute renal failure in animals. Functional toxicity probably results from both vasoconstriction and direct cellular effects. Both organic and inorganic mercurials are toxic in vitro.

Gottschalk and his collaborators (Biber et al., 1968) administered mercuric chloride to rats and then evaluated individual nephron function by micropuncture and structural integrity by microdissection. Nephrotoxic doses produced relatively selective histopathologic and functional alterations in the pars recta of the proximal tubule. They suggested that this localization of effect was consistent with the normal appearance of the surface of the poisoned kidney and the rather modest effect of $HgCl_2$ on glucose excretion (most glucose reabsorption occurs in the convoluted portion of the proximal nephron). The majority of PAH secretion occurs in the pars recta, and PAH transport appears to be extremely sensitive to Hg (Phillips et al., 1977). As the dose of mercury is increased, toxicity occurs throughout the proximal nephron.

The basic biochemical mechanism whereby mercury produces renal cellular damage is not completely clear. However, it is well known that mercury will combine with sulfhydryl groups and inhibit a great number of enzyme systems. Mitochondrial enzyme systems seem to be particularly sensitive to mercury, and the pathophysiologic effects often seen suggest inhibition of oxidative pathways. However, mitochondrial effects of mercury might not be the initiating events in mercury nephrotoxicity. Ganote et al. (1974) attempted to evaluate the time course of the effect of mercuric chloride on the ultrastructure of the kidney and to correlate these changes with several parameters of metabolic integrity. Within 24 hours a low dose of mercuric chloride (1 mg/kg) to rats produced a relatively selective necrosis of proximal tubular cells in the inner cortex, consistent with an effect within the *pars recta*. However, as early as eight hours after the mercury they were able to identify a variety of other morphologic changes including loss of brush border, dispersion of ribosomes, and formation of clumps of smooth membranes in the cytoplasm of the proximal tubule. These changes were followed by the appearance of vacuoles and other changes, including rupture of the plasma membrane and mitochondrial changes characteristic of cell necrosis. As early as eight hours there were alterations in water and ion movement in renal cortical tissue consistent with some of the morphologic changes. However, the ability of the tissue to accumulate PAH was not depressed until after 16 hours. Oxygen consumption of tissue slices was not reduced until 24 hours after the poison, when the cells were frankly necrotic. Thus, these data suggest that mitochondrial injury does not play a primary role in the pathogenesis of mercury toxicity; rather the data suggest that the mitochondrial damage occurred only at about the same time as general disruption of the plasma membrane.

Chromium. Another of the widely studied metal nephrotoxins is chromium, usually administered as potassium dichromate. In sublethal doses, chromium produces a proximal tubular necrosis that is similar to mercury except for its localization. Low doses of chromium produce a relatively specific necrosis of the proximal convoluted tubule. Functionally, this leads to pronounced glucosuria (Fig. 11–4). After low doses of chromium the surface of the kidney shows marked signs of ischemia and tissue damage. As with mercury, when the dose of chromium is increased, toxicity is seen throughout the proximal tubule.

Chromium seems to be directly toxic to the cells of the proximal tubule in that alterations in transport of organic compounds can be seen following *in vitro* addition of the toxin to slice preparations or following administration to animals. Interestingly, Hirsch (1976) saw an apparent stimulation of organic ion (PAH and NMN) accumulation by renal cortical slices following low doses of potassium dichromate *in vivo* or with low concentrations of dichromate

in vitro. As the dose *in vivo* or the concentration *in vitro* was increased, the anticipated decrease in transport capacity was seen. Although the mechanism of the apparent enhanced transport is not clear, Hirsch interpreted these changes as indices of toxicity. At low doses of the poison, uptake of PAH and NMN into the tissue was not depressed. Possibly due to changes in membrane permeability or changes in intracellular protein binding, the ability of PAH or NMN to move out of the slice was reduced. Additionally, some other renal function that normally competes with ion transport for energy could have been inhibited by chromium, thereby removing this competing source of energy, allowing more PAH and NMN transport to occur.

Other Metals. Uranium is another well-known toxic metal that, like mercury and chromium, has been documented to produce massive cellular necrosis in the proximal tubule and subsequent anuria, elevated BUN, and death. Like chromium in low doses, uranium has been shown to enhance organic ion transport (Hirsch, 1976). However, this effect appears to be relatively specific for organic base transport.

Other metals known to be nephrotoxic in animals and man have similarly been shown to be directly cytotoxic. Acute or chronic administration of lead produces tissue damage and decreased transport of PAH and NMN. Similarly, cadmium reduces the ability of the kidney to extract PAH and reduces uptake by renal cortical slices *in vitro*. Renal damage has been obtained following the administration of arsenic, gold, iron, antimony, platinum, and thallium (Maher, 1976). Cadmium is an interesting metal, in that following administration of the metal there is enhanced synthesis in the liver of the metal-binding protein metallothionein. This compound seems to have a paradoxic effect on systemic toxicity of cadmium. Metallothionein appears to bind cadmium, and in this way it protects certain organs such as the testes from cadmium toxicity, yet at the same time metallothionein may enhance cadmium nephrotoxicity, possibly because the cadmium-metallothionein complex is taken up by the kidney more readily than the free ion (Nordberg et al., 1975).

Halogenated Hydrocarbons

Carbon tetrachloride (CCl_4) and chloroform ($CHCl_3$) are both hepatotoxic and nephrotoxic. The magnitude of the nephrotoxicity varies with species, strain, and sex. In male rats, CCl_4 produces a recognizable renal lesion; whereas anesthesia, hepatic necrosis, and death occur after $CHCl_3$ before any marked nephropathy is observable. Male mice are particularly sensitive to the nephrotoxicity of $CHCl_3$ and the degree of sensitivity to the poison varies among several strains. With both hydrocarbons the functional lesion in the kidney appears to be primarily due to proximal tubular damage, although structural alterations are seen in other portions of the nephron as well. Functionally, the nephropathy appears similar to other types of acute renal insult with polyuria, glucosuria, and proteinuria at low doses, leading to anuria and complete renal failure with higher doses. Inhibition of PAH uptake by renal cortical slices appears to be one of the most sensitive indices of toxicity (Watrous and Plaa, 1972).

There is considerable evidence to indicate that in the liver, CCl_4 and $CHCl_3$ are metabolically activated to the toxic species. Suggestions have been made that activation of $CHCl_3$ and CCl_4 by mixed-function oxidases involves formation of a reactive metabolite that covalently binds to hepatic or renal tissue. Prior treatment with a nonlethal dose of CCl_4 will protect the liver against a subsequent challenge, probably because the first dose decreased the drug-metabolizing enzyme systems of the liver. Agents known to enhance drug-metabolizing enzyme activity in the kidney and liver may similarly alter nephrotoxicity of the hydrocarbons. Ilett et al. (1973) administered ^{14}C-$CHCl_3$ to male mice and monitored renal necrosis and covalent binding of ^{14}C to renal protein. $CHCl_3$ produced necrosis primarily in the proximal tubules. Treatment of mice with piperonyl butoxide or phenobarbital reduced the extent of renal necrosis and the binding of ^{14}C to renal proteins in vivo. Covalent binding peaked 6 to 12 hours after $CHCl_3$ administration, while histologic evidence of damage was not apparent until 24 hours after dosing. Striker et al. (1968) have shown in kidneys of rats that early signs of damage occur long after CCl_4 has been eliminated, suggesting that in the kidney, as in the liver, a metabolite of CCl_4 is responsible for inducing tissue damage. Presumably metabolic activations of $CHCl_3$ and CCl_4 are renal phenomena. However, no definitive data are available to rule out the formation of a toxic material in the liver being transported to the kidney.

Other halogenated hydrocarbons such as bromobenzene, trichloroethylene, and trichloroethane have also been shown to be toxic to the kidney, producing effects similar to those of CCl_4 and $CHCl_3$.

Therapeutic Agents

Analgesics. Analgesic mixtures (containing aspirin and phenacetin) taken by man in large doses over prolonged periods produce a classic picture of medullary interstitial nephritis, papillary damage, and chronic renal failure with loss of concentrating ability. Histologically, the kidney demonstrates a loss of renal papillae, a medullary inflammatory response with interstitial fibrosis, and nephron atrophy (Kincaid-Smith, 1978). Proximal tubular damage may also be seen. Considerable controversy has arisen concerning the specific agent in the mixture responsible for the nephrotoxicity. Resolution of the problem has been complicated by the lack of a suitable animal model for experimental studies. Phenacetin or one of its metabolites, primarily N-acetyl-para-aminophenol (APAP, acetaminophen, paracetamol), has been implicated as a major contributor to the toxicity in man; however, removal of phenacetin from analgesic mixtures has not eliminated the problem (Kincaid-Smith, 1978).

In large acute doses to rats, aspirin or phenacetin will produce renal medullary necrosis, often with accompanying proximal tubular damage. Molland (1978) fed rats relatively moderate doses of analgesics for extended times and observed that aspirin had a greater nephrotoxic effect than either phenacetin or APAP, although aspirin toxicity was less alone than in combination with one of the nonsalicylates. Following aspirin alone the earliest changes occurred in the medullary interstitial cells. Interestingly, the cortical lesions did not depend on the presence of papillary necrosis, suggesting that the papillary and cortical damage might be separate events. It was suggested that the early papillary changes might be secondary to ischemia due to vasospasm in the vasa recta. Such an effect is consistent with the ability of aspirin to inhibit prostaglandin synthesis. Theoretically, inhibition of renal medullary prostaglandin synthesis might remove an endogenous vasodilator prostaglandin, leading to localized vasoconstriction. Indeed, Nanra (1974) has observed that not only aspirin, but other inhibitors of prostaglandin synthesis will produce renal medullary lesions in rats.

The reason for localization of the chronic effect of analgesics to the medulla is not completely clear, but it has been suggested that it is due to the trapping of compounds in the medulla by the countercurrent mechanism. However, neither aspirin nor phenacetin has been shown to achieve increased concentrations in the medulla, whereas APAP and its conjugates appear to concentrate in the renal medulla (Duggin and Mudge, 1976). Dehydration of animals leads to maximal concentrations of these materials in the medulla, a fact consistent with the enhanced toxicity that occurs during dehydration.

Anesthetics. Several of the halogenated hydrocarbon anesthetics have been suggested to produce nephrotoxicity, but only one agent, methoxyflurane, has been documented to produce reproducible renal failure. In both animals and man, methoxyflurane produced a high-output renal failure, negative fluid balance, and increases in serum sodium, osmolality, and BUN. Patients or animals were unable to concentrate urine despite fluid deprivation and vasopressin administration, pointing to a defect in the renal concentrating mechanism. This toxicity had not originally been seen in animals studies. When Mazze (1976) and his collaborators studied a series of five rat strains, however, they found that the Fischer-344 and the Buffalo strains metabolized methoxyflurane to a greater extent than the other strains studied. The Fisher-344, with the greatest degree of metabolism, was the only strain that evidenced nephrotoxicity. Methoxyflurane appears to be metabolized primarily to inorganic fluoride and oxalate. Enhanced metabolism and nephrotoxicity were seen following phenobarbital treatment whereas enzyme inhibition decreased metabolism and reduced nephrotoxicity. Subsequent studies indicated that it was the generation of the fluoride ion (acting in the ascending limb of the loop of Henle or in the collecting duct) that rendered the medulla ADH resistant.

Antibiotics. Several antibiotics in high doses have been shown to produce nephrotoxicity. The most common examples occur in the aminoglycoside class of antibiotics. This group includes streptomycin, neomycin, kanamycin, and the newer agents amikacin and gentamicin. Following relatively high doses, or after prolonged therapy in man and laboratory animals, gentamicin produces symptoms of acute renal damage typical of alterations of proximal tubular function (Appel and Neu, 1977b). This is probably a direct cytotoxic effect of the agent, possibly compounded by glomerular changes. Gentamicin has a relatively short half-life in the plasma, but the half-life in the kidney is considerably longer, suggesting that the material is tightly bound to renal tissue. Although there have been suggestions that gentamicin might be actively secreted or reabsorbed, no definitive data are yet available. Nevertheless, it is clear that the material is accumulated within the cells of the proximal tubule, which leads to cellular damage (Appel and Neu, 1977b). A similar phenomenon is produced by the cephalosporin-type antibiotics. The compound most commonly associated with nephrotoxicity is cephaloridine. Like gentamicin, cephaloridine has a relatively short half-life in plasma, although its renal elimination is not particularly high. However, cephaloridine is accumulated by cells of the proximal tubule by an active transport system and then is avidly retained. Accumulation of cephaloridine and the accompanying nephrotoxicity can be attenuated by probenecid and other compounds that block active organic anion transport (Tune, 1975). Similarly, in newborn animals, when development of anionic transport is incomplete, the renal toxicity is low. Enhancement of transport increases toxicity (Wold et al., 1977). There have been several suggestions of an interaction or synergism between cephaloridine and gentamicin nephrotoxicity; however, this has yet to be documented.

Tetracyclines, particularly demeclocycline, have on occasion produced renal medullary toxicity. Outdated tetracyclines may produce proximal tubular damage with polyuria, glucosuria, and aminoaciduria. In man, penicillins and sulfonamides have been implicated in an inflammatory interstitial nephritis that is not dose related. This appears to be due to an immunologic-type mechanism (Appel and Neu, 1977a, 1977b). Amphotericin B has been shown to be markedly nephrotoxic, producing histopathologic changes in the proximal and distal tubules. The functional alteration implicating a distal tubular lesion is decreased acidification of the urine. Decreased PAH transport is an early indication of proximal tubule damage (Appel and Neu, 1977c).

The aminonucleoside of puromycin has been used as an experimental tool to produce an animal model of the nephrotic syndrome in man. Functionally, there appears to be an increased permeability of the glomerulus to proteins such as albumin. Although several hypotheses have been suggested considering the nature of the defect, little has been documented until recently, when Brenner et al. (1977) demonstrated that glomerular permeability to a series of charged dextrans was markedly increased, suggesting that there had been a pathologic alteration in net electrical charge of the glomerular basement membrane (Fig. 11–5).

Environmental Pollutants

A variety of pesticides and herbicides have reached sufficient concentrations in the environment to constitute potential hazards to man and animals. 2,4,5-Trichlorophenoxyacetic acid (2,4,5-T) is a widely used herbicide. This compound has not been shown to be directly nephrotoxic but it may influence renal function. The compound appears to be actively transported by the organic anion secretory system and is capable of inhibiting organic anion transport. Furthermore, in high concentrations the compound appears to inhibit cation transport as well (Berndt, 1976). The herbicide paraquat produces profound pulmonary damage following acute intoxication. In sublethal doses paraquat appears to be actively secreted by the organic cation transport system of the kidney and is fairly rapidly removed from the body. Following high doses, however, paraquat produces direct renal damage, thereby reducing its own elimination. This leads to prolonged high plasma levels of this agent, which enhance the lung damage (Ecker *et al.*, 1975).

A number of industrial and agricultural chemicals may influence kidney function. Several of these compounds have profound metabolic effects on the liver, and it is these abnormalities that have received most attention. However, it is not unlikely that in the future heretofore unrecognized abnormalities in renal function could be attributed to one or more of these agents. Polychlorinated biphenyls (PCBs) are a mixture of chemicals used in a wide variety of manufacturing processes, notably in the plastics industry, and as insulators. These compounds are ubiquitous contaminants of the environment. The PCBs have been shown to have marked stimulating effects on drug metabolism in the liver and to increase liver size and liver weight. PCBs also have been shown to enhance drug-metabolizing enzyme activity in the kidney (Vainio, 1974). The polybrominated biphenyls (PBBs), although not so widespread, are also significant environmental contaminants. The PBBs similarly induce drug-metabolizing enzyme activity in the liver and kidney and thereby present a potential hazard (McCormack *et al.*, 1978). Tetrachlorodibenzo-*p*-dioxin (TCDD) is an extremely toxic agent that has been known to produce a wide variety of toxic symptoms in animals and man. Like the polyhalogenated biphenyls, TCDD has not been shown to have a profound direct toxic effect on the adult kidney but does alter drug metabolism in this organ and could pose a potential hazard (Fowler *et al.*, 1977). The presence of such potential stimulators of drug metabolism in the environment could lead to difficulty in interpreting experimental data. For instance, following accidental exposure to one of these stimulators, a relatively innocuous substance could be metabolically altered within the kidney and produce nephrotoxicity.

Miscellaneous Nephrotoxins

On occasion, chemicals may reach such high concentrations in the tubular urine that they exceed their solubilities and are precipitated as crystals. These crystals may be eliminated from the kidney or may be deposited in the collecting system, leading to the formation of larger crystals or stones. The stones may mechanically obstruct the tubules leading to tubular dilatation, backing up of fluid, and an increase in intratubular pressure. This could lead to diminution in glomerular filtration rate and renal blood flow, resulting in tissue ischemia and subsequent loss of renal tissue. Such effects have been seen with sulfonamide drugs and oxalate (metabolically derived from glycols). In some cases uric acid may form stones (Bluestone *et al.*, 1975). The synthetic amino acid α-methyltyrosine may achieve sufficiently high concentrations to form stones in the kidney (Hook and Moore, 1969).

Dimethylnitrosamine has been reported to produce renal carcinoma in appropriately preconditioned animals (Swann *et al.*, 1976). Diphenylamine has been used as a tool to produce cystic kidneys in adult animals (Gardner *et al.*, 1976). Maleic acid has been used as a tool to study reabsorptive pathways for amino acids and glucose because of its ability to produce reproducible nephropathy in the proximal tubule (Segal and Thier, 1973). A vasopressin-resistant concentrating defect has been produced in animals with 2-amino-4,5-diphenylthiazole (Carone *et al.*, 1974). Recent studies indicate that several mycotoxins produce renal proximal damage (Berndt and Hayes, 1977).

Apparent nephropathy may also be caused as a secondary effect of several pharmacologic agents. For instance, long-term treatment of animals with diuretics may lead to loss of total body potassium resulting in potassium depletion nephropathy. Similarly, drugs that reduce blood pressure or increase renal vascular resistance may produce effects reminiscent of ischemia. Yet the drugs themselves are not directly nephrotoxic (Maher, 1976).

Nephrotoxicity in Newborn

Administration of several chemical agents during the prenatal period has been shown to produce profound alterations in kidney structure at birth. Agents like methyl salicylate and TCDD have been shown to produce teratogenic effects on the kidney, primarily hydronephrosis. Hypervitaminosis A during gestation has been suggested to produce hydronephrosis in offspring. Diphenylamine when fed to pregnant rats has been reported to produce a polycystic kidney in newborn animals. Similarly, large doses of steroid hormones to newborn or weanling rabbits produced polycystic kidney. However, as pointed out by Gibson (1976), these reports must be viewed with some caution in that traditional teratogenic studies are performed on animals derived by cesarean section. An apparent abnormality in structure might not constitute permanent structural damage but only reflect delayed maturation. Considerably more investigation needs to be made into the functional sequelae in newborn animals of prenatal administration of chemicals. Preliminary data have suggested that prenatal dinoseb, paraquat, and TCDD can produce alterations in PAH transport in kidney slices from newborn animals even when no structural lesion is apparent (Gibson, 1976). Further studies are necessary to evaluate the significance of these changes and to determine if they are maintained throughout the life of the animals or if the animals may compensate for these changes during normal growth and development.

REFERENCES

Appel, G. B., and Neu, H. C.: The nephrotoxicity of antimicrobial agents (part 1). *N. Engl. J. Med.*, 296:663–70, 1977a.

Appel, G. B., and Neu, H. C.: The nephrotoxicity of antimicrobial agents (part 2). *N. Engl. J. Med.*, 296:722–28, 1977b.

Appel, G. B., and Neu, H. C.: The nephrotoxicity of antimicrobial agents (part 3). *N. Engl. J. Med.*, 296:784–87, 1977c.

Berndt, W. O.: The effect of potassium dichromate on renal tubular transport processes. *Toxicol. Appl. Pharmacol.*, 32:40–52, 1975.

Berndt, W. O.: Renal function tests: What do they mean? A review of renal anatomy, biochemistry, and physiology. *Environ. Health Perspect.*, 15:55–71, 1976.

Berndt, W. O., and Hayes, A. W.: Effects of citrinin on renal tubular transport functions in the rat. *J. Environ. Pathol. Toxicol.*, 1:93–103, 1977.

Biber, T. U. L.; Mylle, M.; Baines, A. D.; Gottschalk, C. W.; Oliver, J. R.; and MacDowell, M. C.: A study in micropuncture and microdissection of acute renal damage in rats. *Am. J. Med.*, 44:664–705, 1968.

Bluestone, R.; Waisman, J.; and Klinenberg, J. R.: Chronic experimental hyperuricemic nephropathy. *Lab. Invest.*, 33:273–79, 1975.

Brenner, B. M.; Bohrer, M. P.; Baylis, C.; and Deen, W. M.: Determinants of glomerular permselectivity: Insights derived from observations *in vivo*. *Kidney Int.*, 12:229–37, 1977.

Carone, F. A.; Stolarczyk, J.; Krumlovsky, F. A.; Perlman, S. G.; Roberts, T. H.; and Rowland, R. G.: The nature of a drug-induced renal concentrating defect in rats. *Lab. Invest.*, 31:658–64, 1974.

Duggin, G. D., and Mudge, G. H.: Analgesic nephropathy: Renal distribution of acetaminophen and its conjugates. *J. Pharmacol. Exp. Ther.*, 199:1–9, 1976.

Ecker, J. L.; Hook, J. B.; and Gibson, J. E.: Nephrotoxicity of paraquat in mice. *Toxicol. Appl. Pharmacol.*, 34:178–86, 1975.

Fowler, B. A.: Ultrastructural evidence for nephropathy induced by long-term exposure to small amounts of methyl mercury. *Science*, 175:780–81, 1972.

Fowler, B. A.; Brown, H. W.; Lucier, G. W.; and Krigman, M. R.: The effects of chronic oral methyl mercury exposure on the lysosome system of rat kidney. *Lab. Invest.*, 32:313–22, 1975.

Fowler, B. A.; Hook, G. E. R.; and Lucier, G. W.: Tetrachlorodibenzo-*p*-dioxin induction of renal microsomal enzyme systems: Ultrastructural effects on pars recta (S_3) proximal tubule cells of the rat kidney. *J. Pharmacol. Exp. Ther.*, 203:712–21, 1977.

Ganote, C. E.; Reimer, K. A.; and Jennings, R. B.: Acute mercuric chloride nephrotoxicity: An electron microscopic and metabolic study. *Lab. Invest.*, 31:633–47, 1974.

Gardner, K. D., Jr.; Solomon, S.; Fitzgerrel, W. W.; and Evan, A. P.: Function and structure in the diphenylamine-exposed kidney. *J. Clin. Invest.*, 57:796–806, 1976.

Gibson, J. E.: Perinatal nephropathies. *Environ. Health Perspect.*, 15:121–30, 1976.

Gottschalk, C. W.: Osmotic concentration and dilution of the urine. *Am. J. Med.*, 36:670–85, 1964.

Hirsch, G. H.: Differential effects of nephrotoxic agents on renal transport and metabolism by use of *in vitro* techniques *Environ. Health Perspect.*, 15:89–99, 1976.

Hook, J. B., and Moore, K. E.: The renal handling of α-methyltyrosine. *J. Pharmacol. Exp. Ther.*, 168:310–14, 1969.

Ilett, K. F.; Reid, W. D.; Sipes, I. G.; and Krishna, G.: Choroform toxicity in mice: Correlation of renal and hepatic necrosis with covalent binding of metabolites to tissue macromolecules. *Exp. Mol. Pathol.*, 19:215–29, 1973.

Kincaid-Smith, P.: Analgesic nephropathy. *Kidney Int.*, 13:1–4, 1978.

Maher, J. F.: Toxic nephropathy. In Brenner, B. M., and Rector, F. C., Jr. (eds.): *The Kidney*. W. B. Saunders, Philadelphia, 1976.

Mazze, R. I.: Methoxyflurane nephropathy. *Environ. Health Perspect.*, 15:111–19, 1976.

McCormack, K. M.; Kluwe, W. M.; Rickert, D. E.; Sanger, V. L.; and Hook, J. B.: Renal and hepatic microsomal enzyme stimulation and renal function following three months of dietary exposure to polybrominated biphenols. *Toxicol. Appl. Pharmacol.*, 44:539–53, 1978.

Molland, E. A.: Experimental renal papillary necrosis. *Kidney Int.*, 13:5–14, 1978.

Nanra, R. S., and Kincaid-Smith, P.: Chronic effect of analgesics on the kidney. In Edwards, K. D. G. (ed.): *Progress in Biochemical Pharmacology*, Vol. VII: *Drugs Affecting Kidney Function and Metabolism*. S. Karger, Basel, 1972.

Nanra, R. S.: Pathology, aetiology and pathogenesis of analgesic nephropathy. *Aust. N. Z. J. Med.*, 4:602–603, 1974.

Nordberg, G. F.; Goyer, R.; and Nordberg, M.: Comparative toxicity of cadmium-metallothionein and cadmium chloride on mouse kidney. *Arch. Pathol.*, 99:192–97, 1975.

Oken, D. E.: Acute renal failure caused by nephrotoxins. *Environ. Health Perspect.*, 15:101–109, 1976.

Phillips, R.; Yamauchi, M.; Côté, M. G.; and Plaa, G. L.: Assessment of mercuric chloride-induced nephrotoxicity by *p*-aminohippuric acid uptake and the activity of four gluconeogenic enzymes in rat renal cortex. *Toxicol. Appl. Pharmacol.*, 41:407–22, 1977.

Segal, S., and Thier, S. O.: Renal handling of amino acids. In Orloff, J., and Berliner, R. W. (eds.): *Handbook of Physiology. Section 8: Renal Physiology*. American Physiological Society, Washington, D.C., 1973.

Striker, G. E.; Smuckler, E. A.; Kohnen, P. W.; and Nagle, R. B.: Structural and functional changes in rat kidney during CCl_4 intoxication. *Am. J. Pathol.*, 53:769–78, 1968.

Swann, P. F.; Magee, P. N.; Mohr, U.; Reznik, G.; Green, U.; and Kaufman, D. G.: Possible repair of carcinogenic damage caused by dimethylnitrosamine in rat kidney. *Nature (Lond.)*, 263:134–36, 1976.

Tune, B. M.: Relationship between the transport and toxicity of cephalosporins in the kidney. *J. Infect. Dis.*, 132:189–94, 1975.

Vainio, H.: Enhancement of microsomal drug oxidation and glucuronidation in rat liver by an environmental chemical, polychlorinated biphenyl. *Chem. Biol. Interact.*, **9**:379–87, 1974.

Valtin, H.: *Renal Function: Mechanisms Preserving Fluid and Solute Balance in Health.* Little, Brown & Co., Boston, 1973.

Watrous, W. M., and Plaa, G. L.: Effect of halogenated hydrocarbons on organic ion accumulation by renal cortical slices of rats and mice. *Toxicol. Appl. Pharmacol.*, **22**:528–43, 1972.

Wold, J. S.; Joost, R. R.; and Owen, N. V.: Nephrotoxicity of cephaloridine in newborn rabbits: Role of the renal anionic transport system. *J. Pharmacol. Exp. Ther.*, **201**:778–85, 1977.

Chapter 12

TOXIC RESPONSES OF THE RESPIRATORY SYSTEM

Daniel B. Menzel and *Roger O. McClellan*

INTRODUCTION

The primary function of the lung is to provide a means for the exchange of oxygen and carbon dioxide. To achieve this, the mammalian lung has evolved into a complex organ particularly suited for the uptake and excretion of volatile compounds in addition to oxygen and carbon dioxide. The large surface area, the airways, and the minute separation between the air space and capillary circulation make the lung an efficient organ for the absorption of nonvolatile toxicants as well. Toxicants can enter the respiratory system as gases, solids, or liquid aerosols and are readily taken up and transported to other organs. The lung receives all of the cardiac output, speeding distribution to other organs. Because of the vital nature of pulmonary function, direct action of toxicants on the lung can be acutely and chronically important to health. Respirable toxicants need not be absorbed to produce disease, as exemplified by fibrous minerals that produce pulmonary fibrosis and cancer.

Exposure to toxicants via inhalation occurs in all phases of human activity. The importance of inhalation as a route of exposure at the workplace cannot be overemphasized. The workplace often contains dusts, aerosols, and gases that are either direct toxicants or indirect promoters of toxicity. The home is also contaminated with toxicants that can be inhaled. Gas cooking, for example, produces nitrogen dioxide and carbon monoxide which reach measurable and relatively high concentrations around the stove and in the kitchen. The air of most urban areas is contaminated with large concentrations of a myriad of air pollutants. During play and sports, inhalation exposure is increased, leading to higher doses than at rest. The involuntary nature of respiration places a particular burden on the toxicologist to ensure the safety of the air we breathe.

The reported incidence of pulmonary disease is increasing due to inhaled toxicants such as air pollutants, better diagnosis of pulmonary disease, and increased longevity of diseased patients. Patients with chronic lung diseases, such as asthma, bronchitis, emphysema, and pulmonary fibrosis, constitute a large fraction of the population that may be especially at risk from exposure to inhaled toxicants. Chronic pulmonary disease is as crippling and as disabling as the more obvious injuries to limbs and other organ systems.

As a further complication to the study of the toxicology of the lung, it has recently become apparent that the pulmonary capillary network has specialized functions to remove, metabolize, and excrete vasoactive hormones. The lung functions as an exocrine organ regulating angiotensin, biogenic amines, and prostaglandin concentrations in the circulation. Deterioration of these functions is likely to result in loss of local regulation of blood pressure and flow, potentially producing perfusion-ventilation abnormalities impairing gas exchange.

The lung also actively excretes toxicants either inhaled or absorbed through other routes. It possesses an active cytochrome P450 system metabolizing many xenobiotic compounds. The excretion of these toxicants and the potential metabolism by the lung consequently may result in pulmonary toxicity. Clearance or removal is particularly important to proper pulmonary function. Electrolytes and nonionized compounds are rapidly cleared from the lung. Particles are removed by specialized mechanisms combining mucus secretion and ciliary action. The toxicity of the compound will increase in the pulmonary system as well as in other organ systems when diseases or other toxicants have impaired the clearance mechanisms of the lung. A common source of self-intoxication, tobacco smoking, is particularly important to these clearance mechanisms.

In this chapter, a general introduction to inhalation toxicology is presented. Some detail is provided on the structure of the lung, since structure is especially related to function in this organ. The complexity of the cell population of the lung is also emphasized, as specific functions are recognized for the different cell types. Pulmonary damage from a given toxicant may be localized in a specific cell type because of the particular sensitivity of that cell type. A general discussion is also provided on the specialized methodology of inhalation toxicology. A lack of sophistication in this aspect can lead to serious errors in estimating the toxicity of a compound to man or in the assessment of an inhalation hazard. Some specific toxicants are considered in a limited scope. Detailed descriptions of the toxicity of air pollutants appear in Chapter 24 and of inhaled radionuclides in Chapter 19. A basic understanding of pulmonary physiology is assumed in this discussion. Two excellent monographs by West (1974, 1977) provide this information and were used as the basic reference works for pulmonary physiology throughout.

STRUCTURE OF THE RESPIRATORY TRACT

The deposition and retention of inhaled gases and aerosols are influenced by many anatomic features of the respiratory tract, including lung volume, alveolar surface area, and structure and spatial relationships of conducting airways into alveoli. Distribution of deposited material as a function of time, in combination with the location of the over 40 cell types identified in the respiratory tract, determines the cells at risk for any inhaled material.

The respiratory tract may be considered as having three major regions: the *nasopharyngeal,* the *tracheobronchial,* and the *pulmonary.* The nasopharynx begins with the anterior nares and extends back and down to the level of the larynx. The nasal passages are lined with vascular mucous epithelium, which is characterized, except at the entrance, by ciliated columnar epithelium and scattered mucous glands. The nasopharynx filters out large inhaled particles and is the region in which the relative humidity is increased and the temperature of the air is moderated. The trachea, bronchi, and bronchioles serve as conducting airways between the nasopharynx and alveoli, where gas exchange occurs. The conducting airways are lined with ciliated epithelium and coated with a thin layer of mucus secreted by goblet cells and mucus-secreting cells. This mucous covering terminates at the film covering the alveolar membrane. The surface of the airways serves as a mucociliary escalator, moving particles from the deep lung to the oral cavities so they may be swallowed and excreted. The branching patterns and physical dimensions of the airways are critical in determining the deposition of particles and the absorption of gases by the respiratory tract.

Several mathematical models have been developed describing the physical dimensions of the airways (Weibel, 1963; Davies, 1961). The airways tend to be equally bifurcating in man, decreasing in diameter as they divide. The cross-sectional area, however, increases as bifurcation increases. In addition to the axial diffusion of gases along the streamline of the airways, the increase in cross-sectional area also produces a radial diffusion. Gases tend to be diluted by this anatomic feature of the lung, independent of mixing with other inspired gases. Rodent lungs are similar to man's, but have fewer divisions. Each division is sometimes referred to as a generation. The human airways have about 23 generations.

The *acinus* is the basic functional unit of the mammalian lung and is the primary location of gas exchange between the environment and blood. Anatomically, the acini consist of the structures distal to and including the first-order respiratory bronchiole, which is the first bronchiole with alveoli. The acini, of which there are about 200,000 in the adult human, include three or four orders of respiratory bronchioles, several orders of alveolar ducts and alveolar sacs, hundreds of alveoli and associated blood vessels, lymphatic tissues, supportive tissues, and nerve enervations. The anatomy of the acinus is described in detail by Pump (1964), Frasier and Pare (1971), Nagahi (1972), and Phalen et al. (1973). Quantitative anatomic information for these structures includes estimates of airway tube numbers, diameters, and lengths; alveolar numbers and diameters; surface areas; and mean thicknesses for the air-blood barrier (Weibel, 1963; Kliment, 1973).

Respiratory bronchioles are tubular structures with diameters of about 0.5 mm and lengths of about 1.0 mm in the adult human. Bronchioles are lined with low cuboidal epithelium and at times with ciliated epithelium. Their walls contain collagen, smooth muscle, and elastic fibers, but no cartilage, making them quite distensible. One or more aveoli is open to its lumens along one side while the other side is relatively smooth and in contact with branches of the pulmonary artery.

The *alveolar ducts* and *sacs* are thin-walled tubes, literally covered with alveoli on all sides. In adults their diameters are about 0.5 mm and lengths are about 0.7 mm. Alveolar sacs, which are clusters of two or more alveoli terminating in one or more alveoli, branch from alveolar ducts and are essentially closed-end versions of ducts. The total number of alveolar ducts and sacs in man is estimated to be about 10 to 25 million (Weibel, 1963).

Alveoli are thin-walled, polyhedral pouches with one side open to either a respiratory bronchiole, an alveolar duct, or an alveolar sac. Thin, squamous pulmonary epithelial cells form most of the continuous inner lining of the alveolus. More rounded septal cells are also located within the walls, and free, motile phagocytic cells, pulmonary macrophages, often lie in contact with the inner surface of the alveolus. A dense capillary vascular plexus covers the alveolus. In man, the number of alveoli increases rapidly after birth until about eight years of age (Charnock and Doershuk, 1973), when approximately 300 million are present. The value of 300 million alveoli in the adult human is consistently reported, although recent estimates have ranged from 100 million (Kliment, 1973) to over 500 million (Davies, 1961). The alveolus of the adult human, though not strictly spheric, has an equivalent diameter of about 150 to 300 μm, but the range of 250 to 350 μm is probably more realistic (Weibel, 1963). Alveolar dimensions vary also with degree of lung inflation and with the vertical position within the thorax. The total alveolar surface area in the adult human is about 35 m² during expiration, 70 to 80 m² at three-fourths total lung capacity, and 100 m² during deep inspiration (von Hayek, 1960; Weibel, 1963). The thickness of the air-blood barrier is variable, even for a given alveolus. The air-blood barrier consists of endothelium, basement membrane, and alveolar epithelium, with a total thickness of 0.36 to 2.5 μm. The tissue thickness between adjacent alveoli is made up of the thickness of the alveolar wall, basement membrane, interstitium, and any interposed capillary. The capillary diameter is about 8 μm, and 90 to 95 percent of the alveolar surface is covered with capillaries. The mean tissue thickness between alveoli is then about 9 μm.

Well over 40 cell types are required to perform the diverse functions of the respiratory tract. These include 17 types of epithelium, nine types of unspecified connective tissue, two types of bone and cartilage, seven types of cells related to blood vessels, two distinctive types of muscle cells, and five types associated with the pleural or nervous tissue elements. The cells of greatest interest are those that are unique to the respiratory tract, such as ciliated bronchial epithelium, nonciliated bronchiolar epithelium (Clara cells), type I (squamous alveolar) pneumocytes, type II (great alveolar) pneumocytes, and alveolar macrophages. In addition, three other cell types are of special interest: endothelial cells and interstitial cells (fibroblasts and fibrocytes), which constitute the greatest percentage of total cells present; and lining cells of the trachea and bronchi, which account for only a small portion of the mass of the total respiratory tract. These latter three cell types are extremely susceptible to various types of injury.

The ciliated tracheobronchial epithelial cells are the predominant cells in the trachea, bronchi, and bronchioles of airways greater than 1 mm in diameter, where they outnumber goblet or mucus-secreting cells five to one. As the terminal bronchiole diminishes in diameter and terminates in the respiratory bronchiole, the cilia-bearing cells gradually disappear.

The ciliated epithelium functions to move a fluid film and particles deposited on it from the lung to the nasopharynx. Direct observations have shown that transport rates in the trachea or large bronchi in several species range from 1 to 3.5 cm/min. Mucociliary transport is capable of clearing inhaled particles from the conducting airways in a few hours and is a major detoxification mechanism.

Nonciliated bronchiolar cells (Clara cells) are present only in small bronchioles and can be identified by their bulging into the bronchiolar lumen, by the absence of cilia, and by the presence of apical cytoplasmic granules (Cutz and Conen, 1971). The ultrastructural characteristics reveal the presence of plasma membranes that form complex interdigitations, including desmosomes, with adjacent epithelial cells. The function of the Clara cells is not known, although ultrastructural and cytochemical evidence indicates that they are metabolically active, probably secretory, and have characteristics like merocrine-type secretory cells.

The surface of the pulmonary alveoli is largely covered by the continuous, exceedingly attenuated (0.1 to 0.2 μm) cytoplasm of the squamous epithelium, which has nuclei resembling those of capillary endothelium. This cell is located on the epithelial side of the basement membrane and, with the type II cells, completely lines the alveolus. The junction between the type I and type II cells is "tight," forming a *zonulae occludens*. The surface area of the type I cell has been calculated as 2,290 μm² and that of type II as 63 μm². Thus, even though the ratio of type I to type II cells in the alveolus is 2:3, the type I cell makes up most of the barrier of the blood-gas pathway. The cytoplasm of type I cells is barely visible with light microscopy and is equally unimpressive with electron microscopy because of its sparseness and the paucity of organelles. With the exception of pinocytotic vesicles, the cytoplasmic extensions of the type I cell are practically devoid of organelles. Some organelles are concentrated in the perinuclear cytoplasm.

With the light microscope, type II pulmonary epithelial cells are cuboidal. They are usually located in corners of the alveoli. The nucleus is spheric and the cytoplasm abundant with vacuoles. Type II cells from a number of species have basically similar ultrastructures (Sorokin, 1967). The cytoplasm has a loosely ordered granular endoplasmic reticulum, an extensive Golgi apparatus, numerous multivesicular bodies, and many large osmophilic multilamellated inclusions or cytosomes.

Type II cells are strongly implicated as the source of the pulmonary surfactant (Sorokin, 1967). Other functions of these cells have not been documented; however, the type II cells are frequently the proliferative cells in the repair of subtle diffuse injury to the squamous pulmonary epithelium, such as results from beryllium and oxygen toxicity (Kapanci et al., 1969; Carrington and Green, 1970; Bowden and Adamson, 1971). Type II cells have been classified as a renewing cell population by several investigators (Evans and Bils, 1969), with relatively long turnover times ranging from 20 to 84 days. Type II cells mature to type I cells with time.

The elaboration of the pulmonary surfactant by these cells is essential for proper ventilation. Surfactant consists mostly of dipalmitoyl lecithin and, as a thin film, has a very low surface tension characterized by unequal pathways of compression and relaxation. Surfactant lowers the surface tension in small alveoli so that inflation of small and large alveoli occurs at similar pressures. In the absence of surfactant, small alveoli coalesce into large alveoli, reducing the surface area available for gas exchange (respiratory distress syndrome of the premature infant).

Alveolar macrophages are the phagocytic cells of the lung and are found free in the alveoli. With light microscopy, alveolar macrophages in tissue sections are ovoid mononuclear cells, 7 to 10 μm in diameter. The nucleus is 5 to 6 μm in diameter and is round, oval, or kidney shaped. Macrophages washed from the lungs look similar, but they are larger (15 to 25 μm) and flatter and have more definitive cytologic detail.

The major function of alveolar macrophages is the ingestion of inhaled particulate material. Infectious particles are usually killed by the macrophages, except in some chronic bacterial and fungal infections, such as tuberculosis, and in some viral diseases where the virus actually replicates in the macrophage (Green, 1970; Green *et al.*, 1977).

The endothelial cells form a continuous cytoplasmic tube lining the pulmonary vasculature. The adjoining cells become closely approximated or may interdigitate and overlap. The endothelium of the alveolar septa is separated from the epithelium by an interstitial space of variable thickness.

The pulmonary capillary endothelium functions to exchange gases and volatile metabolites between the blood and air. However, these cells may also interact with the blood that perfuses them and perform functions with significant implications. The pulmonary endothelial cells are stem cell, renewing-cell

populations (Evans and Bils, 1969). The turnover time has not been determined but must be long, i.e., a matter of years.

The fibroblast is a cell of mesenchymal origin that is responsible for production of intercellular substances of connective tissues. These are relatively undifferentiated cells, and it is probable that the fibroblasts found in the lung are similar to those found elsewhere in the body.

PULMONARY PHYSIOLOGY

Figure 12–1 is a very simplified diagram of the distribution of volumes and flows within the adult human lung. The role of each of these volumes in respiration can be seen in Figure 12–2, which represents the normal respiratory pattern at rest. The changes in volume and flow are recorded using a spirometer, a lightweight, gastight bell immersed in water. The movement of the bell is recorded with time as the subject breathes. Normally, only a small volume of the lung is ventilated, the *tidal volume*. The tidal volume of 500 ml inhaled over a minute at 15 breaths/min represents the *minute volume* of 7,500 ml/min. Maximal inspiration and expiration are shown and the total volume represents the *vital capacity*. Some gas remains in the lung following maximal expiration and amounts to about 150 ml. This is the *residual volume*. The difference between no gas in the lung and the minimum of the tidal volume represents the *functional residual capacity*.

The difference between the volume of gas entering the lung and the volume not exhaled during normal respiration is *alveolar ventilation*, or the volume of fresh gas available for exchange

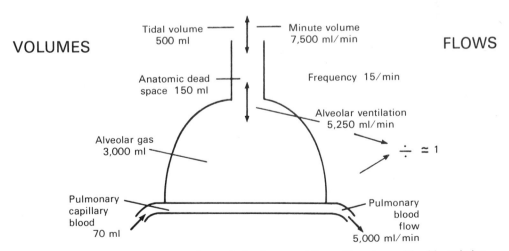

Figure 12–1. Diagram of a lung showing typical volumes and flows. There is considerable variation around these values. (From West, J. B.: *Respiratory Physiology—The Essentials.* © 1974 The Williams & Wilkins Co., Baltimore.)

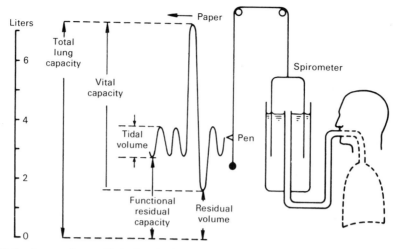

Figure 12–2. Lung volumes. Note that the functional residual capacity and residual volume cannot be measured with the spirometer. (From West, J. B.: *Respiratory Physiology—The Essentials.* © 1974 The Williams & Wilkins Co., Baltimore.)

at the alveolus. In our example the alveolar ventilation is:

(Tidal volume − anatomic dead space) × breaths/min
= (500 ml − 150 ml) × 15 breaths/min, or 5,250 ml/min

The pulmonary blood flow over the same minute is about 5,000 ml. The gas exchanged, or alveolar ventilation, is almost exactly the same volume as the blood perfusing the alveolus. The match of blood perfusion volume to alveolar ventilation is critical for proper gas exchange and oxygenation of the blood. A mismatch in either flow or ventilation actually decreases oxygenation (see West, 1974, for detailed explanation).

The amount of a gaseous toxicant delivered to the lung will be a function of its concentration in the incoming gas and the minute volume. The dose can be integrated over the time period of the exposure to give the total amount of toxicant to which the lung has been exposed. Alterations in the pattern of breathing, such as work or exercise, will alter the total dose received. Similarly, the deposition of aerosols will be a function of the tidal volume and respiratory rate, since these control the velocity of gas as it courses down the airway and the amount of aerosol reaching the lung. Because of the complex anatomy of the lung, flow rates are especially important in determining the rate and site of deposition of aerosols.

The flow of gas from the lung can be used to diagnose pathophysiologic changes in the lung. If the subject inhales and exhales maximally, the *forced vital capacity* (FVC) and *forced expiratory volume at one second* ($FEV_{1.0}$) can be recorded. $FEV_{1.0}$ is a particularly reproducible and sensitive measure of obstructive or restrictive flows in the

lung. Restrictive flows often result from exposure to inhaled toxicants. A detailed discussion of the pulmonary function tests used to discern pathophysiologic changes in the lung is provided in West (1977). Alterations in blood gases are particularly useful in determining perfusion-ventilation abnormalities. Chronic exposure to toxicants often results in either interstitial fibrosis or emphysema. Specific tests are available to determine these and other abnormalities. Similar tests can be conducted on experimental animals, although they are generally more difficult due to the lack of cooperation on the part of the animal in performing the maneuver. Anesthesia or other intervention is sometimes required.

Alterations in pulmonary mechanics produced by acute exposure to irritants or to pharmacologically active agents such as histamine or acetylcholine can be measured quantitatively in unanesthetized guinea pigs. Irritants that affect mainly the larger airways produce predominantly an increase in flow resistance. Irritants that have their action mainly in the peripheral portions of the lung produce predominantly a decrease in compliance. Response to specific irritant air pollutants is discussed in Chapter 24. Drazen (1976) presents an excellent discussion of the use of alterations in pulmonary mechanics to determine the site of toxic reaction. Kessler *et al.* (1973) demonstrated in dogs exposed to *Ascaris* that measurement of pulmonary mechanics to indicate site of action correlated well with localization of constriction demonstrated by tantalum bronchography. Properly interpreted, measurements of pulmonary mechanics are a useful tool of pulmonary toxicology.

Respiratory frequency is simple to measure and has been used to assess the response to irritants. As Drazen (1976) points out, however, a stimulus may have a profound effect upon the lung without altering the respiratory frequency. Given intravenously to guinea pigs, 10 mg/kg acetylcholine produced a response primarily in the small airways and parenchyma (decreased compliance). Increasing the dose to 30 mg/kg caused a response involving the entire lung (a further decrease in compliance and an increase in resistance). The frequency increased the same amount in response to both doses. Had frequency alone been measured, it would have been concluded that the pulmonary response was the same to both doses.

GASES AND VAPORS

Diffusion Dominates Toxicant Uptake

Unlike the exchange of oxygen and carbon dioxide, the uptake of toxic gases occurs throughout the respiratory system, starting with the nasopharyngeal cavity. The dominant driving force in the uptake of toxicants is diffusion. Since toxicants are present at very low concentrations in air, but vanishingly small concentrations in the tissue, the driving force for diffusion is essentially the concentration of the toxic gas in the inspired air. The solubility of the gas in water is generally the major characteristic determining the relative toxicities of gases. Unfortunately, there is no way, at present, by which toxicant concentrations can be measured directly in the airways at different points or within the tissues themselves during inhalation. Only a few attempts have been made to describe quantitatively by mathematical models the transport of inhaled toxicants (Miller *et al.*, 1978), and they are of such complexity as to be beyond the scope of this text. Generally, deposition of gases is much more poorly described than deposition of particles.

Henry's law describes the transfer of a solute from the gas to the liquid-solute phase. The flux or mass transfer is directly proportional to the concentration of the solute in the gas phase and inversely proportional to the diffusional radius of the solute in the liquid phase. The diffusion coefficient is generally not available for most toxicants of interest, but one can approximate it by the quotient of the solubility divided by the square root of the molecular weight. These considerations are of theoretic interest only until mathematical models accounting for the gas transport within the lung become more widely available. One should be aware of such models, as they represent the future predictive role of inhalation toxicology. As computer-based models become more popular and available, calculations of actual doses delivered to the lung will be possible by knowing the ambient concentration of the toxicant.

The airways are lined with protective and functional layers of fluids through which toxic gases must penetrate to reach the underlying lung tissue. The thickness of the liquid layer lining the airways varies from the mucus-secreting upper airway to the surfactant-lined alveolus. Most morphologists believe that mucus secretions are thickest in the upper airway and decrease in a linear manner down the airways toward the alveoli. As discussed above, the human airways are equally bifurcating and the diameter of the airway decreases exponentially with the bifurcations. The total surface area, however, increases due to the increasing number of airways. In rodents, the transitional generations of airways having both conducting and oxygen–carbon dioxide exchange function may be absent or much decreased compared to those present in man.

In laryngectomized patients, mucus production is about 10 ml/24 hr or about 6.9×10^{-3} ml/min. The velocity of transport of the mucus is about 0.02 cm/sec up and out of the airway to be swallowed or expectorated. Similar values have been reported for rats. Mucous layers can be calculated to range in thickness from 5 to 10 μm in man and animals according to these measurements.

The alveoli are lined with the pulmonary surfactant, which is a complex mixture predominantly composed of dipalmitoyl lecithin. Great debate centers around the presence of an aqueous layer between the lipid surfactant layer and the luminal surface of the alveolar cells. The thickness of this layer is estimated to be about 0.5 to 1 μm.

The diffusion of inhaled toxicants into these protective layers will also be a function of the radial and axial diffusion of the gas and its mixture with other nontoxic gases simultaneously inhaled, such as nitrogen, oxygen, carbon dioxide, and water vapor. Since several breaths are required before sufficient toxicant is absorbed, the transport of toxic gases can be treated as reaching a steady state. Naturally, steady state may not be achieved in the presence of very high concentrations of toxic gases such as hydrogen cyanide or hydrogen sulfide, which are lethal within minutes under the proper conditions. Most toxicologic problems today, however, deal with chronic exposures and thus better fit the achievement of a steady state. Breath-by-breath models are needed to provide more quantitative estimates, however. Inhaled gases may react chemically with the components of the mucous or surfactant layer. Since the mucous layer is being constantly renewed and removed by ingestion or expectoration following the upward transport out of the airways by the cilia, dissolution in or reaction with the mucous layer is a mechanism of detoxification.

Other gases, such as anesthetic agents, diffuse through the lung and reach saturation in the blood. They are transported, dissolved in blood, to peripheral tissues where they diffuse into tissues. Concentration and local perfusion rates determine the speed of accumulation in peripheral tissues and their distribution. In these cases, direct effects of the toxicant do not occur in the lung but rather in other organs.

Inhaled toxicants can either react directly with the lung or be transported to other tissues in the blood. For example, nitrogen dioxide, ozone, and sulfur dioxide react directly with pulmonary tissue to produce major effects, whereas the anesthetic gases are readily absorbed and transported to bone marrow to where some may produce aplastic anemia.

When the concentration of the inhaled toxicant is sufficient to provide a measurable flux or mass transfer of toxicant across the protective mucous or surfactant layer to the surface of the pulmonary cells, toxicity to lung tissue will result. Highly reactive anhydrous acids or strong oxidants react directly with the pulmonary cells to cause changes in permeability or death. Less reactive gases such as nickel carbonyl may diffuse through the cells lining the lumen before causing toxic reactions with endothelial cells. Exposure may result in death of capillary endothelial cells without apparent damage to epithelial cells. This is confusing at first glance but only reflects the relative rate of reaction of the toxicant compared to its rate of diffusion.

Relative Permeability of the Lung to Solutes

Toxicants that do not exert immediate toxic effects on the lung may pass through the lung, reach the capillaries, and be transported to other tissues by the blood. The relative permeability of the respiratory tract to a number of solutes has been measured. The administration techniques used are such that it is difficult to determine the site of absorption, since a small volume of solution (either water, saline, or isotonic sucrose) of the toxicant is instilled within the trachea, bathing the upper and lower airways. A number of lipid-insoluble neutral compounds, including urea, erythritol, mannitol, and sucrose, are removed at rates directly proportional to the concentration of the solute (Enna and Schanker, 1972). The relative rates of absorption are ranked in the same order as the diffusion coefficients of the solutes. Simple diffusion appears to account for removal of compounds of this nature. If one assumes diffusional absorption through pores or channels for such lipid-insoluble compounds, three classes of pores can be discerned: the smallest-diameter pores allow passage of urea and not the saccharides; a second allows

passage of erythritol; and a third, all saccharides but not dextrans of 70,000 daltons. Organic cations and anions (sulfanilic acid, tetraethyl ammonium ion, p-aminohippuric acid, p-acetyl-hippuric acid, and procainamide ethobromide) are absorbed by diffusion, presumably through aqueous channels, since their rates of removal are not saturable with increasing concentration of solute and is roughly related to molecular size rather than to their lipid/aqueous partition coefficients. The main barrier for the diffusion of hydrophilic compounds appears to be the alveolar membrane, which has been calculated to have an equivalent pore radius of 8 to 10 Å in the dog (Taylor and Gaar, 1970).

Lipophilic compounds are also removed at diffusion-controlled rates. A number of antibiotics and corticosteroids were found to be removed rapidly, with $t_{1/2}$ of 1.9 to 33 min (Burton and Schanker, 1974a, 1974b). Highly lipophilic pesticides, such as DDT and leptophos, are removed at extremely slow rates, with $t_{1/2}$ of about 300 min in the rat. A comparison of the pulmonary absorption rate with the physical properties of the compound, such as the molecular weight and chloroform/water partition coefficient, suggests that partitioning into the lipid of the lung membrane is the rate-determining factor. The question is not closed and is in need of further investigation.

Specialized absorption systems probably exist in the lung and have been recognized for the absorption of phenol red (Enna and Schanker, 1973). Phenol red is partially absorbed by diffusion, but primarily by a carrier-mediated system. The system is saturated at high concentrations of phenol red and is inhibited by a number of closely related compounds. Organic anions such as benzylpenicillin and cephalothin are also competitors for the phenol red removal system.

A specialized storage or uptake mechanism also exists on the luminal surface of the lung. The herbicide paraquat is highly toxic to the lung and is stored within the lung on ingestion (Clark et al., 1966; Rose et al., 1976; Charles et al., 1978). Paraquat is only poorly transported from the luminal surface of the lung, while the closely related and relatively nontoxic compound diquat is removed at much greater rates ($t_{1/2}$ 356 vs. 75 min). Unlike paraquat, diquat does not produce pulmonary toxicity. Paraquat uptake is both energy and concentration dependent. The site of paraquat storage may be the type II pneumocyte, which may also be the cell type most affected by paraquat poisoning.

Specialized sites of absorption and metabolism also exist in the pulmonary capillary bed. The lung functions in the removal and metabolism of a number of vasoactive hormones, and an appreciation of this nonrespiratory function has only recently become recognized.

The role of inhaled toxicants in the perturbation of this complex function has likewise only recently come to the fore and may be of importance in chronic lung diseases.

Nasopharyngeal Removal

Man is an obligatory mouth breather when exercising at work or play. Most experiments with animals, however, involve exposure to airborne toxicants under conditions in which the animals are obligatory nose breathers. This difference in respiratory pattern is particularly important, since the nasopharyngeal cavity can remove 50 percent or more of inhaled toxicants. The rate of removal of toxicants depends mostly on the water solubility of the toxicant. Anhydrous acid vapors such as SO_2 and NO_2 are more rapidly removed than relatively insoluble compounds such as O_3. The removal of organic vapors by the nasopharyngeal cavity has not been studied but, by analogy with the buccal absorption of drugs, is also likely to occur readily. The entrance of toxic gases into the nasopharyngeal cavity significantly reduces the final concentration to which the upper airways are exposed. The reduction in concentration of the inhaled toxicants is similar to the physiologic need for saturation of incoming air with water vapor prior to reaching the upper airways. While the inhaled vapor concentration is significantly reduced by this mechanism, entrance of toxicants into the body is not prevented. The nasopharynx provides little or no protection from toxicants that produce toxic effects in organs other than the lung. Generally, the lung is much more sensitive to toxic injury than distal organs and is thus protected by the scrubbing action of the nasopharynx.

Upper Airway Deposition

The upper airways are composed of several cell types, two of which, goblet and ciliated cells, are the predominant types lining the luminal side of the airway. The secretion of mucus by the goblet cells is stimulated by acetylcholine, presumably via cyclic GMP as the intracellular messenger. Cholinergic innervation has been suggested but not proven. The secretion of mucus is also a function of the prevalence of goblet cells. Dietary vitamin A determines the maximum number of goblet cells developed in the airways, since ciliated cells and squamous metaplastic cells dominate the upper airway population in vitamin A–deficient or marginally vitamin A–sufficient animals. The chemical composition of airway mucus is not known, but

probably is similar to parotid gland mucus, which is highly glycosidated. The secretion of mucus may be influenced by the inhalation of toxicants, especially if the toxicant has cholinomimetic properties or if disruption of goblet cell integrity results on contact with the toxicant. In man, hyperplasia and probably altered molecular composition of the goblet cell mucus occurs in asthma, bronchitis, and cystic fibrosis. The exact effect of such chronic disease states on the absorption of toxicants from the upper airway is not known but might be greater, since these patients are more sensitive to NO_2, SO_2, and O_3. Bronchoconstriction evoked in bronchitic and asthmatic patients can be partially blocked by prior administration of atropine. Some of the atropine effect may be directly on the smooth muscles of the upper airways.

Bronchoconstriction is one of the most common immediate responses observed on the inhalation of a number of highly reactive gases. Inhalation of solid aerosols of soluble salts, such as sulfuric acid or sulfate salts, also provokes constriction. The constriction may either be due to a direct action of the salt on the airway smooth muscles or occur indirectly through the release of histamine. Histamine release may not be the only factor involved.

After toxicants penetrate the mucous lining of the upper airway and come into contact with the goblet and ciliated cells, cytotoxicity is often observed. Ciliated cells are generally more sensitive to gaseous toxicants than are goblet cells. Cilia are often lost from the cell, and the entire cell may die and leave a denuded area. Fragments of ciliated cells can be found in the mucus as a result. Complex mixtures of gases and particles in cigarette smoke inhibit ciliary action without cytotoxicity.

As in the case of nasopharyngeal removal, gases can be classified as acting on either the upper or lower airways, depending on their relative solubility in water. Anhydrides of acids tend to produce bronchoconstriction and upper airway necrosis, while less water-soluble compounds reach the lower airway to produce alveolar damage.

Undoubtedly, chemical reaction with mucus is a highly important protective factor for the upper airway. An open question is the effect of chemical products of reaction with mucus on the airway itself.

The relative ventilation of different parts of the lung during breathing at rest versus exercise affects the distribution of toxicants within the airways as well. More extensive and smaller airway constriction occurs at exercise than at rest. Detailed studies of the airway response in man on exposure to O_3 and SO_2 have been undertaken,

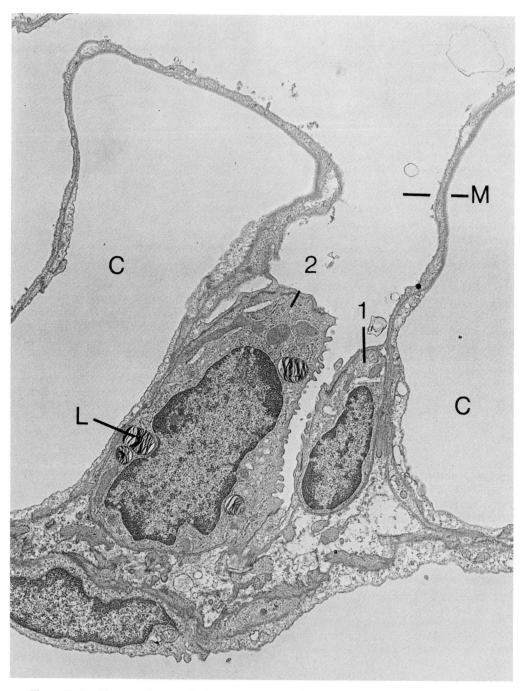

Figure 12–3. Electron micrograph of a rat lung. The alveolus is separated from the blood capillary (*C*) by a thin margin of the type I cell (*1*). Note the closeness of approach of these two compartments at *M*. A type II cell (*2*) can be seen containing lamelli bodies (*L*) presumed to be storage sites for the lung surfactant.

factors in the assessment of their toxic p
Rapid removal lessens the time avai
cause critical damage to the pulmonary tis
to permit systemic absorption of mater
have target organs other than the lung.

Respiratory tract clearance and its cou
retention of inhaled particles, are not co
understood. This is the case because o
accessibility of the respiratory tract, th
character of the various substructures
it is comprised, and the extent to w
structures exist in parallel and are
intermixed beyond the tracheal bif
Perhaps, because of their relatively easi
and the extent to which changes tal
rapidly, clearance from the ciliated su
the tracheobronchial and nasopharyngea
has received much greater attention 1
clearance from the pulmonary region.
discussion of clearance here is inte
supplement the simplified mathemat
scription of clearance developed by t
Group on Lung Dynamics (TGLD) a
in Chapter 19. Detailed coverage of th
may be found elsewhere (Hatch anc
1964; Task Group on Lung Dynamic
Casarett, 1972; Green, 1973; Morro
Kilburn, 1977).

Nasopharyngeal and Tracheobronchia Clearance

Clearance from the ciliated surface
respiratory tract, which extend from the
bronchioles to the nose, is primarily b
ciliary transport. Goblet cells associatec
ciliated epithelial cells produce the
blanket that covers these surfaces. It
suggested that the cilia beat in a serous fl
The tips of the cilia contact the overly
of mucus only when the movement of t
tips is at the maximum forward velocit
ance rates from the ciliated surfaces h
measured in man and laboratory anim
a variety of techniques. Radioactive
have been inhaled, and radioactive or ra
substances have been insufflated, inj
placed directly on the surfaces of int
their rate of clearance observed by
monitoring of the radioactivity or by
raphy.

Particles have been observed to move
7 mm/min in the human nose and tr
1 mm/min in the upper bronchial tre
0.4 to 0.6 mm/min in the lower bron
(Quinlan et al., 1969; Morrow et al., 1
effect of these relatively high velocities
the ciliated surfaces of particles in a
hours. It should be noted, however, tha
and Stirling (1977) have reported th

illustrating these effects. A review of the distribution of gases in the lung with exercise can be found in West (1974).

Lower Airway Deposition

The overall distribution of toxic effects of inhaled gases in the lower airways including the alveoli parallels the ventilation of that section of the lung. The lower lobes of the lung in man are more generally affected than the upper lobes, due to this differential ventilation. West (1974) describes the pulmonary mechanics responsible for these anomalies, which apply equally as well to toxic gases as to oxygen. As a result, from the top to the bottom of the lung, a pH gradient also exists that serves to accentuate differences in exposure to toxic gases and to exacerbate secondary infections resulting from toxic injury and inflammation. Ventilatory differences between the vertical lung of man and the horizontal lung of animals account for the differential effects seen in animals and man. In the interpretation of human effects on the basis of animal exposures, one must be careful to take these basic differences in pulmonary physiology into account. Similarly, the rat, a popular experimental animal, is highly susceptible to pneumonias that are often mistaken for toxic effects of inhaled gases.

Once the toxic gas has reached the level of the alveolus, the uptake of the gas can be treated essentially the same as that for oxygen. The lung is extremely well organized to promote diffusion across the very thin alveolar space into the blood. Figure 12–3 illustrates this intimate association of the airway with the capillary space. Diffusion again dominates the physical processes, accounting for uptake of the inhaled toxic gases. The alveolar region is essentially a sheet of blood interrupted in small regions by the connective tissue supporting the structure.

Certain regions of the lower airway are more affected by inhaled gases that act directly on the lung than by others. The transitional region between the respiratory bronchiole and alveolus bounded by Clara cells is most susceptible to both ozone and nitrogen dioxide. The particular susceptibility can be accounted for on the basis of the total amount of these toxicants delivered to that region of the lung. The mass transfer of toxicant within the lung is a function of its axial and radial diffusion, solubility, and reactivity with upper air mucus and buccal cavity, and with the cyclic nature of respiration. These factors combine to deliver a greater dose of toxicant to the transitional region of the lower lung. This is the same region where pulmonary macrophages penetrate to the lumen to remove particles. Injury to the transitional region may have important consequences.

Another cell type exposed to inhaled toxicants in the alveolar region is the pulmonary macrophage. The macrophage acts mainly to remove from the alveolus particles such as bacteria, viruses, and inorganic and organic substances. The macrophage can be injured and die on exposure, releasing its cellular contents. Because of their phagocytic capacity, macrophages contain acid hydrolases that produce decompartmentalization of the alveolar sacs. The autolysis of the alveolar wall by proteases released from macrophages may be a contributor to emphysema.

The Lung as an Excretory Organ

The lung may be exposed to toxic gases and vapors through its function as an excretory organ. Volatile solvents, such as carbon tetrachloride and benzene, are excreted through the lung. Depending on the rate of metabolism of the compound to more polar, water-soluble substances of higher vapor pressure, excretion in the exhaled breath may be significant. Delayed pulmonary toxicity may occur following the ingestion of such toxicants as they are redistributed from the liver and exhaled. The lung has an active cytochrome P450 system, capable of metabolizing many of these compounds to reactive intermediates that are bound to pulmonary macromolecules to promote necrosis in a fashion similar to that observed in the liver on metabolism of certain drugs.

The pulmonary capillaries are also specialized to take up amines, prostaglandins, and peptide hormones of angiotensin and the kinins. During redistribution of drugs or toxicants absorbed by other routes, the lung may accumulate high concentrations, resulting in pulmonary damage. Inhibition of the regulatory functions of the lung may be highly deleterious.

PARTICULATE MATERIAL

Classification of Particles

Many airborne materials of toxicologic importance can be considered under the generic term "aerosols." An aerosol is a relatively stable suspension of solid particles or liquid droplets in a gaseous medium. Gases or vapors are frequently adsorbed on the surface or dissolved in aerosols. Traditionally, several terms have been used to describe aerosols.

Dusts arise from processes such as grinding, milling, or blasting. They are identical in chemical composition to the parent material. Depending on the process of generation, the size may vary from Ångstrom size to 100 μm in diameter. Fumes are formed by combustion, sublimation, or condensation. Usually the formation of fumes is accompanied by a

tained. The site of deposition a
severity of the consequences of tiss
the respiratory tract, (2) the degree
of systemic toxicants, and (3)
mechanisms available for the ultim
the particles.

Factors Influencing Regional Dep
ure 12–6 illustrates schematically th
interaction of physical and bic
leading to regional deposition. The
ships shown for the various com
not quantitative. They are intenc
indicate the increase in both siz
area that occur with increasing
respiratory tract. The directional
posed on the airflow become less a
velocity decreases as particles
respiratory tract.

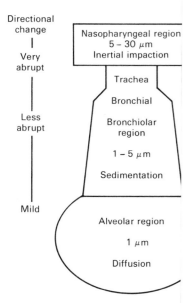

Figure 12–6. Parameters influen
deposition. (From Casarett, L. J.: T
Alveolar clearance mechanisms i
toxicology. In Blood, F. R. [ed.]: *E*
cology, Vol. 3. Academic Press, Inc
1972.)

Particles having an aerodynam
5 to 30 μm are largely deposited
pharyngeal region by impaction. B
size, impaction is an important r
their removal from an airstream.
velocity and the tortuous nature
pharyngeal air passages, forcing
changes in airflow direction, prc
area for impaction. Particles ha
dynamic diameter of 1 to 5 μm ar
the tracheobronchial regions by s

Table 12–1 (*continued*)

TOXICANT	CHEMICAL COMPOSITION	OCCUPATIONAL SOURCE	PULMONARY DAMAGE	NUMBER OF U.S. WORKERS EXPOSED
Osmium tetraoxide	OsO_4	Chemical and metal industry		3,000
Oxides of nitrogen	NO, NO_2, HNO_3	Welding, silo filling, explosive manufacture	Emphysema	1.5 million direct or indirect
Ozone	O_3	Welding, bleaching flour, deodorizing	Emphysema	380,000
Phosgene	$COCl_3$	Production of plastics, pesticides, chemicals	Edema	10,000
Perchloro-ethylene	C_2Cl_4	Dry cleaning, metal de-greasing, grain fumigating	Edema	275,000
Silica	SiO_2	Mining, stone cutting construction, farming, quarrying	Silicosis (fibrosis)	1.2 million non-agricultural workers
Sulfur dioxide	SO_2	Manufacture of chemicals, refrigeration, bleaching, fumigation		5 million
Talc	$Mg_6(SiO_2)OH_4$	Rubber industry, cosmetics	Fibrosis, pleural sclerosis	20,000
Tin	SnO_2	Mining, processing of tin		25,000
Toluene 2,4-diiso-cyanate	$CH_3-C_6H_3(NCO)_2$	Manufacture of plastics	Decrement of pulmonary function (FEV_1)	40,000
Vanadium	VO_5	Steel manufacture	Irritation	10,000
Xylene	$C_6H_4(CH_3)_2$	Manufacture of resins, paints, varnishes, other chemicals, general solvent for adhesives	Edema	140,000

during heavy work reduces the protection provided by the upper respiratory tract and increases potential toxicity. Depth of respiration and minute volume will also influence the dose received by the lung. The added pulmonary stress of cigarette smoking increases the risk of serious disease from occupational exposure to these materials. Many of these agents are also present in polluted urban environments. The concentrations are much lower than in industrial environments, but the exposure may be more prolonged and the population exposed includes the infirm, the elderly, and sensitive individuals. Factors entering into considerations of risk assessment thus differ somewhat from those for occupational situations.

Table 12–2 provides additional information on the toxic action of these industrially important toxic materials. The common name of the resultant pulmonary disease and the site of toxic action within the respiratory system are given. Many agents have an acute effect produced by initial exposure or by shorter exposure to high concentrations. These acute effects are listed, as are the chronic effects resulting from long-term exposure. Except in instances when the con-

centration is sufficient to threaten life or produce residual pulmonary damage, the chronic effects are the more significant clinically.

Direct Airway Irritation

The bronchial tone of the lung is influenced by many inhaled compounds. Cholinergic constriction is immediately induced by inhalation of pharmacologic agents such as aerosols of carbachol or acetylcholine. Bronchodilation is produced by inhalation of aerosols of isoproterenol, which acts on the β-adrenergic receptors of bronchial smooth muscle. The ready accessibility of the bronchial smooth muscles to inhaled agents is used extensively in asthma therapy, especially with isoproterenol.

Ammonia and chlorine are classic examples of irritant gases. Bronchoconstriction occurs immediately on inhalation. Dyspnea (the feeling of an inability to breathe) probably results from the individual's inability to breathe rapidly and deeply enough to satisfy respiratory demands (West, 1977). Ammonia and chlorine are highly water soluble and are, therefore, primarily removed by the upper airways. Both gases are well tolerated in that, unless the concentration is

Table 12–2. SITE OF ACTION AND PULMONARY DISEASE PRODUCED BY SELECTED OCCUPATIONALLY INHALED TOXICANTS

TOXICANT	COMMON NAME OF DISEASE	SITE OF ACTION	ACUTE EFFECT	CHRONIC EFFECT
Asbestos	Asbestosis	Parenchyma		Pulmonary fibrosis, pleural calcification, lung cancer, pleural mesothelioma
Aluminum	Aluminosis	Upper airways, alveolar interstitium	Cough, shortness of breath	Interstitial fibrosis
Aluminum abrasives	Shaver's disease, corundum smelter's lung, bauxite lung	Alveoli	Alveolar edema	Fibrotic thickening of alveolar walls, interstitial fibrosis and emphysema
Ammonia		Upper airway	Immediate upper and lower respiratory tract irritation, edema	Chronic bronchitis
Arsenic		Upper airways	Bronchitis	Lung cancer, bronchitis, laryngitis
Beryllium	Berylliosis	Alveoli	Severe pulmonary edema, pneumonia	Pulmonary fibrosis, progressive dyspnea, interstitial granulomatosis, cor pulmonale
Boron		Alveolus	Edema and hemorrhage	
Cadmium oxide		Alveolus	Cough, pneumonia	Emphysema, cor pulmonale
Carbides of tungsten, titanium, tantalium	Hard metal disease	Upper airway and lower airway	Hyperplasia and metaplasia of bronchial epithelium	Fibrosis, peribronchial and perivascular fibrosis
Chlorine		Upper airways	Cough, hemoptysis, dyspnea, tracheobronchitis, bronchopneumonia	
Chromium (VI)		Nasopharynx, upper airways	Nasal irritation, bronchitis	Lung tumors and cancers
Coal dust	Pneumoconiosis	Lung parenchyma, lymph nodes, hilus		Pulmonary fibrosis
Coke oven emissions		Upper airways		Tracheobronchial cancers
Cotton dust	Byssinosis	Upper airways	Tightness in chest, wheezing, dyspnea	Reduced pulmonary function, chronic bronchitis
Hydrogen fluoride		Upper airways	Respiratory irritation, hemorrhagic pulmonary edema	
Iron oxides	Siderotic lung disease: Silver finisher's lung, hematite miner's lung, arc welder's lung	Silver finisher's: pulmonary vessels and alveolar walls; hematite miner's: upper lobes, bronchi and alveoli; arc welder's: bronchi	Cough	Silver finisher's: subpleural and perivascular aggregations of macrophages; hematite miner's: diffuse fibrosis-like pneumoconiosis; arc welder's: bronchitis
Kaolin	Kaolinosis	Lung parenchyma, lymph nodes, hilus		Pulmonary fibrosis
Manganese	Manganese pneumonia	Lower airways and alveoli	Acute pneumonia, often fatal	Recurrent pneumonia

Table 12–2   (*continued*)

TOXICANT	COMMON NAME OF DISEASE	SITE OF ACTION	ACUTE EFFECT	CHRONIC EFFECT
Nickel		Parenchyma (NiCO), nasal mucosa (Ni_2S_3), bronchi (NiO)	Pulmonary edema, delayed by 2 days (NiCO)	Squamous cell carcinoma of nasal cavity and lung
Osmium tetraoxide		Upper airways	Bronchitis, bronchopneumonia	
Oxides of nitrogen		Terminal respiratory bronchi and alveoli	Pulmonary congestion and edema	Emphysema
Ozone		Terminal respiratory bronchi and alveoli	Pulmonary edema	Emphysema
Phosgene		Alveoli	Edema	Bronchitis
Perchloro-ethylene			Pulmonary edema	
Silica	Silicosis, pneumo-coniosis	Lung parenchyma, lymph nodes, hilus		Pulmonary fibrosis
Sulfur dioxide		Upper airways	Bronchoconstriction, cough, tightness in chest	
Talc	Talcosis	Lung parenchyma, lymph nodes		Pulmonary fibrosis
Tin	Stanosis	Bronchioles and pleura		Widespread mottling of x-ray without clinical signs
Toluene		Upper airways	Acute bronchitis, bronchospasm, pulmonary edema	
Vanadium		Upper and lower airways	Upper airway irritation and mucus production	Chronic bronchitis
Xylene		Lower airways	Pulmonary edema	

sufficient to cause death, the acute effects do not result in chronic residual pulmonary damage (Weill *et al.*, 1969).

Arsenic compounds in industrial applications are usually of a sufficiently large particle size to be deposited in the nasopharyngeal region and the large airways. Irritation of the bronchi results in chronic cough and bronchitis, and laryngitis can result in chronic exposure. The lung also serves as a route of absorption for the more soluble arsenate salts. The toxicity of absorbed arsenic is discussed in Chapter 17.

Cellular Damage and Edema

A variety of materials produce damage to the cells of the airways and alveoli. The resulting increase in permeability leads to the release of edema fluid into the lumen of the airways and alveoli. The production of major edema may take several hours to develop so that seriously damaging or even fatal exposures may occur without the individual's being aware at the time of the extent of the potential damage. The cytotoxicity may be of a general nonspecific nature, but the effects may be localized in the lung and depend on the distribution of the toxic agent within the lung (Miller *et al.*, 1978). One major determinant of site of action is water solubility. As was indicated earlier, if the toxic agent is present as an aerosol, the prime determinant of site of action is the particle size.

Ozone and nitrogen dioxide are examples of toxic agents that produce cellular damage. The water solubility is sufficiently low that the main site of action is at the level of the respiratory bronchioles and alveoli. The most likely mode of action is through peroxidation of cellular membranes. The toxicity of these gases is discussed in detail in Chapter 24.

Phosgene is another irritant capable of producing delayed pulmonary edema. The moisture of the respiratory tract hydrolyzes phosgene to hydrochloric acid and carbon dioxide. A high concentration produces a burning sensation in the nose and upper respiratory passages. The gas that penetrates to the peripheral portions of the lung undergoes *in situ* hydrolysis, producing nascent hydrogen chloride, which destroys the permeability of the cells of the alveolar membranes. Clinically, a delay of approximately 24 hours lapses between exposure and symptomatology. Individuals exposed to phosgene should be under medical surveillance for at least 48 hours so that oxygen and other emergency measures are immediately at hand if major edema results.

Cadmium oxide is produced as a fume of extremely fine particle size that readily penetrates to the alveoli. Edema results and histopathology indicates an interstitial pneumonitis with a marked proliferation of the lining cells of the alveolar spaces. Chronic exposure results in emphysema, characterized by the loss of individual septa or decompartmentalization of the alveoli. The alveolar volume available for respiratory gas exchange is greatly reduced, and disparities between perfusion and ventilation arise in damaged segments. Perfusion-ventilation anomalies are serious impairments that can eventually result in almost total physical disability. The clinical features of emphysema, which is produced by a wide variety of toxic materials, are discussed by West (1977).

The toxicity of nickel compounds and nickel metal to the respiratory tract depends on the physical/chemical properties of the nickel (National Academy of Sciences, 1975). Nickel, nickel subsulfide, and nickel oxide are generated in relatively large particle sizes during the production and mining of nickel and are, thus, associated with damage to the nasal mucosa. Nickel carbonyl is a liquid with a high vapor pressure at room temperature. Exposure to vaporized nickel carbonyl occurs in electroplating, in nickel refining, and in the electronics industry. The highly insoluble vapor penetrates to the alveoli with resultant edema, which has a latent period of about two days. Nickel metal has been detected within alveolar cells following exposure to nickel carbonyl. This suggests that the nickel carbonyl has penetrated the cells, decomposed there to nickel metal, and produced cellular damage.

Paraquat is an example of a toxic agent that can produce direct damage to pulmonary cells when it enters the body by a route other than inhalation. Ingestion of paraquat produces a frothy exudate in the lungs and pulmonary edema (Clark et al., 1966). It is only slowly removed from the lungs, where it appears to be concentrated in the type II cells. Paraquat may exert its toxic action through the generation of superoxide radical anions (O_2^-) or other free radicals. The closely related herbicide diquat is not toxic to the lung and is not retained by the lung (Charles et al., 1978). Both paraquat and diquat are toxic to cultured lung cells. This suggests that the ability to be retained by type II cells is the critical difference in toxicity between the two compounds. The active transport system for paraquat in type II cells has not yet been fully elucidated.

Perchlorethylene and xylene produce effects on the lung typical of organic solvents. These solvents are sufficiently volatile and water insoluble that they reach the alveolar region of the lung. Much of the inhaled dose is removed readily and transported to other organs where it produces its toxic symptoms. Both compounds are acted upon by the cytochrome P450 system of the liver and other organs. Oxygenated intermediaries may be produced in the lung leading to covalent binding. This covalent binding may be the mechanism that produces pulmonary edema through cellular necrosis.

Production of Fibrosis

The incidence of pulmonary fibrosis appears to be on the increase in the United States, but the cause of this increase is not known. This seriously debilitating disease was recognized as one of the earliest forms of occupational disease. Pneumoconiosis is the term applied to this general class of disease in which pulmonary fibrosis is the central factor. The widely publicized coal miner's pneumoconiosis is but one form of the disease. One of the most confusing aspects of pulmonary fibrosis initiated by dust inhalation is the difference in potency of different dusts. This has led to confusion regarding the hazards of dust inhalation and the mechanisms by which fibrosis is initiated. Originally, silica was thought to be the main responsible agent, but it is now recognized that fibrosis can be initiated by a wide variety of particles of different chemical composition. An excellent discussion of the occupational medical aspects of inhalation of dusts is given by Hunter (1969).

Silicosis. Silica (SiO_2) exists in several forms, but only the crystalline materials produce the chronic pulmonary condition termed specifically silicosis. Quartz is the most stable and common crystalline form of silica. Heating produces tridymite or cristobalite, both of which appear to have greater fibrogenic potency than quartz. These minerals occur naturally in some volcanic rock encountered in mining operations. They are also formed when quartz or amorphous silica is heated, for example, in the silica brick industry or in the calcining of diatomaceous earth.

Despite the fact that the incidence of silicosis dates from antiquity, current research still leaves many gaps in our knowledge relating to the precise manner in which the human pulmonary lesion develops, to the relationship of crystal structure and size of silica dust to the production of silicosis, and to the correlation between retained dust load and the degree of pulmonary tissue reaction. Numerous theories based on one or more characteristics of silica particles have been proposed. These have centered mainly on physical shape, solubility, crystalline structure, or cytotoxicity to macrophages. No single theory seems to provide a fully adequate explanation of the fibrotic lesions of silicosis.

The cytotoxic and fibrogenic activity appears related to the rupture of the lysosomal membrane of the macrophage and the release of lysosomal enzymes into the cytoplasm. The macrophage is, thus, digested by its own enzymes. Following lysis of the macrophage, the free silica particles are once again released to be ingested by fresh macrophages in which the cycle is repeated. Perivascular aggregation of lymphoid tissue and fibrosis follow, but the chain of events is not entirely clear. Heppleston (1969) has suggested that the damaged macrophages release factors capable of stimulating collagen formation. Phospholipids released from the dying macrophages cause stimulation of fibroblasts, which leads to collagen formation.

The so-called silicotic nodule is the typical pulmonary lesion that positively identifies silicosis. These are firm nodules of concentrically arranged bundles of collagen fibers, usually 1 to 10 mm in diameter. They appear in lymphatics around blood vessels, beneath the pleura in the lungs, and sometimes in mediastinal lymph nodes. The nodules may fuse, resulting in the condition known as progressive massive fibrosis. The blood vessels in the silicotic nodules become narrowed and blocked by fibrous tissue. Perifocal emphysema frequently occurs around the nodule, with destruction of alveolar walls and an increase in the size of the alveolar ducts and sacs. These changes further decrease the ventilation and blood flow in the lungs. Especially in the past, silicosis was frequently further complicated by tuberculosis.

Asbestosis. "Asbestos" is a general name for a large group of hydrated silicates that, when crushed or milled, separate into flexible fibers. The group is a continuous solid solution series of minerals that represents a small part of a larger mineral group of fibrous minerals, the amphiboles. Chrysotile is the most important commercially and represents some 90 percent of the total usage. Other minerals marketed as asbestos include amosite, crocidolite, anthophyllite, tremolite, and actinolite. Since this class of minerals is a solid solution series, the chemical composition varies considerably from locality to locality and from one class member to another. Tremolite occurs as a contaminant in talc, while others, and the amphiboles in general, occur in practically every other commercial mineral including coal. Use of asbestos is now extensive

and is increasing with the development of greater technology.

Asbestosis was recognized as a respiratory disease very early and led to the development of some of the first standards regulating dust levels in the workplace. Asbestosis in man involves diffuse interstitial fibrosis, calcification and fibrosis of the pleura, bronchogenic carcinoma, and mesothelial tumors. There is some doubt about the relative potency of each mineral type of asbestos to produce all or some of these symptoms. All amphiboles, including those derived from nonasbestos sources, may be capable of initiating symptoms in man. The difficulty stems, in part, from the lack of knowledge of the mechanisms by which asbestos initiates these effects. The organization of the surface of the fibers, their lengths, and their diameters seems critical in the production of biologic effects in experimental animals. In man, bronchogenic carcinoma and mesothelial tumors rarely occur less than 30 years after exposure. Other environmental and personal habits exposing people to other carcinogens or potential carcinogens further complicate the interpretation of the incidence of cancer in man following asbestos exposure. Smoking clearly enhances cancer production. Also, the same mineral type of asbestos may be more or less carcinogenic, depending on the locality and population exposed.

Studies of the increase of asbestos fibers in the human lung indicate that all urban dwellers have retained large numbers of mineral fibers. The proportion of mineral fibers that are found in the lung on autopsy and are classified "asbestos" (e.g., chrysotile) cannot be easily determined. Minerals of a fibrous nature, aside from asbestos, will form "asbestos bodies" or protein-coated inclusions within the lung. This generalized type of reaction around a fibrous mineral particle is best referred to as a ferruginous body. These bodies can be identified with ease by both light and electron microscopy.

The production of interstitial fibrosis from asbestos inhalation is most common in the lower lobes of the lung. Bronchogenic carcinoma is widely distributed and derived from all cell types of the bronchial tree. There does not seem to be any localization within the lung. Mesothelial tumors in man are rare, but appear to be increasingly common. The ability of ingested asbestos to evoke mesothelial tumors is not resolved. Since asbestos fibers occur widely in food through the use of asbestos filters (fruit juices, beer, and wine, for example) and through the presence of asbestos and amphibole fibers in drinking water, the contribution of inhaled asbestos to the total incidence of mesothelial tumors is not clear. Similarly, the calcification of the pleura could be due to either ingested or inhaled fibers.

Exposure of experimental animals to asbestos and similar fibrous minerals generally produces fibrosis. Tumors occur at a low rate of incidence because only a short time period is possible between exposure and sacrifice. Rodent experiments in excess of two years are almost impossible to conduct. Tumor induction appears to require prolonged time periods and possibly multiple exposures, although single exposures at high levels have been reported to produce tumors after a long induction period. This is an example where rodents are not very useful as a model of human disease. Fiber migration clearly takes place by an unknown mechanism that removes inhaled fibers from the airways into the pleural cavity. Direct injection of fibers into the peritoneum evokes more rapid and frequent tumor response.

A critical problem is the relative potency of fibers of differing lengths and diameters. Generators producing experimental asbestos aerosols for animal studies are generally rather crude. The fibers are produced by some grinding process that tends to make a very disperse preparation with respect to both the chemical and physical properties of the fibers, but fibers of 5 μm in length and 0.3 μm in diameter seem to be the most active.

To date, no one has reported a mutagenic activity for these fibers in microbial or cell culture systems. The chemical mechanism (if one exists) for the induction of tumors is not known. The surfaces of these and other fibers are chemically very active, leading to the theory that these fibers produce mutagenesis and carcinogenesis by carrying sorbed chemical carcinogens into the lung. This suggestion is attractive, but still lacks direct evidence and does not explain the carcinogenesis observed with other inorganic compounds such as nickel salts.

The major concern with asbestos stems from the long period between exposure and malignancy as observed in U.S. shipworkers who were exposed, during World War II, to asbestos lagging applied to ship interiors. This group of workers has been identified as having a moderate exposure and has been found to have an increasing incidence of bronchogenic and mesothelial tumors now that 30 years have elapsed. The widespread use of asbestos in building materials, especially after 1940, for fireproofing has increased the total amount of this potential toxicant in the environment. As these buildings are demolished or renovated, much of this material is dispersed into the air, water, and soil. The nature of the dose-response curve in man is unknown. From the experience in occupational exposure of man, lowering the total fibers available for inhalation and decreasing the exposure frequency decrease the incidence of fibrosis and tumors. However, the quantitative relationship between the number and frequency of fibers inhaled and the risk of disease is not known.

Induction of Allergic Response

Bronchoconstriction and chronic pulmonary disease can result from inhalation of a variety of materials that appear to act wholly or partly through an allergic response. This underlying mechanism is demonstrated by the presence of circulating or fixed antibodies to specific components of the inhaled materials. In some instances these reactions are caused by spores of molds or by bacterial contaminants. In other instances, as in the case of cotton dust, they appear to be related to components of the material itself.

Farmer's Lung. A classic example of a pulmonary disease related to inhalation of an organic dust is farmer's lung. The major cause of the disease is the inhalation of spores of thermophilic actinomycetes, organisms that flourish and produce vast numbers of spores when the temperature of damp hay rises to 40° to 60° C. The disease entity is characterized by extrinsic allergic alveolitis. A classic attack of farmer's lung may appear between five and six hours after exposure, but the disease also frequently develops insidiously with no consistent interval between exposure and appearance of symptoms. The disease is characterized by fever, malaise, chills with aches and pains, and weight loss. Severe dyspnea is a more common symptom than cough and is often out of proportion to the crepitant rales observed on examination. Radiologic findings in the chronic disease include evidence of fibrosis and "honeycomb" lung, especially in the upper lobes. Serologic, inhalation, and skin tests may provide a certain amount of valuable diagnostic information, especially when the clear-cut clinical picture of acute farmer's lung is no longer apparent.

Other Disorders. Other forms of extrinsic allergic alveolitis of a similar nature may be caused by microorganisms or fungi. Examples include mushroom picker's lung, maple bark stripper's disease due to a fungus, cheese washer's lung caused by *Penicillium* spores, and a disease resulting from inhalation of spores from moldy sawdust. A more complete discussion of these and other similar diseases is found in Hunter (1969) or in microbiologically oriented pathology texts.

Bagassosis occurs in workers exposed to the dust arising from handling of dried sugar cane that has been allowed to lie around following extraction of the sugar-containing juices. The disease does not arise from exposure to moist sugar cane, but only from the dried material known as bagasse. Signs and symptoms include shortness of breath, production of small amounts of black sputum, fever, chills, and weight loss. The onset may occur after one or two days to a month, depending in part on the dose inhaled. The termination of contact with bagasse dust results in reasonably complete recovery within weeks or months, although some patients may remain symptomatic for a year or longer. Once an individual has had the disease it is advisable to avoid all further contact with bagasse dust. Renewed contact almost invariably produces a relapse; each episode tends to be more severe and prolonged than the last. The cause is proably molds or fungi in the stored bagasse.

Byssinosis arises from the inhalation of cotton, flax, or hemp dusts. The symptoms, in the form of chest tightness and respiratory difficulty, frequently appear after a period of absence from work, either a weekend or a prolonged vacation. Unlike farmer's lung and bagassosis, byssinosis does not seem to result from bacterial or fungal action on the cotton since the disease occurs also in individuals who work with the cotton before it is brought to the factory. The bronchoconstriction results from an agent or agents contained in the fibers or dust of the cotton plant itself, especially the bracts. Agents have been found in cotton that promote the release of histamine and 5-hydroxytryptamine. Heat treatment of the cotton tends to decrease the potency of the dust, which suggests a heat-labile toxicant or allergen. Symptoms are reduced by prior treatment with drugs that prevent degranulation of pulmonary mast cells. Byssinosis and other respiratory problems of cotton workers are reviewed by Harris et al. (1972).

Toluene diisocyanate (TDI), which is widely used in the manufacture of polyurethane plastics, also produces allergic-like symptoms on inhalation. It is a very reactive material that can conjugate with proteins. It may react with pulmonary tissue proteins or serum albumin to produce a hapten to which antibodies are subsequently directed. Some investigators have found a decrement in pulmonary function as assessed by measurement of 1 sec forced expiratory volume ($FEV_{1.0}$). This is observed from Monday to Friday during a work week. The individuals who show the greatest reduction over the course of a week tend also to show a long-term reduction when measurements are repeated one to two years later. Whether this represents the response of sensitized individuals or merely the response of individuals most sensitive to the irritant action per se has been debated. The literature has been recently reviewed in the NIOSH Criteria Document for Diisocyanates (1978).

Production of Pulmonary Cancer

The high incidence of lung cancer in the United States has directed much attention to inhaled toxic materials that produce pulmonary cancer. Without much doubt, cigarette smoking is the main contributor to lung cancer in man. Cigarette smoke is composed of a myriad of compounds, which include recognized carcinogens as well as recognized irritants. The production of tracheobronchial cancer in experimental animals by cigarette smoke inhalation has been difficult. The self-exposure of man has provided sufficient data that demonstration of a similar response in experimental animals is certainly not needed to delineate the hazard of cigarette smoking. Epidemiologic data also indicate that cigarette smoking increases the incidence of cancer in asbestos workers.

Coke oven emissions contain benzo(a)pyrene and a number of other polycyclic aromatic hydrocarbons. These materials can be metabolized by the lung cytochrome P450 system to reactive intermediaries capable of inducing mutations leading to malignant transformation. The action of chromate and nickel salts is less clearly understood. Nickel and nickel compounds produce mainly squamous cell carcinoma of the nasal cavity and the lung, suggesting that the mucus-secreting and cilia basal cells are most sensitive to transformation. Chromate and divalent nickel ions bind easily to DNA, but such binding is far removed from malignant transformation. These issues are discussed in more detail in Chapter 6.

REFERENCES

Anderson, A. A.: New sampler for the collection, sizing, and enumeration of viable airborne particles. *J. Bacteriol.*, **76**:471–84, 1958.

Boecker, B. B.; Aguilar, F. L.; and Mercer, T. T.: A canine inhalation exposure apparatus utilizing a whole body plethysmograph. *Health Phys.*, **10**:1077–89, 1964.

Bowden, D. H., and Adamson, I. Y. R.: Reparative changes following pulmonary cell injury. Ultrastructural, cytodynamic, and surfactant studies in mice after oxygen exposure. *Arch. Pathol.*, **92**:279–83, 1971.

Brunstetter, M.-A.; Hardie, J. A.; Schiff, R.; Lewis, J. P.; and Cross, C. E.: The origin of pulmonary alveolar macrophages. Studies of stem cells using the Es-2 marker of mice. *Arch. Intern. Med.*, **127**:1064–68, 1971.

Burton, J. A., and Schanker, L. S.: Absorption of antibiotics from the rat lung. *Proc. Soc. Exp. Biol. Med.*, **145**:752–56, 1974a.

———: Absorption of corticosteroids from the rat lung. *Steroids*, **23**:617–24, 1974b.

Carrington, C. B., and Green, T. J.: Granular pneumocytes in early repair of diffuse alveolar injury. *Arch. Intern. Med.*, **126**:464–65, 1970.

Casarett, L. J.: The vital sacs: Alveolar clearance mechanisms in inhalation toxicology. In Hayes, W. J., Jr. (ed.): *Essays in Toxicology*, Vol. 3. Academic Press, Inc., New York, 1972, Vol. 3.

Charles, J. M.; Abou-Donia, M. B.; and Menzel, D. B.: Absorption of paraquat and diquat from the airways of the perfused rat lung. *Toxicology*, 9:59–67, 1978.

Charnock, E. L., and Doershuk, C. F.: Development aspects of the human lung. *Pediatr. Clin. North Am.*, 20(2):275–92, 1973.

Clark, D. G.; McElligott, T. F.; and Hurst, E. W.: The toxicity of paraquat. *Br. J. Ind. Med.*, 23:126–32, 1966.

Corn, M.; Montgomery, T. L.; and Esmen, N. A.: Suspended particulate matter: seasonal variation in specific surface areas and densities. *Environ. Sci. Technol.*, 5:155–58, 1971.

Cuddihy, R. G., and Boecker, B. B.: Controlled administration of respiratory tract burdens of inhaled radioactive aerosols in beagle dogs. *Toxicol. Appl. Pharmacol.*, 25:597–605, 1973.

Cuddihy, R. G., and Ozog, J. A.: Nasal absorption of $CsCl$, $SrCl_2$, $BaCl_2$ and $CeCl_3$ in Syrian hamsters. *Health Phys.*, 25:219–24, 1973.

Cuddihy, R. G.; Brownstein, D. G.; Raabe, O. G.; and Kanapilly, G. M.: Respiratory tract deposition of inhaled polydisperse aerosols in beagle dogs. *J. Aerosol Sci.*, 4:35–45, 1973.

Cutz, E., and Conen, P. E.: Ultrastructure and cytochemistry of Clara cells. *Am. J. Pathol.*, 62:127–34, 1971.

Davies, C. N.: A formalized anatomy of the human respiratory tract. In Davies, C. N. (ed.): *Inhaled Particles and Vapours*. Pergamon Press, London, 1961, pp. 82–87.

Drazen, J. M.: Physiologic basis and interpretation of common indices of respiratory mechanical function. *Environ. Health Perspect.*, 16:11–16, 1976.

Drew, R. T., and Laskin, S.: Environmental inhalation chambers. In Gay, W. I. (ed.): *Methods of Animal Experimentation*, Vol. IV: *Environment and the Special Senses*. Academic Press, Inc., New York, 1973, pp. 1–41.

Drew, R. T., and M. Lippmann Calibration of Air Sampling Instruments - II. Production of Test Atmospheres for Instrument Calibration. *Air Sampling Instruments - 4th Edition*, American Conference of Governmental Industrial Hygienists (ACGIH), 1972.

Enna, S. J., and Schanker, L. S.: Absorption of saccharides and urea from the rat lung. *Am. J. Physiol.*, 222:409–14, 1972.

————: Phenol red absorption from the rat lung: Evidence of carrier transport. *Life Sci.*, 12:231–39, 1973.

Evans, M. J., and Bils, R. F.: Identification of cells labeled with tritiated thymidine in the pulmonary alveolar walls of the mouse. *Am. Rev. Respir. Dis.*, 100:372–78, 1969.

Felicetti, S. A.; Silbaugh, S. A.; Muggenburg, B. A.; and Hahn, F. F.: Effect of time post-exposure on the effectiveness of bronchopulmonary lavage in removing inhaled ^{144}Ce in fused clay from beagle dogs. *Health Phys.*, 29:89–96, 1975.

Frasier, R. G., and Pare, J. A. P.: *Structure and Function of the Lung*. W. B. Saunders Co., Philadelphia, 1971.

Green, G. M.: The J. Burns Amberson Lecture—in defense of the lung. *Am. Rev. Resp. Dis.*, 102:691–703, 1970.

————: Alveolobronchiolar transport mechanisms. *Arch. Intern. Med.*, 131:109–14, 1973.

Green, G. N.; Jakab, G. J.; Low, R. B.; and Davis, G. S.: Defense mechanisms of the respiratory membrane. *Am. Rev. Resp. Dis.*, 115:479–514, 1977.

Harris, T. R.; Merchant, J. A.; Kilburn, K. H.; and

Hamilton, J. D.: Byssinosis and respiratory diseases of cotton mill workers. *J. Occup. Med.*, 14:199–206, 1972.

Hatch, T. F., and Gross, P.: *Pulmonary Deposition and Retention of Inhaled Aerosols*. Academic Press, Inc., New York, 1964.

Heppleston, A. G.: The fibrogenic action of silica. *Br. Med. Bull.*, 25:282–87, 1969.

Hinners, R. G.; Burkart, J. K.; and Punte, C. L.: Animal inhalation exposure chambers. *Arch. Environ. Health*, 16:194–206, 1968.

Hunter, D.: *The Diseases of Occupations*, 4th ed. Little, Brown & Co., Boston, 1969.

Kanapilly, G. M.: Alveolar microenvironment and its relationship to the retention and transport into blood of aerosols deposited in the alveoli. *Health Phys.*, 32:89–100, 1977.

Kanapilly, G. M., and Goh, C. H. T.: Some factors affecting the *in vitro* rates of dissolution of respirable particles of relatively low solubility. *Health Phys.*, 25:225–37, 1973.

Kanapilly, G. M.; Raabe, O. G.; Goh, C. H. T.; and Chimenti, R. A.: Measurement of *in vitro* dissolution of aerosol particles for comparison to *in vivo* dissolution in the lower respiratory tract after inhalation. *Health Phys.*, 24:497–507, 1973.

Kapanci, Y.; Weibel, E. R.; Kaplan, H. P.; and Robinson, F. R.: Pathogenesis and reversibility of the pulmonary lesions of oxygen toxicity in monkeys. II. Ultrastructural and morphometric studies. *Lab. Invest.*, 20:101–18, 1969.

Kessler, G.-F.; Austin, J. H. M.; Graf, P. D.; Gamsu, G.; and Gold, W. M.: Airway constriction in experimental asthma in dogs: Tantalum bronchographic studies. *J. Appl. Physiol.*, 35:703–708, 1973.

Kilburn, K. H.: Clearance mechanisms in the respiratory tract. In Lee, D. H. K.; Falk, H. L.; Murphy, S. D.; and Geiger, S. R. (eds.): *Handbook of Physiology, Section 9: Reactions to Environmental Agents*. American Physiological Society, Bethesda, MD, 1977, pp. 243–62.

Kliment, V.: Similarity and dimensional analysis. Evaluation of aerosol deposition in the lungs of laboratory animals and man. *Folia Morphol. (Warsaw)*, 21:59–69, 1973.

Kotrappa, P., and Light, M. E.: Design and performance of the Lovelace aerosol particle separator. *Rev. Sci. Instrum.*, 43:1106–12, 1972.

Lippmann, M.: "Respirable" dust sampling. *Am. Ind. Hyg. Assoc. J.*, 31:138–59, 1970.

————: Filter media for air sampling. In *Air Sampling Instruments for Evaluation of Atmospheric Contaminants*, 4th ed., pp. N2–N21. American Conference of Governmental Industrial Hygienists, 1972.

————: Regional deposition of particles in the human respiratory tract. In Lee, D. H. K.; Falk, H. L.; Murphy, S. D.; and Geiger, S. R. (eds.): *Handbook of Physiology. Section 9: Reactions to Environment Agents*. American Physiological Society, Bethesda, MD, 1977, pp. 213–32.

Lippmann, M.; Albert, I. E.; and Peterson, H. T.: Regional deposition of inhaled aerosols in man. In Walton, W. H. (ed.): *Inhaled Particles and Vapours, III*. Unwin, Old Woking, Surrey, England, 1971, pp. 105–20.

Lundgren, D. A.: An aerosol sampler for determination of particle concentration as a function of size and time. *J. Air Pollut. Control Assoc.*, 17:225–28, 1967.

MacFarland, H. N.: Respiratory toxicology. In Hayes, W. J., Jr. (ed.): *Essays in Toxicology*, Vol. 7. Academic Press, Inc., New York, 1976, pp. 121–54.

Mercer, T. T.: On the role of particle size in the dissolution of lung burdens. *Health Phys.*, 13:1211–21, 1967.

————: *Aerosol Technology in Hazard Evaluation.* Academic Press, Inc., New York, 1973.

Mercer, T. T.; Tillery, M. I.; and Newton, G. J.: A multi-stage, low flow rate cascade impactor. *J. Aerosol Sci.* 1:9–15, 1970.

Miller, F. J.; Menzel, D. B.; and Coffin, D. L.: Similarity between man and laboratory animals in regional pulmonary deposition of ozone. *Environ. Res.*, 17:84–101, 1978.

Morrow, P. E.: Alveolar clearance of aerosols. *Arch. Intern. Med.*, 131:101–108, 1973.

Morrow, P. E.; Gibb, F. R.; and Gazioglu, K. M.: A study of particulate clearance from the human lungs. *Am. Rev. Resp. Dis.*, 96:1209–21, 1967.

Muggenburg, B. A.; Felicetti, S. A.; and Silbaugh, S. A.: Removal of inhaled radioactive particles by lung lavage—a review. *Health Phys.*, 33:213–20, 1977.

Nagahi, C.: *Functional Anatomy and Histology of the Lung.* University Park Press, Baltimore, MD, 1972.

National Academy of Sciences: *Nickel.* Series: Medical and Biological Effects of Environmental Pollutants. NAS-NRC, Washington, D.C., 1975.

Nelsen, F. M., and Eggertsen, F. T.: Determination of surface area. Adsorption measurements by a continuous flow method. *Anal. Chem.*, 30:1387–90, 1958.

NIOSH: *Criteria for a Recommended Standard. Occupational Exposure to Diisocyanates.* DHEW (NIOSH) Publ. No. 78–215, Washington, D.C., 1978.

Patrick, G., and Stirling, C.: The retention of particles in large airways of the respiratory tract. *Proc. R. Soc. London Ser. B.*, 198:455–62, 1977.

Phalen, R. F.: Inhalation exposure of animals. *Environ. Health Perspect.*, 16:17–24, 1976.

Phalen, R. F.; Yeh, H. -C.; Raabe, O. G.; and Velasquez, D. J.: Casting the lungs *in-situ. Anat. Rec.*, 177:255–64, 1973.

Pump, K. K.: The morphology of the finer branches of the bronchial tree of the human lung. *Dis. Chest*, 46:379–98, 1964.

Quinlan, M. F.; Salman, S. D.; Swift, D. L.; Wagner, H. N., Jr.; and Proctor, D. F.: Measurement of mucociliary function in man. *Am. Rev. Resp. Dis.*, 99:13–23, 1969.

Raabe, O. G.: Generation and characterization of aerosols. In Hanna, M. G., Jr.; Nettesheim, P.; and Gilbert, J. R. (eds.): *Inhalation Carcinogenesis.* Proceedings of a Biology Division, Oak Ridge National Laboratory, Conference. U. S. Atomic Energy Commission, Oak Ridge, TN, 1970, pp. 123–72.

Raabe, O. G.; Bennick, J. E.; Light, M. E.; Hobbs, C. H.; Thomas, R. L.; and Tillery, M. I.: An improved apparatus for acute inhalation exposure of rodents to radioactive aerosols. *Toxicol. Appl. Pharmacol.*, 26:264–73, 1973.

Raabe, O. G.; Boyd, H. A.; Kanapilly, G. M.; Wilkinson, C. J.; and Newton, G. J.: Development and use of a system for routine production of monodisperse particles of $^{238}PuO_2$ and evaluation of gamma emitting labels. *Health Phys.*, 28:655–67, 1975.

Rose, M. S.; Lock, E. A.; Smith, L. L.; and Wyatt, I.: Paraquat accumulation: tissue and species specificity *Biochem. Pharmacol.*, 25:419–23, 1976.

Sinclair, D., and Hinchliffe, L.: Production and measurement of submicron aerosols. II. In Mercer, T. T.; Morrow, P. E.; and Stöber, W. (eds.): *Assessment of Airborne Particles.* Charles C Thomas Publisher, Springfield, IL., 1972.

Sorokin, S. P.: A morphologic and cytochemical study on the great alveolar cell. *J. Histochem. Cytochem.*, 14:884–97, 1967.

Sorokin, S. P., and Brain, J. D.: Pathways of clearance in mouse lungs exposed to iron oxide aerosols. *Anat. Rec.*, 181:581–626, 1975.

Stöber, W., and Flachsbart, H.: Size-separating precipitation of aerosols in a spinning spiral duct. *Environ. Sci. Technol.*, 3:1280–96, 1969.

Task Group on Lung Dynamics, Committee II of the International Radiological Protection Commission: Deposition and retention models for internal dosimetry of the human respiratory tract. *Health Phys.*, 12:173–207, 1966.

Taylor, A. E., and Gaar, K. A., Jr.: Estimation of equivalent pore radii of pulmonary capillary and alveolar membranes. *Am. J. Physiol.*, 218:1133–40, 1970.

von Hayek, H.: *The Human Lung.* Hafner, New York, 1960.

Weibel, E. R.: *Morphometry of the Human Lung.* Academic Press, Inc., New York, 1963.

Weill, H.; George, R.; Schwarz, M.; and Ziskind, M.: Late evaluation of pulmonary function after acute exposure to chlorine gas. *Am. Rev. Resp. Dis.*, 99:374–79, 1969.

West, J. B.: *Ventilation/Blood Flow and Gas Exchange.* Blackwell, Oxford, 1970.

West, J. B.: *Respiratory Physiology—The Essentials.* Williams & Wilkins Co., Baltimore, 1974.

————: *Pulmonary Pathophysiology—The Essentials.* Williams & Wilkins, Co., Baltimore, 1977.

Chapter 13

TOXIC RESPONSES OF THE EYE

Albert M. Potts and *Leonard M. Gonasun*

INTRODUCTION

In this chapter the discussion will be limited to the deleterious effects of chemical substances on the globe, adnexa, and optic nerve. We recognize that thermal burns and chemical burns have factors in common and that the effects of ionizing radiation are similar to the effects of some chemicals. We also appreciate that by this stipulation we must consider incompletely the effects of hallucinogens on the visual system as a whole. Further, for our purposes we will make no distinction between substances that have known therapeutic value and those that have none. It is axiomatic that a substance that has some pharmacologic effect will be toxic if a sufficiently high dose is given. Without these stipulations the subject would become even more complex than its present fascinating complexity.

Even within these stipulated limitations it is not intended to be exhaustive. Space limitations would not permit such treatment, for there are enough specific instances of ocular poisons to fill volumes. Such texts exist and should be consulted for details on specific substances (see Galezowski, 1878; Uhthoff, 1911; Lewin and Guillery, 1913; Duke-Elder and MacFaul, 1972; Grant, 1974). References are also given on ocular anatomy and physiology (Duke-Elder and Wybar, 1961; Davson, 1972).

The eye, despite its small mass, contains derivatives of surface ectoderm (corneal epithelium and conjunctiva) and of mesoderm (choroid, iris, and ciliary body stroma). It contains true neural tissue (the inner retinal layer and optic nerve) and a highly specific light-sensitive modification of neural tissue (the photoreceptors). It contains two relatively large avascular areas (the lens and cornea), which are bounded by unique active transport systems responsible for maintaining a steady state of hydration and hence transparency. It contains a small private cerebrospinal fluid system (the aqueous system) where ciliary body processes are analogous to choroid plexus, where the barrier to circulating blood is as specific as that of the brain, and where the outflow system is so critical that loss of sight is the price of dysfunction. Unique chemical substances in significant concentration are the organ-specific lens proteins; the (at least) four photosensitive pigments; and the avid electron acceptor, melanin, present in ocular tissues at higher levels than anywhere else in the human body. These unique features in a small physical compass make for a multiplicity of types of reaction to injury and a potentially high sensitivity to toxic substances.

CORNEA, CONJUNCTIVA, AND NEIGHBORING TISSUES

Special Considerations

The cornea (Fig. 13–1) and its neighboring partial analog, the conjunctiva, are the portions of the eye directly exposed to external insults. The cornea must maintain its transparency to remain functional. A scar, the normal body reparative process, with or without vascularization, is tolerated by other body structures with no adverse effects. In the case of the cornea a scar or vascularization can destroy function completely. Hence a very small amount of corrosive substance—an amount of no consequence elsewhere on the body—can be the cause of blindness if it reaches the cornea.

There is convincing evidence that corneal transparency is maintained by the boundary layers of epithelium and endothelium, which have small mass and relatively high metabolic activity (Maurice, 1969). Thus death of these boundary layers—20 to 25 mg of tissue in the adult eye—is responsible for imbibition of water and loss of transparency. The stoichiometric implications of these minute quantities is impressive.

External Contact Agents

Acids. A splash of acid in the eye is a medical emergency and offers a poor setting for gathering scientific data. We must rely on adequately

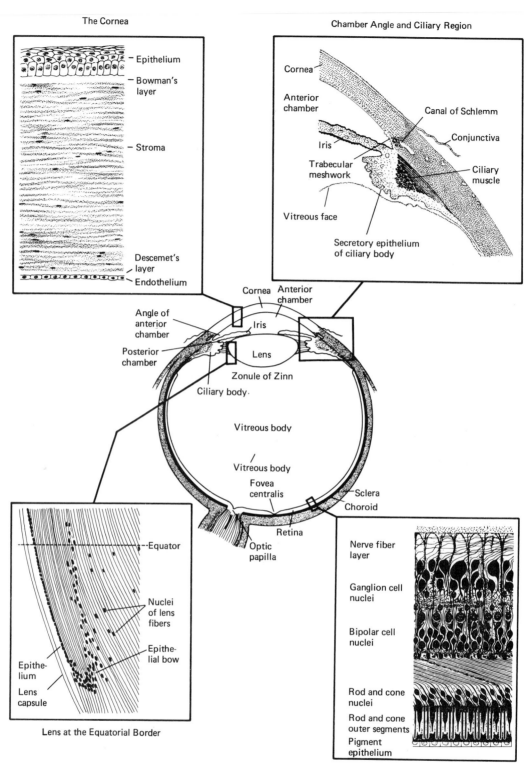

The Cornea

— Epithelium
— Bowman's layer
— Stroma
— Descemet's layer
— Endothelium

Chamber Angle and Ciliary Region

Cornea
Anterior chamber
Iris
Trabecular meshwork
Vitreous face
Canal of Schlemm
Conjunctiva
Ciliary muscle
Secretory epithelium of ciliary body

Cornea
Anterior chamber
Angle of anterior chamber
Iris
Lens
Posterior chamber
Zonule of Zinn
Ciliary body
Vitreous body
Vitreous body
Fovea centralis
Sclera
Choroid
Retina
Optic papilla

Lens at the Equatorial Border

Equator
Nuclei of lens fibers
Epithelial bow
Epithelium
Lens capsule

Cross Section of Retina

Nerve fiber layer
Ganglion cell nuclei
Bipolar cell nuclei
Rod and cone nuclei
Rod and cone outer segments
Pigment epithelium

Figure 13–1. Digrammatic horizontal cross section of the eye, with medium-power enlargement of details in cornea, chamber angle, lens, and retina. (The enlarged retina diagram [lower right] is taken from Polyak, S.: *The Retina*. University of Chicago Press, Chicago, 1941. By permission of Mrs. Stephen Polyak.)

controlled experimental studies for much of our knowledge of corneal burns. An excellent set of studies was performed during World War II under the auspices of the Office of Scientific Research and Development and was reported by Friedenwald and coworkers (Friedenwald *et al.*, 1944, 1946). These authors established standard techniques for applying acids (and bases) to the eye and set standards by which damage could be evaluated. Their results bore out the clinical impression that damage by acid was a dual function of pH and of the capacity of the anion in question to combine with protein. Acid burns vary in severity from those that heal completely to those that cause complete opacity or even perforation of the globe. Their distinctive aspect is that their severity may be assessed early. Unlike the situation with alkali burns, the damage from acid that is visible in the first few hours is a measure of the long-term damage to be expected.

Special aspects of some acids complicate the picture. The dehydrating effect of concentrated sulfuric acid as well as the high heat of hydration adds to its acid properties in determining the severity of the burn. The affinity of the anion for the corneal tissues also plays a role in the severity of damage. Friedenwald and coworkers (1946) showed that buffered solutions of picric, tungstic, and tannic acids produced lesions of significant severity in the rabbit eye and with no great differences in severity from pH 1.5 to pH 9.

This effect was in sharp contrast to hydrochloric acid, which caused severe damage at pH 1 with virtually no effect at pH 3 and above. As the pH of buffered solutions applied to the human eye is decreased from 7.4, the onset of discomfort begins at about pH 4.5. Between pH 4.5. and 3.5 one creates punctate breaks in the corneal epithelium that are stainable with fluorescein but heal in a few hours' time.

Another special instance, more of a hazard in the past than in the present, is that of compressed sulfur dioxide. When many industrial refrigeration plants used SO_2 as the refrigerant, eye damage caused by a high-pressure jet of sulfur dioxide was not uncommon. The anhydrous liquid hitting the cornea a high-pressure jet of sulfur dioxide was not uncommon. The anhydrous liquid hitting the cornea under pressure not only combines with corneal water to form H_2SO_3 but because of its relative fat solubility it penetrates the cornea into the aqueous and hydrolyzes there causing deep keratitis and iritis. Studies on the mechanism of SO_2 injury were done by Grant (1947).

It is universally agreed that the one best treatment for acid burns is rapid irrigation with large volumes of water. The reduction of concentration, including hydrogen ion concentration, by dilution is most important. Mechanical removal from the site of injury by the stream of water is accomplished simultaneously. Attempts to obtain some special buffered solution or mildly alkaline wash only delay the start of treatment. Washing should begin as close in time and place to the site of the accident as possible. All industrial safety personnel should know this fact and be prepared to begin treatment by washing. Even in the case of concentrated sulfuric acid burns, where it is expected that the addition of water will generate heat, the water wash is best, using a large enough volume and a fast enough rate to dissipate heat as well as wash out acid.

Strong Alkalies—Ammonia, Collagenase. In addition to considerations of pH there are several factors specific to alkali burns. First, alkalies in concentrations that can cause serious eye burns exist in many homes. Household ammonia and sodium hydroxide-containing drain cleaners are the chief offenders. The second problem specific to alkalies is the serious late effects of alkali burns. Even burns that at the time of injury appear to be mild can go on to opacification, vascularization, ulceration, or perforation (Hughes, 1946a, 1946b). The photographs presented in Hughes' experimental paper (Hughes, 1946b) are eloquent on this subject. It should be noted that in experimental animals Hughes produced burns of all degrees of severity by exposure of the cornea to isotonic $N/20$ sodium hydroxide. Exposure for 30 seconds followed by washing caused signs that lasted for several weeks only and usually cleared with no residues. Exposure to the same agent for three minutes followed by washing caused severe early opacification, marked vascularization at three months, and residues of opacity, pigment, and vessels after ten months. Irrigation with $N/20$ NaOH for more than three minutes could cause catastrophic changes in the cornea and surrounding tissues leading to complete opacification and purulent infiltration within a week or ten days with ulceration and perforation.

This is a measure of the severity of alkali burns. Apparently with the exceptions to be mentioned below the nature of the cation has relatively little bearing on the severity and end result of the burn. The pH and time of exposure have much more bearing on outcome, complicated somewhat by the resistance of the epithelium to penetration of the base. It should be mentioned that in the absence of epithelium, solutions up to pH 11 applied for ten minutes or less cause minimal and reversible damage (Grant and Kern, 1955). This, of course, corresponds to $N/100$ NaOH. The $N/20$ NaOH of Hughes (pH = 12.7) is 50 times more concentrated.

One of the exceptions to the uniform behavior of alkali cations is that of ammonia. Of all the alkali cations measured, ammonium ion as ammonium hydroxide penetrates epithelium, stroma, and anterior chamber more rapidly than any other. Grant speculates on whether this is due to the fat solubility of nonionized NH_3, to rapid diffusion, or to the ability of NH_4OH to injure corneal epithelium (Grant, 1974). However this may be, it has been shown that ammonia is detectable in the anterior chamber 15 seconds after exposure of the cornea to concentrated NH_4OH (Siegrist, 1920). Uveitis may be an early manifestation in ammonia burns.

The Special Case of Lime Burns. The second exception to the generalizations about cations is the case of calcium oxide, known popularly as unslaked lime. This substance, a component of Portland cement and of most commercial wall plasters, absorbs water to form calcium hydroxide with the liberation of heat. Calcium hydroxide is sparingly soluble in water, but in solution (saturated solution, 0.15 percent, pH = 12.4) causes the usual alkali burn. In addition to the generation of heat, the special problem in lime burns is that lime, plaster, or cement on reaching the eye tends to react with the moisture and protein found there and form clumps of moist compound, very difficult to remove by the usual irrigation. Such clumps tend to lodge deep in the cul-de-sacs inferiorly and superiorly and act as reservoirs for the liberation of $Ca(OH)_2$ over long periods of time. This is why physicians have been especially concerned about lime burns in the past and why special care must be taken in treatment of this condition. This treatment consists of (Grant, 1974) (1) rapid irrigation, to remove as much material as can be quickly washed away; (2) debridement, to remove physically whatever gross particles of lime can be seen on the cornea and in the cul-de-sacs; and (3) use of a complexing agent, preferably ethylenediaminetetraacetic acid disodium salt (EDTA), to remove the remainder of the $Ca(OH)_2$-generating material that cannot be handled grossly. With observation of these extra requirements lime burns can be made to follow the pattern of other alkali burns.

The Late Effects. The fact that early appearance of an alkali burn is not an adequate guide to prognosis and the possible appearance of infiltration, ulceration, and perforation about a week after the injury have caused much speculation about the mechanism of these late serious sequelae. It is generally agreed that a primary or secondary toxic substance is generated by the action of alkali on corneal tissue. What this substance may be is the subject of considerable speculation. Most recently attention has turned to the possibility that formation or liberation of collagenase in the cornea is responsible for ulceration and perforation.

Slansky and coworkers (1968) demonstrated the presence of collagenase in the cornea using an artificial dye-coupled substrate. They showed that damage to the epithelium liberates collagenase and that chelation of calcium by 10^{-3} M ethylenediaminetetraacetic acid (EDTA) inhibits enzyme activity. A year later Brown and associates (1969) described the killing of all of the epithelial cells by an alkali burn and demonstrated that collagenase may be determined in alkali-induced corneal ulcers by incubating 2-mm trephine buttons on reconstituted collagen gel and measuring the area of gel lysis. Brown and coworkers (1970) on the basis of injection of extracts of alkali-burned cornea concluded that the concentration of collagenase found could not be accounted for on the basis of the corneal epithelium and that the collagenase probably came from neutrophils invading the cornea after the burn. The Brown group introduced the use of cysteine as a collagenase inhibitor. They recently described a typical series of human alkali burns treated effectively with cysteine and a soft corneal contact lens (Brown et al., 1972).

It should be appreciated that even with collagenase inhibitors the catastrophe that has been avoided is perforation of the globe. This is important because after perforation visual function is usually beyond repair. However, after a serious alkali burn treated with collagenase inhibitors one is still left with an opaque cornea and light perception only, in the involved eye. The only hope for useful function is a successful corneal transplant—a result made less likely by a seriously burned and opaque recipient cornea.

Organic Solvents. Neutral organic solvents such as ethanol, acetone, ethyl ether, ethyl acetate, hexane, benzol, and toluene may contact the eye in industrial or laboratory accidents. These substances have in common their ability to dissolve fats. As a result they cause pain on contacting the eye, and examination after a generous splash of solvent shows dulling of the cornea. The epithelium will show punctate staining with fluorescein. The damage appears to be scattered loss of epithelial cells due to solution of some of the fats that occur in these cells. The sensation is due to trauma of some of the populous and sensitive corneal nerve endings. Damage is never extensive or long lasting if the splash is at room temperature. Hot solvents of low volatility add the problem of thermal burn to that of solvent action, and the end result is potentially more serious and less predictable.

Detergents. An increasing number of substances are used in technology as detergents, emulsifying agents, wetting agents, antifoaming agents, and solubilizers. They have the common property of lowering the surface tension of aqueous solutions and they possess discrete nonpolar and polar portions in the same molecule. The nonpolar portion is frequently a long aliphatic chain. The polar portion can be cationic, anionic, or nonionic.

Curiously, there appears to be no relation between surface tension-lowering ability and the amount of damage caused by any given detergent, and the mechanism of damage is not at all clear.

In general, cationic detergents are more damaging than anionic agents and both of these more than nonionics. For a rabbit eye test that has become the FDA standard and for a table of the maximum tolerated concentrations of 23 surface-active agents, see Draize and Kelley (1952). It is remarkable that such tolerated concentrations vary from 0.5 percent for the cationic lauryl dimethyl benzyl ammonium chloride through 20 percent for sodium lauryl sulfate to 100 percent for the nonionic sorbitan mono-laurate or mono-oleate. Note that one-third of the animals in the rabbit test have no washing of the eye after instillation of 0.1 ml of test substance, one-third have the eye washed after two seconds, and one-third have the eye washed after four seconds. A "tolerated concentration" is one in which there is no residual irritation after seven days.

Some of the surface-active agents, especially the cationic substances, in higher concentrations can cause severe burns with permanent opacity and vascularization. In human accidents the immediate severe pain leads to rapid washing out of the eye, and only in the most extreme circumstances will permanent damage result. One exceptional circumstance with hazard potential is that some nonionic detergents actually cause topical anesthesia of the cornea (Martin *et al.*, 1962). It is conceivable that if a formulation contains such a surfactant in combination with an anionic or a cationic detergent, the anesthetic surfactant might eliminate the pain warning and allow severe damage to occur.

The Vesicant War Gases. A group of chemical substances have in common the property of causing severe skin burns on contact in very low concentrations. They have been used or their use has been considered as chemical warfare agents—thus the rubric for this section. All of these agents cause severe eye burns on contact with the liquid or vapor. Whereas mass exposures are improbable—witness the absence of chemical warfare agents as combat weapons in World War II—civilian life is not entirely free from potential exposure. Furthermore, entirely new substances with potentially toxic effects, synthesized for reasons unconnected with combat, can be guarded against only if we are aware of potential toxicity.

Two general categories of such vesicants are

$$
\begin{matrix}
\text{I} & & \text{II} \\
& R_1{-}X_1 & \\
& \diagup & \\
R_3{-}Z & & \text{and} \quad X_3{-}R_4{-}As{-}(X_4)_2 \\
& \diagdown & \\
& R_2{-}X_2 &
\end{matrix}
$$

Where $Z = N$ or S

$R_1, R_2, R_3, R_4 =$ Aliphatic groups, saturated, olefinic, or halogenated (R_4 may be aromatic)

$X_1, X_2, X_3, X_4 =$ Halogen

The prototype of compound I is classic mustard gas, β,β-dichlordiethyl sulfide:

$$
\begin{matrix}
& C_2H_4{-}Cl \\
& \diagup \\
S & \\
& \diagdown \\
& C_2H_4{-}Cl
\end{matrix}
$$

And the prototype of compound II is lewisite, chlorvinyl dichlorarsine:

$$Cl{-}CH{=}CH{-}AsCl_2$$

Nitrogen mustards and lewisite analogs such as phenyldichlorarsine have been synthesized and are vesicant.

The two types of substances appear to work in distinctly different ways. The reactivity of the mustard-type compounds depends on their ability to form the highly active sulfonium derivative in solution.

$$
\begin{matrix}
H_2C{-}CH_2 & \\
& \diagdown \\
& S^+ \quad Cl^- \\
& \diagup \\
ClCH_2{-}CH_2 &
\end{matrix}
$$

This substance reacts rapidly with functional groups of proteins—OH, NH_2, and SH groups, alkylating them and changing the functional nature of metabolic proteins such as enzymes. The ion can react with water forming hemi-mustard:

$$
\begin{matrix}
OH{-}CH_2{-}CH_2 & \\
& \diagdown \\
& S \\
& \diagup \\
Cl{-}CH_2{-}CH_2 &
\end{matrix}
$$

and this too can become activated, the second half of the molecule forming the sulfonium ion and allowing the second beta carbon to combine with functional groups. The covalent bonds thus formed are highly stable and, for biologic functional purposes, irreversible. Thus, once the mustards have been allowed to react with tissues, the further course of poisoning must run its course. The only practical antimustard agents are prophylactic substances such as thiosulfate that speed hydrolysis, making reaction with $S_2O_3^{2-}$ preferential to reaction with tissue (Gilman and Philips, 1946).

Unlike the mustards, the lewisite group appears to react by the arsenic combining with the vicinal sulfhydryl groups of proteins. This combination can be reversed by treatment with a vicinal dithiol with greater affinity for trivalent arsenic than protein. Such a substance is 2,3-dimercapto-l-propanol (dimercaprol, British anti-lewisite, BAL) (Peters *et al.*, 1945). It may prevent a burn if applied as late as one hour after exposure to lewisite.

During World War I there was reasonably extensive experience with the eye effects of thio mustard (lewisite was never used in combat) (Beauvieux, 1920; Derby, 1920; Elliott and Soltau, 1923; Anonymous, 1939). It has become customary to express exposure to mustard vapor as "CT", i.e., concentration in mg/m³ × minutes. "Mild" exposures to CTs of 40 to 90 exhibit a symptomless latent period of 2 to 48 hours followed by subjective irritation and signs of conjunctivitis with clearing in one week on symptomatic treatment. Moderately severe burns are caused by a CT of 90 to 100 with incapacitating eye involvement after a latent period of two to ten hours. Then ulcers, opacity, and perforation can result. An unusual result of severe mustard burns is very late recurrent vascularization and ulceration many years after the initial injury. Mann and coworkers made a special study of this phenomenon (Mann *et al.*, 1948). A confirmatory report from the United States is that of Atkinson (1947).

Nitrogen mustards are designated HN1, HN2, and HN3, depending on whether one, two, or three of the substituents on the nitrogen are halogenated. They behave very similarly to thio mustard in experiments on rabbit cornea. Fortunately there is no extensive experience with human exposure, but on the basis of animal work doses of all four substances can be obtained that produce identical effects (Maumenee and Scholz, 1948). Of course, no long-term effects of severe nitrogen mustard corneal burns in humans have been observed.

Without reference to chemical warfare, HN2 is an intermediate in the manufacture of meperidine (Pethidine, Demerol), and eye irritation has been reported among plant personnel (Minton, 1949). Furthermore, numerous variants on nitrogen mustards are now standard therapeutic agents for a number of neoplastic diseases, especially lymphomas and blood dyscrasias. The manufacture and utilization of these drugs will continue to present a finite eye hazard.

For the sake of completeness the vesicant action of some substituted nitrosamines should be mentioned.

$$O{=}N{-}N\begin{array}{c} C_2H_4{-}Cl \\[1em] C{-}OCH_3 \\ \parallel \\ O \end{array}$$

N-Carbomethoxy-*N*-(β-chlorethyl)-nitrosamine is a typical example of a vesicant that like nitrogen mustard is an alkylating agent. Mann and associates (1948) studied this substance experimentally and reported several mild accidental eye burns in human workers.

Lacrimators and Smog. A number of chemically reactive substances in very high dilution are able to stimulate corneal sensory endings and cause reflex tearing. These contrast sharply with the mustards, which show a long latent period for subjective symptoms and then cause severe damage. The lacrimators in threshold concentrations cause instant sensation and no tissue damage. However, in higher concentrations lacrimators can cause chemical burns with loss of corneal epithelium.

Typical lacrimators are as follows:

α-Chloroacetophenone   α-Brombenzyl cyanide

$$C_2H_5{-}OC{-}CH_2I$$

Ethyl iodoacetate

See Jacobs (1942).

Lacrimator eye damage is complicated by the method of delivery. The two most common forms of delivery are the pencil-like tear-gas gun, purchaseable by individuals in many states, and the aerosol can, used by law enforcement agencies under the trade name Mace. The pencil gun has a charge of powdered α-chloroacetophenone propelled by the equivalent of a 22-caliber blank cartridge. When the gun is discharged near the eye, the force of the propellant can drive the powdered lacrimator deep into the cornea. The cartridge wadding can also strike the eye with force causing mechanical injury (Levine and Stahl, 1968). The chemical alone causes mechanical damage and its concentration in the eye exceeds the lacrimatory threshold by many, many times. This type of injury may lead to permanent corneal opacity. A similar but less severe injury can result if an aerosol can containing dissolved chloracetophenone is discharged close to the eye instead of at a distance of several feet or more as recommended by the manufacturer (Thatcher *et al.*, 1971).

The mechanism of action of the lacrimators was investigated during World War II, notably by Dixon (1948) and Mackworth (1948). Their investigations showed that whatever the chemical nature of the lacrimator, they all shared the property of inhibiting sulfhydryl enzymes. They had no effect on enzymes not dependent on SH groups for their activity.

There are a few incongruities not well explained by this theory. Iodoacetate is a sulfhydryl reagent but is not a lacrimator. Lewisite is a good sulfhydryl reagent; even under the conditions of the Dixon experiments it combines with 65 percent of the available SH groups; but it is not a lacrimator. The mustards react with SH groups. Whereas this reaction is a slow one and happens in minutes rather than seconds, the latent period for eye symptoms from the mustards is a matter of hours. Dixon himself pointed to another incongruity in the simple sulfhydryl reaction theory. The instant lacrimation on exposure to above-threshold concentration, the rapid cessation of effect on stopping exposure, the resumption of irritation on restoring the lacrimator, all speak against an irreversible combination of agent with critical tissue constituent. Dixon's suggestion that the nerve might respond to a *change* in -SH seems improbable. However, the whole subject of lacrimators is past due for reinvestigation.

The likely stimulus for such an investigation is the upsurge of an environmental lacrimator that must be dealt with expeditiously. This is photochemical smog. Not to be confused with industrial smog, this entity results from the interaction of automobile exhaust emissions and ultraviolet radiation from sunlight. It was first noticed in the Los Angeles area in the 1940s about the time when the last definitive work on chemical warfare lacrimators reached print. More recently it has appeared in the metropolitan areas of the Southwest and on exceptionally sunny days in the large cities of the East and Midwest. We appear to be dealing with substances formed by ultraviolet-activated oxygen, with oxides of nitrogen, and the olefins, aromatics, and perhaps aliphatic hydrocarbons of automobile exhaust. Of the products the major identified component is the class of peroxyacyl nitrates, which have distinct lacrimator action. This is not the whole story, however, for artificially generated smog used in laboratory studies is several times more active a lacrimator than peroxyacetyl nitrate. For a competent review of this subject, see Jaffe (1967).

Despite increased emission control standards for new cars the smog problem will be with us in the foreseeable future. There will be intensified interest in the whole gamut of lacrimator substances in photochemical smog; how these substances work on the eye; and how the effects can be combatted or prevented. The beneficial fallout from the smog problem may be better understanding of the lacrimators.

Miscellaneous Substances. *Metallic Salts.* Heavy metal ions combine with protein functional groups. In high enough concentration metal salts cause tissue destruction. Thus workers with such materials have the hazard of corneal opacity and ulceration should a splash hit the eye. Adequate protection is indicated.

The more subtle deposition of metal components in the tissues of cornea, conjunctiva, and lids secondary to chronic overuse for therapeutic purposes is a phenomenon of the recent preantibiotic past when heavy-metal salts were the only available antibacterial agents. The tissue discoloration is a striking cosmetic defect. The chief offenders in the United States have been mild silver proteinate and yellow oxide of mercury (Wheeler, 1947; Wilkes, 1953). Outside of the United States there have been reports of argyrosis secondary to a silver-containing eyelash dye (Velhagen, 1953).

Hydroquinone. In many industries a fine dust of particles can be generated and in the absence of adequate exhaust velocity these particles can reach the eye. This set of events can occur in the manufacture of any noxious solid substance. A particularly striking report was that of Anderson (1947) on workers engaged in the manufacture of hydroquinone for many years. The colorless hydroquinone dust on reaching the eye (with a distribution corresponding to the palpebral fissure) oxidizes to brown benzoquinone. This material is stored in large granules in or near the basal layer of the corneal epithelium and in smaller granules in the more superficial epithelium. It is visible as a brown band keratopathy.

Dichloroethane. A remarkable note on species specificity is provided by the reaction of the dog cornea to the systemic administration of 1,2-dichloroethane. Milky-white opacity results after exposure to 1,000 ppm for seven hours. This appears not to be related to direct contact of the eye with the agent but is due to secondary action of the drug or a metabolic product on the corneal endothelium. Of many species of vertebrates tested, only the dog and the fox show the effect. For a report on a number of experiments see the review by Heppel and coworkers (1944).

Lash Lure. In the past when there were few restrictions on the composition of cosmetics in this country, hair dyes and eyelash dyes were sold whose principal ingredient was *p*-phenylenediamine. It was the severe reaction to such a preparation sold under the proprietary name Lash Lure that encouraged more stringent federal regulation. It appears that *p*-phenylenediamine and its analogs can easily sensitize the lid skin and external ocular structures. Continued application of the hapten can cause severe damage to the contacted tissues. Corneal ulceration with loss of vision and even a fatality have been reported. A concentration of papers appeared in the *Journal of the American Medical Association* in 1933 and 1934. For a review, see Linksz (1942).

Corneal Involvement by Internally Administered Substances

Uncommonly a systemic drug may affect the cornea selectively.

Quinacrine. The antimalarial quinacrine

(Atabrine) is such a substance, and the effect is corneal edema. A typical report is that of Chamberlain and Boles (1946). This edema was a relatively rare occurrence in the Pacific theater during World War II where some 25 cases were recognized among many thousands of men taking the usual daily 100-mg prophylactic dose. The precise mechanism of action is unclear, though it is tempting to postulate a specific effect on the corneal endothelium.

Chloroquine. A second antimalarial substance affecting the cornea after oral administration is chloroquine. However, just as with the retinal lesions (see below), chloroquine keratopathy is seen chiefly in patients receiving 250 to 500 mg/day for rheumatoid arthritis or systemic lupus. The subjective symptoms are intolerance to glare and halos around lights. At ordinary levels of illumination vision is not impaired. Slit lamp examination shows grayish turbidity in the deep layers of the epithelium. Biopsy has shown that these particles fluoresce; so they are presumably chloroquine or a metabolic product. The involvement disappears on cessation of drug administration. For a good early report, see Calkins (1958). For retinal effects of chloroquine, see below.

Chlorpromazine. The eye effects of chlorpromazine are minimal, but in patients who have received daily doses of 500 mg or more for at least three years granular deposits have been noted on the corneal endothelium and the lens capsule. These findings were first reported by Greiner and Berry (1964) in 12 of 70 patients. DeLong and coworkers (1965) described an additional series of 49 involved patients in a series of 131. In this latter series only patients who received a cumulative dose of 1,000 g or more of the drug showed corneal changes.

Addendum on Lids and Lacrimal Apparatus

As mentioned in a previous section, the lids are usually involved in heavy-metal pigmentation. Another function that may be disturbed by lid damage is the drainage of tears through the lacrimal puncta at the inner nasal margins of the upper and lower lids. The normal tear flow enters the lacrimal canaliculi in the lid margins via the puncta and continues on through common canaliculus, lacrimal sac, and nasolacrimal duct into the nasopharynx. Action of any of the corrosives discussed above can cause scarring shut of the puncta or canaliculi or both with obstruction of tear flow and annoying epiphora—tears running down the cheek. Indeed the scar need not even obstruct the drainage system. If it distorts lid position enough so that the lacrimal punctum is everted and no longer in contact with the tear film, this is enough to cause epiphora. Because the drainage system of the upper lid is often inefficient, sometimes involvement of the lower lid alone is enough to cause epiphora. Other effects of

scarring can be turning in of the lids (entropion) with abrasion of the cornea by eyelashes. Turning out of the lids (ectropion) can cause desiccation of the cornea if it is exposed. The surgical correction of these scarring effects is difficult and not uniformly successful.

One medication that has the property of lowering intraocular pressure was found after ten years of general use to block the lacrimal drainage system. The structure of the drug, furfuryl trimethyl ammonium iodide (Furmethide), is as follows:

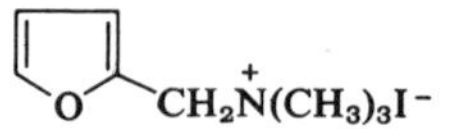

It was introduced to ophthalmic practice by Meyerson and Thau (1940) and was used in 10 percent solution for cases of intractable glaucoma until the report of Shaffer and Ridgway in 1951 described numerous cases of lacrimal obstruction in patients who used the drug continuously for three months or more. The obstruction was caused by nonspecific inflammatory tissue. Biopsy showed such inflammation in conjunctiva and at multiple points in the lacrimal drainage system.

The toxicology of the sclera is peculiar in that for practical purposes it does not exist. Externally applied corrosives reach the cornea before the sclera. Since loss of transparency of the cornea is accomplished by relatively low concentrations of corrosives and since cornea and sclera are equally susceptible to extreme burns that might cause perforation, selective scleral damage by corrosives just does not happen. Similarly, when collagen synthesis is inhibited as in lathyrism, the greater exposure of the cornea makes it more susceptible to perforation, other things being equal.

A new hazard to the eye appears to reside in the drug practolol, used in Great Britain for its properties as a blocker of β-adrenergic activity. In the U.S. propranolol has been used for almost a decade without reliably reported adverse ocular effects.

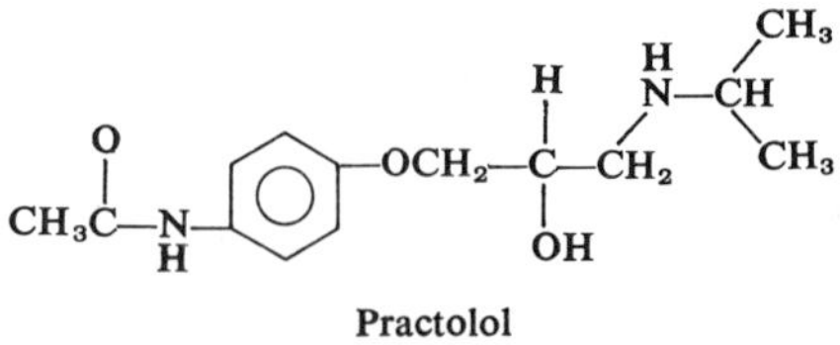

Practolol

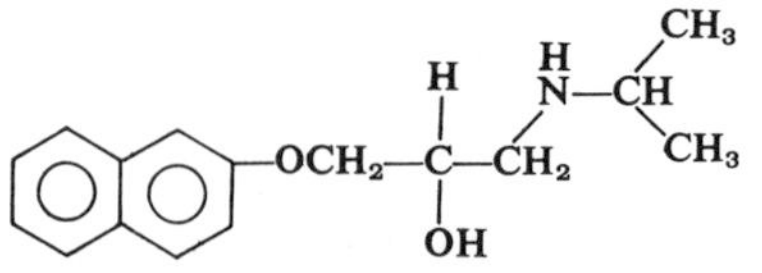

Propranolol

In a limited number of patients practolol causes an "oculocutaneous syndrome" with atrophy of the lacrimal gland, corneal ulceration, and even corneal perforation. Because of its appearance and immunologic behavior the syndrome has been called ocular cicatricial pemphigoid (Van Joost et al., 1976).

Elevated antinuclear antoantibodies have been demonstrated in two laboratories (Garner and Rahi, 1976; Jachuck *et al.*, 1977).

Considering the structure of practolol versus that of innocuous propranolol, it would appear that the β-blocking property is conferred by N-isopropyl propanolamine side chains, ether linked to an aromatic nucleus. This suggests that the disease-producing property of practolol resides in the dissimilar portion of the molecule. The *p*-acetamidophenol of practolol suggests similarity to the sulfonamide moiety, which can cause the oculocutaneous syndrome Stevens-Johnson disease.

Apparently unrelated to hypersensitivity is the cicatricial ectropion reported to occur secondary to prolonged systemic 5-fluorouracil therapy (Straus *et al.*, 1977). The condition is reversible on stopping the drug.

THE IRIS, AN INDICATOR OF AUTONOMIC ACTIVITY

Peripheral Effects

The special aspect of the iris (Fig. 13–1) for pharmacology is its double innervation (sympathetic for dilator and parasympathetic for sphincter) and its being behind a transparent window, the cornea. Thus as one would expect, sympathomimetic and parasympatholytic substances dilate the pupil and parasympathomimetic and sympatholytic substances constrict the pupil—events easily observed in the intact subject. Allowing for the poor ocular penetration of very polar substances and for the co-existence of centrally initiated impulses, the pupil is an excellent indicator of autonomic activity of topically or systemically administered drugs and poisons.

The eye effects of extracts of mandragora and hyoscyamus were known to Galen in the second century A.D. These effects in sixteenth-century Venice gave rise to the plant name belladonna (Matthiolus, 1598). The early experiments of Thomas Fraser on physostigma (Fraser, 1863) and those of T. R. Elliott on epinephrine (Elliott, 1905) utilized observations of the iris in intact animals.

The greatest potential, happily unrealized, for observation of these types of effects in human toxicology is from the effects of so-called "nerve gases" in combat. All of these substances are so-called "irreversible" cholinesterase inhibitors. Di-isopropyl fluorophosphate is an early synthesized example of such compounds. The acetylcholine constantly manufactured at cholinergic nerve endings and unhydrolyzed by normally present cholinesterase causes pupillary constriction in poisoning by these substances.

Since World War II, such cholinesterase inhibitors have been synthesized as insecticides. An occasional accidental toxic episode has been reported—usually concerning a worker standing in a field being dusted

with insecticide from an airplane. Further, the pilot of such a plane may experience visual symptoms from the same cause (Upholt *et al.*, 1956).

A somewhat odd iris effect has been labeled "cornpicker's pupil." It is mydriasis caused by operating farm machinery in a cornfield containing jimson weed, *Datura stramonium*. Enough hyoscyamine and related parasympatholytic substances from the plant reach the eye to dilate the pupil over a period of days (Goldey *et al.*, 1966).

It is understood that accidental poisoning by any of the agents in the autonomic group will, if severe enough, cause pupillary signs that may be helpful in establishing a diagnosis.

Central Effects

Not all pupillary changes due to toxic substances are demonstrably direct effects on the iris. The markedly constricted pupil characteristic of morphine poisoning appears to be due to central reinforcement of the physiologic light reflex. Constriction of the pupil caused by morphine is abolished by section of the optic nerve. The consensual reflex caused in the optic nerve-sectioned eye by light stimulation of the intact eye is enhanced by systemic administration of morphine. There is a small residual pupillary constriction caused by morphine in the absence of light. This may be direct action on the pupillary constrictor center or on the muscle itself, but this effect is small in comparison to light reflex enhancement (McCrea *et al.*, 1942).

Similarly, any drug effects observed in the alert animal are algebraically additive with centrally originating reflexes such as sympathetic dilation in the startle reflex, or pupillary constriction that accompanies concentration on a near object. These tend to be transient and are able to be sorted out from toxic drug effects. Similarly, the effects of general anesthetics in first constricting, then dilating, the pupil are superimposed on other pharmacologic and toxicologic effects.

Inflammatory Iris Reactions

The highly vascular iris is quite sensitive to physical and chemical trauma. Its response to all types of insults is nonspecific and consists primarily of increase in vascular permeability. The result of this is, first, liberation of protein into the normally low-protein aqueous humor. Both serum proteins and fibrin can enter the anterior chamber, and fibrin coagulum can eventually cause blockage of outflow of the aqueous humor (see below). The second reaction to insult is entry of leukocytes from inflamed iris vessels into the aqueous humor. Subsequent fibroblast metaplasia is again a threat to the aqueous outflow system.

Any of the corrosive substances discussed earlier can cause iritis if they reach the cornea in sufficient concentration to penetrate the anterior chamber or if they rapidly destroy the corneal epithelial barrier and then penetrate. In a special category are the relatively fat-soluble bases like ammonia and pyridine and acids or acid anhydrides such as sulfur dioxide, acetic acid, and acetic anhydride. These penetrate intact corneal epithelium rapidly and reach the iris in concentrations high enough to cause iritis.

Some insults to the iris are severe enough to cause loss of cellular integrity. This is most easily observable as liberation of melanin granules from the highly pigmented posterior iris epithelium into the aqueous humor. These granules may contribute to blockage of the aqueous outflow channels with consequent secondary glaucoma. The deposits on corneal endothelium and anterior lens capsule caused by high doses of phenothiazines resemble very tiny pigment granules. It seemed on personal observation by one of us that the white granules reported by others were diffraction halos around the tiny pigment particles as seen in the slit lamp. The remarkable storage of phenothiazines in the pigmented structures of the eye has already been reported (Potts, 1962). It seems highly probable, in view of this storage and in view of the fact that the chlorpromazine opacities are confined to surfaces bathed by the aqueous humor, that (1) the drug is responsible for very chronic and very low-grade loss of posterior pigment epithelial cells of the iris and (2) the pigment granules liberated from these cells accumulate on corneal endothelium and lens capsule and even may be eventually incorporated into these structures, giving rise to the clinical effects of chlorpromazine on the anterior segment.

THE AQUEOUS OUTFLOW SYSTEM

General Considerations

As was mentioned at the beginning of this chapter, the eye, a small segregated portion of the central nervous system, has its own equivalent of the cerebrospinal fluid system. Disturbances of this system are as disastrous to the eye as disturbances of the cerebrospinal fluid system are to the brain. The ocular equivalent of cerebrospinal fluid is the aqueous humor, which is actively secreted into the posterior chamber by the double epithelial layer covering the ciliary processes (Fig. 13–1). The aqueous humor flows between the posterior surface of the iris and the anterior lens surface, enters the anterior chamber through the pupillary aperture, and leaves the eye at the anterior chamber angle via the trabecular meshwork, the canal of Schlemm, and the aqueous veins (Fig. 13–1). Although pathways have not yet been

worked out completely, there appears to be a homeostatic mechanism that maintains normal intraocular pressure within the physiologic limits of approximately 10 to 22 mm Hg. However, the mechanism does not have the capacity for 100 percent modulation, for when the aqueous outflow system becomes severely incompetent due to disease, aqueous secretion is not shut off and intraocular pressure rises. When this pressure exceeds 28 to 30 mm Hg, ischemic damage occurs to the optic nerve fibers just before they pierce the lamina cribrosa to exit from the eye. This damage due to increased intraocular pressure is glaucoma and may lead to complete blindness unless treated.

There are two major mechanisms by which glaucoma may originate. The first involves gradual diminution of the ability of the trabecular meshwork–canal of Schlemm system to pass fluid as with the inflammatory changes discussed in the previous section. This type of disease is characterized by insidious rise in pressure into the 30-to-40-mm-Hg range, absence of pain, and slow loss of peripheral visual field usually unnoticed by the patient. This type of disease is known as "chronic simple glaucoma" or "chronic open-angle glaucoma." When it follows an identifiable inflammatory episode such as a chemical burn it may be called "secondary" but it is still in the open-angle glaucoma category. The second mechanism is operative only in certain susceptible individuals who because of an inherited narrow chamber angle, or an angle narrowed by a swelling cataractous lens, can experience sudden and complete occlusion of the chamber angle filtration system by the most peripheral portion of the iris on iris dilation (cf. Fig. 13–1). This type of disease is characterized by rapid rise in intraocular pressure to 60, 70, or even 100 mm Hg, severe pain, conjunctival and deep scleral injection, and rapid loss of vision. This type of disease is known as "acute congestive" or "angle-closure" glaucoma.

Open-Angle Glaucoma

Glaucoma of the first type, open-angle glaucoma, can occur secondary to any toxic inflammation. Burns by acid, alkali, and vesicant gases have been documented as initiators of open-angle disease (Duke-Elder, 1969). A more unusual cause of open-angle glaucoma is "epidemic dropsy" reported from India. Individuals show edema of the extremities, gastrointestinal disturbances, cardiac hypertrophy as well as glaucoma (Maynard, 1909). The occurrence has been attributed to contamination of cooking oil by oil from the seeds of *Argemone mexicana* and the offending agent has been said to be the alkaloid sanguinarine from the argemone oil (Sarkar, 1926; Sarkar, 1948). Claims have been made in the past that the disease could be reproduced in experimental animals by argemone oil and by sanguinarine administration (Hakim, 1954). A recent reevaluation of the problem suggests that administration of sanguinarine orally, intravenously, or by cardiac puncture to rabbits, cats, and chickens does not reproduce the effects of epidemic dropsy; however, administration of argemone oil to chickens does cause edema of wattles (Dobbie and Langham, 1961). There seems little question that the disease is attributable to contaminated cooking oil. One of the problems is that since the first reports of epidemic dropsy the term "sanguinarine" has changed its meaning from an impure mixture of substances obtained from *Sanguinaria canadensis*, the Canadian bloodroot (Dana, 1828), to a pure chemical substance—a naphthaphenanthridine alkaloid (Manske, 1954). It is by no means impossible that in this process the actual toxic agent of argemone oil has been lost and that we have been defeated by a change in semantics. Thus, although sanguinarine is probably not the toxic agent, some component of argemone oil is. This does not make the problem less real or less deserving of reinvestigation.

Another type of open-angle glaucoma that has been recognized only recently is that caused by long-term topical administration of anti-inflammatory corticosteroids for eye disease (François, 1961; Goldmann, 1962; Armaly, 1963). Armaly showed further that eyes already glaucomatous had greater rises in intraocular tension after corticoids than did normal eyes. Not only can steroid glaucoma be caused by topical application to the eye, but it may be caused by systemic administration as well (see Bernstein *et al.*, 1963a, for early literature references). The additional hazard with systemic administration is that therapy for allergic, rheumatic, and other disease will not be conducted by an ophthalmologist, and the idea of checking intraocular pressure or visual field may not occur to the physician until severe damage has occurred.

Angle-Closure Glaucoma

The second type of glaucoma, angle-closure glaucoma, can be induced in an individual who is susceptible because of a genetically narrow anterior chamber angle or who has an angle narrowed by intraocular changes. This disease is frequently iatrogenic and the precipitating event is often mydriasis for eye examination or for the treatment of iritis. The most commonly offending drug is atropine because of the effectiveness of its action and its difficult reversibility. However, any mydriatic can be the precipitating cause and all have been implicated at one time or another. For a partial list, see Duke-Elder (1969).

THE CILIARY BODY

The ciliary body, which lies just posterior to the root of the iris (Fig. 13–1), is a structure with dual function. By means of the collagenous zonular fibers that stretch from lens to ciliary processes the ciliary body acts as the structure physically supporting the lens. Increase in tension of the radially directed and parasympathetically innervated ciliary muscle allows the tension on the zonular fibers to relax. This in turn allows the natural elasticity of the lens capsule to make the lens more spheric and to change the focus of the retinal image from distant to near objects. This is the mechanism of accommodation that is stimulated by parasympathomimetic agents and paralyzed by parasympatholytic agents. Thus in poisoning by cholinesterase inhibitors the small pupil caused by action of acetylcholine on the iris sphincter is accompanied by spasm of accommodation due to action on the ciliary muscle. This causes blurring of distant objects that were previously in focus. The converse is true in atropine poisoning. The pupil is wide and accommodation is paralyzed making it difficult to see near objects. When atropine or other parasympatholytics are used as medication in gastrointestinal disease, it is rare that the dose is high enough to cause measurable pupillary effects. However, it is not uncommon, particularly in a patient whose accommodation is already limited by presbyopia, that the medication will cause discomfort in near vision.

There are numerous medications said to cause blurring of vision where the mechanism of action is less understandable. One such instance is the blurring experienced from large doses of phenothiazines. It appears to be possible, at least, that the blurring described is due to ciliary muscle weakness secondary to very high concentrations of the drug in ciliary body due to storage of the polycyclic phenothiazine on melanin pigment in the ciliary body.

The second function of ciliary body depends on its vascularity and on the two specialized layers of epithelium that cover it. The epithelium secretes aqueous humor at the rate of approximately 1 μl/min. Although it is problematic whether any substance can increase aqueous secretion, there is evidence that both epinephrine and carbonic anhydrase inhibitors such as acetazolamide can decrease aqueous humor formation. Diuretics based on the property of carbonic anhydrase inhibition can lower intraocular pressure as a side effect, but there is no record of any of them causing serious difficulty such as phthisis bulbi.

THE LENS

Description

Normal Function and Composition. The lens (Fig. 13–1) is an avascular, transparent tissue surrounded by an elastic, acellular, collagenous capsule. It has the property of acting with the transparent cornea as an essential element in the image-forming system of the eye.

The lens is composed of only a single cell type and continually grows throughout life without losing a single cell; growth rate is inversely related to age. The lens can be arbitrarily divided into its anterior and posterior parts with an equatorial region separating the two. On the anterior or corneal side, lying just beneath the capsule, is a layer of cuboidal epithelial cells: the only area where the cells possess the organelles typically found in all cells. The epithelial cells undergo mitosis and migrate toward the equatorial region where they elongate into fibers, become layered over older fibers, and continue migrating toward the anterior and posterior poles. Consequently, the major portion of the lens is composed of long, thin fibers that have a hexagonal cross-section and form closely packed, onion-like layers. The oldest fibers occupy the center of the lens or nucleus, while younger fibers surrounding the nucleus occupy the area known as the cortex. The most superficial cortical cells possess some cytoplasmic organelles, but as the cells continue to differentiate, these organelles gradually disappear, giving way to a low-density fibrillar material, which in turn allows greater transparency. The tips of the fibers differentiating from either side of the anterior pole eventually join and form a special arrangement called suture lines.

Water and protein are the primary chemical constituents of the lens (Paterson, 1972). The fibers are mostly composed of the soluble proteins α-, β-, and γ-crystallins and the insoluble protein albuminoid. These proteins are unique in being organ specific, not species specific, immunologically. With such a great proportion of protein, it is not surprising that the lens actively synthesizes proteins; in fact, lenticular growth and development depend on a continuous and abundant supply of biosynthetic proteins (Waley, 1969). Protein synthesis may also be the prime consumer of energy generated in the lens, which is necessary in the synthetic mechanics itself and in actively transporting amino acids against a concentration gradient from the aqueous humor into the epithelium (Kuck, 1970b).

Maintenance of an ionic equilibrium with a high intracellular K^+/Na^+ ratio through active transport of K^+ across the epithelium into the lens and Na^+ out of the lens expends a large quantity of energy. The flow of these ions through the lens has been attributed to the existence of a "pump-leak" mechanism (van Heyningen, 1969; Kuck, 1970b; Paterson, 1972). The high level of K^+ in the lenticular epithelium as a result of active transport from the aqueous humor favors diffusion of K^+ along a concentration gradient across the posterior capsule and into the vitreous. On the other hand, high vitreal content of Na^+ favors diffusion of Na^+ in the opposite direction proceeding toward the epithelial cell layer where it is actively transported out of the lens and into the aqueous humor. The enzyme presumed to be associated with active transport, Na^+- and K^+-activated adenosine triphosphatase, is almost exclusively located in the epithelium. The energy necessary to drive active transport and other endergonic reactions is derived from the metabolism of glucose and primarily from anerobic glycolysis (van Heyningen, 1969; Kuck, 1970b). However, glucose degradation via the Krebs cycle with subsequent synthesis of ATP by the mitochondrial respiratory chain located solely in the anterior

epithelium and superficial cortical fibers may possibly contribute as much as 30 percent to the total lenticular energy output (van Heyningen, 1969; Trayhurn and van Heyningen, 1971a, 1971b).

Other biochemical reactions important to lenticular metabolism include nucleic acid synthesis in areas undergoing mitosis, pentose shunt pathway supplying reduced nicotinamide adenine dinucleotide phosphate, sorbitol pathway, and the α-glycerophosphate cycle. Other cellular constituents include small amounts of lipids and glycoproteins, ophthalmic acid, and a relatively large quantity of reduced glutathione, whose role in lenticular metabolism has not been fully evaluated. Small amounts of Ca^{2+} are also necessary to maintain membrane integrity.

Cataract. Normal lenses are transparent permitting light to pass through and allowing it to be focused on the retina. Transparency is dependent not only on the highly ordered cellular arrangement, but also on fiber size, uniformity of dimension and shape, molecular structure, and regularity of packing (Kuck, 1970a, 1970c). In fact, the primary function of lenticular metabolism appears to be directed toward maintaining this organized structure and resulting transparency. Interference with normal lens metabolism, interference with active transport across the cell boundaries, breakage of the lens capsule, and many other types of insult cause alteration in optical properties. Such alterations take various morphologic appearances. Layers of cells in anterior or posterior cortex can change refractive index, the axial lens nucleus can change refractive index, or the anterior or posterior subcapsular layers can change refractive index. Although in medical jargon these changes are termed "opacities," they merely represent the change from perfect transparency to translucency. The result is that image quality in the optical system of the eye deteriorates and visual acuity falls. All such changes, whatever the cause, are lumped under the common term "cataract." Cataracts can be caused by a variety of unrelated circumstances (van Heyningen, 1969), for example, senile cataract due to age, congenital cataracts possibly related to immunologic or pathologic infections, inborn errors of metabolism such as in galactosemia, endocrine cataracts as in diabetes, and drug-induced cataracts. It is this latter category that will be described here, although similarities in mechanism may exist in all the above classes.

Cataract Caused by Drugs

2,4-Dinitrophenol. In addition to a variety of toxic effects, systemic administration of 2,4-dinitrophenol (DNP) causes cataracts in some individuals. The classic instances of human dinitrophenol poisoning occurred during

1935 to 1937 when the substance was introduced as an antiobesity agent and was sold without prescription. Several hundred human cataracts resulted. For a review of these events, see Horner (1942). Lenticular opacity first develops in the anterior capsule and eventually spreads to include the cortex and the nucleus. Although cataracts may not develop until after months of treatment or until after drug withdrawal, the subcapsular and the posterior poles of the lens are the more severely affected. Vision is not immediately hindered but rapidly deteriorates as the cataract develops.

Experimental animals are insensitive to the cataractogenic activity of DNP, with the exception of young fowl and rabbits. A reversible cataract can be induced in chicks within one hour after systemic treatment. Analysis of aqueous humor, vitreous humor, and lens after a dose of DNP indicated a higher DNP concentration present in the young animal than in the adult, suggesting a possible explanation for both species and age sensitivity for DNP cataractogenic activity (Gehring and Buerge, 1969b). Within four to six hours after feeding a diet containing 0.25 percent DNP, vacuolization of the anterior lens can be induced in ducklings and chicks. *In vitro* incubation of lens with DNP forms cataracts (Gehring and Buerge, 1969a), with an increase in sodium influx and potassium efflux and swelling prior to cortical opacification (Ikemoto, 1971).

The cataractogenic activity of DNP may be related to its ability to uncouple oxidative phosphorylation, that is, inhibiting ATP synthesis without influencing electron transfer along the mitochondrial respiratory chain. Although experimental studies with other species indicate that lens metabolism is essentially anerobic, with ATP synthesis depending on glycolysis and therefore insensitive to DNP, mitochondrial oxidative phosphorylation in the epithelial cells may play a greater role in ATP synthesis in fowl and human lenses (Kuck, 1970b). As with any cell, removal of sodium ions from the lenticular cells may be the major energy utilizing reaction, in order to maintain proper ionic balances (Trayhurn and van Heyningen, 1971b). Other inhibitors of mitochondrial respiration, such as cyanide and amytal, also lead to increases in lenticular sodium content, which would be followed by decreases in ATP concentration, swelling, and opacification of the fibers.

Steroids. This first controlled study on the cataractogenic activity of corticosteroids was reported in 1960 (Black *et al.*, 1960). Thirty-nine percent of patients receiving prolonged therapy with either cortisone, prednisone, or dexamethasone for rheumatoid arthritis developed posterior subcapsular cataracts. A good correlation existed between cataract formation and dose and duration of therapy. No cataracts were observed in patients receiving low doses for

a year or longer and medium or high doses for less than a year. In this study, there was no serious impairment of vision. Further investigation revealed that corticosteroid-induced cataracts could be distinguished by clinical morphology from cataracts caused by diabetes, 2,4-dinitrophenol, and trauma, but could not be distinguished from cataracts caused by intraocular disease and ionizing radiation (Oglesby *et al.*, 1961b). Later reports confirmed the etiology and morphology and a correlation was clearly established between the incidence of posterior subcapsular opacities and having received 15 mg of prednisone per day or equivalent for a year or longer (Oglesby *et al.*, 1961b; Crews, 1963; Williamson *et al.*, 1969; Williamson, 1970). In contrast, four children developed posterior subcapsular cataracts after receiving 1 to 3 mg of prednisolone or equivalent dose of paramethazone for only three to ten months, suggesting either a genetic or an age-dependent sensitivity (Loredo *et al.*, 1972). The clinical progression of the posterior subcapsular opacity has been graded I to IV by Williamson and coworkers (1969). Once vacuoles have formed, they are not reversible even if the drug is withdrawn during the early phases of opacification, although further progression to advanced stages will not occur (Lieberman, 1968). Grade III has been established as the point where visual difficulties become evident and vacuole extension into the cortex will progress in spite of drug withdrawal (Williamson, 1970). Similar findings have been reported after topical administration of corticosteroids (Becker, 1964). A useful current review is that of Lubkin (1977).

Experimentally, steroidal cataracts were first observed in two out of four rabbits receiving 2 mg of betamethasone subconjunctivally for 41 weeks (Tarkkanen *et al.*, 1966). Long-term topical administration of several steroids also caused lenticular changes that were confined to the anterior subcapsular and cortical areas (Wood *et al.*, 1967) and therefore different from human cataracts. In contrast, short- or long-term systemic administration of prednisone or prednisolone did not result in cataracts when administered alone, although it did potentiate the cataractogenic activity of 2,4-dinitrophenol (Bettman *et al.*, 1964) and galactose (Bettman *et al.*, 1968), but not xylose, triparanol, or radiation. Betamethasome, applied topically, did enhance the formation of galactose cataracts (Cotlier and Becker, 1965).

The mechanism of steroid-induced cataracts has not been sufficiently investigated. *In vitro* studies (Ono *et al.*, 1971, 1972b) indicated that the lens can not only accumulate cortisol but also metabolize it to its sulfate and glucuronide conjugates. Cortisol also binds to the soluble proteins β-crystallin and α-crystallin (Ono *et al.*, 1972b). Alterations in Na$^+$ and K$^+$ ion transport have been reported resulting in increased hydration of the lens (Harris and Gruber, 1962). Inhibition of synthesis of lenticular proteins has been suggested as a possible mechanism of steroidal cataracts (Ono *et al.*, 1972a). It has been known since the work of Axelsson and Holmberg (1966) that long-acting cholinesterase inhibitors cause anterior and posterior subcapsular cataracts. This has been amply confirmed in humans and in monkeys (Shaffer and Hetherington, 1966; Kaufman *et al.*, 1977a). The mechanism of cataractogenesis is unknown. A new and curious finding is that topical application of atropine prevents the experimental cataract in monkeys (Kaufman *et al.*, 1977b).

Chlorpromazine. It was noted in the cornea section above that pigment granules appear on the anterior lens surface as well as the corneal endothelium in individuals who have received large doses of chlorpromazine over long periods of time. Although these granules are almost certainly exogenous to the lens in origin, they become incorporated into lens substance and cause loss of transparency. By these criteria this phenomenon is cataract and should be mentioned here.

Thallium. The soluble salts of thallium acetate and thallium sulfate have been used as insecticides, as rodenticides, and, at one time, as a systemic or topical depilatory agent. Thallous ion (Tl$^+$) is readily absorbed through the skin or gastrointestinal epithelium. Ingestion or application causes a variety of toxic symptoms, such as disturbances of the gastrointestinal tract, hair loss, polyneuritis of feet and legs, weakness or paralysis of the legs, psychic disturbances, neuritis of the optic nerve (described below), and, in rare instances, cataracts Duke-Elder, 1969; (Grant, 1974). Thallium acetate induces cataracts in rats within six weeks after initiating a daily dose of 0.1 mg, appearing first as radial striations in the anterior cortex between the sutures and the equator. While the early phases will remain stationary if thallium administration ceases, development of subcapsular opacities will occur if administration continues. Microscopic examination reveals areas of proliferation or deletion of subcapsular epithelium and accumulation of a homogeneous or granular material axially to the fibers (Duke-Elder, 1969). The nuclear region is spared.

Thallous ion rapidly accumulates in the lens both *in vivo* (Potts and Au, 1971) and *in vitro* (Kinsey *et al.*, 1971) possibly by an active transport mechanism dependent on the action of Na$^+$-K$^+$-ATPase. Thallium especially accumulates in those tissues with high K$^+$ levels, suggesting a competition for the same cellular transport mechanisms. In fact, thallium substitutes for potassium in many enzymes requiring K$^+$ for activity, but is effective at a concentration ten times lower than is needed for K$^+$. Examples of some enzymes studied are the following: (1) brain K$^+$-activated phosphatases (Inturrisi, 1969a), (2) brain microsomal Na$^+$-K$^+$-ATPase (Inturrisi, 1969b), (3) muscle pyruvate kinase (Kayne, 1971), and (4) skin Na$^+$-K$^+$-ATPase (Maslova *et al.*, 1971). Whether any of the above reactions are affected in the lens has not been reported, but substitution for K$^+$ in the frog skin Na$^+$-K$^+$-ATPase results in inhibition of the Na$^+$-pump. Electron microscopic examination of the kidney, liver, and intestine from rats chronically receiving subacute doses (10 to 15 mg Tl$^+$ per kilogram) of thallium acetate reveals a possible primary lesion of the mitochondria, exhibiting swelling, loss of cristae, deposition of granular material, and aggregation of mitochondrial granules (Herman and Bensch, 1967). Additional morphologic changes include disruption of the endoplasmic reticulum and formation of autophagic vacuoles.

Busulfan. Busulfan (Myleran) is a 1,4-bis=(methanesulphonyloxy)-butane alkyating agent used in treating chronic myeloid leukemia.

$$CH_3 \cdot \overset{\overset{O}{\uparrow}}{\underset{\underset{O}{\downarrow}}{S}} \cdot (CH_2)_4 \cdot O \cdot \overset{\overset{O}{\uparrow}}{\underset{\underset{O}{\downarrow}}{S}} \cdot CH_3$$

Busulfan (Myerlan)

Posterior subcapsular opacities or irregularities may result following chronic busulfan therapy (Podos and Canellos, 1969; Ravindranathan *et al.*, 1972; Grant, 1974; Hamming *et al.*, 1976), although the incidence or conditions surrounding these cataracts have not been fully investigated.

Experimentally induced cataracts can be obtained be feeding rats a diet containing 7.5 to 20.0 mg/kg of busulfan. An irreversible cataract is completely developed in five to seven weeks (Solomon *et al.*, 1955; von Sallmann, 1957). The earliest observation includes an increased mitotic activity of the epithelium primarily in the equatorial region, which eventually returns to and drops below normal levels. White dots or small vacuoles appear in the posterior and anterior lens, rapidly followed by opacification progressing from the equator to the posterior and anterior subcapsular zones. Similarities have been drawn between busulfan and ionizing radiation cataracts suggesting that those species with the slowest lens mitotic activity will develop cataracts more slowly (von Sallmann, 1957). The underlying mechanism may involve altered epithelial cell division. Injection of a single 12.5 mg/kg dose intraperitoneally reveals that busulfan acts during the relatively long G phase (Grimes *et al.*, 1964) of the cell cycle (Harding *et al.*, 1971), permitting normal synthesis of DNA but preventing subsequent mitosis. Consequently, the affected epithelial cells accumulate in preprophase, containing bizarre clumps of nuclear chromatin and twice the normal DNA content. Some of these cells undergo nuclear fragmentation and disintegration, while the remainder return to interphase with a tetraploid level of DNA. A similar mechanism occurs after chronic administration of busulfan (Grimes and von Sallmann, 1966). Following each cycle of DNA synthesis, mitosis is inhibited; and since the cells in the equatorial zone have the shortest intermitotic time (19 days), these are affected first. The cells in the equatorial zone normally migrate through the meridional rows and differentiate into lens fibers. However, death of these cells occurs after three days of busulfan treatment, leading to a decrease in cell density and disorganization of the meridional rows, and finally opacification. Continuous administration of this drug results in a depletion in the number of epithelial cells and complete disruption of the equatorial zone.

Triparanol. Triparanol (MER-29) was developed in the late 1950s as a blood cholesterol-lowering agent. Subsequent experiments in rats revealed decreased serum and tissue cholesterol levels and concomitant elevation in desmosterol levels. Triparanol inhibits cholesterol synthesis by inhibiting the $C_{24,25}$ double-bond reduction in desmosterol (Avigan et al., 1960; Steinberg and Avigan, 1960). Two reports published prior to the removal of triparanol from the market due to other toxicities confirmed the development of posterior and anterior subcapsular opacities following a dose of at least 250 mg per day for 15 to 18 months (Kirby et al., 1962; Laughlin and Carey, 1962).

Triparanol can induce cataracts in rats fed a diet containing 0.1 percent of the drug (von Sallmann et al., 1963). Small sudanophilic vesicles form on the fibers and eventually aggregate into large clusters. Prior to central and peripheral opacification, triparanol causes a tenfold increase in lens sodium content, causing hydration and swelling (Harris and Gruber, 1969, 1972). Upon returning to a normal diet, the cataracts are reversed as new fibers are laid down in the periphery, excess Na^+ and water are pumped out, and K^+ levels return to normal. Morphologic alterations have been observed under the electron microscope with other tissues sensitive to triparanol toxicity. Abnormalities consist of crystalloid and membranous intracytoplasmic inclusion bodies in neurons (Schutta and Neville, 1968), mitochondrial swelling, and rupture and fragmentation of the endoplasmic reticulum in the liver (Otto, 1971). Since cholesterol is an essential component of cellular membranes, inhibition of its synthesis could result in an overall inhibition of membrane synthesis (Rawlins and Uzman, 1970), involving all subcellular membranous structures, including mitochondria. Changes in mitochondrial oxidative metabolism (Otto, 1971) could conceivably result in deficiencies of the Na^+-pump mechanism

in extruding intracellular Na^+ from the lens, and consequently lead to Na^+ accumulation in the lens. Further experimental evidence concerning the mechanism of triparanol cataracts is lacking.

Experimental Cataract Formation. *Naphthalene.* In addition to its retinotoxic action, systemic absorption of naphthalene vapor may result in cataracts (Grant, 1974). Oral administration of 1 g/kg/day to rabbits leads to lenticular changes, initially observed as a swelling in the peripheral portion of the lens. Vacuoles form between the epithelium cells within six hours after the first dose, spread toward the nucleus, and within two weeks the whole lens is affected with a mature cataract. Mitosis of the epithelial cells is inhibited after two or three doses, and the cells break down later. After one week, swelling and striations extend into the cortex and mitotic arrest is observed. Finally, after two weeks of naphthalene treatment, the epithelium shows areas of cell duplication, nuclear degeneration, and normal and abnormal mitosis. Since abnormal mitotic areas become partly denuded of cells, cells are irregularly arranged in the periphery (Pirie, 1968). The stages of naphthalene-induced cataract are similar to those that occur in the development of human senile cataract.

The biochemical basis for naphthalene cataract has been investigated (van Heyningen and Pirie, 1967) and shown to be related to the liver metabolite of naphthalene, 1,2-dihydro-1,2-dihydroxynaphthalene. Lenticular catechol reductase metabolizes 1,2-dihydro-1,2-dihydroxynaphthalene to 1,2-dihydroxynaphthalene, which in turn is autoxidized in air at neutral pH to 1,2-naphthoquinone and hydrogen peroxide. Ascorbic acid reverses the latter reaction and forms dehydroascorbic acid, which can be reduced by glutathione. Since ascorbic acid diffuses out of the lens very slowly, it accumulates in the lens of the naphthalene-fed rabbit and in the lens incubated in vitro with 1,2-dihydro-1, 2-dihydroxynaphthalene (van Heyningen, 1970a). The sequence of reactions involves reduction of ascorbic acid by 1,2-naphthoquinone in the aqueous humor to dehydroascorbic acid, which rapidly penetrates the lens and is reduced by glutathione. Oxidized glutathione and 1,2-naphthoquinone may compete for the enzyme glutathione reductase, which normally maintains high lenticular levels of reduced glutathione. A reduction in the concentration of these coupled with the removal of oxygen from the aqueous humor due to the autoxidation of 1,2-dihydroxynaphthalene may make the lens sensitive to naphthoquinone toxicity. Other diols that do not form quinones in similar in vitro experiments do not result in lenticular opacities or increased ascorbic acid levels (van Heyningen, 1970b).

In addition to the reduction of glutathione levels and aqueous humor oxygen content, 1,2-naphthoquinone is a very active compound and reacts with lenticular glutathione, amino acids, and proteins (Rees and Pirie, 1967). Interaction with the structural proteins results in the brown color of the lens characteristic of naphthalene cataracts and insoluble complexes of β- and γ-crystallins. However, combination with these proteins does not inhibit naphthoquinone oxidation of ascorbic acid. Reactions between coenzymes and enzymes and 1,2-naphthoquinone can cause changes in the oxidation/reduction potential of the lens and abnormal metabolic reactions, which either alone or in combination would lead to cellular disruption and, finally, cataracts.

Galactose. An unusual experimental cataract results from feeding animals a diet containing high levels of galactose. The morphologic changes in the lens during galactose feeding were photographed and described by Sippel (1966). Within two days after initiating a diet containing 50 percent galactose, rats showed water clefts situated between lenticular fibers in the anterior equatorial region. After ten days the cortex is almost completely liquefied and more transparent to light as a result of vacuole aggregation. Total lenticular opalescence is complete after 28 days of galactose feeding. Accompanying these changes is an increase in DNA synthesis (Weller and Green, 1969) and mitosis of the epithelial cells (Kuwabara *et al.*, 1969; van Heyningen, 1969) after three days of feeding. Eventually mitosis returns to and drops below normal activity as the cataract progresses.

The mechanism of galactose- and other sugar-related cataracts has been explained by excessive hydration of the lens observed as early as 12 hours after initiating a galactose-enriched diet. Galactose and other sugars are transported across the capsule and epithelial cell membrane by facilitated transport and diffusion (Elbrink and Bihler, 1972), and on entering the lens, galactose is either slowly phosphorylated to galactose-6-phosphate or reduced by the NADPH-dependent aldose reductase to dulcitol. While other sugar alcohols formed by aldose reductase are converted by polyol-NADP oxidoreductase to readily diffusible products, dulcitol is not further metabolized. Since it diffuses out of the lens only very slowly, dulcitol accumulates to high levels and consequently exerts a strong osmotic force drawing water into the lens in order to maintain osmotic equilibrium. Therefore, increases in dulcitol levels are accompanied by a parallel increase in water content (Kinoshita, 1965; van Heyningen, 1971). If dulcitol synthesis is depressed by inhibiting aldose reductase with 3,3-tetramethyleneglutaric acid, water uptake and fiber vacuolization are prevented (van Heyningen, 1971). Furthermore, feeding young Carworth Farms Webster (CFW) mice a galactose-enriched diet does not produce cataracts, since lenses of this strain fail to metabolize galactose to dulcitol (Kuck, 1970c). Therefore, lenticular hydration resulting from the osmotic

force due to dulcitol accumulation and retention explains fiber vacuolization and the initial structural alterations in galactose cataracts. Further investigations verified the lack of or very low activity of other lenticular enzymes that could metabolize dulcitol, e.g., galactokinase or 1-gulonate NADP oxidoreductase (van Heyningen, 1971).

Additional biochemical changes consist of a very early loss in amino acids due to a deficiency in the amino acid-concentrating mechanism and a marked drop in glutathione content (Kinoshita, 1965; Sippel, 1966a; Kinoshita *et al.*, 1969; van Heyningen, 1969, 1971). Both decreases are probably related to increased membrane permeability following swelling. Glycolysis and respiration decrease to 60 percent of normal after two days of galactose feeding but remain at this level of activity as the cataract progresses (Sippel, 1966b). Adenosine triphosphate levels decrease slightly during the early stages, but progressive vacuolization and opacification is accompanied by a 75 percent loss in ATP content (Sippel, 1966b; Kuck, 1970c). Decreased aldolase activity correlates with progressive vacuolization of the cortex and glutathione loss during the first week of galactose diet; however, decreases in glucose-6-phosphate dehydrogenase, lactic acid dehydrogenase, and α-glycerophosphate dehydrogenase activity correlate with protein diminution occurring during the development of nuclear cataract (Sippel, 1967; Kuck, 1970c). Alterations in electrolyte balance do not occur until the late vacuolar stage. Surprisingly, the increased water uptake observed during the initial stages of cataract development is not accompanied by an increase Na^+ uptake and a loss of K^+ ions from the lens. In fact, Na^+ ion is pumped out of the lens during the initial development as effectively as from a normal lens, with only a slight loss in K^+. Only in the late vacuolar stage, with the development of nuclear opacification, does the lens fail to extrude Na^+, suggesting a second dramatic increase in membrane permeability to water during the terminal stages (Kinoshita, 1965). This is in the face of a still very much active cation pump mechanism. Decreases are observed in Mg^{2+}-dependent adenosine triphosphatase activity after six days of feeding a galactose-enriched diet, while Na^+-K^+-activated adenosine triphosphatase activity is markedly depressed after 15 days (Fournier and Patterson, 1971).

The lenticular opacities that develop on galactose feeding can be reversed if the sugar is withdrawn from the diet prior to nuclear involvement. After 10 to 12 days on the galactose diet, membrane permeability alters so that dulcitol leaks out as fast as it is formed. At this time, little if any protein is lost, but there is an increasing concentration of lens amino acids derived from protein, either from proteolysis or from inhibition of protein synthesis (Barber, 1972). As the cataract develops further, amino acids are suddenly reduced. Parallel accumulation of dulcitol and water in the lenticular fibers definitely causes the initial stages of cortical vacuolization and opacification. However, only failure of the lens to synthesize proteins or alterations in enzymic acticity essential in maintaining lens integrity could explain the irreversible nature of the mature nuclear cataract. The entire biochemistry of the lens would be deleteriously affected by the removal of reduced pyridine dinucleotide phosphate (NADPH) consumed during the reduction of galactose to dulcitol catalyzed by aldose reductase. Consequently, the reduced NADPH/NADP ratio alters the oxidation-reduction potential of the lens (Kuck, 1970b).

Experimentally induced galactose cataract has its counterpart in human physiology. Galactosemia is an autosomal recessive genetic deficiency in galactose metabolism. Affected infants on a milk diet show high blood and urine galactose levels, hepatomegaly, splenomegaly, eventual mental retardation, and cataracts. The genetic defect is deficiency in the enzymes galactose-1-phosphate-uridyl transferase or galactokinase (Kinoshita, 1965; Monteleone et al., 1971; Nordmann, 1971; Levy et al., 1972). These enzymes are necessary in transforming unusable galactose into usable glucose-1-phosphate. Galactose or galactose-1-phosphate reaches excessive levels in the blood and aqueous humor triggering dulcitol synthesis in the lens and subsequent fibril vacuolization (van Heyningen, 1969). Removal of galactose from the diet can reverse the symptoms.

THE RETINA AND CHOROID

Nature of the Structure

The retina is the very compact and highly complex neural structure responsible for transducing the ocular light image and doing considerable preprocessing of the neural impulses before sending them toward the brain (Fig. 13–1). The layer of rods and cones—modified neural structures containing photosensitive pigments—is the receptor of the light image. The receptor cells synapse with bipolar cells, which in turn synapse with ganglion cells. In addition, lateral synapses occur with horizontal cells and feedback synapses occur with amacrine cells. The Müller cells, the glia equivalent in retina, have nuclei near the center of the retinal thickness and long processes that extend through the whole retinal thickness. Finally, the single layer of retinal pigmented epithelium underlies the receptors and sends processes that envelop the receptor outer segments. It should be evident from these relationships—all of which exist in the 100 to 500-μm retinal thickness—that studies on the overall biochemistry and physiology of such a structure are likely to be confusing and misleading. To dispel any lingering hope that the retinal layers are uniform metabolically if not morphologically, one need only read below how specific toxic substances affect specific retinal layers. After one has recognized with Warburg (1926) that the retina as a whole is the most actively metabolizing structure in the normal body, one must view metabolic studies on whole retina with healthy skepticism. The extremely compact structure of the retina creates a real

dilemma when one wishes to study a single cell type. One solution is that worked out by Lowry and coworkers (1956, 1961), who microdissected freeze-dried retina and picked out nuclei of each cell type for metabolic studies. Other approaches utilize histochemical techniques on retinas with individual cell layers destroyed by toxic substances. This subject is still very much open for definitive study and its incomplete state will hinder us greatly in reaching satisfying conclusions on the mechanism of action of retinotoxic substances.

The choroid is a vascular layer whose chief constituents in addition to the blood vessels are collagenous connective tissue and cells containing large numbers of melanin granules. The latter are important because of the affinity of melanin for polycyclic aromatic compounds. In primates, which have a well-established retinal blood supply, the choroid is responsible for nutrition of the receptor cell layer only. In lower vertebrates the choroidal vasculature supplies all of the retina.

Because of this dependence and because of physical proximity many diseases primary in the choroid cause retinal damage and some diseases primary in retina cause choroidal damage. Thus, chorioretinitis is a commonly encountered term. It is based on clinical observation and does not imply which structure is primary for the disease process.

Polycyclic Compounds

Chloroquine. The 4-aminoquinoline chloroquine is effective as (1) an antimalarial, requiring

Chloroquine

doses of 500 mg per week for three to four weeks, with maintenance on 250 mg per week, and (2) an anti-inflammatory agent, requiring doses of at least 250 mg per day to be effective. The low-dose therapy used for malaria is essentially free from any toxic side effects; however, the chronic, high-dose therapy used for rheumatoid arthritis, discoid and systemic lupus erythematosus frequently causes a number of side effects, the most serious of which involves an irreversible loss of retinal functions. In 1959, the first cases of chloroquine-induced retinopathy were reported (Hobbs et al., 1959), but since then numerous reports have confirmed the etiology of similar observations as resulting from chloroquine therapy (see reviews by Nylander, 1967; Duke-Elder and MacFaul, 1972). Hydroxychloroquine has also been

reported to cause a similar retinopathy (Crews, 1967; Shearer and Dubois, 1967), although the incidence of toxicity may be less (Shearer and Dubois, 1967; Sassaman *et al.*, 1970).

The clinical findings accompanying chloroquine retinopathy may generally be thought of in terms of early and late phenomena. Among the early findings are (1) a "bull's-eye retina," visualized as a dark, central pigmented area involving the macula, surrounded by a pale ring of depigmentation, which in turn is surrounded by another ring of pigmentation; (2) diminished electrooculogram; (3) possible granular pigmentation of the peripheral retina; and (4) subjective visual disturbances, observed as blurred vision and difficulty in reading, with words or letters missing in long sentences or long words. Late findings are (1) progressive scotoma, (2) constriction of the peripheral fields commencing in the upper temporal quadrant, (3) narrowing of the retinal arteries, (4) color and night blindness, (5) absence of a typical pigment pattern, and (6) abnormal electrooculograms and electroretinograms; these symptoms are irreversible. Indeed, there have been reports of irreversible chloroquine retinopathy where the entire development of the disease has occurred after cessation of the drug (R. P. Burns, 1966). It is generally recognized that the incidence of these chloroquine-induced toxic effects increases as the daily dose, total dose, and duration of therapy increase. The absence of permanent damage has been reported in patients receiving not more than 250 mg of chloroquine or 200 mg of hydroxychloroquine per day (Scherbel *et al.*, 1965). Nevertheless utilization of sensitive testing methods such as "macular dazzling" and retinal threshold tests has indicated some degree of retinal malfunction in all patients receiving even small doses of these drugs (Carr, 1968). Thus, there is a qualitative difference between the depression of visual function observed in all patients and the specific damage seen in relatively few individuals. Approximately 20 to 30 percent of the patients receiving higher doses of chloroquine will exhibit some type of retinal abnormality, while 5 to 10

percent show severe changes in retinal function (Butler, 1965; Crews, 1967; Nylander, 1967). One interesting paradox is worth noting. Despite severe retinopathy and "extinguished" ERG, normal or nearly normal dark adaptation performance is characteristic of chloroquine toxicity. This is in marked contrast to phenothiazine retinopathy (see below) (Krill *et al.*, 1971).

Experimentally induced chloroquine retinopathy was first produced in the cat after long-term, oral administration of subtoxic doses, 1.5 to 6.0 mg daily (Meier-Ruge, 1965a). A light pigmentation appeared in the cat's fundus four to seven weeks after the daily dosage schedule and the retinopathy was fully developed after eight weeks. Histologic and histochemical analysis revealed a thickening of the pigment epithelial cell layer, increases in the mucopolysaccharide and sulfhydryl group content, decreases in enzymatic activity of the pigment epithelium, migration of pigment into the outer nuclear layer, and finally total atrophy of the photoreceptors (Meier-Ruge, 1968). Similar findings were observed in rabbits (Dale *et al.*, 1965; Meier-Ruge, 1965b; François and Maudgal, 1967) and humans (Bernstein and Ginsberg, 1964; Wetterholm and Winter, 1964). Depression of the rabbit ERG (McConnell *et al.*, 1964) and minimal ultrastructural changes in the photoreceptor inner segment consisting of mitochondrial swelling and disorganization of the endoplasmic reticulum without other gross histologic changes (Solze and McConnell, 1970) have been reported.

Because of its high affinity for melanin, the mechanism of chloroquine-induced retinopathy has been related to the extremely high concentrations that are attained in the pigmented eye and that remain at these high levels (Bernstein *et al.*, 1963b; Potts, 1964a, 1964b) long after other tissue levels have been depleted. Both hydroxychloroquine and desethylchloroquine, the major metabolite of chloroquine, behave similarly (McChesney *et al.*, 1965, 1967). Accumulation of chloroquine in the pigmented structures of the human choroid and pigmented epithelium has been reported and the amount depends on dosage and duration of drug therapy (Lawwill *et al.*, 1968). In addition, small amounts of chloroquine and its metabolites are excreted in the urine years after cessation of drug treatment (Bernstein, 1967). The prolonged exposure of the retinal cell layers to chloroquine probably explains the irreversible nature of human retinopathy, which may not only progress (Okun *et al.*, 1963) but also develop after chloroquine has been withdrawn (R. P. Burns, 1966).

Investigations concerning the primary retinotoxic lesion caused by chloroquine have led to two schools of thought. Based on the histologic and histochemical findings and the melanin-binding property of chloroquine described above, one theory indicates a primary biochemical lesion in the pigmented epithelium cell layer of the retina. It is clear that storage in pigment in itself is not a sufficient cause for toxicity.

It is simply that a toxic substance such as chloroquine like any other poison increases its effect as the concentration in tissue multiplied by time of exposure $(C \times T)$ increases. Storage on melanin causes enormous increases in this $C \times T$ factor for the melanin-containing tissue—in this case the retinal pigment epithelium.

Another group of researchers have been impressed by the intracytoplasmic inclusion bodies found in chloroquine-treated animals and in humans (Gleiser et al., 1969; Reinert and Rutty, 1969; Abraham and Hendy, 1970; Gregory et al., 1970; Hodgkinson and Kolb, 1970; Ramsey et al., 1970; Ramsey and Fine, 1972). These myeloid bodies, consisting of tightly packed lamellar structures containing concentric rings, are found primarily in the ganglion cell layer, but may be present in the bipolar cell layer, visual cell layer, and pigmented epithelium cell layer. These myeloid bodies, formed from autophagic vacuoles and containing lysosomal enzymes, are not specific for the retinal ganglion cells, but are found in several different tissues of animals treated with high doses of chloroquine (Read and Bay, 1971). Formation of the membranous cytoplasmic bodies was recently reported to occur in the retinal ganglion cells of monkeys within one week after initiation of chloroquine treatment. However, the ERG and fundus pigment remained normal even after a year of treatment (Kolb et al., 1972). This report, confirmed by unpublished research of one of us (A. M. P.), suggests that myeloid bodies, like the dazzle test, are characteristic of early chloroquine administration—not of chloroquine toxicity.

Many biochemical reactions can be inhibited by chloroquine (reviewed by Bernstein, 1967; Sams, 1967; Mackenzie, 1970), e.g., DNA and RNA synthesis, DNA polymerase, protein synthesis (Roskoski and Jaskunas, 1972), NADH-cytochrome c reductase, and the conversion of α-ketoglutarate to succinate in the tricarboxylic acid cycle. While chloroquine inhibits the above enzymatic pathways in bacterial and extraocular tissue preparations, chloroquine has been demonstrated to inhibit only the NADH-nitro-blue tetrazolium reductase in the retina (Yanoff and Tsou, 1965). Accumulation in lysosomes (Zvailfer, 1964), stabilization and labilization of lysosomal membranes (Filkins, 1969; Ottlecz et al., 1970), and altering the digestive activity of lysosomes by neutralizing the acidic content (Homewood et al., 1971, 1972) have been demonstrated in cellular systems other than the eye. Whether chloroquine exerts similar actions on any of the retinal cell layers has not been documented.

Inhibition of protein metabolism of the pigment epithelium has been proposed as the primary cause for the retinotoxic effects of chloroquine (Meier-Ruge, 1968). In vitro experiments utilizing only whole-pigment epithelial cells have indicated that chloroquine and hydroxychloroquine markedly inhibit amino acid incorporation in protein (Gonasun and Potts, 1972).

Phenothiazines. The potency of phenothiazines as tranquilizers is related to the chemical

constituent attached to the N-atom of the three-ring base: Group I compounds possessing an aminopropyl side chain are least potent; group II compounds with a piperidine group in the side chain are more potent; and group III drugs composed of a piperazine group in the side chain are the most potent antipsychotic drugs (Boet, 1970). Successful remission of psychotic states requires persistent drug therapy at relatively high doses. Therefore, it is not surprising that many side effects are associated

Chlorpromazine
(aminopropyl side chain)

Thioridazine
(piperidyl group in the side chain)

Prochlorperazine
(piperazinyl group in the side chain)

with long-term high-dose phenothiazine therapy. Ocular complications may involve the cornea and the lens, described above, and the retina, described in this section.

The first phenothiazine derivative reported to alter retinal function belonged to group II: piperidyl-chlorophenothiazine (Sandoz NP-207). During clinical trials, the initial symptoms of visual disturbances were observed as impairment to adaptation in dim light. Further disturbances involved reduced visual acuity, constricted visual fields, and abnormal pigmentation of the retina, appearing in the periphery or macula as fine salt-and-pepper clumps of pigment (Kinross-Wright, 1956). Abnormalities in dark adaptation, color vision, and the ERG coupled with severe pigment clumping during the advanced stages indicated toxic effects in both rod and cone receptors. Disturbances of retinal function usually developed within two to three months after receiving 400 to 800 mg of the drug per day and a total of 20 to 30 g. Higher dosages required only 30 days to develop toxic symptoms. On withdrawal of the drug, some symptoms may be reversed although pigment clumping remains visible in the fundus. However, total reversal is not possible and in some cases severe visual loss and blindness result. The strong evidence that NP-207 was the causative agent in these visual disturbances resulted in its removal from clinical study (Boet, 1970).

Replacement of the 2-chlorine of NP-207 with a methylmercapto group yields thioridazine, a phenothiazine derivative effective in treating schizophrenia and nonpsychotic severe anxiety without possessing some of the side effects common to the aminopropyl phenothiazines. Thioridazine also causes pigmentary and visual disturbances similar to those caused by NP-207 but dosages of over 1200 mg per day for 30 days are required to affect retinal function (Weekley et al., 1960). Initially, a loss of visual acuity is observed, followed by night blindness, difficulty in adapting to average light conditions after being exposed to bright sunlight, and finally retinal pigmentary changes. In severe toxicity. excessive pigment deposition and an extinguished ERG are found. Usually, cessation of the medication is accompanied by complete or partial restoration of retinal function, although the pigmentary disturbances remain (Potts, 1968). Additional reports of thioridazine-induced retinopathy have been summarized (Siddall, 1966; Boet, 1970; Cameron et al., 1972). The dosages required to produce these retinopathies are usually in excess of the recommended therapeutic levels. Normal dosages do not cause disturbances in retinal function even after years of treatment.

The group I phenothiazine chlorpromazine is generally free from retinotoxic effects. Rare cases have been reported (Siddall, 1965, 1966, 1968) of a reversible, fine granular pigmentation in the retinal background after 2.4 g of chlorpromazine per day for two years following 1 to 2 g per day for 6 to 28 months. Only one patient recorded heavy pigmentation.

The piperazine derivatives (group III) have not been reported to affect retinal function (Duke-Elder and MacFaul, 1972). Since these drugs are the most potent phenothiazine derivatives, less drug is needed to control the psychotic individual, resulting in a lessening of side effects.

Experimentally induced phenothiazine retinopathy was accomplished by orally administering NP-207 to cats; the initial dose of 10 mg/kg/day was slowly increased to 120 mg/kg/day (Meier-Ruge and Cerletti, 1966; Cerletti and Meier-Ruge, 1967). The first retinal changes appeared as fine grayish-blackish spots on the fundus after four to five weeks of treatment. These fine granules gradually coalesced and formed irregular patches of pigment as the retinopathy became fully developed after six to seven weeks of treatment. A partial explanation for the retinal changes was made by the finding that phenothiazine derivatives accumulate in very high concentrations in the uveal tract (Potts, 1962a, 1962b). Experiments utilizing labeled chlorpromazine, prochlorperazine, and NP-207 have indicated binding of these drugs to the melanin-containing tissues of the eye, allowing high concentrations to accumulate and remain in the eye for extended periods of time (Potts, 1962a, 1962b; Green and Ellison, 1966; Cerletti and Meier-Ruge, 1967). In vitro studies employing isolated choroidal melanin granules or synthetic melanin (Potts, 1964a, 1964b) have indicated that several phenothiazine derivatives bind to melanin, therefore verifying the result obtained in vivo that tissue melanin content is the essential component responsible for concentrating these N-substituted phenothiazines. As stated above for chloroquine, concentration on pigmented structures merely gets the phenothiazine to the tissue in high concentration. Both toxic and nontoxic phenothiazines participate in this effect. After storage the specific toxic activity (possibly one of the effects detailed below) must cause tissue damage.

Histologic examination of retinas from NP-207–treated cats has shown initial posterior vacuolization of outer segments one to two weeks after retinal pigmentation, followed by disorganization of the entire lamellar structure of the disk, and finally atrophy and disintegration of the rods and cones. Other cellular layers appear normal with the exception of a proliferative pigment epithelium (Cerletti and Meier-Ruge, 1967). Histochemical enzymic analysis of the same tissues revealed an increase in lactic acid dehydrogenase activity of the Müller cells, followed shortly by a decrease of this enzyme's activity in the rod and cone ellipsoids, both changes occurring prior to retinal pigmentation and structural changes. Similar but less marked alterations were noted for glutamic dehydrogenase, glucose-6-phosphate dehydrogenase, and 6-phosphogluconate dehydrogenase activities. Loss in enzymic activities of adenosine triphosphatase, succinic acid dehydrogenase, and DPN diaphorase paralleled the loss of rods and cones (Cerletti and Meier-Ruge, 1967). An increased amount of lipid-staining material in the pigment epithelium, due to the disintegration of outer segments, an increase of glycogen in the Müller cells, and a decreased amount of phospholipid-staining material were observed shortly before major morphologic changes.

The phenothiazines, in particular chlorpromazine, influence a variety of biochemical reactions: (1) inhibition of oxidative phosphorylation, (2) reaction with flavin adenine nucleotides, (3) inhibition of hexokinase, (4) inhibition of cholinesterase, (5) inhibition of sodium and potassium transport, (6) direct reaction with cations, and (7) other biochemical reactions (Guth and Spirtes, 1964). In addition, interaction with biologic membranes (Seeman, 1966), depletion of membrane calcium (Kwant and Seeman, 1969a, 1969b), reaction with the photoreceptor cell membrane (François and Feher, 1972), and inhibition of protein synthesis (Raghupathy et al., 1970; Rösner, 1972) have been well documented for chlorpromazine. Cerletti and Meier-Ruge (1967) propose that the phenothiazines interfere with rhodopsin synthesis and the entire energy production of the photoreceptors by reacting with flavin adenine dinucleotide and consequently inhibit oxidative phosphorylation (Reinert and Rutty, 1969). However, while this theory may explain NP-207 and thioridazine retinotoxic effects, it does not explain the lack of retinotoxicity by chlorpromazine. Furthermore, this theory excludes any effect on the pigment epithelium, which may also play an important role and mediate the lesions of the photoreceptor cell layer.

Indomethacin

Administration of the anti-inflammatory drug, indomethacin, in dosages of 50 to 200 mg per day for one to two years may result in decrease of visual acuity, visual field changes, and abnormalities in dark adaptation, ERG, and the EOG (C. A. Burns, 1966, 1968; Henkes and van Lith, 1972; Henkes et al., 1972). In one study of 34 patients (C. A. Burns, 1968), all exhibited a decreased retinal sensitivity, manifested as a lowered ERG or an altered threshold for dark adaptation. Ten of these patients had macular area disturbances, evidenced by paramacular depigmentation varying from mottled depigmentation to areas of pigment atrophy. Greater decreases in the scotopic component of the ERG than in the phototopic component have been

reported (Palimeris et al., 1972). However, except for the pigmentary disturbances, visual function improves upon cessation of drug treatment accompanied by a return to normal amplitudes in the a and b waves of the ERG.

Coupled to its anti-inflammatory properties, indomethacin prevents the release of lysosomal enzymes and stabilizes liver lysosomes when exposed to labilizing conditions (Ignarro, 1972). Inhibition of Ca^{2+} accumulation in injured tissue (Northover, 1972) and Ca^{2+} influx into stimulated smooth muscle by indomethacin (Northover, 1971) have been reported. However, the role of the metabolic reactions on indomethacin-induced retinopathy is unclear, since no experimental studies have been carried out involving indomethacin and the retina.

Oxygen

The therapeutic use of oxygen in concentrations greater than in ambient air has increased during the past several years. Healthy adults can usually tolerate breathing pure oxygen for up to three hours without exhibiting any uncomfortable symptoms; however, further inhalation at atmospheric pressure or short-term inhalation of high concentrations of oxygen at 2 to 3 atmospheres results in bilateral progressive constriction of the peripheral fields, impaired central vision, mydriasis, and constriction of the retinal vasculature (Grant, 1974; Nichols and Lambertsen, 1969; Mailer, 1970). All the symptoms are reversible upon inhalation of air. Although severe retinal damage in adults is rare during hyperoxia, one case was reported concerning an individual suffering from myasthenia gravis who developed irreversible retinal atrophy after breathing 80 percent oxygen for 150 days (Kobayashi and Murakami, 1972). The retinal vasculature was markedly constricted with no blood flowing through both eyes. The vascular disorder was limited only to retinal circulation.

Although there is a dose-dependent vasoconstriction of the retinal vessels and decrease in blood flow during hyperoxia, there is actually an increase in the oxygenation of the retina (Dollery et al., 1969). Since the choriocapillaris can now supply the inner retinal layers with oxygen in addition to the supply from the retinal vessels, toxic levels of oxygen may accumulate and inhibit certain metabolic reactions essential for vision. More importantly, a decrease in the supply of nutrients, and especially glucose, to the visual cells results from the secondary decrease in blood flow, and only when the endogenous supply of nutrients is metabolized and exhausted will deficiencies in vision be noticed (Nichols and Lambertsen, 1969).

A selective effect of hyperoxia on mature visual cells is exemplified by exposing adult rabbits to

Indomethacin

100 percent oxygen for 48 hours. The result is loss of the ERG and visual cell death (Noell, 1955). Further experimentation with rabbits indicated that the centrally located rods, characterized by a low glycogen content and rich choroidal blood supply and therefore analogous to the human macula, are the most sensitive cells to oxygen toxicity (Bresnick, 1970). Peripheral rods and cones are less sensitive and spared from the toxic effects while other retinal layers—the inner nuclear layer, the ganglion cell layer, and the pigmented epithelial layer—appear normal. Rods containing a single synaptic ribbon appear to be more sensitive than rods with multi-synaptic ribbons. The earliest morphologic changes in the outer nuclear layer include the formation of membrane-bound vesicles in the inner segment, swelling of the endoplasmic reticulum and Golgi apparatus followed by nuclear pyknosis, mitochondrial abnormalities, degeneration of the synaptic bodies, and vesiculation of the outer segment (Bresnick, 1970).

Although adults are not seriously affected by breathing high concentrations of oxygen, this is not true for premature infants. Frequently, premature infants are placed in incubators and breathe oxygen in concentrations greater than in air. On removal from hyperoxia, they develop an irreversible bilateral ocular disease known as retrolental fibroplasia. Critical in the development of this oxygen-induced disease is the embryologic nature of the human retinal vasculature. Beginning with the fourth month of gestation, the retinal vascular system develops from the hyaloid vascular stalk in the optic nerve, and by the eighth month, the retina is vascularized only in its nasal periphery. Development into the peripheral retina is not complete until after birth of a full-term infant (Patz, 1969–1970). Only the incompletely developed retinal circulation is susceptible to toxic levels of oxygen, whereas a mature retinal vascular system and other incompletely formed circulations are not sensitive to oxygen toxicity. Within six hours after an infant is placed in a high-oxygen-containing atmosphere, vasoconstriction of the immature vessels occurs, which is reversible if the child is immediately returned to air but is irreversible if hyperoxia therapy is continued (Beehler, 1964). Obliteration of the capillary lumen takes place as the vessel walls adhere to each other. This is followed by degeneration of the capillary endothelial cells and depression of the normal anterior forward growth of the retinal vessels. Immediately after returning to a normal oxygen atmosphere, vessels adjacent to the damaged area rapidly proliferate, invade the retina, penetrate the internal limiting membrane, and enter the vitreous. During the advanced stages, retinal fibrosis may cause retinal detachment. The opaque retrolental mass causes leukocoria (Beehler, 1964; Patz, 1969–1970).

Experimental investigations with kittens have indicated a similar and selective degeneration and proliferation of the developing retinal capillary endothelium. The vasoconstriction and lumen obliteration are directly related to the degree of immaturity of the retinal vascular system and to the concentration and duration of exposure to oxygen (Ashton and Pedler, 1962; Ashton, 1966, 1970; Patz, 1969–1970; Flower and Patz, 1971). While hyperoxia is selectively toxic to the immature retinal vascular system, no toxic effects are evident on the retina itself. Glycolytic and respiratory rates are unchanged (Graymore, 1970). These results contrast with the oxygen-induced photoreceptor atrophy observed in adult animals.

High concentrations of oxygen inhibit a number of enzymatic paths (Davies and Davies, 1965). Inhibition of respiration, electron transport, ATP synthesis, glycolysis, and a number of enzyme and coenzyme functions requiring free sulfhydryl groups for activity has been reported (reviewed by Haugaard, 1965, 1968; Menzel, 1970). The toxicity induced during maturation of the retinal vascular system, causing retrolental fibroplasia, may be explained by any of the above deficiencies, although no specific mechanism has been proposed. However, the toxicity on the mature photoreceptor cells may be explained by inhibition of glycolysis, which is essential for retinal function.

Epinephrine

In eyes that are aphakic, postcataract extraction cystoid macular edema has been described after the use of epinephrine (Kolker and Becker, 1968; Obstbaum et al., 1976). Recovery is expected but not invariable on cessation of use of the drug.

Iodate

In the preantibiotic era of the 1920s attempts were made to combat systemic septic disease, such as septicemia, by intravenous injection of inorganic antiseptics. It was found after the use of one of these—concentrated Pregl solution, known under the trade name of Septojod—that a number of individuals became blind (Riehm, 1927). It was demonstrated by Riehm (1929) that the primary retinal involvement was of the pigment epithelium and that this disease could be induced experimentally by injecting Septojod into pigmented rabbits. Vito (1935) was able to demonstrate that the actual toxic agent involved was sodium iodate. However, the exact way in which iodate causes degeneration and the reason for the particular susceptibility of the pigment epithelium have not been adequately worked out. Although iodate is known to be a relatively stable oxidizing agent, and though the probability of this mechanism of action is reinforced by the fact that the iodate effect can be completely neutralized by the reducing agent, cysteine (Sorsby and Harding, 1960), the effect has not been reproduced by other oxidizing agents, such as manganese dioxide, perborate, and persulfate (Sorsby, 1941). It is true, however, that none of these agents has the relative stability of iodate, and a dose comparable to that of iodate could not be given intravenously without killing the experimental animals.

Various experiments verified a primary effect of iodate on the pigment epithelium cell layer, followed by a secondary lesion and degeneration of the rod outer segments. Within hours after the administration of iodate, the thickness of the pigment epithelium layer is reduced, accompanied by loss of cellular limits, loss of definition, and formation of a granular cytoplasm (Graymore, 1970). Enzymic activity measured histochemically was completely lost from the pigment epithelium within 12 hours after a 24-mg/kg dose to rabbits (Birrer, 1970), followed by swelling of the Müller cells and disruption of outer segment membranes noticeable after 24 hours (Grignolo et al., 1966). A decrease in total rhodopsin content of light-adapted but not dark-adapted animals following iodate administration implied an inhibition in the synthesis of rhodopsin, possibly in the energy-requiring esterification of vitamin A with fatty acids (Grignolo et al., 1966). In fact, the low concentrations of iodate observed localized in the retinal pigment epithelium in vivo (Orzalesi and Calabria, 1967) can inhibit in vitro both glucose uptake and glycolysis by the pigment epithelium without affecting the same metabolic pathways in retinal samples free of the pigment epithelium (Glocklin and Fast, unpublished), although respiration was unaltered by iodate in either tissue sample.

In conclusion, histologic and electron microscopic examination have indicated a primary lesion of the pigment epithelium due to iodate followed by secondary lesions of the rod outer segments. Since the pigment epithelium cell layer lies between the choroidal vasculature and photoreceptors, it is responsible for exchange of nutrients and metabolites from the blood to the visual cells. Iodate-induced interruption in this flow of nutrients by possibly affecting the energy supply of the pigment epithelium or the rhodopsin cycle in the pigment epithelium would subsequently lead to photoreceptor degeneration.

Sparsomycin

The antibiotic sparsomycin, prepared from *Streptomyces sparsogenes*, is useful as an anticancer drug. One report (McFarlane et al., 1966) described two patients who received sparsomycin intravenously and developed pigmentary disturbances corresponding to bilateral ring scotomas. The total dose was 12 and 7.5 mg over a period of 13 and 15 days, respectively. Post-mortem histologic examination of the eyes disclosed primary degeneration of the pigment epithelium and a closely associated secondary degeneration of the rods and cones, with a decrease in the acid mucopolysaccharide content of the damaged areas. As an inhibitor of protein synthesis, sparsomycin exerts its action by inhibiting peptide bond formation in both bacterial, mammalian (Trakatellis, 1968; Goldberg and Friedman, 1971), and human test systems (Neth and Winkler, 1972); but whether a similar effect occurs in the pigment epithelium as part of the sparsomycin-induced visual disturbances is not known.

Experimental Retinopathy

Iodoacetate. An important technique used in examining metabolic interrelationships between the different cell layers in the retina and also in determining which cells contribute to the components of the electroretinogram is to selectively destroy individual cell layers in experimental animals. A most potent tool for such studies is iodoacetate, which in carefully controlled doses rapidly and thoroughly obliterates receptor cells in rabbits (Schubert and Bornschein, 1951; Noell, 1952).

Graymore and Tansley (1959) were able to reproduce the effect in rats with the help of sodium malate in addition to the iodoacetate. Examination of the fundus of rabbits, cats, or monkeys indicates the development of a grayish retinal opacity after the first day of treatment, which persists for about a week. Retinal pigmentation, superficially similar to human retinitis pigmentosa, appears about a week following the initial dose. Electron microscopic examination of rabbit retinas indicates lesions in the rod and cone outer segments within three hours after treatment with iodoacetate in albino rabbits and within 12 hours after iodoacetate treatment in pigmented rabbits with marked disintegration of outer segments in albinos observed after 12 hours (Lasansky and de Robertis, 1959; Birrer, 1970). Disorganization of the outer segment through vesiculation and lysis of the membrane structure is accompanied by swelling and vacuolization of the endoplasmic reticulum and Golgi apparatus in the inner segment, by disintegration of mitochondria in the ellipsoid, by pyknosis of the nuclei, and by lysis of the synaptic vessicles. Widespread capillary closure rapidly follows destruction of the photoreceptor cell layer (Dantzker and Gerstein, 1969). Iodoacetate causes an irreversible decrease in the amplitudes of the a, b, and c-waves of the electroretinogram (Noell, 1959; François et al., 1969a). All the evidence indicates a selective retinotoxic effect of iodoacetate on the photoreceptor cells since even one week after a small dose, both the pigment epithelium and inner nuclear cell layers are intact (Dantzker and Gerstein, 1969).

The mechanism of iodoacetate-induced retinopathy may be twofold. Iodoacetate inhibits glyceraldehyde-3-phosphate dehydrogenase and therefore prevents the conversion of 1,3-diphosphoglyceraldehyde into 1,3-glyceric acid, a necessary reaction in pyruvate and lactate production during the glycolytic catabolism of glucose (Noell, 1959). Glycolysis provides the major source of energy to the photoreceptor cells, and inhibition of this reaction would necessarily lead to cell destruction. Moreover, anerobic glycolysis was inhibited 75 percent after ten minutes of treatment with iodoacetate in a dose that yielded visual cell damage (Graymore, 1970). However, this theory is inconsistent with other experimental observations. The ERG is diminished within minutes after infusion of iodoacetate (Noell, 1959), and decreases in enzyme activity do not always appear prior to morphologic and structural changes of these cells. Alteration in the free sulfhydryl group content of the visual cells has been reported (Reading and Sorsby, 1966) suggesting that damages to the membrane structure of the photoreceptor cells and outer segments may be the primary retinotoxic effect of iodoacetate. An additional effect on glycolysis may contribute to the irreversible nature of iodoacetate toxicity.

Dithizone. Administration of the diabetogenic (Kadota, 1950; Okamoto, 1955) chemical dithizone intravenously to rabbits in doses

Dithizone (diphenylthiocarbazone)

between 17.5 and 40 mg/kg causes retinal lesions (Grignolo et al., 1952; Weitzel et al., 1954; Sorsby and Harding, 1962). Ophthalmoscopic and histologic examination reveal severe retinal edema developing within 24 to 48 hours followed by the appearance of red islets indicating recovery from edema and pigmentary disturbances in the fundus. When the edema finally disappears, usually in six to eight days, the irregular pigmentation has spread throughout the retina (Sorsby and Harding, 1962). While the rabbit receptors appear to be the cell layer most sensitive to dithizone toxicity, there is swelling of the nerve fiber layer. The diffuseness of the lesion is reflected in the decreased amplitudes of the ERG and the EOG (Babel and Ziv, 1957, 1959; François et al., 1969a), initially observed as a suppression of the c-wave (Wirth et al., 1957) and b-wave amplitudes (Babel and Ziv, 1957). Eventually the entire ERG is completely obliterated. Finally, as the retina becomes disorganized, optic atrophy (François et al., 1969b) and proliferation of the pigment epithelium (Karli, 1963) are observed. Pretreatment of rabbits with

cysteine does not protect against the retinotoxic action of dithizone as it does against iodate and iodoacetate poisoning (Sorsby and Harding, 1960, 1962). This suggests a difference in mechanisms between the three retinotoxic agents.

Dithizone-induced retinopathy appears to be species-specific, developing in those species possessing a tapetum, e.g., dogs and rabbits, but not developing in those species lacking a tapetum, e.g., rats, monkeys (Budinger, 1961; Delahunt et al., 1962), and man. A possible relationship, at least in the dog, has been suggested (Weitzel et al., 1954; Budinger, 1961; Delahunt et al., 1962) between the Zn^{++}-chelating properties of dithizone and retinal degeneration. Dithizone depletes the canine tapetum of its rich supply of Zn^{++}, leading to severe tapetal necrosis, retinal edema, and finally loss of retinal structure and function. On the other hand, in the rabbit, an early decrease of ERG amplitude and swelling of the neuroepithelium followed rapidly by complete retinal disorganization suggests that additional factors are involved in dithizone retinopathy. Experiments with ethambutol, another zinc chelator, show that tapetal zinc in dogs is lowered by an amount comparable to the lowering caused by dithizone. The green color of the tapetum is lost but no retinopathy results (Figueroa et al., 1971). Possible interference in the active transport of ions from the choriocapillaris through the pigment epithelium (François et al., 1969b) and alterations in the total and free sulfhydryl group content resulting from protein denaturation (Reading and Sorsby, 1966) have been reported. A similar compound, sodium diethyldithiocarbamate, not only causes tapetal necrosis in dogs but also inhibits oxygen consumption, pyruvate utilization, and citrate synthesis (DuBois et al., 1961) in liver and kidney. Perhaps dithizone exerts a similar inhibitory effect on retinal metabolism.

The diabetogenic activity of dithizone may be unrelated to its retinotoxic effects. However, dogs, which develop tapetal necrosis and retinal degeneration, are insensitive to dithizone's diabetogenic activity (Alcalde et al., 1952). Dissociation of these two actions was further demonstrated by the results of Sorsby and Harding (1962) with rabbits. Low dosages, which caused edema and retinal degeneration, did not produce diabetes, while at higher doses, retinopathy and diabetes occurred independently of one another. Based on the above discussion, no definite conclusions concerning the mechanism of action can be drawn from the available experimental data.

Diaminodiphenoxyalkanes. A set of toxic substances that appear to be specific for pigment epithelium is the family of the diaminodiphenoxyalkanes.

The series, in which $n = 5, 6$, and 7 are the most active, was originally synthesized for schistosomacidal properties. No human use was ever reported, but in susceptible animals—monkey, dog, and cat—a single oral or intravenous dose causes eventual pigmented retinopathy (Edge et al., 1956; Sorsby and Nakajima, 1958) and complete loss of the electroretinogram within a few days (Nakajima, 1958). There is selective action on the pigmented epithelium, but when these cells are destroyed, the overlying receptor cells also degenerate (Ashton, 1957). This is like the iodate situation above.

An approach to the mechanism of toxic action was begun when Glocklin and Potts (1962) showed that uptake of ^{32}P into acid-soluble phosphorus fractions was inhibited by diaminodiphenoxyheptane in pigment epithelium in vitro but not in neuroretina.

THE GANGLION CELL LAYER AND OPTIC NERVE

General Considerations

The attribute that separates the ganglion cell (Figure 13–1) from the remainder of the retina is that it is the cell body of a neuron that extends into the depth of the central nervous system. The axons from the ganglion cell layer form the nerve fiber layer of the retina and exit from the eye at the optic papilla. Most of the fibers, carrying visual information, travel some 120 mm from the globe via optic nerve, optic chiasm, and optic tract to the point where they synapse in the lateral geniculate body of the midbrain. Like any other central nervous system neuron, the optic nerve fiber degenerates in both directions from a cut. Thus the ganglion cell of the retina may be damaged by direct action upon it, the cell body, or it may degenerate secondary to toxic destruction of the optic nerve. Instances of both types of damage will be cited below.

A second unique property of the ganglion cell-optic nerve is its behavior as a physiologically dual structure. The central 5 percent of the field of vision is the sole portion that possesses high visual acuity. This corresponds to an area of retinal receptors of 1.5-mm diameter centered on the fovea centralis. Although there is considerable preprocessing of visual information in the retina, there is still correspondence between receptor location and ganglion cell type or ganglion cell location or both. The result of this is that the information from that central most acute 5 percent of visual field runs in an identifiable bundle of fibers—the so-called papillomacular bundle—whose position can be identified by myelin degeneration stains at each position in the optic nerve and optic tract after

damage to the central retina (Brouwer and Zeeman, 1926). Moreover, this fiber bundle acts as a separate entity in its behavior toward a number of toxic substances as well as toward some diseases.

It is not clear why this should be the case. We do know that papillomacular fibers are predominantly small fibers (Potts et al., 1972). It is possible that these fibers with the greatest ratio of surface area to volume have the highest metabolic demand of all optic nerve fibers. However, in the case of some toxic substances the papillomacular bundle is spared and the peripheral fibers are hit. Thus it appears that specific chemical affinities may play a role. However this may be, some toxic substances affect the ganglion cell body; others affect the fibers of the papillomacular bundle; others affect peripheral fibers only. In each case, death of a portion of the neuron means death of the entire neuron and loss of that specific information transmission channel. To take cognizance of this attribute where damage to a retinal cell body can cause loss of function through an entire tract we will designate this section as dealing with the ganglion cell neuron (GCN).

One other special consideration deals with a clinical entity, pallor of the disk. When any considerable number of optic nerve fibers die, their lack of demand for nutrition is somehow conveyed to the surrounding capillaries. These disappear over a period of months. In the one place where optic nerve capillaries may be inspected with ease, the optic papilla, the nerve head becomes abnormally pale on ophthalmoscopic inspection, owing to loss of capillary supply. There is a very good correlation between the pallor observed after the loss of a large number of fibers and optic atrophy. This has reached the point where many clinicians report "optic atrophy" on ophthalmoscopic examination when they mean "pale disk." Such an examination in marginal cases or done by a poor observer could lead to erroneous results. It is important for the reader of a report on toxicology to know whether the description of optic atrophy is a clinical or a histologic one.

Specific Substances

Methanol. A well-publicized and uniquely American poison affecting the GCN is methanol. The first practical distillation process that created a preparation potable by the unwary and the clinical report of the first 275 cases of methanol poisoning appeared in the United States (Wood and Buller, 1904). Whenever access to ethanol has been restricted, as in prohibition or in wartime, the incidence of methanol poisoning has risen, and epidemics centering on some local source of supply are reported in significant number. The characteristic results of an epidemic are that a third of those exposed to methanol recover with no residues, a third have severe visual loss or blindness, and a third die. Thus in sufficiently high doses methanol has profound systemic effects. Studies in the 1950s showed that methanol poisoning was a primate disease (Gilger and Potts, 1955) and that it was a palimpsest of three different diseases (Potts *et al.*, 1955). Those diseases are (1) organic solvent poisoning (which is the only disease the subprimates show), (2) systemic acidosis, and (3) central nervous system effects, including changes in the eye and the basal ganglia. It was shown that the LD90 for primates gave only transient solvent toxicity signs and that a lucid interval set in, followed by systemic acidosis. Acidosis was enough to kill the animal unless it was combatted with base. If the acidosis was treated, the animal died later of the CNS disease. In many monkeys at the peak of the CNS signs, retinal edema was a common finding. In its most severe form it covered the entire retina and produced the rhesus equivalent of the cherry-red spot.

Because methanol poisoning in humans is a medical emergency and it is usually impossible to determine the dose ingested, this kind of unified picture is difficult to come by. However, all of the phases seen in the rhesus disease are seen in human disease even to the basal ganglion lesion (Orthner, 1950).

The specific eye effects are definite as far as they go. Everyone agrees that nerve head pallor is a constant finding in human cases who recover from methanol poisoning with permanent visual impairment. In monkeys marked demyelination of temporal retina has been demonstrated along with marginal loss of ganglion cells (Potts *et al.*, 1955). Thus, optic atrophy is a definite finding in methanol poisoning but there is some question of whether the disease is primary in the ganglion cell layer. Arguments in favor are the observed retinal edema in the acute phase and the finding of loss of ganglion cells. Arguments against are lack of ganglion cell loss reported by McGregor (1943) and Orthner (1950).

The proximal toxic agent is generally accepted to be the methanol oxidation product formaldehyde (Potts, 1952; Cooper and Kini, 1962). It has now been established after some controversy that the mechanism of oxidation of methanol differs in primates and subprimates. In primates the principal metabolic pathway is via alcohol dehydrogenase (Kini and Cooper, 1961). In subprimates the favored pathway is via the catalase system (Tephly *et al.*, 1963). It is tempting to attribute the primate nature of methanol poisoning to some difference in

availability of formaldehyde from alcohol dehydrogenase oxidation. This does not seem to be the case. In unpublished results from our laboratory equal amounts of ^{14}C label from $^{14}CH_3OH$ are bound to eye and brain in rabbits and monkeys.

The treatment of methanol poisoning involves both combatting acidosis and preventing methanol oxidation. The most effective means for this latter therapy is administration of ethanol, which competes successfully for the enzyme and allows methanol to be excreted via urine or breath without being oxidized. It was suggested by Gilger and coworkers (1956) that treatment for a 70-kg man be 4.5 oz of 50 percent ethanol initially, followed by 3.0 oz every four hours for 48 hours or until blood methanol reached negligible levels. In a number of sporadic cases this has appeared to be effective therapy.

Ethambutol. This substance was found by *in vivo* screening to be most effective against

$$CH_2OH \quad\quad\quad\quad\quad\quad\quad\quad\quad C_2H_5$$
$$HC-HN-(CH_2)_2-NH-CH \quad \cdot 2HCl$$
$$C_2H_5 \quad\quad\quad\quad\quad\quad\quad\quad\quad CH_2OH$$

d-2-2'-(Ethylenediimino)-di-l-butanol dihydrochloride

tuberculosis in mice (Thomas *et al.*, 1961). The drug, because of its relatively good tolerance and its efficacy against isoniazid-resistant tuberculosis, has become an established member of the antituberculosis armamentarium. In some 10 percent of patients receiving 25 to 50 mg/kg/day, loss of vision appears one to seven months after start of dosage (Carr and Henkind, 1962; Place and Thomas, 1963). (For a thorough review of human and animal toxicity, see Leibold, 1966; Place *et al.*, 1966; Schmidt, 1966.)

The typical toxic phenomenon is "retrobulbar neuritis" in the sense that there is visual field involvement without obvious swelling of the nerve head. However, in addition to central scotoma, which is thought of as the typical finding in retrobulbar neuritis, a smaller proportion of patients show loss of peripheral field with preservation of central vision (Leibold, 1966). All visual symptoms are dose-related. Figures collected from various sources in the literature by Citron (1969) suggest:

DOSAGE (mg/kg/day)	CASES	INCIDENCE OF COMPLICATIONS
50	60	15%
> 35	59	18%
< 30	59	5%
25	130	3%
15	—	Negligible

Visual disturbances appear to regress completely on cessation of drug administration.

The mechanism of therapeutic action and the mechanism of toxicity are far from clear. Ethambutol is a chelating agent that will remove zinc from the tapetum lucidum of dogs. However, it does not cause the pigmentary retinopathy that a chelating agent such as dithizone causes (Figueroa *et al.*, 1971). When *Mycobacterium smegmatis* is used as a model for *M. tuberculosis*, ethambutol-inhibited cells become deficient in RNA. As a consequence, protein synthesis is inhibited (Forbes *et al.*, 1965). A recent recommendation of substituting biweekly high-dose therapy for daily intermediate-dose therapy is said to eliminate visual system toxicity (Trumbull *et al.*, 1977).

Carbon Disulfide. This inflammable and volatile liquid (BP = 46.3° C) was important in the past as a solvent for sulfur in the rubber industry and as a solvent for alkali-treated cellulose in the viscose process for rayon and cellophane. The fire hazard and health hazard led first to better personnel protection by ventilation and then to replacement by less hazardous materials and processes. Today the chronic carbon disulfide poisoning that profoundly affected vision is a rarity, but it was quite real for Galezowski (1878). Further, a restudy of the disease in the future promises to give us another clue, however fragmentary, to the dual nature of the optic nerve. Thus there is inducement to not forget the entity of carbon disulfide poisoning because of its larger implications for ophthalmic toxicology.

The earliest cases of chronic carbon disulfide poisoning were described by Delpeche in Paris in 1856. A generalized polyneuritis accompanied by personality changes was observed. The constant visual finding was central scotoma with marked decrease of visual acuity. An inconstant finding was concomitant peripheral constriction of the visual field.

A curious aspect of CS_2 poisoning is the lack of correspondence between anatomic and physiologic findings (Birch-Hirschfeld, 1900; Ide, 1958). One possible reason for this is restriction of the experimental situation to rodents, which do not appear to have a dual optic nerve. Much experimentation will be required to exploit the little we now know of carbon disulfide poisoning.

Thallium. Considerable clinical experience in thallium poisoning has arisen from use of thallous acetate in the 1920s as an epilating agent by dermatologists and its use as a rat poison (Celio Paste) with consequent accidental and intentional poisonings. For a short time in the early 1930s a cosmetic depilatory cream (Koremlu) caused additional chronic cases. (For reviews of this material, see Heyroth, 1947, and Prick *et al.*, 1955.) Systemic symptoms in thallium poisoning include gastroenteritis,

polyneuritis, and allopecia. Ocular involvement is cataract, especially in rats, and optic neuritis in man.

The unifying concept that made the behavior of lens and optic nerve understandable was developed in the 1960s when it became apparent that thallous ion is in many ways a stand-in for potassium ion. For a review of this, see Gehring and Hammond (1967). The University of Chicago laboratory was able to show that lens and optic nerve, two high-potassium tissues, were also able to store Tl^+ (Potts and Au, 1971). The ionic similarities are great enough that Tl^+ can activate (Na^+-K^+) activated ATPase (Britten and Blank, 1968). Kinsey and coworkers (1971) demonstrated that thallous ion accumulation in lens was by active transport and by the alkali metal-transporting system. An additional and unexpected finding was high storage of Tl^+ in melanin-containing eye structures (Potts and Au, 1971). Although Tl^+ can act for K^+ in many systems, it is clear that it cannot do so in every case. It seems logical that accumulation of thallium where potassium should normally be, without its being able to substitute for potassium in every enzyme system, is the basis for thallium toxicity. It is not clear which parts of the GCN are most affected.

Needless to say, prophylaxis is the only practical therapy in thallium poisoning.

Pentavalent Arsenic. Pentavalent arsenicals have been found in the past to be effective against trypanosomiasis (Thomas, 1905).

NaO—As—⟨O⟩—NH₂ with OH above and O below the As

Sodium arsanilate (Atoxyl)

NaO—As—⟨O⟩—NH—CH₂—C with OH above, O below the As, and C bearing O and NH₂

Sodium *N*-(carbamoylmethyl)-arsanilate (Tryparsamide)

The same ability to pass the blood-brain barrier that allowed effectiveness against trypanosomes also made possible treatment of neurosyphilis. Numerous derivatives of sodium arsanilate were synthesized by Ehrlich in his early investigations of trypanocidal and spirochetocidal activity. Tryparsamide, a substance of relatively low toxicity, was synthesized at the Rockefeller Institute (Jacobs and Heidelberger, 1919) and introduced into tropical medicine shortly thereafter (Pearce, 1921). Tryparsamide was then found effective against neurosyphilis (Henrichsen, 1939).

Eye effects were a constant accompaniment of the use of pentavalent arsenicals and were a prime reason for their eventual abandonment. The clinical figures of Neujean and coworkers (1948) suggest that 3 to 4 percent of trypanosomiasis cases treated with tryparsamide show visual effects, and a third of these—i.e., 1 percent of all cases—show peripheral contraction of visual fields. There are anatomic findings to accompany the clinical symptoms, and here the peripheral area of the ganglion cell layer is most severely involved (Birch-Hirschfeld and Köster, 1910). There is considerable evidence that at the cellular level all of the arsenicals reach the same oxidation state, whatever their form at introduction (Ehrlich, 1909). Most animal experimentation has employed rodents, which lack the dual optic nerve (Young and Loevenhart, 1924). Hence, full information on the nature of the dual optic nerve that the arsenicals might contribute has not been obtained. Once more an abandoned drug class leaves a negligible toxic medical hazard. Cessation of investigation has also left unexploited opportunities for learning important facts about the visual system. Note in particular that whereas most of the toxic substances affect the central optic nerve fibers, pentavalent arsenic has a selective effect on the peripheral GCN. It should be a particularly useful category of substances for study.

Quinine Poisoning. Although quinine effects on the eye may be less frequent than generally supposed (Carapancea, 1959), there is often considerable drama involved and the problem has received much attention. Lewin and Guillery (1913) devoted 33 pages to the subject. For clinical details, this section is recommended. Early cases were reported as idiosyncrasy to antimalarial doses. See the list of reactions to total doses from 0.13 to 2.0 g in Duke-Elder and MacFaul (1972). With disuse of quinine as an antimalarial and as a tonic most cases of quinine poisoning stem from its use as an abortifacient or in attempted suicide. One is then dealing with sizable doses whose exact magnitude is usually undetermined.

Rapid loss of vision is not uncommon in quinine poisoning with marked arteriolar constriction and retinal edema as the chief ophthalmoscopic findings. It is unusual that visual loss is permanent, but decreased acuity may last for hours or even days. Permanent loss of peripheral visual field is not uncommon (Lincoff, 1955; Behrman and Mushin, 1968). This loss means death of many peripheral GCN.

The pathophysiology of quinine eye effects is by no means established. Because one sees ophthalmoscopically comparable edema in closure of the central retinal artery or an arterial branch by disease, it is tempting to postulate that the primary event is the observed arteriolar

narrowing (Giannini, 1934). However, some cases of visual loss are manifest before arteriolar constriction is observed or in some cases the constriction never becomes severe (Dejean et al., 1958). Thus a primary vascular etiology is far from proven.

It has been shown on a molecular scale that the acridine antimalarials, the 4-amino quinolines (of which chloroquine is the most notable example), and quinine all inhibit the incorporation of $^{32}PO_4{}^{3-}$ into nucleic acid (Schellenberg and Coatney, 1961). This inhibition of nucleic acid synthesis has been interpreted in the case of chloroquine and quinacrine as being due to intercalation of the small molecules between the component bases of DNA, inhibiting strand separation of the double helix. Since strand separation is essential for replication, these antimalarials appear to work by inhibiting DNA replication. Inhibition of RNA transcription and inhibition of protein synthesis are logical consequences. That these occur in the eye under the influence of quinine is suggested by the vacuolation of the ganglion cell nuclei, observed by many workers in quinine-treated experimental animals.

Assorted therapy has been suggested for quinine amblyopia in the past beginning with von Graefe's (1857) cupping and tending later to vasodilation. However, since eye symptoms do not appear until cell damage begins, avoidance of quinine is the best preventive.

Glutamate. An experimental entity involving the ganglion cell neuron is glutamate poisoning. Lucas and Newhouse (1957) reported that administration of high doses of sodium l-glutamate to suckling mice caused degeneration of the retinal ganglion cell layer and failure of formation of the inner nuclear layer. Freedman and Potts (1962) were able to reproduce this phenomenon in newborn albino rats. They showed that glutaminase I was repressed in the retinas of these animals and postulated this as the mechanism of glutamate toxicity.

It should be noted that for both mice and rats near-lethal concentrations of glutamate were required, and lesser concentrations had no retinal effect. Thus, it is highly improbable that the furor regarding "the Chinese restaurant syndrome" and regarding glutamate seasoning in baby food has any real connection with glutamate retinal damage.

Methyl Nitrosocarbamate. In research performed during World War II on the vesicant methyl nitrosocarbamate (see section on vesicant gases, nitrosamines) it was found that there was selective chromatolysis and destruction of the retinal ganglion cell layer. The experiments were done in cats allowed to inhale the vapor at

$$Cl-CH_2-CH_2-\underset{\underset{N=O}{|}}{N}-\overset{\overset{O}{\parallel}}{C}-OCH_3$$

Methyl *N*-β-chlorethyl-*N*-nitrosocarbamate

a concentration of 50 μg/1 for ten minutes (Gates and Renshaw, 1946). The compound is an alkylating agent like the nitrogen mustards and it alkylates functional groups of proteins and nucleic acids in a more or less random manner. However, there is evidently something special about the composition of the ganglion cell nucleus that makes it more susceptible to damage by this compound than other cells in the body. This tiny clue to specificity, small as it is, may be a starting point for new knowledge about the ganglion cell neuron.

Special mention should be made of the optic nerve damage (accompanying widespread demyelination in the CNS) caused by 7-iodo-5-chloro-8-hydroxyquinoline, iodochlorhydroxyquin known as "Clioquinol," "Entero-Vioform," and "Vioform."

The drug is an effective amebicide and is useful in the treatment of amebiasis when given at the level of 500 to 750 mg three times a day for ten days. An eight-day interval must be observed before a second ten-day course is given.

However, this drug has been available over the counter outside the United States principally to combat "traveler's diarrhea" where a specific diagnosis has not been made and where physician control of dosage is lacking. Particularly in Japan an entity has been recognized and labeled "subacute myelo-opticoneuropathy" (SMON) attributable to use of this substance. It is said that from 1955 to 1970, 10,000 cases of SMON were diagnosed in Japan. A national commission was formed by the Japanese government, and in 1970 the sale of the drug was prohibited. For a bibliography of the Japanese literature see Shigematsu (1975).

The entity is characterized clinically by paresthesias and numbness of the extremities, ataxia, and weakness in the legs. Twenty-seven percent of SMON patients have visual disturbances attributed to demyelination of the optic nerve (Sobue and Ando, 1971).

The extremely high incidence in Japan has not been explained satisfactorily. High dosage levels, additive effects of environmental pollutants, and as-yet-unidentified factors have all been invoked. A representative of the manufacturer claims that since 1935 only 50 cases of SMON with a history of iodochlorhydroxyquin consumption have been identified in the rest of the world (Burley, 1977).

The disease can be reproduced in experimental animals by feeding the drug, and optic nerve demyelination is demonstrable in dogs and cats (Tateishi and Otsuki, 1975).

THE QUESTION OF HALLUCINOGEN ACTION

Attention has been focused in recent years on substances that modify visual perception in the human. Substances such as mescaline, lysergic acid diethylamide (LSD), and tetrahydrocannabinol have this property. If these substances work on cells in the visual system central to the retinal ganglion cell, they are beyond the scope of this chapter. A single research report describes spontaneous potentials from retina and optic nerve after LSD and mescaline in cats (Apter and Pfeiffer, 1956). These potentials must arise from cells within the globe. However, it must be recognized that the doses used in the experiment were extremely high and the mescaline used was an LD100. No more can be said on this subject until clarifying research appears.

REFERENCES

Abraham, R., and Hendy, R. J.: Irreversible lysosomal damage induced by chloroquine in the retinae of pigmented and albino rats. *Exp. Mol. Pathol.*, **12**:185–200, 1970.

Alcalde, V.; Colás, A.; Grande, F.; and Peg. V.: Ineficacia de la ditizona como agente diabetógeno en el perro. *Rev. Esp. Fisiol.*, **8**:175–85, 1952.

Anderson, B.: Corneal and conjunctival pigmentation among workers engaged in the manufacture of hydroquinone. *Arch. Ophthalmol.*, **38**:812–26, 1947.

Anonymous: Gas injuries to the eye. *Lancet*, **2**:756–57, 1939.

Apter, J. T., and Pfeiffer, C. C.: Effect of hallucinogenic drugs on the electroretinogram. *Am. J. Ophthalmol.*, **42**:206–11, 1956.

Armaly, M.: Effect of corticosteroids on intraocular pressure and fluid dynamics. *Arch. Ophthalmol.*, **70**:482–91, 492–99, 1963.

Ashton, N.: Degeneration of the retina due to 1:5-di-(*p*-aminophenoxy) pentane dihydrochloride. *J. Pathol. Bacteriol.*, **74**:103–12, 1957.

———: Oxygen and the growth and development of retinal vessels: *in vivo* and *in vitro* studies. *Am. J. Ophthalmol.*, **62**:412–35, 1966.

———: Some aspects of the comparative pathology of oxygen toxicity in the retina. *Ophthalmologica.*, **160**:54–71, 1970.

Ashton, N., and Pedler, C.: Studies on developing retinal vessels. IX. Reaction of endothelial cells to oxygen. *Br. J. Ophthalmol.*, **46**:257–76, 1962.

Atkinson, W. S.: Delayed mustard gas keratitis (dichlorodiethyl sulfide) a report of two cases. *Trans. Am. Ophthalmol. Soc.*, **45**:81–92, 1947.

Avigan, J.; Steinberg, D.; Vroman, H. E.; Thompson, M. J.; and Mosettig, E.: Studies on cholesterol biosynthesis. I. The identification of desmosterol in serum and tissues of animals and man treated with MER-29. *J. Biol. Chem.*, **235**:3123–26, 1960.

Axelsson, U., and Holmberg, A.: The frequency of cataract after miotic therapy. *Acta Ophthalmol.*, **44**:421–29, 1966.

Babel, J., and Ziv, B.: L'action du dithizone sur la

rétine du lapin étude electrophysiolôgique. *Experientia*, 13:122–23, 1957.

————: L'action du métabolisme des hydrates de carbone sur l'électrorétinogramme du lapin. *Ophthalmologica*, 137:270–81, 1959.

Barber, G. W.: Physiological chemistry of the eye. *Arch. Ophthalmol.*, 87:72–76,1972.

Beauvieux: Les lésions oculaires par les gaz vésicants. *Arch. Ophtalmol. (Paris)*, 37:597–619, 1920.

Becker, B.: Cataracts and topical corticosteroids. *Am. J. Ophthalmol.*, 58:872–73, 1964.

Beehler, C. C.: Oxygen and the eye. *Surv. Ophthalmol.*, 9:549–60, 1964.

Behrman, J., and Mushin, A.: Electrodiagnostic findings in quinine amblyopia. *Br. J. Ophthalmol.*, 52:925–28, 1968.

Bernstein, H. N.: Chloroquine ocular toxicity. *Surv. Ophthalmol.*, 12:415–77, 1967.

Bernstein, H. N., and Ginsberg, J.: The pathology of chloroquine retinopathy. *Arch. Ophthalmol.*, 71:238–45, 1964.

Bernstein, H. N.; Mills, D. W.; and Becker, B.: Steroid-induced elevation of intraocular pressure. *Arch. Ophthalmol.*, 70:15–18, 1963a.

Bernstein, H. N.; Zvaifler, N.; Rubin, M.; and Mansour, Sister A. M.: The ocular deposition of chloroquine. *Invest. Ophthalmol.*, 2:384–92, 1963b.

Bettman, J. W.; Fung, W. E.; Webster, R. G.; Noyes, P. P.; and Vincent, N. J.: Cataractogenic effect of corticosteroids on animals. *Am. J. Ophthalmol.*, 65:581–86, 1968.

Bettman, J. W.; Noyes, P.; and DeBoskey, R.: The potentiating action of steroids in cataractogenesis. *Invest. Ophthalmol.*, 3:459, 1964.

Birch-Hirschfeld, A.: Beitrag zur Kenntnis der Netzhautganglienzellen unter physiologischen und pathologischen Verhältnissen. *Albrecht von Graefes Arch. Ophthalmol.*, 50:166–246, 1900.

Birch-Hirschfeld, A., and Köster, G.: Die Schädigung des Auges durch Atoxyl. *Albrecht von Graefes Arch. Ophthalmol.*, 76:403–63, 1910.

Birrer, L.: Zur Histochemie der Natriumjodat-und Natriumjodazetat Retinopathie. *Ophthalmologica*, 160:176–94, 1970.

Black, R. L.; Oglesby, R. B.; von Sallmann, L.; and Bunim, J. J.: Posterior subcapsular cataracts induced by corticosteroids in patients with rheumatoid arthritis. *J.A.M.A.*, 174:166–71, 1960.

Boet, D. J.: Toxic effects of phenothiazines on the eye. *Doc. Ophthalmol.*, 28:1–69, 1970.

Bresnick, G. H.: Oxygen-induced visual cell degeneration in the rabbit. *Invest. Ophthalmol.*, 9:372–87, 1970.

Britten, J. S., and Blank, W.: Thallium activation of the $(Na^+ - K^+$ activated ATPase of rabbit kidney. *Biochim. Biophys. Acta*, 159:160–66, 1968.

Brouwer, B., and Zeeman, W. P. C.: The protection of the retina in the primary optic neuron in monkeys. *Brain*, 49:1–35, 1926.

Brown, S. I.; Tragakis, M. P.; and Pearce, D. B.: Treatment of the alkali-burned cornea. *Am. J. Ophthalmol.*, 74:316–20, 1972.

Brown, S. I.; Weller, C. A.; and Akiya, S.: Pathogenesis of ulcers of the alkali-burned cornea. *Arch. Ophthalmol.*, 83:205–208, 1970.

Brown, S. I.; Weller, C. A.; and Wassermann, H. E.: Collagenolytic activity of alkali-burned corneas. *Arch. Ophthalmol.*, 81:370–73, 1969.

Budinger, J. M.: Diphenylthiocarbazone blindness in dogs. *Arch. Pathol.*, 71:304–10, 1961.

Burley, D.: Clioquinol: Time to act. *Lancet*, 1: 1256, 1977.

Burns, C. A.: Ocular effects of Indomethacin. Slit lamp and electroretinographic (ERG) study. *Invest. Ophthalmol.*, 5:325, 1966.

————: Indomethacin, reduced retinal sensitivity and corneal deposits. *Am. J. Ophthalmol.*, 66:825–35, 1968.

Burns, R. P.: Delayed onset of chloroquine retinopathy. *N. Engl. J. Med.*, 275:693–96, 1966.

Butler, I.: Retinopathy following the use of chloroquine and allied substances. *Ophthalmologica*, 149:204–208, 1965.

Calkins, L. L.: Corneal epithelial changes occurring during chloroquine (Aralen) therapy. *Arch. Ophthalmol.*, 60:981–88, 1958.

Cameron, M. E.; Lawrence, J. M.; and Obrich, J. G.: Thioridazine (Mellaril) retinopathy. *Br. J. Ophthalmol.*, 56:131–34, 1972.

Carapancea, M.: Étude physio-pathologique clinique et expérimentale sur les troubles oculaires dans l'intoxication quininique. *Arch. Ophtalmol (Paris)*, 19:841–49, 1959.

Carr, R. E.: Chloroquine and organic changes in the eye. *Dis. Nerv. Syst.*, 29 (Suppl.):36–39, 1968.

Carr, R. E., and Henkind, P.: Ocular manifestations of ethambutol. Toxic amblyopia after administration of an antituberculous drug. *Arch. Ophthalmol.*, 67:566–71, 1962.

Cerletti, A., and Meier-Ruge, W.: Toxicological studies on phenothiazine induced retinopathy. In *Toxicity and Side Effects of Psychotropic Drugs. Proc. Eur. Soc. Drug Toxic.*, 9:170–88, 1967.

Chamberlain, W. P., Jr., and Boles, D. J.: Edema of cornea precipitated by quinacrine (Atebrine). *Arch. Ophthalmol.*, 35:120–34, 1946.

Citron, K. M.: Ethambutol: A review with special reference to ocular toxicity. *Tubercle*, 50 (Suppl.):32–36, 1969.

Cooper, J. R., and Kini, M. M.: Biochemical aspects of methanol poisoning. *Biochem. Pharmacol.*, 11:405–16, 1962.

Cotlier, E., and Becker, B.: Topical steroids and galactose cataracts. *Invest. Ophthalmol.*, 4:806–14, 1965.

Crews, S. J.: Posterior subcapsular lens opacities in patients on long-term corticosteroid therapy. *Br. Med. J.*, 1:1644–46, 1963.

————: The prevention of drug induced retinopathies. *Trans. Ophthalmol. Soc. U.K.*, 86:63–76, 1967.

Dale, A. J.; Parkhill, E. M.; and Layton, D. D.: Studies on chloroquine retinopathy in rabbits. *J.A.M.A.*, 193:241–43, 1965.

Dana: Sanguinarin, ein neues organisches Alkali in Sanguinaria. *Mag. Pharm.*, 23:124, 1828.

Dantzker, D. R., and Gerstein, D. D.: Retinal vascular changes following toxic effects on visual cells and pigment epithelium. *Arch. Ophthalmol.*, 81:106–14, 1969.

Davies, H. C., and Davies, R. E.: Biochemical aspects of oxygen poisoning. In Fenn, W. D., and Rahn, H. (eds.); *Handbook of Physiology*, Vol. 2, Sect. 3, American Physiological Society, Washington, D.C., 1965.

Davson, H.: *The Physiology of the Eye*, 3rd ed. Academic Press, Inc., New York and London, 1972.

Dejean, C.; Viallefont, H.; and Boudet, C.: Un cas d'intoxication par la quinine. *Bull. Soc. Ophtalmol. Fr.* (Paris), No. 2, 184–87, 1958.

Delahunt, C. S.; Stebbins, R. B.; Anderson, J.; and Bailey, J.: The cause of blindness in dogs given hydroxypyridinethione. *Toxicol. Appl. Pharmacol.*, 4:286–91, 1962.

DeLong, S. L.; Poley, B. J.; and McFarlane, J. R., Jr.: Ocular changes associated with long-term chlorpromazine therapy. *Arch. Ophthalmol.*, 73:611–17, 1965.

Delpeche, A. L. D.: Accidents produits par l'inhalation du sulfure de carbone en vapeur; expériences sur les animaux. *Gaz. Hebdom. Med. Chir.*, 3:384–85, 1856.

Derby, G. S.: Ocular manifestations following exposure to various types of poisonous gases. *Arch. Ophthalmol.*, **49**:119–20, 1920.

Dixon, M.: Reactions of lachrymators with enzymes and proteins. *Biochem. Soc. Symp.*, **2**:39–49, 1948.

Dobbie, G. C., and Langham, M. E.: Reaction of animal eyes to sanguinarine argemone oil. *Br. J. Ophthalmol.*, **45**:81–95, 1961.

Dollery, C. T.; Bulpitt, D. J.; and Kohner, E. M.: Oxygen supply to the retina from the retinal and choroidal circulations at normal and increased arterial oxygen tensions. *Invest. Ophthalmol.*, **8**:588–94, 1969.

Draize, J. H., and Kelley, E. A.: Toxicity to eye mucosa of certain cosmetic preparations containing surface active agents. *Proc. Sci. Sect. Toilet Goods Assoc.*, **17**:1–4, 1952.

DuBois, K. P.; Raymund, A. B.; and Hietbrink, B. E.: Inhibitory action of dithiocarbomates on enzymes of animal tissues. *Toxicol. Appl. Pharmacol.*, **3**:236–55, 1961.

Duke-Elder, Sir S.: Cataract. In Duke-Elder, Sir S. (ed.): *System of Ophthalmology.* Vol. XI. Diseases of the lens and vitreous; Glaucoma and hypotony. Henry Kimpton, London, 1969.

Duke-Elder, Sir S., and Jay, B.: Diseases of the lens and vitreous; glaucoma and hypotony. In Duke-Elder, Sir S. (ed.): *System of Ophthalmology*, Vol. XI. Henry Kimpton, London, 1969.

Duke-Elder, Sir S., and MacFaul, P. A.: Injuries. In Duke-Elder, Sir S. (ed.): *System of Ophthalmology*, Vol. XIV, Part II, pp. 1011–1356. C. V. Mosby, St. Louis, 1972.

Duke-Elder, Sir S., and Wybar, K. C.: The anatomy of the visual systems. In Duke-Elder, Sir S. (ed.): *System of Ophthalmology*, Vol. II. C. V. Mosby, St. Louis, 1961.

Edge, N. D.; Mason, D. F. J.; Wein, R.; and Ashton, N.: Pharmacological effects of certain diaminodiphenoxy alkanes. *Nature* (*Lond.*), **178**:806–807, 1956.

Ehrlich, P.: Über den jetzigen stand der Chemotherapie. *Ber. Dtsch. Chem. Ges.*, **42**:17–47, 1909.

Elbrink, J., and Bihler, I.: Membrane transport of sugars in the rat lens. *Can. J. Ophthalmol.*, **7**:96–101, 1972.

Elliott, T. R.: The action of adrenalin. *J. Physiol.*, **32**:401–67, 1905.

Elliott, T. R., and Soltau, A. B.: Vesicants, mustard gas. In Macpherson, W. G.; Herringham, W. P.; Elliott, T. R.; and Balfour, A., (eds.): *History of the Great War: Medical Services, Diseases of the War*, Vol. 2, Chapt. 13. His Majesty's Stationery Office, London, 1923.

Figueroa, R.; Weiss, H.; Smith, J. C., Jr.; Hackley, B. M.; McBean, L. D.; Swassing, C. R.; and Halstead, J. A.: Effect of ethambutol on the ocular zinc concentration in dogs. *Am. Rev. Resp. Dis.*, **104**:592–94, 1971.

Filkins, J. P.: Comparison of *in vivo* and *in vitro* effects of effects of chloroquine on hepatic lysosomes. *Biochem. Pharmacol.*, **18**:2655–60, 1969.

Flower, R. W., and Patz, A.: Oxygen studies in retrolental fibroplasia. IX. The effects of elevated oxygen tension in retinal vascular dynamics in the kitten. *Arch. Ophthalmol.*, **85**:197–203, 1971.

Forbes, M.; Kuck, N. A.; and Peets, E. A.: Effect of ethambutol on nucleic acid metabolism in mycobacterium smeginatis and its reversal by polyamines and divalent cations. *J. Bacteriol.*, **89**:1299–1305, 1965.

Fournier, D. J., and Patterson, J. W.: Variations in ATPase activity in the development of experimental cataracts. *Proc. Soc. Exp. Biol. Med.*, **137**:826–32, 1971.

François, J.: Glaucome apparement simple, secondaire à la cortisonothérapie locale. *Ophthalmologica*, (Suppl.), **142**:517–23, 1961.

François, J., and Feher, J.: The effect of phenothiazine on the cell membrane. *Exp. Eye Res.*, **14**:65–68, 1972.

François, J.; Jönsas, C.; and de Rouck, A.: Étude expérimentale sur l'effect de l'iodo-acétate de soude sur l'électro-rétinogramme et l'électro-oculogramme du lapin. *Ann. Ocul.* (Paris), **202**:637–42, 1969a.

———: Experimental studies on the effect of dithizone on the electro-retinogram and the electro-oculogram in rabbits. *Ophthalmologica*, **159**:472–77, 1969b.

François, J., and Maudgal, M. C.: Experimentally induced chloroquine retinopathy in rabbits. *Am. J. Ophthalmol.*, **64**:886–93, 1967.

Fraser, T. R.: On the characters, actions and therapeutical uses of the ordeal bean of Calabar. *Edinburgh Med. J.*, **9**:36–56, 123–32, 235–48, 1863.

Freedman, J. K., and Potts, A. M.: Repression of glutaminase I in the rat retina by administration of sodium-l-glutamate. *Invest. Ophthalmol.*, **1**:118–21, 1962.

Friedenwald, J. S.; Hughes, W. F.; and Herrmann, H.: Acid-base tolerance of the cornea. *Arch. Ophthalmol.*, **31**:279–83, 1944.

———: Acid burns of the eye. *Ibid.*, **35**:98–108, 1946.

Galen: De Methodo Medendi. In Kuhn, C. G. (ed.): *Opera Omnia*, (Lib. III, Cap. 2) Vol. 10, p. 171. Knobloch, Leipzig, 1825.

Galezowski, X.: *Des Amlyopies et des Amauroses Toxiques.* P. Assaebin, Paris, 1878.

Garner, A., and Rahi, A. H. S.: Practolol and ocular toxicity. *Br. J. Ophthalmol.*, **60**:684–86, 1976.

Gates, M., and Renshaw, B.: Chemical warfare agents and related chemical problems. *Sum. Tech. Rep. Div. 9.* NDRC, Washington, D.C., 1946.

Gehring, P. J., and Buerge, J. F.: The cataractogenic activity of 2,4-dinitrophenol in ducks and rabbits. *Toxicol. Appl. Pharmacol.*, **14**:475–86, 1969a.

———: The distribution of 2,4-dinitrophenol relative to its cataractogenic activity in ducklings and rabbits. *Toxicol. Appl. Pharmacol.*, **15**:574–92, 1969b.

Gehring, P. J., and Hammond, P. B.: The interrelationship between thallium and potassium in animals. *J. Pharmacol. Exp. Ther.*, **155**:187–201, 1967.

Giannini, D.: Dell'influenze dei disturbi di circolo sulla patogeenesi della alterazioni funzionali ed anatomiche del uervo ottico e della retina uegli avvelenamenti da chinino. *Ann. Ottal.*, **62**:1069–88, 1934.

Gilger, A. P., and Potts, A. M.: Studies on the visual toxicity of methanol. V. The role of acidosis in experimental methanol poisoning. *Am. J. Ophthalmol.*, **39**:63–86, 1955.

Gilger, A. P.; Potts, A. M.; and Farkas, I.: Studies on the visual toxicity of methanol. IX. The effect of ethanol on methanol poisoning in the rhesus monkey. *Am. J. Ophthalmol.*, **42**:244–52, 1956.

Gilman, A., and Philips, F. S.: The biological actions and therapeutic applications of the β-chlorethyl amines and sulfides. *Science*, **103**:409–15, 1946.

Gleiser, C. A.; Dukes, T. W.; Lawwill, T.; Read, W. K.; Bay, W. W.; and Brown, R. S.: Ocular changes in swine associated with chloroquine toxicity. *Am. J. Ophthalmol.*, **67**:399–405, 1969.

Glocklin, V. C., and Fast, D.: The metabolism of retinal pigment cell epithelium. III. The effect of sodium iodate. Unpublished results.

Glocklin, V. C., and Potts, A. M.: The metabolism of retinal pigment cell epithelium. I. The *in vitro* incorporation of P-32 and the effect of diamino-diphenoxyalkane. *Invest. Ophthalmol.*, **1**:111–17, 1962.

Goldberg, I. H., and Friedman, P. A.: Specificity in the mechanism of action of antibiotic inhibitors of protein and nucleic acid synthesis. *Pure Appl. Chem.*, **28**:499–524, 1971.

Goldey, J. A.; Dick, D. A.; and Porter, W. L.: Corn-picker's pupil: a clinical note regarding mydriasis from Jimson weed dust (Stramonium). *Ohio State Med. J.*, **62**:921, 1966.

Goldmann, H.: Cortisone glaucoma. *Arch. Ophthalmol.*, **68**:621–26, 1962.

Gonasun, L. M., and Potts, A. M.: In vitro inhibition of protein synthesis in the retinal pigment epithelium by chloroquine. *Invest. Ophthalmol. Visual Sci.*, **13**:107–15, 1974.

Gonasun, L. M., and Potts, A. M.: Possible mechanism of chloroquine induced retinopathy. Presented at the Fifth International Congress on Pharmacology, San Francisco, California, July 23–28, 1972.

Grant, W. M.: Ocular injury due to sulfur dioxide. *Arch. Ophthalmol.*, **38**:755–61; 762–74, 1947.

———: A new treatment for calcific corneal opacities. *Arch. Ophthalmol.*, **48**:681–85, 1952.

———.: *Toxicology of the Eye*, 2nd. ed. Charles C Thomas Publisher, Springfield, Ill., 1974.

Grant, W. M., and Kern, H. L.: Action of alkalies on the corneal stroma. *Arch. Ophthalmol.*, **54**:931–39, 1955.

Graymore, C. N.: Biochemistry of the retina. In Graymore, C. N. (ed.): *Biochemistry of the Eye*. Academic Press, Inc., New York and London, 1970.

Graymore, C. N., and Tansley, K.: Iodoacetate poisoning of the rat retina. I. Production of retinal degeneration. *Br. J. Ophthalmol.*, **43**:177–85, 1959.

Green, J., and Ellison, T.: Uptake and distribution of chlorpromazine in animal eyes. *Exp. Eye Res.*, **5**:191–97, 1966.

Gregory, M. H.; Rutty, D. A.; and Wood, R. D.: Differences in the retinotoxic action of chloroquine and phenothiazine derivatives. *J. Pathol.*, **120**:139–50, 1970.

Greiner, A. C., and Berry, K.: Skin pigmentation and corneal and lens opacities with prolonged chlor-promazine therapy. *Can. Med. Assoc. J.*, **90**:663–65, 1964.

Grignolo, A.; Butturini, U.; and Baronchelli, A.: Ricerchi preliminari sul diabete sperimentale da ditizone. III. Manifestazioni oculari. *Boll. Soc. Ital. Biol. Sper.*, **28**:1416–18, 1952.

Grignolo, A.; Orzalesi, N.; and Calabria, G. A.: Studies on the fine structure and the rhodopsin cycle of the rat in experimental degeneration induced by sodium iodate. *Exp. Eye Res.*, **5**:86–97, 1966.

Grimes, P., and von Sallmann, L.: Interference with cell proliferation and induction of polyploidy in rat lens epithelium during prolonged myleran treatment. *Exp. Cell Res.*, **42**:265–73, 1966.

Grimes, P.; von Sallmann, L.; Frichette, A.: Influence of myleran on cell proliferation in the lens epithelium. *Invest. Ophthalmol.*, **3**:566–76, 1964.

Guth, P. S., and Spirtes, M. A.: The phenothiazine tranquilizers: biochemical and biophysical actions. *Int. Rev. Neurobiol.*, **7**:231–78, 1964.

Hakim, S. A. E.: Argemone oil, sanguinarine, and epidemic-dropsy glaucoma. *Br. J. Ophthalmol.*, **38**:193–216, 1954.

Hamming, N. A.; Apple, D. J.; and Goldberg, M. F.: Histopathology and ultrastructure of busulfan-induced cataract. *Albrecht von Graefes Arch. Ophthalmol.*, **200**:139–47, 1976.

Harding, C. V.; Reddan, J. R.; Unakar, N. J.; and Bagchi, M.: The control of cell division in the ocular lens. *Int. Rev. Cytol.*, **31**:215–300, 1971.

Harris, J. E., and Gruber, L.: The electrolyte and water balance of the lens. *Exp. Eye Res.*, **1**:372–84, 1962.

———: The reversal of triparanol induced cataracts in the rat. *Doc. Ophthalmol.*, **26**:324–33, 1969.

———: Reversal of triparanol-induced cataracts in the rat. II. Exchange of ^{22}Na, ^{42}K, ^{86}Rb in cataractous and clearing lenses. *Invest. Ophthalmol.*, **11**:608–16, 1972.

Haugaard, N.: Poisoning of cellular reactions by oxygen. *Ann N.Y. Acad. Sci.*, **117**, Art. 2:736–44, 1965.

———: Cellular mechanisms of oxygen toxicity. *Physiol. Rev.*, **48**:311–73, 1968.

Henkes, H. E., and van Lith, G. H. M.: Retinopathy due to indomethacin. *Ophthalmologica*, **164**:385–86, 1972.

Henkes, H. E.; van Lith, G. H. M.; and Canta, L. R.: Indomethacin retinopathy. *Am. J. Ophthalmol.*, **73**:846–56, 1972.

Henrichsen, J.: Tryparsamide in the treatment of syphilis—a review of the literature. *Venereal Dis. Inform.*, **20**:293–322, 1939.

Heppel, L. A.; Neal, P. A.; Endicott, K. M.; and Porterfield, V. T.: Toxicology of dichloroethane. I. Effect on the cornea. *Arch. Ophthalmol.*, **32**:391–94, 1944.

Herman, M. M., and Bensch, K. G.: Light and electron microscopic studies of acute and chronic thallium intoxication in rats. *Toxicol. Appl. Pharmacol.*, **10**:199–222, 1967.

Heyroth, F. F.: Thallium, a review and summary of medical literature. *Public Health Service Reports* (Suppl.). Printing Office, U.S. Government, Washington, D.C., 1947.

Hobbs, H. E.; Sorsby, A.; and Friedman, A.: Retino-pathy following chloroquine therapy. *Lancet*, **2**:478–80, 1959.

Hodgkinson, B. J., and Kolb, H.: A preliminary study of the effect of chloroquine on the rat retina. *Arch. Ophthalmol.*, **84**:509–15, 1970.

Homewood, C. A.; Warhurst, D. C.; and Baggaley, V. C.: A physico-chemical explanation for the clumping of malaria pigment by chloroquine. *Trans. R. Soc. Trop. Med. Hyg.*, **65**:423–24, 1971.

Homewood, C. A.; Warhurst, D. C.; Peters, W.; and Baggaley, V. C.: Lysosomes, pH, and the anti-malarial action of chloroquine. *Nature* (Lond.), **235**:50–52, 1972.

Horner, W. D.: Dinitrophenol and its relation to formation of cataract. *Arch. Ophthalmol.*, **27**:1097–1121, 1942.

Hughes, W. F.: Alkali burns of the eye. I. Review of literature and summary of present knowledge. *Arch. Ophthalmol.*, **35**:423–49, 1946a.

———: Alkali burns of the eye. II. Clinical and patho-logical course. *Arch. Ophthalmol.*, **36**:189–214, 1946b.

Ide, T.: Histopathological studies on retina, optic nerve and arachnoidal membrane of mouse exposed to carbon disulfide poisoning. *Acta Soc. Ophthalmol. Jap.*, **62A**:85–108, 1958.

Ignarro, L. J.: Lysosome membrane stabilization *in vivo*. Effects of steroidal and nonsteroidal anti-inflammatory drugs on the integrity of rat liver lysosomes. *J. Pharmacol. Exp. Ther.*, **182**:179–88, 1972.

Ikemoto, K.: Effects of cataractogenic compounds, fatty acids and related compounds on cation transport of incubated lens. *Osaka City Med. J.*, **71**:1–18, 1971.

Inturrisi, C. E.: Thallium activation of K^+-activated phosphatases from beef brain. *Biochem. Biophys. Acta*, **173**:567–69, 1969a.

———: Thallium-induced dephosphorylation of a phosphorylated intermediate of the (sodium and thallium-activated) ATPase. *Biochim. Biophys. Acta*, **178**:630–33, 1969b.

Jachuck, S. J.; Stephenson, J.; Bird, T.; Jackson, F. S.; and Clark, F.: Practolol induced autoantibodies and their relation to oculocutaneous complications. *Postgrad. Med. J.*, **53**:75–77, 1977.

Jacobs, M. B.: *War Gases*. Interscience, New York, 1942.

Jacobs, W. A., and Heidelberger, M.: Aromatic arsenic

compounds. II. The amides and alkyl amides of N-arylglycine arsonic acids. *J. Am. Chem. Soc.*, **44**:1587–1600, 1919.

Jaffe, L. S.: Photochemical air pollutants and their effect on men and animals. I. General characteristics and community concentrations. *Arch. Environ. Health*, **15**:782–91, 1967.

Kadota, I.: Studies on experimental diabetes mellitus, as produced by organic reagents. Oxine diabetes and dithizone diabetes. *J. Lab. Clin. Med.*, **35**:568–91, 1950.

Karli, P.: Les dégénérescences rétiniennes spontanées et expérimentales chez l'animal. *Progr. Ophthalmol.*, **14**:51–89, 1963.

Kaufman, P. L.; Axelsson, U.; and Bárány, E. H.: Atropine inhibition of echothiophate cataractogenesis in monkeys. *Arch. Ophthalmol.*, **95**:1262–68, 1977.

———: Induction of subcapsular cataracts in cynomolgus monkeys by echothiophate. *Arch. Ophthalmol.*, **95**:499–504, 1967.

Kayne, F. J.: Thallium (I) activation of pyruvate kinase. *Arch. Biochem. Biophys.*, **143**:232–39, 1971.

Kini, M. M., and Cooper, J. R.: Biochemistry of methanol poisoning. III. The enzymic pathway for the conversion of methanol to formaldehyde. *Biochem. Pharmacol.*, **8**:207–17, 1961.

Kinoshita, J. H.: Cataracts in galactosemia. *Invest. Ophthalmol.*, **4**:786–99, 1965.

Kinoshita, J. H.; Barber, G. W.; Merola, L. O.; and Fung, B.: Changes in the levels of free amino acids and myoinositol in the galactose-exposed lens. *Invest. Ophthalmol.*, **8**:625–32, 1969.

Kinross-Wright, V.: Clinical trial of a new phenothiazine compound NP-207. *Psychiatr. Res. Rep. Am. Psychiatr. Assoc.*, **4**:89–94, 1956.

Kinsey, V. E.; McLean, I. W.; and Parker, J.: Studies on the crystalline lens. XVIII. Kinetics of thallium (Tl$^+$) transport in relation to that of the alkali metal cations. *Invest. Ophthalmol.*, **10**:932–42, 1971.

Kirby, T. J.; Achor, R. W. P.; Perry, H. O.; and Winkelmann, R. K.: Cataract formation after triparanol therapy. *Arch. Ophthalmol.*, **68**:486–89, 1962.

Kobayashi, T., and Murakami, S.: Blindness of an adult caused by oxygen. *J.A.M.A.*, **219**:741–42, 1972.

Kolb, H.; Rosenthal, A. R.; Juxsoll, D.; and Bergsma, D.: Preliminary results on chloroquine induced damage to retina of rhesus monkey. Presented at Association for Research in Vision and Ophthalmology, Sarasota, Florida, Spring, 1972.

Kolker, A. E., and Becker, B.: Epinephrine maculopathy. *Arch. Ophthalmol.*, **79**:552–62, 1968.

Krill, A. E.; Potts, A. M.; and Johanson, C. E.: Chloroquine retinopathy. Investigation of discrepancy between dark adaptation and electroretinographic findings in advanced stages. *Am. J. Ophthalmol.*, **71**:530–43, 1971.

Kuck, J. F. R., Jr.: Chemical constituents of the lens. In Graymore, C. N. (ed.): *Biochemistry of the Eye.* Academic Press, Inc., New York and London, 1970a.

———: Metabolism of the lens. In Graymore, C. N. (ed.): *Biochemistry of the Eye.* Academic Press, Inc., New York and London. 1970b.

———: Cataract formation. In Graymore, C. N. (ed.): *Biochemistry of the Eye.* Academic Press, Inc., New York and London. 1970c.

———: Response of the mouse lens to high concentrations of glucose and galactose. *Ophthalmic Res.*, **1**:166–74, 1970d.

Kuwabara, T.; Kinoshita, J. H.; and Cogan, D. G.: Electron microscopic study of galactose-induced cataract. *Invest. Ophthalmol.*, **8**:133–49, 1969.

Kwant, W. O., and Seeman, P.: The membrane concentration of a local anesthetic (chlorpromazine). *Biochim. Biophys. Acta*, **183**:530–43, 1969a.

———: The displacement of membrane calcium by a local anesthetic (chlorpromazine). *Biochim. Biophys. Acta*, **193**:338–49, 1969b.

Lasansky, A., and de Robertis, E.: Submicroscopic changes in visual cells of the rabbit induced by iodoacetate. *J. Biophys. Biochem. Cytol.*, **5**:245–50, 1959.

Laughlin, R. C., and Carey, T. F.: Cataracts in patients treated with triparanol, *J.A.M.A.*, **181**:339–40, 1962.

Lawwill, T.; Appleton, B.; and Altstatt, L.: Chloroquine accumulation in human eyes. *Am. J. Ophthalmol.*, **65**:530–32, 1968.

Leibold, J. E.: The ocular toxicity of ethambutol and its relation to dose. *Ann. N. Y. Acad. Sci.*, **135**:904–909, 1966.

Levine, R. A., and Stahl, C. J.: Eye injury caused by tear-gas weapons. *Am. J. Ophthalmol.*, **65**:497–508, 1968.

Levy, N. S.; Krill, A. E.; and Beutler, E.: Galactokinase deficiency and cataracts. *Am. J. Ophthalmol.*, **74**:41–48, 1972.

Lewin, L., and Guillery, H.: *Die Wirkung von Arzneimitteln und Giften auf das Auge*, Vols. 1 and 2. A. Hirshwald, Berlin, 1913.

Lieberman, T. W.: Prolonged pharmacology and the eye. Ocular effects of prolonged systemic drug administration. *Dis. Nerv. Syst.*, **29** (Suppl.): 44–50, 1968.

Lincoff, M. A.: Quinine amblyopia—report of a case. *Arch. Ophthalmol.*, **53**:382–84, 1955.

Linksz, A.: Applied pharmacology of the skin in the ophthalmologists everyday practice. *Arch. Ophthalmol.*, **28**:959–82, 1942.

Loredo, A.; Rodriguez, R. S.; and Murillo, L.: Cataracts after short-term corticosteroid treatment. *N. Engl. J. Med.*, **286**:160, 1972.

Lowry, O. H.; Roberts, N. R.; and Lewis, C.: The quantitative histochemistry of the retina. *J. Biol. Chem.*, **220**:879–92, 1956.

Lowry, O. H.; Roberts, N. R.; Schulz, D. W.; Clow, J. E.; and Clark, J. R.: Quantitative histochemistry of retina. II. Enzymes of glucose metabolism. *J. Biol. Chem.*, **236**:2813–20, 1961.

Lubkin, V. L.: Steroid cataract—a review and a conclusion. *J. Asthma Res.*, **14**:55–59, 1977.

Lucas, D. R., and Newhouse, J. P.: The toxic effect of sodium l-glutamate on the inner layers of the retina. *Arch. Ophthalmol.*, **58**:193–201, 1957.

McChesney, E. W.; Banks, W. F., Jr.; and Fabian, R. J.: Tissue distribution of chloroquine, hydroxychloroquine and desethylchloroquine in the rat. *Toxicol. Appl. Pharmacol.*, **10**:501–13, 1967.

McChesney, E. W.; Banks, W. F., Jr.; and Sullivan, D. J.: Metabolism of chloroquine and hydroxychloroquine in albino and pigmented rats. *Toxicol. Appl. Pharmacol.*, **7**:627–36, 1965.

McConnell, D. G.; Wachtel, J.; and Havener, W. H.: Observations on experimental chloroquine retinopathy. *Arch. Ophthalmol.*, **71**:552–53, 1964.

McCrea, F. D.; Eadie, G. S.; and Morgan, J. E.: The mechanism of morphine miosis. *J. Pharmacol. Exp. Ther.*, **74**:239–46, 1942.

McFarlane, J. R.; Yanoff, M.; and Scheie, H. G.: Toxic retinopathy following sparsomycin therapy. *Arch. Ophthalmol.*, **76**:532–40, 1966.

McGregor, I. S.: Study of histopathologic changes in the retina and late changes in the visual field in acute methanol poisoning. *Br. J. Ophthalmol.*, **27**:523–43, 1943.

Mackenzie, A. H.: An appraisal of chloroquine. *Arthritis Rheum.*, **13**:280–91, 1970.

Mackworth, J. F.: The inhibition of thiol enzymes by lachrymators. *Biochem. J.*, **42**:82–90, 1948.

Mailer, C. M.: Paradoxical differences in retinal vessel diameters and the effect of inspired oxygen. *Can. J. Ophthalmol.*, **5**:163–68, 1970.

Mann, I.; Pirie, A.; and Pullinger, B. D.: An experimental and clinical study of the reaction of the anterior segment of the eye to chemical injury with special reference to chemical warfare agents. *Br. J. Ophthalmol. Suppl.*, **13**:1–171, 1948.

Manske, R. H. F.: α-Napthaphenanthredine alkaloids. In Manske, R. H. F., and Holmes, H. L. (eds.): *The Alkaloids, Chemistry and Physiology*, Vol. IV. Academic Press, Inc., New York, 1954, pp. 253–63.

Martin, G.; Draize, J. H.; and Kelley, E. A.: Local anesthesia in eye mucosa produced by surfactants in cosmetic formulations. *Proc. Sci. Sect. Toilet Goods Assoc.*, **37**:2–3, 1962.

Maslova, M. N.; Natochin, Y. V.; and Skulsky, I. A.: Inhibition of active sodium transport and activation of Na^+-K^+-ATPase by ions Tl^+ in frog skin. *Biokhimiia*, **36**:867–69, 1971.

Matthiolus, P. A.: *Commentarius in sex libros super Dioscorides*. N. Baseus, 1598.

Maumenee, A. E., and Scholz, R. O.: The histopathology of the ocular lesions produced by the sulfur and nitrogen mustards. *Bull. Johns Hopkins Hosp.*, **82**:121–47, 1948.

Maurice, D. M.: The cornea and the sclera. In Davson, H. (ed.): *The Eye*, Vol. I, 2nd ed. Academic Press, Inc., New York and London, 1969.

Maynard, F. P.: Preliminary note on increased intraocular tension met within cases of epidemic dropsy. *Indian Med. Gaz.*, **44**:373–74, 1909.

Meier-Ruge, W.: Experimental investigation of the morphogenesis of chloroquine retinopathy. *Arch. Ophthalmol.*, **73**:540–44, 1965a.

———: Die Morphologie der experimentellen Chlorochinretinopathie des Kaninchens. *Ophthalmologica*, **150**:127–37, 1965b.

———: The pathophysiological morphology of the pigment epithelium and its importance for retinal structure and function. *Med. Probl. Ophthalmol.*, **8**:32–48, 1968.

Meier-Ruge, W., and Cerletti, A.: Zur experimentellen Pathologie der Phenothiazin-Retinopathie. *Ophthalmologica*, **151**:512–33, 1966.

Menzel, D. B.: Toxicity of ozone, oxygen, and radiation. *Annu. Rev. Pharmacol.*, **10**:379–94, 1970.

Meyerson, A., and Thau, W.: Ocular pharmacology of furfuryl trimethyl ammonium iodide with special reference to intraocular tension. *Arch. Ophthalmol.*, **24**:758–60, 1940.

Minton, J.: *Occupational Eye Diseases and Injuries*. Grune & Stratton, Inc., New York, 1949, p. 46.

Monteleone, J. A.; Beutler, E.; Monteleone, P. L.; Utz, C. L.; and Casey, E. C.: Cataracts, galactosuria and hypergalactosemia due to galactokinase deficiency in a child. *Am. J. Med.*, **50**:403–407, 1971.

Nakajima, A.: The effect of amino-phenoxy-alkanes on rabbit ERG. *Ophthalmologica*, **136**:332–44, 1958.

Neth, R., and Winkler, K.: Proteinsynthese in menschlichen Leukocyten. II. Wirkung einiger Antibiotica auf die Proteinsyntheseleistung von Zellsuspensionen und auf die Peptidyltransferase-Aktivität in zellfreien Systemen. *Klin. Wochenschr.*, **50**:523–24, 1972.

Neujean, G.; Weyts, E.; Bacq, Z. M.: Action du B.A.L. sur les accidents ophthalmologiques de la thérapeutique à la tryparsamide. *Bull. Acad. R. Med. Belg.*, **13**:341–50, 1948.

Nichols, C. W., and Lambertsen, C. J.: Effects of high oxygen pressures on the eye. *N. Engl. J. Med.*, **281**:25–30, 1969.

Noell, W. K.: The impairment of visual cell structure by iodoacetate. *J. Cell Comp. Physiol.*, **40**:25–45, 1952.

———: Metabolic injuries of the visual cell. *Am. J. Ophthalmol.*, **40**:60–70, 1955.

———: The visual cell: electric and metabolic manifestations of its life processes. *Am. J. Ophthalmol.*, **48**:347–70, 1959.

Nordmann, J.: L'oculiste et la detection preventive systematique de la galactosemie. *Ophthalmologica*, **163**:129–35, 1971.

Northover, B. J.: Mechanism of the inhibitory action of indomethacin on smooth muscle. *Br. J. Pharmacol.*, **41**:540–51, 1971.

———: The effects of indomethacin in calcium, sodium, potassium and magnesium fluxes in various tissues of the guinea pig. *Br. J. Pharmacol.*, **45**:651–59, 1972.

Nylander, U.: Ocular damage in chloroquine therapy. *Acta Ophthalmol.*, **92** (Suppl.):1–71, 1967.

Obstbaum, S. A.; Galin, M.A.; and Poole, T. A.: Topical epinephrine and cystoid macular edema. *Ann. Ophthalmol.*, **8**:455–58, 1976.

Oglesby, R. B.; Black, R. L.; von Sallmann, L.; and Bunim, J. J.: Cataracts in rheumatoid arthritis patients treated with corticosteroids. *Arch. Ophthalmol.*, **66**:519–23, 1961a.

———: Cataracts in patients with rheumatic diseases treated with corticosteroids. *Arch. Ophthalmol.*, **66**:625–630, 1961b.

Okamoto, K.: Experimental pathology of diabetes mellitus. (Report II) I. Experimental studies on production and progress of diabetes mellitus by zinc reagents. *Tohoku J. Exp. Med.*, **61** (Suppl. III):1–35, 1955.

Okun, E.; Gouras, P.; Bernstein, H.; and von Sallmann, L.: Chloroquine retinopathy. *Arch. Ophthalmol.*, **69**:59–71, 1963.

Ono, S.; Hirano, H.; and Obara, K. O.: Absorption of cortisol-4-¹⁴C into rat lens. *Jap. J. Exp. Med.*, **41**:485–87, 1971.

———: Presence of cortisol-binding protein in the lens. *Ophthalmic Res.*, **3**:233–40, 1972a.

———: Study on the conjugation of cortisol in the lens. *Ophthalmic Res.*, **3**:307–10, 1972b.

Orthner, H.: *Methanol Poisoning*. Springer, Berlin, 1950.

Orzalesi, N., and Calabria, G. A.: The penetration of I^{131} labeled sodium iodate into the ocular tissues and fluids. *Ophthalmologica*, **153**:229–38, 1967.

Ottlecz, A.; Horpacsy, G.; and Karady, S.: Biphasic effect of chloroquine treatment on the lysosomal enzyme activity into urniquet shock. *Enzyme*, **11**:491–96, 1970.

Otto, H. F.: Tierexperimentelle Untersuchungen zur Hepato-Toxizität von Triparanol. *Beitr. Pathol.*, **142**:177–93, 1971.

Palimeris, G.; Koliopoulos, J.; and Velissaropoulos, P.: Ocular side effects of indomethacin. *Ophthalmologica*, **164**:339–53, 1972.

Paterson, C. A.: Distribution and movement of ions in the ocular lens. *Doc. Ophthalmol.*, **31**:1–28, 1972.

Patz, A.: Retrolental fibroplasia. *Surv. Ophthalmol.*, **14**:1–29, 1969–70.

Pearce, L.: Studies on the treatment of human tyrpanosomiasis with tryparsamide (the sodium salt of N-phenylglycineamide-*p*-arsonic acid). *J. Exp. Med.*, **34** (Suppl. 1):1–104, 1921.

Peters, R. A.; Stocken, L. A.; and Thompson, R. H. S.: British Anti-Lewisite (BAL). *Nature (Lond.)*, **156**:616–19, 1945.

Pirie, A.: Pathology in the eye of the naphthalene-fed rabbit. *Exp. Eye Res.*, **7**:354–57, 1968.

Place, V. A.; Peets, E. A.; Buyske, D. A.; and Little, R. R.: Metabolic and special studies of ethambutol in normal volunteers and tuberculous patients. *Ann. N.Y. Acad. Sci.*, **135**:775–95, 1966.

Place, V. A., and Thomas, J. P.: Clinical pharmacology of ethambutol. *Am. Rev. Resp. Dis.*, **87**:901–904, 1963.

Podos, S. M., and Canellos, G. P.: Lens changes in chronic granulocytic leukemia. *Am. J. Ophthalmol.*, **68**:500–504, 1969.

Potts, A. M.: Methyl alcohol poisoning. *ONR Resp. Rev.*, pp. 4–9, Nov., 1952.

——: The concentration of phenothiazines in the eyes of experimental animals. *Invest. Ophthalmol.*, 1:522–30, 1962a.

——: Uveal pigment and phenothiazine compounds. *Trans. Am. Ophthalmol. Soc.*, 60:517–52, 1962b.

——: Further studies concerning the accumulation of polycyclic compounds on unveal melanin. *Invest. Ophthalmol.*, 3:399–404, 1964a.

——: The reaction of uveal pigment *in vitro* with polycyclic compounds. *Invest. Ophthalmol.*, 3:405–16, 1964b.

——: Agents which cause pigmentary retinopathy. *Dis. Nerv. Syst.*, 29 (Suppl.):16–18, 1968.

Potts, A. M., and Au, P. C.: Thallous ion and the eye. *Invest. Ophthalmol.*, 10:925–31, 1971.

Potts, A. M.; Hodges, D.; Shelman, C. B.; Fritz, K. J.; Levy, N. S.; and Mangnall, Y.: Morphology of the primate optic nerve. III. Fiber characteristics of the foveal outflow. *Invest. Ophthalmol.*, 11:1004–16, 1972.

Potts, A. M.; Praglin, J.; Farkas, I.; Orbison, L.; and Chickering, D.: Studies on the visual toxicity of methanol. VIII. Additional observations on methanol poisoning in the primate test object. *Am. J. Ophthalmol.*, 40:76–82, 1955.

Prick, J. J. G.; Sillevis-Smitt, W. G.; and Muller, L.: *Thallium Poisoning*. Elsevier Publishing Co., New York, 1955.

Raghupathy, E.; Peterson, N. A.; and McKean, C. M.: Effects of phenothiazines on *in vitro* cerebral protein synthesis. *Biochem. Pharmacol.*, 19:993–1000, 1970.

Ramsey, M. S.; Bloodworth, J. M. B.; and Engerman, R. L.: Chloroquine retinopathy in rabbit. *Can. J. Ophthalmol.*, 5:264–73, 1970.

Ramsey, M. S., and Fine, B. S.: Chloroquine toxicity in the human eye. Histopathologic observations by electron microscopy. *Am. J. Ophthalmol.*, 73:229–35. 1972.

Ravindranathan, M. P.; Paul, V. J.; and Kuriakose, E. T.: Cataract after busulphan treatment. *Br. Med. J.*, 1:218–19, 1972.

Rawlins, F. A., and Uzman, B. G.: Retardation of peripheral nerve myelination in mice treated with inhibitors of cholesterol biosynthesis. A quantitative electron microscopic study. *J. Cell Biol.*, 216:505–17, 1970.

Read, W. K., and Bay, W. W.: Basic cellular lesion in chloroquine toxicity. *Lab. Invest.*, 24:246–59, 1971.

Reading, H. W., and Sorsby, A.: Retinal toxicity and tissue—SH levels. *Biochem. Pharmacol.*, 15:1389–93, 1966.

Rees, J. R., and Pirie, A.: Possible reactions of 1,2-naphthaquinone in the eye. *Biochem. J.*, 102: 853–63, 1967.

Reinert, H., and Rutty, D. A.: Mechanisms of chloroquine and phenothiazine retinopathies. *Toxicol. Appl. Pharmacol.*, 14:635–36, 1969.

Riehm, W.: Ueber Presojod-Schädigung des Auges. *Klin. Monatsbl. Augenheilkd.*, 78:87, 1927.

——: Akute Pigmentdegeneration der Netzhaut nach Intoxikation mit Septojod. *Arch. Augenheilkd.*, 100-101:872–882, 1929.

Røe, O.: The ganglion cells of the retina in cases of methanol poisoning in human beings and experimental animals. *Acta Ophthalmol. Scand.*, 26:169–82, 1948.

Roskoski, R., Jr., and Jaskunas, S. R.: Chloroquine and primaquine inhibition of rat liver cell-free polynucleotide-dependent polypeptide synthesis. *Biochem. Pharmacol.*, 21:391–99, 1972.

Rösner, H.: Untersuchungen zur Wirkung von Chlorpromazin im ZNS von Teleosteern. I. Einfluss auf das Normalverhalten sowie den Einbau von ^{3}H-Uridin und ^{3}H-Histidin. *Psychopharmacologia*, 23:125–35, 1972.

Sams, W. M., Jr.: Chloroquine: mechanism of action. *Mayo Clin. Proc.*, 42:300–309, 1967.

Sarkar, S. L.: Katakar oil poisoning. *Indian Med. Gaz.*, 61:62–63, 1926.

Sarkar, S. N.: Isolation from argemone oil of dihydrosanguinarine and sanguinarine: Toxicity of sanguinarine. *Nature (Lond.)*, 162:265–66, 1948.

Sassaman, F. W.; Cassidy, J. J.; Alpern, M.; and Maaseidvaag, F.: Electroretinography in patients with connective tissue diseases treated with hydroxychloroquine. *Am. J. Ophthalmol.*, 70:515–23, 1970.

Schellenberg, K. A., and Coatney, G. R.: The influence of antimalarial drugs on nucleic acid synthesis in plasomodium gallinaceum and plasomodium berghei. *Biochem. Pharmacol.*, 6:143–52, 1961.

Scherbel, A. L.; Mackenzie, A. H.; Nousek, J. E.; and Atdjian, M.: Ocular lesions in rheumatoid arthritis and related disorders with particular reference to retinopathy. A study of 741 patients treated with and without chloroquinine drugs. *N. Engl. J. Med.*, 273:360–66, 1965.

Schmidt, I. G.: Central nervous system effects of ethambutol in monkeys. *Ann. N.Y. Acad. Sci.*, 135:759–74, 1966.

Schubert, G., and Bornschein, H.: Spezifische Schädigung von Netzhautelementen durch Jodazetat. *Experientia*, 7:461–62, 1951.

Schutta, H. S., and Neville, H. E.: Effects of cholesterol synthesis inhibitors on the nervous system. A light and electron microscopic study. *Lab. Invest.*, 19:487–93, 1968.

Seeman, P. M.: Membrane stabilization by drugs: tranquilizers, steroids, and anesthetics. *Int. Rev. Neurobiol.*, 9:145–221, 1966.

Shaffer, R. N., and Hetherington, J.: Anticholinesterase drugs and cataracts. *Am. J. Ophthalmol.*, 62:613–28, 1966.

Shaffer, R. N., and Ridgway, W. L.: Furmethide iodide in the production of dacryostenosis. *Am. J. Ophthalmol.*, 34:718–20, 1951.

Shearer, R. V., and Dubois, E. L.: Ocular changes induced by long-term hydroxychloroquine (plaquenil) therapy. *Am. J. Ophthalmol.*, 64:245–52, 1967.

Shigematsu, I.: Subacute myelo-optico-neuropathy (SMON) and clioquinol. *Jap. J. Med. Sci. Biol.*, 28 (Suppl.):35–55, 1975.

Siddall, J. R.: The ocular toxic findings with prolonged and high dosage chlorpromazine intake. *Arch. Ophthalmol.*, 74:460–64, 1965.

——: Ocular toxic changes associated with chlorpromazine and thioridazine. *Can. J. Ophthalmol.*, 1:190–98, 1966.

——: Ocular complications related to phenothiazines. *Dis. Nerv. Syst.*, 29 (Suppl.):10–13, 1968.

Siegrist, A.: Konzentrierte Alkali-und Säurewirkung auf das Auge. *Z. Augenheilkd.*, 43:176–94, 1920.

Sippel, T. O.: Changes in water, protein, and glutathione contents of the lens in the course of galactose cataract development in rats. *Invest. Ophthalmol.*, 5:568–75, 1966a.

——: Energy metabolism in the lens during development of galactose cataract in rats. *Invest. Ophthalmol.*, 5:576–87, 1966b.

——: Enzymes of carbohydrate metabolism in developing galactose cataracts of rats. *Invest. Ophthalmol.*, 6:59–63, 1967.

Slansky, H. H.; Freeman, M. I.; and Itoi, M.: Collagenolytic activity in bovine corneal epithelium. *Arch. Ophthalmol.*, 80:496–98, 1968.

Sobue, I., and Ando, K.: Myeloneuropathy with abdominal symptoms—5 clinical features and diagnostic criteria. *Clin. Neurol.*, 11:244–48, 1971.

Solomon, C.; Light, A. E.; and De Beer, E. J.: Cataracts

produced in rats by 1,4-dimethanesulfonoxybutane (myleran). *Arch. Ophthalmol.*, 54:850–52, 1955.

Solze, D. A., and McConnell, D. G.: Ultrastructural changes in the rat photoreceptor inner segment during experimental chloroquine retinopathy. *Ophthalmic Res.*, 1:140–48, 1970.

Sorsby, A.: The nature of experimental degeneration of the retina. *Br. J. Ophthalmol.*, 25:62–65, 1941.

Sorsby, A., and Harding, R.: Protective effect of cysteine against retinal degeneration induced by iodate and iodoacetate. *Nature (Lond.)*, 187:608–609, 1960.

———: Experimental degeneration of the retina. VIII. Dithizone retinopathy. Its independence of the diabetogenic effect. *Vision Res.*, 2:149–55, 1962.

Sorsby, A., and Nakajima, A.: Experimental degeneration of the retina. IV. Diaminodiphenoxyalkanes as inducing agents. *Br. J. Ophthalmol.*, 42:563–71, 1958.

Steinberg, D., and Avigan, J.: Studies on cholesterol biosynthesis. II. The role of desmosterol in the biosynthesis of cholesterol. *J. Biol. Chem.*, 235:3127–29, 1960.

Straus, D. J.; Mausolf, F. A.; Ellerby, R. A.; and McCracken, J. D.: Cicatricial ecotropion secondary to 5-fluorouracil therapy. *Med. Pediat. Oncol.*, 3:15–19, 1977.

Tarkkanen, A.; Esila, R.; and Liesmaa, M.: Experimental cataracts following long-term administration of corticosteroids. *Acta Ophthalmol.*, 44:665–68, 1966.

Tateishi, J., and Otsuki, S.: Experimental reproduction of SMON in animals by prolonged administration of clioquinol: Clinico-pathological findings. *Jap. J. Med. Sci. Biol.*, 28 (Suppl.):165–86, 1975.

Tephly, T. R.; Parks, R. E., Jr.; and Mannering, G. J.: Methanol metabolism in the rat. *J. Pharmacol. Exp. Ther.*, 143:292–300, 1963.

Thatcher, D. B.; Blaug, S. M.; Hyndiuk, R. A.; and Watzke, R. C.: Ocular effects of chemical Mace in the rabbit. *Clin. Med.*, 78:11–13, 1971.

Thomas, H. W.: Some experiments in the treatment of trypanosomiasis. *Br. Med. J.*, 1:1140–43, 1905.

Thomas, J. P.; Baughn, C. O.; Wilkinson, R. G.; and Shepard, R. G.: A new synthetic compound with antituberculous activity in mice: ethambutol dextro-2,2′ ethylenediimino di-l-butanol. *Am. Rev. Resp. Dis.*, 83:891–93, 1961.

Trakatellis, A. C.: Effect of sparsomycin on protein synthesis in the mouse liver. *Proc. Natl. Acad. Sci., U.S.A.*, 59:854–60, 1968.

Trayhurn, P., and van Heyningen, R.: The metabolism of glutamate, aspartate and alanine in the bovine lens. *Biochem. J.*, 124:72P–73P, 1971a.

———: Aerobic metabolism in the bovine lens. *Exp. Eye Res.*, 12:315–27, 1971b.

Trumbull, G. C.; Sbarbaro, J. A.; and Iseman, M.: (Correspondence) High dose ethambutol. *Am. Rev. Resp. Dis.*, 115:889–90, 1977.

Uhthoff, W.: Die Augenstörungen bei Vergiftungen. In Graefe-saemisch *Handbuch der Gesamten Augenheilkunde*, 11:1–180, Engelmann, Leipzig, 1911.

Upholt, W. M.; Quinby, G. E.; Batchelor, G. S.; and Thompson, J. P.: Visual effects accompanying TEPP-induced miosis. *Arch. Ophthalmol.*, 56:128–34, 1956.

van Heyningen, R.: The lens: Metabolism and cataract. In Davson, H. (ed.): *The Eye, Vegetative Physiology and Biochemistry*, Vol. 1, 2nd ed. Academic Press, Inc., New York and London, 1969.

———: Ascorbic acid in the lens of the naphthalene-fed rabbit. *Exp. Eye Res.*, 9:38–48, 1970a.

———: Effect of some cyclic hydroxy compounds on the accumulation of ascorbic acid by the rabbit lens *in vitro. Exp. Eye Res.*, 9:49–56, 1970b.

———: Galactose cataract: a review. *Exp. Eye Res.*, 11:415–28, 1971.

van Heyningen, R., and Pirie, A.: The metabolism of naphthalene and its toxic effect on the eye. *Biochem. J.*, 102:842–52, 1967.

Van Joost, T. H.; Crone, R. A.; and Overdijk, A. D.: Ocular cicatricial pemphigoid associated with practolol therapy. *Br. J. Dermatol.*, 94:447–50, 1976.

Velhagen, K.: Zur Hornhautargyrose. *Klin. Monatsbl. Augenheilkd.*, 122:36–42, 1953.

Vito, P.: Contributo allo studio della degenerazione pigmentaria della retina indotta dalla soluzione iodica di Pregl. *Boll. Ocul.*, 14:945–57, 1935.

von Graefe, A.: Fälle von Amaurose nach Chiningebrauch. *Albrecht von Graefes Arch. Ophthalmol.*, 3:396–405, 1857.

von Sallmann, L.: The lens epithelium in the pathogenesis of cataract. *Am. J. Ophthalmol.*, 44:159–70, 1957.

von Sallmann, L.; Grimes, P.; and Collins, E.: Triparanol induced cataract in rats. *Arch. Ophthalmol.*, 70:522–30, 1963.

Waley, S. G.: The lens: function and macromolecular composition. In Davson, H. (ed.): *The Eye*, Vol. 1, 2nd ed. Academic Press, Inc., New York and London, 1969.

Warburg, O.: *Über den Stoffwechsel der Tumoren.* f. Springer, Berlin, 1926, p. 138.

Weekley, R. D.; Potts, A. M.; Reboton, J.; and May, R. H.: Pigmentary retinopathy in patients receiving high doses of a new phenothiazine. *Arch. Ophthalmol.*, 64:65–74, 1960.

Weitzel, G.; Strecker, F. J.; Roester, U.; Buddecke, E.; and Fretzdorff, A. M.: Zink im tapetum lucidum. *Hoppe Seylers Z. Physiol. Chem.*, 296:19–30, 1954.

Weller, C. A., and Green, M.: Methionyl-tRNA synthetase detected by [^{75}Se]-selenomethionine in lenses from normal and galactose-fed rats. *Exp. Eye Res.*, 8-84–90, 1969.

Wetterholm, D. H., and Winter, F. C.: Histopathology of chloroquine retinal toxicity. *Arch. Ophthalmol.*, 71:82–87, 1964.

Wheeler, M. C.: Discoloration of the eyelids from prolonged use of ointments containing mercury. *Trans. Am. Ophthalmol. Soc.*, 45:74–80, 1947.

Wilkes, J. W.: Argyrosis of cornea and conjunctiva. *J. Tenn. Med. Assoc.*, 46:11–13, 1953.

Williamson, J.: A new look at the ocular side-effects of long-term systemic corticosteroid and adenocorticotrophic therapy. *Proc. R. Soc. Med.*, 63:791–92, 1970.

Williamson, J.; Paterson, R. W. W.; McGavin, D. D. N.; Jasani, M. K.; Boyle, J. A.; and Doig, W. M.: Posterior subcapsular cataracts and glaucoma associated with long-term oral corticosteroid therapy. In patients with rheumatoid arthritis and related conditions. *Br. J. Ophthalmol.*, 53:361–72, 1969.

Wirth, A.; Quaranta, C. A.; and Chistoni, G.: The effect of dithizone on the electroretinogram of the rabbit. *Bibl. Ophthalmol.*, 48:66–73, 1957.

Wood, C. A., and Buller, F.: Poisoning by wood alcohol. Cases of death and blindness from Columbian spirits and other methylated preparations. *J.A.M.A.*, 43:972–77; 1058–62; 1117–23; 1213–21; 1289–96, 1904.

Wood, D. C.; Contaxis, I.; Sweet, D.; Smith, J. C., II; and Van Dolah, J.: Response of rabbits to corticosteroids. I. Influence on growth, intraocular pressure and lens transparency. *Am. J. Ophthalmol.*, 63:841–49, 1967.

Yanoff, M., and Tsou, K-C.: A tetrazolium study of whole eye. *Arch. Ophthalmol.*, 59:808, 1965.

Young, A. G., and Loevenhart, A. S.: The relation of the chemical constitution of certain organic arsenical compounds to their action on the optic tract. *J. Pharmacol. Exp. Ther.*, 23:107–26, 1924.

Zvailfer, N. J.: The subcellular localization of chloroquine and its effect on lysosomal disruption. *Arthritis Rheum.*, 7:760–61, 1964.

Chapter 14

TOXIC RESPONSES OF THE BLOOD

Roger P. Smith

INTRODUCTION

For many years hematology concerned itself exclusively with the study of the formed elements of the blood. An immense body of knowledge has accrued from the microscopic study of smears of peripheral blood (Bessis, 1977), which constitutes a complex organ at least as large as the liver. Gradually the field expanded to include other essential parts of the system such as the bone marrow, spleen, lymph nodes, and the reticuloendothelial tissue consisting of phagocytic macrophages in the reticulum of various organs and lining many sinuses. Obviously, the formed elements have a functional interrelationship with the blood plasma and with the heart and the lungs. Most of the biochemical and hematologic parameters indicated in this chapter apply to man; Mitruka and Rawnsley (1977) have compiled an anthology of reference values for normal experimental animals.

HEMATOPOIESIS

In the human fetus several organs are involved in the production of the formed elements of the blood. For a very brief period the yolk sac produces nucleated red cells containing a special embryonic hemoglobin designated as $\alpha_2\epsilon_2$. Subsequent crops of red cells are furnished by the liver, the spleen, and eventually the bone marrow. These cells are not nucleated, but they contain fetal hemoglobin, $\alpha_2\gamma_2$. The oxygen affinity of human fetal blood is higher than that of human adult blood although that difference does not extend to the purified hemoglobins. At birth only the marrow is still producing red cells. A slow conversion from the synthesis of fetal to adult hemoglobin ($\alpha_2\beta_2$) begins at that time and it is usually completed by the fourth to sixth month of age. Up to the age of about four years hepatic and splenic red cell production can be reactivated in response to the normal demands of growth, but beyond that age these extramedullary sites are activated only in pathophysiologic states.

The Bone Marrow

Bone marrow contains stem cells, which are the immature precursors of the formed elements of the blood (Fig. 14–1). This multipotential stem cell pool is stimulated to differentiate into unipotential (or committed) cells, which eventually mature into red cells (erythrocytes), platelets (thrombocytes), or one of several series of white cells (leukocytes). Decreased numbers of these elements in peripheral blood are referred to respectively as anemia, thrombocytopenia, and leukopenia. Stimulation of the stem cell pool is carried out by blood-borne factors called "poietins." It is highly likely that each circulating cell type has its own poietin.

Erythropoiesis refers to the process by which red cells are produced. It is initiated by the release of an erythropoietic factor from the kidney and perhaps other organs or tissues. By mechanisms as yet poorly understood, hyperoxia and polycythemia (abnormally increased number of red cells in the blood) suppress the release of the renal erythropoietic factor (REF) whereas hypoxia, anemia, and cobalt increase REF release. The REF is an enzyme that acts on proerythropoietin, a blood protein released from the liver, to convert it to active erythropoietin. Polycythemia is one of the signs of cobalt toxicity. It was regularly observed in the epidemics of beer drinker's cardiomyopathy in the 1960s. The onset of these epidemics coincided with the introduction of minute amounts of cobalt into some brands of beer for the purpose of stabilizing the foam (e.g., Gosselin *et al.*, 1976).

In the marrow erythropoietin apparently acts on the differentiation process at the stage in which a stem cell is converted to a proerythroblast and then to a basophilic erythroblast (Fig. 14–1). Therefore, erythropoietin may be thought of as regulating the size of the committed red cell pool. After several additional stages, the immature red cell is released from the marrow as a reticulocyte. By then the cell has lost its nucleus and ability to divide. It still possesses an endoplasmic

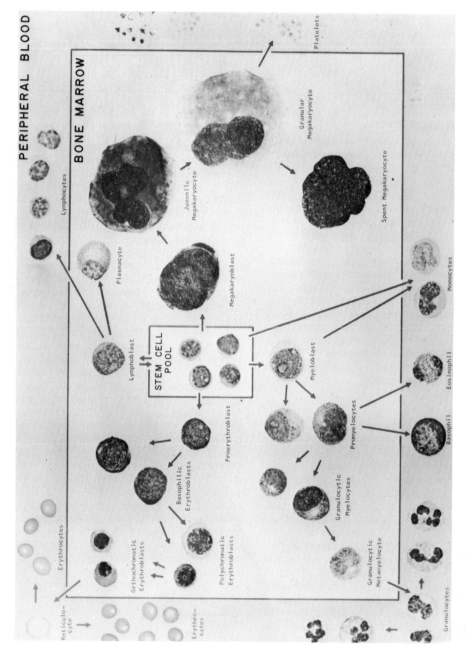

Figure 14–1. The normal morphology of the hematopoietic cells. (From Erslev, A. J., and Gabuzda, T. G.: *Pathophysiology of Blood.* W. B. Saunders Co., Philadelphia. 1975.)

reticulum (hence its name), and it can synthesize small amounts of hemoglobin. Cytochrome systems and the tricarboxylic acid cycle are still functional in the reticulocyte, but all of these are absent in the mature mammalian red cell. Birds, fish, amphibians and reptiles, however, always have nucleated red cells (Prankerd, 1961).

Presence of an abnormally large number of reticulocytes in the peripheral blood (more than 1 percent of the erythrocytes) is called reticulocytosis, and it indicates an accelerated replacement function of the bone marrow such as might occur in chronic hemolytic disease or several days following an acute episode of intravascular hemolysis. Reticulocytes are easily distinguished after supravital staining of peripheral blood smears. It is common to correct the crude percentage count of reticulocytes for any abnormality in the hematocrit or to present the absolute count where the normal is about 60,000/mm^3. The presence of nucleated "blast" forms in peripheral blood may indicate an even greater demand for replacement. Megaloblastic anemia may also be a sign of either vitamin B_{12} or folic acid deficiency. Folic acid antagonist drugs used in cancer chemotherapy (methotrexate) or as antimalarials (pyrimethamine, chlorguanide) may induce megaloblastic anemia as a side effect because they interfere with DNA but not RNA or protein synthesis (Stebbins and Bertino, 1976). Traditionally megaloblastic anemia is thought of as being associated with red cells, but all formed elements can be shown to be affected.

Similarly, chemicals toxic to the bone marrow can result in a decrease in the circulating numbers of all three major groups of formed elements, a condition known as pancytopenia. Agents regularly associated with pancytopenia provided that the exposure is sufficiently intense include ionizing radiation, benzene, antimetabolites, mustards, arsenic, chloramphenicol, trinitrotoluene, gold, hydantoin derivatives, and phenylbutazone (Harris and Kellermeyer, 1970).

The damage to the bone marrow may be so severe that it fails to proliferate, a condition described in morphologic terms as aplastic anemia. On the other hand, the marrow can have a normal cellularity or even hypercellularity but still fail to deliver normal formed elements or normal numbers of formed elements. Anemia of bone marrow failure is a functional description of a normal-appearing but unresponsive marrow. In addition to direct cytotoxic effects of chemicals on the marrow, which are usually mediated through disturbances in DNA structure or function, bone marrow damage may have an allergic basis involving antibodies to precursor cells and a sensitizing chemical. Chloramphenicol-induced bone marrow damage may sometimes involve immune mechanisms. Although the liver and the spleen can serve as a reserve erythropoietic effort, they cannot support life in the event of bone marrow failure; thus, chemical or physical damage to this vital organ is always a grave threat to survival.

Thrombocytes. Differentiation into thrombocytes, the smallest of the formed elements of the blood, is a unique process because it involves the largest cell type in the marrow, the megakaryocyte. One megakaryocyte results in the release of large numbers of thrombocytes. The spent form of this giant cell is then phagocytized in the marrow.

Platelets are the first line of defense against accidental blood loss. They accumulate almost instantaneously where vascular injury has exposed collagen fibers. Within seconds the normally nonsticky circulating platelets will adhere to these fibers, undergo degranulation, and release ADP, which in turn causes adhesion and aggregation of new platelets. In addition, another platelet factor is unmasked on the thrombocyte surface that augments thrombin formation. The platelet plug is then coated with fibrin resulting in a white thrombus. This process of intravascular coagulation also involves many other plasma factors as well.

Increasing knowledge about the mechanism of clot formation has suggested that the control of platelet aggregation by drugs may be useful in preventing the thromboembolic complications of such diseases as atherosclerosis and hypertension. Considerable interest has been focused on aspirin since epidemiologic evidence has suggested that its use may prevent a second myocardial infarction in patients who have already experienced one. Aspirin inhibition of platelet aggregation may depend on its ability to suppress prostaglandin synthesis since prostaglandins are known to have varied effects on the process.

A normal platelet count in man is about 250,000/mm^3. Thrombocytopenia is manifested by hemorrhagic disorders the most common of which is leakage from capillaries following minor injury (purpura). Petechiae, prolonged bleeding time, and impaired clot retraction are also consequences. Thrombocytopenia accompanies a bewildering array of congenital and acquired disorders, but drugs are the most common cause. The myelosuppressive anticancer drugs may cause thrombocytopenia as part of a generalized depression of bone marrow function, but cytosine arabinoside is said to affect platelet production somewhat specifically. Quinidine and phenacetin are widely recognized as causes of autoimmune thrombocytopenia, which results in increased peripheral platelet destruction. Thrombocytosis (an increased number of circulating platelets) has not as yet been associated with chemical injury.

Leukocytes. Leukocytes have the most complex organization and functions of the formed elements. They differ from other formed elements in that they perform important functions outside of the vascular compartment. Although each subtype seems to have some separate functions, the primary purpose for their existence appears to be to defend the body against "foreignness." Defense against foreign organisms or extraneous materials involves two mechanisms: (1) phagocytosis as carried out by the phagocytic series, and (2) antibody production as carried out by the immunocytic series (Fig. 14–2).

Phagocytes. The phagocytic series can be divided into the granulocytes (neutrophils, eosinophils, and basophils) and the monocyte-macrophages. Subdivision of the granulocytes can be accomplished on the basis of their reaction with Wright's stain, but these distinctions would be more valuable if their various functions were more clearly understood. Eosinophilia occurs in some allergic diseases and in infestations with large parasites whereas basophilia occurs in polycythemia vera, but the significance of these associations is unknown.

Granulocytes spend less than a day in the circulation before they become marginated (attached to blood vessel walls); they then pass between vascular epithelial cells by diapedesis and are disposed of in various tissues. Specific leukotaxines that increase capillary permeability are released from inflammatory lesions, and these induce local migration of granulocytes. The actual bactericidal activity appears to involve a destruction of bacterial membranes, and the release of lysosomal enzymes, pyrogens, and other degradation products may temporarily exacerbate the local inflammation. It is interesting that one effect of pharmacologic doses of glucocorticoids is to decrease the number of granulocytes that will diapedese and enter an exudate. Presumably this phenomenon accounts for increased susceptibility to infections of patients on steroids without a decrease in their rate of granulocyte production.

Monocytes exist in the blood for three to four days. After they migrate into reticuloendothelial tissues like liver, spleen, and bone marrow, they are called macrophages, and they survive in these sites for several months. Macrophages play a role in the phagocytic response to inflammation and infection, but they are also responsible for the ongoing destruction of senile blood cells. Denatured plasma proteins and plasma lipids are disposed of by pinocytosis. Macrophages are also involved in iron metabolism and possess inducible heme oxidase activity for the catabolism of hemoglobin.

The term "granulocytopenia" is used when the absolute granulocyte count is less than $3,000/mm^3$. When the count reaches $1,000/mm^3$, the patient becomes vulnerable to infection and at $500/mm^3$ the risk is very serious. The confusing term "agranulocytosis" is reserved for the serious granulocytopenias in which both the marginated pool and the bone marrow are devoid of neutrophils (also called neutropenia).

Granulocytopenia to varying degrees is the

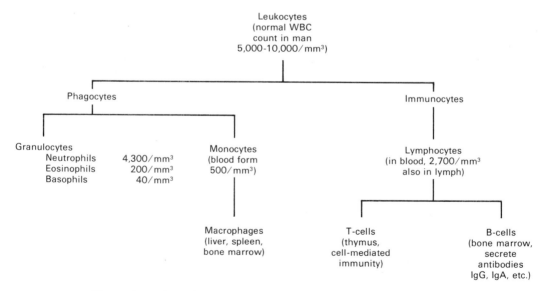

Figure 14–2. A classification of leukocytes and their normal values in man.

most common manifestation of chemically induced bone marrow damage, and many drugs as well as ionizing radiation can induce the reaction. Alkylating agents and antimetabolites regularly cause granulocytopenia, and phenothiazines, nonsteroidal anti-inflammatory drugs, antithyroid drugs, and some anticonvulsants sometimes elicit the reaction (Pisciotta, 1974). Peripheral destruction of granulocytes although an uncommon reaction has occurred via drug haptens after exposure to aminopyrine, phenylbutazone, and methyluracil. Granulocytes coated with the antigen-antibody complex are destroyed by the reticuloendothelial system.

An excess of granulocytes (granulocytosis) occurs transiently after the administration of epinephrine, cortisone, and some endotoxins, but it is not believed to be of any physiologic significance. Chronic granulocytosis has not been associated with exposure to specific chemicals. Granulocytosis is the term used when the granulocyte count is greater than 10,000/mm^3. When the count is greater than 30,000/mm^3, the term "leukemia" is employed. In patients far advanced with the disease the white cell "crit" may actually exceed the red cell "crit" and the blood will appear pale in accord with the German origins of the name. Chronic granulocytic leukemia has a better prognosis than the acute form of the disease. The former more commonly occurs in middle age, and although chemicals are suspected as etiologic agents, clear-cut associations have been difficult to make. The acute leukemias are often rapidly fatal in the absence of chemotherapy. They are usually classified into two groups: (1) acute lymphocytic leukemia (below) and (2) the acute myelogenous leukemias, which include all other bone marrow–derived leukocytes. Benzene, chloramphenicol, and phenylbutazone have been associated with acute myelogenous leukemia.

Neither monocytosis nor monocytopenia appears to be specifically induced by chemical injury, but either can be part of a generalized syndrome of bone marrow damage.

Immunocytes. The immunocytic series of leukocytes work in concert with the phagocytic series to defend the body against foreign invaders. Both the bone marrow and the thymus are primary lymphocyte-producing organs, and from these sites the cells are dispatched to populate secondary lymphatic tissue in the gastrointestinal tract (Peyer's patches) and the bursa in birds. Circulating pools of lymphocytes exist in both blood and lymph.

Immunocytic defense mechanisms are of two types. One is associated with the cell itself as in the case of the thymus lymphocytes (T cells). The other is humoral in the form of antibodies as in the case of the bone marrow–derived lymphocytes (B cells). Other characteristics distinguish between these cells such as the bizarre "hairy" appearance of B lymphocytes when viewed by scanning electron microscopy. Perhaps these structures are associated with the greater complement of surface immunoglobulins and receptors for antigen-antibody complexes of B cells. T cells can be distinguished by their ability to stick to sheep red cells and form rosettes.

T cell–mediated immunity is responsible for delayed hypersensitivity, homograft rejection, graft vs. host reactions, and defense against viral, fungal, bacterial, and, perhaps, neoplastic invasion. After receiving a specific antigenic stimulus, T cells are activated to perform several functions: (1) they appear to inhibit the migration of macrophages from the area, (2) they secrete cytotoxic factors, (3) they recruit other T cells, and (4) they form subpopulations of small nondividing lymphocytes that may remain dormant over the lifetime of the host but retain a "memory" of the event and can respond on reexposure to the initial antigen.

B cells must also be programmed with a specific antigen, and T cells appear to cooperate in the activation of B cells to plasma cells. Plasma cells cannot divide, but they can initiate antibody synthesis. A family of five immunoglobulins is produced of which IgG is by far the major type (Fig. 14–2), yet these five molecules exhibit both remarkable diversity and specificity in terms of antigenic reactions.

Lymphocytopenia is induced transiently by corticosteroids, but the significance of that response is unknown. Lymphocytosis and acute lymphocytic leukemia have not been associated with specific chemical insults.

Erythrocytes. No cell type in the human body has been studied as extensively as the red blood cell (Surgenor, 1975). This unique disk-shaped element has a diameter of about 8 μm, and its biconcave sides make it more than twice as thick at the periphery (about 2.4 μm) as it is in the center. Although devoid of intracellular organelles, special techniques in combination with scanning electron microscopy suggest that an internal structure may exist. As much as 30 percent of the wet weight of red cells consists of hemoglobin, which, in turn, is the most extensively studied protein in the world.

Normal human blood contains about 4.9 $\times$ 10^6 red cells/mm^3, which perform the essential function of transporting oxygen from the alveoli of the lungs to peripheral tissue, where it is used to support aerobic metabolism. Nor is the return trip wasted, since it serves as the means for the transport of waste carbon dioxide for excretion via the lungs. A small amount of carbon dioxide is transported in simple solution within the cell, but the bulk (75 percent) is transported as bicarbonate anion by virtue of the activity of carbonic anhydrase in the red cell. It is of interest that the remainder combines directly with free amino groups on hemoglobin to form carbamino-hemoglobin (Hb-NH-COOH). An analogous reaction occurs with cyanate, which can carbamylate the N-terminal valine residues resulting in a hemoglobin with an increased oxygen affinity (Cerami and Manning, 1971). Hemoglobin can also accept hydrogen ions, and it accounts for about 85 percent of the buffer capacity of the blood.

Acute damage to the red cell or its hemoglobin content can result in an impairment of oxygen transport with consequent peripheral hypoxia. The signs and symptoms in such cases are due secondarily to damage to the central nervous system and/or the heart, the organs most sensitive to oxygen lack. Normally the human erythrocyte remains in the blood for an average of 120 days before it ends its life in the spleen. Common laboratory animals (rabbits, rats, and especially guinea pigs and mice) have much shorter red cell survival times than man (Prankerd, 1961).

Anemia can arise if for any reason the rate of red cell destruction in peripheral blood exceeds the normal rate of production in bone marrow. Some chemicals are recognized as having acute and direct hemolytic effects *in vivo*, e.g., saponin, phenylhydrazine, arsine, and naphthalene. Other chemicals, such as primaquine among many others, produce hemolysis only in red cells congenitally deficient in glucose-6-phosphate dehydrogenase (cf. Fig. 14–5). Finally, peripheral destruction of red cells may involve an allergic mechanism (autoimmune hemolytic anemia) after sensitization by a chemical such as acetanilid.

ANEMIC HYPOXIA

Hypoxia refers to any condition in which there is an inadequate supply of oxygen to the tissues, but it is often useful to classify hypoxias on the basis of three quite different causes. Arterial or anoxic hypoxia is characterized by a lower-than-normal P_{O_2} in arterial blood when the oxygen capacity and rate of blood flow are normal or elevated. In toxic insults this type of hypoxia results from exposure to pulmonary irritants or drugs that depress the respiration. Anemic hypoxia is characterized by a lowered oxygen capacity when the arterial P_{O_2} and rate of blood flow are normal or elevated. Stagnant (hypokinetic) hypoxia is characterized by a decreased rate of blood flow. Sometimes a fourth condition, histotoxic hypoxia, is included in the classification (see below).

Oxygen Binding to Hemoglobin

Hemoglobin is an oligomeric protein with four separate peptide chains: two alpha chains and two beta chains ($\alpha_2\beta_2$); its molecular weight is about 67,000 daltons. Each peptide chain has a porphyrinic heme group bound in a non-covalent linkage (Fig. 14–3). The protein chains (globin) have irregularly folded conformations that enclose the heme group in a hydrophobic pocket. Hemoglobin is one of a handful of proteins for which the complete tertiary structure is known (Perutz *et al.*, 1968).

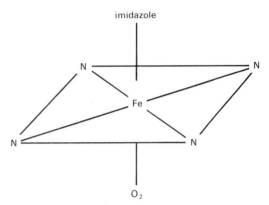

Figure 14–3. A stylized representation of a single heme group.

The structure of a single heme group may be represented diagrammatically as a square planar complex with the four nitrogens of the porphyrin ring at the angles. The central iron atom has a hexavalent coordination shell analogous to the inorganic iron complex, ferrocyanide. Of the two remaining coordination bonds, one is closely associated with an imidazole residue from the particular globin chain to which the heme group is attached. The remaining bond is available for reversible combination with molecular oxygen. No ligand is known to occupy this latter site in the case of deoxyhemoglobin. The reversible binding of oxygen by hemoglobin is called oxygenation, and the tertiary structures of the oxygenated and deoxygenated forms of hemoglobin are known to differ. Since conformational changes do not occur on oxygenation of a single globin chain-heme unit such as myoglobin, it follows that there are interactions between the four subunits comprising a hemoglobin molecule. These interactions are referred to as cooperativity.

A large body of experimental evidence now supports the concept that the deoxygenation process occurs in four separate steps, each with a different dissociation constant because of co-operativity changes that accompany the release of each successive oxygen molecule:

$$Hb_4O_8 \longrightarrow Hb_4O_6 + O_2 \quad K_1$$
$$Hb_4O_6 \longrightarrow Hb_4O_4 + O_2 \quad K_2$$
$$Hb_4O_4 \longrightarrow Hb_4O_2 + O_2 \quad K_3$$
$$Hb_4O_2 \longrightarrow Hb_4 + O_2 \quad K_4$$

It has not yet been possible to determine the exact values for each individual dissociation constant, K_1 through K_4. Both dissociation and association constants are defined here as equilibrium constants, the distinction between the two being merely the way in which the chemical equation is written. For the first equation shown above the dissociation constant has the value:

$$K_1 = \frac{[Hb_4O_6][O_6]}{[Hb_4O_8]}$$

with units of moles. The association constant would be the reciprocal expression with units of $moles^{-1}$. Obviously, the smaller the dissociation constant (or the larger the association constant), the more tightly the oxygen is bound and the more stable is the complex.

When the hemoglobin molecule is fully saturated, all of the oxygens are thought to be equivalent, and any one of them may be the first to be released in response to a fall in the ambient P_{O_2}. The release of the first oxygen, however, triggers a cooperativity change that greatly facilitates the release of the second oxygen molecule. Thus, K_1 is considerably smaller than K_2. In the same manner the release of the second oxygen facilitates the release of the third oxygen. Release of the fourth oxygen does not occur under normal physiologic conditions.

The above sequence of events is responsible for the sigmoid shape of the normal oxygen dissociation curve (Fig. 14–4). Since the total oxygen content of normal blood is about 20 ml/100 ml, the release of 5 ml/100 ml (or $\frac{1}{4}$ of the total) is analogous to the release of one oxygen molecule from a single hemoglobin tetramer. That release requires a change in the P_{O_2} of about 60 mm Hg (from point a to point V). The release of an additional 5 ml/100 ml, which is analogous to the dissociation of the second oxygen molecule, requires a further decrease in the P_{O_2} of only about 15 mm Hg (from about 40 down to 25 mm Hg) because of cooperativity. The release of the third increment of 5 ml/100 ml blood can then be effected by a decrease in the P_{O_2} of only 10 mm Hg. Thus, the properties of the hemoglobin molecule facilitate the loading and unloading of large amounts of oxygen over a physiologically critical range of P_{O_2}.

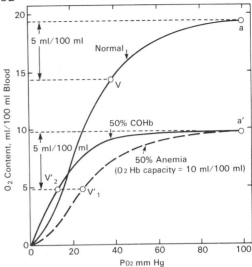

Figure 14–4. Normal oxyhemoglobin dissociation curve and curves for the case of a 50 percent anemia and the case of a 50 percent carboxyhemoglobinemia. The delivery of 25 percent of the total oxygen content of fully oxygenated arterial blood (5 ml/100 ml blood) requires a drop in the P_{O_2} of about 60 mm Hg (from point a to point V on the normal curve). Delivery of a comparable volume of oxygen in the case of a 50 percent anemia requires a drop in the P_{O_2} of more than 75 mm Hg (from point a' to point V_1'), but an even greater fall in the P_{O_2} is required to deliver the same volume of oxygen in the case of the curve distorted by the presence of carboxyhemoglobin (from point a' to point V_2'). See text for an explanation for this phenomenon. (From Bartlett, D., Jr.: Effects of carbon monoxide in human physiological processes. *Proceedings of the Conference on Health Effects of Air Pollutants*, Washington, D.C. U.S. Government Printing Office, Serial 93–15, pp. 103–26, Nov., 1973).

Carbon Monoxide Binding to Hemoglobin

Carbon monoxide is the best-known example of an agent that can decrease the oxygen transport capability of the blood and produce an anemic hypoxia. The elucidation of its mechanism of action by Claude Bernard in 1865 is a classic example of the successful application of the experimental method.

Claude Bernard's deductions about the mechanism of action of carbon monoxide were formalized by Douglas and the Haldanes in 1912. The so-called Haldane equation quantitatively defines the competition between oxygen and carbon monoxide for the same ferrous heme-binding sites on hemoglobin:

$$\frac{[COHb]}{[HbO_2]} = M \frac{[P_{CO}]}{[P_{O_2}]}$$

The constant, M, has the value of 220 at pH 7.4 for human blood. Therefore, if the $P_{CO} = 1/220 \times P_{O_2}$, the blood at equilibrium will be half-saturated with oxygen and half-saturated with carbon monoxide. Since air contains 21 percent oxygen by volume, it is obvious that exposure to a gas mixture of 0.1 percent carbon monoxide in air would result in a 50 percent carboxyhemoglobinemia in man at sea level. For this reason carbon monoxide is potentially dangerous at very low concentrations. However, the rate at which the arterial blood approaches equilibrium with the inspired concentration depends on such factors as the diffusion capacity of the lungs and the alveolar ventilation both of which in turn depend on the level of exercise of the subject.

Some species variation is recognized with respect to the value of M, but this is not necessarily a major determinant of the species sensitivity to carbon monoxide. For example, the well-known sensitivity of the canary to carbon monoxide is more likely due to its higher rate of aerobic metabolism. Other factors being equal, a high metabolic rate renders the species more sensitive to hypoxic stress. Moreover, such species tend to have faster rates of alveolar gas exchange to support their metabolic demands and approach equilibrium saturation of their hemoglobin more rapidly (Spencer, 1961).

If, instead of oxygen, hemoglobin is exposed to pure carbon monoxide, a gradual decrease in the P_{CO} would allow one to describe a series of dissociation constants for carboxyhemoglobin analogous to those for oxyhemoglobin. If the absolute value for each of the latter were known, the former could be derived, e.g., $K_{1O_2}/220 = K_{1CO}$, by correcting for the more tenacious binding of carbon monoxide. In actual experience this principle holds as a first approximation. Thus, the hemoglobin molecule has no intrinsic mechanism for distinguishing between oxygen and carbon monoxide, and carboxyhemoglobin exhibits the phenomenon of cooperativity as does oxyhemoglobin.

When carbon monoxide and oxygen are present together, another phenomenon is observed that has profound physiologic significance (Fig. 14–4). If deoxyhemoglobin is exposed to a gas mixture in which the $P_{CO} = 1/220\ P_{O_2}$, at equilibrium half the heme groups will be occupied by carbon monoxide and half by oxygen. The distribution of the two ligands among the four heme groups on any one hemoglobin molecule, however, is random. Thus, the blood will contain a distribution of hybrid species in which most molecules will contain both oxygen and carbon monoxide. Chance would dictate that the most common species would be a molecule with two oxygens and two carbon monoxides, e.g., $Hb_4(O_2)_2(CO)_2$.

In Figure 14–4 the experimental conditions have been contrived in such a way that the P_{CO} is held constant while the P_{O_2} can be reduced. Therefore, half the total number of heme-binding sites are always occupied by carbon monoxide irrespective of the degree of oxygen saturation. For the most common hybrid species, $Hb_4(O_2)_2$-$(CO)_2$, only two oxygen molecules are available for dissociation, and there can be only one opportunity for cooperativity to facilitate the dissociation of oxygen. In effect, only the top half of the dissociation curve can be called into play, and it is displaced downward because of the loss of half the total oxygen capacity. Since cooperativity cannot be utilized to facilitate the dissociation of a third oxygen molecule, the result is an apparent increase in the mean binding strength for oxygen (a shift to the left of the curve) and a distortion in the shape of the curve from its normal sigmoid appearance. The physiologic significance of this phenomenon may be grasped from Figure 14–4, where a change in the P_{O_2} of about 75 mm Hg is required to deliver 5 ml O_2/100 ml of blood to peripheral tissue in the case of a 50-percent anemia. Here the residual hemoglobin functions normally with respect to the influence of cooperativity even though the total oxygen content is only half that of normal. In the case of a 50-percent carboxyhemoglobinemia, however, a change of 85 mm Hg or more in the P_{O_2} is required to deliver the same 5 ml O_2/100 ml of blood. Obviously, the latter individual would be more severely compromised in terms of peripheral hypoxia.

Carbon Monoxide Poisoning. Although the above model is felt to be useful for understanding the molecular events at work in carbon monoxide poisoning, other factors influence the course of events in intact animals and man. Lower portions of the oxygen dissociation curve will be forced into play, and changes in regional blood flow will shunt the perfusion toward the more critical organs. Changes in ventilation will result in changes in the rate of hemoglobin saturation with carbon monoxide. Exposure to very high ambient concentrations can result in sufficient hemoglobin saturation to produce death in minutes with almost no premonitory signs, but equilibrium between hemoglobin saturation and ambient P_{CO} occurs slowly on exposure to low concentrations of the gas. For these reasons a poor correlation exists between the blood content of carboxyhemoglobin and signs and symptoms in poisoned humans.

The presence of carboxyhemoglobin can result in a significant decrease in the oxygen content of blood, but the ambient concentration is rarely high enough to result in a detectable decrease in the arterial P_{O_2}. Thus, chemoreceptor mechanisms may not be triggered, and the usual respiratory parameters may remain within normal limits. Peripheral vasodilation in response to a slowly developing hypoxia may exceed the compensatory ability to increase the cardiac output. For this reason fainting is more common than dyspnea in victims of carbon monoxide poisoning, and consciousness may be lost for long periods before death. Tachycardia and ECG changes suggestive of hypoxia have been observed at carboxyhemoglobin saturations of 30 percent or even lower. Other symptoms include headache, weakness, nausea, dizziness, and dimness of vision. Lactic acidemia may result from impaired aerobic metabolism. Unconsciousness, coma, convulsions, and death are associated with 50-to-80-percent saturation.

Carbon monoxide is not a cumulative poison in the usual sense. Carboxyhemoglobin is fully dissociable, and, once an acute exposure has been terminated, the pigment will eventually revert to oxyhemoglobin and the carbon monoxide will be excreted via the lungs. Certain individuals occupationally exposed to carbon monoxide, such as garage workers or traffic policemen, may suffer acute recurring toxic episodes during each working day. Without an adequate medical history, the unwary physician may be presented with a baffling symptom complex. Eventually in cases such as these and in cases of single massive exposure, permanent sequelae may result from hypoxic damage to neural structures.

Carboxyhemoglobin is a cherry red color, and its presence in high concentrations in capillary blood may impart an abnormal red color to the skin, mucous membranes, and fingernails. Carbon monoxide combines with other heme proteins such as myoglobin and cytochromes, including P_{450}, but these reactions have no significance in acute poisoning. This point was made by Haldane in 1895 by placing mice in a high concentration of carbon monoxide together with 2 atmospheres of oxygen. Even though the circulating blood pigment in these animals was totally in the form of carboxyhemoglobin enough oxygen was carried in physical solution in their blood to prevent signs of poisoning.

Management of Carbon Monoxide Poisoning. The obvious and specific antagonist to carbon monoxide is oxygen. After termination of the exposure, respirations must be supported artificially if necessary. By increasing the ambient P_{O_2}, advantage can be taken of the mass law to increase significantly the rate of conversion of carboxyhemoglobin to oxyhemoglobin *in vivo*. For example, the half-recovery time in terms of blood carboxyhemoglobin levels for resting adults breathing air at 1 atmosphere is 320 minutes.

When oxygen is given at 1 atmosphere, the time is decreased to 80 minutes. By the use of hyperbaric chambers developing 3 atmospheres of oxygen, this time can be further reduced to 23 minutes, although such measures carry some risk of oxygen poisoning. Exchange transfusion has also been used for moribund victims.

The addition of 5 to 7 percent carbon dioxide to oxygen to serve as a respiratory stimulant (with precautions against rebreathing) does hasten the pulmonary excretion of carbon monoxide. At the same time it entails some risk of compounding the metabolic acidosis arising from tissue hypoxia. (Gosselin *et al.*, 1976).

Endogenous and Environmental Carbon Monoxide. Nonsmoking human adults normally do not have more than 1 percent of their total circulating blood pigment in the form of carboxyhemoglobin, but heavy smokers may show values as high as 5 to 10 percent saturation. Combustion and automobile exhaust (4 to 7 percent carbon monoxide) are other key environmental sources. For many years it was presumed that environmental exposure was responsible for the low levels of carboxyhemoglobin found in the general population, but in 1967 Coburn and coworkers established that carbon monoxide is generated endogenously in normal humans. A major source of this endogenous carbon monoxide arises from the catabolism of heme proteins, principally hemoglobin, although catalase and cytochromes contribute small amounts.

The alpha-methene bridge of the heme porphyrin is the group metabolized, and carbon monoxide is generated in amounts that are equimolar to the bile pigment produced or to the heme catabolized. The average rate of production (0.4 ml/hr) is increased in hemolytic disease because of increased heme catabolism. The physiologic significance of this source in combination with environmental exposure is not well defined at present. Indeed, the entire subject of chronic low-level exposure to carbon monoxide is being subjected to an intensive reexamination. (National Academy of Sciences, 1977a).

Methemoglobinemia

The heme iron of hemoglobin is susceptible to a true chemical oxidation involving a valence change from the ferrous to the ferric state. The resulting pigment is called methemoglobin. It is greenish brown to black in color, and it cannot combine reversibly with oxygen or with carbon monoxide. Therefore, methemoglobinemia is another potential cause of anemic hypoxia. As in the oxidation of simple inorganic coordination complexes like ferrocyanide, the oxidation of the heme iron does not change the total number (six) of the bonds in the coordination shell (Fig. 14-3). The additional positive charge on the heme iron itself is satisfied in physiologic solutions by hydroxyl or chloride anions. The ferric heme iron can also combine with a variety of nonphysiologic anions, a property that has been exploited for therapeutic purposes.

Methemoglobin has at least one additional property that is of toxicologic interest, namely, its ability to dissociate complete heme groups as units. When methemoglobin is free in plasma instead of in intact red cells, the transfer of heme groups to albumin results in methemalbumin, an abnormal pigment found during acute hemolytic crises such as transfusion reactions, severe malaria, paroxysmal nocturnal hemoglobinuria, and poisonings by some chemicals such as chlorate salts.

Spontaneous Hemoglobin Oxidation. Although the rate of hemoglobin oxidation is greatly increased by exposure to a variety of chemicals, heme group oxidation occurs spontaneously in air. Presumably spontaneous or autoxidation accounts for the very low concentrations (less than 2 percent) found in normal circulating blood. As studied *in vitro* autoxidation appears to be a first-order process with respect to the concentrations of the ferrous forms of either hemoglobin or myoglobin. The first-order rate constants, however, depend in a complex manner on the partial pressure of oxygen. The rate constants are maximal at partial pressures of oxygen that correspond to half-saturation of the heme groups. Since a reaction mechanism in which a deoxygenated molecule (or heme group) interacts with an oxygenated one would not exhibit first-order kinetics, a multistep mechanism is inferred. The quasi-first-order kinetics can then be explained as arising from an algebraic artifact rather than any single intramolecular, rate-determining step. The complexity of these reactions is illustrated by studies on their stoichiometry. Both myoglobin and hemoglobin oxidation consume many times more oxygen than can be accounted for on the basis of the reduction of an appropriate amount of oxygen to water (Smith and Olson, 1973).

Methemoglobin-Generating Chemicals. Some chemicals capable of mediating the oxidation of hemoglobin are active both *in vivo* and *in vitro*. Others are active only *in vivo*, and a third group are active only in lysates or solutions of hemoglobin. Among chemicals active both *in vivo* and *in vitro*, sodium nitrite is the best known. Inorganic hydroxylamine has some similarities to nitrite, but these two agents appear to oxidize hemoglobin by different mechanisms (Cranston and Smith, 1971).

The mechanism of the reaction between hemoglobin and nitrite is still not understood. Under strictly anaerobic conditions 1 mole of nitrite yields 1 mole of ferric heme and 1 mole of the ferroheme-NO complex. Under physiologic conditions and in the presence of an excess of nitrite complete conversion to methemoglobin occurs, but the heme oxygen is largely consumed. After a lag phase, the reaction proceeds with a pronounced autocatalytic phase that is not observed when nitrite reacts with deoxyhemoglobin (e.g., Smith and Olson, 1973). Nitrite is also included among those anions that can complex with ferric heme groups. Thus, excess nitrite first generates methemoglobin then forms a nitrite-methemoglobin complex. The latter has significance for the spectrophotometric determination of methemoglobin (van Assendelft and Ziljstra, 1965), and it may account for the uniquely protracted nitrite methemoglobinemia observed in some species as compared with other chemicals active *in vivo* (Smith, 1967).

Organic compounds active both *in vivo* and *in vitro* include some simple aminophenols and certain *N*-hydroxyarylamines (Kiese, 1974). As tested in mice, phenylhydroxylamine, *N*-hydroxy-*p*-aminotoluene, and *N*-hydroxy-*p*-acetophenone were all about equipotent, i.e., generated equivalent peak concentrations of methemoglobin at equal doses. At the same time all these were ten or more times more potent than nitrite, hydroxylamine, or simple aminophenols (Smith *et al.*, 1967). It is now clear that intraerythrocytic recycling accounts for the high potency of phenylhydroxylamine relative to other compounds. According to Kiese (1974), phenylhydroxylamine and hemoglobin react to form methemoglobin and nitrosobenzene. In the intact normal red cell provided with substrate, mechanisms exist for the reduction of nitrosobenzene to regenerate phenylhydroxylamine. The requirement of this reaction for glucose (as opposed to lactate) suggests that some component of the pentose phosphate shunt such as NADPH is involved in the cycle (cf. Fig. 14-5). Although phenylhydroxylamine is active in lysates, under those conditions it is no more potent than nitrite. Similarly aminophenols and inorganic hydroxylamine are not recycled in red cells so they are equipotent in intact red cells and in lysates.

Among agents active only *in vivo* the aromatic amines and arylnitro compounds are best known. Amyl nitrite and other aliphatic nitrites and nitrates are weakly active at best. Obviously these substances must be metabolized *in vivo* to active forms presumably by mixed-function oxidase activity in the liver. It has long been suspected that the active metabolites are either aminophenols or *N*-hydroxy derivatives. For some compounds such as aniline and nitrobenzene the relative importance of these two possible metabolites still has not been clarified. In contrast, conclusive evidence has established

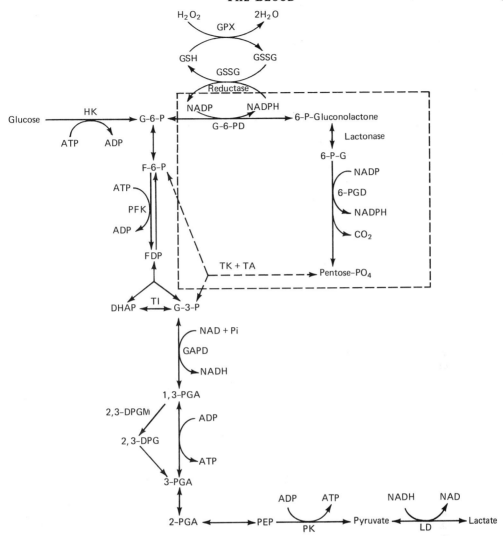

Figure 14–5. The metabolic resources of the mature mammalian red cell. *GSH*, reduced glutathione; *GSSG*, oxidized glutathione; *G-6-P*, glucose-6-phosphate; *F-6-P*, fructose-6-phosphate; *FDP*, fructose-1,6-diphosphate; *DHAP*, dihydroxyacetone phosphate; *G-3-P*, glyceraldehyde-3-phosphate; *LD*, lactic dehydrogenase; *NADP*, oxidized triphosphopyridine nucleotide; *NADPH*, reduced triphosphopyridine nucleotide; *NAD*, oxidized diphosphopyridine nucleotide; *NADH*, reduced diphosphopyridine nucleotide; *6-P-G*, 6-phosphogluconate; *G-6-PD*, glucose-6-phosphate dehydrogenase; *TK*, transketolase; *TA*, transaldolase; *Pi*, inorganic phosphate; *ADP*, adenosine diphosphate; *ATP*, adenosine triphosphate; *PEP*, phosphoenolpyruvate; *PK*, pyruvic kinase; *1,3-PGA*, 1,3-phosphoglyceric acid; *3-PGA*, 3-phosphoglyceric acid; *2-PGA*, 2-phosphoglyceric acid; *2,3-DPG*, 2,3-diphosphoglyceric acid; *6-PGD*, 6-phosphogluconate dehydrogenase; *PFK*, phosphofructokinase; *HK*, hexokinase; *TI*, trioseisomerase; *GPX*, glutathione peroxidase; *GAPD*, glyceraldehyde-3-phosphate dehydrogenase; *2,3-DPGM*, 2,3-diphosphoglycerate mutase. (Modified from Harris, J. W., and Kellermeyer, R. W.: *The Red Cell—Production, Metabolism, Destruction: Normal and Abnormal*, rev. ed. Harvard University Press, Cambridge, Mass., 1970.)

that the active metabolite of *p*-aminopropiophenone (PAPP) in several species is the *N*-hydroxy metabolite. Thus, the high potency of PAPP can be ascribed to the intraerythrocytic mechanism for the recycling of the active metabolite. The case of PAPP is exceptionally

well documented. For most agents active *in vivo* the methemoglobin-generating metabolites are still not known with certainty. In the case of nitrobenzene recent evidence suggests that the active metabolite in rats is generated by nitroreductases in the intestinal microflora rather than in the liver (Reddy *et al.*, 1976). For this group of chemicals prominent species differences may be anticipated that depend on differences in the rates of activation and detoxication of the parent compounds.

Two compounds with widely different chemical properties are active chiefly or only in lysates. The first of these is potassium ferricyanide, which cannot penetrate the intact red cell membrane. Even so, it is widely used in the laboratory as a reagent for generating methemoglobin standards in solution. One mole of ferricyanide mediates the oxidation of one mole of heme whether or not oxygen is present. If oxyhemoglobin is used, the heme oxygen is quantitatively released. Ferrocyanide is generated, which can bind tenaciously to the globin moiety of the methemoglobin.

An interesting contrast with phenylhydroxylamine is the paradoxic methemoglobin-generating activity of methylene blue, which is prominent only in lysates (Smith and Thron, 1972). The products of this reaction are methemoglobin and leucomethylene blue. The latter is spontaneously reoxidized by molecular oxygen so that a cyclic mechanism is established in this case also. The potency of methylene blue as a methemoglobin-generating agent in lysates is roughly equivalent to that of phenylhydroxylamine in intact cells provided with substrate. Conversely, as already noted, phenylhydroxylamine is only weakly active in lysates whereas methylene blue in intact cells provided with substrate actively reduces methemoglobin (see below).

Susceptibility of Mammalian Hemoglobins to Oxidation. Inherent differences are recognized among hemoglobins in their susceptibility to oxidation by various agents (Bartels *et al.*, 1963). Such differences undoubtedly reflect structural or conformational variations, but their contribution to the overall methemoglobinemic response seems necessarily small. For example, Smith and Beutler (1966a) found the conversion half-times in minutes for hemoglobin solutions exposed to identical concentrations of nitrite to be about 2 for sheep, goat, and bovine hemoglobin, 3 for human hemoglobin, 4 for equine hemoglobin, and up to 7 for porcine hemoglobin. Such differences cannot play a major role since even in species resistant to nitrite an acute methemoglobinemia can be expected to last for several hours.

Pathophysiology of Methemoglobinemias. Impairment of the oxygen transport capability of the blood is not the only analogy between carboxyhemoglobin and methemoglobin. The presence of a certain fraction of methemoglobin distorts the oxygen dissociation curve of residual hemoglobin in a manner analogous to the presence of a certain fraction of carboxyhemoglobin. Presumably this analogy extends also to the mechanism for the distortion, as discussed above for carbon monoxide. The distortion with a given fraction of methemoglobin, however, is said to be less drastic than with an identical fraction of carboxyhemoglobin.

As an experimental tool for the study of the effects of peripheral hypoxia, methemoglobinemia is less satisfactory than simulated altitude, oxygen replacement, or exposure to carbon monoxide. Unless the methemoglobin-generating chemical is continuously infused, it is impossible to maintain stable circulating levels of the pigment for prolonged periods of time. If death does not intervene, a variety of intraerythrocytic reductive mechanisms are activated to reduce methemoglobin back to hemoglobin. With a single dose of the agent, methemoglobin levels tend to rise abruptly and then decline toward normal at rates that vary widely with the species. These fluctuating levels of circulating methemoglobin undoubtedly lead to wide variations in peripheral oxygen tensions.

Moreover, all chemical agents used to generate methemoglobin have additional toxic effects, and, unlike carbon monoxide, these side effects may make profound contributions to the toxic syndrome. Some aromatic amino and nitro compounds, such as aniline and nitrobenzene, have central and prominent cardiac effects that in some species, including man, appear to be the proximal cause of death. Chlorate salts produce intravascular hemolysis, and the "methemoglobin" formed appears to be largely extracellular. Inorganic salts of nitrite and organic nitrates and nitrites also act directly as peripheral vasodilators. A stagnant (hypokinetic) hypoxia due to orthostatic hypotension, reflex tachycardia, circulatory inadequacy, and cardiovascular collapse certainly compound the effects of a nitrite methemoglobinemia. Unsubstituted hydroxylamine and even *p*-aminopropiophenone in large doses produce Heinz bodies, sulfhemoglobin, and hemolysis as well as methemoglobin (Cranston and Smith 1971).

It is doubtful that any chemical agent produces an otherwise uncomplicated methemoglobinemia, although PAPP in moderate doses appears to approach this experimental ideal. Large differences among various agents can be shown to exist for the methemoglobin levels measured at the time of death, even when tested in a single species (Smith and Olson, 1973). Therefore, it is inappropriate and misleading to suggest that there is a "lethal level of methemoglobin" without account to the particular agent and species involved.

Metabolic Resources of the Mature Mammalian Red Cell. Unlike carboxyhemoglobin, which spontaneously dissociates in accord with the ambient partial pressures of oxygen and carbon monoxide metabolic energy must be expended by the red cell to reduce methemoglobin to hemoglobin. Indeed, a major share of the total metabolic energy of the red cell is directed toward that end and toward the maintenance of the integrity of the cell membrane. As shown in Figure 14–5, however, the metabolic resources of the mature mammalian red cell are rather limited. Only two anaerobic alternatives are available for glucose metabolism: (1) the Embden-Meyerhof (glycolytic) pathway and (2) the pentose phosphate (phosphogluconic acid, hexosemonophosphate) shunt (enclosed by dashed lines in Figure 14–5).

The enzyme glucose-6-phosphate dehydrogenase occupies a key position in red cell metabolism. It introduces the shunt and participates in the reduction of NADP. An additional mole of NADP is reduced in the next reaction by 6-phosphogluconate dehydrogenase. Since the shunt is the only source of NADPH in the mature human red cell, the appropriate selection of substrates can thwart NADP reduction while permitting NAD reduction. If lactate is substituted for glucose, NADH is generated via the activity of lactic dehydrogenase. In some mammalian erythrocytes stereospecificity of glucose-6-phosphate dehydrogenase prevents the utilization of galactose as a substrate in the shunt although it is available for glycolysis (Smith and Beutler, 1966b).

Methemoglobin Reducing Systems. *Spontaneous Methemoglobin Reduction.* The major system responsible for methemoglobin reduction in mammalian red cells (to the extent of at least 60 percent) is methemoglobin reductase or diaphorase. As indicated in Figure 14–6, this intracellular enzyme requires NADH as a cofactor.

Chronic methemoglobinemia in rare individuals without exposure to suspect chemicals has been recognized for more than a century. In 1959 Scott and Griffith demonstrated that the erythrocytes of some chronically methemoglobinemic individuals were deficient in NADH-methemoglobin reductase. From 10 to 50 percent of their total circulating blood pigment existed as methemoglobin, whereas in the general population values rarely exceed 2 percent. Since their methemoglobin levels remain at a steady state throughout life, alternative mechanisms for methemoglobin reduction must be available but deficient individuals are extremely sensitive to methemoglobin-generating chemicals. So are newborns, although high concentrations of fetal hemoglobin may contribute as much to their sensitivity as the recognized transient deficiency in NADH-reductase.

The congenital methemoglobinopathies due to abnormal amino acid substitutions in the globin chain constitute a separate disease entity. These abnormalities as in hemoglobin M or H apparently enhance heme dissociation, rendering the iron more

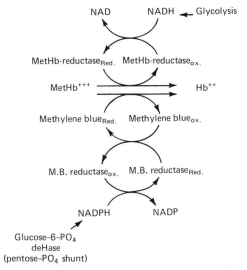

Figure 14–6. The spontaneous (*NADH*) and the dormant (*NADPH*) methemoglobin reductase systems. Methemoglobin (*MetHb*) reductase is active in intact red cells in the presence of substrates that can provide for NAD reduction. The NADPH system requires intact red cells, glucose or its metabolic equivalent, a functioning pentose phosphate shunt, and methylene blue (*M.B.*). M.B.-reductase reduces M.B., which in turn nonenzymatically reduces MetHb.

susceptible to molecular oxygen. Such individuals are also sensitive to oxidant chemicals despite a normal NADH-reductase activity.

The duration of a methemoglobinemia after an acute challenge with sodium nitrite is largely determined by the methemoglobin reductase activity in the erythrocytes of that species. As shown in Table 14–1, a greater than tenfold difference exists among the listed species with respect to methemoglobin reductase activity. It is presumed that these data represent primarily NADH-reductase activity, although the contributions from alternative pathways for the most part have not been evaluated. In each case glucose was the substrate, and the data have been expressed as a ratio of the species activity to that in human cells. In order to place these ratios in some perspective, estimates of the reduction half-time for high (80 to 100 percent) levels of methemoglobin in normal human red cells under similar conditions range from 6 to about 24 (Bolyai et al., 1972) hours. In general, rates of reduction tend to decrease with decreasing methemoglobin levels.

Table 14–1 shows that pig and horse red cells have considerably lower rates of methemoglobin reduction than human red cells. Both of these species are said to utilize plasma lactate in preference to glucose to drive reduction (Rivkin and Simon, 1965; Robin and Harley, 1967). Rat, guinea pig, mouse, and rabbit red cells have relatively high rates of methemoglobin reductase activity. The significance of these differences remains unknown.

Table 14-1. SPONTANEOUS METHEMOGLOBIN REDUCTASE ACTIVITY OF MAMMALIAN ERYTHROCYTES*

SPECIES	INVESTIGATORS (1)	(2)	(3)	(4)	(5)
	Activity in Species/Activity in Man				
Pig	0.37	0.37		0.09	
Horse	0.75	0.50		0.64	
Cat		0.50	0.85	1.2	1.0
Cow	0.80	0.75		1.1	
Goat	1.1	0.75			
Dog		0.88	1.4	1.3	1.0
Sheep	1.4	1.0		2.1	
Rat		1.4	1.3	1.9	5.0
Guinea pig		1.2	2.4	1.9	4.5
Rabbit		3.5	3.3	3.8	7.5
Mouse					9.5

* Data from various investigators using nitrited red cells with glucose as a substrate have been normalized by making a ratio of the activity of the species to the activity in human red cells. The indicated investigators are: (1) Smith and Beutler, 1966a; (2) Malz, 1962; (3) Kiese and Weis, 1943; (4) Robin and Harley, 1966; (5) Stolk and Smith, 1966; Smith *et al.*, 1967; Bolyai *et al.*, 1972.

The Dormant NADPH-Reductase System. Normal human and most mammalian erythrocytes possess a second reductive system that requires NADPH as a cofactor. The physiologic role of this system is not understood. In most species the system appears to be dormant, and it is activated only in the presence of exogenously added electron carriers such as methylene blue. According to Sass and coworkers (1969), the enzyme involved reduces methylene blue to the leuco form, which in turn nonenzymatically reduces methemoglobin (Fig. 14–6).

The evidence that this system plays no important physiologic role in methemoglobin reduction is compelling. What may be an extremely rare congenital deficiency of this enzyme has been found (Sass *et al.*, 1967), and the propositus had normal levels of methemoglobin. Moreover, in cases of a far more common congenital deficiency, namely that of glucose-6-phosphate dehydrogenase, individuals are not methemoglobinemic despite decreased shunt activity and impaired NADP-reductive capacity. Although this system plays no physiologic role, its therapeutic activation is an important procedure for

the management of acute acquired methemoglobinemia. It cannot be activated, however, in either of the deficiency states noted above.

Species differences are also recognized in terms of the magnitude of the response to added methylene blue (Table 14–2), but all species tested responded to the dye (1 to 2×10^{-5} M) by an increase in reductase activity over that observed with glucose alone. The data are expressed as a ratio of the species increase to the increase observed in human cells under the same conditions. To place these ratios in some perspective, estimates of the reduction half time of high (70 to 90 percent) levels of methemoglobin in normal human red cells with methylene blue range from 45 to 90 minutes (Layne and Smith, 1969). A certain parallelism is noted between Tables 14–1 and 14–2 in that species with high spontaneous rates of reductase activity respond more vigorously to methylene blue, with the possible exception of the rabbit. The nucleated red cells of reptiles and birds have both NADH and NADPH reductase activity, but in this case the tricarboxylic acid cycle appears to be the source of the NADH (Board *et al.*, 1977).

Table 14-2. STIMULATION OF METHEMOGLOBIN REDUCTASE ACTIVITY OF MAMMALIAN ERYTHROCYTES BY METHYLENE BLUE*†

SPECIES	INVESTIGATORS (1)	(2)	(3)	(4)	(5)
	Increased Activity, Species/Increased Activity, Man				
Pig	0.05	0.03		0.15	
Horse	0.10	0.06		0.25	
Goat	0.50	0.03			
Sheep	0.38	0.28		0.45	
Cow	0.42	0.34		1.0	
Cat		0.69	0.16	0.65	1.0
Dog		0.41	0.24	0.85	1.0
Rabbit		0.50	1.4	0.70	0.50
Mouse					1.1
Guinea pig		1.3	0.94	2.4	
Rat		2.1	1.0	2.2	1.9

* Data from various sources using nitrited red cells with glucose as a substrate have been normalized by the ratio:

$$\frac{(\text{activity M.B. and glucose} - \text{activity glucose})_{species}}{(\text{activity M.B. and glucose} - \text{activity glucose})_{human}}$$

† See footnote to Table 14–1 for literature citation.

Minor Pathways for Methemoglobin Reduction. Several minor pathways exist in red cells for methemoglobin reduction, which are at least in part nonenzymatic. Reduced glutathione slowly reduces methemoglobin, but it can account only for 12 percent of the total erythrocyte reductive capacity (Scott et al., 1965) Ascorbic acid (vitamin C) has been used to reduce methemoglobin levels in individuals with NADH-reductase deficiency, but this reaction is too sluggish to be of value in an acute methemoglobinemic crisis. It accounts for no more that 16 percent of the reductive effort of the red cell. Methemoglobinemia is not found in subjects with frank ascorbate deficiency (scurvy) or in subjects with abnormally low levels of reduced glutathione in their red cells (glucose-6-phosphate dehydrogenase deficiency). The guinea pig is one of the few non-primate mammals unable to synthesize ascorbate. Oddly, methemoglobinemic guinea pig red cells do not respond to ascorbate as do human red cells (Bolyai et al., 1972). NADH, NADPH, cysteine, and ergothioneine also have limited capacities for direct methemoglobin reduction.

Management of Chemical Methemoglobinemias. Although all methemoglobin-generating chemicals have additional toxic effects, it is generally agreed that a reduction in the circulating titer of the abnormal pigment is a desirable therapeutic goal. For agents that produce hemolysis as well as methemoglobin and methemalbumin (e.g., chlorate salts) exchange transfusion is the only present approach to that goal. If the methemoglobin is contained within intact and functional erythrocytes, the intravenous administration of methylene blue (1 to 2 mg/kg) usually evokes a dramatic response (Gosselin et al., 1976). Although a spectrum of efficacy can be shown experimentally in human red cells exposed to various agents, methylene blue provides unequivocal protection against death in animals, with all methemoglobin generating agents tested. (Smith and Layne, 1969).

A suggested alternative that would bypass the lesion in the oxygen-transport function of the blood is hyperbaric oxygen. Although recommended on empirical grounds for many years, this procedure has only recently been investigated experimentally. Goldstein and Doull (1971) found that oxygen at 4 atmospheres decreased mortality and methemoglobin levels after nitrite in rats. After PAPP in rats, however, methemoglobin levels were actually increased (Goldstein and Doull, 1973). Since PAPP is a model for compounds metabolized to N-hydroxylarylamines, hyperbaric oxygen would appear to be contraindicated for related structures. The mechanism of the effect on nitrite is not understood, but hyperbaric oxygen seems to block acetylation of PAPP, which is a major route for its detoxification. In reversing nitrite poisoning in mice, methylene blue and hyperbaric oxygen appear to have at least additive effects (Way and Sheehy, 1971).

Oxidative Hemolysis

Sulfhemoglobin. The term "sulfhemoglobin" was coined more than a century ago to describe a pigment generated *in vitro* by exposing oxyhemoglobin to high concentrations of hydrogen sulfide. This phenomenon plays no role in acute hydrogen sulfide poisoning, which is described below. When generated *in vitro* as described, sulfhemoglobin is unstable and solutions are so turbid that visible absorption spectra must be derived indirectly (Drabkin and Austin, 1935–1936). It appears to have a weak absorption maximum at about 620 nm, which overlaps to some extent the absorption maximum of methemoglobin at about 635 nm. This similarity was responsible for much confusion in the early literature. In contrast to methemoglobin, however, the absorption band for sulfhemoglobin is not abolished by the addition of cyanide, and this difference serves as the basis for methods for determining both pigments in the same solution (Evelyn and Malloy, 1938; Van Kampen and Ziljstra, 1965). In recent years so-called sulfhemoglobins of high purity have been generated with hydrogen sulfide under special conditions (e.g., Nichol et al., 1968), but their relationship to the originally described phenomenon has not been clarified.

When the criteria of an absorption band at 620 nm, which is stable toward cyanide, were applied to large numbers of human blood samples in clinical laboratories, positive results were encountered in some patients (Evelyn and Malloy, 1938). By definition these patients were said to have "sulfhemoglobinemia" even though no source of exposure to hydrogen sulfide could be documented and even though all previous attempts to generate sulfhemoglobin *in vivo* by exposure to hydrogen sulfide had failed. In retrospect it appears likely that two unrelated phenomena have been identified for years by the same name because of a coincidence in the position of an absorption maxima and its failure to shift with cyanide (National Academy of Sciences, 1977b).

Over the years the term "sulfhemoglobin" has come to be used almost exclusively in the literature for the abnormal pigment(s) generated *in vivo* in the apparent absence of hydrogen sulfide. This phenomenon, which might better be called pseudosulfhemoglobinemia, is associated with at least three clinical situations: (1) the ingestion of "oxidant" drugs, which may also generate methemoglobin in normal subjects, (2) the presence of an abnormal hemoglobin (Tönz, 1968) such as one of the hemoglobins M, and (3) the exposure of individuals congenitally deficient in glucose-6-phosphate dehydrogenase to certain drugs or chemicals. It is reasonable to assume that three such widely different conditions cannot be generating "sulfhemoglobin" by the same mechanism. Thus, it also seems likely that the phenomenon represents nonspecific oxidative damage, perhaps including a transient methomoglobinemia and partial hemoglobin denaturation (Beutler, 1969). The use of spectrophotometric techniques for the alleged quantitative determination of such a mixture is probably not justified.

No mechanisms exist in the red cell for the reversal of a sulfhemoglobinemia. Because it is irreversible, sulfhemoglobinemia would appear to constitute a more serious toxicologic threat than methemoglobinemia. Sulfhemoglobin, however, has never been generated in sufficient concentrations *in vivo* to constitute a serious threat to life. The disorder is either self-limiting as damaged cells are replaced by erythropoiesis, or it forms one part of a more serious condition as indicated below.

Heinz Bodies. Heinz bodies (Fig. 14–7) are dark-staining, refractile granules found in red cells. They are thought to consist of denatured hemoglobin, possibly sulfhemoglobin. Heinz bodies lie on or near the interior surface of the red cell membrane and appear to be firmly attached to membrane thiol groups. Sulfhydryl groups on the denatured hemoglobin may form disulfide bonds with the membrane surface (Jacob *et al.*, 1968). This process leads to an impairment of membrane functions involving active and passive ion transport. Hyperpermeability and hemolysis may result due to osmotic pressure. Actual distortion in the shape of the cell may occur, resulting in premature splenic capture (see below). Sulfhemoglobin, Heinz bodies, and hemolysis may, therefore, be regarded as a continuum of oxidative stress to the red cell.

According to Jandl and coworkers (1960), however, this process is preceded by a transient methemoglobinemia. Not all authorities agree that methemoglobin is an obligatory or even an important

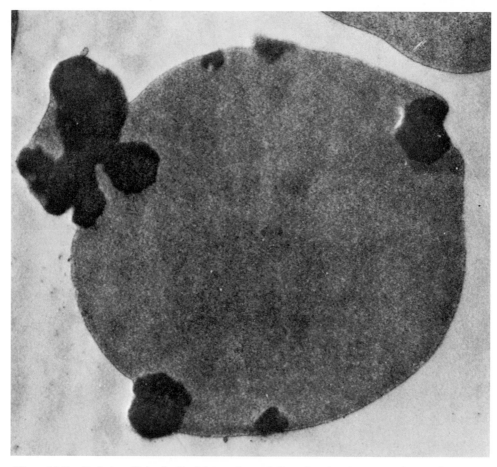

Figure 14–7. End-stage Heinz bodies lying under and distorting the plasma membrane of a mature erythrocyte. × 26,000. (From Rifkind, R. A., and Danon, D.: Heinz body anemia—an ultrastructural study. I. Heinz body formation. *Blood*, **25**:885–96, 1965.)

precursor. There is a rather poor correlation (almost an inverse one) between the ability of a given chemical to generate methemoglobin and its ability to produce Heinz bodies (Rentsch, 1968), although some overlap is recognized. Methemoglobinemia per se does not lead to hemolysis (Beutler, 1969) but in some cases this may simply be a matter of dose or concentration. The presence of molecular oxygen is required. The hydroxylamine-deoxyhemoglobin reaction results only in methemoglobin formation, whereas the hydroxylamine-oxyhemoglobin reaction results in both methemoglobin and sulfhemoglobin (Cranston and Smith, 1971).

Mechanisms of Heinz Body Formation. Congenital Heinz body hemolytic anemia occurs in individuals who have hemoglobins with certain abnormal amino acid substitutions. A rather convincing body of evidence (Jacob et al., 1968; Rieder, 1970) now indicates that in such cases dissociation of the heme group is enhanced in these abnormal pigments. This instability may also be related to the mild methemoglobinemia also associated with the syndrome. Dissociation of heme presumably results in decreased solubility and precipitation of the pigment as a Heinz body. Stabilization of the heme group by the addition of cyanide or carbon monoxide inhibits Heinz body formation *in vitro*.

Heme dissociation, however, has not been convincingly demonstrated in acquired Heinz body anemias, such as the reaction of normal erythrocytes to phenylhydrazine or the reaction of glucose-6-phosphate dehydrogenase-deficient cells to primaquine. Heme loss did not occur during hemoglobin denaturation by hydroxylamine although it was observed to a limited extent with ferricyanide (Cranston and Smith 1971).

According to Cohen and Hochstein (1964) oxidant drugs like phenylhydrazine generate peroxide in the red cell either by reaction with molecular oxygen or by a coupled reaction with oxyhemoglobin. Hydrogen peroxide is detoxified by glutathione peroxidase (Fig. 14–5), resulting in the oxidation of reduced glutathione. Oxidized glutathione is reduced by the activity of glutathione reductase, which requires the NADPH generated by glucose-6-phosphate dehydrogenase. These three enzymes work in concert, and a deficiency in any one of them carries with it an increased sensitivity to oxidant chemicals. A necessary part of this hypothesis is that glutathione peroxidase plays the major role in red cell disposal of peroxide instead of catalase, which is also present in abundance.

The peroxide hypothesis is attractive because, whether the reaction is induced in normal or in glucose-6-phosphate dehydrogenase-deficient cells, an early event is a precipitous fall in red cell levels of reduced glutathione. Allen and Jandl (1961) suggest that oxidized glutathione forms mixed disulfides with free thiol groups on hemoglobin, contributing to its instability and denaturation.

Agents Producing Heinz Bodies. As in the case of methemoglobin-generating agents, prominent species differences are recognized or are to be expected because of different patterns of metabolism of suspect Heinz body-producing chemicals. The nature of the active metabolites of agents producing Heinz bodies only *in vivo* is no more clear than for methemoglobin formers. Aromatic amino (aniline) and nitro (nitrobenzene) compounds produce Heinz bodies in many species, but nonnitrogenous structures have also been implicated: phenols, ascorbic acid, sulfite, dichromate, arsine, stibine, and others. Hydroxylamine and chlorate salts were among the earliest agents to be recognized as eliciting the response. At present no single unifying hypothesis links these diverse structures to red cell damage. It is not known, for example, whether all these are capable of generating hydrogen peroxide in the red cell.

Species Differences. Cat, mouse, dog, and human erythrocytes are said to be particularly susceptible to Heinz body formation, whereas rabbit, monkey, chick, and guinea pig are among the least responsive. These impressions, however, are based on a variety of compounds, some of which were not tested in all species. Moreover, they are based at least in part on *in vivo* observations, which have the limitations mentioned above. This question undoubtedly deserves reexamination with emphasis on the *in vitro* approach.

The morphology and ultrastructure of Heinz bodies also show some variations with species and with agents. Under certain conditions a large number of small bodies are seen. It has been suggested that these eventually coalesce into larger and perhaps multibodied inclusions. In the nucleated turkey erythrocyte, phenylhydrazine Heinz bodies were smaller than those produced under identical conditions in dog or horse red cells, and they were present in both the nucleoplasm and the cytoplasm. Extraerythrocytic Heinz bodies were observed with suspensions of horse erythrocytes but not dog or turkey red cells (Simpson, 1971). Such differences among agents and species and the absence of an unambiguous method for assessing the extent of the damage promise to impede further advances in this area.

The Spleen. Although many lines of evidence indicate that the red cell normally ends its life in the spleen, splenectomy in man does not result in a significant increase in red cell survival time. Thus, other segments of the reticuloendothelial system such as the bone marrow and liver, in addition to the spleen, must play important roles in senescent red cell destruction.

With respect to the spleen, however, its anatomic ultrastructure appears particularly well suited to the above task. Numerous fine arterial vessels arise from the central splenic artery and form a rich plexus in the white pulp. These appear to run to the periphery of the white pulp and terminate in the marginal zone or the contiguous red pulp, although some communicate with cordal vessels. The latter are vascular spaces in the red pulp and lie between the splenic sinuses, which collect blood for the venous return. The splenic cords communicate with the sinuses through mural apertures or fenestrations smaller than the diameter of a red cell. The apertures are lined with reticular cells that have a phagocytic function. Red cells are believed to move through these apertures by diapedesis.

At this point senescent or damaged erythrocytes may be trapped and phagocytized. This concept is supported by the demonstration that red cell deformability has a metabolic dependence (Weed *et al.*, 1969). Thus, cells with impaired metabolic resources or physical impediments may be subject to hemolysis. After hemolysis, hemoglobin is catabolized and the heme groups degraded to bilirubin. Splenic engorgement is, therefore, another sign of hemolytic disease where there is an increased demand for these functions.

The spleen is an example of a site for extravascular destruction of red cells, but cells are also subject to intravascular hemolysis where the cell contents are released into the plasma. In such cases, hemoglobin (or its heme groups) are rapidly trapped by albumin, haptoglobin, or hemopexin (Müller-Eberhard, 1970) and then transported to the reticuloendothelial system. If the rate of hemolysis is such as to saturate these carrier protein systems, free hemoglobin may be excreted in the urine, and hemoglobinuria is a further sign of an acute hemolytic crisis.

HISTOTOXIC HYPOXIA

Semantic purists object to the term histotoxic "hypoxia" since the critical lesion does not involve an inadequate supply of oxygen to peripheral tissues. Instead the peripheral tissue P_{O_2} is often normal or even greater than normal, but the cells are unable to utilize oxygen. Two chemicals are thought to act by this mechanism: hydrogen sulfide and hydrogen cyanide. The biochemical lesion is illustrated for the case of cyanide in Figure 14–8, but sulfide probably has the same mechanism of action. The undissociated acid, hydrogen cyanide, interrupts electron transport down the cytochrome chain by inhibiting at the cytochrome a–cytochrome a_3 step. Since these cytochromes are isolated as a single unit, they are referred to as cytochrome aa_3 or cytochrome oxidase. As a result of cyanide inhibition, oxidative metabolism and phosphorylation are compromised. Electron transfer from cytochrome a_3 to molecular oxygen is blocked,

peripheral tissue oxygen tensions begin to rise, and the unloading gradient for oxyhemoglobin (Fig. 14–8) is decreased. Sometimes high concentrations of oxyhemoglobin are found in the venous return, imparting a flush to skin and mucous membranes.

Cyanide directly stimulates the chemoreceptors of the carotid and aortic bodies with a resultant hyperpnea. Cardiac irregularities are often noted, but the heart invariably outlasts the respirations. Death is due to respiratory arrest of central origin. It can occur within seconds or minutes of the inhalation of high concentrations of hydrogen cyanide gas. Because of slower absorption, death may be more delayed after the ingestion of cyanide salts, but the critical events still occur within the first hour.

Two other sources of cyanide have been responsible for human poisoning. One of these is amygdalin, a cyanogenic glycoside found in apricot, peach, and similar fruit pits and in sweet almonds. Amygdalin is a chemical combination of glucose, benzaldehyde, and cyanide from which the latter can be released by the action of β-glucosidase or emulsin. Although these enzymes are not found in mammalian tissues, the human intestinal microflora appears to possess these or similar enzymes capable of effecting cyanide release resulting in human poisoning. For this reason amygdalin may be as much as 40 times more toxic by the oral route as compared with intravenous injection. Amygdalin is the major ingredient of Laetrile, and this alleged anticancer drug has also been responsible for human cyanide poisoning. An ethical drug that may also cause cyanide poisoning in overdose is the potent vascular smooth muscle relaxant sodium nitroprusside. Although nitroprusside is related chemically to ferricyanide, unlike the latter it penetrates into erythrocytes and reacts with hemoglobin to release its cyanide (Smith and Kruszyna, 1974). Fortunately, the therapeutic margin for nitroprusside appears to be quite large.

Treatment of Cyanide Poisoning

The treatment regimen consists first of the intravenous injection of sodium nitrite (300 mg for an adult). A modest and tolerable fraction of the circulating blood pigment is converted to methemoglobin (Fig. 14–8). The newly generated ferric heme groups act as competitors with cytochrome a_3 for cyanide by complexing with the ionic form. The affinity of methemoglobin for cyanide exceeds that of cytochrome a_3, leading to a dissociation of the cyanide-cytochrome complex and a resumption of oxidative metabolism. Obviously, in the intact animal or man this competition for free cyanide occurs across a

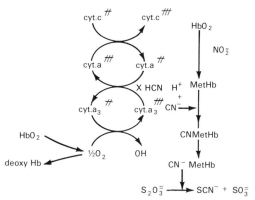

Figure 14–8. Principles of the therapeutic management of cyanide poisoning. Although the exact chemical details are still unknown, the undissociated form (HCN) appears to block electron transfer in the cytochrome a-a_3 complex, which is isolated *in vitro* as a single unit. As a consequence oxygen utilization is decreased and oxidative metabolism may slow to the point that it cannot meet metabolic demands. At the level of the brainstem nuclei this effect may result in central respiratory arrest and death. On injection of sodium nitrite methemoglobin is generated, which can compete effectively with cytochrome aa_3 for free cyanide. Note that it is the ionic form that complexes with methemoglobin. The injection of thiosulfate provides substrate for the enzyme rhodanese, which catalyzes the biotransformation of cyanide to thiosulfate.

number of biologic barriers, yet it is rapidly efficacious.

At this point a certain fraction of the total circulating hemoglobin exists as cyanmethemoglobin, which is inert in terms of oxygen transport. Although the cyanide is bound very tenaciously, cyanmethemoglobin is a somewhat dissociable complex, and there is some risk of the release of free cyanide. Therefore, the second prong of the therapeutic approach involves the intravenous administration of sodium thiosulfate. Thiosulfate serves as a substrate for the enzyme rhodanese, which mediates the conversion of cyanide to the much less toxic thiocyanate, which is excreted in the urine. Although ubiquitously distributed in the body, liver rhodanese probably plays the major role in cyanide detoxification. It is an endogenous mechanism for cyanide metabolism, but the provision of exogenous sulfur greatly accelerates the rate of the reaction. Methemoglobin is restored to functional blood pigment by the intracellular reductase systems (Fig. 14–6).

From the principles summarized in Figure 14–8, it would appear that the administration of oxygen in

cyanide poisoning would serve no useful purpose. Since the lesion is one of oxygen utilization instead of oxygen transport, peripheral tissue oxygen tensions are normal or even supranormal. It has been demonstrated that even hyperbaric oxygen has no effect on cyanide poisoning in mice (Way *et al.*, 1972). However when oxygen at 1 atmosphere is given in combination with nitrite and thiosulfate, a significantly greater protective effect is obtained than when the two chemicals are given in combination with air at the same pressure (Way *et al.*, 1966). Oxygen and thiosulfate provide significantly greater protection against death than do air and thiosulfate, whereas the combination of oxygen and nitrite is only slightly better than the combination of air and nitrite (Sheehy and Way, 1968). The major effect of oxygen appears to be on the rhodanese reaction, although the enzyme itself is not known to be sensitive to oxygen.

Hydrogen Sulfide Poisoning

Hydrogen sulfide is also an established inhibitor of cytochrome oxidase *in vitro*. Signs and symptoms of poisoning on exposure to hydrogen sulfide gas or after the administration of soluble sulfide salts to animals are similar in almost all respects to those produced by cyanide. The only notable exceptions are due to the irritancy of hydrogen sulfide, which on chronic exposure to low concentrations may produce conjunctivitis (gas eye) or occasionally pulmonary edema.

The hydrosulfide anion (HS^-) also forms a complex with methemoglobin known as sulfmethemoglobin, which is analogous to cyanmethemoglobin. Sulfmethemoglobin is a well-characterized entity as distinct from the confusion noted above surrounding the nature of sulfhemoglobin. The dissociation constant for sulfmethemoglobin has been estimated as 6×10^{-6} moles/liter whereas the dissociation constant for cyanmethemoglobin is about 2×10^{-8} moles/liter. Despite the lower binding affinity for sulfide, an induced methemoglobinemia provides unequivocal protection against death from acute sulfide poisoning in animals (Smith and Gosselin, 1964). The induction of methemoglobinemia was successful in the resuscitation of one human severely poisoned by hydrogen sulfide (Stine *et al.*, 1976). No rationale is seen for the use of thiosulfate in sulfide poisoning. As in the case of cyanide, oxygen does not affect the course of acute sulfide poisoning (Smith *et al.*, 1976), but oxygen would be specifically indicated if pulmonary edema occurs.

Because of its ability to react with disulfide bonds under physiologic conditions, the hydrosulfide anion can be inactivated by oxidized glutathione and other simple disulfides (Smith and Abbanat, 1966). Sulfide *in vivo* is metabolized rapidly to sulfate and other sulfur oxides. Human hydrogen sulfide poisoning is invariably the result of occupational exposure to the gas. It is encountered in some natural gas deposits and in volcanic gases in high concentrations. A synonym, sewer gas, refers to the presence of hydrogen sulfide wherever organic matter undergoes putrefication. It is a pollutant in the atmosphere in the proximity of industrial paper plants using the kraft process. The leather industry uses sodium sulfide to remove the hair from hides prior to tanning, and ton quantities are employed in the production of heavy water for nuclear reactors (National Academy of Sciences, 1977b).

REFERENCES

Allen, D. W., and Jandl, J. H.: Oxidative hemolysis and precipitation of hemoglobin. II. Role of thiols in oxidant drug action. *J. Clin. Invest.*, 40:454–75, 1961.

Bartels, H.; Hilpert, P.; Barbey, K.; Betke, K.; Riegel, K.; Lang, E. M.; and Metcalfe, J.: Respiratory functions of blood of the yak, llama, camel, Dybowski deer, and African elephant. *Am. J. Physiol.*, 205:331–36, 1963.

Bernard, C.: *An Introduction to the Study of Experimental Medicine* (first published in 1865). Reprinted by Dover, New York, 1957.

Bessis, M.: *Blood Smears Reinterpreted*, translated by G. Brecher. Springer-Verlag, Berlin, 1977.

Beutler, E.: Drug-induced hemolytic anemia. *Pharmacol. Rev.*, 21:73–103, 1969.

Board, P. G.; Agar, N. S.; Gruca, M.; and Shine, R.: Methaemoglobin and its reduction in nucleated erythrocytes from reptiles and birds. *Comp. Biochem. Physiol.*, 57B:265–67, 1977.

Bolyai, J. Z.; Smith, R. P.; and Gray, C. T.: Ascorbic acid and chemically induced methemoglobinemias. *Toxicol. Appl. Pharmacol.*, 21:176–85, 1972.

Cerami, A., and Manning, J. M.: Potassium cyanate as an inhibitor of the sickling of erythrocytes *in vitro. Proc. Natl. Acad. Sci.*, 68:1180–83, 1971.

Coburn, R. F.; Williams, W. J.; White, P.; and Kahn, S. B.: The production of carbon monoxide from hemoglobin *in vivo. J. Clin. Invest.*, 46:346–56, 1967.

Cohen, G., and Hochstein, P.: Generation of hydrogen peroxide in erythrocytes by hemolytic agents. *Biochemistry*, 3:895–900, 1964.

Cranston, R. D., and Smith, R. P.: Some aspects of the reactions between hydroxylamine and hemoglobin derivatives. *J. Pharmacol. Exp. Ther.*, 177:440–46, 1971.

Douglas, C. G.; Haldane, J. S.; and Haldane, J. B. S.: The laws of combination of haemoglobin with carbon monoxide and oxygen. *J. Physiol.* (Lond.), 44:275–304, 1912.

Drabkin, D. L., and Austin, J. H.: Spectrophotometric studies. II. Preparations from washed blood cells; nitric oxide hemoglobin and sulfhemoglobin. *J. Biol. Chem.*, 112:51–65, 1935–1936.

Evelyn, K. A., and Malloy, H. T.: Microdetermination of oxyhemoglobin, methemoglobin and sulfhemoglobin in a single sample of blood. *J. Biol. Chem.*, 126:655–62, 1938.

Gleason, M. N.; Gosselin, R. E.; Hodge, H. C.; and Smith, R. P.: *Clinical Toxicology of Commercial Products. Acute Poisoning*, 3rd ed. Williams & Wilkins Co., Baltimore, 1969.

Goldstein, G. M., and Doull, J.: Treatment of nitrite-induced methemoglobinemia with hyperbaric oxygen. *Proc. Soc. Exp. Biol. Med.*, 138:137–39, 1971.

———: The use of hyperbaric oxygen in the treatment of p-aminopropiophenone-induced methemoglobinemia. *Toxicol. Appl. Pharmacol.*, 26:247–52, 1973.

Gosselin, R. E.; Hodge, H. C.; Smith, R. P.; and Gleason, M. N.: *Clinical Toxicology of Commercial Products. Acute Poisoning*, 4th ed. Williams & Wilkins Co., Baltimore, 1976.

Haldane, J.: The relation of the action of carbonic oxide to oxygen tension. *J. Physiol.*, 18:201–17, 1895.

Harris, J. W., and Kellermeyer, R. W.: *The Red Cell Production, Metabolism, Destruction: Normal and Abnormal*, rev. ed. Harvard University Press, Cambridge, Mass., 1970.

Jacob, H. S.; Brain, M. C.; and Dacie, J. V.: Altered sulfhydryl reactivity of hemoglobins and red blood cell membranes in congenital Heinz body hemolytic anemia. *J. Clin. Invest.*, 47:2644–77, 1968.

Jandl, J. H.; Engle, L. K.; and Allen, D. W.: Oxidative hemolysis and precipitation of hemoglobin. I. Heinz body anemias as an acceleration of red cell aging. *J. Clin. Invest.*, 39:1818–36, 1960.

Kiese, M.: *Methemoglobinemia: A Comprehensive Treatise*. CRC Press, Cleveland, 1974.

Kiese, M., and Weis, B.: Die Ruduktion des Hämiglobins in den Erythrocyten verschiedener Tiere. *Naunyn Schmiedebergs Arch. Pharmacol.*, 202:493–501, 1943.

Layne, W. R., and Smith, R. P.: Methylene blue uptake and the reversal of chemically induced methemoglobinemias in human erythrocytes. *J. Pharmacol. Exp. Ther.*, 165:36–44, 1969.

Malz, E.: Vergleichende Untersuchungen über die Methämoglobinreduktion in kernhaltigen und kernlosen Erythrozyten. *Folia. Haematol.* (*Leipz.*), 78:510–15, 1962.

Mitruka, B. M., and Rawnsley, H. M.: *Clinical Biochemical and Hematological Reference Values in Normal Experimental Animals*. Masson Publishing USA, Inc., New York, 1977.

Müller-Eberhard, U.: Hemopexin. *N. Engl. J. Med.*, 283:1090–94, 1970.

National Academy of Sciences: *Carbon Monoxide*. Committee on Medical and Biological Effects of Environmental Pollutants, National Research Council, Washington, D.C., 1977a.

National Academy of Sciences: *Hydrogen Sulfide*. Committee on Medical and Biological Effects of Environmental Pollutants, National Research Council, Washington, D.C., 1977b.

Nichol, A. W.; Hendry, I.; and Morell, D. B.: Mechanism of formation of sulphhaemoglobin. *Biochim. Biophys. Acta*, 156:97–108, 1968.

Perutz, M. F.; Muirhead, H.; Cox, J. M.; and Goaman, L. C. G.: Three-dimensional Fourier synthesis of horse oxyhaemoglobin at 2.8 Å resolution: The atomic model. *Nature* (*Lond.*), 219:131–39, 1968.

Pisciotta, A. V.: Immune and toxic mechanisms in drug-induced agranulocytosis. *Semin. Hematol.*, 10:279–310, 1973.

Prankerd, T. A. J.: *The Red Cell. An Account of Its Chemical Physiology and Pathology*. Blackwell Scientific Publications, Oxford, England, 1961.

Reddy, B. G.; Pohl, L. R.; and Krishna, G.: The requirement of the gut flora in nitrobenzene-induced methemoglobinemia in rats. *Biochem. Pharmacol.*, 25:1119–22, 1976.

Rentsch, G.: Genesis of Heinz bodies and methemoglobin formation. *Biochem. Pharmacol.*, 17:423–27, 1968.

Rieder, R. F.: Hemoglobin stability: Observations on the denaturation of normal and abnormal hemoglobins by oxidant dyes, heat and alkali. *J. Clin. Invest.*, 49:2369–76, 1970.

Rivkin, S. E., and Simon, E. R.: Comparative carbohydrate catabolism and methemoglobin reduction in pig and human erythrocytes. *J. Cell. Comp. Physiol.*, 66:49–56, 1965.

Robin, H., and Harley, J. D.: Factors influencing response of mammalian species to the methaemoglobin reduction test. *Aust. J. Exp. Biol. Med. Sci.*, 44:519–26, 1966.

———: Regulation of methaemoglobinaemia in horse and human erythrocytes. *Aust. J. Exp. Biol. Med. Sci.*, 45:77–88, 1967.

Sass, M. D.; Caruso, C. J.; and Axelrod, D. R.: Mechanism of the TPNH-linked reduction of methemoglobin by methylene blue. *Clin. Chim. Acta*, 24:77–85, 1969.

Sass, M. D.; Caruso, C. J.; and Farhangi, M.: TPNH-methemoglobin reductase deficiency: A new red-cell enzyme defect. *J. Lab. Clin. Med.*, 70:760–67, 1967.

Scott, E. M.; Duncan, I. W.; and Ekstrand, V.: The reduced pyridine nucleotide dehydrogenases of human erythrocytes. *J. Biol. Chem.* 240:481–85, 1965.

Scott, E. M., and Griffith, I. V.: Enzymatic defect of hereditary methemoglobinemia: The diasphorase. *Biochim. Biophys. Acta*, 34:584–86, 1959.

Sheehy, M., and Way, J. L.: Effect of oxygen on cyanide intoxication. III. Mithridate. *J. Pharmacol. Exp. Ther.* 161:163–68, 1968.

Simpson, C. F.: The ultrastructure of Heinz bodies in horse, dog, and turkey erythrocytes. *Cornell Vet.*, 61:228–38, 1971.

Smith, J. E., and Beutler, E.: Methemoglobin formation and reduction in man and various animal species. *Am. J. Physiol.*, 210:347–50, 1966a.

———: Anomeric specificity of human erythrocyte glucose-6-phosphate dehydrogenase. *Proc. Soc. Exp. Biol. Med.*, 122:671–73, 1966b.

Smith, R. P.: The nitrite methemoglobin complex—its significance in methemoglobin analyses and its possible role in methemoglobinemia. *Biochem. Pharmacol.*, 16:1655–64, 1967.

Smith, R. P., and Abbanat, R. A.: Protective effect of oxidized glutathione in acute sulfide poisoning. *Toxicol. Appl. Pharmacol.*, 9:209–17, 1966.

Smith, R. P., and Gosselin, R. E.: The influence of methemoglobinemia on the lethality of some toxic anions. II. Sulfide. *Toxicol. Appl. Pharmacol.*, 6:584–92, 1964.

Smith, R. P.; Alkaitis, A. A.; and Shafer, P. R.: Chemically induced methemoglobinemias in the mouse. *Biochem. Pharmacol.*, 16:317–28, 1967.

Smith, R. P., and Layne, W. R.: A comparison of the lethal effects of nitrite and hydroxylamine in the mouse. *J. Pharmacol. Exp. Ther.*, 165:30–35, 1969.

Smith, R. P., and Olson, M. V.: Drug-induced methemoglobinemia. *Semin. Hematol.*, 10:253–68, 1973.

Smith, R. P., and Thron, C. D.: Hemoglobin, methylene blue and oxygen interactions in human red cells. *J. Pharmacol. Exp. Ther.*, 183:549–58, 1972.

Smith, R. P., and Kruszyna, H.: Nitroprusside produces cyanide poisoning *via* a reaction with hemoglobin. *J. Pharmacol. Exp. Ther.*, 191:557–63, 1974.

Smith, R. P.; Kruszyna, R.; and Kruszyna, H.: Management of acute sulfide poisoning. Effects of oxygen, thiosulfate, and nitrite. *Arch. Environ. Health*, 31:166–69, 1976.

Spencer, T. D.: Effects of carbon monoxide on man and canaries. *Ann. Occup. Hyg.*, 5:231–40, 1962.

Stebbins, R., and Bertino, J. R.: Megaloblastic anemias produced by drugs. *Clin. Haematol.*, 5:619–30, 1976.

Stine, R. J.; Slosberg, B.; and Beacham, B. E.: Hydrogen sulfide intoxication. A case report and discussion of treatment. *Ann. Intern. Med.*, 85:756–58, 1976.

Stolk, J. M., and Smith, R. P.: Species differences in methemoglobin reductase activity. *Biochem. Pharmacol.*, 15:343–51, 1966.

Surgenor, D. M.: *The Red Blood Cell*, 2nd ed. Academic Press, Inc., New York, Vol. I, 1974; Vol. II, 1975.

Tönz, O.: *The Congenital Methemoglobinemias. Physiology and Pathophysiology of the Hemiglobin Metabolism.* S. Karger, Basel, 1968. Published simultaneously as Bibliotheca Haematologica No. 28.

van Assendelft, O. W., and Zijlstra, W. G.: The formation of haemiglobin using nitrites. *Clin. Chim. Acta*, 11:571–77, 1965.

van Kampen, E. J., and Zijlstra, W. G.: Determination of hemoglobin and its derivatives. In Sobotka, H., and Stewart, C. P. (eds.): *Advances in Clinical Chemistry*, Vol. 8. Academic Press, Inc., New York, 1965.

Way, J. L.; Gibbon, S. L.; and Sheehy, M.: Effect of oxygen on cyanide intoxication. I. Prophylactic protection. *J. Pharmacol. Exp. Ther.*, 153:381–85, 1966.

Way, J. L., and Sheehy, M. H.: Antagonism of sodium nitrite intoxication. *Toxicol. Appl. Pharmacol.*, 19:400–401, 1971.

Way, J. L.; End, E.; Sheehy, M. H.; de Miranda, P.; Feitknecht, U. F.; Bachand, R.; Gibbon, S. L.; and Burrows, G. E.: Effect of oxygen on cyanide intoxication. IV. Hyperbaric oxygen, *Toxicol. Appl. Pharmacol.*, 22:415–21, 1972.

Weed, R. I.; LaCelle, P. L.; and Merrill, E. W.: Metabolic dependence of red cell deformability. *J. Clin. Invest.*, 48:795–809, 1969.

Chapter 15

TOXIC RESPONSES OF THE REPRODUCTIVE SYSTEM

Robert L. Dixon

INTRODUCTION

Survival of any species depends on the integrity of its reproductive system. Genes located in the chromosomes of the germ cells transmit genetic information from previous generations and control cell differentiation and organogenesis. Under normal circumstances germ cells ensure the maintenance of structures and functions in the organism in its own lifetime and from generation to generation. But human beings now live in an environment in which at least 10,000 chemicals are prevalent and to which some 700 to 1,000 new compounds are added each year. And it is the potential toxicity of such chemicals to human beings during their most vulnerable stages of development—conception to birth—that is among the least understood toxicologic phenomena.

The toxic effects of drugs and environmental chemicals on the human reproductive system have become a major health concern; incidences of chemically induced germ cell damage and sterility appear to be on the increase. Recently, in the United States, male factory workers occupationally exposed to 1,2-dibromo-3-chloropropane (DBCP) became sterile, evidencing oligospermia, azoospermia, and germinal aplasia. Factory workers in battery plants in Bulgaria, lead mine workers in the state of Missouri, and workers in Sweden who handle organic solvents (toluene, benzene, and xylene) suffer from low sperm counts, abnormal sperm, and varying degrees of infertility. Diethylstilbestrol (DES), hexafluoracetone (HFA), borax, cadmium, methylmercury, and many cancer chemotherapeutic agents have been shown to be toxic to the male and female reproductive system and possibly capable of inflicting genetic damage to germ cells (Lucier *et al.*, 1977; Harbison and Dixon, 1978).

The effects of chemicals on human reproduction and the risks from exposure are difficult to assess because of the complexity of the reproductive process and the long span of years required for reproductive maturation. Moreover, the developmental defects actually seen may not be adequate indices of the effects of chemical exposure, for, in the human, it is estimated that over one-third of early embryos die and about 15 percent of recognized pregnancies abort spontaneously. Among the surviving fetuses at birth, approximately 3 percent have developmental defects (not always anatomic), and with increasing age over twice that many become detectable. Twenty to thirty percent of these defects have a major genetic etiology; up to 6 percent are due to known environmental agents. The remaining defects are of unknown cause, perhaps representing a combination of genetic and environmental components.

Given these complexities, for one to understand better the basis of reproductive toxicity, attention should be given to the entire spectrum of reproductive events and processes that must function normally to produce a healthy offspring (Diczfalusy *et al.*, 1977). They are as follows:

Preservation of the germ line: Study the possibility of nonlethal mutation retention.

Gametogenesis: Study effects on germ cell production (spermatogenesis and oogenesis).

Release and transport of gametes: Determine effects on normal muscular, ciliary, and secretory activity.

Fertilization: Examine for direct effects on zygote and alterations of the uterine environment that affect implantation.

Cleavage and blastocyst (preimplantation) states: Determine chemical penetration; effect is usually embryolethality rather than teratogenesis at this stage.

Implantation: Study effects on endometrium, uterine fluids, and motility.

Metabolic changes in the pregnant mother: Study altered susceptibility of maternal organism during pregnancy.

Embryonic period: Determine teratogenic

effects that occur during tissue differentiation and organogenesis.

Fetal period, prenatal growth, and functional maturation: Examine for adverse influences —growth retardation, prematurity.

Placental functions and maternal-conceptus relationship: Define adverse influences on blood flow, nutrient exchange, and endocrine function.

Birth and adjustment to postnatal existence: Study binding, metabolism, distribution, etc.; Organism at this stage is usually highly susceptible.

Lactation and maternal care of offspring: Examine for adverse influences on lactation, altered appearance of milk, quantity or composition of milk, and chemicals secreted in milk.

Postnatal growth and maturation of offspring: Determine postnatal effects of gestational chemical exposure; central nervous and endocrine systems are particularly important areas.

Of these events and processes, this chapter will consider the effects of toxic factors on the processes of gametogenesis, spermatogenesis, and oogenesis. However, it will also discuss general pharmacologic and toxicologic principles, procedures for evaluating the reproductive toxicity of chemical and other toxic factors, and regulatory requirements. And finally, research needs in the area of reproduction as identified by the Second Task Force for Research Planning in Environmental Health Science will be mentioned (Nelson *et al.*, 1977).

GENERAL REPRODUCTIVE BIOLOGY

Organogenesis: Urinary and Genital Systems

Because of the developing gonads' unique sensitivity to chemical insult and the reproductive organs' potential for teratogenic alterations, toxicologists should be generally familiar with the major aspects of urinary and genital organogenesis (Hoar, 1978). During development, the genital and urinary systems, which together compose the urogenital system, are closely associated; they are united both through inductive interactions and, especially in the male, through the utilization of a common discharge duct, the penile urethra. Having acknowledged this close association, for the sake of clarity, the two systems are generally discussed separately.

Urinary System. The urinary system develops within the intermediate mesoderm, which occupies a position lateral to the aorta and anterolateral to the developing vertebral column and its musculature. Three different overlapping kidney systems develop in rapid succession, appearing in a craniocaudal progression in the intermediate mesodermal ridge between the third and fourth weeks of gestation. The pronephros is transitory and of little importance.

The appearance of the mesonephros is characterized by a single Bowman's capsule for each segmentally arranged excretory tubule and a longitudinal collecting duct, the mesonephric duct. The mesonephric duct at first ends blindly just short of the cloaca and then fuses with it. The ureteric bud, an outgrowth of the mesonephric duct close to its entrance into the cloaca, then penetrates the intermediate mesodermal ridge and induces the metanephros or definitive kidney. The ureteric bud gives rise to the collecting system while the metanephric mesoderm forms the filtering system. In the human, these events occur between the seventh and tenth weeks, culminating in functional capacity early in the second half of pregnancy.

The urorectal septum separates the primitive urogenital sinus from the anorectal canal by the seventh week. The primitive urogenital sinus is now modified further into a bladder and two structures, the pelvic part of the urogenital sinus and the definitive urogenital sinus, whose final determination awaits the expression of the sex of the embryo.

Genital System. During the sixth week in the human, the primordial germ cells complete their migration from the yolk sac into the genital ridge, establishing the gonad. At this time also two pairs of genital ducts are completed and the embryo is in an indifferent bisexual state. The mesonephric duct (wolffian duct), now in close association with the gonad and emptying into the urogenital sinus, is free to become the main genital duct of the male, the ductus deferens. The paramesonephric duct (mullerian duct), from which the oviducts and uterus will develop, is also in close proximity to the developing gonad.

Depending on the sex of the embryo, one of these two duct systems will complete its development and the other will disappear almost completely. In the male the paramesonephric duct (mullerian duct) disappears, and the mesonephric duct (wolffian duct) differentiates into its several components: the epididymis, seminal vesicles, and ductus deferens. In the female the mesonephric duct disappears almost completely, and the paramesonephric duct differentiates into the oviduct with its ostium and the corpus and cervix of the uterus.

By the end of the sixth week, the external genitalia of the male and female are essentially identical. During the seventh week the cloacal folds are divided by the urorectal septum into anal and urethral folds. In the female, the genital tubercle enlarges slightly to become the clitoris; the urethral folds do not fuse, becoming the labia minora, while the genital swellings enlarge to become the labia majora. The definitive urogenital sinus is modified slightly to form the urethra and the vestibule.

At about the ninth week the vagina begins its development from that portion of the urogenital sinus in the region of the fused paramesonephric ducts. By the fifth month the vaginal outgrowth is canalized but remains separated from the urogenital sinus by the hymen.

In the male the genital tubercle elongates into a phallus, drawing the urethral folds into a long urethral groove that fuses and by the end of third

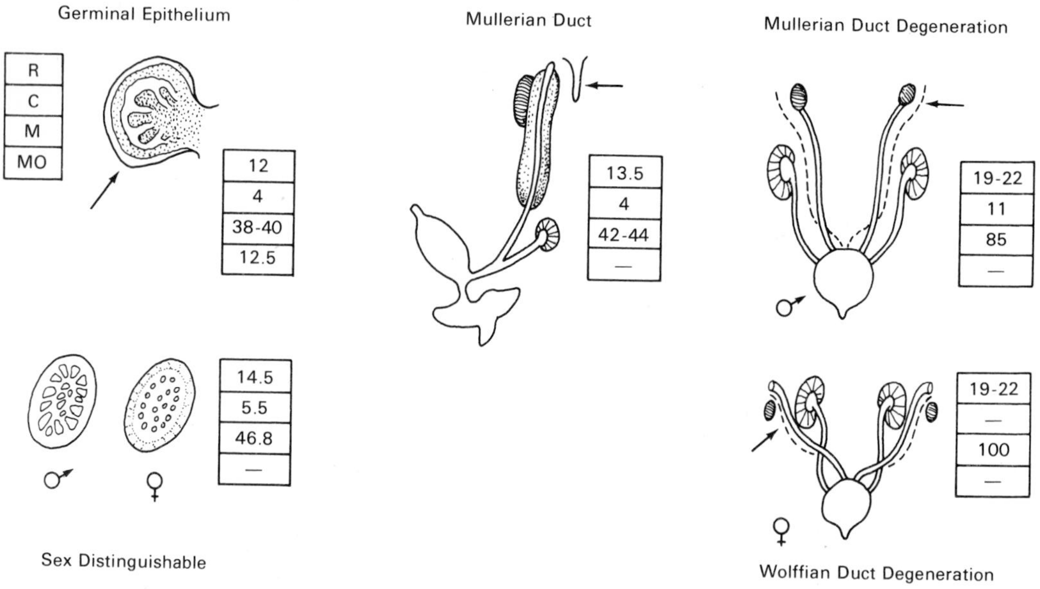

Germinal Epithelium | Mullerian Duct | Mullerian Duct Degeneration

| R |
| C |
| M |
| MO |

| 12 |
| 4 |
| 38-40 |
| 12.5 |

| 13.5 |
| 4 |
| 42-44 |
| — |

| 19-22 |
| 11 |
| 85 |
| — |

| 14.5 |
| 5.5 |
| 46.8 |
| — |

| 19-22 |
| — |
| 100 |
| — |

Sex Distinguishable

Wolffian Duct Degeneration

Figure 15–1. Various developmental stages of the reproductive system accompanied by the age in days on which a particular event occurs in the rat (*R*), mouse (*MO*), and man (*M*) based on fertilization age and in the chick (*C*) based on incubation age. (Modified from Hoar, R. M.: Comparative developmental aspects of selected organ systems: II. Gastrointestinal and urogenital systems. *Environ. Health Perspect.*, **18**:61–66, 1976.)

month forms the penile portion of the urethra. The pelvic part of the urogenital sinus becomes the prostatic and membranous urethra. The genital swellings enlarge, moving caudally and fusing to form the scrotum. These scrotal swellings are prepared for the descending testes during the third month, but the testes do not complete their descent into the scrotum until between the seventh month of development and birth.

Figure 15–1 presents the age in days on which a particular event occurs in the organogenesis of man, rat, and mouse based on fertilization age and in the chick according to its incubation age. These figures are approximations included to create a clearer picture of the time involved during organogenesis. Because vertebrates have such widely variant periods of development, it is often easier to compare them on the basis of developmental stages that attempt to eliminate all the variables such as length of gestation and growth rate.

Gametogenesis

Following their common origin in the germinal ridge, the mammalian primitive cells undergo a number of differentiation processes. Gametogenesis involves three phases: a period of proliferation during which the primitive germ cells divide repeatedly, a period of growth marked by rapid enlargement of cells produced by division, and a final period of maturation limited to two final divisions that involve fundamental nuclear changes.

The maturation of the oocyte takes place primarily before birth; oogenesis is, therefore, an abbreviated event in postnatal life compared to spermatogenesis. In the male the earliest cell of the germ line, the gonocyte, appears in the fetal gonad and persists throughout intrauterine life. Gonocytes transform into the spermatogonia of postnatal life. The ovum is functionally mature at the end of maturation; the male cells must develop through an additional stage before they become motile sperm.

Spermatogenesis. The formation of sperm, termed "spermatogenesis", is a unique process in which timing and direction of the stages of development from a primordial cell are known with a considerable degree of certainty. Neatly coordinated "cycles" with discrete stages can be readily identified by relatively simple histologic procedures. Although various cell types have been identified, distinguishing between spermatogonia, spermatocytes, spermatids, and sperm seems sufficient for most investigations in reproductive toxicology.

Spermatogenesis is a continuous rather than a cyclic event and different levels of spermatogenesis can be seen in the tubules at all times. The length of time involved in the conversion of the human primitive germ cell to mature sperm is about two months.

The sperm is among the smallest cells in man. In humans, its length is about $50 \mu m$ or only about half the diameter of the ovum, the largest cell of the female organism; its relative volume is about 1/100,000 that of the egg. The sperm has head, middle piece, and tail, which correspond, respectively, to the following functions: activation and genetics, metabolism, and motility. The ultramicroscopic structure of the human sperm is presented in Figure 15–2.

Whereas only a few hundred ova are released as cells ready for fertilization, millions of motile sperm are formed in the spermatogenic tubules each day

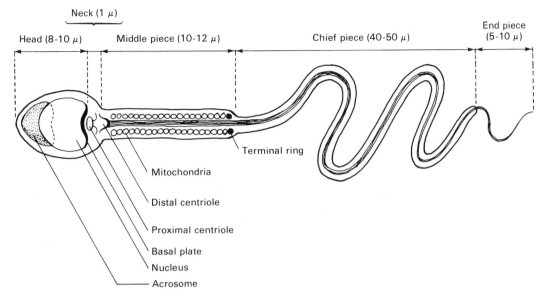

Figure 15–2. Ultramicroscopic structure of human sperm.

(Fig. 15–3). Another fundamental difference between ova and sperm can be noted in Figure 15–3, the unequal duration of meiosis in the two sexes. In the male, meiosis comes about within several days. In the female, the process is begun during fetal life but is suspended for a considerable time, indeed for about a dozen years until puberty.

Spermatogenesis starts at puberty and continues almost throughout life. The primitive male germ cells are spermatogonia, which are situated next to the basement membrane of the seminiferous tubules. Following birth, spermatogonia are dormant until puberty when proliferative activity begins again. The onset of spermatogenesis accompanies functional maturation of the testes. Two major types of spermatogonia are present—type A, which generates other spermatogonia, and type B, which become mature sperm. The latter type develop into primary spermatocytes, which undergo meiotic divisions, divide into secondary spermatocytes having the haploid number of chromosomes and then mature into spermatids (Fig. 15–4).

In contrast to mitosis and its four phases (prophase, metaphase, anaphase, and telophase), the process of meiosis results in the reduction of the normal complement of chromosomes (diploid) to half this number (haploid). Meiosis ensures the biologic necessity of evolution through the introduction of controlled variability; although each gamete must receive one of each pair of chromosomes, whether it receives the maternal or paternal chromosome is a matter of chance. This is true for each of the 23 pairs of chromosomes in man; the possible number of recombinations of the chromosomal pairs is enormous. Meiosis is one of the most susceptible stages for chemical toxicity.

The spermatids complete their development into sperm by undergoing a period of transformation (spermiogenesis) that involves extensive nuclear and cytoplasmic reorganization. The nucleus condenses and becomes the sperm head; the two centrioles give rise to the flagellum or axial filament; part of the Golgi apparatus becomes the acrosome; and the mitochondria concentrate into a sheath located between two centrioles.

The time required for the spermatogenic testicular phase is about 48 days in rats, 34 days in mice, and 62 days in man. The total time from the stem cell to ejaculated sperm is about 52 days for the rat, 41 days for the mouse, and 83 days for man.

The physiologic changes that have been observed in sperm of various species as they pass along the tubules of the testes and epididymides of rodents include increasing capacity for fertility, changes in motility, progressive dehydration of the cytoplasm, decreased resistance to cold shock, changes in metabolism, and variations in membrane permeability.

As many as five hundred million sperm are ejaculated at one time. Each ejaculate contains a spectrum of normal sperm as well as those which are either abnormal or immature.

Oogenesis. As already mentioned, the ovaries are derived during embryogenesis from the germinal ridge and descend into the pelvis in the early part of fetal life. A variety of endogenous and exogenous factors can influence embryonic development. During the fetal period, primordial cells or oogonia proliferate within the cortex of the fetal ovary and subsequently become surrounded by epithelial cells to form the primary follicle. Shortly after birth, oogonia cease to proliferate and become oocytes, which continue to increase in size. Primary oocytes are about seven times as large as the oogonia and are surrounded by a multicellular layer of cuboidal cells.

In humans, between 300,000 and 400,000 follicles are present at birth in each ovary. After birth many

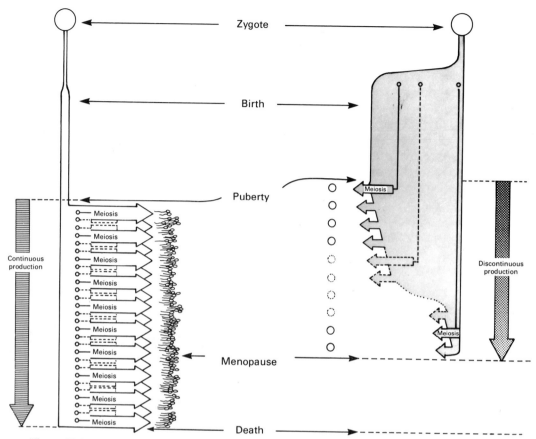

Figure 15-3. Chronology of gametogenesis. (Modified from Tuchmann-Duplessis, H.; David, G.; and Haegel, P.: *Illustrated Human Embryology*: *Embryogenesis*, Vol. I. Springer-Verlag, New York, 1972.)

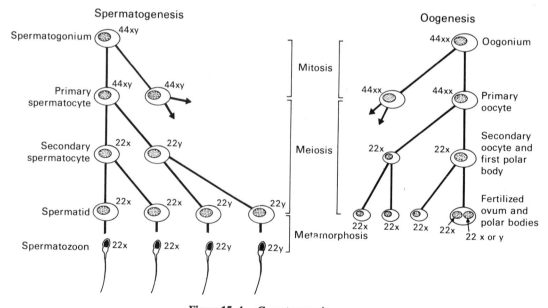

Figure 15-4. Gametogenesis.

336

of these die (atresia), and those that survive are continuously reduced in number. Any agent that damages the oocytes will accelerate the depletion of the pool and can lead to reduced fertility in females. About half the number of oocytes present at birth remain at puberty; the number is reduced to about 25,000 by 30 years of age. About 400 primary follicles will yield mature ova during the life of a woman (Fig. 15–3).

In mammalian species, germ cells are formed in females before birth. Shortly after birth, all germ cells in the ovary are arrested at the primary oocyte stage, diplotene. The oocytes remain in this meiotic state until just before they are ovulated. During the 30 years or more that constitute the reproductive periods, follicles in various stages of growth can always be found. After menopause; follicles are no longer present in the ovary.

The follicles remain in a primary follicle stage following birth until puberty when a number of follicles start to grow during each ovarian cycle. However, most fail to achieve maturity. For the follicles that continue to grow, the first event is an increase in size of the primary oocyte. During this stage, fluid-filled spaces appear among the cells of the follicle, which unite to form a cavity or antrum. This type of development is characteristic of mammals and represents the stage of vesicular or graafian follicle. As the growth of the follicle continues, the oocyte becomes situated more and more off center in the enlarging antrum and is buried in a mound of follicle cells, termed the cumulus oophorus or egg-bearing hillock.

The primary oocyte undergoes two specialized nuclear divisions, which result in the formation of four cells containing half the number of chromosomes. In the first stage of meiosis the primary oocyte is actively synthesizing DNA and protein in preparation for entering prophase (Fig. 15–4). The DNA content doubles as the prophase chromosomes have each produced their mirror image. Each doubled chromosome is attracted to its homologous mate to form tetrads; chromosomes of the same parental origin are connected to one another by their centromeres. The members of the tetrads synapse or come to lie side by side. Before separation, the homologous pairs of chromosomes exchange genetic material by a process known as crossing-over, which accounts for most of the qualitative differences between the resulting gametes. The subsequent meiotic stages distribute the members of the tetrads to the daughter cells in such a way that each cell receives the haploid number of chromosomes. At telophase, one secondary oocyte and a polar body have been formed, which are no longer genetically identical since the members of the chromosomal pairs as well as parts of chromosomes may have been exchanged.

The secondary oocyte enters the next cycle of division very rapidly; each chromosome splits longitudinally; the ovum and the three polar bodies now contain the haploid number of chromosomes and half the amount of genetic material. Although the words "egg" and "ovum" are often used interchangeably, ovum actually refers to only the final stage with the haploid number of chromosomes.

Although the nuclei of all four eggs are equivalent, the cytoplasm is divided unequally. The end products are one large ovum and three rudimentary ova known as polar bodies, which subsequently degenerate. The ovum is released from the ovary at the secondary oocyte stage; the second stage of meiotic division is triggered in the oviduct by the entry of the sperm.

Fertilization

In the process of fertilization (Fig. 15–5), the ovum contributes the maternal complement of genes to the nucleus of the fertilized egg. The ovum rejects all sperm but one and provides food reserves for the early embryo. The innermost envelope of the egg is the vitelline membrane. Outside of the ovum proper (approximately 0.14 mm in diameter) lies a thick, tough, and highly refractile capsule termed the zona pellucida, which increases the total diameter of the human ovum to 0.15 mm. Beyond the zona pellucida is the corona radiata derived from the follicle; it surrounds the ovum during its passage in the oviduct.

The formation, maturation, and meeting of a male and female germ cell are all preliminary to their actual union into a combined cell or zygote. Penetration of ovum by sperm and the coming together and pooling of their respective nuclei constitute the process of fertilization.

Union depends on a proper state of maturity of both male and female germ cells. In almost all mammals, the first polar body must be extruded and the second polar body in a state of arrest before penetration of the sperm can take place.

The second meiotic division continues to completion only during the preliminary events of fertilization. The sperm to be successful must possess high motility and must be in the functionally potent phase like the egg. Both egg and sperm must reside in the oviduct for about five hours before they are fully capacitated or prepared for fertilization.

The act of fertilization can be divided arbitrarily into three phases: penetration of the egg by the sperm; activation of the egg; and union of egg and sperm nuclei.

In the great majority of animals, only one sperm finds its way into the egg. At the moment of attachment of the fertilizing spermatozoon to the egg, rapid changes take place in cortical structure of the egg, which reduces the possibility of penetration of a second sperm but does not make the egg completely impenetrable. Within the next minute, a sperm-impermeable layer forms at the egg surface.

Mammalian sperm secrete hyaluronidase, an enzyme probably localized in the acrosome, capable of dissolving the egg membrane to provide a route through the cells of the corona radiata. Hyaluronic acid is the intracellular cement. The zona pellucida is later denuded by the dispersal of corona cells.

From the single fertilized cell (the zygote), cells proliferate and differentiate until more than a trillion cells of about 100 different types are present in the adult organism. Cell multiplication continues in most tissues throughout life replenishing the dying cells; every 24 hours almost 1 percent of our cells are discarded and renewed. Various tissues are characterized by their cell turnover rates. Throughout

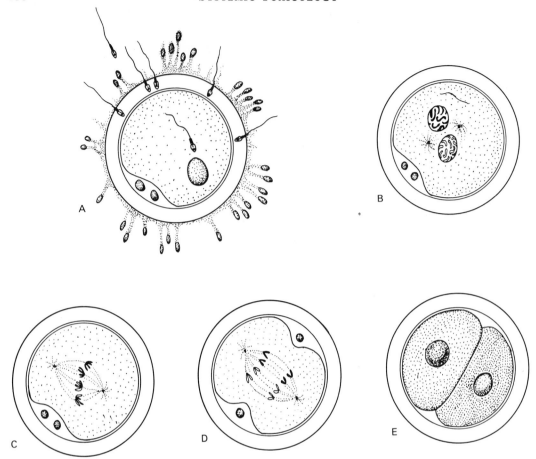

Figure 15–5. Morphologic changes in fertilization: (*A*) The sperm has just penetrated the ovum; the second polar body is extruded (the division of the first polar body is not shown here). (*B*) Formation of the two pronuclei. (*C*) Metaphase of the first cleavage mitosis: the normal chromosome stock is reconstituted. (*D*) Anaphase of the first cleavage mitosis. (*E*) The first two blastomeres, still surrounded by the zona pellucida.

the male's reproductive lifespan of more than six decades, approximately a quadrillion sperms are produced. In contrast, the female is born with only about 350,000 oocytes arrested at the diplotene phase—a population that decreases rapidly due to ovulation and the atretic process (atresia).

Cells of every animal species contain a definite and characteristic number of chromosomes. Chromosomes are circles of DNA approximately 1,000 times the length of the cell. The chromosome number is identical for all somatic cells as well as immature sex cells. The smallest possible chromosome number is two and is found in a form of roundworms; the largest number is found in a moth, which has more than 200. In humans, the total number of chromosomes is 46, distributed in 23 pairs. With one exception, each member of a chromosome pair is morphologically and functionally similar to its mate. In the female, there are 23 pairs of different kinds of chromosomes; the male has one pair, which contains two different chromosomes, resulting in 24 different

kinds. The number of genes varies greatly from one chromosome to another within the nucleus, but the general distribution is the same throughout the species. Human chromosomes contain 30,000 pairs or more of genes, which are the focus of mutagenic events. A mutation is a permanent change in genetic structure that is transmitted to the progeny.

GENERAL PHARMACOLOGIC PRINCIPLES

Most reproductive toxicologists seek to determine the effects of chemicals or other factors on male and female reproductive function using rather simple measures and observations. The design of the experiment is based on the anticipated amounts and patterns of consumption (or exposure) for a substance as well as its chemical and physical properties; these properties determine the pharmacokinetic parameters for the experiment. Test doses are selected bearing in mind these pharmacokinetic factors; doses must neither be so large that they overwhelm adaptation mechanisms nor be administered so often that they unknowingly accumulate within the experimental animal. The route of administration of the test dose should be the same as the human experiences, and the purity of the test substance must be carefully determined. The value of rather simple pharmacokinetic parameters such as rate of absorption, volume of distribution, biologic half-life, and routes of biotransformation cannot be overstated. Rodents are generally used for routine toxicology tests, while data obtained from larger laboratory animals (monkeys and dogs) are also sometimes required.

The objective of toxicologic study of a target organ is to elucidate the qualitative and quantitative toxic effects of a chemical on the organ. The ultimate objective is to assess the toxic effects of a chemical in laboratory animals and extrapolate the pertinent experimental data to man. To accomplish these objectives, one must consider the main factors that may influence and modulate the toxic effects of chemicals in the organ. In gonads, such modifying factors are the pharmacokinetic parameters governing the absorption, distribution, activation of indirect-acting chemicals, and detoxication, covalent bindings to macromolecules, and DNA damage as well as DNA repair of damaged germ cells.

When assessing the reproductive and developmental toxicity of a chemical on the male gonad, the blood-testis barrier, the biotransformation mechanisms that can decrease or increase the toxicity of a chemical, and the capacity of the spermatogenic cells to repair DNA damage are all important pharmacokinetic aspects to be considered. A pharmacokinetic model of the testicular compartments is presented in Figure 15–6.

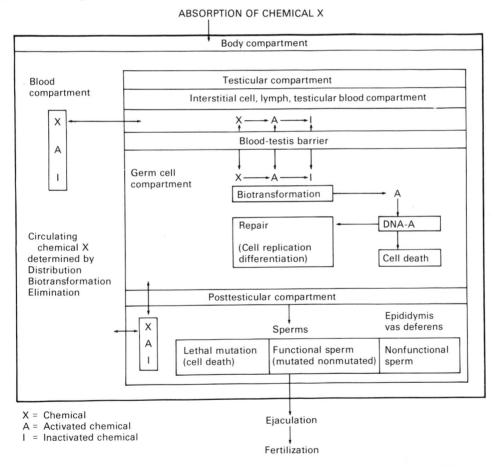

Figure 15–6. A pharmacokinetic model for the male gonad system. (From Lee, I. P., and Dixon, R. L.: Factors influencing reproduction and genetic toxic effects on male gonads. *Environ. Health Perspect.*, **24**:117–27, 1978.)

Blood-Testis Barrier

The blood-testis barrier (BTB) regulates the penetration of exogenous chemicals to male germ cells in the seminiferous tubules (Okumura *et al.*, 1975; Lee and Dixon, 1978). Apparently, permeability of nonelectrolytes across the BTB is dependent on molecular size, suggesting bulk flow through water-filled pores. On the other hand, permeability of ionic drugs with varying pK_a values correlates best with lipid solubility (partition coefficients). The transport of chemicals from blood to seminiferous tubules closely resembles their transport from blood to cerebrospinal fluid (Fig. 15–7). It appears that the BTB is a complex multicellular system composed of membranes surrounding the seminiferous tubules and the several layers of spermatogenic cells organized within the tubules, which restricts the penetrability to the male germ cells of many foreign compounds. This barrier as well as other pharmacokinetic parameters must be borne in mind when extrapolating data from *in vitro* toxicity test systems to man (Dixon and Lee, 1973).

There does not appear to be a blood-ovarian barrier protecting the ovum similar to that which restricts the penetration of chemicals from the blood to the lumen of the seminiferous tubules. However, the ovary does seem to have the capability to biotransform certain exogenous substrates.

Biotransformation

Exogenous chemicals introduced into an organism may undergo chemical transformation, a process termed metabolic transformation or biotransformation. Transformation is accomplished by enzymes and results in either the alteration of the foreign chemical or the formation of conjugated products. The new product may be more toxic than the parent compound. For example, the toxic effects of polycyclic hydrocarbons in tissues other than germ cells have been demonstrated to be due to its metabolite, an epoxide, which interacts with DNA, RNA, and other macromolecules. A steady-state level of epoxide(s) within the cells of a target organ is obviously a function of the metabolite's rate of formation and degradation and the sensitivity of the organ to such toxic metabolite(s). Consequently, the rates of epoxide-forming and detoxifying enzyme activities in various tissues or cells can be an important determinant of tissue specific toxicity.

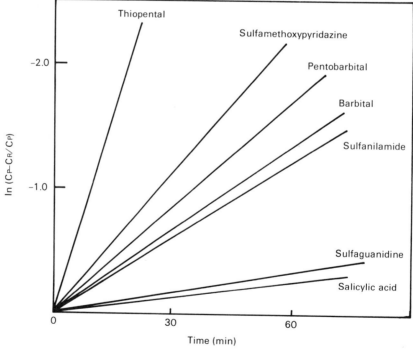

Figure 15–7. Relative rates of transport of various chemicals into the rete-testis fluid. The slope of each line is the rate constant. C_R represents chemicals concentration in the rete-testis fluid, and C_P represents unbound concentration of chemicals in the plasma. (From Okumura, K.; Lee, I. P.; and Dixon, R. L.: Permeability of selected drugs and chemicals across the blood-testis barrier of the rat. *J. Pharmacol. Exp. Ther.*, **194**:89–95, 1975. © 1975 The Williams & Wilkins Co., Baltimore.)

Table 15-1. EPOXIDE HYDRASE, GLUTATHIONE S-TRANSFERASE. AND ARYL HYDROCARBON HYDROXYLASE ACTIVITIES AND CYTOCHROME P-450 CONTENT OF MICROSOMES OR 176,000 g SUPERNATANT FRACTION FROM ADULT RAT TESTIS

ENZYME	SPECIFIC ACTIVITY OR CONTENT MEAN $\pm$ SD(n)	
	Testis	Liver
Glutathione S-transferase, nmole product/min-mg protein with benzo[a]pyrene-4,5-oxide substrate*	19.99 $\pm$ 1.11(8)	41.29 $\pm$ 2.10(4)
Epoxide hydrase, nmole product/min-mg protein with benz[a]pyrene-4,5-oxide substrate†	0.77 $\pm$ 0.06(8)	10.85 $\pm$ 1.68(4)
Aryl hydrocarbon hydroxylase, pmole 3-hydroxybenzo[a]pyrene formed/min-mg protein†	5.17 $\pm$ 0.58(4)	106 $\pm$ 8.3(6)
Cytochrome P-450, nmole/mg protein†	0.125 $\pm$ 0.018(4)	0.85 $\pm$ 0.03(6)

* 176,000 g supernatant.
† Microsomes.

The relative specific activities of aryl hydrocarbon hydroxylase (AHH), epoxide hydroxylase (EH), glutathione S-transferase (GSH-ST), and cytochrome P-450 in adult testes and liver are shown in Table 15–1. Appreciable activities of both mixed-function oxidases and epoxide-degrading enzymes, as well as cytochrome P-450, have been found in testicular tissue. Glutathione S-transferase activity was especially high. The distribution of these enzymes and cytochrome P-450 in the interstitial and germ cell compartment indicates that AHH activity and cytochrome P-450 content of microsomes from the interstitial cells were nearly two-fold greater than those in the tubules (Table 15–2). In contrast, the specific activities of the detoxication enzymes, EH and GSH-ST, in tubules were

twice those in the interstitial cells. Although AHH activity in interstitial cell microsomes was only 5.0 percent that of hepatic microsomes, its close proximity to the germ cells may be important for enzyme-activated toxic chemicals (Bend et al., 1977; Lee and Dixon, 1978).

Factors affecting induction of AHH and cytochrome P-450 probably play a significant role in germ cell toxicity. 2,3,7,8-Tetrachlorodibenzo-p-dioxin (TCDD) and benzo(a)pyrene significantly induce both testicular and prostatic AHH activity and cytochromes. AHH activity induced by TCDD in rat testis and prostate gland was 2 and 150 times that of its controls, respectively. Thus, exposure to environmental chemicals can induce significant levels of activating enzyme systems in male testis

Table 15-2. EPOXIDE HYDRASE, GLUTATHIONE S-TRANSFERASE, AND ARYL HYDROCARBON HYDROXYLASE ACTIVITIES AND CYTOCHROME P-450 CONTENT OF MICROSOMES OR 176,000 g SUPERNATANT FRACTION PREPARED FROM RAT TESTICULAR INTERSTITIAL AND SPERMATOGENIC CELLS

ENZYME	SPECIFIC ACTIVITY OR CONTENT	
	Interstitial Cells	Spermatogenic Cells
Glutathione S-transferase, nmole/min protein*	65.3 $\pm$ 4.8(3)	119 $\pm$ 6.8(3)
Epoxide hydrase, nmole/min-mg protein†	1.09 $\pm$ 0.32(3)	2.36 $\pm$ 0.52(3)
Aryl hydrocarbon hydroxylase, pmole/min-mg protein†	5.98 $\pm$ 0.58(3)	3.18 $\pm$ 0.32(3)
Cytochrome P-450 content nmole mg protein†	0.196(2)	0.084(2)

* 176,000 g supernatant.
† Microsomes.

as well as in the prostate gland, which suggests further modulation of genetic toxicity of germ cells as well as potential tumorigenicity of prostate glands.

DNA Repair

There are many indications that the mammalian cell recognizes and removes DNA damaged as a consequence of exposure to a variety of chemical agents. Moreover, there appear to be two distinct mechanisms by which this repair of mammalian cell DNA can be achieved. The first is referred to as excision repair or "cut and patch repair"; the chemical region in the DNA is recognized by a complex enzyme system that excises the modified base from the DNA, degrades it, resynthesizes a section to reconstitute the original DNA strand, and then inserts this in the preexisting DNA.

The second type of repair in mammalian cells is the so-called postreplication DNA repair, which bypasses damage in the DNA templates. Synthesis takes place only along the undamaged portions of the DNA strands, which are later joined into normal DNA strands following cell replication.

Damage inflicted on the DNA templates, unless repaired, may interfere with transcription and replication resulting in lethal mutations (cell death), mutations that develop into transformed cells, or genetic mutations that in the case of germ cells can be amplified by generations of genetic recombinations. Genetic deficiencies in the DNA repair system are found among people with the disease called xeroderma pigmentosum.

The incorporation of thymidine into DNA following a mutagen challenge is one estimate of unscheduled DNA synthesis or DNA repair. Following treatment with the mutagen methylmethanesulfonate (MMS), thymidine incorporation can be demonstrated in not only spermatogonia but also the leptotene, zygotene, pachytene, and diplotene cells (Fig. 15–8). In contrast, the spermatogenic cells (spermatids and sperm) do not demonstrate thymidine incorporation following MMS suggesting an inability to repair damaged DNA.

Little is known about the ability of ovum in the ovaries to repair their DNA damaged by chemical or physical mutagens. Most reports suggest that this capability is absent until after conception; repair has been demonstrated in preimplantation blastocysts and embryos.

DNA repair capacity appears to be finite and might be saturated with very high test doses of mutagens. Overloading the repair system would result in larger number of affected cells. Repair

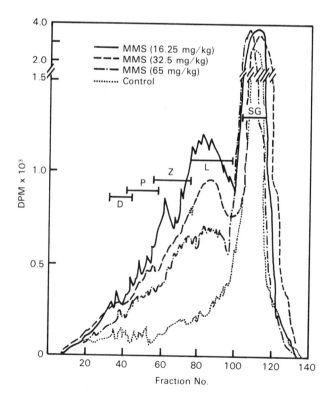

Figure 15–8. Control and MMS-induced changes in the radioactive profiles of various spermatogenic cells after velocity sedimentation cell separation. (From Lee, I. P., and Dixon, R. L.: Factors influencing reproduction and genetic toxic effects on male gonads. *Environ. Health Perspect.*, 24:117–27, 1978.)

rates need to be quantitated and factored into the pharmacokinetic model described (Lee and Dixon, 1978).

GENERAL TOXICOLOGIC PRINCIPLES

The conventional chronic or long-term animal toxicity study is a key feature in the assessment of the safety of most chemicals. The duration of these tests is two to seven years depending on species. Like other areas of toxicology, reproduction must develop more sophisticated approaches to the assessment of toxicity that are more reliable, cheaper, and faster. This chapter will indicate certain experimental approaches that are relatively simple and more quickly yield information regarding reproductive toxicity.

In general, the damage to gonads and their function can result from (1) direct actions of chemicals on germ cells without apparent influence on endocrine glands, (2) actions affecting the accessory secretions of prostate and seminal vesicles in the male, or (3) inhibition of overall hormonal controlling mechanisms at either the gonads or hypothalamic-pituitary level. Evidence suggests that different environmental chemicals might exert their effects via any of these mechanisms.

Experimental results suggest that a large number of chemicals affect male and female reproduction. These are summarized in Tables 15-3 and 15-4. Although the extrapolation from laboratory animals to humans is inexact, a large number of these chemicals do affect human reproduction; almost all require further study.

Testing Male Reproductive Capacity in Laboratory Animals

A variety of morphologic, biochemical, and functional parameters are used to assess toxic effects on male reproductive function. A brief discussion of each parameter follows.

Gross Pathology. A great deal of useful information can be obtained by measuring the weight and the volume of the testis, prostate, seminal vesicles, epididymis, and coagulating glands. Gross changes in the pituitary and adrenal glands are also useful parameters obtained easily. When working with larger animals such as the beagle dog and rhesus monkey, it is important to realize that the dog does not reach puberty until one year of age and the monkey at about three years.

The external appearance of the genitalia is especially important in assessing the postnatal effects of gestational chemical exposure. For example, is the penis hypoplastic, is hypospadias evident? The genitoanal distance is useful in

Table 15-3. INFERRED TOXICITY: MALE REPRODUCTION

Steroids
Natural and synthetic estrogens (antiestrogens), androgens (antiandrogens), and progestins

Chemotherapeutic Agents
Alkylating agents—esters of methanesulfonic acid (MMS, EMS, busulfan); nitrosoureas (CCNU, BCNU, MNU); hydrazines (procarbazine); ethylenimines (TEM, TEPA); nitrogen mustards (cyclophosphamide); others (mitomycin C)
Antimetabolites—folic acid antagonists (methotrexate); nucleic acid analogs (6-MP, 5-FU, azauridine, cytosine arabinoside)
Antitumor antibiotics—dactinomycin, daunomycin, adriamycin, bleomycin
Miscellaneous—vinca alkaloids (vincristine, vinblastine)

Other Therapeutic Agents
Psychopharmacologic agents—reserpine, phenothiazines, monoamine oxidase inhibitors
Adrenergic blocking agents—guanethidine
Diuretics—thiazides, spironolactone
Anti-infective agents—hycanthrone, nitrofuran derivatives
Volatile anesthetics—halothane, methoxyflurane
Oral hypoglycemia agents—chlorpropamide
Chronic alcoholism—tetraethylthiuram disulfide (antabuse)

Trace Elements
Cadmium, mercury, methylmercury, boron, lead

Insecticides
Organochlorine derivatives—O chlorophenothane (DDT), dieldrin, chlordane, benzene hexachloride, chlordecone (kepone)
Organophosphates—chlolinesterase inhibitors
Carbamates—carbaryl

Other Pesticides
Herbicides—chlorinated phenoxyacetic acids (2,4,-D, 2,4,5-T), diquat, paraquat
Fungicides—ethylene dibromide, 1,2 dibromo-3-chloropropane (DBCP), dithiocarbamates
Fumigants—ethylene dibromide

Food Additives and Contaminants
Cyclamate, nitrofuran derivatives, diethylstilbestrol (DES), aflatoxins

Industrial Chemicals
Volatile solvents—benzene, toluene, xylene
Alcohols—ethanol
Monomers—vinyl chloride
Chlorinated hydrocarbons—polychlorinated biphenyls (PCBs), 2,3,7,8-tetrachlorodibenzo-*p*-dioxin (TCDD), hexafluoroacetone

Miscellaneous
Radiation—alpha, beta, and gamma radiation; x-rays
Stable isotopes—deuterium oxide
Physical factors—heat

**Table 15-4. INFERRED TOXICITY:
FEMALE REPRODUCTION**

Steroids

Natural and synthetic estrogens, androgens, and progestins

Miscellaneous Drugs

Reserpine, phenothiazines, amphetamine, serotonin, monamine oxidase inhibitors, antineoplastic agents (cyclophosphamide)

Organochlorine Derivatives

Chlorophenothane (DDT) and derivatives

Organophosphates

Parathion and derivatives (cholinesterase inhibitors)

Carbamate Insecticides

Carbaryl

Food Additives and Contaminants

Cyclohexylamine, nitrosamines, nitrofuran derivatives (AF$_2$), diethylstilbestrol (DES)

Industrial Chemical and Pollutants

Polychlorinated biphenyls (PCBs), phthalic acid esters (DEHP)

---

determining the sex of very young animals. The position of the testes should be determined. Are the testes scrotal or retained? Internal examination should concentrate on anatomic relationships noting retained testes, tumors, or "feminization" (the occurrence of vagina or uterus coexisting with male structures).

Histopathology. Light microscopy of the testes, prostate, seminal vesicle, vas deferens, epididymis, adrenal, and pituitary is essential. Transmission electron microscopy of the testes and pituitary may provide additional information. Scanning electron microscopy has only recently been directed to the male reproductive system, and its usefulness as of yet is undetermined.

Biochemical Parameters. Biochemical indicators of toxicity include a variety of well-established tests. Sperm respiration can be determined by monitoring oxygen consumption and carbon dioxide production. Kinase activity is an important indicator of phosphorylation.

The synthesis rates of nucleic acids as well as total nucleic acid content contribute to the overall toxicologic assessment.

The study of cytoplasmic and nuclear androgen receptors in the target tissues is a rapidly developing area with application to toxicology. Gonadotropin receptors can also be demonstrated in the testes. Affinity constants of these receptors can

be estimated and the effects of various exogenous chemicals determined.

"Marker enzymes" indicative of normal or abnormal cellular differentiation or function have been sought by many investigators. Shen and Lee (1977) studied eight enzymes: hyaluronidase (H), lactate dehydrogenase isoenzyme-X (LDH-X), dehydrogenases of sorbitol (SDH), α-glycerophosphate (GPDH), glucose-6-phosphate (G6PDH), malate (MDH), glyceraldehyde-3-phosphate (G3PDH), and isocitrate (ICDH). Using spectrophotometric kinetic assays, they determined enzyme activities in testicular homogenates and observed two types of enzyme developmental patterns: one involved H, LDH-X, SDH, and GPDH, the other G6PDH, MDH, G3PDH, and ICDH. The pattern for the first group changed from low to high levels with development; the second group changed from high to low levels as spermatogenesis was initiated. The two enzyme patterns crossed at puberty. They also examined distribution of SDH and G6PDH in the epididymis and vas deferens. The epididymis and vas deferens of adult mice were high in SDH and low in G6PDH, whereas the reverse was true in prepubertal mice. Histologic observed alterations correlated well with changes in enzyme activities.

Accessory Cell Function. Among the germinal cells of the seminiferous tubules are Sertoli cells. These relatively large cells apparently provide nourishment for the sperm. They are thought to play a role in establishing the blood-testis barrier and have high levels of α-glutamyl-peptidase and androgen-binding proteins (ABP) to transport androgens into premeiotic germ cells.

The Leydig cells, located in the interstitial tissue between the seminiferous tubules, are rich in 3-β-ketosteroid dehydrogenase and secrete testosterone. Testosterone levels in serum should be determined over time since males have episodic secretion of testosterone. The amplitude of these peaks and their frequency should be determined by collecting plasma samples over short intervals for 24 hours.

Hormonal Status. Several hormones are involved in spermatogenesis. One of the roles of follicle-stimulating hormone (FSH) is to stimulate Sertoli cells to produce androgen-binding (ABP) protein to transport androgens to differentiating germ cells, while the role of luteinizing hormone (LH) is to stimulate and maintain continual synthesis of androgens in the interstitial cells. In addition, for the complete process to occur, testosterone must be secreted by the interstitial cells.

The testis has both hormonal and spermatogenic functions. Androgens are the principal sex hormones produced by the testis. The most important is testosterone secreted by the Leydig cells located in the interstitial tissue between the seminiferous tubules. In the Sertoli cells, the conversion of testosterone to estrogen is thought to take place. Androgens and small amounts of estrogens are also produced by the adrenal cortex of both sexes.

Primary testicular failure is due to direct effects on the organ, while secondary failure involves a failure of the adenohypophyseal-testes interaction.

Sperm Analysis. Sperm count is an important but often unreliable indicator of testicular function. In man, a minimum sperm count is 60 million sperms per millimeter of semen; concentration is more important than total number. Sperm morphology is also a useful indicator of chemical toxicity although the background of abnormal cells is high; as many as 40 percent of human sperms may be abnormal. Motility is measured as the number of sperm actively motile and traveling in a straight line. Methods are also available to determine the viability of sperm. The average of "normal" sperm counts in American men may have dropped over the past 25 years. Semen samples of 1,000 men in 1950 showed 44 percent with sperm counts of 100 million or more; a study published in 1977 revealed that only 22 percent of 2,000 men tested had sperm counts of 100 million or more. The percentage of men with sperm counts in the 20-million-to-40-million range rose from 12 percent in the 1950 study to about 22 percent in 1977.

Although it takes only one sperm to fertilize the ovum, there are normally about 100 million sperm per milliliter of semen. Sperm counts of less than 20 million per milliliter of semen generally constitute sterility. The large number of sperm per ejaculate are necessary to overcome the anatomic and chemical difficulties encountered by the sperm in its journey to the ovum in the oviduct. The sperm travel through the chemically unfavorable vagina and pass through the cervix, uterus, and oviduct in order to reach the ovum and fertilize it. Survival of sperm depends on the sperm concentration and motility as well as the rate of passage. Only a few thousand sperm reach the site of fertilization.

Although the maximal rate of speed is only 3 mm per minute, sperm appear in the oviduct 45 minutes after they have been deposited in the vagina. The female organs obviously play an important role in the transport of sperm.

Seminal plasma is the source of nutrients, a buffer, and a vehicle for sperm. The Cowper's gland (bulbourethral gland) produces only scant secretions. The products of the testis, epididymis, and vas deferens accumulate in the vas deferens.

In man, about 30 percent of the semen volume comes from the prostate while 60 percent is produced by the seminal vesicles. The role of the individual accessory gland secretions is unclear. Pregnancy can be induced in animals with sperm taken directly from the epididymis.

Semen analysis does not play a major role in the assessment of reproductive toxicity using laboratory animals although advances are being made in this area. In the human, the preliminary semen examination concerns volume (usually about 3.5 ml), sperm count, and analyses. Chemical analysis of semen focuses on pH and viscosity (coagulated semen usually liquefies in 20 minutes) as well as prostatic and seminal vesicle secretions. The extended semen analysis described by Eliasson (1978) includes estimates of nuclear maturation, metabolic patterns, survival and motility patterns, and intracellular constituents as well as sperm penetration of cervical mucus.

Prostatic secretions are rich in acid phosphatase, lysozymes, citric acid, aminotransferase, dehydrogenases, zinc, and magnesium. Seminal vesicle secretions are rich in fructose and prostaglandins.

Spermatogenic Cell Separation. The inability to separate physically complex cell populations, such as spermatogenic cells, into their homogenous subpopulations capable of normal function can severely limit the study of biochemical events of individual cell types. Most studies in the past utilized autoradiographic and/or histochemical techniques. However, various investigators have recently described zonal gradient centrifugation, unit gravity velocity sedimentation techniques, or a combination of these to effect separation of the various cell types. Lam and coworkers (1970) introduced the velocity sedimentation technique to isolate cells from suspensions of mouse seminiferous tubules. The velocity cell separation technique was further developed and applied to toxicologic evaluation of male reproductive effects (Lee and Dixon, 1972). The incorporation of thymidine, uridine, and L-leucine by the individual cell types was determined and chemical effects on the utilization of these substrates by spermatogenic cells studied.

Nine types of spermatogenic cells can be tentatively identified: diplotene, pachytene, zygotene, secondary spermatocytes, round spermatids, spermatogonia, early elongated spermatids, late elongated spermatids, and sperm (Fig. 15–9). The diplotene cells have the fastest rate of sedimentation; early elongated spermatids, late elongated spermatids, and sperm, the slowest.

The uptake of thymidine radioactivity is

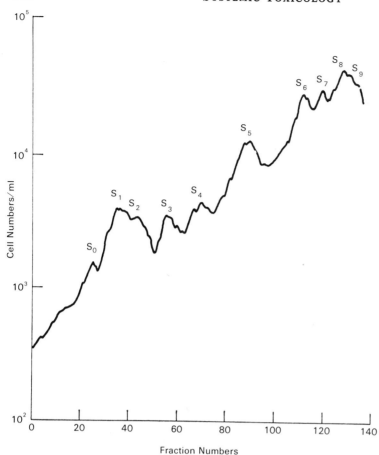

Figure 15–9. Sedimentation pattern of mouse spermatogenic cells. Identification of spermatogenic cells: S_0, unidentified; S_1, diplotene; S_2, pachytene; S_3, zygotene; S_4, secondary spermatocytes; S_5, round spermatids; S_6, spermatogonia; S_7, early elongated spermatids; S_8, late elongated spermatids; S_9, spermatozoa. (From Lee, I. P., and Dixon, R. L.: Antineoplastic drugs effects on spermatogenesis studied by velocity sedimentation cell separation. *Toxicol. Appl. Pharmacol.*, **23**:20–41, 1972.)

confined to a single peak containing predominantly the spermatogonial cell type, indicating that these cells are uniquely involved in normal DNA synthesis.

Following the administration of a mutagenic substance such as methyl methanesulfonate (MMS), thymidine incorporation by various spermatogenic cell types indicates unscheduled DNA synthesis (Fig. 15–8). Because these cell types do not normally incorporate thymidine, they are sensitive indicators of DNA damage that trigger the repair mechanism.

The velocity cell separation technique can also be used to determine the cellular affinity of specific spermatogenic cells for chemicals and trace metals. For instance, both cadmium and zinc are incorporated into the late elongated spermatids, the early elongated spermatids, and the spermatogonia. A competitive binding relationship exists with spermatids between cadmium and zinc with cadmium having greater affinity.

Reproductive Function. The serial mating technique using experimental animals (mice and

rats) is a useful test of dominant lethal mutations as well as male reproductive function. After treatment with the selected chemical, each male is housed singly with a virgin female for a period of seven days. This duration ensures that the female experiences one estrus cycle during the breeding period. During each seven-day period, female animals are examined daily for vaginal plugs to ensure that the treatment does not interfere with ejaculation and mating capability. After seven days the female mouse is replaced. These breeding studies are usually continued for for 70 days (Lee and Dixon, 1972b).

Nine days after the end of the breeding period, when a female could be approximately 12.5 days pregnant, the females are sacrificed, uteri and fetuses are examined, and the number of dead and viable fetuses recorded. Fertility profiles can be drawn from these data and presented in the form of a graph in which the ordinate expresses the percentage or the fraction of the males determined to be fertile as indicated by pregnant females (Fig. 15–10). The relative duration of each main type of spermatogenic stage for mice is

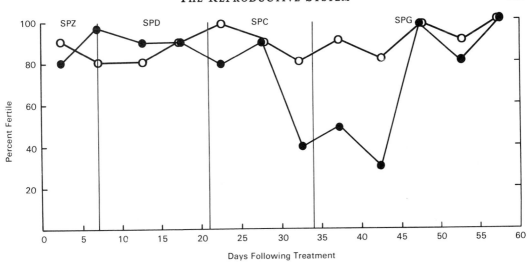

Figure 15–10. Fertility profile expressing the percentage of males determined to be fertile as indicated by pregnant females.

as follows: spermatogonia nine days, spermatocytes 11 days, spermatids 14 days, sperm seven days. Serial mating assesses the biologic functionality of sperm cells and produces fertility patterns that are inversely related in time to the phase of spermatogenesis damaged by the treatment. Thus, the relationship between the environmental agent effect on fertility and the type of spermatogenic stage affected and possible biochemical effect can be estimated.

As an example, the fertility profile presented in Figure 15–10 indicates that the test chemical affected only spermatogonia and perhaps early primary spermatocytes. This unique effect suggests an action on DNA synthesis. The test chemical is, in fact, cytosine arabinoside, an effective inhibitor of DNA polymerase that blocks DNA synthesis. Similarly distinct profiles are produced with chemicals like vincristine that cause mitotic arrest and alkylating agents that affect both replicating as well as nonreplicating (spermatids, sperm) cells.

Serial mating studies have also been widely used in attempts to assess mutagenic events employing intact animals. Objections to this assay are its relative insensitivity to certain known mutagens and the nonheritable nature of the end point. The most reliable indicator of dominant lethality is a statistically significant increase in the number of early embryonic deaths when females are mated to mutagen-treated males. In certain instances, the mutagen induces a lethal mutation only at a specific stage of spermatogenesis.

Reproductive Behavior. One of the first questions to answer in any reproductive study is whether the animals actually are mating. This can

be determined by inspecting females each day for vaginal plugs. The number of mountings, thrusts, and ejaculations can each be quantitated as indicators of reproductive behavior. It is also important to determine whether the male animal is mounting females or other males. If the male copulates and is still sterile, then one must look at the other type of parameters discussed. If he does not copulate, then the emphasis of further investigations must be on behavioral and neuromuscular deficits.

Testing Female Reproductive Capacity in Laboratory Animals

Although less extensive than for the male, a number of morphologic, biochemical, and functional parameters are available to assess toxic effects on female reproductive function.

Gross Pathology. Animals should be inspected for general appearance of the external genitalia. This is especially important when studying the postnatal effects of gestational chemical exposure. The genitoanal distance can be used to determine the sex of newborn animals, the distance in females being shorter than in males. After sacrifice, the animals can be examined internally for conformity of anatomic relationships, cystic ovaries, and other gross abnormalities. Organ weights, especially of the ovaries and adrenal, are important.

Histopathology. Using light microscopy, all organs important to reproduction should be examined. These obviously include the vagina, cervix, uterus, fallopian tubes, ovaries, adrenals, and pituitary. Periodic acid Schiff's (PAS) stain is used to identify mucous-secreting cells in the vagina and uterus. Transmission electron microscopy (TEM) sometimes provides additional information especially with regard to the ovary and pituitary. Scanning electron microscopy (SEM) of luminal surfaces of the vagina, cervix, and uterus may reveal early anatomic changes.

Ovaries are fixed in Bouin's solution and serial sections prepared. Oocyte counts are generally made in every fifth section, and stages of follicular development quantitated and compared. A comparatively simple and sensitive quantitative method for estimating an increase in the normal rate of follicle atresia consists of using serial sections to count the number of the follicles and then calculate the percent of the atretic follicles. This method provides information on the (1) mean number of follicles in a section, (2) percentage of atretic follicles, and (3) relative percentage of primordial, growing, and graafian follicles.

Biochemical Parameters. The study of nuclear and cytoplasmic hormone receptors in target tissues is a rapidly developing field with important toxicologic application. Estradiol and progesterone receptors are especially important as are the chemicals that compete for these receptors or perhaps alter their conformation. Daily injections of estradiol initially stimulate uterine weight increase and progesterone receptor synthesis, and this effect is reversed with progesterone. It has been hypothesized that progesterone antagonizes estrogen action by reducing estrogen receptor levels although others feel that progesterone acts at a point beyond estrogen receptor availability or translocation to antagonize estrogen action.

Steroid receptors may be important in understanding two aspects of reproductive toxicology. On the one hand, the estrogen receptor may play a role in the initial toxicology of many environmental agents. For example, metabolites of DDT, DMBA, PCBs, and similar aromatic foreign chemicals have been reported to bind to the cytoplasmic receptor for estrogen. Thus, interactions between apparently nonhormonal xenobiotics and cellular receptors for endogenous hormones may result in an inadvertent hormonal response (agonist) or depress normal hormonal balance (antagonist); in either case, reproductive abnormalities could result.

On the other hand, the cellular content of hormone receptors may be modified by exposure to foreign chemicals. Such changes in these important cellular regulatory proteins would alter the response of the affected tissues to subsequent hormonal stimulation. Quantitation of cytoplasmic estrogen receptors in human breast cancer has been a useful adjunct to the therapy of this disease; such studies have helped predict those mammary neoplasms that would respond to estrogen therapy.

The biosynthesis of estradiol and its metabolism to estrone and estriol by the ovary are indicators of reproductive competence. The peripheral catabolism of these steroids is chiefly a function of the liver and involves oxidative metabolism as well as conjugation with glucuronic acid. These metabolic pathways are affected in various ways by exogenous chemicals.

Biochemical analysis, including electrophoresis, of vaginal and uterine luminal fluid is somewhat analogous to semen analysis in the male. In species large enough (like the rabbit, monkey, or dog) follicular fluid from the ovary can be analyzed.

Accessory Cell Function. The follicle with its germ cell has a dual origin; the theca or stromal cells arise from fetal connective tissue of the ovarian medulla and the granulosa cells from the cortical mesenchyme. On the basis of their embryonic origin, the theca and granulosa cells in the female would be comparable to the interstitial (Leydig) and nourishing (Sertoli) cells in the male, respectively. The theca and interstitial cells are probably endocrinologically active while the granulosa and Sertoli cells are more likely endocrinologically inert. Granulosa cells can be prepared from the ovaries and cultured, and the effectiveness of the gonadotropin receptors can be determined by the increase in progesterone biosynthesis in response to LH. Endometrial cells can also be prepared by a multistep enzymatic digestion procedure and maintained in culture where their response to hormones can be evaluated.

Hormonal Status. In all of the above studies it is important that special attention be directed to determining the stage of estrus at the time of examination. Estrous cycles are determined by vaginal smear in laboratory animals. Cycles should be determined over a period of time such as one month and the number of cycles in the period determined as well as the length of each stage of the cycle.

Estimation of the different hormone levels involved in the maintenance of normal ovarian function can be utilized to assess gonadotropic activity as well as to detect subtle deviations. FSH and LH are determined with radioimmunoassay; estrogen and progestrone, with a variety of techniques.

The ovaries or female sex organs have a dual function. They produce and release ova and also produce steroid sex hormones. Estrogens and progesterone each play a role in preparing the uterus for pregnancy.

Changes in pituitary and ovarian hormones during the human estrus cycle are presented in

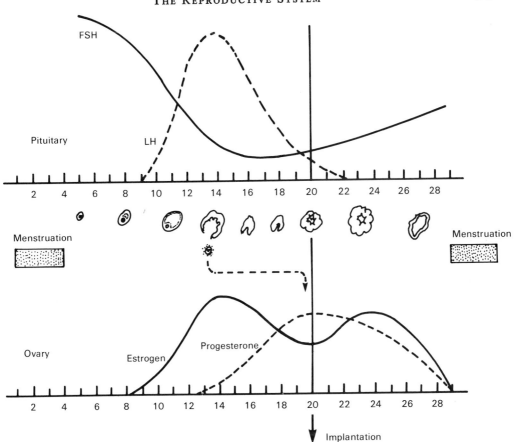

Figure 15–11. Changes in pituitary and ovarian hormones during menstrual cycle. Vertical arrows indicate implantation time of fertilized egg. (Modified from Tuchmann-Duplessis, H.; David, G.; and Haegel, P.: *Illustrated Human Embryology*: *Embryogenesis*, Vol. I. Springer-Verlag, New York, 1972.)

Figure 15–11. Endocrine activity of the ovary is under the control of the anterior lobe of the pituitary, which in human beings secretes two stimulating hormones (gonadotropins). Follicle-stimulating hormone (FSH) is elaborated from the beginning of the cycle. It determines growth of the follicle. Luteinizing hormone (LH) is secreted in the middle of the cycle. It acts synergistically with FSH to provoke ovulation, and it stimulates the development of the corpus luteum. Under the influences of the hypophyseal gonadotropins, endocrine activity of the ovary is disphasic: secretion of estrogen during the first phase, then of estrogen and progesterone during the second phase. Secretion of progesterone is detectable even before formation of the corpus luteum.

The steroid sex hormones also have important regulatory roles in the growth, development, and maintenance of the female sex organs. Among these are the reproductive organs themselves, the oviducts, the uterus and vagina, and secondary sexual characteristics such as the mammary glands, hair, fat distribution, and voice.

The follicles have a triple role. They nurture and expel the mature ovum; secrete estrogen during the growth period of the ovum; and are transformed after maturation and expulsion of the ovum into the corpus luteum, which secretes both estrogens and progesterone. The conceptus somehow prevents the death of the corpus luteum by exerting a luteotropic effect.

Each ovary is in close connection with the fringed end of the oviduct, which leads to the uterus. Rhythmic contractions of the fringed opening aid in directing the recently ovulated ovum into the oviduct. The wall of the oviduct is formed of muscle layers lined internally by ciliated mucosal cells. Both the beating cilia of the tubal lining and the augmented waves in the muscular wall at the time of ovulation are responsible for directing the egg into the oviduct and then transporting it to the uterus. The mucosal cells of the oviduct produce a fluid that increases the fertilizing capacity of the sperm. This process, called capacitation, takes place in the female reproductive tract and continues until the sperm is capable of penetrating the surface of the egg.

The uterus is a muscular organ serving three main functions. It provides the site and conditions necessary for implantation and develops the maternal portion of the placenta necessary for the nourishment and exchange processes of the fetus. The uterus grows and adapts its shape to the rapidly growing fetus and contracts in order to deliver the baby at the end of the gestational period. The uterus has a strong muscular layer, the myometrium, which is lined internally by a mucosa called the endometrium. Both these layers are extremely sensitive to the hormonal secretion of the ovary. The endometrium undergoes cyclic changes in concert with ovarian cycles.

The vagina is lined with a thick layer of stratified squamous epithelium, which undergoes cyclic changes in concert with the ovarian cycle.

A complete reciprocal relationship exists between the two main ovarian hormones, estrogen and progesterone, and the hypophysis, which produces three gonadotropins, follicle-stimulating hormone (FSH), luteinizing hormone (LH), and luteotropic hormone (LTH). These hormones, responding to central nervous system influences, regulate ovulation and the preparation of the endometrium for the nidation and nourishment of the fertilized ovum.

Reproductive Function. Fertility estimation is an integral method for detecting toxic effects on the female reproductive system. The ability to conceive, the outcome of pregnancy, and the viability and postnatal development of the offspring are assessed.

The total reproductive capacity procedure is especially suitable for studying chronic reproductive toxicity in rodents. This type of approach can take advantage of the fact that once the oocytes are lost, they cannot be replaced. Each female is caged permanently with a fertile mature male. Forced breeding is induced by immediate removal of newly born animals from the breeding boxes. Following delivery, the female is immediately receptive to the male. This procedure only provides information concerning whether the fertility of test animals is reduced for whatever reason. The procedure can also be adapted to assess dominant lethality in females.

The forced-breeding technique has been used to study the postnatal effects of diethylstilbestrol (DES), a hormonally active drug and environmental chemical. Following subcutaneous treatment with DES in corn oil on the ninth through sixteenth days of gestation, mice at puberty are subject to the repetitive forced-breeding techniques. A dose-related decrease in reproductive capacity was determined in the female offspring (Table 15-5) (McLachlan and Dixon, 1976).

Over the 32-week period that the animals were observed, the effects ranged from a minimal subfertility (90 percent of controls) at the lowest dose to essential sterility at the two highest doses. It should be pointed out that the highest dose of DES (100 μg/kg) is many times higher than that which might be absorbed in the diet as a result of using DES as a growth promoter.

Ovulation can be induced by the administration of gonadotropins and the quantity and quality of ova examined.

The hormonal responsiveness of the uterus (uterine weight/body weight) can be determined by administering graded doses of estrogen.

Behavioral aspects of reproduction are important and some of the responses, such as lordosis quotients, can be easily obtained.

Table 15-5. FERTILITY OF FEMALE MICE EXPOSED TO DES PRENATALLY*

MATERNAL DES DOSE (μg/kg)	NO. OF OFFSPRING EVALUATED	TOTAL REPRODUCTIVE CAPACITY OF FEMALE OFFSPRING† (% CONTROL)
0	74	100.0
0.001	55	89.4
1	54	76.0
2.5	18	49.4
5	16	22.6
10	61	8.0
100	39	4.3

* Timed pregnant CD-1 mice (at least 20 animals per group) were treated subcutaneously with diethylstilbestrol from days 9 to 16 of gestation.
† Determined by repetitive forced-breeding techniques and expressed as the total number of live young born per mouse over a 32-week interval (McLachlan and Dixon, 1976).

REGULATORY REQUIREMENTS

Tests for Assessing Reproductive Function

Current test procedures for assessing reproductive function are used primarily to meet requirements of the various regulatory agencies. These reproduction studies classically utilize either rats or mice because of their early age of sexual maturity, their short gestational and lactational periods, and ease of handling. Tests are generally conducted to identify general reproductive failures; they usually do not seek information regarding the specific portions of the reproductive sequence involved. Other studies are done routinely for teratogenic or mutagenic effects.

Classically, two different kinds of tests are used: one for drugs, and the other for food additives or pesticides. The two test procedures differ with regard to the way in which either drugs or food additives come in contact with the consuming individual. Drugs are normally taken intentionally at levels that produce biologic effects; therefore, it is assumed their exposure can be controlled. On the other hand, food additives or other environmental contaminants are generally ingested continuously or intermittently at much lower levels, thus not in a directly controllable manner (Tardiff et al., 1977).

Multigeneration Study. An example of a reproductive toxicity test is the multigeneration study. The objective of this experiment is to determine the effect on general reproductive performance of treatment commencing at implantation and continuing through the weaning of F_{2b} litters. Teratology may be included as part of this study.

This protocol offers the advantages of pre-differentiation exposure of the F_1 parental animals without the additional time and costs incurred in a classic two-generation study. If required, pups may be selected from the F_{2b} litters to produce an F_3 generation.

The experiments usually consist of three treatment groups and a control group. Each group consists of 20 sexually mature virgin females mated to a minimum of ten sexually mature males. The highest dosage is a carefully determined maximum tolerated dosage. The two lower dose levels are selected by geometric progression. Test materials are administered orally by gavage, mixed in food, or in drinking water. Treatment of F_0 parental animals may be initiated either on the day of implantation or at the time of pairing. At weaning of the F_{1a} litters, at least ten males and 20 females are randomly selected from each group to become the F_1 parental generation. Body weights and weight gains should be recorded.

When the F_1 parental animals reach sexual maturity, each male is randomly mated with two females from the same group. Successful mating is determined by the presence of a copulation plug or blood in the vagina. If a female does not exhibit additional evidence of copulation at the end of a subsequent estrous cycle, she is returned to her original cage. At the end of two estrous cycles, all males within the same group are rotated and exposed to different females in the same group. No more than three males should be paired with any female during a given breeding cycle. The number of observed copulations, the number of estrous cycles required to obtain a mating, and the number of resulting pregnancies should be recorded. These data are used to calculate mating and fertility indices. The F_{1a} litters are weaned at 21 days postpartum, then sacrificed. After an approximately 15-day rest period, the females are mated again. The above procedure is repeated to obtain the F_{1b} litters. The following indices should be calculated:

Mating index
$$= \frac{\text{Number of copulations}}{\text{Number of estrus cycles required}} \times 100$$

Fecundity index
$$= \frac{\text{Number of pregnancies}}{\text{Number of copulations}} \times 100$$

Male fertility index
$$= \frac{\text{Number of males impregnating females}}{\text{Number of males exposed to fertile non-pregnant females}} \times 100$$

Female fertility index
$$= \frac{\text{Number of females conceiving}}{\text{Number of females exposed to fertile males}} \times 100$$

Incidence of parturition
$$= \frac{\text{Number of parturitions}}{\text{Number of pregnancies}} \times 100$$

All pups (F_{1a}, F_{2a}, and F_{2b}) are examined for physical abnormalities at birth. The numbers of viable, stillborn, and cannibalized members of each litter are recorded. Observations for clinical signs are made daily. The numbers of survivors on days 1, 4, 12, and 21 postparturition are recorded. On the fourth day of lactation, litters with more than ten pups may be reduced to that number by sacrificing randomly selected individuals. A final examination for physical abnormalities is made. Individual body weights are recorded at weaning on lactation day 21. The following survival indices will be calculated:

Live birth index
$$= \frac{\text{Number of viable pups born}}{\text{Total number of pups born}} \times 100$$

24-hour survival index
$$= \frac{\text{Number of pups viable at lactation day 1}}{\text{Number of viable pups born}} \times 100$$

tation cell separation. *Toxicol. Appl. Pharmacol.*, **23**:20–41, 1972a.

Lee, I. P., and Dixon, R. L.: Effects of procarbazine on spermatogenesis studied by velocity sedimentation cell separation and serial mating. *J. Pharmacol. Exp. Ther.*, **181**:219, 1972b.

Lee, I. P., and Dixon, R. L.: Effects of mercury on spermatogenesis studied by velocity sedimentation cell separation and serial mating. *J. Pharmacol. Exp. Ther.*, **194**:171, 1975.

Lee, I. P., and Dixon, R. L.: Factors influencing reproduction and genetic toxic effects on male gonads. *Environ. Health Perspect.*, **24**:117–27, 1978.

Lucier, G. W.; Lee, I. P.; and Dixon, R. L.: Effects of environmental agents on male reproduction. In Johnson, A. D., and Gomes, W. R.: *The Testis.* Advances in Physiology, Biochemistry, and Function, Vol. IV. Academic Press, Inc., New York, 1977, pp. 578–98.

McLachlan, J. A., and Dixon, R. L.: Transplacental toxicity of diethylstilbestrol: A special problem in safety evaluation. In Mehlman, M. A.; Shapiro, R. E.; and Blumenthal, H.: *New Concepts in Safety Evaluation.* Advances in Modern Toxicology, Vol. 1, Part 1. Hemisphere Publishing Co., Washington, D.C., 1976, pp. 423–48.

Nelson, N. (Chairman): *Human Health and the Environment: Some Research Needs.* U.S. Dep. HEW Publ. (NIH) 77–1277, 1977.

Okumura, K.; Lee, I. P.; and Dixon, R. L.: Permeability of selected drugs and chemicals across the blood-testis barrier of the rat. *J. Pharmacol. Exp. Ther.*, **194**:89–95, 1975.

Shen, R. S., and Lee, I. P.: Developmental patterns of enzymes in mouse testis. *J. Reprod. Fertil.*, **48**:301–305, 1977.

Tardiff, R. G. (Chairman): *Principles and Procedures for Evaluating the Toxicity of Household Substances.* National Academy of Sciences. U.S.A., Washington, D.C., 1977.

UNIT III
TOXIC AGENTS

Chapter 16

PESTICIDES

Sheldon D. Murphy

INTRODUCTION

Pesticides occupy a rather unique position among the many chemicals that man encounters daily, in that they are deliberately added to the environment for the purpose of killing or injuring some form of life. Ideally their injurious action would be highly specific for undesirable target organisms and noninjurious to desirable, nontarget organisms. In fact, however, most of the chemicals that are used as pesticides are not highly selective but are generally toxic to many nontarget species, including man, and other desirable forms of life that coinhabit the environment. Therefore, lacking highly selective pesticidal action, the application of pesticides must often be predicated on selecting quantities and manners of usage that will minimize the possibility of exposure of nontarget organisms to injurious quantities of these useful chemicals.

Toxicologic evaluations of the hazard of handling and use of pesticides have for many years focused primarily on preventing injury to man, and common laboratory animals have served as the experimental models for man's biochemical, physiologic, and pathologic responses to these chemicals. Problems of species differences in susceptibility have always left some doubt concerning assignment of safe dosages for man on the basis of studies on common laboratory animals, but this approach appears to have been reasonably successful in protecting the *general population* in that there has not emerged any clear association between increasing use of pesticides and incidence of chronic diseases (Hayes, 1969). However, as discussed subsequently, occupational exposures have resulted in chronic or persistent neurologic disease states in the case of a few compounds.

Acute poisonings by pesticides do occur. They are usually the result of occupational exposures or of careless use, misuse, or mishandling the pesticides. The mortality rate attributed to poisoning by pesticides has been estimated at 0.65 per one million population in the United States, but it has also been estimated that there

are 100 nonfatal poisonings for each fatal one (Hayes, 1969). In spite of the fact that a clear association between chronic diseases and pesticide exposures is not apparent, new and sensitive toxicologic and analytic methods have raised many questions concerning the possibility of subtle effects that would be difficult to recognize unless one directed investigations specifically to reveal them. A review of the status of epidemiologic studies on pesticide toxicology pointed out design and interpretive pitfalls that give cause to question whether our knowledge is adequate to assess the degree of injury or lack of injury to man's health resulting from past or current uses of pesticides (Secretary's Commission on Pesticides, 1969).

Furthermore, increased awareness and concern for ecologic implications of the use of pesticides have begun to direct the attention and research of toxicologists toward studies on wild species as well as on man and domestic animals and laboratory animals that are selected as test models to represent man. The toxicology of pesticides, therefore, must take into account problems relating to both their injurious effects directly upon man and their effects on other species of animals in the environment from which man derives pleasure as well as food or which are essential to maintain a proper ecologic balance.

It is not uncommon for people to equate *pesticides* with *insecticides*. This is erroneous since the term "pesticide" is a general classification and includes a variety of chemicals with different uses. Pesticidal chemicals have in common the capability of destroying life of some form and are classified as pesticides because the organisms against which they are directed are deemed to be undesirable by the person or society that applies them. Indeed, insecticides represent one group of pesticides that are used in large quantities and have a history of causing toxic effects in man, but among the other types of pesticides one can find several potent, injurious agents. In terms of quantities used, the *herbicides*, chemicals used to destroy unwanted plants, rival the insecticides. Another common misconception is that pesticides imply a unity of action, that they all act similarly. This of course is not true. There is as great a diversity in their types of action and primary target tissues as there is diversity in their chemistry and physicochemical properties. There are a large number of pesticides whose acute toxicity is manifested through functional or biochemical action in the central and peripheral nervous systems, but there are others in which nervous system involvement does not occur or is merely secondary to primary effects in other organ systems. The literature on pesticides reveals great disparities in the extent of knowledge concerning specific mechanisms of action. For some groups of compounds the mechanism of toxic action is well understood at the molecular level. For others there is essentially no information concerning mechanisms of toxicity. Similarly the full gamut of toxic dose-response ranges is represented by pesticide chemicals. Even within a similar chemical class, individual compounds ranging from extremely toxic to practically nontoxic may be found. Obviously, therefore, one cannot generalize either qualitatively or quantitatively concerning the toxicity of pesticides.

There is also some misconception that potential health hazards from pesticides are of relatively recent origin. Indeed, some of the most toxic of our current pesticides have been developed in recent years. However, poisoning by pesticides is not a new phenomenon. To illustrate, one can draw upon a case that occurred in the 1920s and is described by John Glaister (1954) in his book *The Power of Poison*. At least 50 homicides involving arsenic poisoning in a small province in Hungary were attributed to one "poisoner for profit." The arsenic was extracted from "flypapers," a common insecticide preparation of the day, and a grocer testified at the trial that more flypapers were sold in the poisoner's village than in the rest of the country. This infamous poisoner-for-profit recognized the fact that the insecticides of the day were a potential, for her a profitable, medium for human destruction. Mrs. Fazekas used insecticides to destroy human pests. Today one of our most-used classes of insecticides, the organic phosphates, are closely allied in their historic development with chemicals developed during World War II whose intended purpose was human destruction.

ECONOMICS AND PUBLIC HEALTH: BENEFITS AND RISKS

As with the use of any potentially injurious chemical substance, the use of pesticides must take into consideration the balance of the benefits that may be expected versus the possible risk of injury to human health or to degradation of environmental quality. It is indeed extremely difficult to quantify the risk-benefit equation relating to the use of pesticides. In some cases the prospect of mass starvation due to destruction of food crops by insects and noxious weeds versus the question of possible injury to a few members of the population as a result of use of insecticides may clearly indicate an advantage of pesticide use in terms of numbers of people whose health and welfare are protected. Similarly where vector-borne diseases represent a major threat to the health of large populations of humans, and where the use of chemical pesticides to destroy the vectors of these diseases is a successful procedure, the application of these chemicals seems to be clearly indicated. On the other hand, widespread distribution of chemicals in the environment to control what may be primarily a nuisance situation raises questions as to whether the benefits to be achieved really justify any risk, however minimal, that human health may be jeopardized.

If one extends these considerations beyond purely a concern for human health and considers the question of ecologic balance, the risk-benefit equation takes on different proportions. In the first case, with the exception of possible exposures of the persons who handle the concentrated pesticides, the human population may not be exposed to any significant quantity of the chemical. However, when these chemicals are distributed over widespread areas of land and aquatic surfaces, there is a distinct possibility that desirable species in the environment, other than man, will receive potentially toxic doses of the chemicals. This may not appear to have any direct effect on man's health and welfare; however, if such effects lead to a serious ecologic imbalance, indirect effects on man are possible. Perhaps the best known of all pesticides, DDT, exemplifies a situation of a product that when introduced as an insecticide in 1942 appeared to hold immense promise of benefit to agricultural economics and protection of public health against vector-borne disease. It was hailed as the miracle insecticide and for two decades was used with little concern for injury, and indeed little evidence that injury was produced. However, during the third decade of its use, effects on the environment, effects in nontarget species other than man, began to raise serious doubts concerning its continued usefulness. Now three decades after its patent many countries of the world have critically restricted the use of DDT because of evidence of environmental damage.

Control of Vector-Borne Disease

Pesticides of various types are used in the control of insects, rodents, and other pests that are involved in the life-cycle of vector-borne diseases such as malaria, filariasis, yellow fever, viral encephalitis, typhus, bubonic plague, Rocky Mountain spotted fever, rickettsialpox etc. The success of DDT in reducing the incidence of malaria in many parts of the world has been dramatic. To cite one example, in the Latina province of Italy in 1944 there were 175 new cases of malaria; in 1945 a DDT spray control program was initiated and by 1947 there were only five new cases of malaria, and by 1949 no new cases of malaria appeared.

This is only one example of a success story for DDT. The story has been repeated and continues to be repeated in some areas. Worldwide estimates of the lives saved by using DDT to destroy insects that transmit malaria and other diseases are numbered in the millions and the illnesses prevented are numbered in the hundreds of millions.

Agricultural Productivity

In many parts of the world excessive loss of food crops to insects and other destructive pests contribute to an obvious health problem—starvation. In these countries use of chemicals for controlling these pests clearly seems to have a favorable cost-benefit relationship. In lands of plenty such a clear health benefit may be less obvious. Then, attempts to evaluate the cost-benefit ratios are often reduced to economic considerations. It has been estimated that in 1963 the use of pesticides in the United States resulted in an increase in the value of farm production of about 1.8 billion dollars. This was achieved with an expenditure of about 0.44 billion dollars for control chemicals and procedures. Thus, one can estimate that the net economic benefit was an approximate 1.4-billion-dollar contribution to the gross national product (Headley and Kneese, 1969).

Urban Pest Control

Although the total usage of pesticides, in terms of pounds applied, is largest in those applications related to agriculture or forestry, these toxic chemicals are also used in urban areas. In addition to the use of pesticides by government service agencies, as in mosquito and rodent control programs and weed control on highways and utility rights of way, there is a rather large use of pesticides by individual home owners and gardeners. For example, during a one-year period in Salt Lake County, Utah, of the total of 200,865 lb of pesticides used, 102,490 lb were used for domestic or household applications. The balance was used by farmers, commercial applicators, fruit growers, and government agencies, and for mosquito abatement, and on livestock. There are, however,

great contrasts in these proportions, as illustrated by the statistics for Arizona. The domestic usage for the state accounted for only about 0.6 percent of the total compared to over 50 percent of the total in Salt Lake County, Utah (Secretary's Commission on Pesticides, 1969).

A study of domestic use in South Carolina indicated that 89 percent of all families used pesticides in some form. In that study 50 percent of the pesticide purchases were made at the grocery store, the same source as the family's food. Lesser retail sources were feed and seed, drug, and general merchandise stores. Ninety percent of the families stored their pesticides in unlocked storage areas; 65 percent of these storage areas were within easy reach of children; about 50 percent of the families stored their pesticides near food or medicine. Moreover, 75 percent of the user families did not take simple precautions such as washing or use of gloves when handling their pesticides. In spite of this almost flagrant violation of precautionary measures, it appeared there was no significant difference in the incidence of a variety of chronic diseases between pesticide user families and nonuser families (Keil et al., 1969). In addition, there are a number of rather subtle possibilities for exposure to pesticides from a wide variety of sources. Pesticides have been incorporated into shelf papers. They are incorporated in some kinds of paints as antifungal agents, they are used in mixtures of swimming pool chemicals for algae control, in various types of automatic dispensers in public buildings and homes, and they have been used in dry-cleaning processes for rugs and other fabrics.

It is clear that the opportunities for exposure to pesticides are great. Because the use of pesticides is associated primarily with agricultural operations, major concern is usually for the food we eat. However, it is quite possible that less controlled and less regulated uses of pesticides may offer the greatest opportunity for exposure to toxicologically significant quantities.

Environmental Contamination

It is apparent that there are many sources of exposure of humans and other nontarget species to pesticides by direct contact with materials at the site of application. In recent years, however, it has become increasingly apparent that exposures to pesticides far remote from the source of application are also possible. This results from the translocation of the chemicals from their sites of application through the various media of the environment. The extent to which translocation within the environment occurs will depend to a large degree on the physicochemical properties of the pesticides. Perhaps one of the most important factors is the extent of and time required for degradation of chemicals to simpler nontoxic forms. Since several of the organo chlorine insecticides and some of the heavy metals are the most persistent types of pesticides, these compounds have been the object of most concern for problems of translocation and biomagnification. For example, DDT is only slowly metabolized by biologic systems. Some of the metabolites are extremely resistant to further degradation, but retain some of the biologic activities of the parent compound. In addition, the partition coefficient for DDT in fat-soluble substances, relative to aqueous media, is very high. Therefore, this chemical will be concentrated through a food chain since it tends to partition into lipoidal biologic materials in increasing concentrations until, at the top of the food chain pyramid, a potentially hazardous concentration may exist.

DDT applied in a mosquito control program in a tropical or subtropical area may ultimately have adverse effects on species in Arctic regions. Thus, small quantities that may be present in mud and surface waters are taken up by plankton and other food sources for phytophagous fish. These fish ingest the plankton containing insecticide and its metabolites at a rate insufficient to poison them, but sufficient to allow storage and concentration in their fatty tissue. The phytophagous fish are eaten by carnivorous fish, again at a rate at which the dosage is not immediately harmful, but partitioning into the fat allows slow accumulation of a high concentration in fat. In turn, these fish may migrate and be ingested by birds in Arctic climates, such as falcons and eagles, in sufficient quantities to contribute doses of the insecticide or its metabolites that can affect avian reproduction (Secretary's Commission on Pesticides, 1969).

Other nonbiologic modes of translocation include vaporization and drift by airborne routes so that the materials are carried by prevailing wind patterns far remote from their site of application. Subsequently, they may be precipitated out by rainfall onto land and surface waters in areas in which the pesticides have not been applied directly. Application to the soil may result, ultimately, in suspension of the pesticides, adsorbed on soil particles, and airborne translocation as dust. The extent to which pesticides will remain in soils after application depends upon a number of factors: such as soil type, moisture, temperature, pH, microorganism content, degradability of the pesticide itself, and the extent of cultivation and cover crops (Lichtenstein, 1966). In general, the organochlorine insecticides are most persistent in soils (with the exception of heavy metals, which of course are not further degraded), followed by certain of the herbicides and with the phosphate insecticides and carbamate insecticides and herbicides being the least persistent. An understanding of the potential for persistence and translocation,

therefore, must take into consideration not only the biologic aspects of pesticides but also an analysis of their behavior under various physical and chemical characteristics of the environment. As will be pointed out subsequently, chemical changes of the parent insecticides that result from either physicochemical reactions in the environment or biologically catalyzed reactions may lead to products with either greater or lesser toxicity and with either greater or lesser potential for biotranslocation.

Production and Use Statistics

Before the mid-1940s the primary pesticides in use were botanical in origin and compounds of heavy metals. Subsequently, there has been a marked increase in total pesticide usage and a rapid proliferation of synthetic organic compounds. There are now approximately 900 chemicals that are registered for sale as pesticides against about 2,000 pest species (Secretary's Commission on Pesticides, 1969). The U.S. production of pesticides in 1971 was approximately 1.2 billion lb (Von Rumker et al., 1975).

The estimated total pesticide purchases by farmers increased from 184 million dollars in 1955 to 1 billion dollars in 1968. This marked increase in sales of pesticides occurred in spite of the fact that the harvested acreage during this period declined from 335 million acres to 294 million acres. In recent years there have been rather dramatic shifts in the types of pesticides used by farmers. For example, until the mid-1960s insecticides were the leading class of pesticides used. Since then herbicides have begun to outpace insecticides. In 1971 the U.S. market for agricultural use of herbicides was estimated at 640 million dollars compared to $225 million for insecticides and $65 million for fungicides (NAS, 1976). Also, in the mid-1960s there was a shift in the types of insecticides used, from the organochlorine to the less stable organophosphate and carbamate classes. In Europe, fungicide sales lead the pesticide market.

Shifts in uses of major classes reflect not only developments in agricultural practice but also the effect of regulatory restrictions and the development of resistance by the pests to certain classes of chemicals.

Human Poisonings

As stated initially, pesticides have a relatively good record in the United States in terms of fatalities resulting from exposure. The United States has escaped major incidents of mass acute fatal poisonings, but this is not the case when one considers the worldwide record (see Table 16-1). There have been several reports of various disease conditions or altered clinical test values resulting from chronic exposure to

Table 16–1. MASS POISONINGS BY PESTICIDES*

KIND OF ACCIDENT	PESTICIDE INVOLVED	MATERIAL CONTAMINATED	NUMBER AFFECTED	NUMBER DIED	LOCATION
Spillage during transport or storage	Endrin	Flour	159	0	Wales
	Endrin	Flour	691	24	Qatar
	Endrin	Flour	183	2	S. Arabia
	Dieldrin	Food	20	0	Shipboard
	Diazinon	Doughnut mix	20	0	U.S.A.
	Parathion	Wheat	360	102	India
	Parathion	Barley	38	9	Malaya
	Parathion	Flour	200	8	Egypt
	Parathion	Flour	600	88	Colombia
	Parathion	Sugar	300	17	Mexico
	Parathion	Sheets	3	0	Canada
	Mevinphos	Plants	6	0	U.S.A.
Eating formulation	Hexachlorobenzene	Seed grain	>3000	3–11%	Turkey
	Organic mercury	Seed grain	34	4	West Pakistan
	Organic mercury	Seed grain	321	35	Iraq
	Organic mercury	Seed grain	45	20	Guatemala
	Warfarin	Bait	14	2	Korea
Improper application	Toxaphene	Collards and chard	7	0	U.S.A.
	Nicotine	Mustard	11	0	U.S.A.
	Parathion	Used as treatment for body lice	>17	15	Iran
	Pentachlorophenol	Nursery linens	20	2	U.S.A.

* From Secretary's Commission on Pesticides, U.S. Department of Health, Education, and Welfare: *Report of the Secretary's Commission on Pesticides and Their Relationship to Environmental Health*, U.S. Governmental Printing Office, Washington, D.C., 1969.

pesticides, but these conditions are generally reversible and thus cannot be classified as true chronic injury. The relatively small numbers of cases in which progressive chronic disease has been associated with pesticide exposure preclude establishment of cause-and-effect relationships and prevent the conclusion that the widespread use of pesticides has contributed to an increasing incidence of chronic disease (Hayes, 1969). This is not to say there is room for complacency in this regard. As new methods of toxicologic evaluation reveal subtle effects previously unknown and as this information is applied to well-designed epidemiologic studies, it may be found that pesticides have produced currently undetected effects on health. In our present state of knowledge, however, we must deal with the evidence at hand and hope that increased awareness on the part of the medical profession and of the public will stimulate further exploration of any possible injurious effects.

Most of the epidemiologic studies that have been conducted to search for possible associations between disease and pesticide exposure have been done on sample populations that would be expected to be high-risk groups, such as persons occupationally exposed in the manufacturing, formulating, or application of the materials. This appears an obvious choice of study groups; however, failure to find effects in

these groups need not preclude that effects occur. For example, persons who experience discomfort or mild illnesses may voluntarily remove themselves from occupations involving the use of pesticides. In addition, as will be discussed later, laboratory animal research has shown that certain types of adaptation occur with continuous and frequent exposures to pesticides. Whether or not this is a factor that can influence the detection of effects in workers with different durations of exposure remains to be demonstrated. As discussed below, however, there is ample evidence that exposure to pesticides has resulted in acute fatal poisonings and reversible illnesses.

Statistical surveys of mortality and morbidity resulting from acute exposures to pesticides reveal that children are the victims of a high percentage of accidental fatal poisonings. Reich and coworkers (1968) reported that during the period of 1956 through 1967 there were 122 fatal cases of documented pesticide poisoning in Dade Country, Florida. Fifty-seven percent of these fatalities were suicidal, 29.8 percent were accidental, homicides accounted for 9.9 percent, and 2.5 percent were occupational. Twenty-seven percent of the fatalities were children under five years of age and the deaths were usually the result of accidental ingestions. Adults over 40 accounted for 48 percent of the cases (mostly suicides) and the route of exposure in 90 percent of these was also oral, with three cases of dermal exposure and five due to inhalation. Of the 122 cases, 65 involved organophosphate insecticides, with parathion as the agent in 53 of these 65. Heavy metals (with arsenic as the prime offender) and white phosphorus were responsible for 27 of the deaths. Succeeding these classes, in order of frequency, were nicotine, organochlorines, cyanide, strychnine, and miscellaneous.

From the period of 1964 to 1967 both mortality and morbidity data were available. Of the 133 cases of documented pesticide poisonings during this period, 47 (35 percent) were fatal. Of the 133 cases, 61 were the result of accidental poisonings with 11 of them fatal. The mean age for accidental poisoning was 8.6 years. There were 25 cases of occupational poisonings, but only one was fatal. There was a 70 percent case fatality rate when pesticides were ingested for suicidal purposes (in 37 of the total 133 poisonings). Of the occupational poisonings 24 of the 25 cases involved organophosphate insecticides. Parathion was the agent in one fatal case of occupational poisoning. Organophosphate insecticides accounted for 72 percent of the total accidental cases and 90 percent of the accidental fatalities, 60 percent of the total suicide attempts, and 51 percent of the successful suicides.

Death records of the California Department of Public Health (1969) for the period 1951 to 1969 revealed that, as in Florida, children accounted for over half (92) of the total (163) accidental deaths due to poisoning by agricultural chemicals. However, only 17 of the fatal childhood poisonings were due to organic phosphates, while arsenic compounds accounted for 48 of the deaths. There were 35 accidental nonoccupational, pesticide poisoning fatalities among adults during this period, 17 of them due to arsenic compounds. Occupational poisonings accounted for 36 of the 163 deaths. Eighteen of the occupational poisonings were due to organophosphate insecticides, seven to methyl bromide, and 13 to other agricultural chemicals. Thus, during the period of 1951 to 1969 arsenic-containing pesticides were involved most frequently in nonoccupational poisonings, while organophosphates were most frequently involved in occupational pesticide poisoning fatalities. It was concluded that organophosphates played a smaller role in fatal poisonings among children in California because state regulations made these agents less readily available for indiscriminate home use. Mortality attributed to accidental poisoning by pesticides in the United States appears to have been declining during the past two decades. Hayes and Vaughn (1977) report that in 1974 there were only 52 fatal accidental poisonings with pesticides, compared to 152 in 1956. During this period the proportion of fatal poisonings in children declined from 61 to 31 percent. This decline was attributed to an increased awareness on the part of poison control centers and pediatricians to the hazards of pesticides to children.

Injuries from occupational exposures reported under the requirements of the State Workmen's Compensation Law in California have provided statistical compilations of the extent of injuries due to pesticides and other agricultural chemicals (California Department of Public Health, 1969). The rate for all occupational disease reports in agricultural workers in 1969 was 8.5 per 1,000 workers, more than three times the rate for all industry (2.6 per 1,000). There were 727 occupational disease reports attributed to agricultural chemicals in California in 1969. Thirty-two percent of these involved organic phosphate insecticides, 10 percent herbicides, 8 percent halogenated hydrocarbon insecticides, 6 percent fertilizers, and 44 percent miscellaneous or unidentified chemicals. Of the 175 cases

Table 16–2. TYPE OF OCCUPATIONAL DISEASE REPORTED CAUSED BY PESTICIDES AND OTHER AGRICULTURAL CHEMICALS IN CALIFORNIA IN 1969*

TYPE OF CHEMICAL	TYPE OF DISEASE				
	Systemic Poisoning	Respiratory Condition	Skin Condition	Other and Unspecified	TOTAL ALL TYPES
Organic phosphate pesticides	140	4	12	75	231
Halogenated hydrocarbon pesticides	9	7	19	22	57
Herbicides	3	9	50	14	76
Fertilizers	—	8	28	7	43
Fungicides	2	3	21	1	27
Phenolic compounds	2	1	10	2	15
Sulfur	1	2	25	3	31
Organomercury compounds	1	—	—	1	2
Lead or arsenic	2	—	2	5	9
Miscell.—specified	5	1	15	7	28
Unspecified	9	12	162	21	204
Total	175	47	345	160	727

* From California Department of Public Health: *Occupational Diseases in California Attributed to Pesticides and Other Agricultural Chemicals, 1969.* Bureau of Occupational Health and Environment Epidemiology, Sacramento, 1969.

diagnosed as systemic poisonings, organophosphate insecticides were responsible for 80 percent, and they were involved in 47 percent of another 160 reports of digestive and other non-localized symptoms of illness. This high contribution of systemic poisonings due to organic phosphates continued the record of several years (from 1956 to 1969 from 125 to 407 reports of systemic occupational poisonings were reported annually in California). Parathion was the agent most frequently involved. Table 16–2 shows the types of disease conditions produced by various agricultural chemicals in California in 1969. Table 16–3 illustrates the industries and occupations in which poisonings by agricultural chemicals occurred. Clearly, workers involved in direct agricultural operations were a high-risk group, and clearly, organophosphorous insecticides were high-risk compounds. Although, as a class herbicides ranked second as a cause of occupational disease, less than 5 percent of these reports involved systemic poisoning.

Reports of studies on workers in the agricultural chemical industry indicate that acute poisonings do occur during the manufacture of insecticides. In a health survey of 300 workers in plants manufacturing toxic organochlorine pesticides (Aldrin, Dieldrin, and Endrin) over a nine-year period, no fatalities or permanent injuries were found but 17 of the workers

had convulsive intoxications, and 5 of the 17 had more than one convulsion (Hoogendam et al., 1965). Moderate to severe chloracne was found in 18 percent of 73 employees engaged in manufacture of the herbicides 2,4-D and 2,4,5-T (Poland et al., 1971). Sixty-six percent of these workers had less severe degrees of acne. No systemic toxicity was found. In a more recent study, 41 workers had chloracne attributed to 3,4,3′4′-tetrachloroazoxybenzene present as a contaminant in the production synthesis of a new herbicide, 2-(3,4-dichlorophenyl)-4-methyl-1,2,4-oxodiazolidine-3,5-dione (Taylor et al., 1977). A five-year study of pesticide workers in a plant in Israel indicated that there was a higher incidence of complaints of symptoms referable to the respiratory, cardiovascular and nervous systems (Wasserman et al., 1970). In that study, 140 workers in the pesticide manufacturing plant were compared with 71 workers from a textile plant as the control group. In contrast to these reports of injury in the manufacture of pesticides, a study of 35 men with a work experience of 11 to 19 years in a plant producing DDT revealed no ill effects that could be attributed to exposure to the DDT, in spite of the fact that fat storage levels ranged from 38 to 647 ppm of DDT-derived material compared to 8 ppm for the general population (Laws et al., 1967).

Since 1949 there have been repeated cases of multiple poisonings among agricultural workers engaged in picking fruits sprayed with the highly toxic organophosphate insecticide parathion (Spear et al., 1975). These poisonings have been correlated with the "dislodgeable" residues of paraoxon, a toxic metabolite and/or weathering product of

Table 16–3. REPORTS OF OCCUPATIONAL DISEASE ATTRIBUTED TO PESTICIDES AND OTHER AGRICULTURAL CHEMICALS IN CALIFORNIA IN 1969*

	TYPE OF INDUSTRY								
TYPE OF CHEMICAL	Agriculture	Manufacturing	Construction	Transportation, Communication, Utilities	Trade	Structural Pest Control	State and Local Government	Other	TOTAL ALL
Organic phosphate pesticides	162	40	1	12	1	1	11	3	231
Halogenated hydrocarbon pesticides	19	15	2	6	2	3	8	2	57
Herbicides	44	4	1	5	—	—	18	4	76
Fertilizers	23	7	1	—	2	—	3	7	43
Fungicides	18	3	1	—	2	—	1	2	27
Phenolic compounds	5	5	3	1	—	—	1	—	15
Sulfur	28	1	1	—	—	—	1	—	31
Organomercury compounds	—	—	—	—	—	—	1	1	2
Lead or arsenic	4	1	1	1	—	—	1	1	9
Carbamates	1	2	—	—	—	—	—	1	4
Miscell.—specified	13	5	1	1	1	1	4	2	28
Unspecified	137	19	1	7	12	3	15	10	204
Total	454	102	13	33	20	8	64	33	727

* Abstracted from California Department of Public Health: *Occupational Diseases in California Attributed to Pesticides and Other Agricultural Chemicals, 1969.* Bureau of Occupational Health and Environmental Epidemiology, Sacramento, 1969.

parathion, on the foliage of the parathion-sprayed fruit trees. An "epidemic" of poisoning due to malathion, an organophosphate that is generally considered safe, occurred among field workers in a malaria control program in Pakistan (Baker et al., 1978). Of 7,500 workers involved in this mosquito control program, 2,800 were estimated to have had at least one episode of malathion intoxication. Five of these were fatal cases. A combination of poor pesticide-handling techniques and the use of unusually toxic formulations (due to the presence of toxic by-products) contributed to this epidemic of poisonings.

Gross negligence in industrial hygiene resulted in poisoning of 76 of 148 exposed workers engaged in the manufacture of chlordecone (Kepone) (Taylor et al., 1978). These workers suffered a syndrome of neurologic effects characterized by tremors, ocular flutter (opsoclonus), hepatomegaly/splenomegaly, rashes, mental changes, and widened gaits. Laboratory tests showed a reduced sperm count and reduced motility of sperm. Other complaints included headache, chest pain, arthralgia, and weight loss. The onset of signs in these workers varied from five days to eight months after the initial exposure to Kepone, and some signs and symptoms persisted for many months after cessation of exposure when the plant involved was closed down. Serious chronic neuropathy has also been reported among several workers involved in the manufacture of the insecticide leptophos (Xintaris et al., 1978). The medical consultant to the company observed a cluster of three cases of suspected "multiple sclerosis," which suggested the possibility of pesticide poisoning. The possibility of concurrent exposure to n-hexane (also neurotoxic) complicated interpretation of these cases of occupational poisonings.

Routes of Exposure

Analysis of residues on masks or on pads placed on exposed skin surfaces of workers involved in pesticide applications indicated that the dermal route offers the greatest potential for occupational exposure (Wolfe et al., 1967). The type of pesticide formulation applied was also a factor in the relative contribution of the respiratory route of exposure. When aerosols were used, an average of 2.87 percent of the total (dermal and respiratory) exposure was by the respiratory route, compared with 0.23 percent for dilute sprays and 0.94 percent for dusts. Different degrees of hazard were associated with different jobs. Thus, indoor house spraying was much more hazardous than outdoor spraying of several types. In an airplane spraying operation the relative hazard differed depending on the particular job. For example in the airplane spraying of a fruit orchard the loader received about three times as much as the pilot and $4\frac{1}{2}$ times as much as the flagman. Of course, the hazard to applicators is dependent not only on the extent and route of exposure, but on several other factors such as the relative rates of absorption from the skin and lungs, particle sizes of dust and aerosols, and the inherent toxicity of the materials. Wolfe and coworkers (1967) found, in their studies of a wide variety of spraying operations involving 11 different pesticides, that the highest mean value for the percentage of toxic dose received per hour of work was 44.2 percent for workers who loaded airplanes with 1 percent TEPP (tetraethyl pyrophosphate) dust. Although there were several illnesses associated with this operation, these authors considered the incidence quite low in view of the relative hazard. They suggested that three factors might account for this: the number of hours per day (or week) that the worker is actually engaged in loading airplanes is low; knowledge of the high toxicity of TEPP may prompt more diligent use of protective clothing and respiratory protective devices; and only a small percentage of the dry dust impinging on exposed skin is likely to be absorbed.

Oral ingestion is the most frequent route of exposure in cases of nonoccupational poisonings. Dermal exposures have resulted in deaths of small children who come in contact with presumably empty containers for highly toxic pesticides. Respiratory exposure (as well as dermal) of the general population is possible as a result of drift from agricultural operations. Household use of pesticide aerosol "bombs," vaporizers, pest strips, and other aerosol or vapor-generating devices is a potential source of respiratory exposure in nonoccupational settings. Hayes (1969) reported that 19 different organophosphorous insecticides are known to have caused poisoning in man. Of the other common types of insecticides that have resulted in human poisonings there were 20 compounds in the organochlorine class, five different carbamates, four botanicals, three inorganic elements, and six miscellaneous compounds for a total of 57 different insecticides. Eight herbicides were responsible for human poisonings, seven fungicides, six rodenticides, one molluscicide, and one nematocide for a total of 80 different compounds. References to the case reports of these poisonings are provided in Hayes's review.

As indicated in Table 16–1, numerous incidents of acute poisoning have resulted from eating food that had become grossly contaminated with pesticides during storage or shipping.

An interesting example is a case of poisoning of seven members of a single family who ingested tortillas prepared from flour that had been contaminated by carbophenothion, an organophosphate insecticide (Oldner and Hatcher, 1969). Although no fatalities resulted, six of the seven individuals required hospitalization and four advanced to coma. The severity of clinical signs and symptoms was related to the number of tortillas eaten. The contaminated food was not detected and discarded until two separate meals had been served (involving different members of the family). When the leftover food was finally discarded it was eaten by, and resulted in the deaths of, a dog, a cat, and eight chickens. The flour had become contaminated, apparently, as the result of carbophenothion contact at some point in storage or shipping. The insecticide had soaked through the paper flour sack. At least one other sack of flour had also been contaminated and was being used by a second family that had not (yet) been poisoned. The reason the first family was poisoned was apparently because they dumped their flour into a can and so had used the contents of the bottom of the sack (the most contaminated, 3220 ppm) first. The second family used their flour from the less-contaminated top of the sack. This case is one illustration of the insidious conditions under which acute pesticide poisonings have occurred.

INSECTICIDES

Only select examples of the various classes of insecticides will be discussed here. For additional discussion of their chemistry and metabolism the reader should consult the extensive report by Menzie (1969). Comprehensive compilations of chemical and common names, structures, and LD50 values in rats may be found in Gaines (1969) and Frear (1969). Acute toxicity data for fish and wildlife are available in several reports (Pickering et al., 1962; Tucker and Crabtree, 1970; Pimental, 1971). Summaries of results of subacute and chronic feeding studies for many compounds have been made available in the monograph by Lehman (1965). Several books and monographs (O'Brien, 1960, 1967, Heath, 1961; Chichester, 1965; Gould, 1966; Secretary's Commission on Pesticides, 1969; Matsumura, 1972; Hayes, 1975; Wilkinson, 1976) that are devoted exclusively to pesticides provide much more extensive coverage than is possible here. Handbooks prepared by Hayes (1963) and by Morgan (1976) provide information on clinical toxicology and emergency treatment for many pesticides.

Organophosphorus Insecticides

As discussed earlier, insecticides (of the several classes of pesticides) have most frequently been involved in human poisonings and organophosphorous compounds have most frequently been the offending agents.

Historic Considerations. The first organophosphate insecticide was tetraethyl pyrophosphate (TEPP). It was developed in Germany as a substitute for nicotine, which was in short supply in that country during World War II. Related extremely toxic compounds such as ethyl N-dimethyl phosphoroamidocyanidate (tabun) and isopropyl methylphosphonofluoridate (sarin) were kept secret by the German government as potential chemical warfare agents. These, and other extremely toxic compounds, are the so-called nerve gas chemical warfare agents.

TEPP, although an effective insecticide, was highly toxic to mammals and was rapidly hydrolyzed in the presence of moisture. Further efforts to find more stable compounds for use in agriculture led to the synthesis by Schrader in 1944 of parathion (E605; O,O-diethyl O-p-nitrophenyl phosphorothioate) and its oxygen analog paraoxon (E600; O,O-diethyl O-p-nitrophenyl phosphate). Because it exhibited a wide range of insecticidal activity and suitable physical and chemical properties such as low volatility and sufficient stability in water and mild alkali, parathion became one of the most widely used organophosphorus insecticides. It continues to be used extensively in agriculture, but because of its high mammalian toxicity, by all routes of exposure, other less hazardous compounds have begun to take its place. Parathion has the dubious distinction of being the pesticide most frequently involved in fatal poisonings. During the last two decades the agricultural chemistry industry has developed many other organic triesters of phosphoric acid and phosphorothioic acid that have been registered for use as insecticides. Summaries of the toxicology of several of these are shown in Table 16–4.

Shortly after parathion became available for study, acute toxicity studies on experimental animals revealed signs of poisoning that resembled excessive stimulation of cholinergic nerves. These could be alleviated by atropine, a cholinergic blocking agent (DuBois et al., 1948). This suggested inhibition of acetylcholinesterase of nerve tissues as the mechanism of toxic action, as had been demonstrated for related organophosphate triesters, and was confirmed by the finding that tissues of rats poisoned by parathion had markedly reduced cholinesterase activity and increased free acetylcholine in their brains (DuBois et al., 1949). Thus, the biochemical basis for acute poisoning by parathion in mammals, i.e., inhibition of the acetylcholinesterase activity of nerve tissue, became known soon after its introduction as an insecticide. Subsequent development and research on other organophosphate insecticides have revealed that they all, in sufficient doses, inhibit acetylcholinesterase *in vivo* and thus share a common mechanism of acute toxic action. The chemical mechanism of cholinesterase inhibition is discussed in more detail later in this chapter and in several extensive reviews and monographs

Table 16–4. TOXICOLOGY OF SOME ORGANOPHOSPHATE INSECTICIDES

COMPOUND	STRUCTURE	LD50 IN MALE RATS (mg/kg)* Oral	Dermal	"NO EFFECT LEVEL"† (mg/kg/day)	ADI‡ (mg/kg)
TEPP	$(C_2H_5O)_2-P(=O)-O-P(=O)-(OC_2H_5)_2$	1.1	2.4	—	—
Mevinphos	$(CH_3O)_2-P(=O)-O-C(CH_3)=CHC(=O)-OCH_3$	6.1	4.7	—	—
Disulfoton	$(C_2H_5O)_2-P(=S)-S-CH_2CH_2-S-CH_2CH_3$	6.8	15	—	—
Azinphosmethyl	$(CH_3O)_2-P(=S)-S-CH_2-N$ (benzotriazinone ring)	13	220	Rat—0.125 Dog—0.125	0.0025
Parathion	$(C_2H_5O)_2-P(=S)-O-C_6H_4-NO_2$	13	21	Rat—0.05 Man—0.05	0.005
Methylparathion	$(CH_3O)_2-P(=S)-O-C_6H_4-NO_2$	14	67	—	—
Chlorfenvinphos	$(C_2H_5O)_2-P(=O)-O-C(=CHCl)-C_6H_3Cl_2$	15	31	Rat—0.05 Dog—0.05	0.002
Dichlorvos	$(CH_3O)_2-P(=S)-O-CH=CCl_2$	80	107	Rat—0.5 Dog—0.37 Man—0.033	0.004
Diazinon	$(C_2H_5O)_2-P(=O)-O-C$ (pyrimidine ring with $CHC(CH_3)_2$, HC, C, CH_3)	108	200	Rat—0.1 Monkey—0.05 Dog—0.02 Man—0.02	0.002
Dimethoate	$(CH_3O)_2-P(=S)-S-CH_2CONHCN_3$	215	260	Rat—0.4 Man—0.04	0.02
Trichlorfon	$(CH_3O)_2-P(=O)-CH(OH)CCl_3$	630	>2,000	Rat—2.5 Dog—1.25	0.01
Chlorothion	$(CH_3O)_2-P(=S)-O-C_6H_3(Cl)-NO_2$	880	1,500–4,500		

* Values obtained in standardized tests in the same laboratory (Gaines, 1969). (continued)
† Maximum rate of intake (usually for three-month to two-year feeding studies) that was tested and did *not* produce significant toxicologic effects (as listed in the monographs issued jointly by the Food and Agriculture Organization of the United Nations and the World Health Organization, as developed by joint meetings of expert panels on pesticide residues held annually, 1965–1972).
‡ Acceptable daily intake (ADI) = the daily intake of a chemical that, during a lifetime, appears to provide the practical certainty that injury will not result (in man) during a lifetime of exposure. Figures taken from World Health Organization (1973).

Table 16–4 (continued)

COMPOUND	STRUCTURE	LD50 IN MALE RATS (mg/kg)*		"NO EFFECT LEVEL"†	ADI‡
		Oral	Dermal	(mg/kg/day)	(mg/kg)
Malathion	$(CH_3O)_2-\overset{\overset{O}{\|\|}}{P}-CHCOOC_2H_5$ $\|$ $CH_2COOC_2H_5$	1,375	> 4,444	Rat—0.5 Man—0.2	0.02
Ronnel	$(CH_3O)_2-\overset{\overset{S}{\|\|}}{P}-O-$ (ring with Cl, Cl, Cl)	1,250	> 5,000	Rat—0.5 Dog—1.0	0.01
Abate	$\left[(CH_3O)_2-\overset{\overset{S}{\|\|}}{P}-O-\bigcirc-S\right]_2$	8,000	> 4,000		

(Heath, 1961; Cohen and Oosterbaan, 1963; O'Brien, 1960, 1967, 1976).

Signs and Symptoms of Acute Poisoning. Signs and symptoms of acute systemic poisoning by organophosphate insecticides are predictable from their biochemical mechanism of action. Thus inhibition of acetylcholinesterase results in accumulation of endogenous acetylcholine in nerve tissue and effector organs with consequent signs and symptoms that mimic the muscarinic, nicotinic, and central nervous system actions of acetylcholine. Acetylcholine is the chemical transmitter of nerve impulses at endings of post-ganglionic parasympathetic nerve fibers, somatic motor nerves to skeletal muscle, preganglionic fibers of both parasympathetic and sympathetic nerves, and certain synapses in the central nervous system.

Muscarinic receptors for acetylcholine are found primarily in smooth muscles, the heart, and exocrine glands. Signs and symptoms of organophosphorus insecticide poisoning that result from stimulation of these receptors include tightness in the chest and wheezing expiration due to bronchoconstriction and increased bronchial secretions, increased salivation and lacrimation, increased sweating, increased gastrointestinal tone and peristalsis with consequent development of nausea, vomiting, abdominal cramps, diarrhea, tenesmus and involuntary defecation, bradycardia that can progress to heart block, frequent and involuntary urination due to contraction of smooth muscle of the bladder, and constriction of the pupils (miosis).

Nicotinic signs and symptoms result from accumulation of acetylcholine at the endings of motor nerves to skeletal muscle and autonomic ganglia. Muscular effects include easy fatigue and mild weakness followed by involuntary twitching, scattered fasciculations and cramps with progression to generalized fasciculations, and muscular weakness that affects the muscles of respiration and contributes to dyspnea and cyanosis. Nicotinic actions at autonomic ganglia may, in severe intoxication, mask some of the muscarinic effects. Thus tachycardia may result from stimulation of sympathetic ganglia to overcome the usual bradycardia due to muscarinic action on the heart. Pallor, elevation of blood pressure, and hyperglycemia also reflect nicotinic action at sympathetic ganglia.

Accumulation of acetylcholine in the central nervous system is believed to be responsible for the tension, anxiety, restlessness, insomnia. headache, emotional instability and neurosis, excessive dreaming and nightmares, apathy, and confusion that have been described after organophosphate poisoning. Slurred speech, tremor, generalized weakness, ataxia, convulsions, depression of respiratory and circulatory centers, and coma are other central nervous system effects.

The immediate cause of death in fatal organophosphate poisonings is asphyxia resulting from respiratory failure. Contributing factors are the muscarinic actions of bronchoconstriction and increased bronchial secretions, nicotinic action leading to paralysis of the respiratory muscles and the central nervous system action of depression and paralysis of the respiratory center.

Localized Effects. Localized effects at the site of exposure may be seen in the absence of obvious signs and symptoms of systemic absorption as described above. Exposure to vapors, dusts, or aerosols can exert local effects on the smooth muscles of the eyes and respiratory tract resulting in early miosis and blurred vision due to spasm of accommodation in the first case and bronchoconstriction in the case of respiratory exposure. Secretory glands of the respiratory tract, as well as smooth muscles, may be affected by minimal inhalation exposure to the organophosphates leading to watery nasal discharge, nasal hyperemia, sensation of tightness in the chest, and prolonged wheezing respiration. Local effects of dermal exposure include localized sweating and fasciculations at the site of contact. Gastrointestinal manifestations are usually the first to appear after oral ingestion and some of them may be due to local anticholinesterase action in the gastrointestinal tract.

Systemic Effects. Systemic effects are, in general, similar irrespective of route of absorption, but the sequence and times may differ. Respiratory and ocular symptoms would be expected first after exposure to airborne organophosphates, while gastrointestinal symptoms and localized sweating would likely be first to appear after oral and dermal exposure, respectively. However, these generalizations may not hold for compounds that must be metabolically activated (see Chapter 4). The onset of symptoms after exposure to organophosphate compounds is usually rapid, within a few minutes to two or three hours. The duration of symptoms is generally from one to five days. In fatal untreated poisonings, deaths usually occur within 24 hours. It should be recognized that, in addition to the usual factors of route of exposure, concentrations of active material, etc., the quality of signs and symptoms, their rate of onset, and their durations may differ markedly for different compounds by virtue of differences in rate of biotransformation, distribution, and affinities for acetylcholinesterase. For example, in five cases of attempted suicide by ingestion of dichlofenthion, severe cholinergic crises did not appear until 40 to 48 hours but they persisted for five to 48 days in the three survivors (Davies *et al.*, 1975). This extremely prolonged course was associated with persistent residues of this insecticide in the blood and fat of the patients. Dichlofenthion has a higher octanol/water partition coefficient than most organophosphorus insecticides, and the prolonged course of the poisonings was due to a slow release of the insecticide from adipose tissue reservoirs.

Organophosphate insecticides in common use are rapidly metabolized and excreted, and subacute or chronic poisoning by virtue of accumulation of the compounds in the body does not occur. However, because several of the organophosphates produce slowly reversible inhibition of cholinesterase *accumulation of this effect* can occur. Signs and symptoms of poisoning that

resemble those produced by a single high dose will occur when the accumulated inhibition of cholinesterase produced by smaller, repeated doses reaches a critical level. Cessation of exposure normally results in complete recovery. Chronic complaints associated with poisoning by organophosphates have been reported as due to sequelae of severe acute poisoning (Tabershaw and Cooper, 1966). A few compounds have produced delayed and persistent peripheral neuropathy, apparently unrelated to anticholinesterase action (see below).

More detailed discussions of organophosphate insecticide poisoning in man may be found in several reviews (Holmstedt, 1959; Grob, 1953; Hayes, 1963, 1975; Namba *et al.*, 1971).

Delayed Neurotoxic Effects. These are produced by several phosphate triesters. Although this can result from a single toxic dose, the neuropathology is generally delayed in onset. Most notorious of the compounds that produce this effect is triorthocresyl phosphate (TOCP) This compound is not a potent anticholinesterase, and it is not used as an insecticide. However, a number of compounds that are used as insecticides can produce this effect and it is common practice to screen for this action in safety evaluation tests. The functional disturbances associated with phosphate triester neuropathy begin in the distal parts of the lower limbs in both man and other sensitive animals. Mild sensory disturbances and motor weakness with ataxia occur, progressing in severity and extent to increased weakness and flaccidity of the legs and varying amounts of sensory disturbance. Upper limbs may also become involved. After several days to a few weeks the peak of the process is reached and thereafter improvement in the functional disturbance begins. Recovery is slow and not always complete.

Histopathologic studies of the peripheral nerves show that the distal fibers are affected earlier and more severely than proximal fibers. There is also a tendency of large-diameter fibers to be affected more than smaller-diameter fibers. The lesion has been described as a "dying-back" process, where the ends of the long nerves, distal to the nerve cell body, are affected first. Axonal degeneration followed by myelin degeneration is observed. These effects are believed to be due to a disturbed metabolism of the nerve cell body in spinal tracts with the consequence that nutrients are not synthesized and transported at a sufficient rate to maintain the long axons of the peripheral nerves (Cavanagh, 1969). Poisonings of this type have occurred in man. Classic cases reported in the United States in the 1930s resulted from drinking ginger liquor that was contaminated with TOCP. The condition was popularly referred to as "ginger jake paralysis." Mass outbreaks of poisoning, again resulting from TOCP, have occurred in

Morocco and other countries as a result of cooking with vegetable oil that had been contaminated with lubricating oil that contained some TOCP. An outbreak of 12 cases of serious peripheral neuropathy (Xintaras *et al.*, 1978) among workers engaged in the manufacture of leptophos, O-(4-bromo-2,5-dichlorophenyl) O-methyl phenylphosphorothioate, was felt to be due to its delayed neurotoxicity, which was demonstrated in hens given single large doses or repeated small doses of this compound (Abou-Donia and Preissig, 1976a, 1976b).

Although hens and man seem to be the most sensitive species to the organic phosphate-triester neuropathy, studies on various compounds have shown that dogs, cats, calves, monkeys, sheep, pigs, horses, pheasants, ducks, and rats will also sustain this effect (Aldridge *et al.*, 1969). For screening for possible production of this effect by pesticides, hens are usually used as the experimental animal. Because of potent anticholinesterase actions of many pesticides, it is often impossible to administer sufficient doses to the animal to produce the neuropathic effect. To overcome this and to screen for the neuropathy, a common procedure is to administer atropine to protect against the acute cholinergic action. Using this procedure Gaines (1969) found that 22 of 30 organophosphorus pesticides tested and three out of nine carbamate insecticides produced leg weakness in atropinized hens under sufficient time and dosage conditions. With all but three of the compounds, however, the onset of leg weakness occurred within 24 hours, and for most compounds the hens recovered within a month. Aldridge and Johnson (1971) consider this rapid onset and relatively rapid recovery to result from a different mechanism than for TOCP and other long-acting neurotoxins.

The precise biochemical action that leads to the paralytic effect and axonal degeneration produced by organophosphorus triesters remains to be determined.

For many years it was considered that the action was related to the antiesterase action of these compounds. Several studies, however, failed to establish an unequivocal correlation between the potency of various compounds to produce peripheral paralytic action and their capacity to inhibit acetylcholinesterase, butyrylcholinesterase, aliesterases, and several other hydrolytic enzymes. Subsequent studies, however, showed that paralytic compounds did have a common property of binding to a specific protein fraction in brains and spinal cords of hens. Although this protein fraction represented only a very small part of the total esterase activity of the nerve tissue, it did possess properties of an esterase and seemed to have a specificity for phenyl phenylacetate (Aldridge *et al.*, 1969). The physiologic role of this membrane-bound protein is unknown. Structure-activity studies with homologs of known paralytic compounds indicate that dimethyl derivatives are weak inhibitors of the "neurotoxic" esterases and have little or no neurotoxic action *in vivo* but that *in vivo* neurotoxicity and the specific antiesterase potency increased progressively with diethyl, dipropyl, and dibutyl derivatives of DFP and mipafox (Aldridge and Johnson, 1971). Refinement of a method for measuring the inhibition of hen's brain neurotoxic esterase has provided some further insight into the mechanism of delayed neurotoxicity and its structure-activity relationships (Johnson, 1975a, 1975b, 1975c). Phosphates, phosphoramidates, and phosphonates were capable of inhibiting neurotoxic esterase and were neurotoxic in intact hens, while phosphinates, sulfonates, and carbamates inhibited the enzyme but were not neurotoxic *in vivo*. In fact, when administered at appropriate times, the latter three types of compounds could prevent the neurotoxicity produced by the former three types. This protection is apparently due to competition for reaction at a critical target site. The determination of whether or not a compound that inhibited neurotoxic esterase would also be neurotoxic or protective appeared to depend on whether an "aged" inhibited neutotoxic esterase could be formed. This "aging" (loss of an alkyl group on the dialkyl phosphorylated enzyme, see Fig. 16–2) is believed to fix an extra charge to a protein whose function must be critical to normal function and integrity of neurons. The identity of the critical protein and its function have not yet been determined, but further research with neurotoxic organophosphate esters will likely provide insight into normal nerve physiology as well as elucidating the mechanism of delayed neurotoxicity of this class of insecticides. Studies with the insecticide EPN (ethyl *p*-nitrophenyl phenylphosphonothionate) demonstrate that optical isomerism may be a determinant of the nature of toxic action of these compounds (Ohkawa, 1977). The racemic ($\pm$), ($+$) isomer, and ($-$) isomer had equal acute toxicity to mice, the ($+$) isomer had three- to fourfold greater insecticidal activity than the ($-$) isomer, while the ($-$) isomer of EPN was the most active in producing delayed neurotoxicity in hens.

Altered neuromuscular function in pesticide workers who did not exhibit other detectable signs and symptoms of poisoning nor depressed blood cholinesterase activity has been detected using electromyographic methods to determine altered peripheral nerve and muscle function (Jager *et al.*, 1970; Drenth *et al.*, 1972). Roberts (1976, 1977) reported on studies of workers in an organophosphorus pesticide factory that indicated that measurements of altered electromyograph patterns and nerve conduction velocities might provide a more sensitive and more meaningful index of excessive occupational exposure to these compounds than measurements of plasma or erythrocyte cholinesterase. Although deviations from "normal" could be detected by these neurophysiologic techniques, their physiologic significance and the mechanisms of their occurrence remain to be demonstrated. These changes most likely differ mechanistically from the severe delayed neuropathy caused by TOCP, leptophos, mipafox, and a few others.

Metabolism-Toxicity Relationships. Several biotransformation reactions that organophosphorous insecticides undergo have been discussed in several reviews and monographs (O'Brien, 1960, 1967; Fukuto and Metcalf, 1969; Menzie, 1969; Dauterman, 1971; Eto, 1974). In this section selected biotransformation reactions are discussed as illustrations of the development of knowledge that has led to an understanding of factors that affect the susceptibility of animals to poisoning by these compounds. The reactions shown in Figure 16–1 can be used as a reference model for this discussion.

Activation. The early organophosphorous anticholinesterases such as TEPP and DFP were phosphate triesters and were potent inhibitors of cholinesterase both *in vivo* and *in vitro*. The development of parathion introduced the phosphorothionates. The majority of compounds now in use as insecticides contain the ($=S$) thiono moiety, and are either phosphorothionates (e.g., parathion, methyl parathion) or phosphorodithioates (e.g., azinphosmethyl, malathion). Early in research on parathion and its oxygen analog, paraoxon, it became apparent that in addition to conferring greater stability against nonenzymatic hydrolysis, substitution of $=S$ for $=O$ on the phosphorus compound altered its toxic properties. Parathion was less toxic to animals than paraoxon, and several factors that altered the toxicity of parathion in rats did not affect paraoxon's toxicity; although both compounds inhibited acetylcholinesterase and produced similar cholinergic signs of poisoning (DuBois *et al.*, 1949). Further studies showed that highly purified parathion did not inhibit cholinesterase *in vitro*, and that the inhibitory activity of less purified samples could be attributed to contamination with the S-ethyl and S-phenyl isomers of parathion or with its oxygen analog, paraoxon (Diggle and Gage, 1951). Subsequently it was demonstrated that paraoxon was the active anticholinesterase formed from parathion in intact rats.

Activation of parathion and other thionophosphorus insecticides that lacked direct (i.e., *in vitro*) anticholinesterase activity could be accomplished by incubating the compounds, aerobically, with liver slices (DuBois *et al.*, 1957). Further studies with a variety of compounds now have established that conversion of phosphorothionate and phosphorodithioate insecticides to their corresponding oxygen analogs is a necessary prerequisite for their action as cholinesterase inhibitors (reaction, I, Fig. 16–1). The enzyme system(s) in liver that catalyzes this reaction belongs to the group of NADPH-dependent mixed-function oxidases of the microsomes (Murphy and DuBois, 1957, 1958; Nakatsugawa and Dahm, 1967; Neal, 1967). Although the liver has by far the greatest capacity to catalyze this reaction in *vitro*,

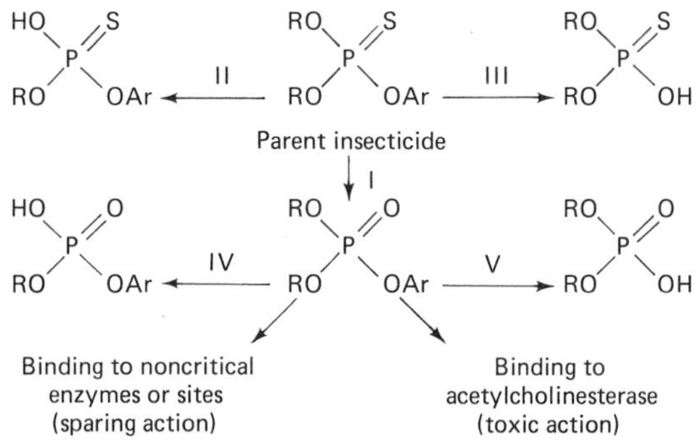

Figure 16–1. General scheme of metabolism and action of dialkyl, aryl phosphorothioate insecticides.

other tissues, including lung and brain, have some activity (Poore and Neal, 1972). Activation of phosphorothionates by extrahepatic tissues, even if only in minimal amounts, may be of great importance if these tissues are critical target organs for acetylcholinesterase inhibition.

There are other activation reactions, involving a few compounds, in which parent insecticides are converted to more potent anticholinesterase agents. They include oxidation of phosphoroamidates and thioether oxidation by mixed-function oxidases.

Inactivation. In addition to the requirement for an oxo ($=O$) group to be present for anticholinesterase activity, metabolic modification of the alkyl and aryl substituents can also influence activity. Reactions II, III, IV, and V (Fig. 16–1) are enzymatic detoxification reactions that yield products that do not inhibit acetylcholinesterase. Largely as a result of *in vitro* studies, it was proposed that reaction V, catalyzed by paraoxonase (A-esterase), was the major pathway of detoxication of parathion. This enzyme is widely distributed among several tissues in rats and other mammals. It does not require addition of cofactors for measurements of activity *in vitro* and probably hydrolyzes several other organophosphates (P=O compounds), but apparently does not hydrolyze the P=S compounds directly. Thus, the proposed enzymatic mechanism of detoxification of parathion and other phosphorothionate insecticides was, for many years, based on the concept that hydrolytic detoxication (reaction V) followed the formation of the oxygen analogs (reaction I). However, studies using ^{32}P-labeled parathion have shown that the aryl-phosphorus bond can be cleaved (reaction III) without prior oxidation to paraoxon (Nakatsugawa and Dahm, 1967; Neal 1967; Poore and Neal, 1972).

This reaction is catalyzed by a microsomal enzyme that, although it requires NADPH and oxygen, appears to be distinct from the enzyme that catalyzes reaction I (Neal, 1967). Alternatively, both microsomal cleavage and sulfur oxidation may pass through a common intermediate step (Ptashne et al., 1971). The rate at which this oxidative cleavage or the combined oxidation-hydrolysis reaction was catalyzed by NADPH-fortified liver homogenates appeared to explain age and sex differences in susceptibility of rats to EPN, O-ethyl O-p-nitrophenyl phenylphosphorothioate (Neal and DuBois, 1965). Adult females were more susceptible to poisoning and had less EPN detoxifying activity in their liver than adult males, and the greater susceptibility of young rats also corresponded to slower rates of enzymatic detoxification by their livers.

Dealkylation reactions II and IV apparently do not occur or occur to only a very minimal extent with parathion (Plapp and Casida, 1958). However, NADPH-dependent oxidative dealkylation has been demonstrated for other compounds. This appears to be a particularly important reaction for determining the toxicity of chlorfenvinphos (Donninger et al., 1972). The relative rates of dealkylation by rat, mouse, rabbit, and dog livers were 1, 8, 24, and 88, respectively. Species with high rates were least susceptible with LD50 values of 10, 100, 500, and > 1200 for rats, mice, rabbits, and dogs, respectively. Oxidative dealkylation also occurred with the dimethyl and diisopropyl analogs. However, the dimethyl compound, tetrachlorvinphos, was preferentially monodealkylated by another system, glutathione alkyltransferase (Hutson et al., 1972). In contrast to the microsomal oxidative dealkylation, glutathione-dependent dealkylation occurred in the soluble fraction of the liver cells and did not show marked species differences in activity.

Glutathione-dependent demethylation yields S-methylglutathione and the corresponding desmethyl phosphate compound. The enzyme system that catalyzes this reaction has been termed *phosphoric acid triester-glutathione S-alkyltransferase* (Hutson et al., 1972). There is considerable evidence that glutathione-dependent demethylation is an important pathway for several other O,O-dimethyl substituted organophosphorus insecticides, e.g., methyl parathion and azinphosmethyl (Plapp and Casida, 1958; Hollingworth, 1972; Benke et al., 1974). It has been demonstrated, in mice, that pretreatment with diethyl maleate and methyl iodide, which reduce liver glutathione levels, potentiated the toxicity of organophosphorous insecticides that are demethylated by glutathionetransferase (Hollingworth, 1970).

Another detoxification pathway (which is not represented in Figure 16–1) involves the hydrolysis of carboxyester or carboxyamide linkages in some insecticides by tissue or plasma carboxylesterases (sometimes called aliesterase). Malathion and dimethoate are examples. Products of the hydrolysis of the carboxyester or amide groups do not inhibit cholinesterase, and enzymatic formation of these products has been demonstrated *in vivo* and in *in vitro* studies (Uchida et al., 1964; Dauterman, 1971). In several species of mammals, this appears to be the major pathway of detoxification for these insecticides, and their selective insecticidal action is due to a relative lack of these hydrolytic enzymes in insects (Krueger et al., 1960). The importance of this reaction in mammals as a detoxification pathway has been demonstrated in studies in which animals pretreated with other organophosphate compounds that strongly inhibit carboxylesterases became more susceptible to the acute toxicity and anticholinesterase action of malathion (DuBois, 1961; Murphy, 1969; Su et al., 1971). Pretreatment with triorthocresyl phosphate (TOCP), a strong inhibitor of carboxylesterase but weak anticholinesterase, reduced the LD50 of malathion in rats from 1100 to 10 mg/kg, a 110-fold potentiation (Murphy et al., 1959).

A "binding" type of inactivation by liver and other tissues has been demonstrated for the oxygen analogs of parathion and malathion, i.e., paraoxon and malaoxon (Lauwerys and Murphy, 1969a; Cohen and Murphy, 1972, 1974). This appears to represent a loss of the active cholinesterase inhibitors to noncritical tissue binding sites, thereby sparing the critical acetylcholinesterase of nerve tissue from inhibition. That this represents an important detoxification mechanism *in vivo* was demonstrated by showing that selective blocking of these binding sites with other compounds *in vivo* potentiated the toxicity of paraoxon (Lauwerys and Murphy, 1969b), and, conversely, that induction of increased binding sites reduced paraoxon's toxicity (Triolo et al., 1970). Although these binding sites have not been identified, there is suggestive evidence, from the studies cited, that they may be nonspecific tissue esterases.

It is apparent from the above discussion that the relationships between enzymatic metabolism and toxicity of organophosphorus insecticides is extremely complex. The toxicity depends upon the net availability of active compound to inhibit acetylcholinesterase at critical sites in nerve tissue, and this in turn is dependent upon the dynamic relationships between activation and inactivation reactions. These are not always predictable from results of measurements of the relative rates of enzyme reactions under optimum conditions *in vitro*, particularly when both activation and inactivation reactions are catalyzed by enzyme systems with common cofactor requirements, tissue distribution, and intracellular location.

Acetylcholinesterase Inhibition and Reversal. There is abundant evidence that both the organophosphorus and carbamate insecticides (discussed subsequently) produce their acute toxic actions by inhibiting acetylcholinesterase. In addition to the fact that it has been demonstrated that many of these compounds are potent inhibitors *in vitro*, several lines of *in vivo* evidence support this mechanism. The consequence of acetylcholinesterase inhibition is accumulation of acetylcholine at effector sites, and the protection against acute poisoning offered by atropine and other cholinergic blocking agents supports the mechanism. Additionally, induced reversal of cholinesterase inhibition by chemical compounds, such as the oxime derivatives, results in alleviation of symptoms of poisoning. A combination of pharmacologic antidotes (atropine) and biochemical antidotes (oximes) is potentiative in its antidotal activity.

A scheme for substrate and inhibitor interactions with acetylcholinesterase is shown in Figure 16–2 for an organophosphorous insecticide, paraoxon, and a carbamate insecticide, carbaryl. The overall reaction can be illustrated by considering the insecticides as substrates:

$$
\underset{\text{(Enzyme)}}{EOH} + \underset{\substack{\text{(Substrate} \\ \text{or} \\ \text{inhibitor)}}}{AX} \underset{k_{-1}}{\overset{k_1}{\rightleftharpoons}} \underset{\substack{\text{(Reversible} \\ \text{complex)}}}{EOH.AX} \overset{k_2}{\longrightarrow} X^- + H
$$

$$
EOA \underset{H_2O}{\overset{k_3}{\longrightarrow}} EOH + A^- + H^+
$$

There are three important steps in the reaction: the first is complex formation and is governed by an affinity constant Ka (i.e., $k-1/k_1$). This is quite small for the carbamate and phosphate insecticides as well as for the natural substrate acetylcholine; therefore, the enzyme substrate or enzyme inhibitor complex (EOH.AX) is favored. With acetylcholine k_2 and k_3 are very fast so that the total reaction occurs rapidly and new enzyme is regenerated. With organic phosphates k_2 is moderately fast, but k_3 is extremely slow; so EOA accumulates while EOX.AX is minimal at any time. With carbamates, Ka is very low, k_2 is slower than for the phosphates; k_3 is slower than k_2 but still significant (and more rapid than for the phosphates). As a result, with carbamates, there are small levels of EOH.AX and large levels of carbamylated enzyme, EOA. If, however, carbamate is removed from the reaction (as by dilution or dialysis) the enzyme recovers rapidly, in part by reversal of the enzyme inhibitor complex and in part by decarbamylation, k_3. Of the three steps— (1) complex formation; (2) acetylation, phosphorylation, or carbamylation; and (3) deacetylation, dephosphorylation, or decarbamylation—the third (k_3) step is the most critical and slowest in each case. Caclulated turnover numbers, the number of molecules hydrolyzed per minute by one molecule of enzyme, have been estimated as 300,000 for acetylcholine, 0.04 for methylcarbamates, and 0.008 for dimethyl phosphates. Therefore, the enzyme rapidly breaks down acetylcholine, but is rather irreversibly inhibited by the organophosphates and markedly slowed by the carbamates (O'Brien, 1967, 1969; Aldridge, 1971).

The rate of recovery of free and active acetylcholinesterase following poisoning by organophosphorous and carbamate insecticides varies with different compounds. In general, the carbamates are usually considered reversible inhibitors of cholinesterase, and their duration of action is relatively short. In addition, because of the reversal of inhibition by dilution of the enzyme (as would occur if one sampled a tissue and diluted it with buffer during preparation for assay), determination of acetylcholinesterase inhibition by carbamates *in vivo* poses some technical difficulties. Unless care is taken, it is quite possible to observe the typical signs of anticholinesterase poisoning following carbamates; but by the time tissues are removed and prepared for assay, decarbamylation or reversal of enzyme-carbamate complex may have occurred and inhibition is undetectable. Therefore, in suspected cases of poisoning, where the history and signs and symptoms suggest a carbamate exposure, but clinical tests show a normal or nearly normal blood cholinesterase value, one must be guided by the history before concluding that the poisoning was not the result of a carbamate insecticide.

The case for organophosphate poisoning is somewhat different in that the compounds are in general much more slowly reversible inhibitors. However, even within this class there are marked differences in the persistence of inhibition following toxic doses of the compound (Table 16–5). Spontaneous reversal of enzyme inhibition

Table 16-5. VARIATION IN TIME TO ONSET AND DURATION OF INHIBITION OF CHOLINESTERASE BY SOME ORGANOPHOSPHATE INSECTICIDES IN RATS*

INSECTICIDE	TIME TO MAXIMUM INHIBITION	TIME FOR COMPLETE REVERSAL
Trichlorfon (Dipterex)	0.25 hours	6 hours
Azinphosmethyl (Guthion)	0.5 hours	24 hours
Disulfoton (Di-Syston)	3.0 hours	120 hours

* Selected from DuBois (1963). The compounds were given at dosages equivalent to 5/8 their LD50s, and all produced 50 percent or greater inhibition of brain of submaxillary cholinesterase activity.

(Fig. 16–2) by organophosphates as well as carbamates can occur at varying rates, depending upon the insecticide, by hydrolysis of the phosphorylated cholinesterase. (Reiner, 1971). The rate of reactivation *in vitro* of mouse brain and diaphragm acetylcholinesterase inhibited *in vivo* was five to ten times greater for azinphosmethyl and parathion-methyl than for

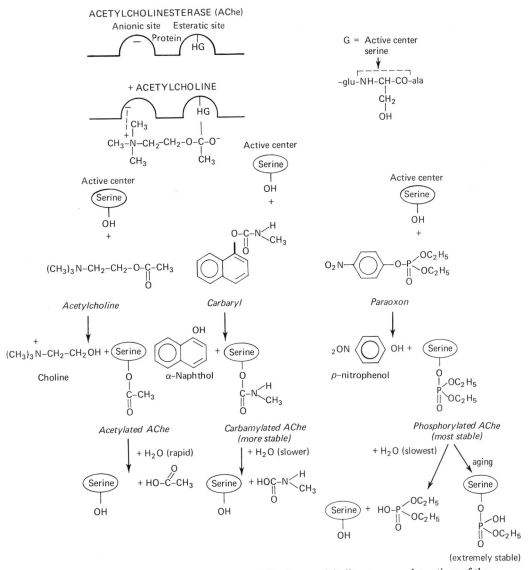

Figure 16-2. Scheme of hydrolysis of acetylcholine by acetylcholinesterase and reactions of the anticholinesterase insecticides carbaryl and paraoxon.

azinphosethyl and parathion-ethyl (Levine and Murphy, 1977a).

With some compounds a phenomenon known as "aging" of the phosphorylated enzyme occurs. This represents a dealkylation of the dialkoxy phosphorylated enzyme. With some compounds dephosphorylation of the inhibited enzymes occurs extremely slowly or not at all. Diisopropyl fluorophosphate (DFP) is one such compound, and the rate of regeneration of the cholinesterase activity of a tissue of a poisoned animal coincides with the rate of resynthesis of new enzyme. For example, in animals poisoned with DFP, plasma cholinesterase activity returns to normal within several days to a few weeks, because it is relatively rapidly replaced by new

enzyme synthesized in the liver. The acetylcholinesterase activity of the erythrocytes, however, remains depressed for the duration of the red cell's life. Erythrocyte cholinesterase activity inhibited by DFP only fully regenerates when there has been a full turnover and replacement of red cells.

Fortunately, there are available chemicals that will accelerate the hydrolysis of the phosphorylated enzyme, and hence accelerate regeneration of active acetylcholinesterase. The most successful compounds are oxime derivatives, and the best known of these is 2-pyridine aldoxime methiodide (2-PAM, pralidoxime) which is now a standard part of the therapy of

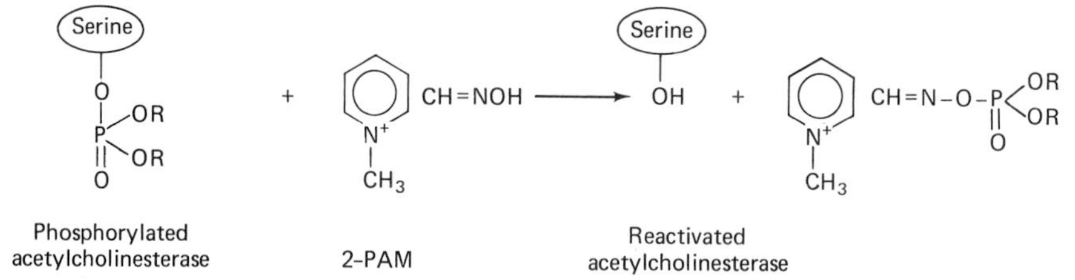

Figure 16–3. Reactivation of phosphorylated acetylcholinesterase by pralidoxime (2-PAM).

organophosphorus poisoning. In addition to the capacity of 2-PAM to accelerate the dephosphorylation of acetylcholinesterase it can also enhance the direct hydrolysis of the active inhibitor at physiologic pH (Fig. 16–3). The effectiveness of 2-PAM in reversing cholinesterase inhibition *in vivo* is dependent upon its early administration following poisoning, because the "aged" phosphorylated enzyme is not reversible by the oximes. The rate of reactivation by oximes appears to vary with both the source of the cholinesterase and the substituents on the phosphorylating group. Diethoxy-phosphorylated enzyme appears to be most readily reactivated as compared with diisopropoxy-phosphorylated and dimethoxy-phosphorylated enzymes. It is believed that the effectiveness of the oximes as dephosphorylating agents is inversely related to the rate of aging of the phosphorylated enzyme. Hence the dimethoxy-phosphoryl enzyme and the diisopropoxy phosphoryl enzyme age more rapidly than the diethoxy phosphoryl enzyme (O'Brien, 1960, 1967; Hobbiger, 1963).

Although 2-PAM and other oximes are effective reversers of unaged phosphorylated acetylcholinesterase, their protective action against poisoning by organophosphates is limited when used alone. Treatment of mice with 2-PAM seldom protected against more than two times the lethal dose of potent inhibitors; however, treatment with both 2-PAM and atropine resulted in a synergistic protective action. For example, 2-PAM alone increased the lethal dose of paraoxon twofold to fourfold. Atropine alone increased the lethal dose by about twofold, but the combination of atropine and 2-PAM increased the lethal dose by 128-fold (O'Brien, 1960). The effectiveness of 2-PAM as an antidote for organophosphate poisoning is partly limited by its poor penetration into the central nervous system. Since it is a quaternary nitrogen derivative it will not readily penetrate the brain and is quite ineffective in reversing inhibition of brain acetylcholinesterase. The aldoxime itself will inhibit cholinesterase at relatively high concentrations by binding to the anionic site of the enzyme. The use of 2-PAM is *contraindicated* in the case of poisoning by carbaryl, a carbamate cholinesterase inhibitor, probably because the reversal of the carbamate inhibited enzyme is so rapid that adding another short-acting though weak inhibitor adds

insult to injury. More extensive discussions of the mechanism of inhibition of cholinesterase by organophosphates and carbamates and its reversal may be found in several reviews (O'Brien, 1960, 1969, 1976; Hobbiger, 1963; Aldridge, 1971; Wills, 1972).

Diagnosis and Treatment of Poisoning. As in any case of poisoning, careful taking of the history of events that led to signs and symptoms is essential. However, the organophosphate insecticides frequently produce poisoning rapidly and, if in sufficient doses, may have a rapid fatal outcome. It is important, therefore, to be guided by the characteristic signs and symptoms and take emergency action even though a complete history may not have been obtained.

In very severe cases the treatment should include (1) artificial respiration, preferably by mechanical means, and (2) atropine sulfate, 2 to 4 mg intravenously as soon as cyanosis is overcome. This may be repeated at five- to ten-minute intervals until signs of atropinization appear. Note that this dosage of atropine is greater than that usually used for other purposes, but because people poisoned by anticholinesterase compounds have increased tolerance for atropine, it is a safe dose, used carefully by an astute physician. (3) Following atropinization, administer 2-PAM, 1 g slowly, intravenously. In very severe cases, it may be necessary to begin treatment before time is spent in decontaminating the skin, stomach, or eyes as may be indicated; however, decontamination must be followed promptly. The skin should be washed with an alkaline soap, which will not only remove, but also help hydrolyze, the phosphate ester. Appropriate clinical procedures for evacuating the stomach and cleansing the eyes may be indicated. A case history of successful treatment of poisoning by dicrotophos, in which a total of 3911.5 mg of atropine and 92 g of pralidoxime chloride was given over a 23-day period, illustrates the importance of vigorous treatment in severe cases of poisoning (Warriner *et al.*, 1977).

In more usual and less severe cases the procedure should be as follows: Administer atropine SO_4, 1 to 2 mg, if symptoms appear. If excessive secretions occur, keep the patient fully atropinized by giving atropine sulfate every hour up to 25 to 50 mg in a day. Proceed with de-contamination of the skin and removal of the poison from the stomach or eyes as the second step in this case. In these less severe poisonings 2-PAM administration should be instituted if the patient fails to respond satisfactorily to atropine, followed, of course, by symptomatic treatment. The doses indicated above are those suggested for adults. Anyone expecting to face the possibility of dealing with severe poisoning by organophosphate insecticides should consult more detailed descriptions of diagnosis and therapy (Durham and Hayes, 1962; Hayes, 1963; Doull, 1976; Morgan, 1976).

Knowledge of the biochemical action of the organophosphate insecticides has provided a means for a relatively specific clinical test for diagnosis of excessive exposure to these compounds. Routine measurements of blood cholinesterase activity are frequently made in workers engaged in occupations where exposure to phosphate insecticides is a possibility. As discussed in several reports (Grob, 1963; Namba, et al., 1971; Wills, 1972), the inhibition of the activity of plasma or red cell cholinesterase is reasonably well correlated with the severity of exposure and poisoning. Measurement of the cholinesterase activity of the blood only indirectly reflects the extent of biochemical lesion at critical sites in nerve tissues or effector organs, however. Depending upon the compound, the relative inhibition of plasma pseudocholinesterase and erythrocyte acetylcholinesterase may differ. Since the red cell enzyme is apparently identical to that in nerve tissue, assays on red cells are usually considered more reflective of nerve tissue activity. Rather marked inhibition of red cell and plasma cholinesterase may be present in the absence of symptoms. Total inhibition of plasma and 60 to 70 percent inhibition in red cell activity has been noted in the absence of overt signs of poisoning. However, the relationship between inhibition of blood cholinesterase activity and symptoms differs with different compounds and may reflect differences in distribution of the inhibitors. Relationships between blood and nerve tissue cholinesterase inhibition and signs of poisoning for various compounds in experimental animals have been reviewed by DuBois (1963) and Wills (1972).

Tolerance to Acute, Sublethal Effects of Some Organophosphates. This has been demonstrated in experimental animals (DuBois, 1965; Stavinoha, et al., 1969). In these experiments the phosphates were administered repeatedly or fed in the diet at sublethal doses for several days. Initially, acute cholinergic signs and symptoms were observed. In time, however, the animals no longer responded with obvious signs after each dose, and their general appearance, growth, and behavior appeared normal. However at sacrifice, these apparently normal animals had markedly inhibited blood and nervous tissue cholinesterase activity and elevated levels of acetylcholine in their brains. Adaptation or compensation to central nervous system and behavioral effects of anticholinesterase insecticides also occurs in rats in spite of continued brain acetylcholinesterase inhibition and elevated acetylcholine levels (Reiter et al., 1973; Bignami et al., 1975).

Experiments by Brodeur and DuBois (1964) suggest that the apparent tolerance involves development of a refractoriness of cholinergic receptor sites. Tolerant animals were resistant to the acute toxicity of carbachol, which has a direct effect on cholinergic receptors. Adaptation to high concentrations of acetylcholine has been observed to occur at the neuromuscular junction and at ganglia within a few minutes to a few hours, in contrast to the several days required for adaptation in the subacute experiments cited above (Kim and Karczmar, 1967). There are also reports that tolerance to reduced cholinesterase activity also occurs in man (Johns and McQuillen, 1966). Stavinoha and associates (1969) found that two different strains of rats that had adapted to low acetylcholinesterase activity in the brain differed with respect to the levels of acetylcholine in the brain; one strain had normal levels of acetylcholine during adaptation while the other had elevated concentrations. They concluded there was no apparent correlation between the concentration of brain acetylcholine and adaptation. Although the mechanism suggested by Brodeur and DuBois (1964) of a refractoriness of cholinergic receptor sites is attractive, other possibilities related to the rate of production, release, and destruction of acetylcholine could be considered.

Carbamate Insecticides

The acute toxicities of the carbamate insecticides also vary through a wide range as shown in Table 16–6. Unlike the organophosphates, most of the aromatic carbamate-ester insecticides have low dermal toxicities. However, one cannot generalize that carbamates are without dermal toxicity as illustrated by the extreme toxicity of aldicarb (Temik) by both the oral and dermal routes. This compound, because of its extreme toxicity, is recommended only for limited use in greenhouse operations. The carbamates are not broad-spectrum insecticides, and some of the common household insect pests such as the housefly and German cockroach are relatively immune (O'Brien, 1967); however, bees are extremely sensitive to these insecticides. For

Table 16–6. EXAMPLES OF RANGE OF ACUTE TOXICITIES OF SOME CARBAMATE INSECTICIDES

		LD50 IN MALE RATS* (mg/kg)	
		Oral	*Dermal*
Baygon (Propoxur)		83	>2,400
Carbaryl		850	>4,000
Mobam		150	>2,000
Temik (Aldicarb)		0.8	3.0
Zectran		37	1,500–2,500

* Values obtained in standardized tests in the same laboratory (Gaines, 1969).

several of the compounds, the LD 50 values for houseflies and German cockroaches are, on a body weight basis, greater than the LD 50s for rats.

Action and Mechanism. The mode of action of the carbamates, like the organophosphates, is inhibition of acetylcholinesterase (Casida, 1963; O'Brien, 1967), and the signs and symptoms of poisoning are typically cholinergic with lacrimation, salivation, miosis, convulsions, and death. As indicated previously, however, the carbamates are relatively rapidly reversible inhibitors of cholinesterase. Atropine sulfate is the recommended antidote for poisoning by carbamate insecticides. Administration of 2-PAM is not recommended and, at least for some

compounds, seems to be specifically contraindicated since there have been reports that it aggravates the toxicity of carbaryl (Carpenter et al., 1961). In addition to the typical cholinergic signs of poisoning, experiments in rats showed that some of the less toxic carbamate insecticides when administered intravenously produced a pronounced anesthetic effect with respiratory failure as the most critical determinant of the intravenous toxicity. This anesthetic action was rapid in onset. However, if artificial respiration was applied for two to five minutes animals resumed spontaneous respiration. Cholinergic signs then gradually developed (Vandekar et al., 1971). No pronounced anesthetic effects were observed with the carbamate insecticides when they were administered by the intraperitoneal or oral routes. This anesthetic effect has also been noted with several organophosphate insecticides (Brown and Murphy, 1971), and also appears to be unrelated to their anticholinesterase action.

Metabolism-Toxicity Relationships. Studies of the correlation between toxicity and *in vitro* anticholinesterase activity of a series of monomethylcarbamates showed that there was good correlation between *in vitro* inhibition and intravenous LD50s in rats, but the *in vitro* anticholinesterase action was poorly correlated with oral LD50s (Vandekar *et al.*, 1971). The carbamate insecticides are direct inhibitors of acetylcholinesterase (i.e., they do not require metabolic activation), and the lack of correlation between the oral toxicity and *in vitro* anticholinesterase activity appeared to reflect differing rates of detoxication of the compounds. Hydrolysis of the carbamic acid ester linkage results in metabolites that lack anticholinesterase activity. The biotransformation pathways for typical carbamate insecticides are shown in Figure 16–4. Although hydrolysis occurs to some extent with all compounds, various oxidation steps that are catalyzed by mixed function oxidases also occur. The products formed by these reactions are not always less toxic than the parent compounds, but the parent compounds themselves, do have anticholinesterase action (Casida, 1963).

Cholinesterase Inhibition and Symptoms. Studies of the relationship between cholinesterase inhibition and signs and symptoms of poisoning in rats showed that with dosages that did not produce any noticeable symptoms (0.25 to 1.0 mg/kg, intramuscularly, of propoxur) the activity of both brain and plasma cholinesterase was reduced as much as 40 percent. The dose at which a very slight tremor occurred (2 mg/kg) reduced the brain and plasma cholinesterase activities to 50 percent of normal level. At higher dosages (10 to 50 mg/kg) the degree of inhibition of both brain and plasma cholinesterase closely followed the severity of symptoms that were produced, with brain cholinesterase being slightly more inhibited than plasma (Vandekar *et al.*, 1971). Studies on human volunteers were also conducted to determine the relationship between the inhibition of erythrocyte cholinesterase and onset of signs of poisoning. The lowest erythrocyte cholinesterase activity (27 percent of normal) was observed at 15 minutes after ingestion of 1.5 mg/kg of propoxur in a 90-kg adult man. At this time no signs were observed, but moderate discomfort, that was described as pressure in the head was present. Blurred vision and nausea developed

three minutes later, and 20 minutes after ingestion the man was pale and his face was sweating, pulse rate was 140 per minute compared to 76 before ingestion, and both systolic and diastolic blood pressures were increased. Following these symptoms, nausea, repeated vomiting, and profuse sweating developed. The symptoms lasted from about the thirtieth until the forty-fifth minute after ingestion, and during this period erythrocyte cholinesterase activity recovered from a level of 50 to 55 percent of its normal value. Sixty minutes after ingestion the patient showed signs of improvement but felt nauseated and tired; pulse and blood pressure were normal. Two hours after ingestion the patient felt completely recovered. This rapid disappearance of symptoms was accompanied by further rapid recovery of erythrocyte cholinesterase activity. Studies on both rats and men indicated that the lethal dose of a carbamate insecticide is a considerably greater multiple of the dose causing the first signs of poisoning than for the organophosphorous insecticides. As a result, overexposure to carbamates might be expected to give early warning of poisoning in the form of appearance of slight symptoms, which, if heeded and exposure terminated, could prevent exposure to acutely dangerous quantities (Vandekar *et al.*, 1971).

Other Actions of Carbamates. One of the least acutely toxic carbamate insecticides, carbaryl, has reportedly produced teratogenic effects in experimental animals. Although in most species the doses for effects on fetuses were near the maternal toxic doses, in beagle dogs the teratogenic dose was found to be only about a tenth of the toxic dose to the mother (Smalley *et al.*, 1968), when given as single daily doses in gelatin capsules. Weil and coworkers (1972) reviewed the considerable literature on studies of reproductive and teratogenic action of carbaryl and concluded that the sensitivity of dogs to teratogenic action was related to the fact that dogs did not metabolize carbaryl to l-naphthol, a major metabolic pathway in most other species including man.

Cloudy swelling of cells in the proximal convoluted tubules of the kidneys was noted in rats and dogs fed 400 ppm of carbaryl in their diets for several months (Carpenter *et al.*, 1961). Of related interest, it has been reported that the urinary amino acid–nitrogen: creatinine ratios were increased in a group of human volunteers who ingested daily doses of carbaryl of 0.12 mg/kg/day for several weeks (Wills *et al.*, 1968). Although the exact relationships between the histologic changes in experimental animals and the biochemical changes in man is not established, they would seem to be related effects and

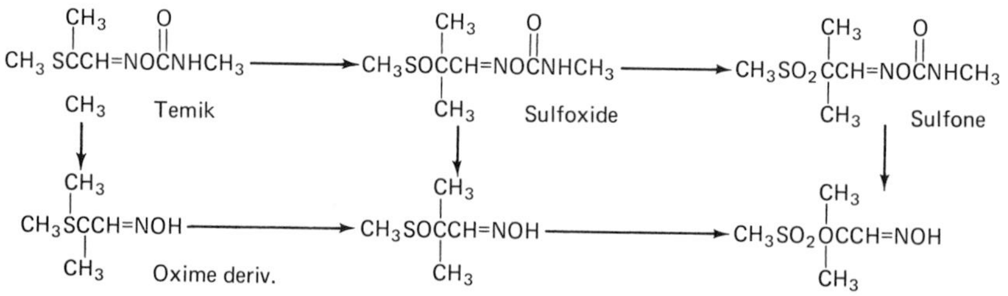

Figure 16–4. Examples of metabolism of carbamate insecticides. *A.* Metabolism of carbaryl pathways within dashed rectangle demonstrated with liver microsomes *in vitro*. Compounds outside rectangle demonstrated urinary metabolites. *B.* Metabolism of Temik. Temik sulfoxide and sulfone are more potent anticholinesterases than the parent compound. Principal urinary metabolites in rats were Temik sulfoxide and the oxime sulfoxide. (Modified from Fukuto, T. R., and Metcalf, R. L.: Metabolism of insecticides in plants and animals. *Ann. N.Y. Acad. Sci.*, **160**:97–113, 1969.)

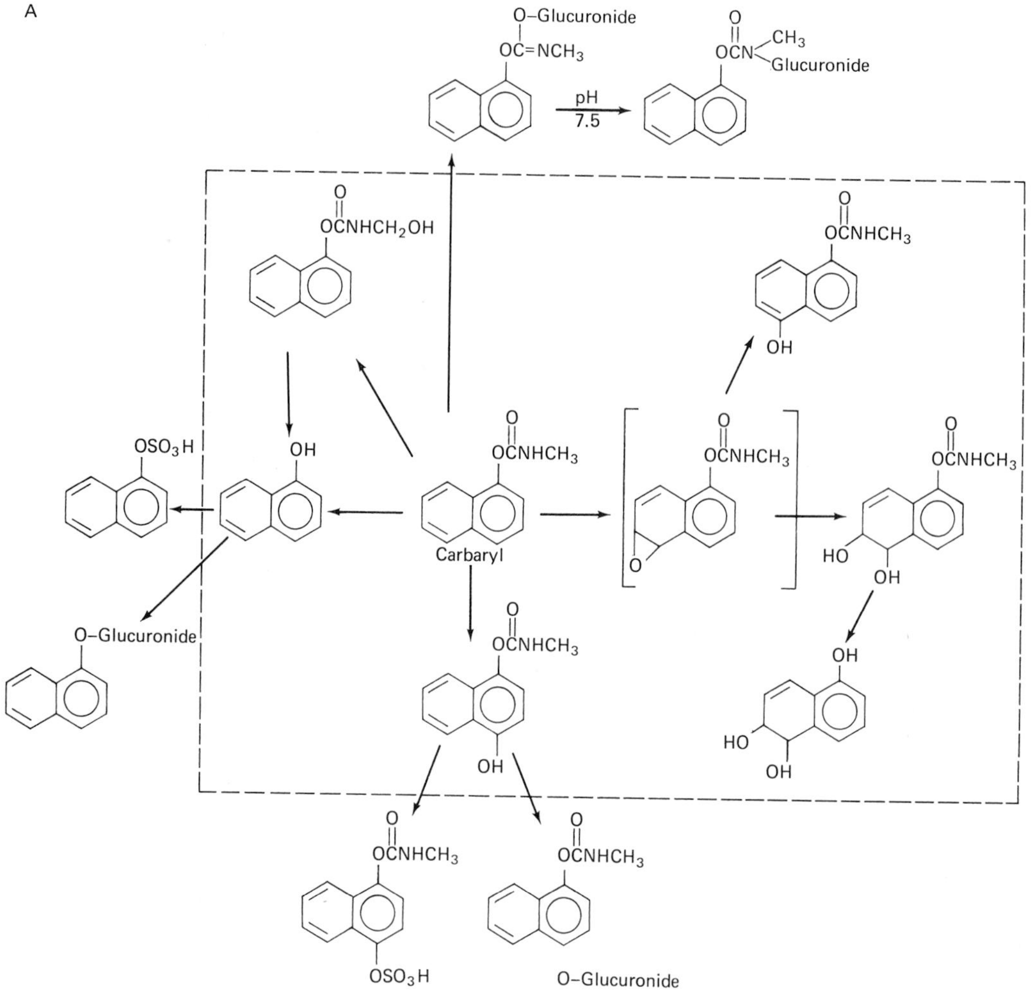

COMPOUND

Chlordane

Lindane

Mirex

including insects. Unli
phosphate insecticides,
after dermal exposure,
in the powder form. Th
the skin probably acco
safety record of DDT
sometimes careless u
formulators (Hayes, 19
   Although the functi
high doses of DDT is
central nervous system
change in the cells ar
nervous system in acut
of the dust results in ir
primary pathologic cl
exposure to high, but
subacute or chronic fee
liver. With large dose
of the liver has been
result in liver enlargen
somewhat characterist
mitochondria themseh
1959). Histologic chan
rats fed diets containin
six months include
bodies, and cytoplas
characteristic type in v
themselves around th
These changes were n

the dosage relationships suggest that man may be much more sensitive to injurious effects of carbaryl on the kidney.

Organochlorine Insecticides

The organochlorine insecticides include the chlorinated ethane derivatives, of which DDT is the best known example; the cyclodienes, which include chlordane, aldrin, dieldrin, hepatachlor, endrin, and toxaphene; and the hexachlorocyclohexanes, such as lindane. From the mid-1940s to the mid-1960s the organochlorine insecticides enjoyed wide use in agriculture, soil, and structure insect control, and in malaria control programs. However, they have, as a class, come into disfavor because they are very persistent in the environment and tend to accumulate in biologic as well as nonbiologic media. As a class the organochlorine insecticides are often considered to be less acutely toxic, but of greater potential for chronic toxicity, than the organophosphate and carbamate insecticides. As shown in Table 16–7, however, there is a wide range of acute toxicities of individual compounds, from extremely toxic to slightly toxic. The organochlorine insecticides can also be classed as neuropoisons. However, their mechanism of action is not the same as that of the phosphates and carbamates. Indeed the precise mechanism is unknown for most of them.

DDT. DDT has been the best known, the cheapest, and probably one of the most effective of the synthetic insecticides. It was synthesized as early as 1874 but its insecticidal effectiveness was not discovered until 1939, and it was patented for this use in 1942. DDT was used extensively during World War II in control of lice and other insects by application directly to humans. There is no evidence that harm to these people resulted from this direct application. Indeed there seems to be no documented, unequivocal report of fatal human poisoning from DDT in spite of its widespread use and availability. Acute, nonfatal poisonings have occurred as a result of accidents or suicide attempts. Statistical associations between levels of storage of DDT and its metabolites and certain types of chronic disease in man have been reported (Casarett et al., 1968; Radomski et al., 1968); however, causal relationships have not been established and other reports indicate no association between tissue DDT levels and chronic disease (Hoffmann et al., 1967; Hayes et al., 1971). There is no question, however, that the general population has sustained exposure to DDT and derivatives, and as a result practically everyone born since the mid-1940s, when DDT was introduced into commerce, has had a lifetime of exposure and storage of some

quantity of this insecticide in fatty tissues (Quimby et al., 1965; Hayes, 1966; Zavon et al., 1969). Thus chronic exposure to DDT has resulted in an accumulation of residues in man and other animals, but the health significance of these residues is not currently apparent and remain to be further evaluated.

On the other hand, there is convincing evidence that DDT and metabolites accumulate in natural food chains by a process of biologic concentration in ecosystems (Dustman and Stickel, 1969; Edwards, 1970). As a result, organisms at the top of these natural food chains may sustain injury from DDT or its metabolites that are present as a result of gradual accumulations of residues in organisms that make up their food sources. Both field and laboratory studies have provided evidence that reproductive success in certain species of wild birds is adversely affected by exposure to DDT or its metabolites (Dustman and Stickel, 1969; Peakall, 1970; Longcore et al., 1971). Additionally, fish and some lower aquatic organisms are extremely sensitive to the acute toxicity of DDT (Pimental, 1971).

The prospect of possible ecologic imbalance from continued use of DDT, the uncertainty as to the effect, if any, of continued prolonged exposure and storage of low levels of DDT in humans, and the development of resistant strains of insects have prompted the Environmental Protection Agency to markedly restrict the use of DDT in the U.S.A. Several other countries have taken similar actions. However, because of its relatively low cost, unavailability of substitutes that are both safe and effective, and its continuing presence as an environmental contaminant in spite of curtailed use, there continues to be interest in its toxicity.

Signs and Symptoms of Acute and Subacute Poisoning. Signs and symptoms of poisoning in man and animals resulting from high doses of DDT include paresthesia of the tongue, lips, and face; apprehension; hypersusceptibility to stimuli; irritability; dizziness; disturbed equilibrium; tremor; and tonic and clonic convulsions. Motor unrest and fine tremors associated with voluntary movements progress to coarse tremors without interruption in moderate to severe poisoning. Symptoms appear several hours after large doses, and in animals poisoned with fatal doses death occurs in 24 to 72 hours. It has been estimated that a dose of 10 mg/kg will cause signs of poisoning in man. Although there are rather marked species differences in susceptibility to acute poisoning by oral ingestion, when the compound is given by intravenous administration, the dose and time required for poisoning are quite similar for a wide variety of species

Table 16-

COMPOUND	
DDT	Se
DDE§	Se
DDA§	Se
Methoxychlor	Se
Aldrin	(
	(
Dieldrin	
	(
Endrin	
	]
	(
Heptachlor	

* Values obtained in :
† Maximum rate of ii
  significant toxicolo
  of the United Nat
  pesticide residues h
‡ Acceptable daily in
  practical certainty
  Health Organizatii
§ Metabolites of DDT
¶ Conditional ADI p

tions concerning the effects of microsoma enzyme inducers on the toxicity of various classes of pesticides. Additional research is necessary to determine the specificities of various inducers (or inhibitors) on the several alternate pathways of metabolism of complex organic pesticides.

Although the above remarks have been primarily restricted to pesticide-pesticide interactions, they apply as well to other pollutant or drug effects on pesticide toxicities. In most cases where such interactions have been detected they appear to have been mediated through altered microsomal enzyme activities. Since at least 200 drugs and chemicals are known inducers of these enzymes, the number of possible interactions is tremendous. Relatively few have been subjected to toxicity tests in intact animals. Durham (1967) has reviewed many additional factors that may affect the toxicity of pesticides.

Pesticide-Drug Interactions. The capacity of organochlorine insecticides and certain herbicides to induce increased activity of liver microsomal enzymes that metabolize a variety of drugs is well established (Conney *et al.*, 1967; DuBois, 1969). However, attempts to correlate the increased capacity of tissues from pesticide-induced animals to metabolize drugs with effects of the pesticides on the intensity and duration of pharmacologic (or toxic) actions of the drugs are relatively few. Hexobarbital sleeping times or zoxazolamine paralysis times are often used as pharmacologic indices of altered drug metabolism *in vivo*, and in a few cases altered blood levels of drugs given to pesticide-treated animals have served as an *in vivo* index of pesticide-drug interactions. Conney and coworkers (1971) found that workers in a DDT factory had significantly higher excretion of 6-β-hydroxy-cortisol and a significantly reduced phenylbutazone half-life. This study suggests that at least occupational exposures can alter drug and steroid metabolism in man as well as experimental animals.

Unlike the organochlorine insecticides, OP insecticides have been shown to inhibit steroid metabolism by rat liver microsomes (Conney *et al.*, 1967). Pesticide "synergists" of the methylenedioxyphenyl type such as piperonyl butoxide have been shown to inhibit or induce microsomal drug-metabolizing enzymes and to prolong or reduce hexobarbital sleep time and to potentiate or antagonize phosphorothioate insecticides (Kamienski and Murphy, 1971) depending on the dose and time of pretreatment with the "synergist." When mice were pretreated with piperonyl butoxide, under conditions favorable to inhibition of microsomal oxidases, they were slightly more susceptible to the diethyl-

substituted phosphorothionates, parathion and azinphosethyl, but were markedly resistant to the corresponding dimethyl-substituted compounds. The mechanism for this appeared to be, in part, due to the fact that glutathione alkyl transferase could serve as an alternate (to oxidation) pathway of detoxification of the dimethyl but not the diethyl-substituted compounds. Additionally, a rapid rate of reversal of dimethylphosphorylated cholinesterase (as compared to the diethyl compounds) allowed for reversal of injury to keep pace with the piperonyl butoxide–induced oxidative production of the active anticholinesterase metabolites (Levine and Murphy, 1977a, 1977b).

The effect that microsomal enzyme induction or inhibition will have on the toxicity and action of a particular drug or chemical will depend not only upon the degree to which the enzyme activity is changed, but also upon the extent to which the enzymatic metabolism of the drug is the limiting factor in determining its intensity and duration of action and the relative influence on possible alternate pathways of metabolism.

Carcinogenic, Teratogenic, and Mutagenic Properties of Pesticides

Since other chapters have been specifically devoted to these pathologic processes, they have not, with a few exceptions, been considered in detail in this chapter. The report of the Secretary's Commission on Pesticides (1969) contains discussion and summaries of data on carcinogenicity, mutagenicity, and teratogenicity of pesticides. The subject has also been reviewed by Durham and Williams (1972).

Pesticides that the Panel on Carcinogenesis of the Secretary's Commission on Pesticides (1969) considered "positive" for tumor induction on the basis of tests conducted adequately in one or more species, the results being significant at the 0.01 level, included aldrin, aramite, chlorbenzilate, p,p'-DDT, dieldrin, mirex, strobane, and heptachlor (all registered for use on food crops), and amitrole, avadex, bis(2-chloroethyl) ether, N-(2-hydroxyethyl)-hydrazine, and PCNB. The recommendation of the panel was that human exposures to these compounds be minimized and that their use be restricted to purposes for which there was a clear health benefit. Many other pesticides were given priorities for further testing because the panel felt that they had not been adequately evaluated in experimental animals. Only three pesticides were considered to have been proven negative to tumor induction on the basis of "adequate" tests in experimental animals. Obviously this report has provoked much controversy, and the purpose of including these summary comments here is to make the reader aware of the problems. The situation for DDT is a case in point. The extensive use of this compound in industrial countries has not been associated with an increase in hepatic cancer in human populations, but many years ago Fitzhugh and Nelson (1947) reported that DDT fed in high doses to rats caused slight increases in hepatic cell tumors. Innes and associates (1969) reported a statistically significant increase in hepatomas in two strains of mice. Hepatic cell tumors in trout and tumors of several sites in F_2 and following generations of mice have followed DDT exposure (Halver, 1967; Tarjan and Kemény, 1969). Additional studies sponsored by the International Agency of Research in Cancer confirmed the hepato-carcinogenicity of DDT in mice (IARC, 1974a); hepatomas were also increased in mice fed 250 ppm of DDE or DDD. While some oncologists feel that hepatoma induction is indicative of carcinogenesis, others feel that hepatomas are reversible lesions. The daily dosages ingested by animals in the experimental demonstrations of hepatomas are considerably greater than the dosage rate that man would receive, based on analyses of residues in typical meals. This, plus the failure of epidemiologic studies to demonstrate associations between DDT exposure and cancer in man, the controversy as to whether hepatoma production represents true carcinogenesis, and the fact that DDT has indeed been of great benefit in the control of malaria and other insect-borne diseases and in enhancing agricultural production, makes the administrative decision of whether or not to ban or greatly restrict its use especially difficult. It is not only a challenge to our scientific capabilities to adequately assess safety, but a challenge to social responsibility as well. Tomatis (1976) reviewed the program on the evaluation of the carcinogenic risk of chemicals to man of the International Agency for Research on Cancer. There were no pesticides among the 17 chemicals that he listed as having been found to have carcinogenicity in man or for which there was a strong suspicion of such action. Ten of the ninety-four chemicals, which the agency had determined to be carcinogenic in experimental animals only, were pesticides. These were amitrole, aramite, BHC, chlorobenzilate, DDD, DDE, DDT, dieldrin, lindane, and Mirex. Tomatis's review covered only compounds that IARC had reviewed by 1975. Both that agency and the U.S. National Cancer Institute have reported several additional pesticides as animal carcinogens since then, some of which are discussed in previous sections of this chapter. The NCI bioassay program will no doubt continue to identify additional pesticides with carcinogenic potential and may exonerate

some that IARC or others have branded as carcinogens. This is an area of great concern and one in which the compounds of greatest interest will likely continue to change.

Durham and Williams (1972) reviewed studies in experimental animals in which at least some mammalian species at some testable dosage of the following pesticides were reported to have produced teratogenic effects: carbaryl, captan, folpet, difolatan, organomercury compounds, 2,4,5-T, pentachloronitrobenzene (PCNB), and paraquat. Human consumption of organomercury compounds by pregnant women is known to have caused serious neurologic disorders in their offspring, which might be considered functional teratogenicity (or perhaps fetal toxicity). Other than this there is no confirmed relationship between exposure to pesticides and human terata. In the positive experimental studies the production of terata was usually demonstrated to be dose dependent, and the doses required were far in excess of what humans might be expected to receive under usual conditions. As with other toxic effects, pesticide teratogenicity and its relationship to human health must be considered from a dose-response standpoint and is subject to the same problems of interpretation and extrapolation as other dose-related effects, albeit a serious and tragic effect.

Recently proposed guidelines by the EPA for evaluating safety of pesticides include a battery of tests for mutagenicity. Durham and Williams (1972) reviewed the submammalian and mammalian tests available and commented on the problems of interpretation of these tests. Epstein and coworkers (1972) reported results of an extensive series of tests for mutagenic action of chemicals as determined by the dominant lethal assay in mice. Twenty-eight common pesticides were included in those tests. None of them was among the 16 chemical agents (out of a total of 174) that produced "unequivocal effects" on early fetal deaths and/or total implants, although TEPA (phosphine oxide, tris[1-aziridinyl]) and METEPA (phosphine oxide, tris[2-methyl-1-aziridyl]), which have been *proposed* as insect chemosterilants were positive. Durham and Williams (1972) reviewed reports of several pesticides that were mutagenic in nonmammalian systems (plants, bacteria, time culture, etc.), and they concluded that "from the present state of knowledge, it must be agreed that no firm conclusions can be drawn as to whether pesticides represent a mutagenic hazard." Considerable sophistication in mutagenicity testing has evolved since then, as described in Chapter 7, and the near future will likely see a resolution in the value of these tests in hazard evaluation.

Comparative Toxicology

A high degree of selective toxicity to target organism is a desirable goal in the development of useful pesticides. Metcalf (1972) has reviewed

Table 16-9. RELATIVE TOXICITY OF VARIOUS INSECTICIDES TO RATS AND HOUSEFLIES*

CLASS	COMPOUND	MSR†
Organochlorines	DDT	59
	DDD	174
	Methoxychlor	668
	Chlordane	72
	Aldrin	27
	Dieldrin	24
	Endrin	2.4
	Heptachlor	72
	Lindane	107
Organophosphates	Parathion	4
	Methyl parathion	20
	Malathion	37.7
	Azinphosmethyl	4.1
	Chlorothion	85
	Dimethoate	390
	Ronnel	1,315
Carbamates	Aldicarb	0.175
	Carbaryl	0.60
	Zectran	0.60
	Propoxur	4.5
	Mobam	10.0

* Data from Metcalf (1972).
† Mammalian selectivity ratio (MSR) is the ratio of the oral LD50 in rats to the topical LD50 in female houseflies in mg/kg for both species. Ratios of less than 1 indicate that per unit of body weight rats are more susceptible than houseflies.

toxicity data for a large number of insecticides and calculated mammalian selectivity ratios, MSRs (mouse oral LD50/female housefly topical LD50). Several of these are shown in

Table 16–9. Considering only these two species and only acute toxicity it is apparent that there is an extremely wide range of relative toxicities. The situation becomes infinitely more complex when one considers a broader spectrum of non-target species, as illustrated by only a few examples shown in Table 16–10.

There are indeed occasional marked differences in susceptibilities of common laboratory test animals, but even more striking are species differences noted among wild animals of the same vertebrate class. For example, Hayes (1967a) compared reported single-dose LD50 values for 20 pesticides in five mammalian species commonly used in safety evaluation studies. The range of susceptibilities generally varied within a factor of less than tenfold. All species were not compared for all 20 compounds, but in the majority of cases rats were more susceptible than mice, guinea pigs, rabbits, or dogs. Comparing the smallest single doses required to produce a serious effect in rats and man, man was more sensitive than rats (usually by factors of tenfold or less). In a similar comparison of reported acute insecticide toxicity values for five species of fish, Murphy (1972), calculated LD50 ratios of least to most sensitive of 2.7 for DDT, 4.7 for dieldrin, 246 for Guthion (azinphosmethyl), 49 for parathion, and 430 for malathion. A similar calculation for ten avian species gave least to most sensitive species ratios of 45 for dieldrin and 192 for parathion. The mechanisms of these species differences have received relatively little research, but there is evidence that they include both differences in sensitivity of target enzymes as well as differences in rates of biotransformation to either more or less toxic metabolites. Certainly, for a class of toxic chemicals that become as widespread in the environment as pesticides, concern for

Table 16–10. COMPARATIVE ACUTE TOXICITIES OF COMMON INSECTICIDES IN VERTEBRATES*

| PESTICIDES | MALE RATS—LD50 | | MALLARDS—LD50 | BLUEGILLS |
| | *Oral* | *Dermal* | *Oral* | 96-HR TLM |
	(mg/kg)		(mg/kg)	(µg/L)
DDT	113	>2,510	>2,240	16
Dieldrin	46	90	381	7.9
Methoxychlor	6,000	—	>2,000	62
Parathion	13	21	2.13	95
Methyl parathion	14	67	10	1,900
Guthion	13	220	136	5.2
Malathion	1,375	>4,444	1,485	90
Carbaryl	850	>4,000	>2,179	5,300

* From Murphy, S. D.: The toxicity of pesticides and their metabolites. In *Degradation of Synthetic Organic Molecules in the Biosphere*. ISBN 0–309–02046–8, Proceedings of a Conference. National Academy of Sciences, Washington, DC., 1972.

effects on a broad spectrum of nontarget species is reasonable. Since it is clearly unrealistic to expect all pesticides to be tested for safety to all nontarget species that might be exposed, the only reasonable approach appears to be to attempt to understand basic mechanisms of species differences in susceptibility and, with this information base, to select or design compounds that will not only be safe for man but also be least likely to affect other nontarget organisms present in the specific areas in which they are applied. An impossible task? Perhaps. A worthwhile objective? Certainly.

REFERENCES

Abbot, D. C.; Goulding, R.; and Tatton, J. O'G.: Organochlorine pesticide residues in human fat in Great Britain. *Br. Med. J.*, 3:146–49, 1968.

Abou-Donia, M. B., and Preissig, S. H.: Delayed neurotoxicity of leptophos: Toxic effects on the nervous system of hens. *Toxicol. Appl. Pharmacol.*, 35:269–82, 1976a.

Abou-Donia, M. B., and Preissig, S. H.: Delayed neurotoxicity from continuous low-dose oral administration of leptophos to hens. *Toxicol. Appl. Pharmacol.*, 38:595–608, 1976b.

Aldridge, W. N.: The nature of the reaction of organophosphorus compounds and carbamates with esterases. *Bull. WHO*, 44:25–30, 1971.

Aldridge, W. N.; Barnes, J. M.; and Johnson, M. K.: Studies on delayed neurotoxicity produced by some organophosphorus compounds. *Ann. N.Y. Acad. Sci.*, 160:314–22, 1969.

Aldridge, W. N., and Johnson, M. K.: Side effects of organophosphorus compounds: delayed neurotoxicity. *Bull. WHO*, 44:259–63, 1971.

Alumot, E.: The mechanism of ethylene dibromide action on laying hens. *Residue Rev.*, 41:1–11, 1972.

Armstrong, R. W.; Eichner, E. R.; Klein, D. E.; Barthel, W. F.; Bennett, J. V.; Jonsson, V.; Bruce, H.; and Loveless, L. E.: Pentachlorophenol poisoning in a nursery for newborn infants. II, Epidemiologic and toxicologic studies. *J. Pediatr.*, 75:317–25, 1969.

Autor, A. P. (ed.): *Biochemical Mechanisms of Paraquat Toxicity*. Academic Press, Inc., New York, 1977.

Baker, E. L.; Zack, M.; Miles, J. W.; Alderman, L.; Warren, M.; Dobbin, R. D.; Miller, S.; and Teeters, W. R.: Epidemic malathion poisoning in Pakistan malaria workers. *Lancet*, 1:31–34, 1978.

Benke, G. M.; Cheever, K. L.; Mirer, F. E.; and Murphy, S. D.: Comparative toxicity, anticholinesterase action and metabolism of methyl parathion and parathion in sunfish and mice. *Toxicol. Appl. Pharmacol.*, 28:97–109, 1974.

Bidstrup, P. L., and Payne, D. J. H.: Poisoning by dinitro-*ortho*-cresol: report of eight fatal cases occurring in Great Britain. *Br. Med. J.*, 2:16–19, 1951.

Bignami, G.; Rosic, N.; Michalek, H.; Milošević, M.; and Gatti, G. L.: In Weiss, B., and Laties, V. (eds.): *Behavioral Toxicology*. Plenum Press, New York, 1975, pp. 155–209.

Boyd, E. M., and Krijnen, C. J.: Toxicity of captan and protein-deficient diet. *J. Clin. Pharmacol.*, 8:225–34, 1968.

Brockmann, J. L.; McDowell, A. V.; and Leeds, W. G.: Fatal poisoning with sodium fluoroacetate. *J.A.M.A.*, 159:1529–32, 1955.

Brodeur, J., and DuBois, K. P.: Studies on acquired tolerance by rats to 0,0-diethyl S-2-(Ethylthio) ethyl phosphorodithioate (Di-Syston). *Arch. Int. Pharmacodyn.*, 149:560–70, 1964.

Brown, D. R., and Murphy, S. D.: Factors influencing dimethoate and triethyl phosphate induced narcosis in rats and mice. *Toxicol. Appl. Pharmacol.*, 18:895–906, 1971.

Brown, V. K. H.; Hunter, C. G.; and Richardson, A.: A blood test diagnostic of exposure to aldrin and dieldrin. *Br. J. Ind. Med.*, 21:283–86, 1964.

Bus, J. S.; Cagen, S. Z.; Olgaard, M.; and Gibson, J. E.: A mechanism of paraquat toxicity in mice and rats. *Toxicol. Appl. Pharmacol.*, 35:501–13, 1976.

Buser, H. R.: Analysis of polychlorinated dibenzo-p-dioxins and dibenzofurans in chlorinated phenols by mass fragmentography. *J. Chromatogr.*, 107:295–310, 1975.

California Department of Public Health: *Occupational Disease in California Attributed to Pesticides and Other Agricultural Chemicals, 1969*. Bureau of Occupational Health and Environmental Epidemiology, Sacramento, 1969.

Campbell, S.: Paraquat poisoning. *Clin. Toxicol.*, 1:245–49, 1968.

Carlson, D. A.; Konyha, K. D.; Wheeler, W. B.; Marshall, G. P.; and Zaylskie, R. G.: Mirex in the environment: Its degradation to kepone and related compounds. *Science*, 194:939–41, 1976.

Carpenter, C. P.; Weil, C. S.; Palm, P. E.; Woodside, M. W.; Nair, J. H., III; and Smyth, H. F., Jr.: Mammalian toxicity of 1-Naphthyl-*N*-methylcarbamate (Sevin insecticide). *J. Agr. Food Chem.*, 9:30–39, 1961.

Casarett, L. J.; Fryer, G. C.; Yauger, W. L., Jr.; and Klemmer, H. W.: Organochlorine pesticide residues in human tissue—Hawaii. *Arch. Environ. Health*, 17:306–11, 1968.

Casida, J. E.: Mode of action of carbamates. *Ann. Rev. Entomol.*, 8:39–58, 1963.

Cavalli, R. D., and Fletcher, K.: An effective treatment for paraquat poisoning. In Autor, A. P. (ed.): *Biochemical Mechanisms of Paraquat Toxicity*. Academic Press, Inc., New York, 1977, pp. 213–28.

Cavanaugh, J. B.: Toxic substances and the nervous system. *Br. Med. Bull.*, 25:268–73, 1969.

Chenoweth, M. B.; Kandel, A.; Johnson, L. B.; and Bennett, D. R.: Factors influencing fluoroacetate poisoning: practical treatment with glycerol monoacetate. *J. Pharmacol. Exp. Ther.*, 102:31–49, 1951.

Chichester, C. O. (ed.): *Research in Pesticides*. Academic Press, Inc., New York, 1965.

Cohen, J. A., and Oosterbaan, R. A.: The active site of acetylcholinesterase and related esterases and its reactivity towards substrates and inhibitors. In Koelle, G. B. (ed.): *Handbuch der Experimentellen Pharmacologie*, XV, "Cholinesterases and Anticholinesterase Agents." Springer-Verlag, Berlin, 1963.

Cohen, S. D., and Murphy, S. D.: Inactivation of malaoxon by mouse liver, *Proc. Soc. Exp. Biol. Med.*, 139:1385–89, 1972.

————: A simplified bioassay for organophosphate detoxification and interactions. *Toxicol. Appl. Pharmacol.*, 27:537–50, 1974.

Cohn, W. J.; Boylan, J. J.; Blanke, R. V.; Fariss, M. W.; Howell, J. R.; and Guzelian, P. S.: Treatment of chlordecone (Kepone) toxicity with cholestyramine. *N. Engl. J. Med.*, 298:243–48, 1978.

Cole, J. F.; Klevay, L. M.; and Zavon, M. R.: Endrin and dieldrin: a comparison of hepatic excretion in the rat. *Toxic. Appl. Pharmacol.*, 16:547–55, 1970.

Collins, R. P.: Methyl bromide poisoning: a bizarre neurological disorder. *Calif. Med.*, 103:112–16, 1965.

Conney, A. H.: Pharmacological implications of microsomal enzyme induction. *Pharmacol. Rev.*, 19:317–66, 1967.

Conney, A. H.; Welch, R. M.; Kuntzman, R.; and Burns, J. J.: Effects of pesticides on drug and steroid metabolism. *Clin. Pharmacol. Ther.*, **8**:2–10, 1967.

Conney, A. H.; Welch, R. M.; Kuntzman,R.; Chang, R.; Jacobson, M.; Munro-Faure, A. D.; Peck, A. W.; Bye, A.; Poland, A.; Poppers, P. J.; Finster, M.; and Wolff, J. A.: Effects of environmental chemicals on the metabolism of drugs, carcinogens, and normal body constituents in man. *Ann. N.Y. Acad. Sci.*, **179**:155–72, 1971.

Conning, D. M.; Fletcher, K.; and Swan, A. A.: Paraquat and related bipyridyls. *Br. Med. Bull.*, **25**:245–49 1969.

Cueto, C.; Page, N.; and Saffiotti, U.: *Report of Carcinogenesis Bioassay of Technical Grade Chlordecone (Kepone R)*. National Cancer Institute, Bethesda, MD, 1976.

Dale, W. E.; Gaines, T. B.; and Hayes, W. J., Jr.: Storage and excretion of DDT in starved rats. *Toxicol. Appl. Pharmacol.*, **4**:89–106, 1962.

Dale, W. E.; Gaines, T. B.; Hayes, W. J., Jr.; and Pearce, G. W.: Poisoning by DDT: relation between clinical signs and concentration in rat brain. *Science*, **142**:1474–76, 1963.

Dalgaard-Mikkelsen, S., and Poulsen, E.: Toxicology of herbicides. *Pharmacol. Rev.*, **14**:225–50, 1962.

Dauterman, W. C.: Biological and nonbiological modifications of organophosphorus compounds. *Bull. WHO*, **44**:133–50, 1971.

Davies, D. S.; Hawksworth, G. M.; and Bennett, P. N.: Paraquat poisoning. *Proc. Eur. Soc. Toxicol.*, **18**:21–26, 1977.

Davies, G. M., and Lewis, I.: Outbreak of food-poisoning from bread made of chemically contaminated flour. *Br. Med. J.*, **2**:393–98, 1956.

Davies, J. E.; Barquet, A.; Freed, V. H.; Haque, R.; Morgade, C.; Sonneborn, R. E.; and Vaclavek, C.: Human pesticide poisonings by a fat-soluble organophosphate insecticide. *Arch. Environ. Health*, **30**:608–13, 1975.

Davies, J. E.; Edmundson, W. F.; Maceo, A.; Baquet, A.; and Cassady, J.: An epidemiologic application of the study of DDE levels in whole blood. *Am. J. Public Health*, **59**:435–41, 1969.

Deichmann, W. B. (ed.): *Pesticides Symposia*. Halos and Associates, Inc., Miami, Florida, 1970.

Deichmann, W. B., and MacDonald, W. E.: Organochlorine pesticides and human health. *Food Cosmet. Toxicol.*, **9**:91–103, 1971.

Deichmann, W. B.; MacDonald, W E.; and Cubit, D. A.: DDT tissue retention: sudden rise induced by the addition of aldrin to a fixed DDT intake. *Science*, **172**:275–76, 1971.

Diggle, W. M. and, Gage, J. C.: Cholinesterase inhibition *in vitro* by OO-diethyl O-p-nitrophenyl thiophosphate (Parathion, E605). *Biochem. J.*, **49**:491–94, 1951.

Donninger, C.; Hutson, D. H.; and Pickering, B. A.: The oxidative dealkylation of insecticidal phosphoric acid triesters by mammalian liver enzymes. *Biochem. J.* **126**:701–7, 1972.

Doull, J.: The treatment of insecticide poisoning. In Wilkinson, C. F. (ed.): *Insecticide Biochemistry and Physiology*. Plenum Press, New York, 1976, pp. 649–67.

Drenth, H. J.; Ensberg, I. F. G.; Roberts, D. V.; and Wilson, A.: Neuromuscular function in agricultural workers using pesticides. *Arch. Environ. Health*, **25**:395–98, 1972.

DuBois, K. P.: New rodenticidal compounds. *J. Am. Pharm. Assoc.*, **37**:307–10, 1948.

————: Potentiation of the toxicity of organophosphorus compounds. *Adv. Pest Control Res.*, **4**:117–51 1961.

————: Toxicological evaluation of the anticholines-terase agents. In Koelle, G. B. (ed.): *Handbuch der Experimentellen Pharmakologie*, XV. Springer-Verlag, Berlin, 1963.

————: Low level organophosphorus residues in the diet. *Arch. Environ. Health*. **10**:837–41, 1965.

————: Combined effects of pesticides. *Can. Med. Assoc. J.*, **100**:173–79, 1969.

DuBois, K. P.; Doull, J.; and Coon, J. M.: Toxicity and mechanism of action of p-nitrophenyl diethyl thionophosphate (E605). *Fed. Proc.*, **7**:216, 1948.

DuBois, K. P.; Doull, J.; Salerno, P. R.; and Coon, J. M.: Studies on the toxicity and mechanisms of action of p-nitrophenyl diethyl thionosphosphate (parathion). *J. Pharmacol. Exp. Ther.*, **95**:79–91, 1949.

DuBois, K. P.; Thursh, D. R.; and Murphy, S. D.: Studies on the toxicity and pharmacologic action of the dimethoxy ester of benzotriazine dithiophosphoric acid to an anticholinesterase agent. *J. Pharmacol. Exp. Ther.*, **119**:572–83, 1957.

Durham, W. F.: The interaction of pesticides with other factors. *Residue Rev.*, **18**:21–103, 1967.

Durham, W. F., and Hayes, W. J., Jr.: Organic phosphorus poisoning and its therapy. *Arch. Environ. Health*, **5**:21–47, 1962.

Durham, W. F., and Williams, C. H.: Mutagenic, teratogenic, and carcinogenic properties of pesticides. *Annu. Rev. Entomol.*, **17**:123–48, 1972.

Dustman, E. H., and Stickel, L. F.: The occurrence and significance of pesticide residues in wild animals. *Ann. N.Y. Acad. Sci.*, **160**:162–72, 1969.

Edwards, C. A.: *Persistent Pesticides in the Environment*. CRC Monoscience Series, Chemical Rubber Co., Cleveland, Ohio, 1970.

Egan, H.; Goulding, R.; Roburn, J.; and Tatton, J. O'G: Organo-chlorine residues in human fat and human milk. *Br. Med. J.*, **2**:66–69, 1965.

Epstein, S. S.; Arnold, E.; Andrea, J.; Bass, W.; and Bishop, Y.: Detection of chemical mutagens by the dominant lethal assay in the mouse. *Toxicol. Appl. Pharmacol.*, **23**:288–325, 1972.

Eto, M.: *Organophosphorus Pesticides: Organic and Biological Chemistry*. CRC Press Inc., Cleveland, 1974.

Fairchild, E. J., II.; Murphy, S. D.; and Stokinger, H. E.: Protection by sulfur compounds against air pollutants, ozone and nitrogen dioxide. *Science*, **130**:386–62, 1959.

Fitzhugh, O. G., and Nelson, A. A.: The chronic oral toxicity of DDT (2,2-bis(p-chlorophenyl-1,1,1-trichloroethane). *J. Pharmacol. Exp. Ther.*, **89**:18–30, 1947.

Frawley, J. P.; Fuyat, H. N.; Hagen, E. C.; Blake, J. R.; and Fitzhugh, O. G.: Marked potentiation in mammalian toxicity from simultaneous administration of two anticholinesterase compounds. *J. Pharmacol. Exp. Ther.*, **121**:96–106, 1957.

Frear, D. E. H.: *Pesticide Index*, 4th ed. College Science Publishers, State College, Pa., 1969.

Fukuto, T. R.: Relationships between the structure of organophosphorus compounds and their activity as acetylcholinesterase inhibitors. *Bull. WHO*, **44**:31–42, 1971.

Fukuto, T. R., and Metcalf, R. L.: Metabolism of insecticides in plants and animals. *Ann. N.Y. Acad. Sci.*, **160**:97–113, 1969.

Cage, J. C.: The action of paraquat and diquat on the respiration of liver cell fractions. *Biochem. J.*, **109**:757–61, 1968.

Gaines, T. B.: Acute toxicity of pesticides. *Toxicol. Appl. Pharmacol.*, **14**:515–34, 1969.

Gaines, T. B., and Kimbrough, R. D.: Oral toxicity of mirex in adult and suckling rats. *Arch. Environ. Health*, **21**:7–14, 1970.

Garrettson, L. K., and Curley, A.: Dieldrin. Studies in a poisoned child. *Arch. Environ. Health*, **19**:814–22, 1969.

Glaister, J.: *The Power of Poison.* Christopher Johnson Publishers, Ltd., London, 1954, pp. 78–86.

Goldstein, J. A.: Effects of pentachlorophenol on hepatic drug metabolizing enzymes and porphyria related to contamination with chlorinated dibenzo-*p*-dioxins and dibenzofurans. *Toxicol. Appl. Pharmacol.,* 37:145–46, 1976.

Good, E. E.; Ware, G. W.; and Miller, D. F.: Effects of insecticides on reproduction in the laboratory mouse: I. Kepone. *J. Econ. Entomol.,* 58:754–56, 1965.

Gould, R. F. (ed.): *Organic Pesticides in the Environment.* Advances in Chemistry Series 60, American Chemical Society, Washington, D.C., 1966.

Grob, D.: Anticholinesterase intoxication in man and its treatment. In Koelle, G. B. (ed.): *Handbuch der Experimentellen Pharmakologie,* XV. Springer-Verlag, Berlin, 1963.

Grossman, H.: Thallotoxicosis: report of a case and a review. *Pediatrics,* 16:868–72, 1955.

Halver, J. E.: Crystalline aflatoxin and other vectors for trout hepatoma. *Bur. Sport Fish. Wldl. Res. Rept.,* 70:78–102, 1967.

Hansen, D. J.; Wilson, A. J.; Nimmo, D. R.; Schimmel, S. C.; Bahner, L. H.; and Huggett, R.: Kepone: Hazard to aquatic organisms. *Science,* 193:528, 1976.

Haq, I. U.: Agrosan poisoning in man. *Br. Med. J.,* 1:1579–82, 1963.

Hayes, W. J., Jr.: The pharmacology and toxicity of DDT. In Muller, P. (ed.): *The Insecticide DDT and Its Importance.* Birkhäuser Verlag, Basel, 1959a.

———: The toxicity of dieldrin to man: report on a survey. *Bull. WHO,* 20:891–912, 1959b.

———: *Clinical Handbook on Economic Poisons.* Public Health Service Publication No. 476. U.S. Government Printing Office, 1963.

———: Monitoring food and people for pesticide content. In *Scientific Aspects of Pest Control.* Pub. No. 1402, National Academy of Sciences. National Research Council, Washington, D.C., 1966, pp. 314–42.

———: The 90-dose LD$_{50}$ and a chronicity factor as measures of toxicity. *Toxicol. Appl. Pharmacol.,* 11:327–35, 1967a.

———: Toxicity of pesticides to man: risks from present levels. *Proc. Roy. Soc. (Biol.),* 167:101–27, 1967b.

———: Pesticides and human toxicity. *Ann. N.Y. Acad. Sci.,* 160:40–54, 1969.

———: Insecticides, rodenticides and other economic poisons. In DiPalma, J. R. (ed.): *Drull's Pharmacology in Medicine,* 4th ed. McGraw-Hill Book Co., New York, 1971, pp. 1256–76.

———: *Toxicology of Pesticides.* Waverly Press, Inc., Baltimore, 1975.

Hayes, W. J., Jr.; Dale, W. E.; and Pirkle, C. I.: Evidence of safety of long-term, high, oral doses of DDT for man. *Arch. Environ. Health,* 22:119–35, 1971.

Hayes, W. J., and Vaughn, W. K.: Mortality from pesticides in the United States in 1973 and 1974. *Toxicol. Appl. Pharmacol.,* 42:235–52, 1977.

Headley, J. C., and Kneese, A. V.: Economic implications of pesticide use. *Ann. N.Y. Acad. Sci.,* 160:30–39, 1969.

Heath, D. F.: *Organophosphorus Poisons.* Pergamon Press, Oxford, 1961.

Hine, C. H.: Methyl bromide poisoning: a review of ten cases. *J. Occup. Med.,* 11:1–10, 1969.

Hobbiger, F.: Reactivation of phosphorylated acetylcholinesterase. In Koelle, G. B. (ed.): *Handbuch der Experimentellen Pharmakologie,* XV. Springer-Verlag, Berlin, 1963, pp. 921–88.

Hodge, H. C.; Boyce, A. M.; Deichmann, W. B.; and Kraybill, H. F.: Toxicology and no-effect levels of aldrin and dieldrin. *Toxicol. Appl. Pharmacol.,* 10:613–75, 1967.

Hoffman, W. S.; Adler, H.; Fishbein, W. I.; and Bauer, F. C.: Relation of pesticide concentrations in fat to pathological changes in tissue. *Arch. Environ. Health,* 15:758–65, 1967.

Hollingworth, R. M.: The dealkylation of organophosphorus triesters by liver enzymes. In O'Brien, R. D., and Yamamoto, I. (eds.): *Biochemical Toxicology of Insecticides.* Academic Press, Inc., New York, 1972.

Holmstedt, B.: Pharmacology of organophosphorus cholinesterase inhibitors. *Pharmacol. Rev.,* 11:567–688, 1959.

Hoogendam, I.; Versteeg, J. P. J.; and DeVlieger, M.: Nine years' toxicity control in insecticide plants. *Arch. Environ. Health,* 10:441–48, 1965.

House, W. B.; Goodson, L. H.; Gadbery, H. M.; and Dockter, K. W.: *Assessment of Ecologic Effects of Extensive or Repeated Use of Herbicides.* Final Report of Midwest Research Institute on Contract No. DAHC15-68-C-0119. U.S. Department of Commerce, 1967.

Huber, J. J.: Some physiological effects of the insecticide Kepone in the laboratory mouse. *Toxicol. Appl. Pharmacol.,* 7:516–24, 1965.

Hutson, D. H.; Pickering, B. A.; and Donninger, C.: Phosphoric acid triester-glutathione alkyltransferase: a mechanism for the detoxification of dimethyl phosphase triesters. *Biochem. J.,* 127:285–93, 1972.

IARC: *Monograph on the Evaluation of Carcinogenic Risk of Chemicals to Man: Vol. 5, Some Organochlorine Pesticides.* International Agency for Research on Cancer, Lyon, France, 1974a.

IARC: *Monographs on the Evaluation of Carcinogenic Risk of Chemicals to Man. Vol. 7, Some Antithyroid and Related Substances, Nitrofurans and Industrial Chemicals.* International Agency for Research on Cancer, Lyon, France, 1974b.

IARC: *Monographs on the Evaluation of Carcinogenic Risk of Chemicals to Man. Vol. 12, Some Carbamates, Thiocarbamates and Carbazines.* International Agency for Research on Cancer, Lyon, France, 1976.

IARC: *Monographs on the Evaluation of Carcinogenic Risk of Chemicals to Man. Vol. 15. Some Fumigants, the Herbicides 2,4,-D and 2,4,5-T, Chlorinated Dibenzodioxins and Miscellaneous Industrial Chemicals.* International Agency for Research on Cancer, Lyon, France, 1977.

Ingle, L.: *A Monograph on Chlordane: Toxicology and Pharmacological Properties.* Library of Congress Card No. 65–28686, 1965.

Innes, J. R. M.; Ulland, B. M.; Valerio, M. G.; Petrucelli, L.; Fishbein, L.; Hart, E. R.; Pallotta, A. J.; Bates, R. R.; Falk, H. L.; Gart, J. J.; Klein, M.; Mitchell, I.; and Peters, J.: Bioassay of pesticides and industrial chemicals for tumorigenicity in mice: a preliminary note. *J. Natl. Cancer Inst.,* 42:1101–14, 1969.

Jager, K. W.; Roberts, D. V.; and Wilson, A.: Neuromuscular function in pesticide workers. *Br. J. Ind. Med.,* 27:273–78, 1970.

Johns, R. J., and McQuillen, M. P.: Syndrome simulating myasthenia gravis: asthenia with anticholinesterase tolerance. *Ann. N.Y. Acad. Sci.,* 135:385–97, 1966.

Johnson, M. K.: The delayed neuropathy caused by some organophosphorus esters: Mechanism and challenge. *CRC Crit. Rev. Toxicol.,* 3:289–316, 1975a.

———: Organophosphorus esters causing delayed neurotoxic effects—mechanism of action and structure/ activity studies. *Arch. Toxicol.,* 34:259–88, 1975b.

———: Structure-activity relationships for substrates and inhibitors of hen brain neurotoxic esterase. *Biochem. Pharmacol.,* 24:797–805, 1975c.

Johnson, R. L.; Gehring, P. J.; Kociba, R. J.; and Schwetz, B. A.: Chlorinated dibenzodioxins and pentachlorophenol. *Environ. Health Perspect.*, **5**:171–75, 1973.

Kamienski, F. X., and Murphy, S. D.: Biphasic effects of methylenedioxyphenyl synergists on the action of hexobarbital and organophosphate insecticides in mice. *Toxicol. Appl. Pharmacol.*, **18**:883–94, 1971.

Keil, J. E.; Finklea, J. F.; Pietsch, R. L. and Gadsden, R. H.: A pesticide use survey of urban households. *Agricultural Chemicals*, **24**:10–12, 1969.

Keplinger, M. L., and Deichmann, W. B.: Acute toxicity of combinations of pesticides. *Toxicol. Appl. Pharmacol.*, **10**:586–95, 1967.

Kim, K. C., and Karczmar, A. G.: Adaptation of the neuromuscular junction to constant concentration of ACh. *Int. J. Neuropharmacol.*, **6**:51–61, 1967.

Kinoshita, F. K., and Kempf, C. K.: Quantitative measurement of hepatic microsomal enzyme induction after dietary intake of chlorinated hydrocarbon insecticides. *Toxicol. Appl. Pharmacol.*, **17**:288, 1970.

Krueger, H. R.; O'Brien, R. D.; and Dauterman, W. C.: Relationship between metabolism and differential toxicity in insects and mice of diazinon, dimethoate, parathion and acethion. *Econ. Entomol.*, **53**:25–31, 1960.

Larson, P. S.; Haag, H. B.; and Silvette, H.: *Tobacco: Experimental and Clinical Studies*. Williams & Wilkins Co., Baltimore, 1961.

Laug, E. P.; Nelson, A. A.; Fitzhugh, O. G.; and Kunze, F. M.: Liver cell alteration and DDT storage in the fat of the rat induced by dietary levels of 1 to 50 p.p.m. DDT. *J. Pharmacol. Exp. Ther.*, **98**:268–73, 1950.

Lauwerys, R. R., and Murphy, S. D.: Comparison of assay methods for studying O,O-diethyl, O-p-nitrophenyl phosphate (paraoxon) detoxication *in vitro*. *Biochem. Pharmacol.*, **18**:789–800, 1969a.

———: Interaction between paraoxon and tri-o-tolyl phosphate in rats. *Toxicol. Appl. Pharmacol.*, **14**:348–57, 1969b.

Laws, E. R., Jr.; Curley, A.; and Boris, F. J.: Men with intensive occupational exposure to DDT: a clinical and chemical study. *Arch. Environ. Health*, **15**:766–75, 1967.

Lehman, A. J.: *Summaries of Pesticide Toxicity*. The Association of Food and Drug Officials of the United States, Topeka, Kansas, 1965.

Levine, B. S., and Murphy, S. D.: Esterase inhibitions and reactivation in relation to piperonyl butoxide–phosphorothionate interactions. *Toxicol. Appl. Pharmacol.*, **40**:379–91, 1977a.

———: Effect of piperonyl butoxide on the metabolism of dimethyl and diethyl phosphorothionate insecticides. *Toxicol. Appl. Pharmacol.*, **40**:393–406, 1977b.

Lichtenstein, E. P.: Persistence and degradation of pesticides in the environment. In *Scientific Aspects of Pest Control*. Publication No. 1402, National Academy of Science, National Research Council, Washington, D.C., 1966.

Lisella, F. S.; Long, K. R.; and Scott, H. G.: Toxicology of rodenticides and their relation to human health. *J. Environ. Health*, **33**:231–37, 361–65, 1971.

Longcore, J. R.; Samson, F. B.; Kreitzer, J. F.; and Spann, J. W.: Changes in mineral composition of eggshells from black ducks and mallards fed DDE in the diet. *Bull. Env. Contam. Toxicol.*, **6**:345–50, 1971.

Lukens, R. J.: *Chemistry of Fungicidal Action*. Springer-Verlag, New York, 1971.

McClosky, W. T., and Smith, M. I.: Studies of the pharmacologic action and the pathology of alpha-naphthylthiourea. I. Pharmacology. *Public Health Rep.*, **60**:1101–1108, 1945.

McLaughlin, J., Jr.; Reynaldo, E. F.; Lamar, J. K.; and

Marliac, J. P.: Teratology studies in rabbits with captan, folpet and thalidomide. *Toxicol. Appl. Pharmacol.*, **14**:641, 1969.

Matsumura, F.; Bousch, G. M.; and Misato, T. (eds.): *Environmental Toxicology of Pesticides*. Academic Press, Inc., New York, 1972.

Matsumura, F., and O'Brien, R. D.: Insecticide mode of action: absorption and binding of DDT by the central nervous system of the American cockroach. *J. Agr. Food Chem.*, **14**:36–39, 1966.

Matsumura, F., and Patil, K. C.: Adenosine triphosphatase: sensitive to DDT in synapses of rat brain. *Science*, **166**:121–22, 1969.

Matsunaka, S.: Propanil hydrolysis: inhibition in rice plants by insecticides. *Science*, **160**:1360–61, 1968.

Menzie, C. M.: *Metabolism of Pesticides*. Bureau of Sport Fisheries and Wildlife Special Scientific Report, Wildlife No. 127, Washington, D.C., 1969.

Metcalf, R. L.: Development of selective and biodegradable pesticides. In *Pest Control Strategies for the Future*. Agricultural Board, Division of Biology and Agriculture, National Research Council, National Academy of Science, Washington, D.C., 1972, pp. 137–56.

Milby, T. H., and Samuels, A. J.: Human exposure to lindane: comparison of an exposed and unexposed population. *J. Occup. Med.*, **13**:256–58, 1971.

Moore, J. A., and Courtney, K. D.: Tetratology studies with the trichlorophenoxyacid herbicides, 2,4,5-T and Silvex. *Teratology*, **4**:236, 1971.

Morgan, D. P.: *Recognition and Management of Pesticide Poisonings*. Publication EPA-540/9-011, U.S. Environmental Protection Agency, 1976.

Murphy, S. D.: Malathion inhibition of esterases as a determinant of malathion toxicity. *J. Pharmacol. Exp. Ther.*, **156**:352–65, 1967.

———: Mechanisms of pesticide interactions in vertebrates. *Residue Rev.*, **25**:201–21, 1969.

———: The toxicity of pesticides and their metabolites. In *Degradation of Synthetic Organic Molecules in the Biosphere*. ISBN 0–309–02046–8, Proceedings of a Conference. National Academy of Sciences, Washington, D.C., 1972, pp. 313–35.

Murphy, S. D.; Anderson, R. L.; and DuBois, K. P.: Potentiation of the toxicity of malathion by triorthototyl phosphate. *Proc. Soc. Exp. Biol. Med.* **100**:483–87, 1959.

Murphy, S. D., and DuBois, K. P.: Enzymatic conversion of the dimethoxy ester of benzotriazine dithiophosphoric acid to an anticholinesterase agent. *J. Pharmacol. Exp. Ther.*, **119**:572–83, 1957.

Murphy, S. D., and DuBois, K. P.: The influence of various factors on the enzymatic conversion of organic thiophosphate to anticholinesterase agents. *J. Pharmacol. Exp. Ther.*, **124**:194–202, 1958.

Nakatsugawa, T., and Dahm, P. A.: Microsomal metabolism of parathion. *Biochem. Pharmacol.*, **16**:25–38, 1967.

Namba, T.; Nolte, C. T.; Jackrel, J.; and Grob, D.: Poisoning due to organophosphate insecticides: acute and chronic manifestations. *Am. J. Med.*, **50**:475–92, 1971.

Narahashi, T.: Mode of action of DDT and allethrin on nerve: cellular and molecular mechanisms. *Residue Rev.* **25**:275–88, 1969.

———: Effects of insecticides on nervous conduction and synaptic transmission. In Wilkinson, C. F. (ed.): *Insecticide Biochemistry and Physiology*. Plenum Press, New York, 1976, pp. 327–52.

NAS: *Pest Control: An Assessment of Present and Alternative Technologies. Vol. V. Pest Control and Public Health*. National Academy of Sciences, Washington, D.C., 1976.

Neal, R. A.: Studies on the metabolism of diethyl 4-nitrophenyl phosphorothionate (parathion) *in vitro*. *Biochem. J.*, **103**:183–91, 1967.

Neal, R. A., and DuBois, K. P.: Studies on the mechanism of detoxification of cholinergic phosphorothioates. *J. Pharmacol. Exp. Ther.*, **148**:185–92, 1965.

O'Brien, R. D.: *Toxic Phosphorus Esters: Chemistry, Metabolism and Biological Effects*. Academic Press, Inc., New York, 1960.

———: *Insecticides, Action and Metabolism*. Academic Press, Inc., New York, 1967.

———: V. Biochemical effects. Phosphorylation and carbamylation of cholinesterase. *Ann N.Y. Acad. Sci.*, **160**:204–14, 1969.

———: Acetylcholinesterase and its inhibition. In Wilkinson, C. F. (ed.): *Insecticide Biochemistry and Physiology*. Plenum Press, New York, 1976, pp. 271–96.

Ohkawa, H.; Mikami, N.; Okuno, Y.; and Miyamoto, J.: Stereospecificity in toxicity of the optical isomers of EPN. *Bull. Env. Cont. Toxicol.*, **18**:534–40, 1977.

Oldner, J. J., and Hatcher, R. L.: Food poisoning caused by carbophenothion. *J.A.M.A.*, **209**:1328–30, 1969.

Olson, W. A.; Habermann, R. T.; Weisburger, E. K.; Ward, J. M.; and Weisburger, J. H.: Induction of stomach cancer in rats and mice by halogenated aliphatic fumigants. *J. Natl. Cancer Inst.*, **51**:1993–95, 1973.

Ortega, P.; Hayes, W. J., Jr.; Durham, W. F.; and Mattson, A.: *DDT in the Diet of the Rat*. Public Health Monograph, No. 43, PHS 484, 1956.

Palmer, J. S., and Radeleff, R. D.: The toxicologic effects of certain fungicides and herbicides on sheep and cattle. *Ann. N.Y. Acad. Sci.*, **111**:729–36, 1964.

Panel on Herbicides: *Report on 2,4,5,-T: A Report of the Panel on Herbicides of the President's Science Advisory Committee*. Executive Office of the President, Office of Science and Technology, U.S. Government Printing Office, Washington, D.C., 1971.

Pattison, F. L. M.: *Toxic Aliphatic Fluorine Compounds*. Elsevier Press, Inc., New York, 1959.

Paulet, G., and Desnos, J.: L'acrylonitrile: toxicite-mecanisme–d'action therapeutique. *Arch. Inst. Pharmacodyn.*, **131**:54–83, 1961.

Peakall, D. B.: Pesticides and the reproduction of birds. *Sci. Am.*, **222**:72–78, 1970.

Pellegrini, G., and Santi, R.: Potentiation of toxicity of organophosphorus compounds containing carboxylic ester functions toward warm-blooded animals by some organophosphorus impurities. *J. Agr. Food Chem.*, **20**:944–49, 1972.

Peters, R. A.: *Biochemical Lesions and Lethal Synthesis*. Macmillan Publishing Co., Inc., New York, 1963.

Petrova-Vergieva, T., and Ivanova-Chemishanska, L.: Assessment of the teratogenic activity of dithiocarbamate fungicides. *Food Cosmet. Toxicol.*, **11**:239–44, 1973.

Pickering, Q. H.; Henderson, C.; and Lemke, A. E.: The toxicity of organic phosphorus insecticides to different species of warmwater fishes. *Trans. Am. Fish. Soc.*, **91**:175–84, 1962.

Pimental, D.: *Ecologic Effects of Pesticides on Non-Target Species*. Report to Executive Office of the President, Office of Science and Technology, U.S. Government Printing Office, Washington, D.C., June 1971, pp. 20–23.

Plapp, F. W., and Casida, J. E.: Hydrolysis of the alkylphosphate bond in certain dialkyl aryl phosphorothioate insecticides by rats, cockroaches, and alkali. *J. Econ. Entomol.*, **51**:800–803, 1958.

Poland, A. P.; Smith, D.; Metter, G.; and Possick, P.: A health survey of workers in a 2,4-D and 2,4,5-T plant with special attention to chloracne, porphyria cutanea tarda, and psychologic parameters. *Arch. Environ. Health*, **22**:316–27, 1971.

Poore, R. E., and Neal, R. A.: Evidence for extrohepatic metabolism of parathion. *Toxicol. Appl. Pharmacol.*, **22**:68, 1972.

Powers, M. B.; Voelker, R. W.; Page, N. P.; Weisburger, E. K.; and Kraybill, H. F.: Carcinogenicity of ethylene dibromide (EDB) and 1,2-dibromo-3-chloropropane (DBCP) after oral administration in rats and mice. *Toxicol. Appl. Pharmacol.*, **33**:171–72, 1975.

Ptashne, K. A.; Woolcott, R. M.; and Neal, R. A.: Oxygen-18 studies on the chemical mechanism of the mixed function oxidase catalyzed desulfuration and dearylation reaction of parathion. *J. Pharmacol. Exp. Ther.*, **179**:380–85, 1971.

Quimby, G. E.; Armstrong, J. F.; and Durham, W. F.: DDT in human milk. *Nature (Lond.)*, **207**:726–28, 1965.

Radomski, J. L.; Deichmann, W. B.; and Clizer, E. E.: Pesticide concentrations in the liver, brain and adipose tissue of terminal hospital patients. *Food Cosmet. Toxicol.*, **6**:209–20, 1968.

Rathus, E. M., and Landy, P. J.: Methyl bromide poisoning. *Br. J. Ind. Med.*, **18**:53–57, 1971.

Reich, G. A.; Davis, J. H.; and Davies, J. E.: Pesticide poisoning in South Florida: an analysis of mortality and morbidity and a comparison of sources of incidence data. *Arch. Environ. Health*, **17**:768–75, 1968.

Reiner, E.: Spontaneous reactivation of phosphorylated and carbamylated cholinesterase. *Bull. WHO*, **44**:109–12, 1971.

Reiter, L.; Talens, G.; and Wooley, D.: Acute and subacute parathion treatment. Effects on cholinesterase activities and learning in mice. *Toxicol. Appl. Pharmacol.*, **25**:582–88, 1973.

Robens, J. F.: Teratogenic activity of several phthalimide derivatives in the golden hamster. *Toxicol. Appl. Pharmacol.*, **16**:24–34, 1970.

Roberts, D. V.: EMG voltage and motor nerve conduction velocity on organophosphorus pesticide factory workers. *Int. Arch. Occup. Environ. Health*, **36**:267–74, 1976.

Roberts, D. V.: A longitudinal electromyographic study of six men occupationally exposed to organophosphorus compounds. *Int. Arch. Occup. Environ. Health*, **38**:221–29, 1977.

Rose, M. S., and Smith, L. L.: Tissue uptake of paraquat and diquat. *Gen. Pharmacol.*, **8**:173–76, 1977.

Roszowski, A. P.: The pharmacological properties of Norbormide, a selective rat toxicant. *J. Pharmacol. Exp. Ther.*, **149**:288–99, 1965.

Rowe, V. K., and Hyman, T. A.: Summary of toxicological information on 2,4-D and 2,4,5-T type herbicides and an evaluation of the hazards to livestock associated with their use. *Am. J. Vet. Res.*, **15**:622–29, 1954.

Saleh, M. A.; Turner, W. V.; and Casida, J. E.: Polychlorobornane components of toxaphene: Structure-toxicity relations and metabolic reductive dechlorination. *Science*, **198**:1256–58, 1977.

Schmid, R.: Cutaneous porphyria in Turkey. *N. Engl. J. Med.*, **263**:397–98, 1960.

Secretary's Commission on Pesticides, U.S. Department of Health, Education, and Welfare: *Report of the Secretary's Commission on Pesticides and Their Relationship to Environmental Health*. U.S. Government Printing Office, Washington, D.C., 1969.

Singleton, S. D., and Murphy, S. D.: Propanil(3,4-dichloropropionanilide) induced methemoglobin formation in mice in relation to acylamidase activity. *Toxicol. Appl. Pharmacol.*, **24**:20–29, 1973.

Sinha, D.; Pascal, R.; and Furth, J.: Transplantable thyroid carcinoma induced by thyrotropin: its similarity to human Hürtle cell tumors. *Arch. Pathol.*, **79**:192–98, 1965.

Smalley, H. E.; Curtis, J. M.; and Earl, F. L.: Terato-genic action of carbaryl in beagle dogs. *Toxicol. Appl. Pharmacol.*, **13**:392–403, 1968.

Smith, P., and Heath, D.: Paraquat. *Crit. Rev. Toxicol.*, **4**:411–45, 1976.

Smith, R. J.: Poisoned pot becomes burning issue in high places. *Science*, **200**:417–18, 1978.

Spear, R. C.; Jenkins, D. L.; and Milby, T. H.: Pesticide residues and field workers. *Environ. Science Technol.*, **9**:308–13, 1975.

Spencer, H. C.; Rowe, V. K.; Adams, E. M.; and Irish, D. D.: Toxicological studies on laboratory animals of certain alkyldinitrophenols used in agriculture. *J. Ind. Hyg. Toxic.*, **30**:10–25, 1948.

Stavinoha, W. B.; Ryan, L. C.; and Smith, P. W.: Bio-chemical effects of an organophosphorus cholinesterase inhibitor on the rat brain. *Ann. N.Y. Acad. Sci.*, **160**: 378–82, 1969.

Street, J. C.; Chadwick, R. W.; Wong, M.; and Phillips, R. L.: Insecticide interactions affecting residue storage in animal tissues. *J. Agr. Food Chem.*, **14**:545, 1969.

Strum, J. M., and Karnovsky, M. J.: Aminotriazole goiter: fine structure and localization of thyroid peroxidase activity. *Lab. Invest.*, **24**:1–2, 1971.

Su, M.; Kinoshita, F. K.; Frawley, J. P.; and DuBois, K. P.: Comparative inhibition of aliesterases and cholinesterase in rats fed eighteen organophosphorus insecticides. *Toxicol. Appl. Pharmacol.*, **20**:241–49, 1971.

Tabershaw, I. R., and Cooper, W. C.: Sequelae of acute organic phosphate poisoning. *J. Occup. Med.*, **8**:5–20, 1966.

Tarjan, R., and Kemény, T.: Multigeneration studies on DDT in mice. *Food Cosmet. Toxicol.*, **7**:215–22, 1969.

Taylor, J. R.; Selhorst, J. B.; Houff, S. A.; and Martinez, A. J.: Chlordecone intoxication in man. 1. Clinical observations. *Neurology*, **28**:626–35, 1978.

Taylor, J. S.; Wuthrich, R. C.; Lloyd, K. M.; and Poland, A.: Chloracne from manufacture of a new herbicide. *Arch. Dermatol.*, **113**:616–19, 1977.

Tomatis, L.: The IARC program on the evaluation of the carcinogenic risk of chemicals to man. *Ann. N.Y. Acad. Sci.*, **271**:396–409, 1976.

Torkelson, T. R.; Sadek, S. E.; Rowe, V. K.; Kodama, J. K.; Anderson, H. H.; Loquvam, G. S.; and Hine, C. H.: Toxicologic investigations of 1,2-dibromo-3-chloropropane. *Toxicol. Appl. Pharmacol.*, **3**:545–59, 1961.

Triolo, A. J.; Mata, E.; and Coon, J. M.: Effect of organochlorine insecticides on the toxicity and *in vitro* plasma detoxication of paraoxon. *Toxicol. Appl. Pharmacol.*, **17**:174–80, 1970.

Tucker, R. K., and Crabtree, D. G.: *Handbook of Toxicity of Pesticides to Wildlife.* United States Depart-ment of Interior, Fish and Wildlife Service, Resource Publication No. 84. Government Printing Office, Washington, D.C., 1970.

Turner, W. A.; Engel, J. L.; and Casida, J. E.: Toxaphene components and related compounds: Preparation and toxicity of some hepta-, octa-, and nonachlorobornanes, hexa- and heptachlorobornenes, and a hexachloro-bornadiene. *J. Agric. Food Chem.*, **25**:1394–1401, 1977.

Uchida, T.; Dauterman, W. C.; and O'Brien, R. D.: The metabolism of dimethoate by vertebrate tissues. *J. Agr. Food Chem.*, **12**:48–52, 1964.

Van Miller, J. P.; Lalich, J. J.; and Allen, J. R.: In-creased incidence of neoplasm in rats exposed to low levels of 2,3,7,8-tetrachlorodibenzo-*p*-dioxin. *Chemo-sphere*, **6**:537–44, 1977.

Vandekar, M.; Plestina, R.; and Wilhelm, K.: Toxicity of carbamates for mammals. *Bull. WHO*, **44**:241–49, 1971.

Verrett, M. J.; Mutchler, M. K.; Scott, W. F.; Reynaldo, E. F.; and McLaughlin, J.: Teratogenic effects of captan and related compounds in the developing chicken embryo. *Ann. N.Y. Acad. Sci.*, **160**:334–43, 1969.

von Rumker, R.; Lawless, E. W.; Meiners, A. F.; Lawrence, K. A.; Kelso, G. L.; and Horay, F.: *Pro-duction, Distribution, Use and Environmental Impact Potential of Selected Pesticides.* EPA Publication 540/1-74-001, Environmental Protection Agency, Washington, D.C., 1975.

Warriner, R. A.; Nies, A. S.; and Hayes, W. J.: Severe organophosphate poisoning complicated by alcohol and turpentine ingestion. *Arch. Environ. Health*, **32**:203–205, 1977.

Wassermann, W.; Wassermann, D.; Imanuel, V.; Israeli, R.; and Frydman, M.: Long term studies on body reactivity in a pesticides plant. *Ind. Med. Surg.*, **39**:35–40, 1970.

Waters, E. M.; Huff, J. E.; and Gerstner, H. B.: Mirex. An overview. *Environ. Res.*, **14**:212–22, 1977.

Weil, C. S.; Woodside, M. D.; Carpenter, C. P.; and Smyth, H. F., Jr.: Current status of tests of carbaryl for reproductive and teratogenic effects. *Toxicol. Appl. Pharmacol.*, **21**:390–404, 1972.

Welch, R. M.; Levin, W.; and Conney, A. H.: Estro-genic action of DDT and its analogs. *Toxicol. Appl. Pharmacol.*, **14**:358–67, 1969.

WHO: 1974 *Evaluations of Some Pesticide Residues in Food.* World Health Organization Pesticide Residue Series, No. 4., pp. 261–263. Geneva, Switzerland, 1975.

Wilkinson, C. F. (ed.): *Insecticide Biochemistry and Physiology.* Plenum Press, New York, 1976.

Williams, C. H., and Jacobson, K. H.: An acylamidase in mammalian liver hydrolyzing the herbicide 3,4-dichloropropionanilide. *Toxicol. Appl. Pharmacol.*, **9**: 495–500, 1966.

Wills, J. H.: The measurement and significance of changes in the cholinesterase of erythrocytes and plasma in man and animals. *CRC Critical Rev. Toxicol.*, March:153–202, 1972.

Wills, J. H.; Jameson, E.; and Coulston, F.: Effects of oral doses of carbaryl on man. *Clin. Toxicol.*, **1**:265–71, 1968.

Wolfe, H. R.; Durham, W. F.; and Armstrong, J. F.: Exposure of workers to pesticides. *Arch. Environ. Health*, **14**:622–33, 1967.

Woodford, E. K., and Evans, S. A.: *Weed Control Handbook*, 4th ed. Blackwell Scientific Publications, Oxford, 1965.

World Health Organization: WHO Technical Report Series No. 525, 1973.

Xintaris, C.; Burg, J. R.; Tanaka, S.; Lee, S. T.; Johnson, B. L.; Cottrill, C. A.; and Bender, J.: *Occupational Exposure to Leptophos and Other Chemicals.* DHEW (NIOSH) Publication No. 78-136. U.S. Government Printing Office, Washington, D.C., 1978.

Zavon, M. R.; Tye, R.; and Latorre, L.: Chlorinated hydrocarbon insecticide content of the neonate. *Ann. N.Y. Acad. Sci.*, **160**:196–200, 1969.

Chapter 17

METALS

Paul B. Hammond and *Robert P. Beliles*

INTRODUCTION

Increasing technologic use of metals is one measure of man's progress since his emergence from the Stone Age. This has posed hazards to health from the time metals were fashioned into spears to present-day exposures to space-age metals, alloys, or salts. High natural concentrations of metals in food or water could have led to the first exposures. Metal leached from eating utensils or metallic cookware increased the risk of exposure. Intentional use of compounds containing toxic metals as pesticides or as therapeutic agents increased the opportunity for hazardous exposures. Although some metals have been known for centuries as industrial poisons, the coming of the industrial age led to more widespread occurrence of occupational disease related to exposure to a variety of toxic metals. In recent years a justifiable concern has arisen in regard to pollution of our environment by toxic metals.

Metals or their salts are also used therapeutically but their use has declined, particularly in the treatment of infectious diseases, with the advent of more effective organic drugs. Certain metal salts such as the mercurial diuretics still have a place in therapy. Recently lithium carbonate has been introduced for use in the treatment of manic-depressive psychosis, and one of the major uses of bismuth is in the manufacture of over-the-counter medications for the treatment of gastrointestinal distress.

Some metals are essential for life. Others have no known biologic function, but are not serious toxic hazards. Still other metals have the potential to produce disease. Metals that are essential nutrients can also exert toxic action if the homeostatic mechanism maintaining them within physiologic limits is unbalanced. Iron, for example, may be purposely included in the diet or given as supplements to correct symptoms of deficiency. Excessive intake of iron, however, is a common cause of accidental poisoning. Iron may also produce industrial disease and, in special cases (e.g., in the Bantus of Africa), it may produce maladies classified as environmental or at least nonoccupational diseases. The metals having the greatest potential for causing disease are those which accumulate in the body.

The daily intake (largely from food) and the body burden of a variety of metals are shown in Table 17-1. Concentrations of aluminum, vanadium, titanium, chromium, strontium, tin, lead, and cadmium in the lung increase up to age 40; these increases are due to the accumulation of insoluble particles. Levels of nickel, tin, strontium, cadmium, lead, and perhaps barium are increased in other tissues as well as in the lungs due to inhalation and relocation (Schroeder, 1970). The tolerance levels for metals in drinking water established by the U.S. Public Health Service along with the results of a survey of concentrations of metals found in drinking water samples are shown in Table 17-2. The survey suggests that significant numbers of people are exposed to the hazards of excess metals in the municipal water supplies.

Although excessive concentrations of metals may occur in water, air, or soil as a result of natural deposits, technologic use of these non-biodegradable materials can lead to their accumulation in the environment. Vanadium may be released into the atmosphere from the combustion of oil. Many metals, including mercury, may be released from the combustion of coal. The use of leaded gasoline has added to the levels of lead in the environment. Table 17-3 shows figures for the concentration of various metals in the atmosphere.

Metals released to the environment may be bioconcentrated and thus enter the food chain. Mercury compounds released with industrial wastes may be converted by microbial systems in aquatic bottom mud to the highly toxic methyl mercury, which is then taken up by fish living in the contaminated waters. Such an incident led to deaths and tragic disabling disease among residents of Minimata, including infants of exposed mothers.

**Table 17-1. BODY BURDEN AND HUMAN DAILY INTAKE
AND CONTENT IN THE EARTH'S CRUST OF
SELECTED ELEMENTS***

ELEMENT	HUMAN BODY BURDEN (mg/70 kg)	DAILY INTAKE (mg)	EARTH'S CRUST (ppm)
Aluminum	100	36.4	81,300
Antimony	<90		0.2
Arsenic	<100	0.7	2
Barium	16	16	400
Boron	<10	0.01–0.02	16
Cadmium	30	0.018–0.20	0.2
Calcium	1,050,000		36,300
Cesium	<0.01		1
Chromium	<6	0.06	200
Cobalt	1	0.3	23
Copper	100	3.2	45
Germanium	Trace	1.5	1
Gold	<1		0.005
Iron	4,100	15	50,000
Lead	120	0.3	15
Lithium	Trace	2	30
Magnesium	20,000	500	20,900
Manganese	20	5	1,000
Mercury	Trace	0.02	0.5
Molybdenum	9	0.35	1
Nickel	<10	0.45	80
Niobium	100	0.60	24
Potassium	140,000		25,900
Rubidium	1,200	10	120
Selenium	15	0.06–0.15	0.09
Silver	<1		0.1
Sodium	105,000		28,300
Strontium	140	2	450
Tellurium	600	0.6	0.002
Tin	30	17	3
Titanium	<15	0.3	4,400
Uranium	0.02		2
Vanadium	30	2.5	110
Zinc	2,300	12	65
Zirconium	250	3.5	70

* Data derived largely from Schroeder, 1965b.

In industrial situations, inhalation is the most important route of exposure. The background of long experience has led to the recommendation of concentrations in the air of the workplace that are deemed safe for eight-hour exposures. These values, which were adapted as Standards by the Occupational Safety and Health Administration (OSHA), are shown in Table 17-4. In some instances (alkyl lead compounds and thallium) the hazards of skin absorption have been taken into consideration as well in establishing the safe level. Other metals, such as nickel, beryllium, and arsenic, include skin changes as part of their spectrum of toxicity. Topical exposure to certain occupational metals may result in irritation of the skin and eyes or sensitization reactions and provide a route of absorption resulting in systemic toxicity. Contact with abraded rather than intact skin can produce serious symptoms of toxicity. While parenteral exposure is generally limited to medicinal use, cases of metal splinters being embedded as the result of industrial use are not unknown.

FACTORS INFLUENCING TOXICITY

Before considering the toxic properties of individual metals, it is useful to call attention to certain general properties of this class of elements that have considerable impact on their toxicity. To begin with, they seldom interface with biologic systems in the elemental form. Rather, they occur as discrete compounds that vary considerably in the ease with which they pass across

Table 17-2.   TOLERANCE LEVELS FOR METALS IN DRINKING WATER AND RESULTS OF SAMPLING OF COMMUNITY WATER SUPPLIES (969) IN 1969*

	LIMITS IN MG/LITER		MAXIMUM CONCENTRATIONS FOUND	NUMBER OF SAMPLES OF A TOTAL OF 2,595 EXCEEDING	
ELEMENT	Mandatory Upper	Desirable Upper		Mandatory	Desirable
Arsenic	0.05	0.01	0.10	5	10
Barium	1.0		1.55	2†	
Boron	5.0	1.0	3.28	0	20
Cadmium	0.01		3.94	4	
Chromium (Cr⁶†)	0.05		0.79‡	5	
Copper		1.0	8.35		42
Iron		0.3	26.0		223
Lead	0.05		0.64	37	
Manganese		0.05	1.32		211
Selenium	0.01		0.07	10	
Silver	0.05		0.03	0	
Uranium (uranyl)§		5.0	Not included		
Zinc		5.0	13.0		8

* From U.S. Public Health Service: *Community Water Supply Study: Analysis of National Survey Findings.* U.S. Department of Health, Education, and Welfare, Washington, D.C., 1970.
† Not measured in all samples.
‡ Total chromium measured.
§ Proposed.

biologic membranes. Soluble salts of metals dissociate readily in the aqueous environment of biologic membranes, facilitating thereby their transport as metal ions. Conversely, insoluble salts are relatively poorly absorbed, particularly if they are presented to absorptive biologic surfaces

Table 17-3.   URBAN AIR METAL PARTICLE CONCENTRATION IN THE UNITED STATES, 1964–1965*

	CONCENTRATION (μg/M³)	
POLLUTANT	Average	Maximum
Antimony	0.001	0.160
Arsenic	0.02	
Beryllium	< 0.0005	0.010
Bismuth	< 0.0005	0.064
Cadmium	0.002	0.420
Chromium	0.015	0.33
Cobalt	< 0.0005	0.060
Copper	0.09	10.0
Iron	1.58	22.0
Lead	0.79	8.60
Manganese	0.10	9.98
Molybdenum	< 0.005	0.78
Nickel	0.034	0.460
Tin	0.02	0.50
Titanium	0.04	1.10
Vanadium	0.050	2.20
Zinc	0.67	58.0
Barium†	0.09	
Samarium†	0.07	

* Data derived from Morgan *et al.*, 1970; Lee *et al.*, 1972.
† 1970 values.

in a polymeric state of aggregation. Even in the case of soluble metallic salts, certain factors modify their absorption. Thus, a soluble salt may interface with an organism in the presence of anions that favor the formation of insoluble salts. As a case in point, a high level of dietary phosphate reduces the gastrointestinal absorption of lead because the highly insoluble lead phosphate salt is formed. Foods have a high capacity for metal binding with consequent reduction of absorption. Thus, absorption is much greater when ingestion occurs during a period of fasting than on a full stomach.

The matter of solubility is particularly important in determining the fate of metals deposited in the airways. The more insoluble the metal compound, the more likely it is to be cleared from the pulmonary bed by retrograde movement to the pharynx with subsequent swallowing. In the course of this retrograde movement, systemic absorption is minimal.

Some metals occur in the environment as alkyl compounds, in which case the metal is firmly bonded to carbon. These alkyl compounds remain largely intact in the biologic environment. They are lipid soluble and pass readily across biologic membranes unaltered by the surrounding medium. Even after their absorption, they are only slowly dealkylated and are, therefore, distributed in the body in accordance with their lipid-soluble characteristics. The most notable examples of this type of organometallic compound are methyl mercury and tetraethyl lead.

Table 17-4. ACCEPTABLE AVERAGE CONCENTRATIONS ($\mu g/M^3$) OF OCCUPATIONAL EXPOSURE BASED ON EIGHT-HOUR EXPOSURES*

Antimony and compounds (as Sb)	500
Stibine (SbH_3)	500 (0.1 ppm)
Arsenic and compounds (as As)	500
Arsine (AsH_3)	200 (0.05 ppm)
Arsenate, calcium	1,000
Arsenate, lead	150
Barium (soluble compounds)	500
Beryllium and compounds	2 (5†)
Boron oxide	15,000
Boron trifluoride	3,000†
Diborane	100
Pentaborane	(0.005 ppm)
Decaborane (skin)	300
Cadmium fume	100 (3,000†)
Cadmium dust	200 (600†)
Chromic acid and chromates	100†
Chromium, soluble salts	500
Chromium, metal and insoluble salts	1,000
Cobalt, metal fume and dust	100
Copper fume	100
Copper, dusts and mists	1,000
Hafnium	500
Iron oxide fume	10,000
Ferbam (ferric dimethyldithiocarbamate)	15,000
Ferrovanadium dust (FeV)	1,000
Lead and its inorganic compounds	200
Lead arsenate	150
Lead, tetraethyl (as Pb—skin)	75
Lead, tetramethyl (as Pb—skin)	75
Lithium hydride	25
Magnesium oxide fume	15,000
Manganese	5,000†
Mercury	100†
Mercury (organo alkyl)	10 (40†)
Molybdenum (soluble compounds)	5,000
Molybdenum (insoluble compounds)	15,000
Nickel, metal and soluble compounds as Ni	1,000
Nickel carbonyl	7 (0.001 ppm)
Osmium tetroxide	2
Platinum (soluble salts as Pt)	2
Rhodium, metal fume and dust as Rh	100
Rhodium (soluble salts)	1
Selenium compounds as Se	20
Selenium, hexafluoride	400
Silver, metals and soluble compounds	10
Tantalum	5,000
Tellurium	100
Tellurium hexafluoride	200 (0.02 ppm)
Thallium (soluble compound—skin as Tl)	100
Tin (inorganic compounds except oxides)	2,000
Tin (organic compounds)	100
Titanium dioxide	15,000
Uranium (soluble compounds)	50
Uranium (insoluble compounds)	250
Vanadium (V_2O_5 dust)	500†
Vanadium (V_2O_5 fume)	100†
Yttrium	1,000
Zinc chloride fume	1,000
Zinc oxide fume	5,000
Zirconium compounds as Zr	5,000

* From *Federal Register*, Vol. 36, No. 157; Friday, Aug. 13, 1971.
† Ceilings.

Their toxicologic properties are quite different from those of inorganic forms, attesting to their integrity in the body as distinct molecular entities.

The strong attraction between metal ions and organic ligands has implications beyond the matter of their availability for absorption. It also influences the disposition of metals in the body and their rate of excretion. Most toxicologically important metals bind strongly to tissues and therefore are only slowly excreted. Consequently, with continuing intake they tend to accumulate to a high degree. Tissue affinities of the various metals are, however, quite dissimilar. Thus, lead and radium have a strong affinity for osseous tissue, whereas cadmium and mercury localize mainly in the kidney.

METAL CHELATION

Because metals persist so strongly in the body, a major therapeutic objective in poisoning is the administration of drugs that enhance their excretion. The concept of enhancing metal excretion by administration of readily excreted complexing agents should probably be credited to Seymour Kety. Starting with the observation that citrate has a powerful solvent action on lead phosphate, he determined by a potentiometric method the high affinity of citrate for ionic lead and suggested the use of citrate as a means of promoting lead excretion (Kety, 1942). The concept was further defined with the development of dimercaptopropanol (British Anti-Lewisite; BAL) as an antidote for arsenic poisoning. Starting with the observation that arsenic has an affinity for sulfhydryl-containing substances, a series of low-molecular-weight sulfhydryl compounds was synthesized and tested for efficacy. Dithiols were found to be more protective than monothiols and, among the dithiols, those with sulfhydryl groups on adjacent carbon atoms were best able to reverse the toxic effects of arsenic. This led to the conclusion that the simultaneous binding of arsenic to two sulfur atoms on adjacent carbon atoms was required to compete successfully with the critical binding site responsible for the toxic effects (Stocken and Thompson, 1946). Further, these observations led to the

prediction that the "biochemical lesion" of arsenic poisoning would prove to be a dithiol with sulfhydryl groups separated by one or more intervening carbon atoms. This prediction was borne out a few years later with the discovery

that arsenic interferes with the function of 6,8-dithiooctanoic acid in biologic oxidation (Gunsalus, 1953).

Since these initial studies, the concept of metal-binding agents as drugs has received considerable attention. Certain principles have emerged and a few more effective agents have been developed. When two or more ligands (e.g., sulfhydryl groups) in a molecule simultaneously form bonds with a metal atom, the donor molecule is properly referred to as a chelating agent. This term is derived from the Greek *chela*, for claw. Multidentate complexes of this type generally are more stable than simple unidentate complexes. The classic ligands are anions of oxo acids, e.g.,

R—C(=O)—O—, or neutral molecules in which the donor atom is nitrogen, e.g., R—NH$_2$. Thiols, such as in dimercaptopropanol, resemble oxo acids in that they coordinate with metal ions by giving up protons. The usual role of these ligands is that they are electron donors. In the process of forming metal chelates, the formation of five- or six-membered rings generally is required for optimal stability.

Chelating agents are generally nonspecific in regard to their affinity for metals. To varying degrees, they will mobilize and enhance the excretion of a rather wide range of metals, including essential metals such as calcium and zinc. Their efficacy depends not solely on their affinity for the metal of interest, but also on their affinity for endogenous metals, mainly Ca, which compete in accordance with their own affinities for the chelator. The affinity constant $\left(K\dfrac{M}{ML}\right)$ for a metal (M) and a ligand donor chelating agent (L) is defined by

$$K\frac{M}{ML} = \frac{[KM]}{[K][M]}$$

The net affinity of the chelator (K'_M) for the metal M is approximated by

$$K'_M = \frac{K^M_{ML}[L]}{\alpha_L + K^{Ca}_{CaL}[Ca^{2+}]}$$

in which α_L is calculated from the affinity of the ligand groups for hydrogen ions at the biologic pH (Catsch, 1961). K'_M is an oversimplified figure of merit. It holds only for 1:1 metal-chelator complexes. For 1:2 complexes the product of the successive formation constants K^M_{ML} and K^M_{ML2} is substituted for K^M_{ML}, giving the net affinity constant:

$$K''_M = \frac{K^M_L\, K^M_{L2}\,[L]^2}{(\alpha_L + K^{Ca}_{CaL}\,[Ca^{2+}])^2}$$

Further, it is obvious that calcium is only one of many metals that compete with toxic metals in the body. However, other metals in the body either form less stable metal chelates or are present in much lower concentrations than calcium.

The most thoroughly studied group of chelating agents is the family of polyaminocarboxylic acids. The most widely used member of this group is ethylenediaminetetraacetic acid (EDTA):

$$\text{HO—C—C} \quad \text{C—C—OH}$$
$$\text{N—C—C—N}$$
$$\text{HO—C—C} \quad \text{C—C—OH}$$

It has been used extensively in the treatment of lead poisoning. The association between metal and chelator probably is usually quadridentate in nature:

$$O=C—O—M—O—C=O$$

Its congener, diethylenetriaminepentaacetic acid (DTPA), has a slightly higher K'_M (Table 17-5). As would be predicted, its lead-mobilizing efficacy is somewhat higher than for EDTA (Hammond, 1971). K^M_{ML}'s, however, are not

Table 17-5. NET AFFINITY CONSTANTS* FOR SOME SELECTED METAL IONS AND CHELATING AGENTS†

METAL ION	EDTA‡	DTPA§	DFOA‖	PA¶
Be^{2+}	−2.3	−1.1		
Fe^{3+}	13.4	15.6	20.7	
Cu^{2+}	7.1	9.6	4.2	8.9 (10.1)
Zn^{2+}	4.6	6.5	1.2	2.4
Ce^{3+}	4.3	8.5		
Hg^{2+}	10.1	14.8		9.9 (11.9)
Pb^{2+}	6.3	7.2		4.8 (5.7)

* Numbers = log K'_M; numbers in parentheses = log K''_M (see text for definitions of K'_M and K''_M).
† Modified from Catsch, A., and Harmuth-Hoene, A.: New developments in metal antidotal properties of chelating agents. *Biochem. Pharmacol.*, 24: 1557–62, 1975.
‡ Ethylenediamine tetraacetate.
§ Diethylenetriamine pentaacetate.
‖ Desferrioxamine.
¶ D-Penicillamine.

always reliable determinants of *in vivo* metal-mobilizing efficacy. Thus, K^M_{ML}'s for mercury suggest that DTPA would be a better mobilizing agent than D-penicillamine (PA) (see Table 17-1), whereas the reverse actually is true (Catsch

and Harmuth-Hoene, 1975). Factors other than relative affinities obviously are involved in *in vivo* metal mobilization. At best, affinity characteristics serve only as a guide to the investigator searching for potential metal mobilizers. Some chelating agents may not be useful because they are rapidly metabolized to inactive forms in the body. Others may bind tightly to a toxic metal but may at the same time remain immobilized at the site of metal complexation by formation of ternary complexes with fixed ligand acceptors in the tissues. See Catsch and Harmuth-Hoene (1975) for an up-to-date review of chelating agents and metal antidotes.

TOXIC EFFECTS

There is very little by way of generalizing principles concerning the mechanisms of action of toxic metals. The very elemental nature of the metals and their diverse affinities for organic ligands in biologic structures are characteristics that discourage any unitarian concepts of toxic actions. Those which have been most thoroughly studied produce a bewildering array of biologic effects. Their toxic actions similarly involve a multiplicity of target organs and systems. In no case can the multiple manifestations of toxicity be assigned to the inhibition of a single enzyme or a single biochemical process.

It is perhaps because of this multiplicity of effects that the concepts of "critical organ" and "critical dose" have evolved in connection with the metals rather than with some other class of poisons (Nordberg, 1976). The term "critical" is used to denote "most sensitive." Thus, the critical organ is the one showing adverse effects at the lowest dose. There is no implication involved as to severity of effect. Other organs and systems may be much more severely affected, but only at higher doses. The concept assumes considerable importance in regard to toxic agents for which a tolerance limit value greater than zero seems necessary because of technologic or economic imperatives. Needless to say, a ranking of effects in accordance with dose has practical meaning only insofar as it can be defined in man or other species for which benefits are an issue. A ranking in laboratory animal species is useful, but only as a first step toward assessment in the species of ultimate concern.

ACQUIRED TOLERANCE

The field of biology owes much of its fascination to the intricacies of adaptation, whether it be on an evolutionary scale or in the moment-to-moment responses of the organism to a changing environment. Tolerance may be viewed as a special form of adaptation in which continued exposure to a chemical agent results in an increased resistance to the noxious consequences of the exposure. In the fields of pharmacology and toxicology, the best-known mechanism of acquired tolerance is induction of the mixed-function oxidase system, wherein certain organic compounds stimulate their own detoxification and that of other organic compounds.

The concept of acquired tolerance to metals has its origins in anecdotal form. Natives of the Austrian Tyrol reputedly acquired a tolerance to arsenic by continuous exposure. No evidence has ever been presented confirming the existence of acquired tolerance to arsenic. Nonetheless, in the case of lead and cadmium at least, there is fragmentary evidence for acquired tolerance. In both cases continued exposure to low doses of the metals results in the elaboration of proteins that strongly bind the metals. The implications of this phenomenon are discussed in more detail under the separate headings for these two metals.

The various aspects of metal toxicology that have been discussed above are not equally understood for all metals. As a matter of fact, the body of knowledge concerning the individual metals is extremely spotty. For a few, notably lead, mercury, and cadmium, a fairly complete picture emerges. For one reason or another, these have been studied most intensively. They serve as models. Admittedly, current and future problems in the toxicology of metals will only be solved by the integration of knowledge drawn from the broad spectrum of biomedical sciences. Nonetheless, the search for knowledge in this area clearly requires an understanding of concepts and phenomena that have evolved in the immediate field of interest. With that thought in mind, the metals whose toxicology is best known will be considered first.

LEAD

Introduction

It is fitting that consideration of individual metals in this chapter should begin with lead. No metal has been more intensively studied from a toxicologic point of view and no metal has presented a broader range of problems, both in regard to the multiplicity of routes of entry, and in regard to the spectrum of organs and systems affected in man, and in domesticated and wild animals as well.

The highest level of exposure occurs principally among people working in lead smelters. The various processes involved in refining lead result in generation of metal fumes and deposition of lead oxide dust in the workers' occupational environment. Conditions are only somewhat better in storage battery factories, where lead oxide dust is a constituent of the battery grids and is likewise an inevitable by-product of grid preparation. Other manufacturing operations, too numerous to describe here, result in varying degrees of lead exposure.

In the general population, the major hazard is for young children who chew and swallow objects contaminated with lead-containing paint, e.g., flaking paint on walls and woodwork or weathered lead paint dust and flakes leaching from the exterior of residential and commercial structures into adjacent soil and dust. For those who are interested in the broad aspects of the environmental significance of lead as a pollutant, there are two good recent reviews (NAS-NRC, 1972; WHO, 1977).

Metabolism

For all practical purposes, there are two forms of lead. The first is inorganic lead, in which the various salts and oxides are considered to act identically once absorbed into the systemic circulation. The second form is alkyl lead, notably tetraethyl lead and tetramethyl lead. These are clearly different from inorganic forms of lead, as to both absorption and disposition in the body. They will therefore be discussed separately.

Metabolism of organic forms of lead has been studied extensively, not only in animal models but also in man. Distinctions are not generally made regarding the disposition of the various inorganic compounds. It is assumed that lead ions dissociate to some degree and are absorbed and distributed in the body in the same manner, regardless of environmental origin. The validity of this assumption has not been tested rigorously, but there is no reason to suspect that lead salts retain their identity as a molecular species during the processes of absorption and subsequent distribution and excretion.

Absorption

The major routes of lead absorption are the gastrointestinal tract and the respiratory system. Small amounts of lead may also be absorbed from the intact or abraded skin when applied in high concentrations (Rastogi and Clausen, 1976; Laug and Kunze, 1948). So far as the general population is concerned, dermal contact with concentrated aqueous solutions of lead is infrequent. This is in contrast to the continual ingestion and inhalation of lead that are experienced to varying degrees by everyone.

In contrast to the relative insignificance of skin as a route of inorganic lead absorption, alkyl lead compounds are absorbed to such a degree that toxicity among handlers of these compounds in the blending of leaded gasoline has

urinary excretion is dominant, as compared to other routes. Approximate contributions to daily lead excretion in adults are as follows:

ROUTE OF EXCRETION	μg Pb EXCRETED PER DAY	%
Urine	36	76
Gastrointestinal secretions	8	16
Epithelial structures and sweat	4	8

Rabinowitz et al., 1973.

On the other hand, from nutritional balance studies it appears that in infants gastrointestinal excretion of lead is somewhat greater than urinary excretion. The pattern of excretion observed in experimental animals resembles that in human infants. The mechanism of urinary lead excretion is not fully known, but the most likely process is glomerular filtration with variable degrees of tubular reabsorption, depending on the filtered load (Vander et al., 1977).

Biologic Effects

Many organs and systems are adversely affected by lead. Some effects have been observed in both man and experimental animals. Others have been observed only in experimental animals. The implications of effects reported only in animal studies often are not known because relevant human studies have not been conducted. The four major target organs and systems are the central nervous system, the peripheral nerves, the kidney, and the hematopoietic system. In all four cases the effects have been observed in man and have been studied extensively.

Central Nervous System. There are numerous reports of a severe, often fatal condition commonly referred to as lead encephalopathy, occurring as a result of chronic or subchronic exposure to high doses of inorganic lead. The major features are dullness, restlessness, irritability, headaches, muscular tremor, ataxia, and loss of memory. These signs and symptoms may progress to convulsions, coma, and death. A high incidence of residual damage is seen, including epilepsy, hydrocephalus, and idiocy. These sequelae are similar to those seen following infectious or traumatic injury to the brain. The pathogenic mechanism leading to these effects is not well understood. Although varying degrees of cerebral vascular damage are common in fatal cases, along with demyelination and axonal damage in neurons, these are not constant findings.

A major concern today is subtle behavioral effects, particularly in children, at levels of exposure below those causing encephalopathy.

Epidemiologic studies suggest that only moderately elevated lead exposure in infants and young children (PbB = 40 to 80) may cause deficits as reflected in psychometric performance tests and in certain neurologic tests (Bornschein et al., 1979).

The toxic effects of alkyl lead compounds on the central nervous system are more of a psychic nature, compared to inorganic lead. Hallucinations, delusions, and excitement are the most common effects. These progress to delirium in fatal cases.

There have been numerous studies utilizing experimental animal models regarding the effects of inorganic lead on the central nervous system. These studies have mainly been concerned with possible effects of lead on certain performance tasks that might reflect effects on cognitive function (learning and memory) or sensorimotor function in the infant animal exposed to lead very early in life or in utero. These studies have not as yet yielded any conclusive, consistent information, but they do tend to confirm observations in children, suggesting subtle effects not accompanied by overt signs of lead poisoning.

The mechanism whereby functional disturbances of the central nervous system occur is poorly understood. Some investigators have studied effects of lead on the action of neurotransmitters using isolated peripheral nerve preparations. Both cholinergic and adrenergic synaptic evoked transmitter release is inhibited by lead. This effect is inhibited by calcium (Kostial and Vouk, 1957; Manalis and Cooper, 1973; Cooper and Steinberg, 1977). The significance of these observations in regard to the brain is highly uncertain at this time.

Peripheral Nervous System. The older literature cites the frequent occurrence of lead palsy among workers in the lead trades. The major manifestation of lead palsy is weakness of the extensor muscles. Sensory disturbances also occur, e.g., hyperaesthesia and analgesia. This peripheral neuropathy has been studied in some detail experimentally. The anatomic lesion is characterized by segmental demyelination and by axonal degeneration. Functionally, nerve conduction velocity is slowed, even in the absence of palsy, an effect seen in both children and adults even with no discernible impairment of myoneural function (Seppäläinen et al., 1975; Feldman et al., 1973).

Kidney. Two distinct types of renal effect have been observed in man. In the first type, the effects are manifestations of damage to the proximal tubules. Tubular reabsorption of glucose, amino acids, and phosphate is depressed. These effects are readily reversible with chelation therapy. The other type of renal effect occurs with

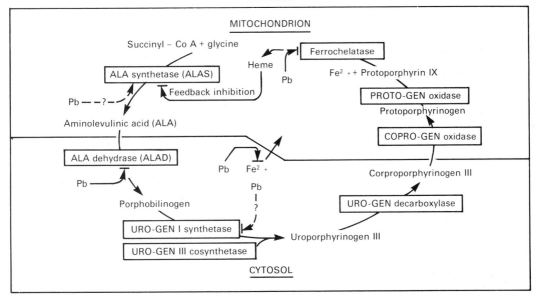

Figure 17–3. Effects of lead on heme metabolism.

prolonged high lead exposure. It is a progressive disease characterized by interstitial fibrosis, sclerosis of vessels, and glomerular atrophy. It occurs mainly among heavy consumers of moonshine whiskey and in workers with high, longterm industrial exposure. Death may ensue due to renal failure. A dramatic example of the slow, progressive nature of this condition was reported from Queensland, Australia. As early as 1897 it was observed that deaths from chronic nephritis in early adulthood were much more common than elsewhere. This excessive death rate was traced to childhood lead poisoning (Henderson, 1958). The most remarkable aspect of this was that the clinical disease occurred many years after termination of the exposure. No comparable incidents have been reported elsewhere, suggesting that unknown ancillary factors were involved. Another interesting feature of this "Queensland disease" was the occurrence of gout, presumably due to reduced renal excretion of uric acid. This condition is occasionally reported in lead poisoning due to moonshine whiskey, but not in occupational lead poisoning.

Most of the toxic effects seen in man have also been observed in experimental animals. There are exceptions. Gout has never been reported in experimental lead poisoning; on the other hand, renal tumors are observed with prolonged lead exposure in rats and mice but not in man. As a matter of fact, excess deaths in industrial lead exposure have been shown only for the categories of cerebrovascular disease and chronic nephritis.

Hematopoiesis and Heme Synthesis. The multiple effects of lead on organs and systems are most vividly apparent here. It has long been known that anemia is one of the early manifestations of lead poisoning. It results from reduction of the lifespan of circulating erythrocytes as well as from inhibition of synthesis of hemoglobin. The shortened lifespan of erythrocytes is inconstant, occurring only in some cases of leadinduced anemia. Erythrocytes exposed to lead *in vitro* show increased osmotic resistance but also show increased mechanical fragility. In addition, it has been shown *in vivo* that, even in moderate lead exposure, erythrocyte Na-K-ATPase is somewhat inhibited, suggesting a loss of cell membrane integrity. This may account for the shortened lifespan of erythrocytes that sometimes occurs.

The actions of lead on the synthesis of hemoglobin are complex. Various effects are seen at different levels of exposure. For example, in some cases of poisoning globin synthesis is impaired. It seems more likely, however, that effects on heme synthesis are of greater importance than effects on globin synthesis, since they occur even at exposure levels below those which result in anemia. At low levels of exposure these effects result in a marginal decrement of hemoglobin concentration. At still lower levels of exposure, some biochemical effects are seen, even in the absence of reduced hemoglobin. In order to understand the interplay of these effects, it is necessary first to understand some major features of heme synthesis. These are summarized in Figure 17-3. The process of heme synthesis begins in the mitochondrion with the formation of δ-aminolevulinic acid (ALA), a process requiring the enzyme δ-aminolevulinic acid synthetase (ALAS). A series of additional steps then takes place, first in the cytoplasm, then again in the mitochondrion, beginning with the condensation of two molecules of ALA to form a pyrrole ring, porphobilinogen, and ending with the insertion of iron into the tetrapyrrole, protoporphyrin IX. The rate-limiting step in the heme biosynthetic pathway is the rate of ALA formation, which, in turn, is dependent on the rate of synthesis of the enzyme ALAS. The end product, heme, regulates ALAS synthesis by negative feedback inhibition. When heme concentration falls, compensatory derepression of ALAS synthesis occurs, with a consequent increase in ALAS-generated ALA synthesis. The several biochemical effects of lead depicted at the bottom of Figure 17-3 are best explained by its known inhibitory effects on the incorporation of iron into protoporphyrin IX. This is either due to its direct inhibition of the enzyme ferrochelatase or to its interference with the entry of iron into the mitochondrion. Both mechanisms are compatible with the rise in erythrocytic protoporphyrin that occurs at a level of lead exposure below the level associated with reduced circulating hemoglobin. The consequent reduction in heme concentration probably triggers the derepression of ALAS, which in turn may explain the rise in urinary ALA and coproporphyrin, effects that occur only at a level of lead exposure greater than is necessary to inhibit conversion of protoporphyrin IX to heme. The evidence in support of

this summary view is admittedly not totally satisfactory. The most puzzling aspect is with regard to inhibition of ALAD. This seems to occur at levels of lead exposure considerably below those involving elevation of its substrate ALA in plasma or urine. The concept of "reserve enzyme" usually is invoked to explain this.

A discussion of the effects of lead on heme synthesis would not be complete without calling attention to the fact that hemoglobin is only one of many hemoproteins essential to normal body function. Others include the cytochromes cytochrome c oxidase and hydroperoxidases, all of which are part of the electron transfer systems requiring heme. The effect of lead on these hemoproteins is poorly understood.

Other Effects. The toxicologic effects of lead are not limited to the systems discussed above. Thus, lead has long been known to cause colic in cases of poisoning. The mechanism is not understood. Lead also causes chromosomal aberrations and, perhaps, abnormal sperm morphology in man. The significance of these effects is at present uncertain.

Dose-Effect and Dose-Response Relationships

The concentration of lead in the blood (PbB) is the best indicator of the dose in the body. Its relationship to effect can be estimated if two conditions can be satisfied. First, the effect must be quantifiable and, second, the time at which the

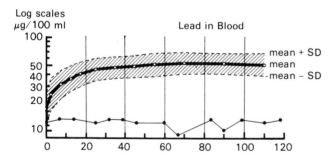

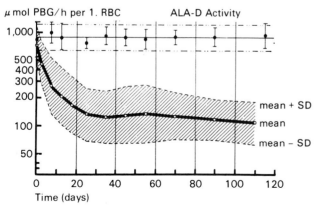

Figure 17–4. Smoothed average blood lead concentrations and ALAD activities plotted against time in semilogarithmic scales. ALAD activities in the control group are presented together with the ALAD curve of the exposed subjects, and the blood lead concentrations in one control subject are presented together with the blood lead curve of the exposed subjects. Shadowed area indicates the standard deviation. (From Tola, S.; Hernberg, S.; Asp, S.; and Nikkanen, J.: Parameters indicative of absorption and biological effect in new lead exposure: A prospective study. *Br. J. Ind. Med.*, 30:134–41, 1973.)

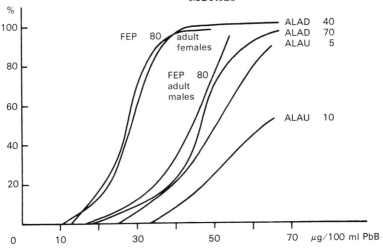

Figure 17–5. Dose-response relationships for effects of lead on heme intermediates. The ordinate represents percent respondents for the various effects.
Effects:
FEP = Concentration of erythrocytic porphyrin concentration, expressed as μg/dl packed cells.
ALAD = Aminolevulinic acid dehydrase activity in blood, expressed as % inhibition.
ALAU = Concentration of aminolevulinic acid in urine, expressed as mg/l.
(From Zielhuis, R. L.: Dose-response relationships for inorganic lead. *Int. Arch. Occup. Health*, 35:1–18, 19–35, 1975.)

dose is measured must correspond to the time at which the effect occurs. Alternatively, the dose must not change during the lag period between occurrence of effect and actual measurement of effect. These conditions are rather difficult to satisfy. As a matter of fact, it can only be done satisfactorily with regard to lead effects on heme synthesis. A good example of how dose and effect change together was provided in a prospective study of newly hired lead workers. As PbB rose, ALAD activity fell more or less concurrently (Fig. 17-4). As would be expected, the response of the workers varied both as to the PbB in the work environment and as to the magnitude of ALAD inhibition. The interindividual variability in response is expressed in the form of dose-response curves. For lead effects on heme synthesis, estimates can be made of the percent respondents. This is illustrated for the major effects of lead on heme synthesis that have been under discussion (Fig. 17-5). The elaboration of dose-response curves is useful only if the particular effect (e.g., FEP > 80) has some health significance.

Treatment of Lead Poisoning

It is extremely difficult to evaluate the benefits of therapeutic regimens for the treatment of lead poisoning, or other metallic poisons for that matter. To begin with, the incidence of frank poisoning and the corresponding amount of clinical experience is low compared to many other diseases, e.g., hypertension or the common

headache. Further, the wide spectrum of manifestations of illness among cases makes it extremely difficult to compare responses to various regimens. In adults and children both, the major specific therapeutic objective is removal of lead from the body using chelating agents. In adults the most widely accepted procedure is intravenous infusion of the calcium salt of disodium ethylenediamine tetraacetate (CaEDTA), 1 to 2 g per day, for 4 to 5 consecutive days. The lead chelate formed by exchange of Ca for Pb is excreted promptly in the urine. Curiously, the major source of lead mobilized in this manner is the bones (Hammond, 1971).

The treatment of lead poisoning in children also entails a course of CaEDTA therapy, either alone or in combination with dimercaptopropanol (BAL). Combined therapy has been found to be more effective than therapy with either drug alone (Chisolm, 1970).

MERCURY

Introduction

It is "the hottest, the coldest, a true healer, a wicked murderer, a precious medicine, and a deadly poison, a friend that can flatter and lie." [Woodall, J.: *The Surgeon's Mate or Military & Domestic Surgery*. London, 1639, p. 256]*

There has always been an aura of magic surrounding mercury. Even the name, shared by a

---

* Quoted from Goldwater, 1972.

Roman god and a distant planet, and the lustrous liquid appearance of this metal suggest magic. Before the time of Christ and even to this day, magic properties have been ascribed to mercury. It occupied a central role among alchemists in the transmutation of base metals into gold. It was carried about as amulets to ward off disease and other evils. At various times down through the centuries it has been used to treat almost every ailment known to man. Even to this day it is used to a limited extent for therapeutic purposes. Its toxic properties, however, were not unappreciated. It has long been widely condemned as being a drug with no reasonable margin of safety, even at a time when it was being used widely, notably for the treatment of syphilis. Even the characteristics of occupational intoxications were described in the Middle Ages.

Man is apparently a poor student of history. Mercury poisoning still occurs to some extent in certain occupations, principally from inhalation of mercury vapor. There also have occurred episodes of environmental contamination with organic forms of mercury, principally methyl mercury. The most widely known such episode occurred in Minamata Bay, Japan, from 1953 into the early 1960s. This was followed by a similar episode in Niigata, Japan. In both cases the cause was consumption by the local inhabitants of fish that were contaminated with mercury from industrial waste. In all, 1,200 cases of poisoning were reported. Even more extensive episodes have resulted from contamination of bread made from cereal grains treated with alkyl-mercury fungicides. The largest of these episodes occurred in Iraq, 1971–1972. It involved some 6,000 cases and 500 deaths.

At the time that outbreaks of methyl mercury poisoning in Japan were under active investigation, Swedish scientists found high concentrations of methyl mercury in freshwater fish. The sources of mercury were mainly chloralkali plants, drainage of fields in which cereal grain seeds had been treated with mercury, and wood pulp plants. Methylation of mercury occurred due to the action of aquatic organisms, leading to transfer and bioconcentration up the food chain to the large carnivorous fish. For more details concerning the environmental significance and toxicology of mercury, there are two good recent reviews (Clarkson, 1972; WHO, 1976).

Metabolism

The chemical form of mercury has a profound influence on its disposition. For all practical purposes there are three general forms of mercury.

1. Elemental mercury—Hg^0. This form is of considerable importance toxicologically because it has a high vapor pressure. A saturated atmosphere at 24° C contains approximately 18 mg/M^3. Of equal significance is the fact that the vapor exists in a monoatomic state. It is therefore distributed primarily to the alveolar bed upon inhalation. Finally, metallic mercury has limited but toxicologically significant solubility in water (20 μg/l) and organic solvents (2.7 mg/l in pentane).

2. Inorganic Mercury—Hg^{1+} and Hg^{2+}. Of these two oxidation states, Hg^{2+} is the more reactive, readily forming complexes with organic ligands, notably sulfhydryl groups. In contrast to $HgCl_2$, which is both highly soluble in water and highly toxic, $HgCl$ is highly insoluble and correspondingly less toxic.

3. Organic Mercury. These compounds are of diverse chemical structure. As the term is used here, organic mercury refers to all compounds in which mercury forms a bond with one carbon atom. For all practical purposes, the group is limited to methyl and ethyl mercury, phenyl mercury, and the family of alkoxyalkyl mercury diuretics.

$$CH_3Hg^+ ; C_2H_5Hg^+ ; C_6H_5Hg^+ ; RCH_2CORCH_2Hg^+$$

These organic cations form salts with inorganic and organic acids, e.g., chlorides and acetates. They also react readily with biologically important ligands, notably sulfhydryl groups. Finally, they pass readily across biologic membranes since they are lipid soluble. The major difference among these various organomercury cations is that the stability of the carbon-mercury bonds *in vivo* varies considerably. Thus, the alkyl mercury compounds are considerably more resistant to biodegradation than either phenyl mercury or the alkoxyalkyl mercury compounds.

Absorption

For elemental mercury the most important route of absorption is the respiratory tract. As would be expected from the mono-atomic nature and lipid solubility of mercury vapor, percent deposition and retention are quite high, of the order of 80 percent in man. Although confirmatory data are not available, monoalkyl mercurials (e.g., methyl mercury) probably also are deposited and retained to a high degree, since they have high vapor pressures and high lipid solubility.

Elemental mercury is very poorly absorbed from the gastrointestinal tract, probably less than 0.01 percent. This may be because, unlike in the lungs, mercury is not in a monoatomic state but, rather, occurs as large globular particles. Inorganic mercury in food is absorbed to the extent of about 7 percent, and organic mercury com-

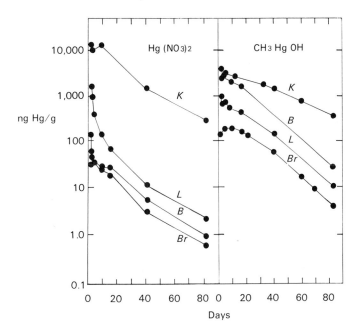

Figure 17–6. The fate of single doses of inorganic mercury and methyl mercury in rats. (Modified from Swensson, Å., and Ulfvarson, U.: Distribution and excretion of mercury compounds in rats over a long period following a single injection. *Acta Pharmacol. Toxicol.*, **26**:273–83, 1968.)

pounds are very efficiently absorbed, owing to their lipid solubility. For example, the absorption of methyl mercury, even mixed with food, is about 95 percent in adults.

As with all metals, the degree of skin absorption in man is not known with any precision. Systemic absorption of alkyl mercurials probably is substantial. People have been poisoned as a result of dermal application of methyl mercury ointments. Some absorption of elemental mercury and even of inorganic salts of mercury occurs. Thus, in experimental animals, 5 percent of an aqueous solution of mercuric chloride was absorbed through the skin of guinea pigs within five hours (Skog and Wahlberg, 1964).

Distribution and Metabolism

The distribution of mercury varies considerably, depending on the chemical form and, to a lesser extent, on the route of administration. Elemental mercury is rapidly oxidized to Hg^{2+} and organic mercury compounds are also to varying degrees metabolized to yield Hg^{2+}. As far as tissue affinity is concerned, the most outstanding single characteristic of mercury is its affinity for the kidney. This is true both for Hg^{2+} and for the organic mercury cation $R–Hg^+$.

The disposition of inhaled elemental mercury vapor is of special interest because of the importance of intoxication by this route. It has long been known that Hg^0 is rapidly oxidized in the erythrocytes to Hg^{2+}, even *in vitro*. Yet, while chronic mercury poisoning due to intake of Hg^{2+} is essentially a renal problem, chronic mercury poisoning due to inhalation of Hg^0 is a disease of

the central nervous system. This apparent paradox is explained by the fact that transfer of the lipid-soluble Hg^0 from the blood to the brain is sufficiently rapid to result in a toxicologically significant differential distribution to that organ (Magos, 1967). The subsequent oxidation of Hg^0 in the brain serves to trap it there. A similar selective distribution occurs in the fetus. The oxidative process is enzyme mediated, with the catalase complex being the most likely site of oxidation.

The disposition of organic mercury compounds is, in general, quite unlike that of Hg^{2+}. This is particularly true of the short-chain alkyl mercury compounds, notably methyl mercury. Figure 17-6 compares the fate of single equal subcutaneous doses of Hg as Hg^{2+} and as methyl Hg. Although both forms of mercury distribute preferentially to the kidney, the concentration in the brain and blood is substantially higher in the case of methyl mercury. Toxic manifestations of inorganic mercury are renal whereas those for methyl mercury poisoning are neurologic.

The disposition of phenyl mercury is essentially the same as for inorganic mercury. This is because the carbon-mercury bond is rapidly cleaved *in vivo*, yielding benzene and Hg^{2+}. The benzene is subsequently oxidized to phenol, conjugated, and excreted. Alkyl and alkoxyalkyl mercury compounds also are subject to some carbon-mercury bond cleavage, but the mechanism whereby this occurs is poorly understood (Gage, 1975). In general, cleavage occurs much more slowly than with phenyl mercury. Rate of clearance from the body varies a great deal. In some cases, as with alkoxyalkyl mercurials used as diuretics, clearance is much faster than for Hg^{2+}. In other cases, as with methyl mercury, clearance is considerably slower than for Hg^{2+}.

Mercury moves readily across the placenta into fetal tissue. Regardless of the chemical form administered, fetal tissues attain concentrations of mercury at least equal to those of the mother. In fact, in the case of exposure to Hg vapor and to methyl mercury, fetal concentrations exceed those of the mother to varying degrees, depending on the species, duration, and absolute level of maternal exposure. Fetal intoxication by way of the mother has been documented in cases of methyl mercury poisoning.

In the earlier section of this chapter dealing with lead, evidence was presented for the existence of a metal-sequestering mechanism, stimulated by the metal itself. Evidence for such a mechanism also exists for mercury. Metallothionein, a low-molecular-weight protein rich in sulfhydryl groups, was originally isolated from horse kidney. It has a high affinity for zinc, cadmium, and mercury. Administration of any one of these metals stimulates the synthesis of metallothionein. The renal concentration of metallothionein is increased as much as sixfold by administration of inorganic mercury. It may serve a protective role for the kidney by sequestering mercury, since the minimal concentration of mercury in kidney associated with toxic effects is considerably greater with chronic administration than with acute administration. The role of metallothionein in toxicology is discussed further in the section on cadmium.

As with lead, the concentration of mercury in the blood has been used as a biologic indicator of exposure. The distribution between blood cells and plasma is dependent on the chemical form. Thus, with methyl mercury exposure the concentration ratio, whole blood/plasma, is approximately 20, while with exposure to mercury vapor the ratio is only slightly above unity (Lundgren *et al.*, 1967). Measurement of mercury in blood has been extremely useful in assessing safe steady-state levels of methyl mercury exposure in man.

The kinetics of methyl mercury disposition are fairly straightforward and simple. Elimination rates as determined in human volunteers receiving single radioactive tracer doses indicate that the clearance of the dose from the body is adequately described by a single exponential elimination constant. The clearance half-time from these studies was found to be about 70 days. This rate of elimination seems to hold over a range of input rates. Thus, the rate of disappearance of mercury from the blood or hair of people who consumed moderate or large amounts of fish or bread contaminated with methyl mercury for long periods of time was quite consistent with the clearance half-time for the amount administered as a tracer dose to volunteers. For other forms of mercury the biologic half-life is not so well described. Limited data suggest, however, that the biologic half-life of inorganic mercury is only about 40 days in man, as contrasted to 70 days for methyl mercury.

Excretion

The relative contribution of urine and feces to the total elimination of mercury is, as with other features of mercury metabolism, quite variable depending on the particular form of mercury in the body. Upon prolonged inhalation of mercury, urinary excretion somewhat exceeds fecal excretion. The same probably applies to mercury administered as Hg^{2+}. The rate of urinary excretion for any one individual fluctuates considerably from day to day even under steady-state exposure conditions but has been found in industry to be roughly proportional to the level of air exposure. The mechanism of renal excretion of mercury is complex. The weight of evidence suggests that glomerular filtration contributes little to the renal excretion of any form of mercury. The mechanisms whereby the tubules release mercury into the lumen of the nephron are not well understood. At nephrotoxic doses of inorganic mercury, however, a substantial excretion occurs by exfoliation of renal cells.

In contrast to the excretion of inorganic mercury, methyl mercury is excreted mainly in the feces. Two separate processes are involved: biliary excretion of methyl mercury and excretion by exfoliation of intestinal epithelial cells move mercury into the intestinal lumen. Intestinal reabsorption of the mercury, however, substantially cancels the biliary contribution to net excretion. A polythiol resin has been developed that short-circuits this enterohepatic recirculation. When the resin is given orally it traps the mercury excreted into the bile and carries a substantial fraction of it out into the feces (Clarkson *et al.*, 1973). This procedure has been demonstrated to accelerate mercury excretion in human cases of poisoning (Bakir *et al.*, 1973).

Biologic Effects

As in the case of lead, mercury has toxic effects involving numerous organs and systems. Some have been clearly shown to occur in man under current and recent circumstances of exposure. Others either are of historic interest or are phenomena that have been demonstrated only in animal models. The relevance of these to the human condition is in many cases uncertain.

Regardless of all that, our present perceptions suggest that, irrespective of the chemical form of mercury, the major target organs are the central nervous system and the kidney. As will be seen, there is no sound basis for concluding that this is because the toxic actions of the various chemical forms can be attributed to a single common metabolite, e.g., Hg^{2+}.

Central Nervous System. The most consistent and pronounced effects of exposure to both elemental mercury vapor and to short-chain alkyl mercury compounds are on the central nervous system. There are similarities but there also are distinct differences. The effects of mercury vapor exposure are strikingly neuropsychiatric in nature whereas those resulting from methyl mercury exposure are largely of a sensorimotor nature. Certain effects are similar in both types of exposure, however, notably tremor. In mercury vapor exposure the tremor progresses in severity with duration of exposure. Initially it involves only the hands but later may spread to other parts of the body. Tremors are triggered by voluntary use of the affected muscles (intentional tremor). Neuropsychiatric signs also occur at relatively low levels of exposure, notably excessive shyness, insomnia, and emotional instability with depressive moods and irritability most frequently reported. This neuropsychiatric complex is known as "erethism."

Tremor also occurs in methyl mercury intoxication, but other effects not seen in mercury vapor exposure occur more consistently and at lower exposure levels. These are sensory in nature. The earliest signs are paresthesias and constriction of the visual field. At somewhat higher levels of exposure other sensory effects occur, such as loss of hearing, of vestibular function, and of the senses of smell and taste. These effects are not known to occur in elemental mercury intoxication. Numerous other neurologic effects occur in methyl mercury intoxication. These are motor effects such as incoordination, paralysis, and abnormal reflexes. It is not clearly known whether motor neurons are uniquely involved. Some of these motor effects, e.g., incoordination, could result from defects in sensory input.

Neuropsychiatric effects, which are so prominent in elemental mercury exposure, are also reported to occur in methyl mercury poisoning, but not so consistently. Further, the effects seem somewhat different from those observed in elemental mercury poisoning. Thus, shyness and irritability are not observed in methyl mercury poisoning but are very prominent in elemental mercury poisoning. On the other hand, spontaneous fits of laughing and crying and intellectual deterioration occur only in methyl mercury poisoning.

The pathogenetic mechanism of neurotoxicity has been investigated intensively in recent years, particularly concerning methyl mercury. The various approaches used reflect the diversity of toxic phenomena exhibited. Thus, the problem has been viewed from the neuroanatomic standpoint as well as from the biochemical, neurophysiologic, and pharmacologic standpoints. Chang (1977) has reviewed these studies and has proposed a tentative pathogenetic mechanism, which applies primarily to methyl mercury because relatively few of the studies have dealt with inorganic mercury or have directly compared effects of the inorganic and alkyl forms.

Both inorganic and alkyl mercury disrupt the integrity of the blood-brain barrier as manifested by extravasation of plasma protein into adjacent cerebral tissue. Since the blood-brain barrier acts to regulate the uptake of amino acids and other metabolites, it is possible that brain metabolism is affected at this point of interface with the circulation. The actions of mercury are probably not limited to the blood-brain barrier, however. Both forms of mercury are widely distributed elsewhere in the central nervous system, but there are quantitative differences. For example, while both forms of mercury localize to a high degree in dorsal root ganglion neurons and nerve fibers, inorganic mercury has a lesser degree of localization in neurons of the calcarine cortex than does methyl mercury. Degenerative changes are widespread in both forms of poisoning, although the nature of the changes differs in certain respects. In general, sensory neurons have been found to be more severely affected than motor neurons. Glial elements actually proliferate in areas of neuronal damage, perhaps to provide metabolic and structural support to the injured neurons. Damage is not limited to the cell bodies. Nerve fibers also are affected. Degeneration of both the axoplasm and the myelin sheath is common.

Biochemical explanations for the various degenerative changes abound. Enzymes along the glycolytic pathway and protein synthesis are inhibited. Inhibition of protein synthesis precedes both changes in anaerobic and aerobic glycolysis as well as neurologic effects. This "silent period" of several days between inhibition of protein synthesis and neurologic effects is seen even with single doses of mercury. It is not certain whether the inhibition is due to reduced amino acid uptake across the blood-brain barrier or whether the inhibition occurs by some other means.

Various neurophysiologic parameters also are altered by mercury. Spike potentials of sensory ganglionic neurons of animals receiving methyl mercury are prolonged, indicating retardation of repolarization. It has also been found that mercury blocks synaptic and neuromuscular transmission. The latter finding is of particular interest since a similar effect occurs in some cases of methyl mercury intoxication in man.

It is not possible at this time to say whether all the varied effects that have been noted experimentally occur as a result of independent actions of mercury or as stages in a chain of related events. Unitarian hypotheses are always attractive. There is none at present that adequately accounts for all the diverse neurologic phenomena that have been observed clinically and experimentally in mercury intoxication.

Kidney. By far the highest concentration of mercury occurs in the kidney, regardless of the chemical form absorbed. Yet, for all that, the kidney is the primary target organ only in the case of inorganic mercury (Hg^{2+}). At least this is so with respect to toxic effects. It is true that the kidney also is the primary target organ for nontoxic effects in the special case of the alkoxyalkyl mercury compounds used therapeutically as diuretics. It is also true that certain morphologic and functional effects are seen with sublethal doses of methyl mercury, but these are of uncertain significance in comparison to effects on the nervous system.

Massive oral doses of inorganic mercury, such as may be taken with suicidal intent, initiate a train of events beginning with anuria, progressing to polyuria, and finally to a recovery of normal renal function. The phase of anuria is the most life-threatening and may last for many days. The pathogenetic mechanism is not well understood. Experimental evidence from animal studies suggests that several factors are involved. These are tubular obstruction, increased back diffusion of tubular filtrate, and preglomerular vasoconstriction.

The phase of polyuria is characterized by decreased renal concentrating capacity. It probably results mainly from a substantial inhibition of proximal tubular sodium reabsorption. In severe poisoning, disturbances in tubular function may persist for several months after poisoning (Valek, 1965).

Acute inorganic mercury poisoning, as described above, is relatively rare. The more usual form of mercury nephrotoxicity occurs with chronic industrial exposure and is characterized by proteinuria. If severe, the nephrotic syndrome is observed, wherein the loss of plasma protein is sufficiently great to cause hypoproteinemia with edema of dependent parts, e.g., the ankles. Surprisingly, very little is known about the nature of the proteins that are excreted in cases of inorganic mercury poisoning. In one recent suicide attempt the proteinuria was mixed. Excretion of both albumin and low-molecular-weight proteins rose concurrently, suggesting both glomerular and tubular damage. Exposure to inorganic mercury at levels sufficient to cause proteinuria does not result in increased amino acid excretion. It appears, therefore, that the renal tubular transport system for reabsorption of α-amino acids is less sensitive than the transport system for absorption of low-molecular-weight proteins.

Information concerning the effects of methyl mercury on renal function in man is nonexistent, except for statements to the effect that even in the presence of neurologic effects the kidney is seldom affected. This is consistent with experimental studies in rats in which subchronic exposure to methyl mercury caused moderate proteinuria only at a level of mercury administration that actually killed a substantial number of the animals.

Other Effects. Although the nervous system and the kidney are the usual major targets for effects of mercury, a variety of other toxic phenomena occur. Some of these are well-known accompaniments of clinical poisoning. Others are effects seen in experimental animals that may prove in the future to have significance for man.

In the case of mercury vapor inhalation, the neuropsychiatric problem resulting from chronic exposure is accompanied by stomatitis, gingivitis, and sometimes excessive salivation and a metallic taste. These tend to occur mainly in people whose oral hygiene is poor. A peculiar discoloration of the anterior surface of the lens in the eye also is frequent ("mercurialentis"). When people are exposed to very high concentrations of mercury vapor, pneumonitis occurs as a result of direct irritation of the lung. In the case of poisoning with inorganic mercury salts by mouth, severe inflammation of the mouth, esophagus, stomach, and small intestine occurs. Following this initial contact inflammation, a secondary inflammatory effect may occur wherein absorbed mercury localizes in the intestinal mucosa. The colon is peculiarly sensitive to this secondary inflammatory action. There also is a disease of infants known as acrodynia or "pink disease" in which inorganic mercury seems to play a role. It is characterized by neuropsychiatric disturbances, peripheral vascular effects, disturbances of sensation of the extremities, stomatitis, and other vague, nonspecific signs. The disease is not uniquely associated with excessive mercury exposure, nor does it occur regularly among children exposed to mercury. See Bidstrup (1964) for a detailed discussion of the role of mercury in this disease.

Dose-Effect and Dose-Response Relationships

It may be recalled that, with lead, it is possible to estimate both dose-effect and dose-response relationships in man. The critical system, the hematopoietic system, is peculiarly amenable to quantitative estimates of effect. Thus, the activity of the enzyme ALAD in blood and the concentration of heme intermediates in blood and urine are readily quantifiable and exhibit clear relationships to the internal dose of lead, as reflected in the concentration of lead in the blood. The situation with mercury is not nearly so simple. To begin with, the critical effects both in the case of poisoning with elemental mercury and with alkyl mercury compounds are neurologic. Such phenomena as tremor, shyness, irritability in the case of elemental mercury and paresthesias and constriction of the visual field in the case of methyl mercury are not readily measured in quantitative terms. It is therefore not possible to construct dose-effect curves. So far as inorganic salts of mercury are concerned, the kidney is the critical organ. It is true that renal function is amenable to quantitative description, but even here there is a problem. The renal effect that seems to be the most sensitive index of mercury toxicity is elevated excretion of protein in the urine, an effect that has not been studied adequately to allow for definition of either dose-effect or dose-response relationships. For these reasons, it is

necessary to forego any thought of estimating dose-effect relationships for any form of mercury in man. As a matter of fact, even dose-response relationships can only be estimated for elemental mercury and methyl mercury exposures.

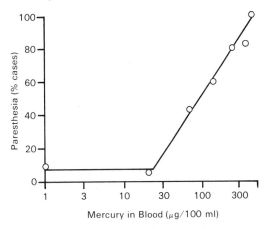

Figure 17–8. Dose-response relationship for methyl mercury, using concentration of mercury in the blood as dose and paresthesia as response. (WHO, 1976. From Bakir, F., *et al.*: Methylmercury poisoning in Iraz. An interuniversity report. *Science*, **181**:230–41, 1973. Copyright 1973 by the American Association for the Advancement of Science.)

In the case of elemental mercury vapor exposure the measurement of dose that seems to correlate best with response is the actual concentration of mercury breathed by the subjects, as contrasted to the concentration of mercury in the blood or urine of the exposed subjects. As the time-weighted average (TWA) air concentration rises above 100 μg Hg/M^3, the frequency of occurrence of classic signs of erethism among workers increases (Smith *et al.*, 1970). On this basis it has been recommended that the TWA limit for workers should be 50 μg Hg/M^3 in order to provide some margin of safety.

In the case of methyl mercury exposure, dose-response relationships have been calculated from the data obtained in the recent large-scale outbreak of poisoning in Iraq, described by Bakir *et al.* (1973). Again, as with elemental mercury exposure, the critical effects measured are those affecting the central nervous system. A hierarchy of response is seen with reference to sensitivity of the central nervous system. The effect occurring at the lowest level of exposure is paresthesia (Fig. 17-7). Both the estimated body burden of mercury (Fig. 17-7) and the concentration of mercury in the blood (Fig. 17-8) are adequate expressions of dose, at least under conditions of long-term intake (months).

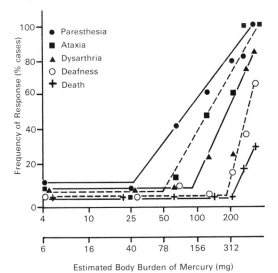

Figure 17–7. Dose-response relationships for methyl mercury. The upper scale of estimated body burden of mercury was based on the authors' actual estimate of intake. The lower scale is based on the body burden, which was calculated based on the concentration of mercury in the blood and its relationship to intake derived from radioisotopic studies of methyl mercury kinetics in human volunteers. (From Bakir, F., *et al.*: Methylmercury poisoning in Iraz. An interuniversity report. *Science*, **181**:230–41, 1973. Copyright 1973 by the American Association for the Advancement of Science.)

Treatment of Mercury Poisoning

As was pointed out in the discussion of the treatment of lead poisoning, data concerning the relative efficacy of various approaches to the treatment of metallic poisoning in general are grossly inadequate. The treatment of mercury poisoning is no exception. Studies of therapeutic regimens conducted on man generally are limited to clinical reports on one or, at most, a few individual cases with one or another selected drug. The reader, and the investigator himself for that matter, are always left to ponder questions concerning what would have happened had the patients not been treated at all, or concerning what would have happened if some alternate drug or regimen had been used. Even when a substantial number of cases is available to a single investigator, ethical considerations severely limit the options. Untreated controls cannot be included in the study if the condition is even moderately severe. Reliance on data from experimental animals is equally unsatisfactory for various reasons. The experimental design may not correspond to the usual human exposure situation or the animal model selected may not behave like man.

Chelating agents are relied upon, as in the case of lead poisoning, to remove mercury from the body. For many years the only chelating agent known to promote the excretion of mercury was dimercaptopropanol (BAL). It has been shown repeatedly that it enhances the excretion of mercury administered experimentally to animals in the inorganic form. It has also been shown to be beneficial in the treatment of inorganic mercury poisoning in man, enhancing the excretion of mercury and effecting substantial improvements in the patients' clinical status. Its efficacy has been attributed to the presence of thiol groups on adjacent carbon atoms, with the presumed participation of both in the binding of divalent mercury as a stable, readily excreted chelate ring.

$$\underset{\displaystyle \underset{\text{Hg}}{S\diagdown\diagup S}}{-C\text{---}C\text{---}C\text{---}OH}$$

Dimercaptopropanol, however, had two drawbacks. It was ineffective when given orally and it was ineffective as an antidote against alkyl mercury compounds. The next major advance was the discovery that the amino acid penicillamine was an effective chelator for mercury, even when administered orally. Its activity as a chelating agent is attributable to ring formation in which the thiol and primary amine groups probably serve as coordination sites.

More recently, the N-acetyl derivative N-acetyl-D,L-penicillamine (NAP) has been discovered to be even more effective and less toxic than D,L-penicillamine. The toxicity of D,L-penicillamine

$$\underset{\displaystyle \underset{\text{Hg}}{S\diagdown\diagup N\diagdown}}{\overset{\displaystyle \overset{\text{CH}_3}{|}}{CH_3\text{---}C\text{-----}C\text{---}COOH}}$$

is attributable to the L-isomer, which inhibits a number of pyridoxine-dependent reactions, probably by reacting with pyridoxal-5-phosphate to form a thiazolidine. By contrast, the L-isomer of NAP is relatively nontoxic. The LD50 of D,L-NAP is considerably greater than for D,L-penicillamine or even than for D-penicillamine.

The concept of ring formation, with the attendant stability of the metal complex, suggests that compounds of the type $R\text{-}Hg^+$, such as methyl mercury, would not form metal chelates with BAL or NAP. Surprisingly, NAP enhances the excretion of methyl mercury to a very substantial degree. It may be speculated that this effect is due only to interaction with Hg^{2+} formed by *in vivo* dealkylation of methyl mercury. This is unlikely, since NAP also removes methyl mercury bound to serum albumin *in vitro* (Aaseth, 1976). An alternate possibility is that NAP first causes a cleavage of the carbon-mercury bond and subsequently reacts with Hg^{2+}. It has been demonstrated that sulfhydryl reagents such as glutathione enhance the cleavage of the carbon-mercury bond of phenyl mercury *in vitro* in the presence of γ-globulin (Gage, 1975). It is not inconceivable, therefore, that NAP might facilitate a similar cleaving action on the carbon-mercury bond of methyl mercury.

In spite of some impressive animal data concerning the efficacy of the penicillamines as mercury chelators, their clinical efficacy in the treatment of methyl mercury poisoning is not impressive (Bakir *et al.*, 1976). To a large extent at least, this is because the neurologic effects of methyl mercury result from irreversible damage to neurons. Even from the more limited point of view of metal-mobilizing efficacy, the results have been equivocal. In some cases there has been essentially no suggestion of metal mobilization, at least insofar as decrease in blood mercury levels is concerned.

CADMIUM

Introduction

Cadmium ranks close to lead and mercury as a metal of current toxicologic concern. It is a relative newcomer, having been identified as a distinct element only in 1817. It occurs in nature in association with zinc and lead. Extraction involves separation and recovery of either zinc and cadmium or of all three metals in a single refinery plant. It quickly found application as an alloy, in electroplating of other metals, and as a pigment. Later it came to be used extensively in the manufacture of alkali storage batteries and plastics. Most early recorded cases of cadmium poisoning were due to inhalation of cadmium fumes or dusts. These cases were generally due to industrial exposure, although the first recorded cases, reported in 1858, were not industrial in nature. Three servants became severely ill from inhaling the dried film of cadmium carbonate that they had applied to silverware as a polishing agent and had subsequently brushed off. It was not until the second or third decade of the present century that the respiratory effects of acute and chronic inhalation of cadmium became recognized as a significant occupational disease entity. Later it was recognized that the kidney also is quite sensitive to cadmium. Friberg first reported in 1948 (Friberg, 1948) the coexistence of renal and lung damage in men working in an alkali storage battery plant.

An event occurred shortly after World War II that stimulated interest in cadmium because it involved relatively low-level exposure of the general population through contamination of food. In 1946, Dr. Hagino, a general practitioner, returned to Fuchu, Japan, from the army to reopen his medical practice. He was visited by numerous patients aged 40 to 70 who complained of severe rheumatic and myalgic pains. He gave this mysterious disease the name *Itai-itai* (pain-pain, or ouch-ouch). Gradually it came to be accepted that cadmium in the local rice played an etiologic role in this disease. The source of the cadmium was the effluent from a Pb-Zn-Cd mine upstream from the rice fields.

Interest in cadmium was further stimulated when Schroeder published a provocative epidemiologic study in 1965 linking dietary cadmium to hypertension in the general population (Schroeder, 1965b). Because of the large number of people potentially affected by hypertension, a great deal of effort has since been expended investigating the effects of cadmium on the cardiovascular system.

The usual sources of cadmium for the general population are mainly food and inhaled tobacco smoke. Among foods, the usual concentration is less than 0.1 μg/g wet weight. The only foods that accumulate excessively high concentrations of cadmium are shellfish, liver, and kidney. In these foods the concentration often exceeds 10 μg/g. Sources of cadmium in foods and other environmental media generated by man are not clearly defined. It is difficult to point to any one or even several sources and to say that it or they are of outstanding significance so far as exposure of any broad segment of the general population is concerned. This is in contrast to mercury, where environmental transport from contaminated waters to fish stands out as a major identifiable concern. Similarly, with lead we know that residues of lead-base paint in old homes and fallout from the air surrounding smelters are major hazards to the general population of children.

For those who have an interest in the broader aspects of cadmium as an environmental pollutant, there are two excellent recent reviews (Friberg *et al.*, 1974; Commission of the European Communities, 1978). Both of these are concerned primarily with man's exposure and with human health effects.

Metabolism

The specific chemical forms of lead and mercury have clearly been shown to exert considerable influence on their disposition in the body. Thus, the valence state of inorganic mercury profoundly influences the degree of absorption and even the pattern of distribution in the body. With both lead and mercury, alkyl compounds are toxicologically significant and exhibit unique toxicologic properties. In contrast, cadmium occurs only in one valence state, +2, and does not form stable alkyl compounds or other organometallic compounds of known toxicologic significance. The solubility of cadmium salts is highly variable. The halogen salts, sulfate, and nitrate are relatively soluble, while the oxide, hydroxide, and carbonate are insoluble in water. Cadmium has a relatively high vapor pressure. Thus, hazardous respirable air concentrations of CdO are readily attained in smelting and refining operations.

Absorption

As with any other aerosol, the pattern of deposition varies greatly with particle size; therefore, no generalizations can be made about fractional deposition. Similarly, no generalizations can be made concerning rate and route of clearance from the respiratory tract. A cadmium chloride aerosol would be cleared predominantly by direct absorption into the systemic circulation because of its high degree of water solubility. The insoluble cadmium oxide, dependent on particle size, would be cleared to a much greater extent by alveolar macrophages or via the mucociliary escalator system and subsequently swallowed.

Absorption of cadmium from the gastrointestinal tract is relatively minor, ranging from 0.5 to 12 percent in various species of animals. Studies of cadmium absorption in man are limited but are consistent with animal studies. Tracer doses of radioactive cadmium administered with food to human volunteers were absorbed to the extent of 4.7 to 7 percent (Rahola *et al.*, 1972). Numerous dietary factors enhance cadmium absorption, notably deficiencies in calcium, iron, and protein. Calcium is actively absorbed by the small intestine. This process requires a low-molecular-weight calcium-binding protein (CaBP), the synthesis of which is stimulated by dietary calcium deficiency. Recent evidence suggests that the increased CaBP activity induced by calcium deficiency may serve to enhance cadmium absorption as well as calcium absorption (Washko and Cousins, 1977). The enhancing effect of CaBP probably is counterbalanced by the influence of metallothionein, a low-molecular-weight protein whose synthesis is induced by cadmium, zinc, and mercury. It has a repressor role in limiting the intestinal absorption of zinc (Richards and Cousins, 1975) and probably exerts a similar effect in regard to cadmium.

As with lead, it has been shown that young animals absorb cadmium to a much greater degree than older animals.

Absorption of cadmium through the intact skin has been investigated only to a very limited extent. Up to 4 percent of the water-soluble chloride salt is absorbed in five hours through the skin of the guinea pig (Skog and Wahlberg, 1964).

Distribution

Cadmium has a strong preferential affinity for the liver and the kidney over a wide range of exposure levels. In general, about 50 percent of the total body burden is found in these two organs. The concentration ratio between the two varies with the total amount in the body. At low doses the concentration in the kidney is approximately ten times greater than in the liver. With increasing levels of exposure the concentration ratio approaches one. In heavy industrial exposure the concentration in the liver may actually exceed the concentration in the kidney. Cadmium is widely distributed elsewhere in the body at low concentrations relative to the liver and kidney. Within the kidney there is a substantial gradation in concentration, progressing downward from outer cortex to inner medulla. Thus, average cortical concentration is about 1.5 times medullary concentration.

Cadmium is highly cumulative. This is suggested by human autopsy data showing concentration rising to a peak in kidney at age 50 and in other organs somewhat earlier in life. This progressive accumulation of cadmium in the body over a major fraction of the lifespan

has also been demonstrated experimentally in animals. Beyond age 50 a decrease in the amount of cadmium in the kidney has been reported by several investigators. Steady-state concentrations of cadmium in blood occur relatively early in life under reasonably constant conditions of exposure. In workers newly exposed to a cadmium-contaminated environment, a new steady-state blood cadmium concentration was attained within one year (Kjellstrom, 1977).

The biologic half-life of cadmium in man has been difficult to determine with any degree of precision because of limited opportunity to do the appropriate experiments on volunteers. From indirect evidence, notably from rates of daily cadmium intake and amounts of cadmium in the body at age 50, the biologic half-life has been estimated to be anywhere from 19 to 38 years (Friberg *et al.*, 1974). In experimental animals such as rats, mice, and dogs, the biologic half-life determined by observing the rate of loss of single tracer doses of radioactive cadmium has been calculated to be of the order of several hundred days. From the standpoint of fraction of lifespan, these estimates in animals correspond roughly to the estimates in man, arrived at using more indirect approaches.

The great disparity in rate and degree of accumulation of cadmium in various organs and systems is not readily explained. Speculation abounds concerning the role of the cadmium-binding protein metallothionein as a determinant of the distribution and retention characteristics of cadmium. This protein, originally isolated from equine kidney by Margoshes and Vallee (1957), was found to contain high concentrations of zinc (2.2 percent) and cadmium (5.9 percent), hence the name metallothionein. It actually consists of two low-molecular-weight proteins (MW ca. 6,500), which differ somewhat as to amino acid composition. Major distinctive features are (1) the absence of aromatic amino acids; (2) high cysteine content; and (3) high affinity for certain metals, notably Cd, Zn, Hg, Ag, and Sn. The strong metal affinity is due to the high sulfhydryl content attributable to cysteine. It is widely distributed in the body of both man and animals, having been isolated from kidney, liver, spleen, intestine, heart, brain, lung, and skin.

Perhaps the most intriguing property of metallothionein is the fact that cadmium induces synthesis of the protein, as do zinc and mercury. Pretreatment of animals with either cadmium or zinc in moderate doses increases tolerance to otherwise lethal single doses of cadmium given later. This effect is accompanied by an increase in hepatic metallothionein (Leber and Miya, 1976). There is some question, however, as to the exact mechanism whereby this protective effect is exerted. Thus, it has been demonstrated that this protective effect is much more transient than the inductive effect and that the metallothionein content of organs other than the liver and perhaps the kidney does not necessarily increase in conjunction with this protective effect (Webb and Verschoyle, 1976). The role of metallothionein as a transport protein is uncertain. During chronic exposure to cadmium more than 90 percent of the circulating cadmium is in the blood cells, partially bound to metallothionein and partially bound to hemoglobin. Cadmium in plasma, however, is not normally bound to metallothionein; rather, it is bound to high-molecular-weight proteins.

Excretion

The major route of cadmium excretion in man is generally stated to be the urine. This conclusion is based on a study of five volunteers who received single oral doses of radioactive cadmium (Rahola et al., 1972). In animals, fecal excretion appears to be greater than urinary excretion. Miscellaneous routes of excretion, principally hair and exfoliated epithelium, have not been evaluated in any meaningful fashion

The urinary excretion of cadmium is of special interest because there is need for a biologic monitoring process whereby the degree of body contamination with cadmium can be assessed. It has already been pointed out that the concentration of cadmium in the blood fails in this regard. Blood cadmium equilibrates with any given level of exposure within a year, while the total amount in the body keeps accumulating over a period of decades. Much the same situation has been noted in regard to the urinary excretion of cadmium. In the general population, there is practically no increase in cadmium excretion with age in spite of strong evidence that the body burden, notably in the kidneys, increases markedly to age 50. By contrast, in heavily exposed population groups urinary excretion does increase with age. A reasonable explanation for this difference has been proposed (Lauwerys et al., 1976). At low levels of exposure, excretion is not proportional to intake because the binding capacity of the accumulative organs is not saturated and may actually increase progressively due to increasing metallothionein levels. At higher levels of exposure the binding capacity more nearly approaches saturation and metallothionein levels may be maximal. Under such circumstances excretion would be greater and more nearly proportional to intake. A substantial rise in the urinary excretion of cadmium is a danger signal. It is associated with renal damage. From animal studies, it has been suggested that the rise in cadmium excretion associated with renal damage is due to presentation of cadmium to the kidney as the metallothionein complex (Goyer et al., 1978). Indeed, cadmium metallothionein administered parenterally is both much more nephrotoxic and much more readily excreted in the urine than cadmium administered as an inorganic salt. It its passage through the kidney, the metallothionein is degraded, and the cadmium released thereby binds to high-molecular-weight renal proteins. Thus, there occurs a somewhat paradoxic situation wherein metallothionein reduces cadmium toxicity under some circumstances and enhances toxicity under other circumstances.

Biologic Effects

In keeping with the policy adhered to in the discussion of lead and mercury, the major focus of this section will be on effects known or suspected to occur in man. Animal data will be cited where they are deemed helpful in explaining or confirming observations in man. As was indicated in the introduction to the subject of cadmium, the major toxic phenomena in man are respiratory and renal toxicity, seen principally in industrial workers; the *itai-itai* disease complex reported from Japan, involving primarily elderly multiparous women; and finally, the highly controversial hypertensive effect suspected to involve a large number of people in the general population. These are all chronic effects. This is not to suggest that there is no such thing as acute cadmium poisoning. Nor is it to suggest that acute poisoning does not deserve a certain amount of attention.

Numerous cases of acute cadmium poisoning have been documented. Many of these have been cases of inhalation of very high concentrations of cadmium. Most other recorded cases have resulted from consumption of beverages and foods contaminated by cadmium transferred from the container. Acute lethal doses by inhalation in man can only be estimated rather crudely. Further, they vary considerably depending on the chemical form, particle size, and period of time over which inhalation occurred. For inhalations occurring within a span of eight hours, the lethal dose of cadmium oxide fumes has been estimated to be approximately 2,600 mg/M^3 for one minute, that is to say that inhalation of 2,600 mg/M^3 for one minute would be fatal, as would any other product of minutes and concentration equaling 2,600, e.g., 26 mg/M^3 for 100 minutes. For cadmium oxide dust the lethal product of time and concentration would be substantially larger and for a cadmium chloride aerosol the product would be substantially lower. Precise numbers are not available, however. The minimal toxic dose for an eight-hour inhalation is probably 1 to 3 mg/M^3 depending on aerosol particle size (Commission of the European Communities, 1978).

The principal toxic effects of cadmium inhalation are attributable to local irritation of the respiratory tract. Death is usually due to massive pulmonary edema. Signs and symptoms are delayed a few hours and consist mainly of irritation of the upper respiratory tract, chest pains, nausea, and dizziness. Gastrointestinal effects, e.g., nausea and diarrhea, may also occur. Long-term or permanent lung damage may occur, taking the form of emphysema and peribronchial and perivascular fibrosis.

Oral lethal doses in man, again, are difficult to estimate and vary considerably depending on the chemical form. Thus, in experimental animals the acute oral LD50 varies from approximately 100 mg/kg for soluble salts of cadmium to several thousand mg/kg for metallic cadmium powder or for the insoluble selenide and sulfide. Estimated lethal doses in man range from 350 to 8,900 mg. The minimal acute toxic dose is probably less than 10 mg. As with inhalation of cadmium, major toxic effects are referable to local irritant effects. In the case of oral intake the manifestations are nausea, vomiting, salivation, diarrhea, and abdominal cramps. Death may occur within 24 hours due to shock and dehydration or may be delayed one or two weeks following onset of various systemic effects, notably renal and cardiopulmonary failure. Extensive damage to the liver also may occur.

Turning to the health effects of long-term exposure, those observed in industrial workers are best understood and least controversial. The principal target organs are the lungs and the kidneys. What follows concerning respiratory effects is documented purely on the basis of cadmium inhalation in workers. By contrast, the renal effects noted in workers are essentially the same as those in cases of *itai-itai* and in other Japanese persons affected as a result of excessive dietary intake of cadmium.

The critical target organ in chronic cadmium exposure is generally held to be the kidneys. That is to say that adverse effects have been detected at lower levels of exposure compared to other organs and systems. The greater sensitivity, however, may be more apparent than real. The techniques used to characterize abnormalities in renal function are unusually sensitive and precise in comparison to those used to study toxic effects in some other organs, notably the lungs. Thus, the specification of the critical organ in the case of cadmium exposure may be somewhat illusory.

The overall consequence of excessive inhalation of cadmium fumes and dusts is loss of ventilatory capacity, with a corresponding increase in residual lung volume. Thus, the disease has the cardinal features of emphysema. Subjective complaints of shortness of breath upon exercise are common. Standard indices of ventilatory capacity are reduced, such as vital capacity and maximal ventilatory capacity. Mean volume of residual air, expressed as percentage of total lung volume, is increased. The most sensitive indices of reduced functional capacity were found recently to be (1) forced vital capacity; (2) forced expiratory volume at one second; and (3) peak expiratory flowrate (Lauwerys *et al.*, 1974). These effects are largely irreversible and are clearly more pronounced with long-term exposure than with short-term exposure. Studies of the anatomic progression of the disease are limited to relatively short-term animal studies, but the pathogenesis as seen in animals is consistent with the functional features of the disease as seen in man. In rats exposed to a cadmium aerosol for 15 days, the initial reaction of the lungs is of an inflammatory nature. This is followed by the appearance of emphysema and, later, of fibrosis (Snider *et al.*, 1973). In the general population, cigarette smoking contributes to the development of emphysema. Although a substantial amount of cadmium is inhaled with cigarette smoke, approximately 3 μg from 40 cigarettes, this amount is quite a bit lower than even the minimal amounts inhaled by workers experiencing emphysema from cadmium. The contribution of this source of cadmium to emphysema therefore is questionable.

The mechanism whereby cadmium causes emphysematous and fibrotic changes in the lungs is not well understood. There have been a number of studies in animals demonstrating that cadmium inhibits pulmonary defense mechanisms against respiratory infection, but the relevance of these studies to the pathogenesis of emphysema and lung fibrosis is not at all clear. Of greater interest is the observation that cadmium inhibits serum α_1-antitrypsin (Chowdhury and Louria, 1976). This effect is specific for cadmium as compared to several other metals studied. There is an association between severe α_1-antitrypsin deficiency of genetic origin and emphysema in man. Proteolytic agents, including papain and trypsin, have been demonstrated experimentally to cause emphysema. Inhibition of α_1-antitrypsin by cadmium may therefore play a role in the pathogenesis of cadmium-induced emphysema.

The current view is that the kidney is the most cadmium-sensitive organ. Toxic effects are noted in man at levels of exposure below those affecting other organs and systems. It must be remembered, however, that the kidney attains much higher concentrations of cadmium than other organs. Thus, it is not really a matter of sensitivity as much as it is a matter of predilection for accumulation.

Attention was first directed to the renal toxicity of cadmium in a report concerning industrial exposure (Friberg, 1948). It was noted that men exposed to cadmium oxide dust in an alkaline storage battery factory exhibited consistent proteinuria and a reduced ability to concentrate urine. It was also noted that the greater the duration of exposure, the greater the incidence of renal damage. We know today that the importance of duration of exposure is in large part due to the highly accumulative character of cadmium. Based on limited renal biopsy studies of affected and nonaffected workers, a threshold concentration for renal toxicity of 200 μg Cd/g kidney cortex has been proposed (Friberg *et al.*, 1974). This threshold has assumed considerable importance in the calculation of acceptable levels of daily cadmium intake (see under Dose-Effect and Dose-Response Relationships). Curiously, with the onset of renal damage the concentration of cadmium decreases somewhat. Perhaps this is due to breakdown in the metallothionein cadmium-sequestering capacity.

Since the initial report of renal damage in cadmium workers, there has been a series of reports that expand on the initial findings. Most recent studies have focused on the nature of cadmium-induced proteinuria. High-molecular-weight proteins are normally filtered but are not reabsorbed by the renal tubules. Thus, increased urinary excretion of these high-molecular-weight proteins, e.g., albumin, is considered to reflect glomerular damage. On the other hand, low-molecular-weight proteins are normally filtered and largely reabsorbed in the course of their passage through the renal tubules. Increased urinary excretion of low-molecular-weight proteins is therefore considered to indicate injury to the tubular reabsorptive mechanism. The effect of cadmium is mixed, in that both low- and high-molecular-weight protein excretion is enhanced (Bernard *et al.*, 1976). There is no question as to the existence of tubular damage in cadmium poisoning. Glycosuria, hypercalciuria, aminoaciduria, and increased uric acid excretion with hypouricemia have all been reported (Kazantzis *et al.*, 1963; Adams *et al.*, 1969). Limited studies indicate that these effects, notably proteinuria, do not disappear following removal from excessive exposure. This is not to be interpreted as indicating that the kidney is irreversibly damaged. Continued malfunction more likely is due to persistence of the cadmium burden in the kidney.

Of all the various effects of cadmium on renal function, the most sensitive appears to be proteinuria. It occurs in a substantial number of cadmium workers who do not have other manifestations of renal damage such as glycosuria and aminoaciduria (Kazantzis *et al.*, 1963).

Chronic cadmium poisoning as described above is of a special character in the sense that the route of intake has a considerable bearing on the nature of the effects. The lungs are prominently affected upon inhalation exposure because they are the first sensitive tissues encountered in the passage of the toxicant from the external environment to the internal environment. *Itai-itai*, the cadmium-induced disease recorded as having occurred in the general population of Japan, presents us with the characteristics of cadmium poisoning resulting from dietary intake. It too, however, is a disease with rather special characteristics. Among the people of the Jintsu River Valley who all consumed similar amounts of cadmium-contaminated rice, middle-aged to elderly multiparous women were mainly affected. The most prominent effects, osteomalacia with attendant spontaneous multiple bone fractures, have seldom been reported in cadmium poisoning of industrial origin. Despite this fact, the role of cadmium in the etiology of this disease is reasonably certain. For one thing, cadmium in the food supply grown in the area was extremely high. Further, the disease featured, in common with the industrial disease, both proteinuria and glycosuria. Finally, the disease has been reproduced experimentally in rats by combining dietary excess of cadmium with calcium deficiency (Itokawa *et al.*, 1974).

Perhaps the most controversial issue of all concerning human health effects of cadmium is the suggestion, first put forth in 1965, that cadmium has a significant role in the etiology of hypertension in the general population (Schroeder, 1965). The initial study was purely epidemiologic. Persons dying from hypertension were found to have significantly higher concentrations of cadmium and higher cadmium-to-zinc ratios in their kidneys than people dying of other causes. Subsequently, Schroeder and his colleagues claimed to have reproduced cadmium hypertension in rats and to have reversed the effect by administration of a polyamino-carboxylic acid chelating agent that removes cadmium from the body (Schroeder *et al.*,

1968b). The role of cadmium in the etiology of hypertension is still not satisfactorily resolved. It has been pointed out that hypertension is not prominent either in industrial cadmium poisoning or in *itai-itai*. On the other hand, several investigators have demonstrated that cadmium has a biphasic effect on blood vessels, wherein at low concentrations it is vasoconstrictive and at higher concentrations produces vasodilation (Perry and Erlanger, 1974; Nechay *et al.*, 1978). Regardless of the ultimate outcome of this particular controversy, it should be pointed out to the student of toxicology that dose-response curves are not necessarily unidirectional.

Numerous other effects of cadmium may be cited, but they are either relatively innocuous or have only been demonstrated to occur in experimental animals. As examples of the former, cadmium causes anosmia and yellow staining of the teeth in heavy industrial exposure. So far as observations of effects in animals is concerned, these are of definite value in that they suggest possible effects in man that require future study. Thus, cadmium causes cerebral and cerebellar damage to newborn animals, whereas adults are resistant to these effects. In addition, cadmium is toxic to the testes of rats and mice, probably as a result of toxicity to the vasculature. Cadmium also causes hyperglycemia and glucose intolerance in animals, possibly as a result of decreased secretory activity of pancreatic beta cells. These and numerous other effects in animals are described and relevant literature is cited in the review articles cited in the introduction to this section.

Dose-Effect and Dose-Response Relationships

As with mercury, it is at present not possible to specify dose-effect relationships in man, and even dose-response relationships are very difficult to develop. The critical organ is generally agreed to be the kidney and the critical effect is proteinuria. In order to develop a dose-effect relationship, it would be necessary to specify the degree of proteinuria, e.g., 10 mg/day, normalized for variable body mass or surface area. For that matter, there is not even any agreement as to the relative contributions of low-molecular-weight proteins (e.g., β_2-microglobulin) and high-molecular-weight proteins (e.g., albumin). The designation of proteinuria in the all-or-none sense for the development of dose-response relationships is beset with similar difficulties. One investigator's definition of proteinuria may be quite different from another investigator's definition. Dose is even more difficult to define than effect, at least so far as application for any practical human monitoring programs is concerned. The concentration of

cadmium in kidney cortex would be a logical index of dose, but it is not accessible for sampling except under very unusual circumstances. Furthermore, there is good evidence that the concentration increases with cumulative exposure only to the point at which renal damage occurs. With the onset of damage a reduction in kidney cadmium occurs coincident with a pronounced rise in urinary excretion of cadmium. Thus, even the concentration of cadmium in the kidney is difficult to interpret, at least following the onset of proteinuria. The concentration of cadmium in the blood is not a good index of internal dose to the kidney. It equilibrates rather rapidly with any given level of external exposure (less than one year), whereas the target organ of interest (the kidney) continues to accumulate cadmium for many years. In a group of workers exposed to fairly constant levels of cadmium for many years, a relationship was found between the incidence of proteinuria and the duration of exposure (Fig. 17-9). This is analogous to a dose-response curve, since the cumulative dose to the kidney was probably somewhat proportional to the number of years of exposure.

Numerous investigators have studied the relationship between urinary cadmium excretion and duration of cadmium exposure or age of the individuals. There does appear to be a correlation between urinary cadmium excretion and duration of cadmium exposure in workers, suggesting that urinary excretion corresponds roughly to the concentration of cadmium in the kidney.

Treatment of Cadmium Poisoning

There is surprisingly little information concerning the management of cadmium poisoning. In the case of *itai-itai*, large doses of vitamin D given over a period of months are effective in relieving painful symptoms and, in some instances at least, therapy reduces the incidence of spontaneous fractures. For a review of the Japanese literature see Friberg *et al.* (1974). There is no therapeutic approach being utilized in the management of industrial cadmium poisoning. Chelating agents have been studied in regard to their efficacy in the mobilization of cadmium. Dimercaptopropanol (BAL) has been shown to increase the uptake of cadmium by the kidney and to increase its nephrotoxicity. A similar effect has been noted regarding EDTA. It too increases both the concentration of cadmium in the kidney and the nephrotoxicity, in spite of an increased urinary excretion of cadmium (Friberg, 1956). In one instance where EDTA was used in the treatment of a man who had swallowed about 5 g CdI_2, the patient died

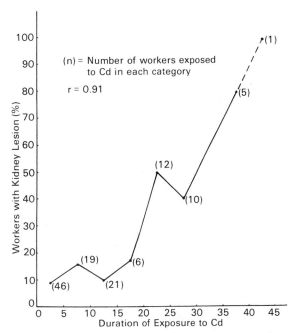

(n) = Number of workers exposed
to Cd in each category

r = 0.91

Figure 17–9. The relationship between duration of cadmium exposure and renal response. The criterion for presence of renal lesion was the presence of an abnormal electrophoretic pattern of urinary proteins. Numbers in parentheses indicate number of men. (From Lauwerys, R. R.; Buchet, J. P.; and Roels, H.: The relationship between cadmium exposure or body burden and the concentration of cadmium in blood and urine in man. *Int. Arch. Occup. Environ. Health*, **36**:275–85, 1976.)

in spite of drug-induced enhancement of cadmium excretion in the urine (Wiśniewska-Knypl *et al.*, 1971). The therapeutic regimen did not prevent extensive damage to the kidney and liver. Based on the experience in animal studies, it may be that the therapeutic regimen actually increased damage to these organs.

ALUMINUM

Occurrence and Use. The principal ore of aluminum is bauxite. Aluminum is widely used as a building material and for other uses where light weight and corrosion resistance are important. Aluminum oxide has industrial uses as an abrasive and catalyst. Medically, various soluble salts of aluminum have been used as astringents, styptics, and antiseptics. The insoluble salts are used as antacids and as antidiarrheal agents. Inhalation of aluminum hydroxide is used as a preventive and curative agent for silicosis.

Absorption, Excretion, Toxicity. The normal blood level of aluminum is 17 μg Al/100 ml and most soft tissues contain between 0.2 and 0.6 ppm (Underwood, 1971). The human body burden of aluminum is 50 to 150 mg and is apparently unaffected by either normal daily intake levels, estimated to be approximately 10 to 100 mg, or considerably higher doses (Browning, 1969). The degree of absorption of ingested aluminum and its compounds is minimal.

Many aluminum salts are converted to the phosphate salt in the gastrointestinal tract and excreted in the feces as such. Milk is a secondary route of excretion. Parenteral injection of aluminum salts results in excretion in both the feces and urine as well as slight increase in the concentration of aluminum in the liver and the spleen.

Massive oral doses of aluminum are reported to be toxic. Interference with phosphate absorption occurs resulting in rickets. Gastrointestinal irritation also occurs following large oral doses of aluminum. The use of aluminum cooking utensils and cans is not enough to contribute significantly to either total body burden or toxic effects (Underwood, 1971).

Shaver's disease is the only aluminum-induced industrial disease. It may result from bauxite fume and the use of abrasive wheels containing aluminum. Exposure to the fume may produce weakness, fatigue, and respiratory distress. Chest x-ray may reveal extensive fibrosis with large blebs. Spontaneous pneumothorax is a frequent complication. Silicon may also play a contributory role in the disease because it is frequently inhaled along with aluminum. Fibrosis has also been noted after aluminum dust inhalation. Similar changes can be reproduced by intratracheal injection in experimental animals (Browning, 1969). One source (AIHA, 1963) has recommended that the maximum atmospheric concentration (eight hours) be 50 million particles per cubic foot.

ANTIMONY

Occurrence and Use. The primary ore of antimony is stibnite (Sb_2S_3). The important uses of this metal are with lead alloys, in storage battery grids, in type alloys, pewter, bearing alloys, rubber, matches, ceramics, enamels, paints, lacquers, and textiles. Antimony may be present in food, resulting from the use of rubber, solders, and tinfoil for packaging. Leaching of antimony from cheap enameled vessels has caused some food contamination. Tarter emetic (antimony potassium tartrate) has been used as an insecticide. Antimony is a common pollutant in urban air.

Antimony or its compounds were used medicinally as early as 4000 B.C. Their popularity in medicine has undergone several cycles of use and disuse. At the present time their use is declining with the advent of newer parasiticides. The therapeutic activity involves reaction with the sulfhydryl groups in enzymes and a selective toxicity due to concentration in the parasite. Both trivalent and pentavalent organic compounds have been administered parenterally for parasiticidal effect; however, based on the hypothesis for the mechanism of effect, the trivalent forms would be expected to have greater efficacy. The probable *in vitro* conversion from the pentavalent to the trivalent forms may well account for the clinical effectiveness of the former. The trivalent compounds have been given orally as emetics and expectorants, but this use has been largely abandoned because of toxicity. The mechanism of emetic activity includes both a local and a central component (Sollmann, 1957).

Absorption, Excretion, Toxicity. Most of the information on the distribution and fate of antimony compounds arises from investigational results of therapeutic compounds. Antimony compounds are slowly absorbed from the gastrointestinal tract and tend to produce vomiting. The distribution of antimony following intravenous or intramuscular administration is somewhat variable and cannot be fully accounted for solely on the basis of valence. The trivalent forms generally concentrate in red blood cells, while the pentavalent compounds are found in the plasma. Trivalent forms accumulate in the liver and are slowly excreted, principally in the feces. In experimental animals significantly high concentrations are found in the thyroid after administration of trivalent compounds. The pentavalent forms tend to concentrate in the liver and spleen and are excreted in the urine. It is noteworthy that repeated dosages of labeled antimony tartar emetic were not accumulated in the body (Browning, 1969; Sollmann, 1957).

Acute poisoning has resulted from accidental or intentional ingestion of antimonials. The symptoms are similar to those of arsenic poisoning and consist of vomiting, watery diarrhea, collapse, irregular respiration, and lowered temperature. Vomiting increases the chance of recovery. In fatal cases death occurs within a few hours after ingestion. Chronic incorporation of potassium antimony tartrate (5 ppm) into drinking water increased the mortality rate and decreased serum glucose levels in rats. The incidence of tumors was not increased; but there was evidence of antimony accumulation in the soft tissue, contrary to what has been reported by other investigators (Schroeder *et al.*, 1970c).

Toxicity data have also been derived in connection with therapeutic use of antimonials. Cardiac effects, in a few cases atrial fibrillation due to a direct effect on the heart and death, liver toxicity, characterized by jaundice and fatty degeneration, pulmonary congestion and edema, and papular skin eruptions have been reported. Occupational poisoning by antimony is often difficult to establish since the antimony used in industry may contain some arsenic. The symptoms of toxicity of antimony and arsenic are similar. The signs ascribed to industrial antimony poisoning include upper respiratory tract irritation, pneumonitis, dizziness, diarrhea, vomiting, and dermatitis.

Antimony miners have developed disabling, but benign forms of silicosis. Some investigators have suggested a relationship between antimony and pulmonary carcinogenesis on the basis of possible antimony-containing abnormal enzyme systems. However, there is no positive evidence that diseased lung tissue contains excess amounts of antimony.

Antimony and antimony compounds may generate stibine (antimony hydride) under reducing conditions. This has occurred during storage battery charging. Although arsine is usually suspected of industrially induced hemolytic anemia, stibine may be involved more frequently than is suspected. The lethal concentration of stibine in the air for mice is about 100 ppm for 1.6 hours, while that of arsine is three hours. Stibine, like arsine, may be expected to cause rapid destruction of red blood cells, hemoglobinuria, and anuria. Subjective signs include headache, vomiting, nausea, and lumbar and epigastric pain (Browning, 1969).

ARSENIC

Occurrence and Use. Arsenic trioxide (As_2O_3) is used as the starting point in the manufacture of most arsenic compounds and is obtained from roasting arsenic-containing ores ($FeAsS$, As_2S_3, and As_2S_2). The major use of arsenic has been in the form of its compounds whose toxicity makes them valuable as insecticides, weed killers, and wood preservatives. Lead-arsenic alloys are also used because they are more rigid than pure lead. Antifouling paints and materials to control sludge formation in lubricating oils also contain arsenic.

Arsenic is ubiquitous in distribution, mostly pentavalent, in soil. Arsenic is a natural constituent of food, although additional amounts may be added by contamination. Sea-foods, pork, liver, and salt may be exceptionally high in arsenic. In general, the naturally occurring arsenic is pentavalent while that added to the environment is trivalent.

Medicinal uses of arsenic have ranged from treatment of leukemia to use as a tonic. Arsenicals act locally and are slow corrosives; they have been used in the treatment of skin cancer. Both trivalent and pentavalent organic arsenic compounds have been used in the treatment of various parasitic diseases (Sollmann, 1957). In the United States there has been a decline in the use of arsenicals in human medicine but the decrease has not been as great in veterinarian or agricultural use.

A certain amount of arsenic is added to the atmosphere by domestic coal use as well as by industrial contaminants. Arsenic is prevalent in small amounts in the water supply (Table 17-2). Some of this arsenic may come from phosphate fertilizers that contain arsenic (Schroeder and Balassa, 1966a).

Absorption, Excretion, Toxicity. Compounds of arsenic may be absorbed after ingestion or by inhalation. It is generally true that trivalent arsenic compounds are more toxic than pentavalent compounds and that natural oxidation favors the conversion of trivalent arsenic to the pentavalent form. It has been shown in some instances, however, that the arsenate is reabsorbed by the proximal renal tubule and excreted as the arsenite (Ginsburg, 1965).

Arsenate is the valence form most prevalent in nature and in this form tends to be rapidly excreted by the kidneys and probably does not accumulate. Arsenate can substitute for phosphate in some enzyme systems without adverse effects.

Arsenites bind to tissue proteins and are concentrated in the leukocytes. They accumulate in the body primarily in the liver, muscles, hair, nails, and skin, perhaps because of combination with sulfhydryl groups. Excretion is via the bile. Arsenite is not found in milk.

The trivalent forms of arsenic are more toxic than the pentavalent forms. To illustrate these differences, single intraperitoneal injections of arsenic salts were administered to mice on days 6, 7, 8, 9, 10, 11, and 12 of gestation. Fetal deaths, resorption, exencephaly, and short jaws were observed among the fetuses. Those dams treated on day 8 of gestation were affected the most. At a dose of 25 mg/kg sodium arsenate was without effect, but at a level of 10 mg/kg sodium arsenite produced embryotoxicity and teratogenic effects (Hood and Bishop, 1972). Chromosomal breaks in human leukocytes have been produced by arsenic *in vitro* (Oppenheim and Fishbein, 1965).

In rats fed sodium arsenate or arsenite at equal arsenic levels, those receiving the arsenate had less severe changes in bile duct enlargement. Similar results in the rats were obtained when growth and survival were used as criteria. In rats, 62.5 ppm of arsenic as arsenite was without effect, while the no-effect level for arsenic as arsenate was 125 ppm. No dogs fed arsenic (125 ppm) as arsenite survived a two-year study. At the same level of arsenic as the arsenate only one of the six dogs died. In neither species was it evident that oral administration of arsenic might be carcinogenic (Byron *et al.*, 1967).

In man the symptom of acute inorganic arsenic poisoning occurring as a consequence of accidental or homicidal ingestion consist of burning and dryness of the oral and nasal cavities, gastrointestinal disturbance, and muscle spasms; vertigo, delirium, and coma may occur. Edema of the face and about the eyelids may also be evident.

Chronic arsenic intoxication is characterized by malaise and fatigue. Gastrointestinal disturbances, hyperpigmentation, and peripheral neuropathy may ultimately occur. Pale bands on the fingernails and toes may develop. Clinical pathology may reveal anemia (slightly hypochromic) and basophilic stippling. Red cell disruption, decreased red cell production, and leukopenia are frequently observed. These signs disappear rapidly when exposure is halted, except for neuropathy, which may regress at a slower rate. Increased arsenic content of hair, nails, and urine is frequently present for long periods after exposure has been discontinued (Kyle, 1970).

Industrial poisoning generally follows the same pattern, although skin changes may occur more frequently than the hematologic changes. Nasal septum ulceration is seen after long industrial exposure (Patty, 1963). While there has been some controversy, the epidemiologic evidence indicates that industrial and agricultural exposure to arsenic is implicated in cancer of the skin and respiratory tract. The individuals at greatest risk are smelter workers, although there is some suggestion that women residing near such operations incur a greater incidence of respiratory cancer (Newman *et al.*, 1976). In experiments, the oral ingestion by animals has not suggested a carcinogenic potential by this route. Epidemiologic studies have implicated ingestion of arsenic as goitrogenic, and this possible effect has been confirmed in animals (Wills, 1966). Epidemiologic studies have suggested that arsenic in drinking water may be related to increased incidence of skin cancer (U.S. Public Health Service, 1962). Extraordinarily high arsenic levels in soil and water have tentatively been linked with a severe form of peripheral arteriosclerosis (blackfoot disease) observed in Taiwan. However, members of the same family, some with blackfoot disease and some without, have similarly high serum arsenic levels (Heydorn, 1970).

Arsine, the hydride of arsenic, is one of the more toxic arsenic compounds. Arsine may be generated when acids are combined with arsenic-containing metals. Poisoning by arsine is the principal source of industrial arsenic poisoning today and has been reported in connection with the refining or processing of tin, lead, and zinc. Poisonings from this source have dire consequences because of the severe hemolytic effect and the inadequacy of available therapy (Foreman, 1962). Arsine, a gas with a slight garlic-like smell detected only above safe levels, produces massive hemolysis and renal failure. Nausea, emesis, diarrhea, disturbance of the vascular bed, pulmonary edema, cyanosis, electrocardiogram abnormalities, hemoglobinuria, and liver dysfunction may occur. There is generally some delay in the onset of symptoms. Exposures as low as 10 ppm have produced delirium, coma, and death. If the exposure is not fatal, the signs of chronic arsenic poisoning may appear. Urine may continue to contain arsenic for some time after poisoning (Parry, 1963; AIHA, 1965).

BARIUM

Occurrence and Use. Barite ($BaSO_4$) and witherite ($BaCO_3$) are the more common mineral forms of barium. Barium is used in various alloys, in paints, soap, paper, and rubber, and in the manufacture of ceramics and glass. Barium fluorosilicate and carbonate have been used as insecticides. Barium sulfate, an insoluble compound, is used as a radiopaque aid to x-ray diagnosis. Barium is relatively abundant in nature and is found in plants and animal tissue. Plants accumulate barium from the soil. Brazil nuts have very high concentrations (3,000 to 4,000 ppm). Some water contains barium from natural deposits.

Absorption, Excretion, Toxicity. The soluble compounds of barium are absorbed and small amounts are retained in the body. Reports indicate the lung has an average concentration of 1 ppm (dry weight). The kidney, spleen, muscle, heart, brain, and liver concentrations are 0.10, 0.08, 0.05, 0.04, 0.03, and 0.03, respectively. Some barium is also found in the skeleton.

Studies suggest that barium may be an essential element inasmuch as rats and guinea pigs maintained on barium-free diets fail to grow normally (Underwood, 1971). The soluble compounds once absorbed are transported by the plasma. The biologic half-life is short (less than 24 hours). Feces appear to be the major excretion route of absorbed barium although some is lost through the kidney. The renal tubules reabsorb barium in the filtrate.

The insoluble forms of barium, particularly barium sulfate, are not toxic by the oral route because of minimal absorption. However, the soluble barium compounds are highly toxic, in contrast to calcium and strontium, the other members of this group in the periodic table.

Accidental poisoning from ingestion of soluble barium salts has resulted in gastroenteritis, muscular paralysis, decreased pulse rate, and ventricular fibrillation and extrasystoles. Potassium deficiency occurs in acute poisoning and the heroic measure, treatment with intravenous potassium, appears beneficial. The digitalis-like toxicity, muscle stimulation, and central nervous system effects have been confirmed by experimental investigation. Baritosis, a benign pneumoconiosis, is an occupational disease arising from the inhalation of barium sulfate (barite) dust and barium carbonate. It is not incapacitating, but does produce radiologic changes in the lungs. The radiologic changes are reversible with cessation of exposure (AIHA, 1962; Browning, 1969).

BERYLLIUM

Occurrence and Use. Beryl ($3BeO \cdot Al_2O_3 \cdot 6SiO_2$) is the chief ore of beryllium. Its industrial uses include the hardening of copper, the manufacture of nonsparking alloys for tools, and the manufacture of lightweight alloys and nuclear reactors. It is also used in the manufacture of ceramics and in the electronics industry (transistors, heat sinks, and x-ray and cathode tubes). Gas lantern mantles, when first ignited, volatilize most of the beryllium they contain. Formerly, beryllium was widely used in the manufacture of fluorescent lights and neon signs. The aerospace industry uses beryllium compounds as propellants, providing a possible source of environmental exposure; however, coal combustion is probably the largest source of environmental beryllium contamination.

Absorption, Excretion, Toxicity. Beryllium is not well absorbed when given by any route. Experimental animals may only absorb 1 percent as a maximum. After inhalation exposure beryllium is retained in the lungs and mobilized slowly. In the bloodstream a colloidal beryllium phosphate is formed. In addition, small amounts may be found in a soluble beryllium-citrate complex that is deposited in the bone or excreted via the urine. The colloidal portion is deposited in the liver, spleen, and bone marrow (Scott and Hodge, 1971).

The skin lesions are the most common sign of the industrial disease. Three distinct types of skin lesions have been described: dermatitis, ulceration, and granulomas. The dermatitis, sometimes accompanied by acute conjunctivitis and corneal ulceration, has been regarded as a hypersensitizing reaction. The finding that victims of chronic beryllium lung disease react positively to patch tests supports this notion and indicates the possible immunologic component of the chronic disease. The ulcer is such that healing will take place only if the offending material is curetted. The granuloma is most frequently the result of broken fluorescent lamps embedding beryllium under the skin. The use of beryllium in this type of lamp has ceased (Stokinger, 1966).

Chronic skin lesions sometimes appear after a long latent period in conjunction with the chronic pulmonary aspect of the disease. Subcutaneous granulomas have been produced in the pig using the beryllium phosphor. Short-term inhalation exposures to levels of soluble beryllium compounds in excess of 100 μg/M^3 result in acute lung distress. A latent period of one day to three weeks may exist. The inflammatory response consists of nasopharyngitis, tracheobronchitis, and, in more severe cases, fulminating pneumonitis. When fulminating pneumonitis is present, chest radiographs show haziness to "snow-flurry" effect. Edema may become so severe that right-side heart failure occurs. The clinical course is four to six weeks in duration although x-ray changes may take longer. The acute pneumonitis is readily reproduced in experimental animals.

Of 124 cases of chronic berylliosis, 11 percent had a history of acute attacks. The symptoms of the chronic form of the disease are dyspnea, chronic cough, weight loss, weakness, fatigue, and chest pain or discomfort. Latent periods of over 20 years have been observed, but a latent period of 10 to 19 years from the first exposure to five to nine years from the termination of exposure is the most common. In those cases in which histologic information from autopsy or biopsy is available, exposure was most frequently in connection with extraction and smelting operations or the manufacture of fluorescent lamps. The development of disease in persons exposed to minimal amounts of beryllium such as those handling a beryllium worker's clothes or living near a plant has been documented. The physical findings show a fine miliary nodulation (ground-

glass appearance). As the fibrosis increases, bleb formation is common and pneumothorax occurs. The striated muscles, liver, spleen, kidneys, and heart may be involved. Lung function and transfer of oxygen may be impaired. Other systemic aspects may include disturbances in nitrogen and calcium metabolism. Differential diagnosis of sarcoidosis and chronic beryllium disease is difficult. The use of the beryllium patch test is helpful but may in fact sensitize the subject. *In vitro* tests utilizing immunologic indicators have been used (Reeves, 1977). A history of beryllium exposure should be sought. While, histologically, granulomatosis pneumonitis is most characteristic of the histologic lung tissue from patients with chronic beryllium disease, 55 of 124 chronic cases had either indistinct or no granuloma formation. However, in many of these cases, the tissue may have been obtained by biopsy rather than at autopsy. The degree of histologic abnormality did not correlate with the lung tissue beryllium content or the length of the latent period (Freiman and Hardy, 1970). There is some indication that early detection of the respiratory changes and reduction of the exposure levels can lead to reversal of the early radiographic abnormalities and to improvement of pulmonary gas exchange (Sprince *et al.*, 1978). A high incidence of hyperuricemia seems to occur in cases of chronic beryllium disease, but the nature of this effect has not been ascertained (Tepper, 1972).

The human disease, chronic pulmonary granulomatosis in the diffuse form, has not been reproduced in experimental animals (Scott and Hodge, 1971). Scattered granulomatous lesions have been produced in rats. Rhesus monkeys react similarly to man when challenged by injection of beryllium oxide powder in the wall of the bronchus or inhalation of beryllium sulfate by development of widespread chronic beryllium pneumonitis with granulomata.

Osteogenic sarcoma has been produced in rabbits and bronchogenic carcinoma has been produced in rats and monkeys. Bony lesions, osteosclerosis in rats and rabbits, rickets in growing rats, and anemia are produced in experimental investigations but seem to be without counterparts in the human disease state (Spiegl *et al.*, 1953; Scott and Hodge, 1971).

BISMUTH

Occurrence and Use. Bismuth is obtained as a by-product of tin, lead, and copper ores. It is used in the manufacture of type alloys, silvering of mirrors, low-melting solders (sometimes used in canning), and heat-sensitive devices such as automatic fire extinguishers. Bismuth telluride is used in the electronics industry as a semiconductor. Bismuth is one of the contaminants measured in urban air (Table 17-3).

Trivalent insoluble bismuth salts are used medicinally to control diarrhea and other types of gastrointestinal distress. Some of these preparations are available without prescription. Various bismuth salts have been used externally for their astringent and slight antiseptic property. Bismuth salts have also been used as radiocontrast agents. Further self-exposure comes from the use of insoluble bismuth salts in cosmetics. Injections of soluble and insoluble salts, suspended in oil to maintain adequate blood levels, have been used to treat syphilis. Bismuth sodium thioglycollate, a water-soluble salt, was injected intramuscularly for malaria (*Plasmodium vivax*). Bismuth glycolyarsanilate is one of the few pentavalent salts that have been used medicinally. This material was formerly used for treatment of amebiasis. Exposure to various bismuth salts for medicinal use has decreased with the advent of newer therapeutic agents.

Absorption, Excretion, Toxicity. Most bismuth compounds to which we are exposed are insoluble and poorly absorbed—either when taken orally or when applied to the skin, even if the skin is abraded or burned. Thus, most of the information on their distribution in the body is related to therapeutic use.

Once the bismuth is absorbed from the site, tissue binding appears minimal. A diffusible equilibrium between tissues, blood, and urine is established. Tissue distribution, omitting injection depots, reveals the kidney as the site of the highest concentration. The liver concentration is considerably lower at therapeutic levels but with massive doses in experimental animals (dogs), the kidney/liver ratio is decreased. Passage of bismuth into the amniotic fluid and into the fetus has been demonstrated. The urine is the major route of excretion. Traces of bismuth can be found in the milk and saliva. The total elimination of bismuth after injection is slow and dependent on mobilization from the injection site.

There have been no reports of industrial poisoning from bismuth (Browning, 1969). Except for strong acidic salts such as bismuth trinitrate or violently reactive compounds such as bismuth tripentafluoride, the bismuth compounds do not present a hazard by dermal application, inhalation, or ingestion. The dermal application of most bismuth compounds does not result in systemic toxicity. Oral administration of bismuth subnitrate produces poisoning through the formation of nitrites. Intravenous injections of bismuth salts were avoided because of toxicity; the soluble salts had a tendency to flocculate. Intramuscular injections tended to be painful, and if sufficient doses were employed, some necrosis was evident at the site of injection. In experimental animals renal and hepatic toxicity have been observed following the achievement of sufficient systemic bismuth levels.

The symptoms of chronic toxicity in man consist of decreased appetite, weakness, rheumatic pain, diarrhea, fever, metal line on the gums, foul breath, gingivitis, and dermatitis. Jaundice and conjunctival hemorrhage are rare, but have been reported. When nephritis does occur in man, albuminuria is used as a signal to discontinue administration (Sollmann, 1957). The renal effects include diuresis and are similar to the effects of mercury. Microscopically, lipid-carbohydrate-protein inclusions containing no bismuth are formed in the renal proximal convoluted tubular cell shortly after treatment with bismuth. They are apparently irreversible (Burr et al., 1965).

BORON

Occurrence and Use. While boron is, strictly speaking, a nonmetal, it is in the group IIIA metals and is of some toxicologic concern (Table 17-4). Boron occurs regularly in natural water supplies (Table 17-2) and in plant and animal tissues. It is essential to plants but apparently not to animals. The average daily intake has been estimated at 10 to 20 mg. Borax ($Na_2B_4O_7$) is the most important mineral. Boric acid is useful medicinally as a mild antiseptic, especially as an eyewash. Borax is used in soldering and welding to remove oxide film, for softening water, in soaps, and in glass, pottery, and enamels.

Absorption, Excretion, Toxicity. Boron in the food, as sodium borate or boric acid, mostly in fruit and vegetables, is almost completely absorbed and is excreted in the urine. Treatment of large burned areas with boric acid results in systemic absorption. Large amounts of absorbed boron cause accumulation in the brain (Underwood, 1971).

In lambs, gastrointestinal and pulmonary disorders have been reported to result from grazing where pasture soils are high in boron content. Industrial poisoning has not been reported from exposure to boron salts except for the boranes. Death has been reported due to dermal application of boric acid for burns and cuts. Central nervous system depression and gastrointestinal irritation are the most severe symptoms. Infants appear to be more susceptible to the toxic effects than adults. Skin irritation has occurred in infants following dermal application.

The boranes diborane, decaborane, and pentaborane are used in high-energy fuels. Decaborane has also been used in vulcanizing rubber. All three are highly toxic. Pentaborane is the most hazardous. Diborane is an irritant to the lungs and kidneys. Decaborane and pentaborane are central nervous system poisons; however, the liver and kidneys may also be damaged if the exposure is severe (Browning, 1969).

CESIUM

Occurrence and Use.   Cesium occurs in nature as pollucite, a hydrous cesium-aluminum silicate. Its main industrial uses are as a catalyst in the polymerization of resin-forming materials and in photoelectric cells. It is useful in this respect because the range of sensitivity is approximately that of the human eye. Radioactive cesium is a constituent of nuclear fallout.

Absorption, Excretion, Toxicity.   Cesium is absorbed after oral administration and is bound within the cells of the soft tissues such as kidney and muscle. It is found in the red blood cells and may in some circumstances be able to replace potassium. The urine is the main route of excretion. Increased potassium levels facilitate cesium excretion. The radioactive material is found in milk.

No cases of industrial injury related to the chemical toxicity of cesium have been reported. It is likely that replacement of potassium by cesium would produce ill effects in man, probably neuromuscular in nature, as has been demonstrated in experimental animals (Browning, 1969).

CHROMIUM

Occurrence and Use.   Chromite ($FeCr_2O_4$) is the most important chrome ore. Chromium plating is one of the major uses of this metal. Steel fabrication, paint and pigment manufacturing, and leather tanning constitute other major uses of chromium. The medicinal uses of chromium are limited to external application of chromium trioxide as a caustic and intravenous sodium radiochromate to evaluate the life-span of red cells.

Absorption, Excretion, Toxicity.   Chromium exists in several valence states. Only the trivalent and hexavalent are biologically significant. While conversion from trivalent to hexavalent and other states is important chemically, the inner conversion from chromic to chromate does not apparently occur biologically. The conversion of hexavalent to trivalent does take place in the body.

Trivalent chromium is an essential element in animals. It plays a role in glucose and lipid metabolism. Chromium deficiency mimics diabetes mellitus and produces aortic plaques in rats. Chromium supplementation improves or normalizes glucose tolerance in diabetics, older people, and malnourished children. It has been suggested that chromium deficiency may be a basic factor in atherosclerosis (Mertz, 1969; Schroeder et al., 1970c). A deficiency of trivalent chromium apparently increases the toxicity of lead (Schroeder et al., 1965).

The major environmental exposure to chromium occurs as a consequence of its presence in food. Brown sugar and animal fats, especially butter, are chromium-rich foods. Chromium is found in urban air (Table 17-3). The concentration in natural water supplies is below 10 ppb; however, in municipal drinking water concentrations of 35 ppb have been reported (Table 17-2). The daily intake has been estimated at 60 μg (30 to 100 μg), 10 μg of which is due to water concentrations (Table 17-1). However, the absorption is limited to approximately 1 percent (Schroeder et al., 1962b). The occurrence of chromium in food or water has not been shown to produce any significant adverse effects in either man or experimental animals (U.S. Public Health Service, 1962; Kanisawa and Schroeder, 1969; Schroeder and Mitchener, 1971).

The total chromium body burden of man has been estimated at less than 6 mg (Table 17-1). Chromium is transported across the placenta and concentrated in the fetus. The tissue concentrations tend to decline rapidly with age except for the lung concentration, which tends to increase. The decline of chromium levels with age does not occur in rats. Wide geographic variations in tissue concentration, presumably due to differences in dietary intake and atmospheric concentration, have been reported (Schroeder et al., 1970d).

Water-soluble chromates disappear from the lungs into the circulatory system after intratracheal application, while the trivalent chromic chloride remains largely in the lungs. Oral administration of trivalent chromium results in little chromium absorption. The degree of absorption is slightly higher following administration of hexavalent compounds. Once absorbed, Cr^{3+} is bound to the plasma proteins. Under normal conditions the body contains stores of chromium in the skin, lungs, muscle, and fat. The bone contains chromium, but this is not due to selective deposition. The caudate nucleus has been reported to have high concentrations. Hexavalent chromium is reduced to the trivalent form in the skin. In the blood little hexavalent chromium can be detected. The reticuloendothelial system, liver, spleen, testes, and bone marrow have an affinity for chromite, possibly as the result of phagocytosis of colloidal particles formed at higher tissue concentrations. On the other hand, chromates are bound largely to the red blood cells. Subcellular distribution studies have indicated that the nuclear fraction contains almost one-half the intracellular chromium. Urinary excretion accounts for about 80 percent of injected chromium. However, elimination via the intestine may also play a role in chromium excretion. Milk is another secondary route of excretion (Mertz, 1969). Average urinary and blood concentrations are 0.4 and 2.8 μg/100 g, respectively (Imbus et al., 1963).

Occupational exposure to chromium compounds (Cr^{6+}) causes dermatitis, penetrating ulcers on the hands and forearms, perforation of the nasal septum, and inflammation of the larynx and liver. The dermatitis is probably due to an allergenic response, although persons sensitive to Cr^{6+} also respond to large amounts of Cr^{3+} (Fregert and Rossman, 1964). The ulcers are believed to be due to chromate ion and not related to sensitization. Chromic acid, and, to a lesser extent, chromate, are presumably the causative agents in perforation of the nasal septum (Browning, 1969). Epidemiologic studies indicate that chromate is a carcinogen with bronchogenic carcinoma as the principal lesion. The latent period appears to be 10 to 15 years. The relative risk of chromate plant workers for respiratory cancer is 20 times greater than that of the general population. Experimental studies have suggested that calcium chromate may be the specific carcinogenic agent (Enterline, 1974). However, some investigators have produced cancer in experimental animals with injections of either the trivalent or hexavalent form (Hueper and Payne, 1962). Incorporation of hexavalent chromium (5 ppm) into the drinking water of mice over their lifetimes produced a slightly higher incidence of malignant tumors than in the controls. Trivalent chromium (chromium acetate) given to rats under similar conditions produced no such effect (Schroeder and Mitchner, 1971; Kanisawa and Schroeder, 1969).

COBALT

Occurrence and Use. Cobalt is a relatively rare metal produced primarily as a by-product of other metals, chiefly copper. It is used in high-temperature alloys and in permanent magnets. Its salts are useful in paint driers, as catalysts, and in the production of numerous pigments. It is an essential element in that 1 μg of vitamin B_{12} contains 0.0434 μg of cobalt. Vitamin B_{12} is essential in the prevention of pernicious anemia. If other requirements exist, they are not well understood. Deficiency diseases of cattle and sheep caused by insufficient natural levels of cobalt are characterized by anemia and loss of weight or retarded growth.

Absorption, Excretion, Toxicity. Cobalt salts are generally well absorbed after oral ingestion, probably in the jejunum. Despite this fact, increased levels tend not to cause significant accumulation. About 80 percent of the ingested cobalt is excreted in the urine. Of the remaining, about 15 percent is excreted in the feces by an enterohepatic pathway, while the milk and sweat are other secondary routes of excretion. The total body burden has been estimated as 1.1 mg.

The muscle contains the largest total fraction, but the fat has the highest concentration. The liver, heart, and hair have significantly higher concentrations than other organs, but the concentration in these organs is relatively low. The normal levels in human urine and blood are about 98 and 0.18 μg/l, respectively. The blood level is largely in association with the red cells.

Significant species differences have been observed in the excretion of radiocobalt. In rats and cattle 80 percent is eliminated in the feces (Schroeder et al., 1967b).

Polycythemia is the characteristic response of most mammals, including man, to ingestion of excessive amounts of cobalt. Toxicity resulting from overzealous therapeutic administration has been reported to produce vomiting, diarrhea, and a sensation of warmth. Intravenous administration leads to flushing of the face, increased blood pressure, slowed respiration, giddiness, tinnitus, and deafness due to nerve damage (Browning, 1969).

High levels of chronic oral administration may result in the production of goiter. Epidemiologic studies suggest that the incidence of goiter is higher in regions containing increased levels of cobalt in the water and soil (Wills, 1966). The goitrogenic effect has been elicited by the oral administration of 3 to 4 mg/kg to children in the course of sickle cell anemia therapy (Browning, 1969).

Cardiomyopathy has been caused by excessive intake of cobalt, particularly in beer to which cobalt was added to enhance its foaming qualities. The onset of the poisoning occurred about one month after cobalt was added in concentrations of 1 ppm. Why such a low concentration should produce this effect in the absence of any similar change when cobalt is used therapeutically is unknown. The signs and symptoms were those of congestive heart failure. Autopsy findings revealed a tenfold increase in the cardiac levels of cobalt. Alcohol may have served to potentiate the effect of the cobalt (Morin and Daniel, 1967).

Hyperglycemia due to alpha cell pancreatic damage has been reported after injection into rats. Reduction of blood pressure has also been observed in rats after injection and has led to some experimental use in man (Schroeder et al., 1967b).

Industrial exposure to cobalt salts leads to respiratory effects, although there is some question as to whether cobalt is the sole agent responsible for these effects. Most industrial exposure comes from the cemented carbide industry where exposure to 1 to 2 mg/M³ has produced pulmonary effects. Sensitization may be an important part of this effect. Experimental studies in animals, however, confirm the lung-irritant effect of the metal as used in this industry but not of other cobalt compounds. Skin and eye lesions similar to allergic dermatitis have also been reported. Skin tests show positive sensitization to cobalt but not to other material used in the cemented carbide industry. Gastric disturbances occurring shortly after daily exposure to cobalt acetate that progress to epigastric pain, pain in the limbs, hematuria, and occult blood in the stool have been reported. Recovery was complete in three weeks (AIHA, 1966a; Browning, 1969).

COPPER

Occurrence and Use. Copper occurs in several oxides, carbonate, and sulfide ores as well as native copper. It is widely used in industry because of its conductivity, malleability, and durability. Copper is widely distributed in nature and is an essential element. Copper deficiency is characterized by hypochromic, microcytic anemia resulting from defective hemoglobin synthesis. Oxidative enzymes, such as catalase, peroxidase, cytochrome oxides, and others, also require copper. Medicinally, copper sulfate is used as an emetic. It has also been used for its astringent and caustic action and as an anthelmintic. Water purification processing has included the use of copper to remove algae. Copper sulfate mixed with lime has been used as a fungicide. Copper salts have also been used as a food additive to give a bright green color to canned peas (Sollmann, 1957). Since copper proteins in the blood of many shellfish act as oxygen carriers, the concentration is frequently high (American oysters, 1,500 ppm).

Absorption, Excretion, Toxicity. The intestinal mucosa acts to some extent as a barrier to the absorption of ingested copper. Most cuprous salts are insoluble in water but they tend to oxidize to the cupric form. Copper is initially bound to serum albumin and later more firmly bound to alpha-ceruloplasmin, where it is exchanged in the cupric form. The normal serum level of copper is 120 to 145 μg/l. The bile is the normal excretory pathway and plays a primary role in copper homeostasis. The liver and bone marrow are the storage organs for excess copper. The amount of copper in milk is not enough to maintain the copper levels in the liver, lung, and spleen of the newborn. The levels decline up to about ten years of age, remaining relatively constant thereafter. Brain levels, on the other hand, tend to almost double from infancy. The ratios of newborn to adult liver-copper show considerable species difference: man, 15:4; rat, 6:4; and rabbit, 1:6. Since urinary copper levels may be increased by soft water, under these conditions concentrations of approximately 60 μg/l are not uncommon.

While copper is an essential element in most organisms, the range between deficiency and toxicity is low in those without effective barriers to controlled absorption, for example, algae, fungi, and some invertebrates. Fish are sensitive to copper, apparently because their gills do not provide an effective barrier against absorption. Ruminants are more sensitive to copper than monogastric mammals. Copper toxicity in sheep and cattle is characterized by excessive hepatic stores, hemolysis, and hemoglobinuria. Other mammals, including man, are less sensitive to copper, presumably because of a better-developed homeostatic mechanism. It is generally felt that excessive copper exposure in normal persons does not result in a chronic disease. While there is no increase in copper tissue stores with age, serum copper levels do increase (Schroeder *et al.*, 1966b). This has led to the speculation that increased serum copper levels may accelerate atherosclerosis (Harman, 1965).

Industrial exposure to copper does not appear responsible for acute or chronic poisoning, except for "brass chills," which is another form of metal fume fever. Whether the responses ascribed to copper are due to this metal or to some other factor is controversial (Browning, 1969). The increased incidence of lung cancer in coppersmiths is not generally accepted as being significant evidence of this metal's carcinogenicity (Furst, 1971).

Acute poisoning resulting from ingestion of excessive amounts of oral copper salts, most frequently copper sulfate, may produce death. The symptoms are vomiting, sometimes with a blue-green color observed in the vomitus, hematemesis, hypotension, melena, coma, and jaundice. Autopsy findings have revealed centrilobular hepatic necrosis (Chuttani *et al.*, 1965). Few cases of copper intoxication as a result of burn treatment with copper compounds have resulted in hemolytic anemia. Copper poisoning producing hemolytic anemia has also been reported as the result of using copper-containing dialysis equipment (Manzler and Schreiner, 1970). Whether increased serum and liver-copper concentrations elicited after insertion of a copper wire into the uterus of rats

**Table 17-6. INTERRELATIONSHIP OF COPPER, IRON, AND LEAD IN THE
DEVELOPING ERYTHROCYTE***

	IRON DEPOSITION			
	Reticulocyte		Erythroblast	
TREATMENT	Vesicles	Mitochondria	Vesicles	Mitochondria
Copper supplemented	+	0	+	0
Copper deficient	+	0	+	0
Copper supplemented + Pb	+ + + +	+ + +	+	0
Control diet + Pb	+ +	+ +	+	+
Copper deficient + Fe	+ + + +	0	+ +	0
Copper deficient + Pb	+ +	0	+ +	0
Copper deficient + Fe + Pb	+ +	0	+	0

* Modified from Goodman, J. R., and Dallman, P. R.: Role of copper in iron localization in developing
erythrocyte. *Blood*, **6**: 747–53, 1969.

will be indicative of difficulties as a result of
using copper-containing intrauterine devices is
open to speculation (Okereke *et al.*, 1972).

A complex interrelationship of copper, iron,
and lead exists in the developing erythrocyte.
The results obtained in rats are summarized in
Table 17-6. These results indicate that excesses
in copper and lead increase the iron content of
the reticulocyte, but that copper deficiency in the
presence of excess lead alters the intracellular
distribution of iron.

GALLIUM

Occurrence and Use. Gallium is obtained as
a by-product of copper, zinc, lead, and aluminum. It is used in high-temperature thermometers, as a substitute for mercury in arc lamps,
in the manufacture of alloys, and as a seal for
glass and vacuum equipment. The metal is a
liquid at temperatures greater than 29.9° C.
Radioactive gallium has been used as a diagnostic tool for the localization of bone lesions.

Absorption, Excretion, Toxicity. Gallium is
not readily absorbed by the oral route, but
occurs in bone at concentrations less than 1 ppm.
Increasing intake produces slight increases in
gallium levels in the liver, spleen, kidney, and
bone. The urine is the major route of excretion.

There are no reported adverse effects of gallium following industrial exposure. Therapeutic
use of radiogallium has produced some effects,
chiefly dermal and gastrointestinal in nature. The
bone marrow depression reported may be due
largely to the radioactivity. In animals gallium
acts as a neuromuscular poison and causes renal
damage. Photophobia, blindness, and paralysis
have been reported in rats. Renal damage ranging from cloudy swelling to necrosis has been
reported. In dogs aplastic changes in the bone
marrow have been observed (Browning, 1969).

GERMANIUM

Occurrence and Use. Germanium occurs in
some mineral ores but is produced in the United
States primarily as a by-product of zinc. It is a
semiconductor and is used in electronics, in fine
lenses, in certain aluminum alloys, and as a
catalyst. However, only small amounts are
actually used industrially; for example, only 7.5
tons were produced in the world in 1964. Germanium is present in most foods. Raw clams,
tuna, baked beans, and tomato juice have significant amounts. The average daily intake has
been estimated at 1,500 μg, but wide variations
may occur. One would expect significant
amounts of germanium to be in the urban atmosphere as a result of relatively high (1.6 to 7.5
percent) germanium concentration in coal.

Absorption, Excretion, Toxicity. Sodium ger-
manite is rapidly absorbed from the gastrointestinal tract—96 percent in eight hours. It is
transported at low serum levels unbound to
plasma proteins. Some is also found in the red
blood cells. Levels of 0.65 and 0.29 mg/ml have
been reported as normal values for red blood
cells and serum, respectively. In dogs 90 percent
of radiogermanium oxide is excreted in the urine
in 72 hours. The normal range of human urine
concentration may be 0.40 to 2.16 μg/ml; milk
and feces are secondary routes of excretion. In
mice continuous feeding of germanium causes
accumulation in the spleen; however, the same
apparently does not hold true for the rat
(Schroeder and Balassa, 1967). Inhalation exposure of rats to germanium and germanium
oxide revealed rapid removal from the lung
tissue (Browning, 1969).

The toxicity of germanium and its compounds
is low. The most widely studied is germanium
oxide. The acute effects reported in animals are
hypothermia, listlessness, diarrhea, respiratory

and cardiac depression, edema, and hemorrhage in the lungs and gastrointestinal tract. The gaseous hydride, like other metal hydrides, is more toxic and causes hemolysis.

Chronic administration to rats in food at 1000 ppm or in water at 100 ppm of germanium oxide caused growth inhibition and mortality. The survivors appeared to develop a tolerance. The cause of the mortality was not apparent. Exposure to germanium is not considered an industrial hazard, nor has it been implicated in any chronic diseases of man (Schroeder and Balassa, 1967; Browning, 1969).

GOLD

Occurrence and Use. Gold is rather widely distributed in small quantities, but the major economically-usable deposits occur as the free metal in quartz veins or alluvial gravel. It may be naturally alloyed as sylvanite $(AuAg)Te_2$. Sea water contains 3 to 4 mg per ton, and small amounts, 0.03 to 1 mg percent, have been reported in many foods. Gold is used in jewelry, for other ornamental uses, and for special industrial purposes where its properties of electrical and heat conductivity, malleability, and ductility outweigh its expense. While gold and its salts have been used for a wide variety of medicinal purposes, their present uses are limited to the treatment of rheumatoid arthritis and rare skin diseases such as discoid lupus.

Absorption, Excretion, Toxicity. Gold salts are poorly absorbed from the gastrointestinal tract. The majority of the information we have concerning the distribution of gold salts originates from its therapeutic use or through experimental studies. Normal urine and fecal excretions of 0.1 and 1 mg per day, respectively, have been reported. After injection of most of the soluble salts, gold is excreted via the urine, while the feces account for the major portion of insoluble compounds. Gold seems to have a long biologic half-life, and detectable blood levels can be demonstrated for ten months after the cessation of treatment. Most of the retained gold salts are found in the kidney; less is present in the liver and other organs, including the spleen. Colloidal gold may be collected by the reticuloendothelial system and larger amounts are found in the liver.

The toxicity of gold and its salts seems to be largely associated with its therapeutic use rather than its industrial use. Dermatitis is the most frequently reported toxic reaction, and stomatitis may accompany this reaction. The skin lesions tend to disappear after the cessation of therapy. Nephritis with albuminuria, encephalitis, gastrointestinal damage, hepatitis, and blood dyscrasia, including leukopenia, agranu-locytosis, thrombopenia, or aplastic anemia have been reported with less frequency (Freyberg, 1966; Dale and Patterson, 1967).

Animal experiments confirm the toxicity of gold salts reported from medical studies. In addition, hypothalamic damage in mice results in obesity after administration of large amounts of gold thioglucose (Sollmann, 1957).

HAFNIUM

Hafnium is one of the rarer metals and has limited commercial use. It is found in most minerals containing zirconium. Hafnium has been used in radio tubes, television tubes, incandescent lights, and as a cathode in x-ray tubes.

There are no reports of human toxicity. In animals the principal toxic effect is the production of nonhealing ulcers following dermal application (hafnyl chloride) to abraded skin. In a 90-day feeding study, 1 percent produced slight liver changes (Haley et al., 1962).

INDIUM

Occurrence and Use. Indium is produced as a by-product in the manufacture of other metals, chiefly zinc, but also tin and lead. Its industrial uses are in electroplating of nontarnishing silver and copper plate, corrosion-resistant alloys, glass manufacture, in nuclear energy processes, and in the manufacture of containers for foodstuffs.

Absorption, Excretion, Toxicity. Indium is poorly absorbed from the gastrointestinal tract. It is excreted in the urine and feces. Its tissue distribution is relatively uniform. The kidney, liver, bone, and spleen have relatively high concentrations. Intratracheal injections produce similar concentrations, but the concentration in the tracheobronchial lymph nodes is increased.

No industrial injury has been reported from the use of indium. While absorption from indium-plated silver in utensils may occur, this is without known toxic effect.

The knowledge of indium toxicity is based largely on results of animal experiments. Subcutaneous and intravenous injection is followed by hindleg paralysis, convulsions, and death. The liver and kidneys are affected. Congestion, hemorrhage, and necrosis are produced in the liver. Hemorrhage and necrosis of the kidneys have been reported. Muscle degeneration has also been reported (Browning, 1969).

IRON

Occurrence and Use. The principal ores of iron are oxides. The industrial uses of iron are many, mainly in the fabrication of steel. Urban air and water may contain significant amounts of iron from industrial or geologic sources. Iron carbonate is a trace mineral and is added to foods. Ferbam, ferric dimethyldithiocarbamate, is an iron-containing fungicide. It has a relatively high threshold limit value of 10 mg/M³. However, when it is heated, it decomposes and emits highly toxic fumes.

Iron is widely distributed in food, animal tissues tending to have considerably more than plants. Iron is an essential element; its major function in the animal body is the formation of hemoglobin (see Chap. 14). However, enzymes also contain iron; these include cytochrome and xanthine oxidase (Beal, 1971).

Iron has been used therapeutically since at least 1500 B.C. Its medicinal uses have included treatment of acne, alopecia, hemorrhoids, gout, pulmonary diseases, excessive lacrimation, weakness, edema, and fever, to name a few. The primary therapeutic use of iron salts today is in the treatment of iron-deficiency anemia. Iron is available in nonprescription forms. Parenteral dosage forms, generally iron carbohydrate complexes, are available for treating iron deficiency that does not respond to oral treatment and for physiologic anemia due to rapid growth, for example, anemia of baby pigs.

Every tissue of the body contains iron. Under normal conditions the body burden is about 4 g. Hemoglobin is the major iron compound in the body and is highly concentrated in the erythrocytes. Sixty-seven percent of the total iron is contained in hemoglobin. Twenty-seven percent is stored as ferritin mainly in the liver, or as hemosiderin, in cases of excess intake.

Absorption, Excretion, Toxicity. The oral absorption of iron is very complicated and the intestinal mucosa is the principal site for limiting the absorption of iron. In this homeostatic mechanism the divalent form is absorbed into the gastrointestinal mucosa and converted to the trivalent form and attached to ferritin. The ferritin passes into the bloodstream and is then converted to transferrin where the iron remains in the trivalent form or is transported to the liver or spleen for storage as ferritin or hemosiderin. The absorption of iron from the gastrointestinal tract may be dependent upon hepatic and pancreatic secretions. The adequacy of iron stores in the body, however, seems to be the major controlling factor in the absorption of iron by the gastrointestinal tract (Fairbanks et al., 1971).

Iron has been shown to cross the placenta and concentrate in the fetus. The concentration of the iron in the fetus may serve a valuable physiologic purpose, inasmuch as it prevents anemia caused by rapid growth in the absence of sufficient supplies of iron in the mother's milk. Under normal circumstances the iron contained in food is not well absorbed in nonanemic persons. With increases in iron beyond the physiologic limits, most is excreted in the feces, but small amounts may accumulate. Some iron may be excreted via the bile. In cases of overload, iron is excreted in the urine, and the presence of high urinary iron concentrations is indicative of excessive iron. Normally, significant quantities of iron are excreted by loss of epithelial cells of the gastrointestinal tract. Women tend to be more anemic than men; menstrual bleeding may account for this tendency (Beal, 1971).

Acute poisoning from accidental ingestion of ferrous sulfate tablets occurs more frequently in children than in adults. About 2,000 such cases occur annually. Only acute intoxications from aspirin, other unknown medications, and phenobarbital occur more frequently than acute iron poisoning (Greengard and McEnery, 1968). Prior to the advent of deferoxamine, the death rate in children was higher from this form of intoxication than from acetylsalicylic acid (Sisson, 1960).

Acute toxicity from oral iron preparations is largely due to the irritation of the gastrointestinal tract; vomiting may be the first sign. There may be some gastrointestinal bleeding, lethargy, restlessness, and gray cyanosis. This may be followed by a short period of recovery, which takes place from several hours to one or two days after the poisoning. This is followed by a third phase of acute iron toxicity in which signs of pneumonitis and convulsions may occur. Gastrointestinal bleeding generally continues throughout this entire period, and some neurologic manifestations, including coma, are predominant during this phase. Signs of hepatic toxicity, such as jaundice, may be observed. Most deaths occur during this time. In those patients surviving three or four days, recovery is generally rapid. Pyloric constriction and gastric fibrosis have been observed, in rare instances, six weeks after the acute phase of iron poisoning. Marked leukocytosis may also occur.

Acute iron poisoning in rabbits produces prolongation of coagulation time and prothrombin time, increased thrombocyte count, and qualitative changes in fibrin formation. Serum glutamic oxalacetic and glutamic pyruvic transaminase are increased. The severity of the clinical course seems to be proportional to the increase in the serum iron concentration. It has been hypothesized that the severe gastrointestinal necrosis facilitates direct access of the iron into the bloodstream, circumventing the mucosal block. Electron microscopic examinations have found livers of rabbits experimentally poisoned with large intravenous doses of iron to have degenerative mitochondria

day, five days a week for 100 da
brain manganese concentration
fold but produced no hematolo
or histologic effects (Martone,
mental chronic oral intake of
rabbits, pigs, and cattle at lev
5,000 ppm has been reported to
mulation and utilization of iro
in manganese contain only slig
100 ppm. Thus, it is difficult to se
reported in animals could apply
1967).

MOLYBDENUM

Occurrence and Use. The
mineral source of molybdenum
(MoS_2). The United States is th
producer of molybdenum. The in
this metal include the manufa
temperature resistant steel alloy:
turbines and jet aircraft engines
catalysts, lubricants, and dyes.
widely distributed in nature, bei
element. It is a cofactor for the en
oxidase and aldehyde oxidase.
necessary for bacterial fixing
nitrogen at the start of protein syr
of these functions it is ubiquitou:
plankton tend to concentrate n
times that of sea water, shellfisl
high concentrations of molybder
num is added in trace amounts
stimulate plant growth. The avera
intake in food is approximatel
concentration of molybdenum i
minimal (Table 17-3).

Fresh water has about 0.35 pp
certain areas the content may be
der et al., 1970a).

The use of molybdenized ferr
been tried for the treatment of
anemia. However, beneficial effec
molybdenum were minimal, an
appeared to have gastrointestin
equal to or greater than those of
(Bothwell and Finch, 1962).

Absorption, Excretion, Toxicit:
lybdenum exists in various valer
logic differences with respect to
clear. The soluble hexavalent c
well absorbed from the gastrointe:
the liver. Increased molybdenum
perimental animals has been sho
tissue levels of xanthine oxidase.

In man molybdenum is contail
in the liver, kidney, fat, and
approximate total of 9 mg in the
concentrated in the liver, kidney
omentum. The molybdenum lev

accompanying the marked hepatic degeneration. Fatty degeneration of the myocardium and masses of granular material in the kidneys have been reported.

Iron poisoning has been treated by dimercaprol (British antilewisite; BAL), diethylenetriaminepentaacetate (DTPA), and ethylenediaminetetraacetate (EDTA). However, these agents have been completely supplanted by deferoxamine.

Chronic excessive intake of iron may lead to hemosiderosis or hemochromatosis. Hemosiderosis refers to a condition in which there is generalized increased iron content in the body tissues, particularly the liver and reticuloendothelial system. Hemochromatosis, on the other hand, indicates demonstrable histologic hemosiderosis and diffused fibrotic changes of the affected organ.

Excessive dietary iron intake appears to be the cause of abnormal iron accumulation in the notable condition occurring in South Africa known as "Bantu siderosis." Bantu siderosis is more frequent in men than in women. The disease probably results from the use of iron pots in food preparation and the brewing of beer in iron containers. This type of disease is marked by iron accumulations in the Kupffer cells of the liver and in the reticuloendothelial cells of the spleen and bone marrow. In addition, a glucose test indicates that 20 percent of the patients with hemochromatosis have abnormal glucose metabolism. Increase in heart disease may also accompany hemochromatosis. It has been reported that high dietary iron intake from other sources, for example red wine, may also play a role in the etiology of hemochromatosis in some areas of the world.

In addition, Kaschin-Beck disease, an unusual disorder, has been reported in Asia. This has been ascribed, perhaps in error, to the consumption of drinking water with excessive iron content and results in an arthritic-type disease.

Numerous investigators have attempted to produce hemochromatosis in experimental animals by chronic parenteral or oral administration of iron in large doses. Although it is possible to induce hemosiderosis in the liver and other viscera, fibrosis has not been clearly demonstrated. In experimental animals the production of hemosiderosis, accompanied by cellular injury and fibrosis, apparently requires a cholinedeficient diet. Administration of folic acid to rats receiving a choline-deficient diet has prevented cellular necrosis and fibrosis.

Parenteral iron preparations are generally given intramuscularly, although some may be used intravenously. Staining at the site of intramuscular injection is a problem with these

materials owing to the iron deposition in man and pigs. Iron dextran, administered by subcutaneous injection, has been shown to cause a high incidence of sarcoma in rats. It has been pointed out that the dose used in some of the studies was 200 to 300 times greater than the therapeutic dose in man on a weight basis. There is a high degree of species specificity in the incidence of sarcomas. The incidence is considerably higher in the rat than in the mouse. Iron dextran was removed from the U.S. market in 1960 because of these effects in animals and returned to the market in 1963 (Fairbanks et al., 1971). Further investigations have revealed that high doses of injectable iron preparations administered intravenously to various species of experimental animals produced teratogenic changes (hydrocephalus, anophthalmia) in the fetuses. The effect was reduced when deferoxamine was administered.

Long-term inhalation exposure to iron, particularly to iron oxide, has resulted in mottling of the lungs, a condition referred to as siderosis. This is considered a benign pneumoconiosis and does not ordinarily cause significant physiologic impairment (Stokinger, 1963). However, hematite miners have been reported in certain areas to have from 50 to 70 percent higher death rates attributable to lung cancer. It has been suggested that at least part of the increased incidence may be due to radioactivity in the mine fields surveyed (Boyd et al., 1970).

LANTHANONS (RARE EARTHS)

Occurrence and Use. The lanthanons comprise the elements with atomic numbers 57 through 71; yttrium and scandium are included because of similar characteristics. The lanthanons occur in monozite sand, a phosphate mineral, in combination with thorium. Various special chemical methods are available for the separation of cerium. The "heavy" lanthanons, samarium through lutetium, are separated by ion exchange. The "light" elements are separated by conventional crystallization procedures. Before these separation techniques were available, their main use was in mantels for gas lights. However, they are now used in control rods for atomic reactors, in alloys with nickel and chrome, in microwave devices, lasers and masers, and in television sets.

Neodymium and several other rare earths have been tried clinically as anticoagulants. Cerium oxalate has been used to remedy vomiting during pregnancy, and other salts of this element have been used as central nervous system depressants, astringents, and antiseptics.

Absorption, Excretion, Toxicity. Only small amounts of the stable rare earths are absorbed

and its compounds are use
alloys, dry cell batteries, elec
ics, matches, glass, dyes, in
rods, as oxidizing agents, ar
additives. The primary uses
antiseptics and germicides. F
ganate ($KMnO_4$) is applied
effects and for its slight astri
is virtually the only mangar
medical use at the present
chloride was administered
schizophrenia, but was aband
of effect and the danger of fl

Manganese is an essential
cofactor in a number of en:
particularly those involved in
cholesterol, and fatty acids syn
is present in all living organ
present in urban air (Table
water supplies (Table 17-2), th
of the intake is derived from
the germinal portions of grain
and some spices are rich in m

Absorption, Excretion, To
burden has been estimated at 2
The liver, kidney, intestine, anc
the highest concentrations.
changes in tissue concentratio
except that tissues that have
concentrations in adults tend
amounts in the newborn. The l
mulate manganese with age
concentrations in urban air.
manganese is rapid. Injected
quickly disappears from the t
concentrated in the mitochondi
pancreas. Administration of sta
any valence state promotes ra
radiomanganese. Serum mang
about 2.5 μg/l, increases after
occlusion and is claimed to be
index of myocardial infarctio
oxalacetic transaminase (Schro

Recent studies suggest that t
excretion is the gastrointestinal
and that the excretion of ma
regulated by a homeostatic sy:
relatively constant tissue lev
apparently involves the liver,
intestinal mechanisms for
manganese, and perhaps the ad
tinchamps et al., 1966; Britt
1966; Hughes et al., 1966; Pa
1966).

This regulating mechanism, p
for extremely large doses of m:
cause gastrointestinal irritation,
lack of systemic toxicity follow
stration or dermal application.

(Browning, 1969; Schroeder et al., 1970a). There are no data documenting molybdenum toxicity in man due to industrial exposure.

NICKEL

Occurrence and Use. In its principal ores nickel is found in combination with iron or copper. The main uses of nickel are in electronics, coins, steel alloys, batteries, food processing (Ni-Cu Monel), and stainless steel.

Nickel is a constituent of urban air (Table 17-3), possibly as a result of fossil fuel combustion. Incinerators also contribute to the nickel content in the atmosphere. Nickel is not a normal constituent of water. While some nickel is found as a contaminant from food processing (gelatin and baking powder), relatively large amounts occur naturally in vegetables, legumes, and grains. While in vitro nickel will activate enzymes, no functional action has been described in the intact animals.

Absorption, Excretion, Toxicity. The average body burden has been estimated at < 10 mg (Table 17-1), but wide geographic variations occur. Nickel is present in the lung, liver, kidney, and intestine of most stillborn infants. The concentration in the lung increases with age. In rats the bones accumulate a major portion of increased intake. Excretion is largely via the feces. Nickel has been found in bile. A mechanism for limiting intestinal absorption has been suggested. Many nickel salts have astringent and irritant properties that limit their absorption. Normal urine values of about 2.3 μg/100 ml have been reported (Schroeder et al., 1962a).

Dermatitis (nickel itch) is the most frequent effect of exposure to nickel. This occurs from direct contact with metals containing nickel such as coins and costume jewelry. It has been estimated that of all eczema, 5 percent is caused by nickel or nickel compounds. The dermatitis is a sensitization reaction, and contact may, in some cases, produce paroxysmal asthmatic attacks and pulmonary eosinophilia (Sunderman, 1971).

Nickel carbonyl ($Ni[CO]_4$) is the most toxic of nickel compounds. It has been estimated to be lethal in man at atmospheric exposures of 30 ppm for 20 minutes (AIHA, 1968a). This material is formed by nickel or its compounds in the presence of carbon monoxide. The initial symptoms of toxicity consist of headache and vomiting. These are relieved by fresh air. Delayed symptoms occurring in 12 to 36 hours include dyspnea, cyanosis, leukocytosis, and increased body temperature. Delirium and other central nervous system signs usually appear. Acute chemical pneumonitis results. Death may occur between the fourth and eleventh days.

While dietary nickel is excreted largely in the feces, inhalation of nickel carbonyl results in the appearance of significant increases in urinary nickel, both with respect to concentration and relative to that in the stools. The increase of nickel in the urine has been used clinically to confirm exposure, and levels above 0.5 mg/l are considered serious. Diethyldithiocarbamate trihydrate (Dithlocarb), a metal binding agent, has been used successfully to treat acute poisoning.

Chronic exposure to nickel carbonyl has been implicated epidemiologically in cancer affecting the lungs and nose. These findings have been confirmed by inhalation exposures in experimental animals. In addition, it has been reported that cigarette smoke contains significant amounts of nickel carbonyl (Sunderman, 1970).

There are no epidemiologic studies that confirm the systemic toxicity of nickel or its compounds (except $Ni[CO]_4$). Doses of nickel sulfate (0.1 to 0.5 mg/kg for 161 days) have induced myocardial and liver damage. High doses of the soluble salts induce giddiness and nausea. Inhalation exposure to nickel and nickel oxide dusts have produced malignant pulmonary neoplasms in guinea pigs and rats. The increase of serum nickel in humans after myocardial infarction is of unknown significance (AIHA, 1966b).

NIOBIUM

Occurrence and Use. Niobium (columbium) is found with tantalum in the primary ore of tantalite and columbite. It is used in the manufacture of high-temperature steel alloys, corrosion-resistant chromium-steel alloys, and in electronic equipment. It has a low thermal neutron cross-section and has growing use in nuclear energy and chemistry.

Niobium appears to be ubiquitous in nature. Most grains, meats, and dairy products contain significant amounts of niobium. Fats and oils, of both vegetable and animal origin, tend to have the highest concentrations of niobium.

Absorption, Excretion, Toxicity. Intake from water is about 20 μg. A little less than half the daily intake is absorbed; this is excreted in the urine. In the body niobium is carried mainly in the red blood cells. The total body burden is approximately 100 mg. The red blood cells, liver, kidney, fat, hair, lungs, and pancreas contain the highest concentration, but niobium is found in most other organs. The "normal" concentrations in the red blood cells, serum, and urine are about 5, 0.7, and 0.25 μg/g, respectively (Schroeder and Balassa, 1965). Niobium is present in the newborn and in milk. Inhalation studies in rats have shown that the largest amounts were retained in the lungs with secondary deposition in the bones. The biologic half-life was 120 days (Thomas et al., 1967).

Incorporation of niobium in the drinking water of mice at 5 ppm plus 1.62 mg/g in the diet caused liver degeneration (Schroeder *et al.*, 1968a). *In vitro* studies have suggested that inhibition of adenosine triphosphatase may be involved with the biologic activity of niobium [(Stokinger, 1963). There are no reports of niobium toxicity in man.

Intravenous administration of 30 mg/kg niobium as potassium niobate to dogs and rats produced severe nephrotoxic effects. Tubular epithelial damage was predominant in the convoluted tubule (Wong and Downs, 1966). Niobium pentachloride produces moderate transient irritation of the eye and severe dermal irritation (Downs *et al.*, 1965).

PLATINUM-GROUP METALS

Occurrence and Use. These metals may be grouped together because of their similar chemical properties. Ruthenium (Ru), rhodium (Rh), and palladium (Pd) are the lighter triad, while osmium (Os), iridium (Ir), and platinum (Pt) are the heavier. They are found together in very sparsely distributed deposits. These rare metals are obtained from such deposits or as a by-product of refining other metals, chiefly nickel and copper.

The chief use of ruthenium is as a hardener in platinum and palladium alloys used in jewelry and electrical contacts. Rhodium is used in the manufacture of rhodium-platinum alloys, in electroplating, electronic components, movie projectors, and in reflectors for searchlights. Although rhodium is reported to have slight chemotherapeutic activity against certain mouse viruses (Browning, 1969), it is not used medicinally at present. The industrial uses of palladium include alloys (especially those used in the communication industry), as a catalyst, for decoration and jewelry, dental alloys, and in cigarette lighters. Palladium in colloidal form has been given medicinally for tuberculosis, gout, and obesity. These uses were without significant benefits. Osmium is used in the hard points of fountain pens and engraving tools, in staining tissues for electron microscopy, and in fingerprinting. Formerly it was used in the manufacture of electrical lights. Iridium is used to harden platinum jewelry and as an alloy with osmium for hard points of fountain pens and engraving tools. Platinum is widely used as a catalyst in the chemical industry and in electronics. It is alloyed with other metals and used in jewelry.

Absorption, Excretion, Toxicity. Intratracheal injections of radioruthenium chloride are retained in the lungs, suggesting that ruthenium might also be retained after inhalation exposure. Toxicologic information is limited to references in the literature indicating that fumes may be injurious to eyes and lungs (Browning, 1969).

Rhodium trichloride produced death in rats and rabbits within 48 hours after intravenous administration at doses near the LD50 (approximately 200 mg/kg). Histologic evaluation revealed no changes; however, it was suggested that death was attributable to central nervous system effects (Landolt *et al.*, 1972).

In a single study, incorporation of rhodium (rhodium chloride) or palladium (palladous chloride) into the drinking water of mice at a concentration of 5 ppm over the lifetime of the animals produced a minimally significant increase in malignant tumors. Most of these tumors were classified as of the lymphomaleukemia type (Schroeder and Mitchener, 1971).

When administered orally, palladium is excreted in the feces. Intravenous administration results in rapid and almost complete excretion in the urine. Palladium chloride is not readily absorbed from subcutaneous injection. No adverse effects have been reported from industrial exposure. Subcutaneous injection of palladium chloride in rabbits leads to gray-brown discoloration at the site of injection. Intravenous administration in lethal doses causes loss of appetite, hemolysis, renal deposits, and bone marrow injury. Colloid palladium ($Pd[OH]_2$) is reported to increase body temperature, produce discoloration and necrosis at the site of injection, decrease body weight, and cause slight hemolysis.

Osmium metals and most of its salts are of little toxicologic significance. Osmium tetroxide, produced by heating the metal, is toxic. Its action is mainly on the eyes. Lacrimation and halo vision occur, probably owing to effects on the cornea. Irritation of the respiratory tract and headache may occur. One fatal case due to pulmonary irritation has been reported. Some renal toxicity has also been ascribed to osmium tetroxide exposure (AIHA, 1968b).

No reports implicating iridium as an industrial hazardous agent have appeared (Stokinger, 1963).

Platinum metal itself is generally harmless, but an allergic dermatitis can be produced in susceptible individuals. Skin changes are most common between the fingers and in the antecubital fossae. Symptoms of respiratory distress, ranging from irritation to an "asthmatic syndrome" with coughing, wheezing, and shortness of breath, have been reported following exposure to platinum dust. The skin and respiratory changes are termed platinosis. They are mainly confined to persons with a history of industrial exposure to soluble compounds such as sodium chloroplatinate, although cases resulting from wearing platinum jewelry have been reported.

Metallic platinum dust itself is reported not to cause these changes.

Toxicity studies of complex platinum bases indicate these are much more toxic than platinum itself. Diamminedichloroplatinum ($Pt[NH_3]_2Cl_2$), given subcutaneously to experimental animals, produces epileptic-type convulsions and death, preceded by coma. Hyperirritability and cardiac effects, due to action on the vagus center, have also been observed with smaller doses (Browning, 1969).

RHENIUM

Occurrence and Use. Rhenium is obtained as a by-product of molybdenum and copper processing. It is used in the electrical industry for electronic tubes and in marine engine magnetos, especially because of its resistance to salt corrosion. It is also used as a heater element.

Absorption, Excretion, Toxicity. Rhenium is excreted primarily in the urine. Although rhenium tends to accumulate in the thyroid, it does not bind there as does iodine. No toxic effects have been reported (Browning, 1969).

RUBIDIUM

Occurrence and Use. Rubidium is a by-product of potassium and molybdenum production. Its chief industrial use is in the manufacture of photoelectric cells. It is widespread in nature at trace levels and it is found in tomatoes, beef, beans, and barley at significant levels. Rubidium is also found in most animal tissues.

Absorption, Excretion, Toxicity. Rubidium seems to be an acceptable substitute for potassium in many physiologic processes. While rubidium will prevent kidney and muscle lesions characteristic of potassium depletion, there is no evidence that rubidium itself is an essential element (Underwood, 1971).

Rubidium is fairly well absorbed after oral administration. The highest concentrations are in the heart and skeletal muscles, while bone contains almost none. The muscle acts as the primary storage site under conditions of excess. In the blood the largest amount is partitioned in the red blood cells. The urine is the major route of excretion. The feces are of secondary importance in excretion.

There is no evidence that rubidium is toxic to man. Rubidium in excess is toxic, especially in animals on potassium-deficient diets. Under this condition hyperirritability, muscle spasms, convulsions, and failure of the young to survive to the weanling stage have been demonstrated. Frequent development of ventricular extrasystoles has also been demonstrated (Browning, 1969).

SELENIUM

Occurrence and Use. Selenium is principally obtained as a by-product of copper refining. Tellurium is also frequently present in these sulfide ores, and some industrial hazards may be due to the combination of these related materials. Selenium is used in the electronics industry for rectifiers, photo cells, and solar batteries, in glass and ceramic manufacturing, as a vulcanizing agent for rubber, in steel manufacturing, and in paints and varnishes. In chemical manufacturing selenium dioxide is used in rare instances as an oxidizing agent and selenium as an oxidant in lubricating and other oils. Selenium has also been used in fungicides, in insecticides, and as an insect repellent. Selenium is used medicinally as an antidandruff agent.

Selenium accumulates in certain plants in sufficient quantities to produce selenium toxicity in livestock. On the other hand, selenium is considered an essential element. Selenium-deficient diets cause liver necrosis in rats and multiple-organ (liver, heart, kidneys, skeletal muscle, and testes) necrosis in mice. In chicks, pancreatic fibrosis, exudative diathesis, and alopecia are responsive to selenium supplementation of deficient diets. Selenium-responsive diseases in the young turkey include muscle (cardiac, skeletal, and smooth-gizzard) myopathies. Lambs and calves suffer from a muscle disease called stiff lamb disease and white muscle disease when raised in selenium-deficient ranges. In addition, embryo mortality in ewes from selenium-deficient areas is reversed by supplementation. Young pigs also may be supplemented with selenium to good effect if maintained on deficient diets to prevent necrotic liver degeneration and cardiac myopathy (mulberry heart). While the role of selenium as an essential mineral seems well established in animals, the same is not so in man, although that possibility seems likely.

The apparent roles of selenium in metabolic chemistry are many. Either as a replacement for vitamin E, or in conjunction with this vitamin, selenium has a significant role in the biosynthesis of ubiquinone (coenzyme Q). Furthermore, the enzyme glutathione peroxidase, important in maintaining erythrocyte integrity, contains selenium as an essential constituent. These roles for selenium and vitamin E in controlling lipid peroxide formation are perhaps the basis for its appearing essential in the diet. Further cellular roles of selenium involve DNA-RNA, control, at least in part, of ion fluxes across cell membranes, maintenance of the integrity of keratins, and stimulation of antibody synthesis. The reaction of selenium with thiol groups may be the primary source of selenium toxicity (Diplock, 1976).

The concentration of selenium in foodstuffs provides another source of exposure. Seafoods, especially shrimp, meat, milk products, and grains, provide the largest amounts in the diet. River water levels of selenium vary depending on environmental and geologic factors; 0.02 ppm has been reported as a representative estimate. Selenium has also been detected in urban air, presumably from sulfur-containing materials. The calculated human dose from urban air is about 0.02 μg/day.

Absorption, Excretion, Toxicity. Elemental forms of selenium are probably not absorbed from the gastrointestinal tract. The average human body burden is approximately 14.6 mg. The greatest concentration is found in the kidney. The level in the liver is approximately one-half that observed in the kidney. Selenium, like arsenic, is reported to accumulate in the hair. Human blood samples contain selenium with an erythrocyte:plasma ratio of approximately 3:1. Selenium is present in the infant, but selenium levels do not increase with age. Human milk contains selenium. Selenium is excreted in the urine, which normally contains about twice as much as the feces. Increased urinary levels provide a reasonable index of excessive exposure. Normal selenium urinary output is 0.0 to 15 μg/100 ml.

Excretory products appear in sweat and expired air. The latter may have a garlicky odor due to dimethyl selenide. Within certain physiologic limits the body appears to have a homeostatic mechanism for retaining trace amounts of selenium and excreting the excess material. Selenium toxicity occurs when the intake exceeds the excretory capacity (McConnell and Portman, 1952; Schroeder et al., 1970b).

Industrial exposure to hydrogen selenide, occurring as a result of a reaction to acid or water with metal selenides, produces "garlic" breath, nausea, dizziness, and lassitude. Eye and nasal irritation may occur. In experimental animals 10 ppm is fatal. Selenium oxychloride, a vesicant, presents an industrial hazard. In rabbits 0.01 ml applied dermally resulted in death. Percutaneous absorption increased blood and liver selenium concentrations.

Acute selenium poisoning produces central nervous system effects, which include nervousness, drowsiness, and sometimes convulsions. Symptoms of chronic inhalation exposure may include pallor, coated tongue, gastrointestinal disorders, nervousness, "garlic" breath, liver and spleen damage, anemia, mucosal irritation, and lumbar pain. It has been suggested that some of these symptoms are due to tellurium impurities (Patty, 1963).

"Blind staggers" caused by excess selenium in livestock consuming 100 to 1,000 ppm is characterized by impairment of vision, weakness of limbs, and respiratory failure (Moxan and Rhian, 1943). Clear evidence of chronic selenium toxicity in man occurs only in seleniferous areas when the local foods are processed. These signs of intoxication may include discolored or decayed teeth, skin eruptions, gastrointestinal distress, lassitude, and partial loss of hair and nails. Livestock foraging on plants containing about 25 ppm suffer from "alkali" disease, which is characterized by lack of vitality, loss of hair, sterility, atrophy of hooves, lameness, and anemia. Fatty necrosis of the liver is frequent. In rats given 3 ppm of the material in drinking water, selenite has been reported to be more toxic than selenate. Selenite produced increased numbers of aortic plaques and was found to be more toxic in female than male mice. Selenium has produced loss of fertility and congenital defects and is considered embryotoxic and teratogenic on the basis of animal experiments (Moxan and Rhian, 1943; Schroeder et al., 1970b). A recent report has also suggested that selenium causes fetal toxicity and teratogenic effects in humans (Robertson, 1970). Chronic toxicity in experimental rodents consists of hepatic cirrhosis and, in the hands of several investigators, evidence of carcinogenesis, primarily in the liver. There has been considerable discussion as to the significance of these findings, and the lack of human selenium-induced carcinogenesis or increased cancer in livestock in seleniferous areas has led to questioning the significance of the results obtained in rodents (Muth, 1967).

In more recent studies, epidemiologic investigations have indicated a decrease in human cancer death rates (age and sex adjusted) correlated with increasing selenium content of forage crops (Shamberger et al., 1976). In addition, recent experimental evidence supports the antineoplastic effect of selenium with regard to benzo(a)pyrene- and benzanthracene-induced skin tumors in mice, N-2-fluorenylacetamide- and diethylaminoazobenzene-induced hepatic tumors in rats, and spontaneous mammary tumors in mice. A possible mechanism of the protective effects of selenium has been postulated to involve the inhibition of the formation of malonaldehyde, a product of peroxidative tissue damage, which is carcinogenic.

Although the mechanism of toxicity of selenium is not well understood, several related factors are very interesting. First, selenium may have the ability to replace sulfur in certain tissues, i.e., nails and hooves, and as selenate, it may have an inhibiting effect on many sulfhydryl enzymes. Second, many of the signs of toxicity can be prevented by high-protein diets, and by methionine in the presence of vitamin E (Sellers *et al.*, 1950; Schroeder *et al.*, 1970b).

In addition to the apparent protective effect against some carcinogenic agents, selenium is an antidote to the toxic effect of other metals. At appropriate levels, mutual detoxification of selenium and mercury, selenium and thallium, selenium and copper, selenium and arsenic, and selenium and cadmium has been demonstrated (Frost and Lish, 1975). The case of silver differs from other selenium-metal interactions in that silver precipitates the symptoms of selenium deficiency in vitamin E–deficient animals, perhaps by the formation of a silver-selenium complex, thereby reducing the effectively available selenium required for normal cellular processes.

SILVER

Occurrence and Use. Silver occurs in many ores. The primary silver ore is argentite (Ag_2S). Silver is also obtained as a by-product of copper, lead, and other metals. Silver is used in electrical applications because of its excellent properties of conduction. Jewelry, coins, and eating utensils are some of the principal uses of the metal. Silver halides are used in photography; silver nitrate is used for making indelible inks and for medicinal purposes. The use of silver nitrate for prophylaxis of ophthalmia neonatorum is a legal requirement in some states. Other medicinal uses of silver salts are as a caustic, germicide, antiseptic, and astringent.

Absorption, Excretion, Toxicity. Silver does not occur regularly in animal or human tissue. The major effect of excessive absorption of silver is local or generalized impregnation of the tissues, a condition referred to as argyria. Silver can be absorbed from the lungs and gastrointestinal tract. Some of the absorbed silver is retained in the cells of the gastrointestinal tract. Intravenous injection produces accumulation in the spleen, liver, bone marrow, lungs, muscle, and skin. The major route of excretion is via the gastrointestinal tract. Urinary excretion has not been reported to occur even after intravenous injection.

Industrial argyria, a chronic occupational disease, has two forms, local and generalized. The local form involves the formation of gray-blue patches on the skin or may manifest itself in the conjunctiva of the eye. In generalized argyria the skin shows widespread pigmentation, often spreading from the face to most uncovered parts of the body. In some cases the skin may become black with a metallic luster. The eyes may be affected to such a point that the lens and vision are disturbed. The respiratory tract may also be affected in severe cases.

Large oral doses of silver nitrate cause severe gastrointestinal irritation due to its caustic action. Lesions of the kidneys and lungs and the possibility of arteriosclerosis have been attributed to both industrial and medicinal exposures. Large doses of colloidal silver administered intravenously to experimental animals produced death due to pulmonary edema and congestion. Hemolysis and resulting bone marrow hyperplasia have been reported. Chronic bronchitis has also been reported to result from medicinal use of colloidal silver (Sollmann, 1957; Browning, 1969).

STRONTIUM

Occurrence and Use. Strontianite ($SrCO_3$) is the principal mineral form of strontium. The metallurgic uses are limited to the addition of small amounts in alloys of tin and lead. Strontium is also used as a deoxidizer in copper and bronze. Various strontium salts are used in paints and rubber, in the refinement of sugar from beets, and in freezing mixtures and refrigerators. Strontium has also been used as a depilatory and in tooth pastes. Some drinking water supplies naturally contain levels as high as 50 ppm. Some plants tend to concentrate strontium from the soil and levels as high as 26,000 ppm have been reported.

Absorption, Excretion, Toxicity. The biologic action and physiologic function of strontium resemble those of calcium, especially with regard to the bone. There is some evidence that strontium is essential for the growth of animals and especially for the calcification of bones and teeth. Apparently a homeostatic balance between calcium and strontium exists that favors the absorption of calcium and the preferential excretion of strontium.

Strontium is absorbed from the gastrointestinal tract in limited amounts, although the rate is somewhat dependent on dietary calcium levels. About one-fourth of the ingested strontium is excreted in the feces, while the remainder is eliminated in the urine. Milk is also a secondary route of excretion. Excess strontium tends to be stored in the teeth and bones, which are the primary storage sites under normal conditions. The normal concentration in the bone is estimated at about 360 ppm. Human fetuses are reported to contain lower concentrations than adults.

The concern over adverse effects of strontium intake is based on the radiation damage, since radiostrontium is a nuclear fallout contaminant. Chemically, toxicity from strontium is almost nil. No adverse effects from industrial use have been reported.

Electrocardiographic changes have been produced after intravenous injection of massive doses. Increased salivation, nausea, diarrhea, and death due to respiratory paralysis have been produced experimentally (Browning, 1969; Underwood, 1971).

TANTALUM

Occurrence and Use. Tantalum is found with niobium in tantalite or columbite. It is used in electronics, in tungsten cutting alloys, in chemical manufacturing as a catalyst, and for acid-resistant materials. Tantalum is used as a supporting gauze in the repair of hernias, as a dressing for burns, in prosthetic appliances, and in local radiation for bladder cancer after neutron activation.

Absorption, Excretion, Toxicity. Oral salts of tantalum are poorly absorbed. After intramuscular injection the liver, bone, and kidney contain significant amounts (Durbin, 1960).

A few animal experiments have suggested that after inhalation, tantalum may produce some pulmonary effects, benign and nonfibrotic in nature (Stokinger, 1963). No adverse effects have been reported as a result of industrial exposure. Implantation of tantalum has not shown any adverse tissue reaction in either man or experimental animals (Browning, 1969).

TELLURIUM

Occurrence and Use. Tellurium is found in various sulfide ores along with selenium and is produced as a by-product of metal refineries. Its industrial uses include applications in the refining of copper and in the manufacture of rubber. Tellurium vapor is used in "daylight" lamps. It is used in various alloys as a catalyst and is a semiconductor.

Condiments, dairy products, nuts, and fish have high concentrations of tellurium. Food packaging contains some tellurium; higher concentrations are found in aluminum cans than tin cans. Some plants, such as garlic, accumulate tellurium from the soil. Potassium tellurate has been used to reduce sweating.

Absorption, Excretion, Toxicity. Of the 600 mg of average body burden in man (Table 17-1), the majority is in the bone. The kidney is the highest in content among the soft tissues. Some data suggest that tellurium also accumulates in the liver (Schroeder *et al.*, 1967a). Soluble tetravalent tellurites, absorbed into the body after oral administration, are reduced to tellurides, partly methylated, and then exhaled as dimethyl telluride. The latter is responsible for the garlic odor in persons exposed to tellurium compounds, but does not account for a high percent of the excreted tellurium. Tellurium in the food is probably in the form of tellurates. The urine and bile are the principal routes of excretion. Sweat and milk are secondary routes of excretion.

Tellurates and tellurium are of low toxicity, but tellurites are generally more toxic. Acute inhalation exposure results in decreased sweating, nausea, a metallic taste, and sleeplessness. The typical garlic breath is a reasonable indicator of exposure to tellurium by the dermal, inhalation, or oral route. Serious cases of tellurium intoxication from industrial exposure have not been reported (AIHA, 1964b). In rats, chronic exposure to high doses of tellurium dioxide has produced decreased growth and necrosis of the liver and kidney (Cerwenka and Cooper, 1961; Patty, 1963; Browning, 1969).

Sodium tellurite at 2 ppm in drinking water or potassium tellurate at 2 ppm of tellurium plus 0.16 μg/g in the diet of mice for their lifetime produced no effects in the tellurate group. The females of the tellurite (tetravalent) group did not live as long (Schroeder and Mitchener, 1972). In rats, 500 ppm in the diet of pregnant females induced hydrocephalus in the offspring (Duckett, 1970). Abnormalities of and reduction in numbers of mitochondria were thought to be possible cellular causes of the transplacental effect.

One of the few serious recorded cases of tellurium toxicity resulted from accidental poisoning by injection of tellurium into the ureters during retrograde pyelography. Two of the three victims died. Stupor, cyanosis, vomiting, garlic breath, and loss of consciousness were observed in this unlikely incident (Keall *et al.*, 1946).

Dimercaprol treatment for tellurium increases the renal damage. While ascorbic acid decreases the characteristic garlic odor, it may also adversely affect the kidneys in the presence of increased amounts of tellurium (Amdur, 1958).

THALLIUM

Occurrence and Use. Thallium is obtained as a by-product of iron, cadmium, and zinc. It is used as a catalyst, in certain alloys, optical lenses, jewelry, low-temperature thermometers, dyes and pigments, and scintillation counters. It has been used medicinally as a depilatory. Thallium compounds, chiefly thallous sulfate, have been used as rodenticides and insecticides.

Absorption, Excretion, Toxicity. Thallium is not a normal constituent of animal tissues. It is absorbed through the skin and gastrointestinal tract. After parenteral administration it can be identified in the urine within a few hours. The highest concentrations after poisoning are in the kidney and urine. The intestines, thyroids, testes, pancreas, skin, bone, and spleen have lesser amounts. The brain and liver concentrations are still lower. Thallium is excreted slowly. Following the initial exposure, large amounts are excreted in the urine during the first 24 hours. After that period the feces may be an important route of excretion.

There have been many cases of poisoning from both the medicinal and the rodenticide use of thallium. Acute poisoning is characterized by gastrointestinal irritation, acute ascending paralysis, and psychic disturbances. Acute toxicity studies in rats have indicated that thallium is quite toxic. It has an oral LD50 of approximately 30 mg/kg. The estimated lethal dose in humans, however, is 8 to 12 mg/kg. Rat studies also indicate that thallium oxide, while relatively insoluble, is more toxic orally than by the intravenous or intraperitoneal route (Downs et al., 1960). The acute cardiovascular effects of thallium ions probably result from the exchange against cellular potassium.

The signs of subacute or chronic thallium poisoning in rats were hair loss, cataracts, and hindleg paralysis occurring with some delay after the initiation of dosing. Renal lesions were observed at gross necropsy. Histologic changes revealed damage of the proximal and distal renal tubules. The central nervous system changes were most severe in the mesencephalon where necrosis was observed. Perivascular cuffing was also reported in several other brain areas. Electron microscope examination indicated that the mitochondria in the kidney may have been the first organelles affected. Liver mitochondria also revealed degenerative changes. The livers of newborn rats whose dams had been treated throughout pregnancy showed these changes. Similar mitochondrial changes were observed in the intestine, brain, seminal vesicle, and pancreas. It has been suggested that thallium may combine with the sulfhydryl groups in the mitochondria and there interfere with oxidative phosphorylation (Herman and Bensch, 1967). A teratogenic response to thallium salts characterized as achondroplasia (dwarfism) has been described in rats (Nogami and Terashima, 1973).

In man fatty infiltration and necrosis of the liver, nephritis, gastroenteritis, pulmonary edema, degenerative changes in the adrenals, degeneration of peripheral and central nervous system, alopecia, and in some cases death have been reported as result of long-term systemic thallium intake. These cases usually are caused by the contamination of food or the use of thallium as a depilatory. Industrial poisoning is a special risk in the manufacture of fused halides for the production of lenses and windows. Loss of vision plus the other signs of thallium poisoning have been related to industrial exposures (Browning, 1969).

TIN

Occurrence and Use. Cassiterite (SnO_2) is the only important ore of tin. It is used in the manufacture of tinplate, in food packaging, and in solder, bronze, and brass. Stannous and stannic chlorides are used in dyeing textiles. Organic tin compounds have been used as fungicides, bactericides, and slimicides, as well as in plastics as stabilizers.

Absorption, Excretion, Toxicity. Effective absorption after oral administration of even soluble tin salts such as sodium stannous tartrate is limited. Ninety percent of the tin administered in this manner is recovered in the feces. The small amounts absorbed are reflected by increases in the liver and kidneys. Injected tin is excreted by the kidneys, with smaller amounts in the bile. The normal urine level is about 14 μg/100 ml. The majority of inhaled tin or its salts remains in the lungs, most extracellularly, with some in the macrophages, in the form of SnO_2. The organic tins, particularly triethyltin, may be somewhat better absorbed. The tissue distribution of tin from this material shows highest concentrations in the blood and liver, with smaller amounts in the muscle, spleen, heart, or brain. Tetraethyltin is converted to triethyltin in vivo.

Chronic inhalation of tin in the form of dust or fumes leads to benign pneumoconiosis. Tin hydride (SnH_4) is more toxic to mice and guinea pigs than is arsine; however, its effects appear mainly in the central nervous system and no hemolysis is produced. Orally, tin or its inorganic compounds require relatively large doses (500 mg/kg for 14 months) to produce toxicity. The use of tin in food processing seems to demonstrate little hazard. The average U.S. daily intake, mostly from foods as a result of processing, is estimated at 17 mg. Inorganic tin salts given by injection produce diarrhea, muscle paralysis, and twitching.

Organic tin compounds tend to be considerably more toxic. An outbreak of almost epidemic nature took place in France due to the oral ingestion of organic tin compounds used for skin disorders. One hundred deaths resulted from this incident (Barnes and Stoner, 1959). Excessive industrial exposure to triethyltin has been reported to produce headaches, visual defects, and EEG changes that were very slowly reversed (Prull and Rompel, 1970). Experimentally, triethyltin produces depression and cerebral edema. The resulting hyperglycemia may be related to the centrally mediated depletion of catecholamines from the adrenals

(Robinson, 1969). Acute burns or subacute dermal irritation has been reported among workers as a result of tributyltin (Stokinger, 1963). Triphenyltin has been shown to be a potent immunosuppressant (Verschuuren *et al.*, 1970). Inhibition in the hydrolysis of adenosine triphosphate and uncoupling of oxidative phosphorylation taking place in the mitochondria have been suggested as the cellular mechanisms of tin toxicity (Moore and Brody, 1961).

TITANIUM

Occurrence and Use. Rutile (TiO_2) and ilmenite ($FeTiO_3$) are the primary ores of titanium. Its industrial uses are as a deoxidizer, in permanent magnets, in corrosion-resistant alloys, in pigments, in welding rods, in electrodes and lamp filaments, and in surgical appliances. Titanium dioxide salve has been used in the treatment of burns. Titanium has been detected in some foods: butter, corn oil, shrimp, lettuce, pepper, and other condiments. Titanium is found in North American rivers at levels of 2 to 107 μg/l. The mean concentration in municipal U.S. drinking water is 2.1 μg/l. Titanium is also a contaminant of urban air (Table 17-3).

Absorption, Excretion, Toxicity. Approximately 3 percent of an oral dose of titanium is absorbed. The majority of that absorbed is excreted in the urine. The normal urine concentration has been estimated at 10 μg/l (Schroeder *et al.*, 1963a).

The estimated body burden of titanium is about 15 mg. Most of it is in the lungs, probably as a result of inhalation exposure. Inhaled titanium tends to remain in the lungs for long periods. It has been estimated that about one-third of the inhaled titanium is retained in the lungs. The geographic variation in lung burden is to some extent dependent on air concentration. For example, concentrations of 430, 1,300, and 91 ppm in ashed lung tissue have been reported for the U.S., Delhi, and Hong Kong, respectively. The mean concentrations of 8 and 6 ppm for the liver and kidney, respectively, were reported in the United States. Newborns have little titanium. Lung burdens tend to increase with age.

Slight fibrosis of lung tissue has been reported following inhalation exposure to titanium dioxide pigment, but the injury was not disabling. Otherwise, titanium dioxide has been considered physiologically inert by all routes (ingestion, inhalation, dermal, and subcutaneous) (AIHA, 1966c). The metal and other salts are also relatively nontoxic except for titanic acid, which, as might be expected, will produce irritation (Browning, 1969).

TUNGSTEN

Occurrence and Use. Wolframite ($[Fe,Mn]WO_4$) and scheelite are the chief ores of tungsten. It is used in making high-speed tool steel and in other alloys. In addition, tungsten is used in filaments for x-ray tubes, radio tubes, and light bulbs as well as in pigments and waterproofing textiles.

Absorption, Excretion, Toxicity. Tungsten is not a normal complement of animal tissues. It is absorbed to some extent from the gastrointestinal tract and retained largely in the bone, although smaller amounts have been assayed in the spleen, liver, and kidney.

The oral toxicity of tungsten compounds varies depending on the salt. The signs of toxicity by oral and parenteral administration are nervous prostration, diarrhea, coma, and death due to respiratory paralysis. Oral toxicity is apparently not a significant problem in man.

Some controversy exists over the effects of tungsten by inhalation. It is difficult to ascertain whether tungsten or cobalt is the causative agent in the pneumoconiosis of the tungsten carbide tool industry. Animal experiments suggest that the effects on the lungs are due not so much to tungsten itself as to other components, especially cobalt.

Tungsten has been shown experimentally to interact with two other elements. The addition of soluble tungsten to the diet reduced the mortality and liver lesions characteristic of high levels of selenium intake. Increased tungsten intake also decreased molybdenum deposition in the liver of rats and reduced intestinal xanthine oxidase. Sufficient amounts of tungsten caused molybdenum deficiency in chicks (Browning, 1969).

URANIUM

Occurrence and Use. The chief raw material of uranium is pitchblende or carnotite ore. This element is largely limited to use as a nuclear fuel.

Absorption, Excretion, Toxicity. The uranyl ion is rapidly absorbed from the gastrointestinal tract. About 60 percent is carried as a soluble bicarbonate complex, while the remainder is bound to plasma protein. Sixty percent is excreted in the urine within 24 hours. About 25 percent may be fixed in the bone (Chen *et al.*, 1961). Following inhalation of the insoluble salts, retention by the lungs is prolonged.

Uranium tetrafluoride and uranyl fluoride can produce a typical toxicity because of hydrolysis to HF. Skin contact (burned skin) with uranyl nitrate has resulted in nephritis (AIHA, 1969a).

The soluble uranium compound (uranyl ion) and those that solubilize in the body by the formation of a bicarbonate complex produce systemic toxicity in the form of acute renal damage. The classic impairment of renal function by uranium may result in death. However, if exposure is not severe enough, the renal tubular epithelium is regenerated and recovery occurs. Renal toxicity with the classic signs of impairment, including albuminuria, elevated blood urea nitrogen, and loss of weight, is brought about by filtration of the bicarbonate complex through the glomerulus, resorption by the proximal tubule, liberation of uranyl ion, and subsequent damage to the proximal tubular cells (Voegtlin and Hodge, 1949–1951; Passow et al., 1961).

Inhalation exposure of rats, dogs, and monkeys to uranium dioxide dust at a concentration of 5 mg U/M^3 for up to five years produced accumulation in the lungs and tracheobronchial lymph nodes that accounted for 90 percent of the body burden. No evidence of toxicity was observed despite the unusually long duration of the experimental investigation (Leach et al., 1970).

VANADIUM

Occurrence and Use. Vanadium occurs in several ores. Carnolite is one of commercial importance from which the metal is usually obtained. Vanadium can also be obtained as a by-product of petroleum refinement. Vanadium pentoxide is used as a catalyst in the production of various materials, of which sulfuric acid may be the most important. It is used in the hardening of steel, the manufacture of pigments, in photography, and in insecticides.

Various salts of vanadium have been used medicinally as an antiseptic, as a spirochetocide, as antituberculosis and antianemia agents, and as a general tonic. These uses are without proven efficacy (Sollmann, 1957). Vanadium is a ubiquitous element. It is common in many foods; significant amounts are found in milk, seafoods, cereals, and vegetables. Vanadium has a natural affinity for fats and oils; food oils have high concentrations. Municipal water supplies may contain on the average about 1 to 6 ppb. Urban air contains some vanadium, perhaps due to the use of petroleum products or from refineries (Table 17-3).

There has been some suggestion that vanadium is useful, if not essential, in various biologic systems. A hematopoietic effect has been postulated. Iron-deficient rats respond more rapidly to added iron in the diet when vanadium is also present. Vanadium also decreases cholesterol and phospholipid content in livers of experimental animals. An anticaries activity of vanadium has also been demonstrated under experimental conditions (Browning, 1969).

Absorption, Excretion, Toxicity. The average body burden of vanadium has been estimated at about 30 mg. The largest single compartment is the fat. Bone and teeth stores contribute to the body burden. It has been postulated that some homeostatic mechanism maintains the normal levels of vanadium in the face of excessive intake, since the element, in most forms, is moderately absorbed. The principal route of excretion of vanadium is the urine. The normal serum level is 35 to 48 μg/100 ml. When excess amounts of vanadium are in the diet, the concentration in the red cells tends to increase. Parenteral administration increases levels in the liver and kidney, but these increased amounts may only be transient. The lung tissue may contain some vanadium, depending on the exposure by that route, but normally the other organs contain negligible amounts (Schroeder et al., 1963b; Browning, 1969).

The toxic action of vanadium is largely confined to the respiratory tract. Bronchitis and bronchopneumonia are more frequent in workers exposed to vanadium compounds. In industrial exposures to vanadium pentoxide dust a greenish-black discoloration of the tongue is characteristic. Irritant activity with respect to the skin and eyes has also been ascribed to industrial exposure. Gastrointestinal distress, nausea, vomiting, abdominal pain, cardiac palpitation, tremor, nervous depression, and kidney damage, too, have been linked with industrial vanadium exposure.

Medicinal use of vanadium compounds (V_2O_5) produced gastrointestinal disturbances, slight abnormalities of clinical chemistry related to renal function, and nervous system effects. Acute vanadium poisoning in animals is characterized by marked effects on the nervous system, hemorrhage, paralysis, convulsions, and respiratory depression. Short-term inhalation exposure of experimental animals tends to confirm the effects on the lungs as well as the effect on the kidney. In addition, experimental investigations have suggested that the liver, adrenals, and bone marrow may be adversely affected by subacute exposure at high levels (Hudson, 1964; Browning, 1969). It has been postulated that heart disease is related to vanadium air pollution and it may act with cadmium to produce these adverse effects (Hickey et al., 1967).

ZINC

Occurrence and Use. The principal ore of zinc is sphalerite (largely ZnS). The principal uses of zinc are in the manufacture of galvanized iron, bronze, white paint, rubber, glazes, enamel, glass, and paper and as a wood preservative, $ZnCl_2$, for its fungicidal action.

Zinc is ubiquitous and is considered an essential trace element. Its necessary roles involve enzymes and enzymatic functions, protein synthesis, and carbohydrate metabolism. It is necessary for normal growth and development in mammals and birds. Human dwarfism and lack of sexual development have been related to zinc deficiency (Halsted *et al.*, 1974). Zinc is present in a number of metalloenzymes, including carbonic anhydrase, carboxypeptidase, alcohol dehydrogenase, glutamic dehydrogenase, lactic dehydrogenase, and alkaline phosphatase (Vallee, 1959).

Therapeutically, zinc compounds are used as topical astringents, dermal products, antiseptics, and emetics. The total exposure to zinc is increased through the widespread use of zinc undecylenate preparations for athlete's foot and zinc pyridinethione in antidandruff shampoos. Zinc is also contained in medicinal preparations of insulin and in zinc bacitracin. Veterinary uses of zinc are similar. In addition, zinc is used as a nutritional supplement to prevent or treat parakeratosis, a disease of pigs caused by zinc deficiency.

Zinc is omnipresent in the environment, being found in water, in air, and in all living organisms. In both natural and contaminated states it is almost always accompanied by cadmium. The zinc : cadmium ratio plays a vital role in the effect zinc has on living organisms. Zinc is found in natural water supplies, but the content may be increased if the water flows through galvanized, copper, or plastic pipes. Seafoods, meats, whole grains, dairy products, nuts, and legumes are high in zinc content. Vegetables are lower. Zinc applied to the soil is taken up in growing vegetables. Zinc atmospheric levels are increased over industrial areas. The average American daily intake is approximately 12.6 mg, mostly from food. Geographic variations in zinc tissue levels may be due to the reduction of zinc by the refining of grains (Schroeder *et al.*, 1967c).

Absorption, Excretion, Toxicity. Under normal conditions, not all of the zinc in the diet is absorbed. Phytate (inositol hexaphosphate) present in cereal grains markedly impairs the absorption of zinc, probably by forming an insoluble calcium-zinc-phytate complex in the upper small intestine. Normally, the muscle, liver, kidney, and pancreas contain large amounts. Relatively high concentrations of zinc are also found in the male reproductive system and the epididymis, prostate, and testes of various species. The eyes also contain high concentrations. The zinc in the blood is largely contained in the red blood cells. Data indicate that there are high levels of zinc in the newborn, but that the level decreases with age. Injection of ^{65}Zn has shown that the liver stores large amounts initially, but the red blood cells and the bone also tend to accumulate zinc. There is a correlation

between zinc plasma and bone concentrations, but the zinc concentrations of the kidney and liver may not be decreased in zinc deficiency.

Zinc is eliminated principally by the gastrointestinal tract. The pancreatic fluid contains significant amounts, while additional quantities are found in the bile. The urine contains significantly less than the feces (about 20 percent of fecal amounts). Milk also contains significant concentrations of zinc (Vallee, 1959; Schroeder *et al.*, 1967c).

The antagonistic action between cadmium and zinc in the rat with respect to increased growth, prevention of dermal lesions, interaction with copper metabolism, testicular damage, teratogenic changes, and maintenance of circulation and body temperature by adequate intake of zinc has been demonstrated. Therefore, it was suggested that, in a sense, cadmium could be considered as an antimetabolite of zinc (Petering *et al.*, 1971). Similar interactions between iron, copper, or molybdenum versus zinc have been suggested, but are not well documented.

Accidental oral poisoning has been reported in humans as a result of consuming acidic food or beverages from galvanized containers. The symptoms of such intoxications consist of fever, vomiting, stomach cramps, and diarrhea. These signs are typical of ingestion of large doses of soluble zinc compounds (Underwood, 1971). However, because these signs, especially the ones related to gastroenteritis, are similar to those resulting from ingestion of cadmium and the zinc in galvanized pans containing 1.0 percent cadmium, it was postulated that some of these cases may be due to cadmium (Schroeder *et al.*, 1967c).

With regard to industrial exposure, the metal fume fever resulting from inhalation of freshly formed fumes of zinc oxide presents the most significant effect. Only the freshly formed material is potent, presumably because of flocculation in the air, thereby preventing deep penetration into the lungs. After the initial response resulting in "chills," repeated exposures often cause no reaction. Workers have noted that this effect appears most frequently on Mondays or after holidays. The primary symptom, fever, has been reproduced in rabbits, and it was postulated that the increased body temperature is due to the action of the fumes on endogenous pyrogen in the leukocytes. Even in the most severe cases recovery is usually complete in 24 to 48 hours. There is no evidence that chronic effects have resulted from oxide inhalation (AIHA, 1969b). While zinc oxide fumes are the most common cause of metal fume fever, inhalation of other metal oxides may induce this reaction.

Dermal toxicity following exposure to $ZnCl_2$

has resulted from consistently handling these salts, and inhalation of mists or fumes may give rise to irritation of the gastrointestinal or respiratory tract. A gray cyanosis, dermatosis, and ulceration of the nasal passages have resulted from the inhalation of this caustic material.

The ocular hazard of zinc salts varies with the salt. Zinc chloride, while used as an astringent in eye drops at 0.2 to 0.5 percent, may cause damage at higher concentrations. Zinc sulfate in concentrations as high as 20 percent has been applied to the cornea for therapeutic purposes (Sollmann, 1957; Browning, 1969).

Attempts to produce zinc toxicity by incorporation of as much as 0.25 percent in the diet of rats have not been successful. At levels above this the homeostatic mechanism breaks down; growth retardation, hypochromic anemia, and defective mineralizations of bone occur. Displacement of copper and altered phosphatase activity are perhaps the mechanisms of action (Schroeder *et al.*, 1967c).

Zinc 2-pyridinethiol-oxide, an antidandruff agent, provides an example of a unique species-specific toxicity. This material in dogs causes blindness, resulting from retinal detachment, following nine oral daily doses of 25 mg/kg. Further studies did not reveal such effects at similar doses in monkeys or rodents. This effect in dogs is judged to be related to the chelation of zinc, which could be accomplished with sodium pyridinethione and hydroxypyridinethione in the tapetum lucidim of the dogs, a structure not present in man or monkeys. However, during the course of these investigations it was revealed that this zinc salt caused a cholinergic-like effect. Antidotal treatment of pyridoxine and nicotinic acid was lifesaving in the dog, but not in primates, suggesting different routes of metabolism (Snyder *et al.*, 1965; Winek and Buehler, 1966).

Testicular tumors have been produced by direct intratesticular injection in rats and chickens. This effect is probably related to the concentration of zinc normally in the gonads and may be hormonally dependent. Other routes have not produced carcinogenic effects by zinc salts (Sunderman, 1971).

ZIRCONIUM

Occurrence and Use.   Zircon ($ZrSiO_2$) is the primary ore of zirconium. It is used in the nuclear industry as a shielding material, in metal alloys, as a catalyst in organic reactions, in the manufacture of water-repellent textiles, in dyes, in pigments on ceramics, in abrasives, and cigarette lighter flints. The metallurgic difficulties probably prevent even wider application. Zirconium oxychloride has been used as an anti-

perspirant. Zirconium carbonate and oxide are used for dermatitis. Intravenous injection of zirconium has been advocated for prophylactic use to prevent skeletal deposition of certain radioelements, especially plutonium.

The daily oral intake in man has been estimated at 3.5 mg. Lamb, pork, eggs, dairy products, and grains contain the highest concentrations. Plant uptake of zirconium from soil and fertilizer has been demonstrated. Zirconium has been detected in rivers at 0.1 ppb. Because the common salts are insoluble, the water concentrations are of small and doubtful significance in urban water supplies.

Absorption, Excretion, Toxicity.   The average body burden is 250 mg. Fat, gallbladder, aorta, liver, red blood cells, diaphragm, lung, kidney, muscle, brain, pancreas, stomach, spleen, and testes have concentrations ranging from 18.7 in fat to 1.88 in testes in terms of micrograms per gram of tissue (wet weight). Zirconium is excreted by the intestine, probably in the bile. Zirconium levels are negligible in the urine. Milk is a secondary route of excretion. Significant amounts of zirconium are found in fetuses. While metabolism studies are lacking, tissue concentrations indicate that significant amounts of zirconium may be absorbed orally. It has been suggested that some homeostatic mechanism exists with respect to zirconium (Schroeder and Balassa, 1966b).

Inhalation exposure to water-soluble $ZrOCl_2$ indicated that the highest concentrations of zirconium occurred in the lungs and pulmonary lymph nodes. Deposition and retention in the bone (femur) were greater than in the liver (Spiegl *et al.*, 1956).

Granulomatous lesions, probably of allergic epithelioid origin, have been observed following the use of deodorant sticks and poison ivy lotions containing zirconium. Rabbits developed pulmonary granulomata following zirconium lactate exposure (Prior *et al.*, 1960; Epstein and Allen, 1964).

Inhalation exposure of $ZnCl_4$ (6 mg Zr/M^3) for 60 days produced slight decrease in hemoglobin and red blood count in dogs and increased mortality in rats and guinea pigs. Zirconium oxide at 75 mg/M^3 caused no effect (Spiegl *et al.*, 1956).

The oral toxicity of zirconium compounds is low. No evidence of industrial disease related to zirconium exposure has been documented (Stokinger, 1963; Browning, 1969).

REFERENCES

Aaseth, J.:   Mobilization of methyl mercury *in vivo* and *in vitro* using N-acetyl-DL-penicillamine and other complexing agents. *Acta Pharmacol. Toxicol.*, **39**:289–301, 1976.

Adams, R. G.; Harrison, J. F.; and Scott, P.: The development of cadmium-induced proteinuria, impaired renal function, and osteomalacia in alkaline battery workers. *Quart. J. Med.*, **38**:425–43, 1969.

Amdur, M. L.: Tellurium oxide. An animal study in acute toxicity. *Arch. Ind. Health*, **17**:665–67, 1958.

American Industrial Hygiene Association: Barium and its inorganic compounds. *Hygienic Guide*. Southfield, Mich., 1962.

——: Aluminum and aluminum oxide. *Hygienic Guide*. Southfield, Mich., 1963.

——: Lithium hydride. *Hygienic Guide*. Southfield, Mich., 1964a.

——: Tellurium. *Hygienic Guide*. Southfield, Mich., 1964b.

——: Arsine. *Hygienic Guide*. Southfield, Mich., 1965.

——: Cobalt. *Hygienic Guide*. Southfield, Mich., 1966a.

——: Nickel. *Hygienic Guide*. Southfield, Mich., 1966b.

——: Titanium dioxide. *Hygienic Guide*. Southfield, Mich., 1966c.

——: Nickel carbonyl. *Hygienic Guide*. Southfield, Mich., 1968a.

——: Osmium and its compounds. *Hygienic Guide*. Southfield, Mich., 1968b.

——: Uranium (natural and its compounds). *Hygienic Guide*. Southfield, Mich., 1969a.

——: Zinc oxide. *Hygienic Guide*. Southfield, Mich., 1969b.

Bakir, F.; Al-Khalidi, A.; Clarkson, T. W.; and Greenwood, R.: Clinical observations on treatment of alkylmercury poisoning in hospital patients. In Conference on Intoxication Due to Alkylmercury-treated Seed. *Bull. W.H.O.* (Suppl.), **53**:87–92, 1976.

Bakir, F.; Damluji, S. F.; Amin-Zaki, L.; Murtadha, M.; Khalidi, A.; Al-Rawi, N. Y.; Tikriti, S.; Dhahir, H. I.; Clarkson, T. W.; Smith, J. C.; and Doherty, R. A.: Methylmercury poisoning in Iraq. An interuniversity report. *Science*, **181**:230–41, 1973.

Barltrop, D., and Khoo, H. E.: The influence of nutritional factors on lead absorption. *Postgrad. Med. J.*, **51**:795–800, 1975.

Barnes, J. M., and Stoner, H. B.: Toxicology of tin compounds. *Pharmacol. Rev.*, **11**:211–31, 1959.

Barry, P. S. I.: A comparison of concentrations of lead in human tissues. *Br. J. Ind. Med.*, **32**:119–39, 1975.

Beal, R. W.: Hematinics I: Patho-physiological and clinical aspects. *Drugs*, **2**:190–206, 1971.

Bernard, A.; Roels, H.; Hubermont, G.; Buchet, J. P.; Masson, P. L.; and Lauwerys, R. R.: Characterization of the proteinuria in cadmium-exposed workers. *Int. Arch. Occup. Environ. Health*, **38**:19–30, 1976.

Bertinchamps, A. J.; Miller, S. T.; and Cotzias, G. C.: Interdependence of routes excreting manganese. *Am. J. Physiol.*, **211**:217–24, 1966.

Bidstrup, P. L.: *Toxicity of Mercury and Its Compounds*. Elsevier Publishing Company, London, 1964.

Bolanowska, W.; Piotrowski, J.; and Trojanowska, B.: The kinetics of distribution and excretion of lead (Pb^{210}) in rats. *Proceedings of the 14th International Congress of Occupational Health*, Madrid, Sept. 16–21, 1963. Excerpta Medica International Congress Series, No. 62, Vol. II, pp. 420–22.

Bornschein, R.; Reiter, L.; and Pearson, D.: Behavioral effects of moderate lead exposure in children and animal models. *Crit. Rev. Toxicol.*, **8**: issue 1 and 2, 1980.

Bothwell, T. H., and Finch, C. A.: *Iron Metabolism*. Little, Brown & Co., Boston, 1962.

Boyd, J. T.; Doll, R.; Faulds, J. S.; and Leiper, J.: Cancer of the lung in iron ore (hematite) miners. *Br. J. Ind. Med.*, **27**:97–105, 1970.

Britton, A. A., and Cotzias, G. C.: Dependence of manganese turnover on intake. *Am. J. Physiol.*, **211**:203–206, 1966.

Browning, E.: *Toxicity of Industrial Metals*, 2nd ed. Butterworths, London, 1969.

Burr, R. E.; Gotto, A. M.; and Beaver, D. L.: Isolation and analysis of renal bismuth inclusions. *Toxicol. Appl. Pharmacol.*, **7**:588–91, 1965.

Byron, W. R.; Bierbower, G. W.; Brouwer, J. B.; and Hansen, W. H.: Pathologic changes in rats and dogs from two-year feeding of sodium arsenite or sodium arsenate. *Toxicol. Appl. Pharmacol.*, **10**:132–47, 1967.

Catsch, A.: Radioactive metal mobilization. *Fed. Proc.*, **20**(3) Part II, Suppl. **10**:206–19, 1961.

Catsch, A., and Harmuth-Hoene, A.: New developments in metal antidotal properties of chelating agents. *Biochem. Pharmacol.*, **24**:1557–62, 1975.

Cerwenka, E. A., and Cooper, W. C.: Toxicology of selenium and tellurium and their compounds. *Arch. Environ. Health*, **3**:189–200, 1961.

Chamberlain, A. C.; Clough, W. S.; Heard, M. J.; Newton, D.; Stott, A. N. B.; and Wells, A. C.: Uptake of lead by inhalation of motor exhaust. *Proc. R. Soc. Lond.*, B., **192**:77–110, 1975.

Chang, L. W.: Neurotoxic effects of mercury—a review. *Environ. Res.*, **14**:329–73, 1977.

Chen, P. S.; Terepka, R.; and Hodge, H. C.: The pharmacology and toxicology of the bone seekers. *Anu.: Rev. Pharmacol.*, **1**:369–93, 1961.

Chisolm, J. J., Jr.: Treatment of acute lead intoxication—choice of chelating agents and supportive therapeutic measures. *Clin. Toxicol.*, **3**:527–40, 1970.

Choie, D. D.; Richter, G. W.; and Young, L. B.: Biogenesis of intranuclear lead-protein inclusions in mouse kidney. *Beitr. Pathol.*, **155**:197–203, 1975.

Chowdhury, P., and Louria, D. B.: Influence of cadmium and other trace metals on human α_1-antitrypsin: an *in vitro* study. *Science*, **191**:480–81, 1976.

Chuttani, H. K.; Gupti, P. S.; and Gultati, S.: Acute copper sulfate poisoning. *Am. J. Med.*, **39**:849–54, 1965.

Clarkson, T. W.: The pharmacology of mercury compounds. *Annu. Rev. Pharmacol.*, **12**:375–406, 1972.

Clarkson, T. W.; Small, H.; and Norseth, T.: Excretion and absorption of methyl mercury after polythiol resin treatment. *Arch. Environ. Health*, **26**:173–76, 1973.

Cole, J. F., and Lynam, D. R.: ILZRO's research to define lead's impact on man. *Proceedings of the International Symposium, Environmental Health Aspects of Lead*, Amsterdam, Oct. 2–6, 1972. Commission of the European Communities, Luxembourg, 1973, pp. 169–87.

Commission of the European Communities: *Criteria (Dose/Effect Relationships) for Cadmium*. Pergamon Press, Oxford, England, 1978.

Cooper, G. P., and Steinberg, D.: Effects of cadmium and lead on adrenergic neuro-muscular transmission in the rabbit. *Am. J. Physiol.*, **232**:C128–31, 1977.

Cotzias, G. C.; Papavasiliou, P. S.; Ginos, J.; Stechk, A.; and Duby, S.: Metabolic modification of Parkinson's disease and of chronic manganese poisoning. *Annu. Rev. Med.*, **22**:305–26, 1971.

Cremer, J. E.: Toxicology and biochemistry of alkyl lead compounds. *Occup. Health Rev.*, **17**(3):14–19, 1965.

Dale, P. W., and Patterson, M. B.: EEG findings in chronic rheumatoid arthritics receiving gold therapy. *Electroenceph. Clin. Neurophysiol.*, **23**:493–501, 1967.

Davis, G. K.: Toxicity of the essential minerals. In Food Protection Committee: *Toxicants Occurring Naturally in Foods*. National Academy of Sciences, Publ. No. 1354, Washington, D.C., 1966, pp. 229–35.

Davis, J. M., and Fann, W. E.: Lithium. *Annu. Rev. Pharmacol.*, 11:285–98, 1971.

Diplock, A. T.: Metabolic aspects of selenium action and toxicity. *Crit. Rev. Toxicol.*, 4:271–329, 1976.

Downs, W. L.; Scott, J. K.; Caruso, F. S. C.; and Wong, L. C. H.: The toxicity of niobium salts. *Am. Ind. Hyg. Assoc. J.*, 26:237–46, 1965.

Downs, W. L.; Scott, J. K.; Steadman, L. T.; and Maynard, E. A.: Acute and subacute toxicity studies of thallium compounds. *Am. Ind. Hyg. Assoc. J.*, 21:399–406, 1960.

Duckett, S.: Fetal encephalopathy following ingestion of tellurium. *Experientia*, 26:1239–41, 1970.

Enterline, P. E.: Respiratory cancer among chromate workers. *J. Occup. Med.*, 16:523–26, 1974.

Epstein, W. L., and Allen, J. J.: Granulomatous sensitivity after use of zirconium-containing poison oak lotions. *J.A.M.A.*, 190:940–43, 1964.

Fairbanks, V. F.; Fahey, J. L.; and Beutler, E.: *Clinical Disorders of Iron Metabolism*, 2nd ed. Grune & Stratton, Inc., New York, 1971.

Feldman, R. G.; Haddow, J.; Kopito, L.; and Schwachman, H: Altered peripheral nerve conduction velocity. Chronic lead intoxication in children. *Am. J. Dis. Child.*, 125:39–41, 1973.

Forbes, G. B., and Reina, J. C.: Effect of age on gastrointestinal absorption (Fe, Sr, Pb) in the rat. *J. Nutr.*, 102:647–52, 1972.

Foreman, H.: Toxicology: Inorganic. *Annu. Rev. Pharmacol.*, 2:341–62, 1962.

Fregert, S., and Rossman, H.: Allergy to trivalent chromium. *Arch. Dermatol.*, 90:406–11, 1964.

Freiman, D. G., and Hardy, H. L.: Beryllium disease. The relation of pulmonary pathology to clinical course and prognosis based on a study of 130 cases from the U.S. beryllium case registry. *Hum. Pathol.*, 1:25–44, 1970.

Freyberg, R. H.: Gold therapy for rheumatoid arthritis. In Hollander, J. L. (ed.): *Arthritic and Allied Conditions*, 7th ed. Lea & Febiger, Philadelphia, 1966.

Friberg, L.: Proteinuria and emphysema among workers exposed to cadmium and nickel dust in a storage battery plant. *Proc. Int. Cong. Ind. Med.*, 9:641–4, 1948.

————: Edathamil calcium-disodium in cadmium poisoning. *Arch. Ind. Health*, 13:18–23, 1956.

Friberg, L.; Piscator, M.; Nordberg, G. F.; and Kjellstrom, T. (eds.): *Cadmium in the Environment*, 2nd ed. CRC Press Inc., Cleveland, 1974.

Frost, D. V., and Lish, P. M.: Selenium in biology. *Annu. Rev. Pharmacol.*, 15:259–84, 1975.

Furst, A.: Trace elements related to specific chronic disease: cancer. In Cannon, H. L., and Hoops, H. C. (eds.): *Environmental Geochemistry in Health and Disease*. Geological Society of America, Boulder, CO., 1971, pp. 109–30.

Gage, J. C.: Mechanisms for the biodegradation of organic mercury compounds: the actions of ascorbate and soluble proteins. *Toxicol. Appl. Pharmacol.*, 32:225–38, 1975.

Ginsburg, J. M.: Renal mechanism for excretion and transformation of arsenic in the dog. *Am. J. Physiol.*, 208:832–40, 1965.

Goldwater, L. J.: *Mercury. A History of Quicksilver.* York Press, Baltimore, MD, 1972, p. xi.

Goodman, J. R., and Dallman, P. R.: Role of copper in iron localization in developing erythrocytes. *Blood*, 34:747–53, 1969.

Goyer, R. A.; Cherian, M. G.; and Richardson, L. D.: Renal effects of cadmium. *Proc. 1st International Cadmium Conference*, San Francisco, CA. Metal Bulletin Books Ltd., London, 1978, pp. 183–85.

Gralla, E. J., and McIlhenny, H. M.: Studies in pregnant rats, rabbits, and monkeys with lithium carbonate. *Toxicol. Appl. Pharmacol.*, 21:428–33, 1972.

Greengard, J., and McEnery, J. T.: Iron poisoning in children. *GP*, 37:88–93, 1968.

Gross, S. B.; Pfitzer, E. A.; Yeager, D. W.; Kehoe, R. A.: Lead in human tissues. *Toxicol. Appl. Pharmacol.*, 32:638–51, 1975.

Gruden, N.: Lead and active calcium transfer through the intestinal wall in rats. *Toxicology*, 5:163–66, 1975.

Gunsalus, I. C.: The chemistry and function of the pyruvate oxidation factor (lipoic acid). *J. Cell. Comp. Physiol.*, 41 (Suppl. 1):113–36, 1953.

Haley, T. J.: Pharmacology and toxicology of the rare earth elements. *J. Pharmacol. Sci.*, 54:663–70, 1965.

Haley, T. J.; Raymond, K.; Komesu, N.; and Upham, H. C.: Toxicologic and pharmacologic effect of hafnium salts. *Toxicol. Appl. Pharmacol.*, 4:238–46, 1962.

Halsted, J. A.; Smith, J. C., Jr.; and Irwin, M. I.: A conspectus of research on zinc requirements of man. *J. Nutr.*, 104:345–78, 1974.

Hammond, P. B.: The effect of chelating agents on the tissue distribution and excretion of lead. *Toxicol. Appl. Pharmacol.*, 18:296–310, 1971.

Harman, D.: The free radical theory of aging: Effect of age on serum copper levels. *J. Gerontol.*, 20:151–53, 1965.

Herman, M. M., and Bensch, K. G.: Light and electron microscopic studies of acute and chronic thallium intoxication in rats. *Toxicol. Appl. Pharmacol.*, 10:199–222, 1967.

Heydorn, K.: Environmental variation of arsenic levels in human blood determined by neutron activation analysis. *Clin. Chem. Acta*, 28:349–57, 1970.

Hickey, A. J.; Schoff, E. P.; and Clelland, R. C.: Relationships between air pollution and certain chronic disease death rates. *Arch. Environ. Health*, 15:728–38, 1967.

Hood, R. D., and Bishop, S. L.: Teratogenic effects of sodium arsenate in mice. *Arch. Environ. Health*, 24:62–65, 1972.

Hudson, T. F. F.: *Vanadium*. Elsevier, Amsterdam, 1964.

Hueper, W. C., and Payne, W. W.: Experimental studies in metal carcinogenesis. Chromium, nickel, iron, arsenic. *Arch. Environ. Health*, 5:445–562, 1962.

Hughes, E. R.; Miller, S. T.; and Cotzias, G. C.: Tissue concentrations of manganese and adrenal function. *Am. J. Physiol.*, 211:207–10, 1966.

Imbus, H. R.; Cholak, J.; Miller, L. H.; and Sterling, T.: Boron, cadmium, chromium, and nickel in blood and urine. A survey of American working men. *Arch. Environ. Health*, 6:286–95, 1963.

Itokawa, Y.; Abe, T.; Tabei, R.; and Tanaka, S.: Renal and skeletal lesions in experimental cadmium poisoning. *Arch. Environ. Health*, 28:149–54, 1974.

Kanisawa, M., and Schroeder, H. A.: Life time studies on the effect of trace elements on spontaneous tumors in mice and rats. *Cancer Res.*, 29:892–95, 1969.

Kazantzis, G.; Flynn, F. V.; Spowage, J. S.; and Trott, D. G.: Renal tubular malfunction and pulmonary emphysema in cadmium pigment workers. *Q. J. Med.*, 32:165–92, 1963.

Keall, M. H. H.; Martin, N. H.; and Turnbridge, R. E.: Three cases of accidental poisoning by sodium tellurite. *Br. J. Ind. Med.*, 3:175–76, 1946.

Kehoe, R. A.: On the toxicity of tetraethyl lead and inorganic lead salts. *J. Lab. Clin. Med.*, 12:554–60, 1927.

————: The metabolism of lead in man in health and disease. The Harben Lectures, 1960. *J. R. Inst. Pub. Health Hyg.*, 24:101–20, 1961.

Kety, S. S.: The lead citrate complex ion and its rôle in the physiology and therapy of lead poisoning. *J. Biol. Chem.*, 142:181–92, 1942.

Kjellstrom, T.: Accumulation and renal effects of cadmium in man. Ph.D. thesis. Karolinska Institute, Stockholm, Sweden, 1977.

Kostial, K., and Vouk, V. B.: Lead ions and synaptic transmission in the superior cervical ganglion of the cat. *Br. J. Pharmacol. Chemother.*, 12:219–22, 1957.

Kostial, K.; Šimonović, I.; and Pišonić, M.: Lead absorption from the intestine in newborn rats. *Nature*, 233:564, 1971.

Kyle, R. A.: Inorganic arsenic intoxication. In Sunderman, F. W., and Sunderman, F. W., Jr. (eds.): *Laboratory Diagnosis of Disease Caused by Toxic Agents.* Warren Green, Inc., St. Louis, MO, 1970, pp. 367–70.

Landolt, R. R.; Berk, H. W.; and Russell, H. T.: Studies on the toxicity of rhodium trichloride in rats and rabbits. *Toxicol. Appl. Pharmacol.*, 21:589–90, 1972.

Laug, E. P., and Kunze, F. M.: The penetration of lead through the skin. *J. Ind. Hyg. Toxicol.*, 30:256–59, 1948.

Lauwerys, R. R.; Buchet, J. P.; Roels, H. A.; Brouwers, J.; and Stanescu, D.: Epidemiological survey of workers exposed to cadmium. Effect on lung, kidney, and several biological indices. *Arch. Environ. Health*, 28:145–48, 1974.

Lauwerys, R. R.; Buchet, J. P.; and Roels, H.: The relationship between cadmium exposure or body burden and the concentration of cadmium in blood and urine in man. *Int. Arch. Occup. Environ. Health*, 36:275–85, 1976.

Leach, L. J.; Maynard, E. A.; Hodge, H. C.; Scott, J. K.; Yuile, C. L.; Sylvester, G. E.; and Wilson, H. B.: A five year inhalation study with uranium dioxide (UO₂) dust. I. Retention and biologic effect in the monkey, dog and rat. *Health Phys.*, 18:599–612, 1970.

Leber, A. P., and Miya, T. S.: A mechanism for cadmium- and zinc-induced tolerance to cadmium toxicity: Involvement of metallothionein. *Toxicol. Appl. Pharmacol.*, 37:403–14, 1976.

Lee, R. E.; Goranson, S. S., Enrione, R. E.; and Morgan, G. B.: The national air surveillance cascade impactor network. Part II. Size distribution measurements of trace metal components. Presented at American Chemical Society 163rd Meeting, Boston, MA, 1972.

Lundgren, K.-D.; Swensson, Å.; Ulfvarson, U.: Studies in humans on the distribution of mercury in the blood and the excretion in urine after exposure to different mercury compounds. *Scand. J. Clin. Lab. Invest.*, 20:164–66, 1967.

Magos, L.: Mercury-blood interaction and mercury uptake by the brain after vapor exposure. *Environ. Res.*, 1:323–37, 1967.

Manalis, R. S., and Cooper, G. P.: Presynaptic and postsynaptic effects of lead at the frog neuromuscular junction. *Nature*, 243:354–55, 1973.

Manzler, A. D., and Schreiner, A. W.: Copper-induced acute hemolytic anemia. A new complication of hemodialysis. *Ann. Intern. Med.*, 73:409–12, 1970.

Margoshes, M., and Vallee, B. L.: A cadmium protein from equine kidney cortex. *J. Am. Chem. Soc.*, 79:4813–14, 1957.

Martone, M. T.: A study of the effects of chronic inhalation of manganese dioxide in pigeons and rats. M.S. thesis. University of Rochester, 1964.

Matsusaka, N.; Inaba, J.; Ichikawa, R.; Ikeda, M.; and Ohkubo, Y.: Some special features of nucleotide metabolism in juvenile mammals. In Sikov, M. R., and Mahlum, D. D. (eds.): *Radiation Biology of the Fetal and Juvenile Mammal.* U.S. Atomic Energy Commission, 1969.

McConnell, K. P., and Portman, O. W.: Excretion of dimethyl selenide by the rat. *J. Biol. Chem.*, 195:277–82, 1952.

Mena, I.; Meurin, O.; Feunzobda, S.; and Cotzias, G. C.: Chronic manganese poisoning. Clinical picture and manganese turnover. *Neurology*, 17:128–36, 1967.

Mena, I.; Kazuko, H.; Burke, K.; and Cotzias, G. C.: Chronic manganese poisoning. Individual susceptibility and absorption of iron. *Neurology*, 19:1000–1006, 1969.

Mertz, W.: Chromium occurrence and function in biological systems. *Physiol. Rev.*, 49:163–239, 1969.

Moore, K. E., and Brody, T. M.: Effect of triethyltin on mitochondrial swelling. *Biochem. Pharmacol.*, 6:134–42, 1961.

Morgan, G. B.; Ozolins, G.; and Tabor, E. C.: Air pollution surveillance systems. *Science*, 170:289–96, 1970.

Morin, Y., and Daniel, P.: Quebec beer-drinkers cardiomyopathy: etiological considerations. *J. Can. Med. Assoc.*, 97:926–31, 1967.

Moxan, A. L., and Rhian, M.: Selenium poisoning. *Physiol. Rev.*, 203:305–37, 1943.

Muth, O. H. (ed.): *Symposium: Selenium in Biomedicine.* 1st International Symposium. Oregon State University, 1966. Westport, CT, 1967.

National Research Council: *Lead: Airborne Lead in Perspective.* National Academy of Sciences, Washington, D.C., 1972.

Nechay, B. R.; Williams, B. J.; Sleinsland, O. S.; and Hall, C. E.: Increased vascular response to adrenergic stimulation in rats exposed to cadmium. *J. Toxicol. Environ. Health*, 4:559–67, 1978.

Neff, N. H.; Barrett, R. E.; and Costa, E.: Selective depletion of caudate nucleus dopamine and serotonin during chronic manganese dioxide administration. *Experientia*, 25:1140–41, 1969.

Newman, J. A.; Archer, V. E.; Saccomanno, G.; Kuschner, M.; Auerbach, O.; Grondahl, R. D.; and Wilson, J. C.: Histologic types of bronchogenic carcinoma among members of copper-mining and smelting communities. *Ann. N.Y. Acad. Sci.*, 271:260–68, 1976.

Nogami, H., and Terashima, Y.: Thallium induced achondroplasia in the rat. *Teratology*, 8:101–102, 1973.

Nordberg, G. F. (ed.): *Effects and Dose-Response Relationships of Toxic Metals.* Elsevier Scientific Publishing Co., New York, 1976.

Okereke, T.; Sternlieb, I.; Morell, A. G.; and Sheinberg, I. H.: Systemic absorption of intrauterine copper. *Science*, 177:358–60, 1972.

Oppenheim, J. J., and Fishbein, W. N.: Induction of chromosome breaks in cultured normal human leukocytes by potassium arsenite, hydroxyurea and related compounds. *Cancer Res.*, 25:980–85, 1965.

Papavasiliou, P. S.; Miller, S. T.; and Cotzias, G. C.: Role of liver in regulating distribution and excretion of manganese. *Am. J. Physiol.*, 211:211–16, 1966.

Passow, H. A.; Rothstein, A.; and Clarkson, T. W.: The general pharmacology of the heavy metals. *Pharmacol. Rev.*, 13:185–224, 1961.

Patty, F. A.: Arsenic, phosphorous, selenium, sulfur, and tellurium. In Fassett, D. W., and Irish, D. D. (eds.): *Industrial Hygiene and Toxicology*, 2nd ed. Interscience, New York, 1963, pp. 871–910.

Pentschew, W.; Ebner, F. F.; and Kovatch, R. M.: Experimental manganese encephalopathy in monkeys. *J. Neuropathol. Exp. Neurol.*, 22:488–99, 1963.

Perry, H. M., Jr., and Erlanger, M. W.: Metal-induced hypertension following chronic feeding of low doses of cadmium and mercury. *J. Lab. Clin. Med.*, 83:541–47, 1974.

Petering, H. G.; Johnson, M. A.; and Slemmer, K. O.: Studies of zinc metabolism in the rat. *Arch. Environ. Health*, 23:93–101, 1971.

Prior, J. T.; Cronk, G. A.; and Ziegler, D. D.: Pathological changes associated with the inhalation of sodium zirconium lactate. *Arch. Environ. Health*, 1:297–300, 1960.

Prull, G., and Rompel, K.: EEG changes in acute poisoning with organic tin compounds. *Electroenceph. Clin. Neurophysiol.*, 29:215–22, 1970.

Rabinowitz, M.: Lead contamination of the biosphere by human activity. A stable isotope study. Ph.D. thesis. University of California at Los Angeles, 1974.

Rabinowitz, M. B.; Wetherill, G. W.; and Kopple, J. D.: Lead metabolism in the normal human: Stable isotope studies. *Science*, 182:725–27, 1973.

Rahola, T.; Aaran, R. K.; and Miettinen, J. K.: Half-time studies of mercury and cadmium by whole body counting. In *Assessment of Radioactive Contamination in Man*. International Atomic Energy Agency, Vienna, 1972.

Rastogi, S. C., and Clausen, J.: Absorption of lead through the skin. *Toxicology*, 6:371–76, 1976.

Reeves, A. L.: Beryllium in the environment. *Clin. Toxicol.*, 10(1):37–48, 1977.

Richards, M. P., and Cousins, R. J.: Mammalian zinc homeostasis: Requirement for RNA and metallothionein. *Biochem. Biophys. Res. Comm.*, 64:1215–23, 1975.

Robertson, D. S. E.: Selenium—a possible teratogen. *Lancet*, 1:518–19, 1970.

Robinson, I. M.: Effects of some organic tin compounds on tissue amine levels in rats. *Food Cosmet. Toxicol.*, 7:47–51, 1969.

Shamberger, R. J.; Tytko, S. A.; and Willis, C. E.: Antioxidants and cancer. Part VI. Selenium and age-adjusted human cancer mortality. *Arch. Environ. Health*, 31:231–35, 1976.

Schroeder, H. A.: The biological trace elements. *J. Chronic Dis.*, 18:217–28, 1965a.

————: Cadmium as a factor in hypertension. *J. Chronic Dis.*, 18:647–56, 1965b.

————: A sensible look at air pollution by metals. *Arch. Environ. Health*, 21:798–806, 1970.

Schroeder, H. A., and Balassa, J. J.: Abnormal trace metals in man: Niobium. *J. Chronic Dis.*, 18:229–41, 1965.

————: Abnormal trace elements in man: Arsenic. *J. Chronic Dis.*, 19:85–106, 1966a.

————: Abnormal trace metals in man: Zirconium. *J. Chronic Dis.*, 19:573–86, 1966b.

————: Abnormal trace metals in man: germanium. *J. Chronic Dis.*, 20:211–24, 1967.

Schroeder, H. A., and Mitchener, M.: Scandium, chromium (VI), gallium, yttrium, rhodium, palladium, indium in mice. Effects on growth and life span. *J. Nutr.*, 101:1431–38, 1971.

————: Selenium and tellurium in mice. *Arch. Environ. Health*, 24:66–71, 1972.

Schroeder, H. A.; Balassa, J. J.; and Tipton, I. H.: Abnormal trace metals in man: Nickel. *J. Chronic Dis.*, 15:51–65, 1962a.

————: Abnormal trace metals in man: Chromium. *J. Chronic Dis.*, 15:941–64, 1962b.

————: Abnormal trace metals in man: Titanium. *J. Chronic Dis.*, 16:55–69, 1963a.

————: Abnormal trace metals in man: Vanadium. *J. Chronic Dis.*, 16:1047–71, 1963b.

————: Essential trace metals in man: Manganese. *J. Chronic Dis.*, 19:545–71, 1966a.

————: Essential trace metals in man: Molybdenum. *J. Chronic Dis.*, 23:481–99, 1970a.

Schroeder, H. A.; Balassa, J. J.; and Vinton, W. H.: Chromium, cadmium, and lead in rats. Effects on life span, tumors, and tissue levels. *J. Nutr.*, 86:51–66, 1965.

Schroeder, H. A.; Buckman, J.; and Balassa, J. J.: Abnormal trace elements in man: Tellurium. *J. Chronic Dis.*, 20:147–61, 1967a.

Schroeder, H. A.; Frost, D. V.; and Balassa, J. J.: Essential trace metals in man: Selenium. *J. Chronic Dis.*, 23:227–43, 1970b.

Schroeder, H. A.; Mitchener, M.; Balassa, J. J.; Kanisawa, M.; and Nason, A. P.: Zirconium, niobium, antimony, and fluorine in mice. Effects on growth, survival and tissue levels. *J. Nutr.*, 95:95–101, 1968a.

Schroeder, H. A.; Mitchener, M.; and Nason, A. P.: Zirconium, niobium, antimony, vanadium, and lead in rats. Life term studies. *J. Nutr.*, 100:59–68, 1970c.

Schroeder, H. A.; Nason, A. P.; and Mitchener, M.: Action of a chelate of zinc on trace metals in hypertensive rats. *Am. J. Physiol.*, 214:796–800, 1968b.

Schroeder, H. A.; Nason, A. P.; and Tipton, I. H.: Essential trace metals in man: Cobalt. *J. Chronic Dis.*, 20:869–90, 1967b.

————: Essential metals in man: Magnesium. *J. Chronic Dis.*, 21:815–41, 1969.

————: Chromium deficiency as a factor in atherosclerosis. *J. Chronic Dis.*, 23:123–42, 1970d.

Schroeder, H. A.; Nason, A. P.; Tipton, I. H.; and Balassa, J. J.: Essential trace metals in man: Copper. *J. Chronic Dis.*, 19:1007–34, 1966b.

————: Essential trace metals in man: Zinc. Relation to environmental cadmium. *J. Chronic Dis.*, 20:179–210, 1967c.

Scott, J. K., and Hodge, H. C.: Nonabsorbable dusts. In DiPalma, J. R. (ed.): *Drill's Pharmacology in Medicine*, 4th ed. McGraw-Hill Book Co., New York, 1971, pp. 1249–52.

Sellers, E. A.; You, R. W.; and Lucas, C. C.: Lipotropic agents in liver damage produced by selenium or carbon tetrachloride. *Proc. Soc. Exp. Biol. Med.*, 75:118–21, 1950.

Seppäläinen, A. M.; Tola, S.; Hernberg, G.; and Kock, B.: Subclinical neuropathy at "safe" levels of lead exposure. *Arch. Environ. Health*, 30:180–83, 1975.

Sisson, T. R. C.: Acute iron poisoning in children. *Q. Rev. Pediatr.*, 15:47–49, 1960.

Skog, E., and Wahlberg, J. E.: A comparative investigation of the percutaneous absorption of metal compounds in the guinea pig by means of the radioactive isotopes: ^{51}Cr, ^{58}Co, ^{65}Zn, ^{110m}Ag, ^{115m}Cd, ^{203}Hg. *J. Invest. Dermatol.*, 43:187–92, 1964.

Smith, R. G.; Vorwald, A. J.; Patil, L. S.; and Mooney, T. F.: Effects of exposure to mercury in the manufacture of chlorine. *Am. Ind. Hyg. Assoc. J.*, 31:687–700, 1970.

Snider, G. L.; Hayes, J. A.; Korthy, A. L.; and Lewis, G. P.: Centrilobular emphysema experimentally induced by cadmium chloride aerosol. *Am. Rev. Resp. Dis.*, 108:40–48, 1973.

Snyder, F. H.; Buehler, E. V.; and Winek, C. L.: Safety evaluation of zinc 2-pyridinethiol 1-oxide in a shampoo formulation. *Toxicol. Appl. Pharmacol.*, 7:425–37, 1965.

Sollmann, T.: *Manual of Pharmacology*. W. B. Saunders Co., Philadelphia, 1957, pp. 1191–1354.

Spiegl, C. J.; Calkins, M. C.; DeVoldre, J. J.; Scott, J. K.; Steadman, L. T.; and Stokinger, H. E.: Inhalation toxicity of zirconium compound. I. Short term studies. Univ. Rochester Atomic Energy Report No. UR 460, 1956.

Spiegl, C. J.; LaFrance, L.; and Ashworth, B. J.: Blood and urine changes in experimental beryllium poisoning. *Arch. Ind. Hyg. Occup. Med.*, 7:319–25, 1953.

Sprince, N. L.; Kanarek, D. J.; Weber, A. L.; Chamberlin, R. I.; and Kazemi, H.: Reversible respiratory disease in beryllium workers. *Am. Rev. Resp. Dis.*, 117:1011–17, 1978.

Stocken, L. A., and Thompson, R. H. S.: British Anti-Lewisite. 2. Dithiol. compounds as antidotes for arsenic. *Biochem. J.*, 40:535–54, 1946.

Stokinger, H. E.: The metals (excluding lead). In Fassett, D. W., and Irish, D. D. (eds.): *Industrial Hygiene and Toxicology*, Vol. II. Interscience, New York, 1963, pp. 987–1194.

Stokinger, H. E. (ed.): *Beryllium: Its Industrial Hygiene Aspects*. Academic Press, Inc., New York, 1966.

Sunderman, F. W., Jr.: Nickel poisoning. In Sunderman, F. W., and Sunderman, F. W., Jr. (eds.): *Laboratory Diagnosis of Diseases Caused by Toxic Agents*. Warren Green, Inc., St. Louis, 1970, pp. 389–95.

————: Metal carcinogenesis in experimental animals. *Fed. Cosmet. Toxicol.*, 9:105–20, 1971.

Swensson, Å., and Ulfvarson, U.: Distribution and excretion of mercury compounds in rats over a long period following a single injection. *Acta Pharmacol. Toxicol.*, 26:273–83, 1968.

Tepper, L. B.: Beryllium. *Crit. Rev. Toxicol.*, 1:261–81, 1972.

Tersinger, J.: Biochemical responses to provocative chelation by edetate disodium calcium. *Arch. Environ. Health*, 23:280–93, 1971.

Thomas, R. G.; Thomas, R. L.; and Scott, J. K.: Distribution and excretion of niobium following inhalation exposure of rats. *Am. Ind. Hyg. Assoc. J.*, 28:1–7, 1967.

Tola, S.; Hernberg, S.; Asp, S.; and Nikkanen, J.: Parameters indicative of absorption and biological effect in new lead exposure: A prospective study. *Br. J. Ind. Med.*, 30:134–41, 1973.

Underwood, W. J.: *Trace Elements in Human and Animal Nutrition*. Academic Press, Inc., New York, 1971.

U.S. Public Health Service: *Public Health Service Drinking Water Standards*. U.S. Government Printing Office, Washington, D.C., 1962.

————: *Community Water Supply Study: Analysis of National Survey Findings*. U.S. Department of Health, Education and Welfare, Washington, D.C., 1970.

Valek, A.: Acute renal insufficiency in intoxication with mercury compounds. I. Aetiology, clinical picture, renal function. *Acta Med. Scand.*, 177:63–67, 1965.

Vallee, B. L.: Biochemistry, physiology and pathology of zinc. *Physiol. Rev.*, 39:443–90, 1959.

Vander, A. J.; Taylor, D. L.; Kalitis, K.; Mouw, D. R.; and Victery, W.: Renal handling of lead in dogs: clearance studies. *Am. J. Physiol.*, 233(6):F532–38, 1977.

Verschuuren, H. G.; Ruitenberg, E. J.; Peetoom, F.; Helleman, P. W.; and VanEsch, G. J.: Influence of triphenyltin acetate on lymphatic tissue and immune response in guinea pigs. *Toxicol. Appl. Pharmacol.*, 16:400–10, 1970.

Voegtlin, C., and Hodge, H. C. (eds.): *The Pharmacology and Toxicology of Uranium Compounds*, Vols. 1–4. McGraw-Hill Book Co., New York, 1949–1951.

Washko, P. W., and Cousins, R. J.: Role of dietary calcium and calcium binding protein in cadmium toxicity in rats. *J. Nutr.*, 107:920–28, 1977.

Webb, M., and Verschoyle, R. D.: An investigation of the role of metallothioneins in protection against the acute toxicity of the cadmium ion. *Biochem. Pharmacol.*, 25:673–79, 1976.

WHO, Task Group on Environmental Health: *Environmental Health Criteria. 1. Mercury*. World Health Organization, Geneva, 1976.

————: *Environmental Health Criteria. 3. Lead*. World Health Organization, Geneva, 1977.

Wiśniewska-Knypl, J. M.; Jablońska, J.; and Myślak, Z.: Binding of cadmium on metallothionein in man: An analysis of a fatal poisoning by cadmium iodide. *Arch. Toxicol.*, 28:46–55, 1971.

Wills, J. H., Jr.: Goitrogens in foods. In Food Protection Committee: *Toxicants Occurring Naturally in Foods*. National Academy of Sciences Publication No. 1354, Washington, D.C., 1966, pp. 3–17.

Winek, C. L., and Buehler, E. V.: Intravenous toxicity of zinc pyridinethione and several zinc salts. *Toxicol. Appl. Pharmacol.*, 9:269–73, 1966.

Wong, L. C. K., and Downs, W. L.: Renal effects of potassium niobate. *Toxicol. Appl. Pharmacol.*, 9:561–70, 1966.

Ziegler, E. E.; Edwards, B. B.; Jensen, R. L.; Mahaffey, K. R.; and Fomon, S. J.: Absorption and retention of lead by infants. *Pediatr. Res.*, 12:29–34, 1978.

Zielhuis, R. L.: Dose-response relationships for inorganic lead. *Int. Arch. Occup. Health*, 35:1–18, 19–35, 1975.

Chapter 18

SOLVENTS AND VAPORS

Herbert H. Cornish

INTRODUCTION

Organic solvents and their vapors are a common part of our modern environment, both at work and in the home. Incidental exposures may be of short duration and to low levels of solvent vapor and, thus, for the most part may be undetected. This would include such normally minimal exposures to gasoline vapors, lighter fluids, aerosol sprays of various types, and spot removers. More serious exposures may develop with the individual use of paint removers, floor and tile cleaners, and other solvents in the home, as well as industrial situations where large quantities of solvents may be used in manufacturing and processing operations. Information on sources of industrial exposure to various types of solvents and vapors may be found in numerous publications (Browning, 1953; Patty, 1963). Since organic solvents number in the hundreds, an attempt will be made here to cover the toxicity and metabolism of only commonly used solvents representing a variety of chemical structures.

Several points relevant to the discussion of solvents and vapors should be made at this time. Vapors are the gaseous form of volatilized liquids, and concentrations are usually expressed in parts per million (ppm) in air. In contrast to the common use of ppm to designate weight ratios in solids or liquids, when ascribed to air concentrations the term represents volumes of vapor per million parts, by volume, of the contaminated air at 25° C and 760 mm Hg pressure. Thus, 1 mole of any vapor (equal volume) distributed in a given volume of air represents equivalency in ppm although the weights of the vaporized materials could be considerably different. For a description of appropriate calculations and conversion from grams per liter of air to ppm, it is recommended that one refer to a textbook of industrial hygiene and toxicology such as that by Patty (1958).

Since one of the major areas of concern with respect to solvent toxicity and vapor inhalation is industrial workers, considerable effort has gone into both animal and human studies in attempts to determine safe levels of exposure for the work environment (see Chap. 28). The compilation and evaluation of these data have been undertaken by the American Conference of Governmental Industrial Hygienists (ACGIH) and have resulted in the yearly publication of their guide entitled *Threshold Limit Values of Airborne Contaminants* (1977). They indicate that "threshold limit values (TLVs) refer to airborne concentrations of substances and represent conditions under which it is believed that nearly all workers may be repeatedly exposed, 8 hours a day, without adverse effects. Threshold limit values refer to time-weighted concentrations for a 7- or 8-hour workday and 40-hour workweek. They should be used as guides in the control of health hazards and should not be used as fine lines between safe and dangerous concentrations." For the toxicologist, it is important to remember that TLVs do not necessarily relate directly to systemic toxicity but may also be set on the basis of eye or skin irritation, narcosis, nuisance, or other forms of stress that would be undesirable in the work environment. Thus, it would be dangerous to attempt to utilize TLVs as a basis for comparison of the systemic toxicity of chemicals without a thorough understanding of the information incorporated into the setting of the individual guidelines.

Where individuals may be exposed to mixtures of vapors, the combined effect may be additive, antagonistic, or potentiating depending on the mechanism of toxicity. Where the toxic response to two chemicals may be similar (i.e., anesthesia), the effects can be considered additive and suitable calculations utilized to estimate a TLV value for the mixture (ACGIH, 1977). Where antagonistic or potentiating effects are known to occur between two chemicals (as with ethanol and carbon tetrachloride), the combined toxicity can only be determined experimentally.

Many of the early effects of inhaled vapors relate to effects on the central nervous system, which has not, to date, lent itself to easy measurement and interpretation of data in experimental animals. However, the development of new toxicologic techniques and the accumulation of fundamental knowledge on the biochemistry of behavior should soon make a most valuable contribution to our understanding of the effects of inhaled vapors on the central nervous system.

ALIPHATIC HYDROCARBONS (PARAFFINS)

The straight-chain hydrocarbons with less than four carbon atoms are gases and are present in natural gas (methane, ethane) and in bottled gas (propane, butane). Methane and ethane are simple asphyxiants and do not produce general systemic effects. The higher-molecular-weight aliphatic hydrocarbons are liquids, and inhalation of the vapor produces central nervous system depression resulting in dizziness and incoordination. Extremely high levels of C_5 to C_8 hydrocarbon vapor (pentane, hexane, heptane, octane) levels produce death in experimental animals (Gerarde, 1960).

A number of widely used commercial products are mixtures of hydrocarbons. These include gasoline, kerosene, and a number of industrial solvents such as Stoddard solvent.

C_5 to C_8 Aliphatic Hydrocarbons

Recent studies of exposure to the C_5 to C_8 hydrocarbon vapors suggest that some of them may not be quite as innocuous as previously reported. Pentane, hexane, heptane, and octane occur in solvents not only as straight-chain hydrocarbons but also in a variety of isomeric forms. Pentane is a major constituent of gasoline while hexane, heptane, and octane have extensive use as general solvents and in glues, varnish, inks, and fat extraction procedures. Inhalation of the vapor from these solvents produces central nervous system depression resulting in dizziness and incoordination. Extremely high levels of exposure may produce death in experimental animals (Gerarde, 1960).

Yamamura (1969) in a study of sandal production in Japan reported 93 workers with polyneuropathy. All of these workers had been engaged in the home production of sandals utilizing a glue whose solvent contained at least 60 to 70 percent of n-hexane. The effects noted were muscular weakness and sensory impairment of the extremities. In a biopsy study of the anterior tibial muscles, Yamamura noted demyelination and axonal degeneration of the peripheral nerves.

In a later study, Iida et al. (1973) reported that after two years 51 of the 93 patients had recovered and after four years 82 had recovered completely.

Subsequently, several investigators have reported symptoms of polyneuropathy in workers exposed to aliphatic solvents containing high concentrations of n-hexane (Yamada, 1972; Yoshida, 1974). Several additional cases of polyneuropathy in industrial workers have been reported where the mixed solvent exposure, although containing n-hexane, has been primarily to other alkanes (Galtier, 1973; Abbritti et al., 1976). Animal studies tend to confirm the neurologic effects of n-hexane. Miyagaki (1967) exposed mice to commercial hexane (65 to 70 percent n-hexane) for 24 hours a day, six days a week for one year. Exposure levels ranged from 100 to 2,000 ppm. Atrophy and degeneration of the hind leg muscle fibers was present in animals exposed to 1,000 and 2,000 ppm. Physiologic measurements showed effects at 250 and 500 ppm. Only the 100-ppm-exposed group failed to show neurologic effects in mice.

Truhaut (1973) reported that both hexane (2,000 ppm) and heptane (1,500 ppm) exposures for one to six months produced neurophysiologic effects in Wistar rats and retractions of the myelin nerve sheaths and in some instances rupture of Schwann cell membranes. Technical grade solvents were used in these studies. Metabolic studies (DeVincenzo, 1976) suggest that n-hexane and the neurotoxin methyl butyl ketone share a number of common metabolites, including 5-hydroxy-2-hexanone and 2,5-hexanediol, which have been shown to be neurotoxic (Spencer and Schaumburg, 1977).

Gasoline and Kerosene

Gasoline and kerosene are primarily mixtures of hydrocarbons, including not only aliphatic hydrocarbon but, particularly in the case of gasoline, a variety of branched and unsaturated hydrocarbons, as well as aromatic hydrocarbons.

In spite of the widespread use of gasoline and the intermittent vapor exposure encountered by gas station attendants and the home auto mechanic, toxic effects do not normally occur under these conditions. Some types of gasoline contain a considerable amount of benzene and could present a hazard that would be difficult to assess in the exposed population.

Extremely high-level exposures to gasoline vapor may result in dizziness, coma, collapse, and death. Exposure to high nonlethal levels is usually followed by complete recovery, although cases of permanent brain damage following massive exposure have been reported (Machle, 1941). Gerarde (1963) suggests that atmospheric concentrations of approximately 2,000 ppm are not safe to enter for even a brief time. No threshold limit value (TLV) has been set for gasoline since its composition varies widely. In general, the toxicity is related to the content of benzene and other aromatic hydrocarbons. Other additives could also alter the overall toxicity of gasoline.

Stoddard Solvent

Stoddard solvent is a typical mixture of primarily aliphatic hydrocarbons, with some naphthenes and benzene derivatives, which is used extensively in degreasing operations and as a paint thinner. Its toxicologic effects are similar to those discussed for gasoline.

All of the liquid hydrocarbons are fat solvents and, as such, defat the skin resulting in dryness, scaling, and dermatitis. Dermatitis is the most common industrial problem associated with the use of such solvents.

An important toxicologic problem associated with the hydrocarbon solvents is the inadvertent or intentional ingestion of gasoline, kerosene, or paint thinners. Although in most instances the acute toxicity of these compounds is quite low, small amounts may be aspirated into the lungs during ingestion, during attempts to induce vomiting, or while pumping the stomach. The response of the lung to small quantities of hydrocarbon solvents is rapid and severe. Relatively small amounts will spread in a thin layer over the large moist surfaces of the lung resulting in pneumonitis, pulmonary edema, and hemorrhage (Gerarde, 1963). Thus, depending on the nature of the solvent and the clinical condition of the patient, it may be unwise to attempt to remove small quantities of such solvents from the stomach.

HALOGENATED HYDROCARBONS, ALIPHATIC

The excellent solvent power of these materials, combined with generally low flammability, has resulted in their being among the most widely used industrial solvents. While the common biologic effect of these compounds is anesthesia, they also vary from practically nontoxic (freons) to those with rather marked vapor toxicity (carbon tetrachloride).

Methylene Chloride (Methylene Dichloride, Dichloromethane, CH_2Cl_2)

Methylene chloride is a volatile solvent with wide general applications as an aerosol propellant, paint stripper, degreasing solvent, and fat extractant. In common with other low-molecular-weight halogenated hydrocarbons, methylene chloride is a central nervous system depressant and may be fatal at high concentrations.

The fatal exposure level (seven hours) for mice is approximately 17,000 ppm (Svirbely, 1947). Heppel

et al. (1944) exposed dogs, rabbits, rats, and guinea pigs to 5,000 ppm, seven hours per day, five days a week for periods up to six months. Three of fourteen guinea pigs and one exposed rat died during the exposure period. At termination of the study kidney, liver, and central nervous system function appeared unaltered. After similar exposures at 10,000 ppm moderate centrilobular congestion and fatty degeneration were noted in two of four exposed dogs. Haun et al. (1972) exposed 200 mice at 100 and 25 ppm for 100 days. The authors report decreased levels of cytochrome P-450 at 100 ppm, with cytochrome b5 and P-420 reduced at 30 days but elevated at 90 days. At 25 ppm these parameters were comparable to those of unexposed control rats.

Human controlled exposure to methylene chloride has demonstrated decreased performance in psychomotor tasks at approximately 300, 500, and 750 ppm after three to four hours (Winneke, 1974). Exposure at 50 or 100 ppm was without effect. The epidemiologic data of exposed workers as recently reviewed (NIOSH, 1976) cite evidence of exposed individuals reporting malaise, insomnia, headache, and heart palpitations. Clinical and laboratory examinations were negative. Unfortunately, these individuals were, in all instances, exposed to mixtures of solvents in the work atmosphere, and the exposure levels are not usually known. Certainly there are no reports of generalized health problems associated with the controlled use of this solvent in industry. As with all central nervous system depressant solvents, there are individual case reports of extreme overexposure resulting in hospitalization and death (Moskowitz and Shapiro, 1952; Stewart and Hake, 1976).

Stewart et al. (1972) made the interesting discovery of elevated carboxyhemoglobin (COHb) levels in an individual using a paint stripper containing methylene chloride. In subsequent human studies, maximum COHb levels of 5.7 percent were observed in nonsmokers exposed to 100 ppm for 7.5 hours (Stewart et al., 1973). Exposure to 500 ppm for 7.5 hours resulted in maximum COHb levels of approximately 12 percent. Daily exposure on the same schedule normally resulted in maximum values at the end of the daily exposure period. Residual COHb levels did not return to baseline values by the following morning.

Several reports indicate that experimental animals also convert methylene chloride to CO. Fodor et al. (1973) reported that a three-hour exposure to 100 ppm of methylene chloride produced 6.2 percent COHb while a similar exposure to 1,000 ppm resulted in a COHb level of 12.5 percent. When a CO exposure of 100 ppm was simultaneous with the three-hour methylene chloride exposure, the COHb levels were essentially additive, the CO exposure alone accounting for a COHb level of 10.9 percent. Hogan (1976) reported a similar finding and in addition noted that the rat reached a maximal COHb level of approximately 7 percent even though methylene chloride exposure was continually increased.

This presumably represents a saturation of the metabolic pathway leading to CO formation or possibly a feedback inhibition of a CO-sensitive pathway (Hogan, 1976). Rodkey and Collison (1977a) have reported that in a closed rebreathing system utilizing $^{14}CH_2Cl_2$, as much as 47 percent was found as ^{14}CO and only 29 percent as $^{14}CO_2$ after a 15-hour period, thus providing further evidence that the CO arises directly from methylene chloride rather than by a stimulation of endogenous CO production. These investigators also noted that several other dihalomethanes, including CH_2Br_2, CH_2BrCl, and CH_2I_2, are metabolized to CO in the rat (Rodkey and Collison, 1977b).

Although early reports in the literature were somewhat confusing with respect to the site of metabolism of methylene chloride, more recent data have confirmed that the conversion to CO does occur through the mixed-function oxidase system (Kubic and Anders, 1975; Hogan, 1976).

Chloroform (CHCl₃)

The primary effect of chloroform is central nervous system depression with inebriation, anesthesia, and narcosis.

Chloroform can be absorbed through the lung, from the gastrointestinal tract, and to some extent through the skin. The inhalation route is, of course, the primary source of chloroform absorption in man. Inhalation toxicology of $CHCl_3$ in animals has been summarized by von Oettingen (1955). Mice exposed to 8,000 ppm of $CHCl_3$ died after three hours of exposure, rabbits died after a two-hour exposure to 12,500 ppm, while dogs survived much higher concentrations. Acute chloroform exposure may result in death by respiratory arrest. The primary toxic response at lower levels of exposure is hepatotoxicity leading to fatty liver and centrilobular necrosis.

Kidney damage may also occur in animals after acute poisoning, primarily in the convoluted tubules, but it may also affect the epithelium of Henle's loops.

Watrous and Plaa (1972) demonstrated that chloroform as well as carbon tetrachloride partially inhibited the accumulation of p-aminohippuric acid in rat kidney slices, indicating an effect of these solvents on the active transport of p-aminohippuric acid after small doses were given to rats one day prior to sacrifice. Cohen and Hood (1969), utilizing low-temperature autoradiography, demonstrated the long-term retention of $CHCl_3$ in body fat, with an increased radioactivity occurring in liver during the postexposure period. Thin-layer chromatography also established the presence of two nonvolatile metabolites in liver.

Van Dyke and coworkers (1964) had demonstrated that after a single injection of ^{14}C-labeled chloroform, $^{14}CO_2$ appeared in the expired air 12 hours later, with 4 to 5 percent of the total dose being exhaled as $^{14}CO_2$, and up to 2 percent of ^{14}C-labeled metabolites appearing in the urine. This represents considerable metabolism of a type of compound usually thought of as biologically stable. In this same study utilizing ^{36}Cl-labeled chloroform, measurable but variable quantities of labeled compounds appeared in the urine, largely in the inorganic form.

Dingell and Heimberg (1968) reported a 40 percent inhibition of microsomal drug-metabolizing enzyme activity in rats fed 1.05 ml/kg of $CHCl_3$ 24 hours prior to sacrifice. This may be related to the degree of hepatic necrosis produced by $CHCl_3$ or to a more subtle effect on the microsomal enzyme system. That this oxidizing system is involved in the metabolism of $CHCl_3$ would be expected because of its structural relationship to CCl_4, where considerable evidence has been developed that implicates this enzyme system with metabolism and toxicity. In the case of $CHCl_3$, Scholler (1970) also reports that the hepatotoxicity of $CHCl_3$ in rats is markedly enhanced by pretreatment with phenobarbital, a known inducer of the microsomal oxidizing system.

It is becoming more apparent that, in a number of instances, the toxic response to seemingly inert chemicals may be related to the metabolism of these compounds and the production of small quantities of unknown metabolites that can have a profound effect on important biologic processes.

Carcinogenicity of chloroform has been evaluated in several animal species. A National Cancer Institute study (1976a) was conducted utilizing B6C3F mice and Osborne-Mendel rats.

Animals were dosed orally five times a week for 78 weeks. Male rats received doses of 90 or 180 mg/kg body weight while female rats were started at 125 or 250 mg/kg and reduced to 90 and 180 mg/kg after 22 weeks. At sacrifice the most significant findings were kidney epithelial tumors in male rats as follows: 0 percent in controls, 8 percent in the low-dose, and 24 percent in the high-dose group. No statistical differences were found between the incidence of kidney tumors in treated female rats and the control group. The mice were started at 35 days of age and initially dosed at 100 and 200 mg/kg for males and 200 and 400 mg/kg for females. After 18 weeks these levels were increased to 150 and 300 mg/kg for males and 238 and 477 mg/kg for females. At sacrifice (92 to 93 weeks) a high incidence of hepatocellular carcinoma was noted. At the high dose, a 98 percent and 95 percent incidence for males and females was noted, and a 36 percent and 80 percent incidence for males and females at the low dose was found, compared with 6 percent in control males, and 0 percent to 1 percent in control females and colony control females. Nodular hyperplasia of the liver was observed in many low-dose animals that had not developed hepatocellular carcinoma. These studies indicate that chloroform has the potential to produce cancer in experimental animals, and this potential biologic activity must be taken into account when attempting to develop safe levels of exposure for man.

Carbon Tetrachloride (CCl₄)

This compound has been more extensively studied than any other chlorinated aliphatic hydrocarbon. It is relatively inexpensive and an excellent solvent, and these factors led originally to its widespread industrial use and its common occurrence in spot removers and other household solvents. However, CCl_4 is now being restricted in its use as a household solvent and will be found primarily in industrial situations. In industry too, it is being replaced in many instances by less toxic solvents.

Carbon tetrachloride, like chloroform, has anesthetic properties leading to confusion, incoordination, and coma. Liver damage may result from either acute or chronic exposure. Characteristically, fatty liver develops first in animals exposed to low levels of CCl_4. A greater exposure results in centrilobular necrosis, and in man this is at times followed by kidney failure, which may be the ultimate cause of death.

The relative ease with which CCl_4 produces fatty liver and liver necrosis in experimental animals has led to its widespread rise as a tool in biochemical studies of liver function and liver damage (see Chap. 10). As a result, a great volume of literature has become available on its hepatotoxicity in various species (Klaassen and Plaa, 1966; Judah, 1969; Fowler, 1970; Grice *et al.*, 1971). Studies of the biochemical events that lead to cellular necrosis (Slater, 1968; Srinivasan and Recknagel, 1971) and development of a variety of techniques to measure the extent of hepatotoxicity of CCl_4 have been published (Cornish and Block, 1960a; Klaassen and Plaa, 1966).

An extensive toxicologic study in rats, guinea pigs, rabbits, and monkeys was reported by Adams and coworkers (1952) and provides the following information. A seven-hour exposure, five days a week, to 400 ppm resulted in more than 50 percent mortality in rats and guinea pigs during a 127-day exposure study. Increased liver and kidney weight was evident. Fatty degeneration and cirrhosis of the liver were noted on histologic examination, along with slight degeneration of kidney tubular epithelium. In exposure of rats, rabbits, guinea pigs, and monkeys to 100 ppm of CCl_4 for 146 to 163 exposures, histopathologic changes were found in liver, being borderline in the monkey. At exposure levels of 10 ppm, rats and guinea pigs showed mild fatty liver develop-

ment and increased liver weights, while rabbits were normal.

In a study of repeated daily exposure of rats to CCl_4 vapor (Cornish and Block, 1960b), it was shown that after several days' exposure to relatively low levels of CCl_4, rats would suddenly develop transient elevations of serum glutamic-oxaloacetic transaminase (SGOT) activity, which would return to normal within 24 hours even though exposure was continued. This suggests a possible accumulation of CCl_4 in tissues, resulting in a concentration that becomes sufficient to bring about the release of cellular enzymes from damaged cells into the bloodstream where they can be conveniently utilized as a measure of hepatotoxicity (Cornish, 1971). In these studies, it was also apparent that the female rat was more susceptible to CCl_4-induced hepatotoxicity than was the male rat.

Klaassen and Plaa (1966) reported comparative studies of a series of halogenated hydrocarbons in mice. CCl_4 and $CHCl_3$ were reported to produce moderate to severe hepatic dysfunction, 1,1,2-trichloroethane produced moderate dysfunction, and mild dysfunction could be demonstrated with 1,1,1-trichloroethane, trichloroethylene, and tetrachloroethylene only when these solvents were administered at near-lethal doses. Renal dysfunction was found only in mice treated with $CHCl_3$ and 1,1,2-trichloroethane. A study of dogs (Klaassen and Plaa 1967) produced somewhat similar findings with CCl_4 producing liver dysfunction at doses less than any of the other halogenated hydrocarbons. Chloroform, 1,1,2-trichloroethane, and tetrachloroethylene produced altered renal function in dogs. In rat kidney slices (Watrous and Plaa, 1972) CCl_4, $CHCl_3$, and 1,1,2-trichloroethane partially inhibited the accumulation of p-aminohippuric acid in rat kidney slices. This could be demonstrated with doses of CCl_4 as low as 0.005 ml/kg of body weight injected into the rat one day prior to sacrifice.

For detailed review and historic development of the study of mechanisms of CCl_4 toxicity, one should consult the extensive reviews available in the literature (Judah and Rees, 1959; Plaa and Larson, 1964; McLean *et al.*, 1965; Recknagel, 1967). The brief summary presented here is based on these reviews and more recent publications.

The development of fatty liver as a result of CCl_4 exposure has been a focal point of interest for many years. Early studies attempted to determine whether fatty liver resulted from increased mobilization from fat depots, increased rate of triglyceride synthesis, decreased ability to release triglyceride from liver into the bloodstream, or a decreased rate of lipid oxidation (Recknagel *et al.*, 1958; Lombardi and Ugazio, 1965; Poggi *et al.*, 1965). Early reports of CCl_4 toxicity demonstrated an effect on the tricarboxylic acid cycle in liver mitochondria both *in vivo* and *in vitro* (Christie and Judah, 1954) along with uncoupling of oxidative phosphorylation (Dianzani, 1954). Effects of CCl_4 on mitochondria, *in vivo* and *in vitro*, have also been demonstrated by electron microscopy (Artizzu *et al.*, 1963; Ashworth *et al.*, 1963). Mitochondria from livers of rats exposed to CCl_4 showed, along with uncoupling of oxidative phosphorylation, altered oxidative pathways and ATP-ase activation (Recknagel and Anthony, 1957; Calvert and Brody, 1958; Recknagel and Anthony, 1959; Reynolds *et al.*, 1962). Fatty acid metabolism was also impaired (Recknagel and Anthony, 1959; Reynolds *et al.*, 1962). That impairment of the oxidative capacity of mitochondria was a prerequisite to fatty liver development was seriously questioned by the finding that fatty liver development occurred very early after CCl_4 exposure during time periods when liver mitochondrial activity appeared to be maintained (Recknagel and Lombardi, 1961).

Triglyceride accumulation in liver as a result of massive discharge of the sympathetic nervous system was first proposed by Brody (1959) as a possible mechanism to account for both CCl_4-induced fatty liver and necrosis. Additional supporting evidence led to the suggestion that diminished hepatic blood flow and subsequent centrilobular hypoxia, coupled with enhanced fatty acid mobilization from lipid depots, would adequately account for CCl_4-produced fatty liver (Brody, 1963). Remarkable protection against CCl_4 toxicity had resulted from spinal cord transection. Larsson and Plaa (1965) demonstrated that loss of temperature control with resulting hypothermia and decreased oxygen consumption accompanied protection in cord-sectioned animals. Cord-sectioned animals maintained at room temperature were not protected against CCl_4 toxicity; conversely, normal animals whose body temperature had been lowered by immersion in cold water were protected in a manner comparable to that of cord-sectioned animals. Thus, the catecholamine hypothesis could not, of itself, account for fatty liver development in CCl_4-treated animals.

With respect to the correlation between plasma fatty acid elevation and hepatic triglyceride levels after CCl_4 treatment, the data indicate that plasma elevation is not well correlated with liver accumulation suggesting that lipid mobilization of itself does not account for fatty liver development (Maximchuk and Rubinstein, 1963; Rees and Shotlander, 1963; Stern *et al.*, 1965). Additional data reviewed by Recknagel also lead to this conclusion (1967).

Studies of the impairment of hepatic secretion of triglycerides into the bloodstream received new emphasis from reports that a variety of studies had shown that CCl_4 markedly reduced the transfer of triglycerides from liver to plasma (Recknagel *et al.*, 1960; Rees and Shotlander, 1963; Poggi and Paoletti, 1964; Poggi *et al.*, 1965). With the injection of palmitate-1-^{14}C into rats, Maling and associates (1962) demonstrated their rapid incorporation into liver triglycerides but their relatively low level in the plasma triglycerides of CCl_4-treated rats, also suggesting an impaired triglyceride release from liver. The demonstration that hepatic triglyceride synthesis is still functional after carbon tetrachloride poisoning strengthens liver synthesis and impaired

release as the apparent mechanism accounting for fatty liver development (Recknagel, 1967). Since triglycerides are released from the liver as low-density lipoproteins, evidence for the early inhibition of protein synthesis by carbon tetrachloride led support to the theory that failure of lipoprotein synthesis might account for the failure of the liver to properly release triglycerides (Smuckler *et al.*, 1962; Seakins and Robinson, 1963). Recknagel (1967) reviews in detail the data relating to the role of protein synthesis and lipoprotein release from the liver. He concludes that, although depression of protein synthesis is an early and prominent feature of carbon tetrachloride damage, it does not appear that protein synthesis is the major factor in hepatic triglyceride accumulation. Rather, he suggests a possible effect on the coupling of triglyceride and acceptor protein in the formation of hepatic lipoprotein.

With respect to the mechanism by which CCl_4 produces its toxic effects, there is growing evidence that activation of CCl_4 is a prerequisite to hepatotoxicity. McCollister and coworkers (1951) and Rubinstein and Kanics (1964) demonstrated that CCl_4 is metabolized to CO_2 in experimental animals. Butler (1961) demonstrated the *in vitro* conversion of CCl_4 to chloroform by rat liver and suggested the formation of free radicals that might then react with enzymes or other tissue constituents. The free radical mechanism has been further advanced, and it is suggested (Recknagel, 1967) that the early changes noted as a result of carbon tetrachloride toxicity, including morphologic alteration of endoplasmic reticulum (Bassi, 1960; Ashworth *et al.*, 1963), effect on drug-metabolizing enzymes (Dingell and Heimberg, 1968; Sasame *et al.*, 1968; Davis *et al.*, 1971), loss of glucose-6-phosphate activity (Recknagel and Lombardi, 1961), and effects on protein synthesis (Smuckler *et al.*, 1962), are at least in part the result of a primary attack by split products of CCl_4 metabolism on lipoidal elements of the endoplasmic reticulum. Fowler and Alexander (1969) reported a new metabolite of carbon tetrachloride as being CCl_3CCl_3. The presence of such a metabolite could most likely be accounted for by condensation of two free radicals ($\cdot CCl_3$) resulting from carbon tetrachloride metabolism. The suggested effect of free radical metabolites on lipid peroxidation as a major initiator of biochemical toxicity does not preclude the effect of such free radicals or other metabolites directly on proteins or other biologic systems.

That carbon tetrachloride toxicity is related to metabolism is further supported by studies such as those of Dambrauskas and Cornish (1970) that demonstrated a marked resistance to CCl_4 exposure in animals that had received a previous exposure. Glende (1972) in subsequent studies found that low doses of carbon tetrachloride resulted in a 75 percent inhibition of the activity of the microsomal aminopyrine demethylase enzyme system, and at this time the animals were quite resistant to carbon tetrachloride toxicity. This is taken as further evidence of the relationship of the microsomal mixed-function oxidase system or a related system to the metabolism of carbon tetrachloride and the production of toxic metabolites. At present there is no direct evidence for the *in vivo* homolytic cleavage of carbon tetrachloride to yield free radicals, but the experimental evidence cited above makes this hypothesis a most attractive one. It is also consistent with evidence that antioxidants offered some protection against carbon tetrachloride poisoning (Gallagher, 1962) and with the peroxidation of lipid that has been reported in rat liver after carbon tetrachloride administration (Recknagel and Ghoshal, 1966; Klaassen and Plaa, 1969).

Further evidence of the effect of carbon tetrachloride on the microsomal enzyme system is reported by Sasame and coworkers (1968), who demonstrated a decrease in the amount of cytochrome P-450 in the liver of carbon tetrachloride-treated rats. This decrease was not attributable to destruction of liver cells, but to more subtle effects on cytochrome P-450. Subsequently, Davis and associates (1971) confirmed the reduction in cytochrome P-450 in livers of carbon tetrachloride-treated rats, accompanied by an inhibition of ethylmorphine demethylase activity. In animals pretreated with phenobarbital, the inhibitory effect was enhanced. Diaz Gomez *et al.* (1975) have recently shown in five animal species that a better correlation exists between irreversible $^{14}CCl_4$ binding to cellular components than between lipid peroxidation and the development of liver necrosis.

The cumulative data on the metabolism of carbon tetrachloride, its oxidant effects, and its relationship to alterations in activity of the microsomal enzyme system all support the hypothesis that metabolism is a prerequisite to carbon tetrachloride hepatotoxicity.

Data on the carcinogenic potential of carbon tetrachloride have recently been summarized in a National Academy of Sciences report (1977). Recent long-term studies by the National Cancer Institute (1976b) have shown significant increases in hepatocellular carcinomas in both male and female rats at the high dose levels, after 78 weeks of oral dosing at 0, 47, and 94 mg/kg/day for males and 0, 80, and 150 mg/kg/day for females. Thus, carbon tetrachloride does have carcinogen potential as demonstrated in experimental animals. In treated animals marked hepatotoxicity with fibrosis, bile duct proliferation, and regeneration was observed. In male and female mice (B6C3F1) receiving 1,250 or 2,500 mg CCl_4/day/kg body weight the incidence of hepatocellular carcinoma was nearly 100 percent.

Methyl Chloroform (1,1,1-Trichloroethane, Cl₃CCH₃)

Methyl Chloroform (1,1,1-Trichloroethane, Cl_3CCH_3)

Methyl chloroform has received widespread acceptance as an industrial solvent since it has many of the solvent and volatility characteristics of carbon tetrachloride. Like the other halogenated hydrocarbons solvents, methyl chloroform has a depressant action on the central nervous system.

Irish (1963) reports that humans exposed to 2,000 ppm exhibited drunkenness and incoordination. Exposures at 1,000 ppm showed no significant response in individuals exposed for as long as 70 minutes. Irish also reports that only two fatal cases are known and they occurred in a tank where the concentration may well have been close to saturation. Acute vapor exposures in animals, as reported by Adams and coworkers (1950), indicated that rats could survive a seven-hour exposure at 8,000 ppm. At 3,000 ppm, rabbits and monkeys showed no abnormal response over a two-month period. The acute LD50 in male rats is approximately 12 g/kg and in female rats approximately 10 g/kg. Experimental human exposures to 500 ppm of methyl chloroform for 6.5 to 7 hours per day for five days gave no evidence of abnormal organ function as measured by a variety of clinical laboratory tests. Ability to perceive the odor decreased during the exposure period. The subjective responses obtained during the exposure were mild and inconsistent except for the complaint of drowsiness (Stewart *et al.*, 1969).

Studies of the comparative toxicity of a series of halogenated hydrocarbons (Klaassen and Plaa, 1969; Watrous and Plaa, 1972) have demonstrated that in experimental animals, near-lethal doses of 1,1,1-trichloroethane are required to produce a measurable hepatotoxic response to a single dose. As shown in these same reports, 1,1,2-trichloroethane is considerably more toxic than 1,1,1-trichloroethane; thus it is apparent that one must be certain of the correct identification of chemical compounds in order to prevent confusion and error in defining their toxicity.

1,1,1-Trichloroethane has considerable use as an aerosol propellant; thus, the potential for overexposure due to misuse of such products needs to be considered. Reinhardt *et al.* (1973) recently reported on the epinephrine-induced cardiac arrhythmia potential of a number of common halogenated solvents, including 1,1,1-trichloroethane. In a recent report in dogs, Egle *et al.* (1976) reported that 1,1,1-trichloroethane did not cause cardiac sensitization at exposure concentrations of 5,000 ppm used in their study. This solvent, however, has been shown to be a cardiac depressant at extremely high exposure levels (approximately 50,000 ppm) (Taylor *et al.*, 1976).

The metabolism of 1,1,1-trichloroethane is also somewhat different from that of 1,1,2-trichloroethane in that it is partially metabolized to trichloroethanol and to a lesser extent to trichloroacetic acid (Ikeda and Ohtsuji, 1972). The overall metabolism of 1,1,1-trichloroethane was considerably less than that of trichloroethylene. Although some metabolism of 1,1,2-trichloroethane was apparent, the low levels made identification of the products uncertain.

Trichloroethylene $Cl_2C{=}CHCl$

Trichloroethylene is widely used as an industrial solvent in degreasing and extraction processes as well as in the dry-cleaning industry. The toxicity of trichloroethylene has been included in a number of reviews (Browning, 1965; Smith, 1966).

Overexposure to trichloroethylene produces central nervous system depression resulting in mental confusion, incoordination, and insomnia. The acute response of experimental animals to trichloroethylene vapor has been reported by Adams and co-workers (1951). At 3,000 ppm, a six-month daily exposure resulted in increased liver and kidney weights. Rats and rabbits exposed for a six-month period to 200 ppm showed no effect. Baker (1958) reported severe changes in the cerebellum, particularly in the Purkinje cell layers in dogs chronically exposed to trichloroethylene. Fatal cases of trichloroethylene exposure reported by Kleinfeld and Tabershaw (1954) showed no tissue abnormalities at autopsy. Death was evidently due to cardiac arrhythmia resulting from the potentiation of endogenous epinephrine by trichloroethylene. Comparative studies on the hepatotoxicity of chlorinated hydrocarbons demonstrated that large, near-fatal acute doses were required to produce mild hepatic dysfunction. In this respect, the acutely toxic response was comparable to that seen with 1,1,1-trichloroethane.

Butler (1949) indicated that trichloroacetic acid, trichloroethanol, and small amounts of chloroform and monochloroacetic acid were the metabolic products of trichloroethylene. Several early reports had attempted to relate the concentration of trichloroacetate in urine to the inhalation exposure to trichloroethylene in man (Ahlmark and Forssman, 1951).

Additional studies on the metabolism of trichloroethylene (Bartonicek, 1962; Stewart et al., 1970a) confirm the major metabolites of trichloroethylene as trichloroacetic acid (TCA) and trichloroethanol (TCE). In general, considerably more TCE is excreted than TCA. For example, in animal studies (Ikeda and Ohtsuji, 1972) rats excreted five to seven times more TCE than TCA after being exposed to trichloroethylene. With respect to the toxicity of these metabolites, Mikiskova and Mikiska (1966) demonstrated that trichloroethanol had a pronounced depressant effect on the central nervous system and suggested that the rate of metabolism of trichloroethylene appeared sufficient for trichloroethanol to play a role in its depressant action.

Since trichloroethylene has a rather long biologic half-life (Stewart et al., 1970a; Ikeda et al., 1972), major consideration must be given to cumulative effects of this compound. The report of Ikeda and coworkers (1972) points out that at a daily exposure level of approximately 100 ppm,

only one-third of the retained trichloroethylene (calculated) is excreted as metabolites in the urine during the work day. Stewart and associates (1970a) had also reported that metabolite excretion gradually increased during repeated daily exposures suggestive of a cumulative effect.

The study of individuals in 17 workshops (Ikeda et al., 1972) demonstrates that urinary excretion of TCE was proportional to the atmospheric concentration of trichloroethylene, confirming reports of its usefulness in following exposure of individuals to this vapor. TCA excretion in urine was proportional to exposure with vapor concentrations up to 50 ppm but not at higher levels of exposure. Thus, it appears that measurement of metabolites in urine may be a useful index of exposure, but as with most measurements of this type, they should be utilized in addition to air analyses of the workroom and adequate control of the exposure.

A long-term oral feeding study of trichloroethylene was carried out by the National Cancer Institute (1976b). Osborne-Mendel rats and B6C3F1 mice, both sexes, were used in the study. Male and female rats received 1,097 or 549 mg/kg while male mice received 2,339 mg/kg or 1,169 mg/kg and female mice received 1,739 or 869 mg/kg body weight. Animals were given the solvent in corn oil, five days a week for 78 weeks. Neither male nor female rats demonstrated any carcinogenic potential associated with trichloroethylene when they were sacrificed 90 weeks after initial treatment. However, in mice, at both low and high dose levels, in both sexes, there was a highly significant increase in hepatocellular carcinomas. For males, 26/50 low-dose and 31/48 high-dose animals had hepatocellular carcinomas compared to 1/20 matched controls and 5/77 colony controls. For females 4/50 low-dose and 11/47 high-dose animals had hepatocellular carcinomas compared with 0/20 in matched controls and 1/80 in colony controls.

Schwetz et al. (1975) exposed rats to 300 ppm of trichloroethylene, seven hours per day on days 6 through 15 of gestation. No teratogenic effects were found in this study.

Tetrachloroethylene (Perchloroethylene, $CCl_2{=}CCl_2$)

Tetrachloroethylene has considerable use in degreasing operations and in dry cleaning. Although relatively few industrial problems appear to arise from the use of this compound, there have been reports of hepatotoxicity as well as the central nervous system effects (Irish, 1963).

In chronic inhalation studies (Carpenter, 1937; Rowe et al., 1952) daily exposure to 1,600 ppm in air resulted in kidney and liver enlargement within one week. In daily exposures over a period of months to levels below 100 ppm, no effects were noted except for an increase in liver weight in the guinea pig, which seemed to be unusually susceptible to this solvent. At approximately 500 ppm, pathologic changes were present in both liver and kidney. At 400 ppm for 130 seven-hour exposures over 183 days, no evidence of damage was seen in the monkey, rabbit, or rat. However, the guinea pig had increased liver weight. In comparative studies of acute toxicity (Klaassen and Plaa, 1966), hepatic dysfunction was found only with the administration of near-lethal single acute doses of tetrachloroethylene and was quite comparable to trichloroethylene in this respect.

Tetrachloroethylene is excreted largely by the lungs (Stewart *et al.*, 1970b). The metabolism of tetrachloroethylene is relatively slow with only a few percent of the dose being excreted as metabolites, the major one being trichloroacetic acid (Ikeda and Ohtsuji, 1972).

A long-term inhalation study by Rampy *et al.* (1977) at exposure levels of 300 to 600 ppm tetrachloroethylene resulted in some deaths in the high-level-exposure male rat group. Although tumors were present in a number of animals, the incidence was not different in control and exposed animals.

Recently, the National Cancer Institute has reported the results of its long-term carcinogenicity study in mice and rats (1977). B6C3F male mice were fed tetrachloroethylene for 78 weeks at 536 or 1,072 mg/kg/day while female mice received 386 or 772 mg/kg/day for the same period. More than 50 percent of the male mice and 40 percent of the female mice developed hepatocellular carcinoma. Similar cancers developed in 12 percent or less of the vehicle treated and untreated control groups. In the same study, Osborne-Mendel rats showed no significant increase in cancer incidence under comparable experimental procedures. A high incidence of kidney damage was noted in both rats and mice in this study.

ALIPHATIC ALCOHOLS

The aliphatic alcohols are straight or branched-chain alcohols that have a wide application as industrial solvents. It is interesting that, of this series, only ethanol has the appropriate physiologic effect, metabolic pathway, and general low order of toxicity that has resulted in its widespread use as an alcoholic beverage. As a result of this use, ethanol has been extensively studied in both man and animals, and thus there is a massive literature relating to all aspects of its metabolism and its biologic effects. For this reason, and particularly because of the close relationship of ethanol and methanol metabolism, ethanol will be considered first in this series.

Ethanol (Ethyl Alcohol, C_2H_5OH)

Ethanol has widespread use as an industrial and laboratory solvent, but human exposure resulting from its use in these situations is insignificant compared with the vast quantities ingested as alcoholic beverages. Thus, although in unusual work situations the inhalation of ethanol could result in symptoms of alcohol intoxication, in most situations resulting in on-the-job injuries, the source of ethanol is not job related.

Ethanol is rapidly absorbed from the gastrointestinal tract and normally metabolized and excreted in a relatively few hours. The review by Kalant (1971) discusses the absorption, distribution, and elimination of ethanol and the role these factors may play in metabolic studies of ethanol.

An additional recent review (Hawkins and Kalant, 1972) points out that in studies measuring the rate of metabolism of ethanol, a variety of techniques may be utilized. These include (1) the measurement of the rate of $^{14}CO_2$ production from ^{14}C-labeled ethanol, which depends not only on the conversion of ethanol to acetaldehyde and acetate but also on the rate of acetate oxidation to CO_2 and thus should be utilized under carefully controlled and restricted conditions; (2) measurement of residual ethanol in tissues after controlled dosage; and (3) the rate of disappearance of ethanol from blood. All these techniques suffer from certain inherent difficulties that make it difficult to compare the data obtained on the rate of metabolism of ethanol in different species and under different conditions. Similar difficulties arise in the interpretation of data obtained by *in vitro* techniques with a variety of animal species and under varying conditions of oxygenation, substrate concentrations, and cofactor additions. Videla and Israel (1970) point out that incubation of liver slices under oxygen (90 to 100 percent) results in a considerable increase in the rate of ethanol metabolism over that obtained at 16 percent oxygen and that the effect may be due to an indirect effect of oxygen on the reoxidation of cofactors required for ethanol metabolism.

Studies of a clinical nature in man, particularly those involving alcoholics, seem to generally agree that the alcoholic shows less of a response to a given dose of ethanol, or to the same blood level of ethanol, than does the nonalcoholic. Clinical studies, however, have also varied widely in the choice of subjects, dose of ethanol or whiskey, nutritional state, and measurements of response. Nevertheless, the development of tolerance to ethanol has been well documented (Mello and Mendelson, 1970). Considerable study has gone into attempts to understand the mechanism by which tolerance develops. Two major alternatives have been proposed to account for alcoholic tolerance: an increased rate of alcohol metabolism and a decreased cellular response to ethanol. In addition to tolerance development, physical dependence also apparently develops in chronic alcoholism. A report by Davis and Walsh (1970) suggested an unusual mechanism for the development of physical dependence. Incubations of rat brainstem homogenates with dopamine, ascorbic acid, NAD$^+$, and ethanol or acetaldehyde in phosphate buffer resulted in an increased production of the alkaloid tetrahydropapaveroline (THP). The authors make the suggestion that alcoholism may be true addiction resulting from the role of ethanol or acetaldehyde in the *in vivo* formation of morphine-type alkaloids.

Metabolism of Ethanol. A number of excellent reviews contain information on the metabolism of ethanol (Wallgren and Barry, 1970; Kalant, 1971; Lundquist, 1971a; Hawkins and Kalant, 1972).

Hepatic alcohol dehydrogenase (ADH) is considered the enzyme primarily responsible for the oxidation of ethanol to acetaldehyde. This particular enzyme has been extensively investigated with respect to its structure and reaction mechanisms (Theorell, 1967; Wong and Williams, 1968). The reaction catalyzed by ADH is as follows:

$$CH_3CH_2OH + NAD^+ \longrightarrow$$
$$NADH + H^+ + CH_3CHO$$

Thus, the reaction requires nicotine adenine dinucleotide (NAD$^+$), which is reduced during the oxidation of ethanol to acetaldehyde.

ADH is a zinc-containing enzyme, with horse liver ADH containing four atoms of zinc. Removal of two atoms of zinc by dialysis or chemical techniques abolishes enzymatic activity (Weiner, 1969). Two sulfhydryl (—SH)-containing polypeptide chains give an overall dimer structure that can be dissociated into two inactive units and recombined to yield several isoenzymes (Jornvall and Harris, 1970). Atypical variants of ADH, having different pH optima, have been reported in human liver (Smith *et al.*, 1971), and possible relationships of such variants to alcohol metabolism and alcoholism are being investigated (Edwards and Evans, 1967). An important aspect of the metabolism of ethanol is the conversion of NAD$^+$ to NADH$_2$, which results in a significant decrease in the overall NAD$^+$/NADH$_2$ ratio in liver (Slater *et al.*, 1964). This shift in ratio may play a most important role in critical biochemical reactions, thus accounting for some of the metabolic effects of ethanol. Other mechanisms that have been implicated in the metabolism of ethanol are the enzyme catalase and the microsomal oxidizing systems (MOS).

Catalase, coupled with a hydrogen peroxide-generating system, will oxidize ethanol directly to acetaldehyde. This reaction will take place in rat liver homogenates (Griffaton and Lowry, 1964) and will oxidize not only ethanol, but methanol and other alcohols. The *in vivo* functioning of this system may, however, be limited by the slow rate of formation of hydrogen peroxide in tissues (Lundquist, 1970). Catalase inhibition by 3-amino-1,2,4-triazole does not alter the rate of metabolism of ethanol *in vivo*, further evidence that catalase is not an important factor in ethanol metabolism under normal conditions (Smith, 1961).

It has also been reported that a microsomal oxidizing system can oxidize both methanol and ethanol to their corresponding aldehydes. Hawkins and Kalant (1972) review these findings in considerable detail and point out that much of the evidence concerning the role of this oxidizing system in ethanol metabolism depends on the specificity of the various inducers (Lieber and DeCarli, 1970a) and inhibitors (Isselbacher and Carter, 1970; Khanna *et al.*, 1970; Lieber and DeCarli, 1970b) that have been used and that none are sufficiently specific to permit a definitive answer.

Induction of the microsomal oxidizing system by phenobarbital failed to increase the rate of ethanol metabolism *in vivo* (Tephly *et al.*, 1969; Khanna and Kalant, 1970). The chronic administration of ethanol has been reported to increase the amount of smooth endoplasmic reticulum (SER) in liver (Rubin *et al.*, 1968) and increases the activity of the microsomal oxidizing system. Consistent with these findings is the report of a greater rate of ethanol disappearance from the blood of rats receiving ethanol on a chronic basis (Lieber and DeCarli, 1970b) without a change in ADH or catalase activity.

Thus, the data regarding the role of the microsomal enzyme system are somewhat conflicting with considerable evidence showing that stimulation of liver microsomal enzyme activity by several inducers does not necessarily increase the rate of ethanol metabolism. A thorough consideration of these data is contained in the review by Hawkins and Kalant (1972).

At the present time, the evidence still indicates that ADH is the major enzyme involved in the conversion of ethanol to acetaldehyde. Nevertheless, the role of ethanol as an inducer or inhibitor of the microsomal oxidizing system is of great importance because of possible effects on the metabolism of drugs and other chemicals by acute or chronic ethanol ingestion. Indeed, such interactions of ethanol with drugs are already well documented (Rubin and Lieber, 1971). Ethanol potentiation of the toxicity of carbon tetrachloride and chloroform is also well known (Cornish and Adefuin, 1966).

Maling *et al.* (1975) report that pretreatment with ethanol enhanced the hepatotoxic response to subsequent doses of carbon tetrachloride, thioacetamide, or dimethylnitrosamine. The ethanol pretreatment did not alter the hepatic concentration of carbon tetrachloride or its metabolite chloroform one hour after carbon tetrachloride administration. Covalent binding of $^{14}CCl_4$ to liver protein and lipid *in vivo* was significantly greater at 6 and 24 hours, but not at three hours, after ethanol pretreatment. *In vitro* binding of labeled chloroform, carbon tetrachloride, or bromotrichloromethane to hepatic microsomal protein was enhanced in alcohol-pretreated rats. Isopropanol reacted in a similar manner with respect to carbon tetrachloride toxicity. Ethanol, but not isopropanol, potentiated the hepatotoxicity of thioacetamide and dimethylnitrosamine. For further discussion of the role of alcohols in potentiation of toxicity see Chapter 10.

Although the conversion of ethanol to acetaldehyde has been intensively investigated, the second step in the metabolism of ethanol, the oxidation of acetaldehyde to acetate, is equally important. The conversion of acetaldehyde to acetate is carried out by aldehyde dehydrogenase (Büttner, 1965), which has a four- to fivefold greater activity in liver and kidney than does ADH; thus acetaldehyde does not normally tend to accumulate during ethanol metabolism. Several other enzymes in liver are also capable of metabolizing acetaldehyde, but their *in vivo* role in the metabolism of ethanol has not been established (Hawkins and Kalant, 1972). The inhibition of aldehyde dehydrogenase by tetraethylthiuram disulfide (disulfiram) results in the accumulation of acetaldehyde in blood (Truitt and Duritz, 1967). The clinical use of disulfiram in man enhances the symptoms of ethanol and acetaldehyde toxicity—nausea, vomiting, headache, and weakness—and has considerable popularity as a voluntary means of assisting the alcoholic in his attempts to refrain from drinking.

The effect of ethanol and ethanol metabolism on a host of metabolic processes has been recently reviewed (Israel, 1970; Mendelson, 1970; Lundquist, 1971b; Hawkins and Kalant, 1972). Needless to say, the effects of excessive ingestion of ethanol are profound, on both an acute and a chronic basis. In both animal and human studies, the effect of ethanol is apparently influenced by other biologic parameters, including nutritional state, and pretreatment and posttreatment procedures.

Ethanol ingestion in man in the postadsorptive state results in an early hyperglycemic response followed by hypoglycemia (Vartia *et al.*, 1960). This has been interpreted as an initial glycogenolysis followed by hypoglycemia subsequent to the depletion of glycogen stores. The hyperglycemic response to ethanol could be prevented in rabbits by ganglionic blockade suggesting an adrenomedullary origin (Perman, 1962). Masten (1972) has recently suggested a role of acetaldehyde in the hyperglycemic response to ethanol. There is also evidence that ethanol has a direct inhibitory effect on hepatic gluconeogenesis (Krebs *et al.*, 1969).

Ethanol ingestion, both acute and chronic, has an effect on lipid metabolism that does result in the accumulation of lipid, primarily triglycerides, in the liver (Lieber, 1967). The synthesis of triglycerides from fatty acids and glycerol has been shown to increase after ethanol ingestion (Nikkila and Ojala, 1963). An increased incorporation of glycerol into liver phosphatidylcholine has also been reported in the ethanol-fed rat (Mendenhall *et al.*, 1969). Ethanol, both *in vivo* and *in vitro*, decreases the rate of fatty acid oxidation by liver (Mendenhall *et al.*, 1969). Although the availability of acetate, as a product of ethanol metabolism, may tend to depress the rate of fatty acid oxidation, the inhibitory effect of ethanol on fatty acid oxidation may also be due to inhibition of other metabolic pathways. Ethanol-induced release of catecholamines and corticosteroids (Ellis, 1966) results in enhanced mobilization from fat depots (Poggi and DeLuzio, 1964), resulting in elevated levels of plasma fatty acids (Mallov, 1961) and increased deposition of liver triglycerides.

Thus, the effect of ethanol on fatty liver development is a complex series of biochemical events that are influenced by a variety of factors including dosage regimen, nutritional state, and to a great extent the experimental techniques involved in the study. Additional uncontrolled conditions complicate the assessment of factors involved in fatty liver development in the alcoholic.

Methanol (Methyl Alcohol, CH_3OH)

Methyl alcohol was commonly called wood alcohol because its primary source was from the distillation of wood. Synthetic methods of production from oxides of carbon and hydrogen now account for a large share of production. It has wide industrial use as a solvent and is extensively employed as a paint and varnish remover, as a chemical intermediate, and in the preparation of stains, enamels, plastics, and films.

Toxic manifestations may occur following absorption through the skin, by inhalation, or by ingestion. Industrial exposures are primarily vapor exposures, and although there may also be opportunity for skin absorption, this can be more readily controlled. A number of reports of severe industrial exposures date back to the early twentieth century, prior to the time of improved industrial control methods. Treon (1963) mentions a number of these in his review of the industrial toxicity of methyl alcohol. He also summarizes the literature on a large number of animal inhalation studies carried out on cats, dogs, mice, rats, rabbits, and monkeys. A great species variation in toxicity appears to exist, although the methods of study, concentration, and length of exposure are so variable that realistic comparisons are difficult.

The monkey appears to be more susceptible than most other species. Dogs exposed to 450 to 500 ppm for 379 consecutive days showed no significant changes from normal in growth rate, behavior, biochemical parameters, or gross and microscopic examination of tissues at autopsy. Histopathologic changes in animals resulting from exposure to higher levels of methanol vapor include petechial hemorrhages in the lung, pulmonary edema, mild fatty infiltration of the liver parenchyma, fatty infiltration of the kidney, fatty degeneration of heart muscle, degenerative changes in the central nervous system, and in the eye, retinal edema, and early signs of degeneration of ganglionic cells of the retina and nerve fibers.

Methyl alcohol, since it resembles ethanol in odor and taste and is tax free, has caused considerable problems as an adulterant, both accidental and intentional, in alcoholic beverages. The symptoms of methanol toxicity in man may begin with inebriation as with ethanol, followed 6 to 24 hours later by vomiting, abdominal pain, visual disturbances, shortness of breath, delirium, unconsciousness, coma, and death. The severity of symptoms appears to vary, not only with dose, but also from individual to individual.

Several instances of mass poisoning from methanol in alcoholic beverages have been reported. In 1951, one incident resulted in 41 deaths with a total involvement of over 300 people (Cooper et al., 1952).

The acute toxicity of this alcohol and attempts to relate metabolic products to the toxic response have been the basis for continual study. A number of reviews have been published on this topic (Harger and Forney, 1967; Watkins, 1971).

Methanol is metabolized more slowly than ethanol and, in the rat over a two-day period, was excreted as carbon dioxide (65 percent) and unchanged methanol (14 percent) in the expired air, and as formate (3 percent) and methanol (3 percent) in the urine. In the rabbit, methylglucuronide has also been found as a methanol metabolite (Parke, 1968). The actual distribution of metabolites varies greatly with the dose with considerable urinary excretion of methanol occurring at high dosages. The large quantity excreted as CO_2 in the rat indicates that methanol is largely metabolized, at least in this species. Other studies in rabbit, dog, and man support these findings (Ritchie, 1970).

There seems to be general agreement that the stepwise metabolism of methanol parallels that of ethanol with the formation of formaldehyde and its subsequent conversion to formate. The toxic effects of methanol are thought to be related to the formation of these metabolites.

Early studies indicated that a partially purified preparation of alcohol dehydrogenase converted both ethanol and methanol to the corresponding aldehydes. Ethanol, however, was metabolized about nine times more rapidly than methanol. Theorell and Bonnischen (1951) showed that with a purified alcohol dehydrogenase preparation, ethanol and a variety of other aliphatic alcohols, but not methanol, were converted to the corresponding aldehydes. Thus, other mechanisms for the oxidation of methanol were investigated. Early studies had suggested a peroxidative enzyme system that was capable of carrying out the oxidation of alcohols. These authors showed that catalase carried out the oxidation of methanol and other alcohols by means of a coupled oxidation involving the utilization of hydrogen peroxide, which is normally generated by a variety of oxidative enzymes. A review (Mannering et al. 1969) discusses in detail the role of the intracellular distribution of hepatic catalase in the peroxidative oxidation of methanol.

Makar and coworkers (1964) reported that the peroxidative system involving hepatic catalase played a major role in the oxidation of methanol in the rat but that in the monkey, the peroxidative mechanism did not appear to be particularly active. Supporting data for this conclusion included the fact that ethanol was a more effective inhibitor of methanol oxidation in the intact monkey than in the rat, suggesting that alcohol dehydrogenase probably played a more important role in metabolism of methanol in the monkey than it did in the rat. In a similar manner, 1-butanol was also a better inhibitor of methanol oxidation in the monkey than one would anticipate if a peroxidative enzyme system were involved. Aminotriazole, a potent inhibitor of hepatic catalase, markedly reduced methanol oxidation in the rat but not in the monkey. Additional in vivo studies included the fact that ethylene glycol stimulated the rate of metabolism of methanol in the rat but not in the monkey. It was suggested that the oxidation of ethylene glycol probably resulted in increased hydrogen peroxide production, thus stimulating the peroxidative system in the rat but not in the monkey where alcohol dehydrogenase is apparently the major metabolic pathway.

The study of Watkins (1971) showed that pyrazole, an inhibitor of alcohol dehydrogenase, markedly inhibited the oxidation of both ethanol and methanol in the monkey. In the rat, pyrazole markedly inhibited ethanol oxidation and produced a modest but significant inhibition of methanol oxidation. These data support the concept that hepatic alcohol dehydrogenase is the major pathway in ethanol and methanol oxidation in the monkey and the major pathway for ethanol oxidation in the rat. These data also

In a recent study of continuous 24-hour exposure to 12 mg/M³ of ethylene glycol, moderate to severe eye irritation occurred in rabbits, and corneal opacity and apparent blindness in rats within eight days of initial exposure (Coon *et al.*, 1970).

The metabolism of a number of glycols was studied by Gessner and coworkers (1960), and the metabolism of ¹⁴C-labeled ethylene glycol was reported by the same authors in 1961 (Gessner *et al.*, 1961). These authors reviewed the earlier literature, which suggests that the only well-established metabolite of ethylene glycol in man and other animals is oxalic acid, which usually accounts for less than 2 percent of the dose. Glycolic acid has also been reported to be a metabolite in rabbits, and unchanged ethylene glycol is excreted by dogs and humans.

The paper by Gessner and associates (1961) reported that in the rabbit, after a dose of 0.1 g/kg, about 40 percent of the glycol was eliminated as CO_2 in the expired air within 24 hours and as much as 60 percent excreted as CO_2 over a three-day period. The major compounds excreted in urine were unchanged ethylene glycol, with oxalic acid as a minor metabolite. In liver slice studies, glycolaldehyde and glyoxylic acid were detected as intermediates in the metabolism of ethylene glycol. More recent metabolic studies in animals have been reported by McChesney and coworkers (1971), and an effect of ethylene glycol on mitochondria has been demonstrated by Bachmann and Golberg (1971).

Clay and Murphy (1977) have recently reported on the severe metabolic acidosis produced by ethylene glycol in the dog and pigtail monkey. This is consistent with clinical reports of human poisoning. The fact that inhibition of alcohol dehydrogenase by alcohol (Wacker *et al.*, 1965) or pyrazole (Mundy *et al.*, 1974) prevents the development of metabolic acidosis demonstrates the role of metabolites or the metabolic process in the acidosis. These studies demonstrate that the accumulation of the metabolite glycolic acid after ethylene glycol administration is sufficient to account for the metabolic acidosis that develops. The contribution of other possible metabolites was considered negligible.

Gershoff and Andrus (1962) studied the role of pyridoxine, magnesium, and combinations of these two materials with respect to their effects on the toxicity of ethylene glycol. On the basis of histopathologic examination, pyridoxine gave partial protection, high magnesium intake could prevent renal lesions, and when both were used, not only were renal lesions prevented, but growth rates in treated animals were returned essentially to normal. With the use of ¹⁴C-labeled ethylene glycol, it was demonstrated that increased levels of pyridoxine in the diet markedly increased the CO_2 production from ethylene glycol but did not alter CO_2 production from labeled glycerol. Thus the partial protection against ethylene glycol toxicity provided by excess pyridoxine may be related to a stimulated rate of metabolism. The magnesium effect may be related to altered solubility properties, thus partially preventing deposition of oxalate crystals.

Bove (1966) studied the renal pathology in a series of rats given ethylene glycol or its metabolites, including glycoaldehyde, glycolic acid, and glyoxylic acid. In animals given single large doses of ethylene glycol (9 to 12 g/kg), striking oxalate formation was present in renal tubules. Crystals appeared throughout the proximal and distal convoluted tubules and were less numerous in the collecting tubules. In only one rat, oxalate crystals were present in the brain, as has also been reported (Pons and Custer, 1946) in human poisoning. Oxalate crystals were also present in renal tubules of animals receiving glycoaldehyde, glycolic acid, and glyoxylic acid, although the renal oxalosis was less extensive with glycoaldehyde. The three proposed intermediates were all more toxic on an acute basis than was ethylene glycol since a number of animals died within eight hours of receiving 5 to 6 g/kg of body weight of the metabolites. Renal tubular pathology was not always accompanied by crystal formation, and the author concludes that cytotoxicity rather than simple mechanical obstruction is largely responsible for renal failure.

Studies by von Wartburg and coworkers (1964) demonstrated that human liver alcohol dehydrogenase metabolized ethylene glycol as well as ethanol, methanol, and other alcohols. Ethanol, which is a much better substrate for alcohol dehydrogenase than is ethylene glycol, is thus a potent competitive inhibitor of ethylene glycol metabolism.

Experimental studies in animals (Peterson *et al.*, 1963) have shown that ethanol markedly inhibits the metabolism of ethylene glycol *in vivo* and protects against the acute toxicity resulting from its metabolism. The oral LD50 in rats was found to be 5.8 ml/kg for ethylene glycol and 10.5 ml/kg when animals received ethanol 15 minutes after the intraperitoneal injection of ethylene glycol.

With this information as background, clinical cases of ethylene glycol poisoning have been treated with ethanol. Wacker and associates (1965) reported two cases of individuals who had ingested 250 to 1,000 ml of ethylene glycol antifreeze. Gastric lavage was not undertaken until admission to the hospital, some six to nine hours after the antifreeze was ingested; thus large quantities were presumably absorbed into the general circulation. Both patients were treated with ethanol infusion, which resulted in a prompt disappearance of oxaluria, and adequate urinary output was maintained. These individuals made uneventful recoveries from these rather massive ingestions of ethylene glycol. This treatment is, of course, consistent with the therapy proposed for methanol poisoning and is based on the same mechanism of substrate competition for alcohol dehydrogenase.

Diethylene Glycol ($HOCH_2CH_2OCH_2CH_2OH$)

Diethylene glycol is used in the lacquer industry, in cosmetics, in permanent antifreeze formulations, in lubricants, as a softening agent, and as a plasticizer. It presents little hazard during industrial handling at ordinary temperatures. Where mists are generated or where operations are carried out at high temperatures, industrial hygiene control methods should be followed to eliminate repeated prolonged inhalation (Rowe, 1963). The major hazard from diethylene glycol occurs following the ingestion of relatively large single doses. Impetus for the study of the toxicity of diethylene glycol was provided by 105 fatalities among 353 people who ingested a solution of sulfanilamide in an aqueous mixture containing 72 percent diethylene glycol (Ruprecht and Nelson, 1937; Smyth, 1952). The symptoms included nausea, dizziness, and pain in the kidney region. This was followed in a few days by oliguria and anuria with death resulting from uremic poisoning.

From the information provided in this episode of human poisoning, it has been estimated that the single oral dose lethal for man is approximately 1 ml/kg.

A long-term rat-feeding study by Fitzhugh and Nelson (1946) showed that 1-percent diethylene glycol in the diet over a two-year period resulted in slight growth depression, a few calcium oxalate bladder stones, minimal kidney damage, and occasional liver damage. At the 4-percent dietary level, there was increased mortality, a marked depression of growth rate, bladder stones, severe kidney damage, and moderate liver damage. In addition, bladder tumors appeared rather frequently. Rowe (1963) suggests that since the purity of the diethylene glycol utilized in this study was not determined, some of the effects noted may not be attributable to the diethylene glycol.

Studies reported by Weil and colleagues (1967) attempted to answer the question of whether diethylene glycol bladder tumors resulted from irritation by stones or whether the chemical was a true carcinogen. Bladder implantations of calcium oxalate stones and of glass beads, along with sham-operated animals as controls, were utilized in this phase of the study. Also included in the study were animals receiving as much as 4 or 6 percent diethylene glycol in the diet. The development of bladder stones and tumors was relatively low in these studies compared with others previously reported.

The authors concluded that bladder tumors never developed in the experimental rats without the preceding or concurrent presence of a foreign body. They suggest that diethylene glycol is not a primary carcinogen but, when fed in very high concentrations, does result in the formation of calcium oxalate bladder stones and subsequent rare bladder tumors.

Propylene Glycol (1,2-Propanediol, $CH_3CHOHCH_2OH$)

Propylene glycol is used as a solvent in pharmaceuticals, cosmetics, and food materials, as a plasticizer, in antifreeze formulations, heat exchangers, and hydraulic fluids. Propylene glycol has a low order of toxicity and is used in food products, cosmetics, and pharmaceutical products with no apparent difficulty.

Acute oral LD50 values in rats, rabbits, and dogs are approximately 32, 18, and 9 ml/kg, respectively. Early studies demonstrated that the rat can tolerate 10 percent propylene glycol in drinking water without physiologic impairment. Robertson and co-workers (1947) exposed monkeys and rats to atmospheres saturated with propylene glycol vapor and found no adverse effects in animals after periods of 12 to 18 months.

Ruddick (1971) reported a low order of toxicity in the rat and chick with the major metabolic product being lactate and/or pyruvate. Dean and Stock (1974) found that two daily ip injections of 4 ml/kg body weight for three days resulted in an increased rate of liver microsomal metabolism of aniline and p-nitroanisole, a significant decrease in aminopyrine demethylation, and no change in cytochrome P-450 levels. Since propylene glycol has been suggested as a drug solvent in studies of the microsomal mixed-function oxidase system, these potential effects of the solvent should be recognized.

GLYCOL ETHERS

These solvents have rather widespread industrial use, particularly since they are both water soluble and soluble in organic solvents. Thus, they find use in many oil-water combinations. They are also used as solvents for resins, paints, varnish, lacquer, dyes, soaps, and cosmetics. There are a large number of these industrial solvents available, depending on the substituent group used to form the ether of mono-, di-, or triethylene glycol. Most of the commonly used ethers are the lower-molecular-weight aliphatic ethers, such as methyl, ethyl, propyl, diethyl, and butyl. However, higher-molecular-weight ethers such as the phenyl ether of diethylene glycol are also available.

Ethylene Glycol Monomethyl Ether (Methyl Cellosolve $HO\text{-}CH_2\text{-}CH_2\text{-}O\text{-}CH_3$)

This compound has a relatively low toxicity with respect to single oral dose (Carpenter et al., 1956).

Repeated injections of ethylene glycol monomethyl ether in guinea pigs showed that five daily injections of either 0.5 or 1.0 ml/kg resulted in prostration and the death of the guinea pigs. Rabbits died after seven ingestions of 1 ml/kg. Several additional reports including Carpenter *et al.* (1956) demonstrated that when a 25 percent solution was given intravenously, hemolysis of the erythrocytes occurred in the rat and that daily injections of 2 ml in rabbits and 6 ml per day in dogs resulted in anuria, urinary casts, lung edema, irritation of the bladder mucosa, and liver and testicular damage.

Since the major route of entry of the glycol ethers is by inhalation, a number of animal studies have utilized this route of entry. These studies are summarized by Rowe (1963).

Irritation of the respiratory tract, hematuria, albuminuria, and casts appeared in the urine of animals exposed to 800 to 1,600 ppm of ethylene glycol monomethyl ether. Werner's (1943a) studies with dogs exposed to 750 ppm for seven hours a day, five days a week for 12 weeks, indicated that the most significant changes were in the peripheral blood. The red cell count, hemoglobin, and cell volumes were all decreased, accompanied by hypochromia and microcytosis. This was accompanied by increased numbers of immature white cells. Measurements of urinary excretion of oxalic acid, methanol, and formic acid in the urine of rabbits injected with ethylene glycol monomethyl ether did not show any increases in these possible metabolites, suggesting that this ether is not hydrolyzed to ethylene glycol and methanol.

For a guide to safe industrial use of this solvent, see the Hygienic Guide Series (American Industrial Hygiene Association, 1970).

A number of instances of human intoxication from exposure to ethylene glycol monomethyl ether have been reported in the literature.

A woman exposed to a solution composed of ethylene glycol monomethyl ether, isopropanol, and cellulose acetate complained of headache, weakness, drowsiness, loss of weight, forgetfulness, memory lapse, disorientation, and lethargy. Two additional cases of intoxication reported predominant symptoms of fatigue, loss of weight, and lethargy. A macrocytic anemia was present and the white blood cell count was depressed. In another report (Greenberg *et al.*, 1938) all exposed individuals had symptoms of excessive fatigue, abnormal reflexes, and tremors, as well as an abnormal blood picture, suggesting macrocytic anemia. More recently, Zavon (1963) reported five cases of individuals exposed to methyl cellosolve in the printing department of a plant making plastic materials. The methyl cellosolve was the commonly used cleaning agent to remove pigments and ink from the floor and equipment. The major findings in these individuals were related to the effects on the central nervous system with ataxia, tremors, slurred speech, and personality changes. The degree of anemia was variable, although the red cell count was approximately 4 million or less in the four individuals for whom it was reported. One of these individuals had a red cell count of 2.9 million.

A report of two individuals who had ingested large amounts of ethylene glycol monomethyl ether (approximately 100 ml) indicated renal failure and oxaluria in one individual (Witter-Hauge, 1970). The author points out that this one individual excreted up to 1,000 mg per day of oxalate during the first week, suggesting the hydrolysis to ethylene glycol and methanol, with methanol being responsible for the metabolic acidosis. Both patients were treated by intravenous infusion of bicarbonate and ethyl alcohol. The ethanol was given to prevent further oxidation of both ethylene glycol and methanol by providing an alternative substrate for alcohol dehydrogenase. The puzzling aspect of this report is that only one patient excreted increased quantities of oxalate. Such a metabolic fate in man would be in contrast to that reported in animals where no cleavage of this ether was demonstrated. Further human data will be necessary to clarify this aspect of the metabolic fate of methyl cellosolve in man.

Although relatively few instances of chronic overexposure to methyl cellosolve have been reported, the neurologic symptoms and the macrocytic anemia and, in some instances, the abnormal leukocyte counts suggest that this material can be a significant hazard in the absence of appropriate control measures.

Ethylene Glycol Monoethyl Ether (Cellosolve $HOCH_2CH_2OCH_2CH_3$)

This glycol ether in general appears to have a somewhat lower order of toxicity than the monomethyl ether. At high dose levels, it produces kidney injury and hematuria in animals when given by the oral route.

Ninety-day feeding studies (Smyth *et al.*, 1951) reported that the maximum dose having no effect was 0.21 g/kg/day. Higher dose levels resulted in decreased growth rate, elevated liver and kidney weight, and microscopic lesions of both liver and kidney. Werner and associates (1943b) exposed rats to 370 ppm of ethylene glycol monoethylether seven hours a day, five days a week for five weeks, and found only minimal effects in the blood. Dogs exposed to 840 ppm on a similar schedule for 12 weeks showed a slight decrease in hemoglobin and red cells and a greater number of immature white cells.

In contrast to the methyl cellosolve, cellosolve has not provided reports of difficulties encountered during industrial exposures.

Ethylene Glycol Monobutyl Ether (Butyl Cellosolve $HOCH_2CH_2OCH_2CH_2CH_2CH_3$)

This material is moderately toxic orally, appreciably irritating and injurious to the eyes, readily absorbed through the skin, and moderately toxic when inhaled (Rowe, 1963). In animal studies, hematuria and kidney damage were common findings along with increased osmotic fragility of the erythrocytes. This was accompanied by reductions in the number of circulating red cells and in hemoglobin levels. Carpenter and coworkers (1956) have shown that butoxy acetic acid is a metabolite of ethylene glycol monobutyl ether in the rat, rabbit, guinea pig, dog, rhesus monkey, and man. In the same study, it was determined that butyl cellosolve is rapidly absorbed through the skin of rabbits leading to systemic toxicity. Red blood cell fragility was increased within an hour after a single three-minute contact with 0.56 ml/kg on 4.5 percent of the total skin surface area of the rabbit. Thus, absorption through the skin could be a significant route of entry for this material.

Dioxane (1,4-Dioxane $C_4H_8O_2$)

Dioxane is a cyclic compound that can be synthesized by the dehydration of two molecules of ethylene glycol or by the dimerizing of ethylene oxide. This material has widespread use as a solvent for lacquers, varnish, paint, plastics, dyes, waxes, and resins. It is irritating to the skin and eyes on prolonged exposure and can be absorbed through the skin in sufficient quantities to produce systemic toxicity.

The symptoms of acute oral toxicity are weakness, depression, coma, and death, as reported by Laug and associates (1939) for mice, rats, and guinea pigs. Kidney and liver injury occurs in rabbits and guinea pigs after repeated application of dioxane to the skin. At high levels of exposure, 5,000 to 10,000 ppm, marked irritation of the mucous membranes and death from lung injury was a common occurrence. Liver and kidney injury occurred following repeated exposures to dioxane at levels ranging from 1,000 to 10,000 ppm.

Fatal cases of industrial poisoning by dioxane have been reported. These reports are summarized by Rowe (1963). Autopsy showed lung and brain congestion and liver and kidney injury. Death apparently resulted from the kidney damage.

Epidemiologic studies in a number of industries utilizing dioxane have been reported and recently reviewed (NIOSH, 1977). The information suggests that at the level of industrial exposure encountered dioxane appeared to present a negligible health hazard.

Chronic animal studies in rats (Argus et al., 1965)

and guinea pigs (Hoch-Legeti and Argus, 1970) showed the presence of hepatomas and lung epithelial hyperplasia. Squamous cell carcinomas in the nasal cavity of six test animals (Hoch-Ligeti et al., 1970) was noted in a 13-month rat-feeding study with dioxane in the water. Four of these rats also had liver tumors (120 total test animals). No tumors were present in the liver or nasal cavity of 30 control rats. Kociba et al. (1974) fed dioxane, 0.01, 0.1, 1.0 percent in drinking water, to groups of 60 male and 60 female Sherman strain rats for up to 716 days. Rats that received 1 percent or 0.1 percent dioxane demonstrated renal tubular, hepatocellular, and epithelial degeneration and necrosis. There was also evidence of hepatic regeneration as indicated by hepatocellular hyperplastic nodule formation and renal tubular regeneration indicated by increased tubular epithelial activity. Nasal cell carcinomas were observed in 3 of 66 rats in the 1 percent dioxane group. In the same group, 10 of 66 rats had hepatocellular carcinomas. No effects were noted in the 0.01 percent dioxane-water intake group. In the control group of 106 rats, one had a hepatocellular carcinoma, one had a cholangiosarcoma, and two had hepatic tumors. Holmes (1976) reported a two-year dioxane-in-drinking-water study in rats and mice. Renal and hepatic toxicity was severe. Squamous cell carcinoma of the nasal cavity was present in 23/57 in the 0.5 percent group, 23/51 in the 1 percent group, and 0/32 in control rats. Other tumor types as well as metastases, mainly to the brain, were also reported. In the mice, hepatocellular carcinomas were present in 4/99 controls, 24/94 in the 0.5 percent group, and 44/87 in the 1 percent group.

Since the usual route of exposure to dioxane is by inhalation, Torkelson et al. (1974) had carried out a two-year exposure study: 111 ± 5 ppm dioxane for seven hours per day, five days per week, with 192 male and 192 female rats being exposed. The TLV value in 1974 was 100 ppm. No hepatic or nasal tumors were present in either control or test animals. All other parameters such as activity, body weight, hematology, and biochemical measurements were comparable in control and test animals. The authors point out that these negative findings are consistent with the hypothesis that liver injury is a prerequisite for tumor development in that organ.

Braun and Young (1977) reported that the proposed metabolites, diglycolic and oxalic acids, could not be confirmed in the urine of rats dosed orally with 1,4[^{14}C] dioxane. However, the major metabolite found in the urine was β-hydroxyethoxyacetic acid with most of the remainder present as unchanged dioxane. The role of metabolism in the toxicity of dioxane has not been established.

AROMATIC HYDROCARBON SOLVENTS

Benzene (Benzol, C_6H_6)

Benzene, the simplest of the aromatic hydrocarbons, containing only a single benzene nucleus, should not be confused with benzine, which is a petroleum distillate containing a mixed group of primarily aliphatic hydrocarbons.

Benzene is produced as a by-product of the petroleum and coke oven industries. It has widespread use in the chemical and drug industries and as a solvent for paints, resins, lacquers, and plastics. It is a constituent of motor fuels, and large quantities are utilized as a starting material in the synthesis of a variety of aromatic products. For example, nitration of benzene yields nitrobenzene, which can be utilized as such or reduced to aniline and other related products. These, in turn, can be converted to nitroso compounds, which can be coupled to form complex dyes and dye materials. Benzene can also be sulfonated, chlorinated, or alkylated to be used as a starting material for various other more complex chemicals. Extensive reviews of the sources, uses, and toxicology of the aromatic hydrocarbons are contained in reports of Swinyard (1970) and Truhaut (1971).

In addition to its excellent solvent properties, the relatively high volatility and rapid drying of this solvent account for its use in certain applications, such as printing, or as a fat solvent in the extraction of seeds and nuts. The overall hazards, however, associated with the use of benzene would suggest that wherever the possibility of human exposure exists, the substitution of other less hazardous solvents would be preferred.

Due to its volatility, the major route of entry of benzene is by vapor inhalation. Gerarde reports (1960) that the ingestion of liquid benzene causes local irritation of the mucous membranes and that the subsequent absorption of benzene leads to symptoms of systemic toxicity. He also states that the ingestion of about 15 ml of benzene has been known to cause collapse, bronchitis, and pneumonia. Aspiration of benzene into the lung results in pulmonary edema and hemorrhage at the site of contact. For man, an exposure of 20,000 ppm is usually fatal within five to ten minutes. Symptoms of intoxication are drowsiness, dizziness, headache, and loss of consciousness. Death is apparently due to respiratory failure and circulatory collapse.

Thus, in its acute stages, benzene toxicity appears to be due primarily to its effect on the central nervous system. Recovery from an acute exposure to benzene depends on the initial severity of the exposure. Symptoms may persist for two to three weeks. A most important point was made that chronic effects of benzene intoxication may arise and persist long after an acute exposure occurs. It would appear that individual response to either acute or chronic benzene exposure is quite variable.

It is in chronic benzene exposure that, although central nervous system and gastrointestinal effects may be present, the important toxic manifestations may be related to injury of the blood-forming tissues. Cases of benzene poisoning resulting in hematologic effects have been reported from repeated exposure to concentrations ranging down to 60 ppm (Hardy and Elkins, 1948) and 105 ppm (Wilson, 1942).

Greenberg and associates (1939), in a study of 102 workmen exposed to benzene vapor, reported chronic benzene poisoning of varying severity in 74 of these individuals. The hematologic findings were variable with effects noted on erythrocyte count, hemoglobin, mean corpuscular volume of red cells, platelet counts, and leukocyte counts. The development of blood abnormalities occurred in some individuals during a 60-day period after the benzene exposure. Aksoy and colleagues (1972) also reported inconsistent blood pictures in 32 patients with varying degrees of benzene poisoning.

Of major concern has been the potential relationship between chronic benzene exposure and leukemia. No animal model has been shown to develop leukemia as a response to benzene. However, case histories and epidemiologic studies have raised this question with respect to man.

Aksoy *et al.* (1974) reported that 26 patients among 28,500 shoeworkers chronically exposed to benzene developed leukemia or preleukemia over a seven-year period. This was an annual incidence of 13/100,000 compared with 6/100,000 in the general population. Thorpe (1974), in a study of 38,000 petroleum workers exposed to low levels of benzene exposure, found the incidence of leukemia no greater than in the general populations used for comparative purposes. In a study of the rubber industry, McMichael *et al.* (1975) reported that the risk of death from lymphatic leukemia in medium- and low-solvent-exposure jobs appeared to be twice that of unexposed workers. This study also suggested a possible relationship between solvent exposure and lymphosarcoma, Hodgkin's disease, and myeloid leukemia.

The early symptoms of chronic benzene poisoning may be rather vague, consisting of headache, fatigue, and loss of appetite, symptoms that are common to many other types of chemical exposures. Early blood examinations may show only slight abnormalities in a variety of different ways, as previously mentioned. The most common blood abnormality appears to be a fall in total white cell count, which may or may not be accompanied by a relative lymphocytosis, and a macrocytic, normochromic, or slightly hyperchromic anemia, as well as thrombocytopenia. The bone marrow changes may be rather nonspecific at this time. As the disease progresses, the bone marrow may become aplastic or hyperplastic in a manner that does not always correlate with the peripheral blood picture (Deichmann et al., 1963; Aksoy et al., 1972). Blood abnormalities include anemia, leukopenia, and thrombocytopenia.

In animals, leukopenia appears to be the most consistent response to benzene poisoning.

Deichmann and coworkers (1963) reported a significant leukopenia after two to four weeks' exposure of rats to 831, 65, or 61 ppm of benzene. Definite leukopenia resulted from the exposure of rats to 47 and 44 ppm of benzene over a five- to eight-week period. The erythrocyte count and hemoglobin levels in the circulating blood were not affected by these levels of exposure. Exposure of rats to 31 ppm of benzene for four months, 29 ppm for three months, and 15 ppm for seven months did not produce measurable effects in the circulating blood.

On the basis of human exposure experience, as well as animal studies with benzene vapor, there is no doubt that benzene is an insidious and unpredictable toxicant. Gerarde (1960) indicates that benzene may be rather unique among the hydrocarbon solvents as a bone marrow toxicant. Although there have been a number of studies of the metabolism of benzene (Cornish and Ryan, 1965), attempts to relate the metabolic fate of this compound to its effect on bone marrow have not been successful to date. It is interesting to note that alkyl substitution of the benzene ring markedly alters the metabolic pathway and also apparently largely removes the potential for bone marrow toxicity.

Benzene is readily absorbed into the blood during vapor exposure and, because of its lipid solubility, tends to distribute itself largely in fatty tissues. Thus, although equilibrium may be rapidly reached between the atmosphere and the blood, the saturation of tissues may not be complete until after several days of exposure. Gerarde (1963) states that the average concentration of benzene in the blood is 2.1 mg/liter for each 100 ppm of benzene in the inhaled air when equilibrium is reached. Elimination of benzene from the animals requires release of benzene into the atmosphere through the lung along with continuous reestablishment of an equilibrium between blood and tissues that have previously stored considerable quantities of benzene. About 40 percent of a single oral dose of benzene given to the rabbit is eliminated from the lungs as unchanged benzene over the immediate 72-hour period after dosing. Most of the benzene is metabolized by the liver to more water-soluble phenolic compounds, which may be excreted as sulfates or as glucuronides (Parke, 1968).

Although a small amount of benzene is excreted as the mercapturic acid, the primary pathway appears to be the oxidation of the benzene ring to form phenol, which in turn is largely converted to the sulfate and excreted in the urine. For discussion of conjugation mechanisms, one is referred to Fishman (1970a, 1970b). A smaller portion of the phenol may be further oxidized to dihydroxybenzenes such as hydroquinine and pyrocatecol. Pyrocatecol may then be further oxidized to trihydroxy derivatives such as hydroxyhydroquinone. In addition the benzene ring is broken to yield the unusual metabolite trans-trans-muconic acid. Trace quantities, less than 1 percent, of several other metabolic products have also been reported. These include dihydrodihydroxybenzene.

Studies on the mechanisms of enzymatic hydroxylation of benzene and other aromatic compounds have proceeded rapidly since the report of Posner and coworkers (1961), which demonstrated the enzymatic hydroxylation of benzene and a variety of other aromatic compounds.

Cornish and Ryan (1965) reported that 23 percent of an 88-mg intraperitoneal dose of benzene was excreted in the urine as phenols, either free or conjugated, in the subsequent 24-hour period. Only 4 mg of the benzene was present as a corresponding glucuronide. However, in rats fasted for 24 hours prior to dosing, approximately 36 percent of the dose was excreted in the urine, but the pattern of metabolites was shifted from organic sulfates to the corresponding glucuronide. This study demonstrates the ability of animals to utilize alternate pathways of metabolism depending on the biologic availability of various components necessary for the formation of conjugates. In addition, the treatment of animals with SKF-525A partially inhibited hydroxylation of benzene resulting in an overall reduced excretion of phenolic products. In a more recent study by Snyder and associates (1967), the metabolism of benzene in rabbit liver homogenates or in the 9,000-g supernatant from rat liver homogenate was markedly stimulated by pretreatment of the animals with phenobarbital, or by pretreatment of the rabbits with a single dose of benzene. The stimulation of benzene metabolism by prior injection of benzene was accompanied by a stimulation of amino acid incorporation into microsomal protein suggesting a true induction of benzene-metabolizing enzymes. Ikeda and Ohtsuji (1971) recently reported that pretreatment with phenobarbital partially protected rats against benzene toxicity.

Snyder and Kocsis (1975) have thoroughly reviewed studies on the metabolism of benzene and the potential role of metabolites in toxicity. Lee et al. (1974), utilizing radiolabeled iron, have been able to demonstrate the effect of benzene on the development of the erythrocyte in bone marrow. These studies suggest that benzene inhibits the early stages of erythrocyte development but does not affect the incorporation of iron into heme. There is some conflicting evidence on the role of benzene metabolism in toxicity. The report by Ikeda and Otsuji (1971) that phenobarbital partially protected rats against the leukopenic effects of benzene could be interpreted to suggest that benzene itself may be the toxic agent. Drew and Fouts (1974) have shown that on an acute LC50 or LD50 basis toxicity of benzene was not altered by pretreatment with either phenobarbital, 3-methylcholanthrene, or chlorpromazine. They point out, however, that this study does not relate to more chronic effects of benzene.

Snyder and Kocsis (1975) point out the difficulty of interpreting such studies since "the increased rate of metabolism brought about by microsomal enzyme inducers may have either detoxified benzene or may have hastened the removal of a toxic intermediate." An additional factor is that the real criteria for the role of toxic effects of benzene or its metabolites must be studies carried out on the bone marrow. The effects of altered rates of liver metabolism may not be reflected by altered levels of exposure of bone marrow cells to metabolites produced at some distant site. The intracellular formation of benzene metabolites in developing red cells still needs additional work. The approach of Lee *et al.* (1974) in studying benzene effects on developing red cells has opened up this area of research. Snyder and Kocsis (1975) in their review point out the difficulties of studies directly in bone marrow but also suggest that "there is no more direct approach to studying the disease process than to investigate it in the organ where it occurs."

Since a considerable portion of inhaled benzene is excreted in the urine as the organic sulfate, which is formed at the expense of available inorganic sulfate, a measure of integrated exposure can be arrived at by determining the ratio of inorganic to organic sulfate in a sample of urine collected near the end of the day's exposure. Inorganic sulfate normally comprises approximately 85 percent or more of the total sulfate present in urine. Upon exposure to benzene, the ratio of inorganic to total sulfate decreases upon the severity of the exposure and may reach a point where nearly all of the sulfate is being excreted as organic sulfate.

Elkins (1959) reports that exposure of individuals for eight hours to concentrations of benzene ranging from 40 to 75 ppm results in a urinary sulfate ratio of approximately 60 percent, 75 to 100 ppm benzene concentration results in a urinary sulfate ratio of approximately 40 percent, while exposures from 100 to 200 ppm result in urinary sulfate ratios below 40 percent. Urinary phenol levels exceeding 20 mg/liter are considered excessive and indicative of minimal exposure to benzene, while a concentration of 100 mg of phenol per liter of urine would correlate approximately with an eight-hour exposure to 30 ppm of

benzene. A determination of benzene in blood, urine, or expired air is more direct evidence of benzene exposure, and Teisinger and Bergerová-Fiserová (1955) have suggested that 50 μg of benzene per liter of urine indicates slight exposure, while levels of 4,000 μg/liter indicate severe benzene exposure.

All of the biologic measurements of benzene or its metabolites mentioned above have been suggested only as attempts to evaluate the degree of individual exposure. These measurements in themselves do not suggest the presence of clinical or biochemical abnormalities resulting from benzene exposure. In addition, the measure of metabolites in urine may be somewhat unreliable in individuals with hepatic disease or individuals utilizing drugs that may induce microsomal enzymes responsible for hydroxylation of the benzene ring. With an unpredictable toxicant such as benzene, it is essential that human exposure be kept to a minimum.

Toluene (Methylbenzene, $C_6H_5CH_3$)

Toluene is widely used as an industrial solvent in paints, varnishes, glues, enamels, and lacquers, as well as a chemical intermediate in the synthesis of organic compounds.

Since at one time toluene was frequently contaminated with variable quantities of benzene, much of the early industrial exposure to toluene was probably a mixed-solvent exposure. Toluene is a narcotic, and symptoms of fatigue, weakness, and confusion have been reported in humans exposed to 200 to 300 ppm for eight hours (von Oettingen *et al.*, 1942). Similar but more exaggerated symptoms occurred after an eight-hour exposure to 600 ppm with pronounced incoordination and nausea, and symptoms still present on the following day. The same authors report a rapid equilibrium of toluene with the blood resulting in a concentration of 7.3 mg of toluene per liter of blood in men exposed to 300 ppm of toluene in air. Skin absorption does occur, but this is not a major route of entry in most situations. In contrast to benzene, there is no definitive evidence to link toluene exposure to permanent hematologic damage.

Since toluene is a solvent for glue, it may be encountered as one of the solvents involved with solvent and glue-sniffing episodes.

O'Brien and associates (1971) report that such a "glue sniffer," who had been sniffing glue and liquid cleaner over a three-year period, demonstrated severe hepatic and renal injury after an acute episode of sniffing "cleaner" from a rag, was jaundiced, and had elevated serum bilirubin and alkaline phosphatase levels. Blood urea nitrogen was elevated and proteinuria was present. The patient was treated by peritoneal dialysis and eventually recovered. Gas chromatography of the cleaner produced 12 peaks, many in very small quantity. The major peak, however, was toluene, and the toluene peak coincided with the ether-extracted material from the patient's blood. The concentration of toluene in blood was 160 ppm (160 mg/liter). The patient has also ingested alcoholic beverages, and this raises the question of the possibility of potentiation of toxicity, particularly with respect to the unidentified products also present in the solvent.

Although some absorbed toluene may be re-exhaled by the lung, the major excretory pathway is the rapid oxidation of toluene to benzoic acid, which is conjugated with glycine and excreted as hippuric acid in the urine (Williams, 1959). Many studies have been undertaken to relate the extent of toluene exposure to the amount of hippuric acid excreted in the urine (Ogata et al., 1970, 1971). These reports all tend to show that within reasonable limits, the excretion of hippuric acid in the urine is proportional to the exposure. An exposure to 200 ppm of toluene resulted in the excretion of 3.5 gm hippuric acid per liter of urine (specific gravity 1.016). Ogata's recent study (Ogata et al., 1971) with human volunteers showed that 68 percent of a calculated dose was excreted as hippuric acid with exposures up to 200 ppm of toluene.

CONCLUSIONS

The inhalation route of entry is the most important with respect to acute and chronic toxicity of solvents and vapors. It is also a portal of entry by which individuals may be overexposed to toxic chemicals without being aware of the extent of the exposure or the hazard involved. Thus, it is doubly important that information on the toxicity of inhaled vapors become increasingly available, and that our understanding of the biologic mechanisms by which these materials produce their toxic response be developed as rapidly as possible.

The major hazard from aliphatic hydrocarbons such as gasoline and Stoddard solvent arises from accidental or intentional oral ingestion of such materials and the entry of small quantities into the lung where they may cause rapid and massive pneumonitis. The presence of aromatic additives may increase the hazard from inhalation or ingestion of such materials.

Two relatively common chlorinated hydrocarbon solvents that may produce severe liver injury are carbon tetrachloride and chloroform. The available evidence now suggests that the hepatotoxicity of these compounds is related to their metabolic fate. Other chlorinated aliphatic hydrocarbon solvents such as trichloroethylene, 1,1,1-trichloroethane, and tetrachloroethylene do not possess the severe hepatotoxic potential particularly attached to carbon tetrachloride.

However, they should not be considered innocuous compounds.

Of most recent concern is the continuing trend for the halogenated hydrocarbon solvents to be found to be animal carcinogens on the basis of the present long-term, maximum-tolerated-dose regimen, often in a tumor-susceptible strain of animals. There is no doubt that carcinogenicity testing has placed investigators in a difficult position. On one side is the legitimate argument that in order to carry out such tests with limited numbers of animals, one must use a very high dose if these data are to be statistically related to potential human exposure. Opposing arguments suggest that animals receiving continuous heavy insult to a particular organ, thus increasing the rate of cell division during the repair process, are bound to have an increased incidence of tumors in that organ. Additionally, the doses used are such that metabolic pathways may be overwhelmed or alternate pathways utilized resulting in an exposure not consistent with that of an animal, or human, receiving a much lower dose. Certainly an urgent need exists for the development of faster, more appropriate testing procedures for carcinogenicity.

Although ethanol is often ingested in sufficient quantity to allow the individual to place himself in many hazardous situations, the major toxicologic problem related to the aliphatic alcohols is provided by methanol. The metabolism of both of these alcohols has been extensively investigated, and it is apparent that the metabolism of methanol makes a major contribution to its toxicity. The inhibition of methanol metabolism by the use of an alternative substrate such as ethanol may offer considerable protection against its toxic effects. The glycols (polyhydric alcohols) present little exposure hazard at ordinary temperatures because of their low volatility. Ethylene and diethylene glycol when ingested are partially converted to oxalic acid, which may deposit in the proximal convoluted tubules, producing severe kidney damage. Propylene glycol, on the other hand, has a low order of toxicity and animals have tolerated large doses on a chronic basis without apparent physiologic impairment.

The glycol ethers, because of their solubility characteristics, find their way into many oil-water combinations. Skin absorption of these compounds is sufficiently rapid that it may contribute substantially to systemic toxicity. The organ most often affected by toxic dose levels is the kidney, although anemia has also been reported as a result of chronic exposure to several of the ethylene glycol ethers.

With respect to the aromatic hydrocarbon solvents, benzene is rather unique in that it is an unpredictable toxicant and, in some individuals, may produce irreversible bone marrow damage. Thus, wherever possible, exposure to benzene should be avoided. Attempts to relate the toxicity of benzene to its metabolic products have not been successful. Toluene is less toxic than benzene and is rapidly metabolized to benzoic acid, conjugated with glycine, and excreted as hippuric acid.

A great deal of effort has gone into studies of carbon tetrachloride, methanol, ethanol, benzene, and other solvents in an attempt to determine their effects on basic biochemical pathways that culminate in the response of the whole animal to the toxicant. Although these goals have not been completely achieved, such studies have provided new information concerning cellular and biochemical responses to toxicants in general and have also provided new insights into functions of the normal cell.

Information on the biochemical activity and metabolic fate of chemical compounds is also essential if one is to develop a logical basis for therapy. This can often be achieved before details of toxic action are known. For example, the utilization of ethanol in the treatment of methanol or ethylene glycol poisoning developed out of an understanding of their common metabolic pathway and the potential use of competitive substrate inhibitors.

Recent study of the ability of the liver microsomal enzyme system to metabolize a wide variety of chemicals has provided a great integrating force between fundamental biochemistry and studies of the biochemical response to toxicants. Such a merger of interests cannot help but serve to increase the rate at which information in biochemical toxicology will become available. The rapid development of such basic knowledge in toxicology will help to protect both man and his environment from the misuse of chemical compounds by providing a rational basis on which to evaluate and predict the toxicity of chemical agents.

REFERENCES

Adams, E. M.; Spencer, H. C.; Rowe, V. K.; and Irish, D. D.: Vapor toxicity of 1,1,1-trichloroethane (methylchloroform) determined by experiments on laboratory animals. *Arch. Ind. Hyg. Occup. Med.*, 1:225–36, 1950.

Adams, E. M.; Spencer, H. C.; Rowe, V. K.; McCollister, D. D.; and Irish, D. D.: Vapor toxicity of trichloroethylene determined by experiments on laboratory animals. *Arch. Ind. Hyg. Occup. Med.*, 4:469–81, 1951.

———: Vapor toxicity of carbon tetrachloride determined by experiments on laboratory animals. *Arch. Ind. Hyg. Occup. Med.*, 6:50–66, 1952.

Ahlmark, A., and Forssman, S.: Evaluating trichloroethylene exposures by urinalyses for trichloroacetic acid. *Arch. Ind. Hyg. Occup. Med.*, 3:386–98, 1951.

Aksoy, M.; Erdem, S.; and Dincol, G.: Leukemia in shoe-workers exposed chronically to benzene. *Blood*, 44:837–41, 1974.

Aksoy, M.; Dincol, K.; Erdem, S.; Akgun, T.; and Dincol, G.: Details of blood changes in 32 patients with pancytopenia associated with long-term exposure to benzene. *Br. J. Ind. Med.*, 29:56–64, 1972.

Albritti, G.; Siracusa, A.; Ciachetti, C.; Coli, G.; Curradi, F.; Perticoni, G.; and DeRosa, F.: Shoemaker's polyneuropathy in Italy—The aetiological problem. *Br. J. Ind. Med.*, 33:92–99, 1976.

American Conference of Governmental Industrial Hygienists: *Threshold Limit Values of Airborne Contaminants*, 1977. Copyright 1977 by American Conference of Governmental Industrial Hygieniate.

American Industrial Hygiene Association: Hygienic Guide Series, Ethylene glycol monomethyl ether (2-methoxyethanol). *Am. Ind. Hyg. Assoc. J.*, 31:517–20, 1970.

Argus, M. F.; Arcos, J. C.; and Hoch-Ligeti, C.: Studies on the carcinogenic activity of protein-denaturing agents—hepatotoxicity of dioxane. *J. Natl. Cancer Inst.*, 35:949–58, 1965.

Artizzu, M.; Baccino, F. M.; and Dianzani, M. V.: The action of carbon tetrachloride on mitochondria *in vitro. Biochim. Biophys. Acta*, 78:1–11, 1963.

Ashworth, C. T.; Luibel, F. J.; Sanders, E.; and Arnold, N.: Hepatic cell degeneration. Correlation of fine structure with chemicals and histochemical changes in hepatic cell injury produced by carbon tetrachloride in rats. *Arch. Pathol.*, 75:212–25, 1963.

Bachmann, E., and Golberg, L.: Reappraisal of the toxicity of ethylene glycol. 3. Mitochondrial effects. *Food Cosmet. Toxicol.*, 9:39–55, 1971.

Baker, A. B.: The nervous system in trichloroethylene intoxication. *J. Neuropathol. Exp. Neurol.*, 17:649–55, 1958.

Bartonicek, V.: Metabolism and excretion of trichloroethylene after inhalation by human subjects. *Br. J. Ind. Med.*, 19:134–41, 1962.

Bassi, M.: Electron microscopy of rat liver after carbon tetrachloride poisoning. *Exp. Cell Res.*, 20:313–23, 1960.

Blood, F. R.: Chronic toxicity of ethylene glycol in the rat. *Food Cosmet. Toxicol.*, 3:229–34, 1965.

Blood, F. R.: Elliot, G. A.; and Wright, M. S.: Chronic toxicity of ethylene glycol in the monkey. *Toxicol. Appl. Pharmacol.*, 4:489–91, 1962.

Bove, K. E.: Ethylene glycol toxicity. *Am. J. Clin. Pathol.*, 45:46–50, 1966.

Braun, W. H., and Young, J. D.: Identification of hydroxyethoxyacetic acid as the major urinary metabolite of 1,4-dioxane in the rat. *Toxicol. Appl. Pharmacol.*, 39:33–38, 1977.

Brody, T. M.: Discussion on Judah, J. D., and Rees, K. R., Mechanism of action of carbon tetrachloride. *Fed. Proc.*, 18:1017–19, 1959.

———: Some aspects of experimental carbon tetrachloride induced hepatotoxicity. *Ann. N.Y. Acad. Sci.*, 104:1065–73, 1963.

Browning, E.: *Toxicity of Industrial Organic Solvents.* Chemical Publishing Co., New York, 1953.

———: Toxicology of organic compounds of industrial importance. *Ann. Rev. Pharmacol.*, 1:397–430, 1961.

———: *Toxicity of Metabolism of Industrial Solvents.* Elsevier Publishing Co., Amsterdam and London, 1965, pp. 189–212.

Butler, T. C.: Metabolic transformations of trichloroethylene. *J. Pharmacol. Exp. Ther.*, 97:84–92, 1949.

———: Reduction of carbon tetrachloride *in vivo* and reduction of carbon tetrachloride and chloroform *in vitro* by tissues and tissue constituents. *J. Pharmacol. Exp. Ther.*, 134:311–19, 1961.

Büttner, H.: Aldehyde-und Alkolhydrogenase-Aktivitat in Leber und Niere der Ratta. *Biochem. Z.*, **341**:300–14, 1965.

Calvert, D. N., and Brody, T. M.: Biochemical alterations of liver function by the halogenated hydrocarbons. I. *In vitro* and *in vivo* changes and their modification by ethylenediamine tetraacetate. *J. Pharmacol. Exp. Ther.*, **124**:273–81, 1958.

Carpenter, C. P.: Chronic toxicity of tetrachloroethylene. *J. Ind. Hyg. Toxicol.*, **19**:323–36, 1937.

Carpenter, C. P.; Pozzani, V. C.; Weil, C. S.; Nair, J. H.; Keck, G. A.; and Smyth, H. F.: The toxicity of butyl cellosolve solvent. *Arch. Ind. Health*, **14**:114–31, 1956.

Christie, G. S., and Judah, J. D.: Mechanism of action of carbon tetrachloride on liver cells. *Proc. Roy. Soc.*, Ser. B, **142**:241–57, 1954.

Clay, K. L., and Murphy, R. C.: On the metabolic acidosis of ethylene glycol intoxication. *Toxicol. Appl. Pharmacol.*, **39**:39–49, 1977.

Clay, K.; Murphy, R.; and Watkins, W. D.: Experimental methanol toxicity in the primate. Analysis of metabolic acidosis. *Toxicol. Appl. Pharmacol.*, **34**:49–61, 1975.

Cogan, D. G., and Grant, W. M.: An unusual type of keratitis associated with exposure to *N*-butyl alcohol (butanol). *Arch. Ophthalmol.*, **33**:106–109, 1945.

Cohen, E. N., and Hood, N.: Application of low temperature autoradiography to studies of the uptake and metabolism of volatile anesthetics in the mouse. I. Chloroform. *Anesthesiology*, **30**:306–14, 1969.

Coon, R. A.; Jones, R. A.; Leukins, L. J.; and Siegel, J.: Animal inhalation studies of ammonia, ethylene glycol, dimethylamine, and ethanol. *Toxicol. Appl. Pharmacol.*, **16**:646–55, 1970.

Cooper, M. N.; Mitchell, G. W., Jr.; Bennett, I. L., Jr.; and Cary, F. N.: Methyl alcohol poisoning: an account of the 1951 Atlanta epidemic. *J. Med. Assoc. Ga.*, **41**:48–51, 1952.

Cornish, H. H.: Problems posed by observations of serum enzyme changes in toxicology. *CRC Crit. Rev. Toxicol.*, **1**:1–32, 1971.

Cornish, H. H., and Adefuin, J.: Ethanol potentiation of halogenated aliphatic solvent toxicity. *Am. J. Ind. Hyg.*, **27**:57–61, 1966.

Cornish, H. H., and Block, W. D.: A study of carbon tetrachloride. I. The effect of carbon tetrachloride inhalation on rat serum enzymes. *Arch. Ind. Health*, **21**:549–54, 1960a.

————: A study of carbon tetrachloride. II. The effect of carbon tetrachloride inhalation on serum and tissue enzymes. *Arch. Environ. Health*, **1**:96–100, 1960b.

Cornish, H. H., and Ryan, R.: Metabolism of benzene in nonfasted, fasted, and aryl-hydroxylase inhibited rats. *Toxicol. Appl. Pharmacol.*, **77**:767–71, 1965.

Dambrauskas, T., and Cornish, H.: Effect of pretreatment of rats with carbon tetrachloride on tolerance development. *Toxicol. Appl. Pharmacol.*, **17**:83–97, 1970.

Davis, D. C.; Schroeder, D. H.; Gram, T. E.; Reagan, R. L.; and Gillette, J. R.: A comparison of the effects of halothane and carbon tetrachloride on the hepatic drug metabolizing system. *J. Pharmacol. Exp. Ther.*, **177**:556–66, 1971.

Davis, V. E., and Walsh, M. J.: Alcohol, amines, and alkaloids: A possible biochemical basis for alcohol addiction. *Science*, **167**:1005–1006, 1970.

Dean, M. E., and Stock, B. H.: Propylene glycol as a drug solvent in the study of hepatic microsomal metabolism in the rat. *Toxicol. Appl. Pharmacol.*, **28**:44–52, 1974.

Deichmann, W.; MacDonald, W.; and Bernal, E.: The hemapoietic tissue toxicity of benzene vapors. *Toxicol. Appl. Pharmacol.*, **5**:201–204, 1963.

DeVincenzo, G.; Kaplan, C.; and Dedinas, J.: Characterization of the metabolites of methyl n-butyl ketone, methyl isobutyl ketone, methyl ethyl ketone in guinea pig serum and their clearance. *Toxicol. Appl. Pharmacol.*, **36**:511–22, 1976.

Dianzani, M. V.: Uncoupling of oxidative phosphorylation in mitochondria from fatty livers. *Biochem. Biophys. Acta*, **14**:514–32, 1954.

Diaz Gomez, M. I.; DeCastro, C. R.; D'Acosta, N.; DeFenos, O. M.; DeFerreya, E. C.; and Castro, A. J.: Species differences in carbon tetrachloride-induced hepatotoxicity: The role of CCl_4 activation and of lipid peroxidation. *Toxicol. Appl. Pharmacol.*, **34**:102–14, 1975.

Dingell, J. V., and Heimberg, M.: The effects of aliphatic halogenated hydrocarbons on hepatic drug metabolism. *Biochem. Pharmacol.*, **17**:1269–78, 1968.

Drew, R. T., and Fouts, J. R.: The lack of effects of pretreatment with phenobarbital and chlorpromazine on the acute toxicity of benzene in rats. *Toxicol. Appl. Pharmacol.*, **27**:183–93, 1974.

Edwards, J. A., and Evans, D. A.: Ethanol metabolism in subjects possessing typical and atypical liver alcohol dehydrogenase. *Clin. Pharmacol. Ther.*, **8**:824–80, 1967.

Egle, J. L.; Long, J. E.; Simon, G. S.; and Borzelleca, J.: An evaluation of cardiac sensitizing potential of a fabric protector in aerosol form, containing 1,1,1-trichloroethane. *Toxicol. Appl. Pharmacol.*, **38**:369–77, 1976.

Elkins, H. B.: *The Chemistry of Industrial Toxicology*, 2nd ed. John Wiley & Sons, Inc., New York, 1959.

Ellis, F. W.: Effect of ethanol on plasma corticosterone levels. *J. Pharmacol. Exp. Ther.*, **153**:121–27, 1966.

Fishman, W. H.: *Metabolic Conjugation and Metabolic Hydrolysis*, Vol. I. Academic Press, Inc., New York, 1970a.

————: *Metabolic Conjugation and Metabolic Hydrolysis*, Vol. II. Academic Press, Inc., New York, 1970b.

Fitzhugh, O. G., and Nelson, A. A.: Comparison of the chronic toxicity of triethylene glycol with that of diethylene glycol. *J. Ind. Hyg. Toxicol.*, **28**:40–43, 1946.

Fodor, G.; Prasjsnar, D.; and Schlipkoter, H.: Endogenous CO formation by incorporated halogenated hydrocarbons of the methane series. *Staub-Reinhalt Luft*, **33**:260–61, 1973.

Fowler, J. S.: Chlorinated hydrocarbon toxicity in fowl and duck. *J. Comp. Pathol.*, **80**:465–71, 1970.

Fowler, J. S., and Alexander, F.: A new metabolite of carbon tetrachloride. *Br. J. Pharmacol.*, **36**:181P, 1969.

Gallagher, C. H.: The effect of antioxidants on poisoning by carbon tetrachloride. *Aust. J. Exp. Biol. Med. Sci.*, **40**:241–54, 1962.

Galtier, M.; Rancurel, G.; Piva, C.; and Efthymoic, M.: Polyneuritis and aliphatic hydrocarbons. *J. Eur. Toxicol.*, **6**:294–96, 1973 (Fr).

Gerarde, H. W.: *Toxicology and Biochemistry of Aromatic Hydrocarbons*. Elsevier Publishing Co., New York, 1960.

————: The aliphatic (open chain, acyclic) hydrocarbons. In Patty, F. A. (ed.): *Industrial Hygiene and Toxicology*, Vol. II, 2nd ed. Interscience, New York, 1963.

Gershoff, S. N., and Andrus, S. B.: Effect of vitamin B_6 and magnesium on renal deposition of calcium oxalate by ethylene glycol administration. *Proc. Soc. Exp. Biol. Med.*, **109**:99–102, 1962.

Gessner, P. K.; Parke, D. V.; and Williams, R. T.: Studies in detoxication. *Biochem. J.*, **74**:1–5, 1960.

————: Studies in detoxication. *Biochem. J.*, **79**:482–89, 1961.

Glende, E. A., Jr.: Carbon tetrachloride induced protection against carbon tetrachloride toxicity. *Biochem. Pharmacol.*, **21**:1697–1702, 1972.

Greenberg, L.; Mayers, M. R.; Goldwater, L. J.; Burke, W. J.; and Moskowitz, S.: Health hazards in the manufacture of "fused collars." I. Exposure to ethylene glycol monoethyl ether. *J. Ind. Hyg. Toxicol.,* 20:134–47, 1938.

Greenberg, L.; Mayers, M. R.; Goldwater, L. J.; and Smith, A.: Benzene (Benzol) poisoning in the rotogravure printing industry in New York City. *J. Ind. Hyg. Toxicol.,* 21:395–420, 1939.

Grice, H. C.; Barth, M. L.; Cornish, H. H.; Foster, G. V.; and Gray, R. H.: Correlation between serum enzymes, isozyme pattern, and histological detectable organ damage. *Food Cosmet. Toxicol.,* 9:847–55, 1971.

Griffaton, G., and Lowry, R.: Oxydation de l'ethanol *in vitro* par un hemogenat de foie de rat. *C. R. Seances Soc. Biol.,* 158:998–1003, 1964.

Hardy, H., and Elkins, H.: Medical aspects of maximum allowable concentrations: benzene. *J. Ind. Hyg. Toxicol.,* 30:196–200, 1948.

Harger, R. N., and Forney, R. B.: Aliphatic alcohols. In Stolman, A. (ed.): *Progress in Chemical Toxicology,* Vol. 3. Academic Press, Inc., New York, 1967, pp. 20–21.

Haun, C.; Vernot, E.; Darmer, K., Jr.; and Diamond, S.: Continuous animal exposure to low levels of dichloromethane. AMRL-TR-130, Proceedings of 3rd Annual Conf. on Environ. Toxicology. Wright-Patterson Air Force Base, Ohio, Aerospace Medical Research Laboratory, 1972, pp. 199–208.

Hawkins, R. D., and Kalant, H.: The metabolism of ethanol and its metabolic effect. *Pharmacol. Rev.,* 24:67–157, 1972.

Henson, E. V.: The toxicology of some aliphatic alcohols—Part II. *J. Occup. Med.,* 2:497–502, 1960.

Heppel, L.; Neal, P.; Perrin, T.; Orr, M.; and Posterfield, V.: Toxicology of dichloromethane (methylene chloride). I. Studies on effects of daily inhalation. *J. Ind. Hyg. Toxicol.,* 26:8–16, 1944.

Hoch-Ligeti, C., and Argus, M. F.: Effect of carcinogens on the lung of guinea pigs. Nettesheim, P.; Hanna, M. G., Jr.; and Deatherage, J. W., Jr. (eds.): *Morphology of Experimental Respiratory Carcinogenesis.* Atomic Energy Commission, Office of Information Services, 1970, pp. 267–79.

Hoch-Ligeti, C.; Argus, M. F.; and Arcos, J. C.: Induction of carcinomas in the nasal cavity of rats by dioxane. *Br. J. Cancer,* 24:164–67, 1970.

Hogan, G.: The metabolic conversion of dichloromethane to carbon monoxide. Doctoral thesis, U. of Michigan, Ann Arbor, Mich., 1976.

Holmes, P. A.: Reported in NIOSH Criteria Document-Dioxane. Nat. Inst. for Occup. Safety & Health Pub. No. 77–226, 1976.

Iida, M.; Yamamoto, H.; and Sobue, I.: Prognosis of n-hexane polyneuropathy-follow-up studies on mass outbreak in F district of Mie prefecture. *Igaku No Ayumi,* 84:199–201, 1973 (Jap.).

Ikeda, M.; Hatsue, O.; Imamura, T.; and Komoike, Y.: Urinary excretion of total trichloro-compounds, trichloroethanol, and trichloroacetic acid as a measure of exposure to trichloroethylene and tetrachloroethylene. *Br. J. Ind. Med.,* 29:328–33, 1972.

Ikeda, M., and Ohtsuji, H.: Phenobarbital induced protection against toxicity of toluene and benzene in the rat. *Toxicol. Appl. Pharmacol.,* 20:30–43, 1971.

———: A comparative study on the excretion of Fujiware reaction-positive substances in the urine of humans and rodents given trichloro- or tetrachloro-derivatives of ethane and ethylene. *Br. J. Ind. Med.,* 29:94–104, 1972.

Irish, D. D.: Halogenated hydrocarbons. I. Aliphatic. In Patty, F. A. (ed.): *Industrial Hygiene and Toxicology,* Vol. II, 2nd ed. Interscience, New York, 1963.

Israel, Y.: Cellular effects of alcohol. A review. *Q. J. Stud. Alcohol,* 31:293–316, 1970.

Isselbacher, K. J., and Carter, E. A.: Ethanol oxidation by liver microsomes: Evidence against a separate and distinct enzyme system. *Biochem. Biophys. Res. Commun.,* 39:530–37, 1970.

Jornvall, H., and Harris, J. I.: Horse liver alcohol dehydrogenase. On the primary structure of the ethanol active isoenzyme. *Eur. J. Biochem.,* 13:565–76, 1970.

Judah, J. D.: Biochemical disturbances in liver injury. *Br. Med. Bull.,* 25:274–77, 1969.

Judah, J. D., and Rees, K. R.: Mechanism of action of carbon tetrachloride. *Fed. Proc.,* 18:1013–16, 1959.

Kalant, H.: Absorption, diffusion, distribution and elimination of ethanol. Effects on biological membranes. In Kissen, B., and Begleiter, H. (eds.): *The Biology of Alcoholism.* Plenum Press, New York, 1971, pp. 1–62.

Kersting, E. J., and Nielsen, S. W.: Experimental ethylene glycol poisoning in the dog. *Am. J. Vet. Res.,* 27:574–82, 1966.

Khanna, J. M., and Kalant, H.: Effect of inhibitors and inducers of drug metabolism on *in vivo* ethanol metabolism. *Biochem. Pharmacol.,* 19:2033–41, 1970.

Khanna, J. M.; Kalant, H.; and Liu, G.: Metabolism of ethanol by rat liver microsomal enzymes. *Biochem. Pharmacol.,* 19:2493–99, 1970.

Kini, M. M. and Cooper, J. R.: Biochemistry of methanol poisoning. 4. The effect of methanol and its metabolites on retinal metabolism. *Biochem. J.,* 82:164–72, 1962.

Kini, M. M.; King, D. W., Jr.; and Cooper, J. R.: Biochemistry of methanol poisoning. V. Histological and biochemical correlates of effects of methanol and its metabolites on the rabbit retina. *J. Neurochem.,* 9:119–24, 1962.

Klaassen, C. D., and Plaa, G. L.: Relative effects of various chlorinated hydrocarbons on liver and kidney function in mice. *Toxicol. Appl. Pharmacol.,* 9:139–51, 1966.

———: Relative effects of various chlorinated hydrocarbons on liver and kidney function in dogs. *Toxicol. Appl. Pharmacol.,* 10:119–34, 1967.

———: Comparison of the biochemical alterations elicited in livers from rats treated with carbon tetrachloride, chloroform, 1,1,2-trichloroethane, and 1,1,1-trichloroethane. *Biochem. Pharmacol.,* 18:2019–27, 1969.

Kleinfeld, M., and Tabershaw, I. R.: Trichloroethylene toxicity. *Arch. Ind. Hyg. Occup. Med.,* 19:134–41, 1954.

Kociba, R. J.; McCollister, S. B.; Park, S.; Torkelson, T. R.; and Gehring, P. J.: 1,4-Dioxane- I. Results of a two-year ingestion study in rats. *Toxicol. Appl. Pharmacol,* 30:275–86, 1974.

Krebs, H. A.; Freeland, R. A.; Hems, R.; and Stubbs, M.: Inhibition of hepatic gluconeogenesis by ethanol. *Biochem. J.,* 112:117–24, 1969.

Kubic, V., and Anders, M.: Metabolism of dihalomethanes to carbon monoxide. II. *In vitro* studies. *Drug Metab. Dispos.,* 3:104–12, 1975.

Larson, R. E., and Plaa, G. L.: A correlation of the effects of cervical cordotomy, hypothermia, and catecholamines on carbon tetrachloride-induced hepatic necrosis. *J. Pharmacol. Exp. Ther.,* 147:103–11, 1965.

Laug, E. P.; Calvery, H. O.; Morris, H. J.; and Woodard, G.: The toxicity of some glycols and derivatives. *J. Ind. Hyg. Toxicol.,* 21:173–201, 1939.

Lee, E.; Kocsis, J.; and Snyder, R.: Acute effects of benzene on ^{59}Fe incorporation into circulating erythrocytes. *Toxicol. Appl. Pharmacol.,* 27:431–36, 1974.

Lieber, C. S.: Metabolic derangement induced by alcohol. *Annu. Rev. Med.,* 18:35–54, 1967.

Lieber, C. S., and DeCarli, L. M.: Ethanol oxidation by hepatic microsomes: adaptive increase after ethanol feeding. *Science*, 162:917–18, 1968.

————: Effect of drug administration on the activity of the hepatic microsomal ethanol oxidizing system. *Life Sci.*. 9:267–76, 1970a.

————: Hepatic microsomal ethanol oxidizing system. *In vitro* characteristics and adaptive properties *in vivo*. *J. Biol. Chem.*, 245:2505–12, (May-June) 1970b.

Lombardi, B., and Ugazio, G.: Serum lipoproteins in rats with carbon tetrachloride-induced fatty liver. *J. Lipid Res.*, 6:498–505, 1965.

Lundquist, F.: Enzymatic pathways of ethanol metabolism. In Tremolieres, J. V. (ed.): *International Encyclopedia of Alcohol and Alcoholism*, Vol. 1. Pergamon, Oxford, 1970, sec. 20, pp. 95–116.

————: The metabolism of alcohol. In Israel, Y., and Mardoves, J. (eds.): *Biological Basis of Alcoholism*. John Wiley & Sons, Inc., New York, 1971a, pp. 1–52.

————: Influence of ethanol on carbohydrate metabolism. A review. *Q. J. Stud. Alcohol*, 32:1–12, 1971b.

McChesney, E. W.; Goldberg, L.; Parekh, C. K.; Russell, J. C.; and Min, B. H.: Reappraisal of the toxicity of ethylene glycol. II. Metabolism studies in laboratory animals. *Food Cosmet. Toxicol.*, 9:21–38, 1971.

McCollister, D. D.; Beamer, W. H.; Atchison, G. J.; and Spencer, H. C.: Distribution and elimination of radioactive CCl_4 by monkeys upon exposure to low vapor concentration. *J. Pharmacol. Exp. Ther.*, 102:112–24, 1951.

McLean, A. E. M.; McLean, E.; and Judah, J. D.: Cellular necrosis in the liver induced and modified by drugs and other agents. *Int. Rev. Exp. Pathol.*, 4:127–57, 1965.

Machle, W.: Gasoline intoxication. *J.A.M.A.*, 117:1965–71, 1941.

Makar, A. B.; Tephly, T. R.; and Mannering, G. J.: Methanol metabolism in the rat. *J. Pharmacol. Exp. Ther.*, 143:292–300, 1964.

Maling, H.; Stripp, B.; Sipes, I.; Highman, B.; Saul, W.; and Williams, M.: Enhanced hepatotoxicity of carbon tetrachloride, thioacetamide, and dimethylnitrosamine by pretreatment of rats with ethanol and some comparisons with potentiation by isopropanol. *Toxicol. Appl. Pharmacol.*, 33:291–308, 1975.

Maling, H. M.; Frank, A.; and Horning, M. G.: Effect of carbon tetrachloride on hepatic synthesis and release of triglycerides. *Biochim. Biophys. Acta*, 64:540–45, 1962.

Mallov, S.: Effect of ethanol intoxication on plasma free fatty acids in the rat. *Q. J. Stud. Alcohol*, 22:250–53, 1961.

Mannering, G. J.; Van Harken, D. R.; Makar, A. B.; Tephly, T. R.; Watkins, W. D.; and Goodman, J. I.: Role of the intracellular distribution of hepatic catalase in the peroxidative oxidation of methanol. *Ann. N.Y. Acad. Sci.*, 168:265–80, 1969.

Masten, L.: The role of acetaldehyde in selected acute toxic responses to ethanol in the rabbit. Doctoral thesis, University of Michigan, 1972.

Maximchuk, H. J., and Rubinstein, D.: Lipid mobilization following carbon tetrachloride accumulation. *Can. J. Biochem. Physiol.*, 41:525–28, 1963.

McMichael, A.; Spirtas, R.; Kupper, L.; and Gamble, J.: Solvent exposure and leukemia among rubber workers: An epidemiological study. *J. Occup. Med.*, 17:234–39, 1975.

Mello, N. K., and Mendelson, J. H.: Experimentally induced intoxication in alcoholics: A comparison between programmed and spontaneous drinking. *J. Pharmacol. Exp. Ther.*, 173:101–16, 1970.

Mendelson, J. H.: Biological concomitants of alcoholism. *N. Engl. J. Med.*, 283:24–32, 1970.

Mendenhall, C. L.; Bradford, R. H.; and Furman, R. H.: Effect of ethanol on glycerolipid metabolism in rat liver. *Biochim. Biophys. Acta*, 187:501–509, 1969.

Mikiskova, H., and Mikiska, A.: Trichloroethanol in trichloroethylene poisoning. *Br. J. Ind. Med.*, 23:116–25, 1966.

Miyagaki, H.: Electrophysiological studies on the peripheral neurotoxicity of n-hexane. *Jpn. J. Ind. Health*, 9:660–71, 1967.

Morris, H. J.; Nelson, A. A.; and Calvery, H. O.: Observations on the chronic toxicities of propylene glycol, ethylene glycol, diethylene glycol, ethylene glycol mono-ethylether, and diethylene glycol monoethyl-ether. *J. Pharmacol. Exp. Ther.*, 74:266–73, 1942.

Moskowitz, S., and Shapiro, H.: Fatal exposure to methylene chloride vapor. *Arch. Ind. Hyg. Occup. Med.*, 6:116–23, 1952.

Mundy, R. L.; Hall, L. M.; and Teague, R. S.: Pyrazole as an antidote for ethylene glycol poisoning. *Toxicol. Appl. Pharmacol.*, 28:320–22, 1974.

National Academy of Sciences: *Drinking Water and Health*. Washington, D.C., 1977, pp. 939.

National Cancer Institute: Report on carcinogenic bioassay of chloroform. Carcinogenesis Program, Division of Cancer Cause and Prevention, National Cancer Institute, National Institutes of Health, Bethesda, MD, 1976a.

National Cancer Institute: Carcinogenesis Technical Report Series No. 2, Feb. 1976. Carcinogenesis bioassay of trichloroethylene, CAS No. 79-01-6, NCI-CG-TR-2. U.S. Dept. of Health, Education, and Welfare, Public Health Service, National Institutes of Health, 1976b.

National Cancer Institute: Bioassay of tetrachloroethylene for possible carcinogenicity. Pub. No. (NIH) 77-813. U.S. Dept. of Health, Education, and Welfare, Public Health Service, National Institutes of Health, National Cancer Institute, Bethesda, Maryland, 1977.

National Institute for Occupational Safety and Health: Criteria for a recommended standard . . . occupational exposure to methylene chloride. U.S. Dept. Health, Education, and Welfare, Public Health Service. HEW Publication No. (NIOSH) 76–138, 1976.

National Institute for Occupational Safety and Health: Criteria for a recommended . . . occupational exposure to dioxane. U.S. Dept. Health, Education, and Welfare, Public Health Service, DHEW (NIOSH) Publication No. 77-226, 1977.

Nikkila, E. A., and Ojala, K.: Role of L-alpha-glycerophosphate and triglyceride synthesis in production of fatty liver by ethanol. *Proc. Soc. Exp. Biol. Med.*, 113:814–17, 1963.

Nitter-Hauge, S.: Poisoning with ethylene glycol monomethyl ether. Report of two cases. *Acta Med. Scand.*, 188:277–80, 1970.

O'Brien, E. T.; Yeoman, W. B.; and Hobby, J. A.: Hepatorenal damage from toluene in a "glue sniffer." *Br. Med. J.*, 3:29–30, 1971.

Ogata, M.; Takatsuka, Y.; and Tomokuni, K.: Excretion of hippuric acid and *m*- or *p*-methylhippuric acid in the urine of persons exposed to vapours of toluene and m- or p-xylene in an exposure chamber and in workshops, with specific reference to repeated exposures. *Br. J. Ind. Med.*, 28:383–85, 1971.

Ogata, M.; Tomokuni, K.; and Takatsuka, Y.: Urinary excretion of hippuric acid and *m*- and *p*-methylhippuric acid in the urine of persons exposed to vapours of toluene and m- and p-xylene as a test of exposure. *Br. J. Ind. Med.*, 27:43–50, 1970.

Parke, D. V.: *The Biochemistry of Foreign Compounds*. Pergamon Press, London, 1968.

Patty, F. A. (ed.): *Industrial Hygiene and Toxicology*, Vol. I., 2nd ed. Interscience, New York, 1958.

————: *Industrial Hygiene and Toxicology*, Vol. II, 2nd ed. Interscience, New York, 1963.

Perman, E. S.: The effect of ethy alcohol on the secretion from the adrenal medulla of the cat. *Acta Physiol. Scand.*, 48:323–28, 1960.

————: Effect of ethanol on oxygen uptake and on blood glycose concentrations in anaesthetized rabbits. *Acta Physiol. Scand.*, 55:189–202, 1962.

Peterson, D. I.; Peterson, J. E.; Hardinge, M. D.; and Wacker, E. C.: Experimental treatment of ethylene glycol poisoning. *J.A.M.A.*, 186:955–57, 1963.

Plaa, G. L., and Larson, R. E.: Carbon tetrachloride induced liver damage. *Arch. Environ. Health.*, 9:536–43, 1964.

Poggi, M., and DiLuzio, H. R.: The role of·liver and adipose tissue in the pathogenesis of the ethanol-induced fatty liver. *J. Lipid Res.*, 5:437–41, 1964.

Poggi, M.; Fumagilli, R.; Sabatini-Pellegrini, A.; and Paoletti, R.: Investigations on the early effects of CCl_4 on lipid transport. Proc. of the 2nd International Pharmacol. Meetings, Prague, Aug. 20–30, 1963. Pergamon Press, New York, 1965, pp. 363–70.

Poggi, M., and Paoletti, R.: A new insight on carbon tetrachloride effect on triglyceride transport. *Biochem. Pharmacol.*, 13:949–54, 1964.

Pons, C. A., and Custer, R. P.: Acute ethylene glycol poisoning. *Am. J. Med. Sci.*, 211:544–52, 1946.

Posner, H. S.; Mitoma, C.; and Udenfriend, S.: Enzymic hydroxylation of aromatic compounds. II. Further studies of the properties of the microsomal hydroxylating system. *Arch. Biochem. Biophys.*, 94:269–79, 1961.

Rainsford, S. G., and Davis, T. A.: Urinary excretion of phenol by men exposed to vapour of benzene: A screening test. *Br. J. Ind. Med.*, 22:21–26, 1965.

Rampy, L. W.; Quast, J. F.; Leong, B. K.; and Gehring, P. J.: Results of long term inhalation toxicity studies on rats of 1,1,1-trichloroethane and perchloroethylene formulations. Abstract. International Congress of Toxicology, Toronto, Canada, 1977.

Recknagel, R. O.: Carbon tetrachloride hepatotoxicity. *Pharmacol. Rev.*, 19:145–208, 1967.

Recknagel, R. O., and Anthony, D. D.: Effects of CCl_4 on enzyme systems of rat liver mitochondria. *Fed. Proc.*, 16:456, 1957.

————: Biochemical changes in carbon tetrachloride fatty liver: separation of fatty changes from mitochondrial degeneration. *J. Biol. Chem.*, 234(1):1052–59, 1959.

Recknagel, R. O., and Ghoshal, A. K.: Quantitative estimation of peroxidative degeneration of rat liver microsomal and mitochondrial lipids after carbon tetrachloride poisoning. *Exp. Mol. Pathol.*, 5:413–26, 1966.

Recknagel, R. O., and Lombardi, B.: Studies of biochemical changes in subcellular particles of rat liver and their relationship to a new hypothesis regarding the pathogenesis of carbon tetrachloride fat accumulation. *J. Biol. Chem.*, 236:564–69, 1961.

Recknagel, R. O.; Lombardi, B.; and Schotz, M. C.: A new insight into the pathogenesis of carbon tetrachloride fat infiltration. *Proc. Soc. Exp. Med.*, 104:608–10, 1960.

Recknagel, R. O.; Stadler, J.; and Litteria, M.: Biochemical changes accompanying development of fatty liver. *Fed. Proc.*, 17:129, 1958.

Rees, K. R., and Shotlander, V. L.: Fat accumulation in acute liver injury. *Proc. Roy. Soc.*, Ser. B., 157:517–35, 1963.

Reinhardt, C.; Mullin, L.; and Maxfield, M.: Epinephrine-induced cardiac arrhythmia potential of some common industrial solvents. *J. Occup. Med.*, 15:953–55, 1973.

Reynolds, E. S.; Thiers, R. E.; and Vallee, B. L.: Mitochondrial function and metal content in carbon tetrachloride poisoning. *J. Biol. Chem.*, 237:3546–51, 1962.

Ritchie, J. M.: The aliphatic alcohols. In Goodman, L., and Gilman, A. (eds.): *The Pharmacological Basis of Therapeutics*, 5th ed. Macmillan Publishing Co., Inc., New York, 1975.

Roberts, J. A., and Seibold, H. R.: Ethylene glycol toxicity in the monkey. *Toxicol. Appl. Pharmacol.*, 15:624–31, 1969.

Robertson, O. H.; Loosli, C. G.; Puck, T. T.; Wise H.; Lemon, H. M.; and Lester, W., Jr.: Tests for the chronic toxicity of propylene glycol and triethylene glycol on monkeys and rats by vapor inhalation and oral administration. *J. Pharmacol. Exp. Ther.*, 91:52–76, 1947.

Rodkey, F. L., and Collison, H. A.: Biological oxidation of [^{14}C] methylene chloride to carbon monoxide and carbon dioxide by the rat. *Toxicol. Appl. Pharmacol.*, 40:33–38, 1977a.

Rodkey, F. L., and Collison, H. A.: Effect of dihalogenated methanes on the *in vivo* production of carbon monoxide and methane by rats. *Toxicol. Appl. Pharmacol.*, 40:39–47, 1977b.

Røe, O.: The roles of alkaline salts and ethyl alcohol in the treatment of methanol poisoning. *Q. J. Stud. Alcohol*, 11:107–12, 1950.

Rowe, V. K.: Glycols. In Patty, F. A. (ed.): *Industrial Hygiene and Toxicology*, Vol. II, 2nd ed. Interscience, New York, 1963.

Rowe, V. K.; McCollister, D. D.; Spencer, H. C.; Adams, E. M.; and Irish, D. D.: Vapor toxicity of tetrachloroethylene for laboratory animals and human subjects. *Arch. Ind. Hyg. Occup. Med.*, 5:566–79, 1952.

Rubin, E.; Hutterer, F.; and Lieber, C. S.: Ethanol increases hepatic smooth endoplasmic reticulum and drug metabolizing enzymes. *Science*, 159:1469–70, 1968.

Rubin, E., and Lieber, C. S.: Alcoholism, alcohol, and drugs. *Science*, 172:1097–1102, 1971.

Rubinstein, D., and Kanics, L.: The conversion of carbon tetrachloride and chloroform to carbon dioxide by rat liver homogenates. *Can. J. Biochem. Physiol.*, 42:1577–85, 1964.

Ruddick, J. A.: Toxicology, metabolism, and biochemistry of 1,2-propanediol. *Toxicol. Appl. Pharmacol.*, 21:102–11, 1971.

Ruprecht, H. A., and Nelson, I. A.: Preliminary toxicity reports on diethylene glycol and sulfanilamide. V. Clinical and pathologic observations. *J.A.M.A.*, 109(2):1537, 1937.

Sasame, H. A.; Castro, J. A.; and Gillette, J. R.: Studies on the destruction of liver microsomal cytochrome P-450 by carbon tetrachloride administration. *Biochem. Pharmacol.*, 17:1759–68, 1968.

Scholler, K. L.: Modification of the effects of chloroform on the rat liver. *Br. J. Anaesth.*, 42:603–605, 1970.

Schwetz, B. A.; Leong, B. K.; and Gehring, P. J.: The effect of maternally inhaled trichloroethylene, perchloroethylene, methyl chloroform and methylene chloride on embryonal and fetal development in mice and rats. *Toxicol. Appl. Pharmacol.*, 32:84–96, 1975.

Seakins, A., and Robinson, D. S.: The effect of the administration of carbon tetrachloride on the formation of plasma lipoproteins in the rat. *Biochem. J.*, 86:401–407, 1963.

Slater, T. F.: The inhibitory effects *in vitro* of phenothiazines and other drugs on lipid-peroxidation systems in rat-liver microsomes, and their relationship to the liver necrosis produced by carbon tetrachloride. *Biochem. J.*, 106:155–60, 1968.

Chapter 19

RADIATION AND RADIOACTIVE MATERIALS

Charles H. Hobbs and *Roger O. McClellan*

INTRODUCTION

Radiation toxicology is a specialized area of toxicology of considerable breadth and depth. Obviously it cannot be covered in great detail in a book such as this. Nonetheless, its importance related to the increasing use of radiation in the modern world dictates that certain basic elements of radiation toxicology be presented in this chapter. The manner of presentation then is of a survey nature with emphasis on providing both specific and general references that will assist the interested reader in obtaining a more detailed understanding of the subject.

BASIC PHYSICAL CONCEPTS

Ionizing radiation is a term applied to radiations that give rise, directly or indirectly, to ionizations when they interact with matter. Ionizing radiations comprise electromagnetic radiation, such as gamma and x-rays, and particulate or corpuscular radiation, such as alpha particles, beta particles, electrons, positrons, neutrons, and protons. The absorption of the energy of ionizing radiations in cells involves ionization of atoms and the production of ions within the cells. Although the exact mechanism of action of ionizing radiation is not known, radiation injury is considered to be related in some way to the production of ions within the cell.

The electromagnetic ionizing radiations, gamma and x-rays, are part of the electromagnetic spectrum with characteristic wavelengths and photon energies as illustrated in Figure 19–1. These rays have penetrating power that is generally directly related to the energy of the photon. For example, gamma or x-rays with energies of 300 Kev would be more penetrating than those with energies of 50 Kev.

X-rays originate outside the nucleus of atoms. In x-ray machines, they are produced by applying a high positive voltage between the source of electrons and a collecting terminal within a vacuum tube. When the electrons strike a suitable target, such as tungsten, their energy is partly converted into x-ray photons.

Gamma rays originate from unstable atomic nuclei releasing energy to gain stability. They have definite energies, characteristic of the nuclide from which they are emitted. Gamma and x-rays ionize materials largely indirectly through a variety of mechanisms that involve ejection of high-speed electrons from the atoms by which they are absorbed. The three primary types of interactions of gamma and x-rays following absorption by matter are photoelectric effect, Compton scattering, and pair production.

The alpha particle (α) is identical to a helium nucleus consisting of two neutrons and two protons. It results from the radioactive decay of heavy elements such as uranium, plutonium, radium, and thorium. Alpha particles have a large mass as compared to most other types of particulate radiations, such as neutrons and electrons. Decay of alpha-emitting radionuclides may result in the emission of several different alpha particles, each with its own discrete energy rather than a continuous distribution of energies. Because of their double positive charge, α particles have great ionizing power but their large size results in very little penetrating power. Their range in tissues is measured in micrometers.

Beta particles (β^-) are electrons resulting from the conversion of a neutron to a proton in the nucleus of an atom. They are identical to electrons from other sources such as those from tubes and heated filaments. Electrons that arise from outside the nucleus by internal conversion and the so-called Auger electrons are also identical but usually are designated by "C" rather than "B." Beta particles are not emitted with discrete energy levels, but rather a continuous spectrum of energy levels from a maximum value characteristic of each beta emitter down to zero. The decay emission of a beta particle generally results from atoms with large values of the ratio of neutrons to protons in the nucleus. Electrons have a greater range and penetrating power but much less ionizing power than alpha particles.

The positron (β^+) is a particle with the same mass as an electron but possesses a single positive

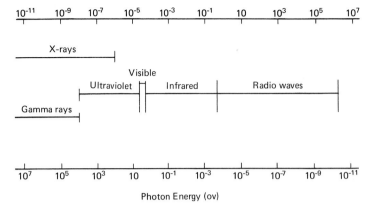

Figure 19–1. Approximate wavelengths and photon energies of major types of electromagnetic radiation. (From Casarett, A. P.: *Radiation Biology.* © 1968 by U.S. Atomic Energy Commission, Washington, D.C. Reprinted by permission of Prentice-Hall, Inc., Englewood Cliffs, N.J.)

charge. The emission of a positron from the nucleus is equivalent to converting a proton to a neutron and is the preferred mode of decay of unstable atoms with a small ratio of neutrons to protons in the nucleus. Electron capture is another way in which electron-deficient nuclei convert protons to neutrons by capturing orbital electrons into the nucleus. An annihilation reaction results when positrons and electrons interact resulting in the formation of two photons each with an energy of 511 Kev.

The neutron is a particle consisting of an electron and a proton. Neutrons may be released from elements that decay by spontaneous fission and from those fission products that possess metastable states with respect to neutron emission. The process of fission results in the release of from one to three neutrons. Due to their mass, neutrons have great kinetic energy, and because they have no charge, they penetrate readily. Neutrons produce ionization indirectly. In biologic materials this usually results from the ejection of protons from the nuclei of hydrogen atoms. These recoil nuclei are charged and are directly ionizing. Neutrons also activate hydrogen and other elements by neutron capture, which results in the release of gamma rays. Free neutrons are unstable and will undergo beta decay with half-lives of about 9 to 30 minutes if uncaptured.

Protons are identical to hydrogen nuclei and are produced in tissues by the interactions of neutrons. Their charge and mass make them potent ionizers.

The radiations discussed above all produce ionizations. The directly ionizing particles are charged and, by virtue of their mass and motion, possess the energy to produce ionizations along their path as a result of impulses imparted to orbital electrons via electrical forces between the charged particles and orbital electrons. Indirectly ionizing radiations are not charged and penetrate through a medium with no interaction

with electrons until they collide with elements of the atom and liberate energetically charged particles that are ionizing.

Radioactive decay occurs from unstable natural and artificially produced isotopes of elements decaying by the emission of subatomic particles and gamma or x-ray photons. In the case of very heavy elements, there is a pronounced tendency to decay by the emission of alpha particles. In the case of lighter elements, beta emission is the most frequent decay process. As discussed previously, beta decay occurs when there is an excess in the neutron-to-proton ratio. A less frequent mode of decay is by positron emission, which is favored by a small neutron-to-proton ratio in the nucleus. Gamma rays often accompany the emission of alpha and beta particles from a nucleus due to an excess in energy in the daughter nucleus following the alpha or beta decay.

The half-life of a radionuclide is the time required for the number of atoms present to decrease by one-half. The disintegration of radioactive nuclei is a random process and the rate of disintegration is directly proportional to the number of radioactive atoms present. Thus, when half the atoms in a sample have decayed, the rate of decay will have decreased by 2. The mathematical expression of radioactive decay is the exponential equation

$$N_t = N_0 e^{-\lambda t} \tag{1}$$

where

N_t = number of nuclei present at any time (t)
N_0 = number of nuclei present initially
λ = the radioactive decay constant
e = base of natural logarithms

The half-life of a radionuclide is then represented by

$$\frac{N_0}{2} = N_0 e^{-\lambda t} 1/2 \tag{2}$$

which can be solved to give

$$T_{1/2} = \frac{\ln 2}{\lambda} = \frac{0.693}{\lambda} \qquad (3)$$

The unit used to express radioactivity is the curie (Ci). The curie was originally related to the activity of 1 g of radium but is now defined as 3.7×10^{10} nuclear disintegrations per second or 2.22×10^{12} disintegrations per minute. A millicurie (mCi), microcurie (μCi), nanocurie (nCi), and picocurie (pCi) are $1/10^3$, $1/10^6$, $1/10^9$, and $1/10^{12}$ curies, respectively. The specific activity of a sample is the total radioactivity of a given radionuclide per given mass of a compound, element, or radioactive nuclide. This activity is usually expressed in curies per gram and may be calculated by

$$\frac{1.308 \times 10^8}{(T_{1/2})(\text{atomic weight})}$$

where

$T_{1/2}$ is the half-life in days

The roentgen (R) is a unit of exposure related to the amount of ionization caused in air by gamma or x-radiation. One roentgen equals 2.58×10^{-4} coulomb per kilogram of air. In the case of gamma radiation over the commonly encountered range of photon energy, the energy deposition in tissue for a dose of 1 R is about 0.0096 joules/kg.

The rad is the unit of radiation-absorbed dose and is a measurement of energy deposition in any medium by all types of ionizing radiation. One rad is equal to 100 ergs/g or 0.01 J/kg in any medium. The rad has more application than the R and should be used whenever the absorbed dose is known.

The dose equivalent, expressed as rem, takes into consideration such modifying factors of dose (in rads) as the quality of the irradiation. The rem is the product of the absorbed dose in rads times the unitless quantities of radiation quality and any other factors such as dose distribution within the target tissue. In practice the latter factors are still so uncertain that they are generally assigned a value of 1 so that the dose equivalent in rems is equal to the rad dose times the quality factor. The terms of the dose equivalent and qualifications of its use have recently been defined and discussed (ICRU, 1971, 1973, 1976; ICRP, 1977).

The quality factor for the various types of ionizing radiation is based on the linear energy transfer (LET) of the type of radiation. The LET is the rate at which charged particles transfer their energies to the atoms in a medium and is a function of the energy and velocity of the charged particle. For example, alpha particles with their large mass, $+2$ charge, and slow speed impart much more energy over their path than do electrons. The damage produced in tissue by absorption of a given amount of energy is generally greater as the distance over which this energy is imparted decreases, that is, the LET increases. In general, the higher the LET of the radiation, the greater the injury for a given absorbed dose. Values of the quality factor for various types of ionizing radiation are given in Table 19–1.

The term relative biologic effectiveness (RBE) is used to denote the experimentally determined

Table 19–1.   QUALITY FACTORS

1. X-rays, electrons, and positrons of any specific ionization

   QF = 1
2. Heavy ionizing particles

AVERAGE LET IN WATER (Mev/cm)	QF
35 or less	1
35 to 70	1 to 2
70 to 230	2 to 5
230 to 530	5 to 10
530 to 1,750	10 to 20

For practical purposes, a QF of 10 is often used for alpha particles‡ and fast neutrons and protons up to 10 Mev. A QF of 20 is used for heavy recoil nuclei.

The following values for quality factors may be used for neutrons when the neutron energy spectrum is known:

NEUTRON ENERGY (Mev)	QF
Thermal	2
0.0001	2
0.001	2.5
0.1	7.5
0.5	11
1.0	11
10	6.5

* From Shapiro, J.: *Radiation Protection.* Harvard University Press, Cambridge, Mass., 1972, p. 52.
† Data from ICRP, 1963; NCRP, 1971a; NCRP, 1971.
‡ The ICRP (ICRP, 1977) has recently recommended a quality factor of 20 for alpha particles.

ratio of the absorbed dose from one radiation type to the absorbed dose of a reference radiation required to produce an identical biologic effect under the same conditions. Gamma rays of ^{60}Co and 200 to 250 Kev x-rays have been used as reference standards. The term RBE has been restricted to experimental radiobiology and the quality factor is used in calculations of dose equivalents (NCRP, 1971b; ICRP, 1977).

It should be noted that the question of the appropriate quality factor for neutrons and alpha particles is under question. The ICRP has recently recommended the use of a quality factor of 20 for alpha particles and uncharged particles. Rossi (1975) in postulating a theory of dual radiation action has suggested that the relative biologic effectiveness for neutrons may approach 100 in some cases. Thus, there is also the need to reexamine the appropriate quality factor for use with neutrons.

In order to conform to the International System of Units (SI) most of the currently used radiation units will probably change over the next ten years. These changes have been recommended by the International Commission on Radiation Measurements and Units (ICRU) and two units have been approved by the International Committee on weights and measures (Linden, 1976). The ICRU now recommends that the rad, the roentgen, the curie and the rem be replaced by the SI units the gray (Gy), the Coulomb per kilogram (C/kg), the becquerel (Bq), and the sievert (Sv), respectively. Unfortunately, the old and new units may not be used interchangeably as explained below.

The SI unit, the joule per kilogram when used for ionizing radiation, is the gray with the symbol Gy; 1 Gy = 100 rad = 1 J/kg. The SI unit of one per second (reciprocal second) for activity is the becquerel with the symbol Bq; 1 Bq = 1/sec ~ 2.703×10^{-11} Ci. The SI unit proposed by ICRU for the rem is the sievert (Sv). As the dose equivalent is the product of the absorbed dose in grays times the unitless modifying factors such as the quality factor

1 Sv = 1 J/kg (= 100 rem)

For a more complete discussion of the above concepts the reader should refer to texts on radiation protection, radiation physics, and radiobiology. Some of the more recent of these are Elkind and Whitmore (1967), Casarett (1968), Altman, Gerber and Okada (1970), Hendee (1970), Fabrikant (1972), Martin and Harbison (1972), and Andrews (1974). For a review of radioactivity measurements, procedures, and radiation monitoring methods the reader is referred to recent publications of the National Council on Radiation Protection and Measurements (NCRP, 1978a, b, and c).

SOURCES OF IONIZING RADIATION EXPOSURE

The sources for exposure of man and animals to ionizing radiation can be broken down into four major groups: (1) natural sources of irradiation, both external and internal; (2) medical sources, such as diagnostic or therapeutic x-irradiation, and radiopharmaceuticals; (3) nuclear reactions, such as nuclear power reactors and nuclear weapons; and (4) other sources, such as industrial x-ray machines. Exposure to natural sources of irradiation is unavoidable for the most part, but the degree of exposure to man-made sources is subject to change, depending on intelligent and judicial use of such sources.

Natural Background Radiation

Exposure to natural sources of external ionizing radiation results from the levels of cosmic and terrestrial x-irradiation present in the environment. Cosmic irradiation at the earth's surface is affected by altitude and geomagnetic latitude. It increases by a factor of 3 in going from sea level to an altitude of 10,000 ft and by 10 to 20 percent in going from 0° to 50° geomagnetic latitude. Estimates of the annual average whole-body dose from cosmic radiation range from 38 mrem/year in Florida to about 75 mrem/year in Wyoming with an average for the United States of about 44 mrem/year (BEIR Report, 1972). Man is also exposed to external gamma radiation from concentrations of radioactive materials in soils and rocks. The dose level for this source of radiation varies markedly depending on the mineral content of the area and other factors such as the types of building materials used. Estimates of the annual dose for this type of exposure vary from about 15 to 140 mrem/year for various parts of the United States with an average of about 40 mrem/year (BEIR Report, 1972a). A more recent report (NCRP, 1975a) has placed the average dose from cosmic radiation in the United States at 28 mrem/year and that from external terrestrial radiation at 26 mrem/year.

Internally deposited, naturally occurring radioactive materials also contribute to the natural radiation dose. Potassium-40 is the most predominant radioactive element of normal foods and human tissues. Annual dose rates of 18 mrem/year (BEIR Report, 1972) or 24 mrem/year have been estimated for internally deposited radioactive materials. Thus, for all sources of natural radiation, the average annual dose rate has been estimated to be about 80 to

100 mrem/year in the United States (BEIR Report, 1972; NCRP, 1975a). This dose rate, however, can vary markedly depending on geographic location and other factors.

It should be noted that the dose to the organs from these sources is not uniform. The dose to the lung from natural sources has been estimated to be 180 mrem/year and that to bone surfaces 120 mrem/year compared to a dose for the bone marrow (whole-body) of 80 mrem/year (NCRP, 1975a). Most of the larger dose to the lung is attributable to the inhalation of the alpha-emitting daughters of the naturally occurring radionuclide ^{222}Rn. Also the dose equivalent rates to the lungs of smokers may be up to three times higher than for nonsmokers due to inhalation of ^{210}Po and ^{210}Pb from the cigarette. Some of the lung dose is also received from radionuclides released during combustion of fossil fuels, which contain small quantities of naturally occurring radionuclides.

Health Science Applications

The use of radiation by the healing arts is recognized as the largest man-made component of the radiation dose to the population of developed countries such as the United States. The main source of this exposure is the medical use of diagnostic x-radiation with lesser contributions from dental x-radiation, radiopharmaceuticals, and therapeutic irradiation. An estimated average annual dose rate of about 70 mrem/year (abdominal dose) has been made (BEIR Report, 1972). In the case of this type of exposure, however, the average dose to the population may have little meaning as the dose is not equally distributed among the population. For example, the average vertebral marrow dose for a diagnostic upper gastrointestinal examination on a patient was reported to be 1.6 rads at midfield (Margulis, 1973). Substantial reductions in the dose to individuals and the population could be made by restricting the radiographic examinations to those in which a high yield of diagnostic information is obtained and by the use of the best available equipment and techniques (Margulis, 1973).

There has been a recent marked increase in the use of various radiopharmaceuticals for diagnostic purposes. Current information based on sales of radiopharmaceuticals has indicated an annual increase of 25 percent per year and an estimate of a fivefold increase in use of these compounds in the 1960s with an estimated sevenfold increase in their use over the next ten years (BEIR Report, 1972). Thus, these compounds are becoming an important source of exposure of man to radiation. A series of reports by the Medical Internal Radiation Dose Committee (MIRD) of the Society of Nuclear Medicine has detailed the physical, chemical, and biochemical characteristics, the biologic distribution, and absorbed-dose calculations for various radiopharmaceuticals (MIRD Reports, 1968, 1969, 1971, 1975a, 1975b).

Nuclear Reactions

After the discovery of nuclear fission, the first nuclear reactor was developed toward the end of 1942 by Fermi and associates. This was followed by the Manhattan Project, which developed the first atomic weapons by the end of World War II. Nuclear fission follows the capture of a single neutron by the nucleus of a fissionable material such as ^{235}U or ^{239}Pu. The fission releases one to three neutrons and, if additional fissionable material is present in sufficient quantity and in the right configuration, a chain reaction results and the reaction is said to be critical. Slow or thermal neutrons are the most efficient for the production of nuclear fission from ^{235}U and ^{238}U mixtures. Thus, materials such as graphite, heavy water, beryllium, and organic chemicals are used as moderators to slow the neutrons. The enrichment of natural uranium with ^{235}U has lessened the need to slow the neutrons, and the operation of reactors with ordinary water as the moderator or with no moderator is now possible. Control rods of neutron-absorbing materials such as cadmium and boron control the chain reaction in many types of nuclear reactors. The process of nuclear fission, in addition to the liberation of from one to three neutrons from the nucleus, produces fission fragments or products with atomic mass numbers of 72 to 160. These fission products have unstable nuclei and decay by beta decay often with gamma emission. In the process of nuclear fission, there is a decrease in total mass, which results in a corresponding gain in energy that is released in a nuclear weapon detonation or is harnessed in a reactor for the production of power.

Most of the world's present-day supply of uranium contains only about 0.7 percent ^{235}U and about 99 percent ^{238}U. ^{238}U as well as ^{232}Th is said to be a fertile substance in that it cannot itself sustain a chain reaction but can be converted into fissionable material following neutron capture. One possible breeding reaction is represented by the following equation:

$$^{238}_{92}\text{U} + ^{1}_{0}\text{N} \longrightarrow ^{239}_{93}\text{U} \xrightarrow[23\,\text{min}]{\beta^-} ^{239}_{93}\text{Np} \xrightarrow[23\,\text{min}]{\beta^-} ^{239}_{94}\text{Pu}$$

Nuclear reactors in which the ratio of conversion to fission is greater than 1 are said to be breeder reactors. The breeder reactors now in the most advanced stages of development use ^{238}U as the fertile material. In addition, ^{239}Pu will be used as fuel. Thorium, which is estimated to be more abundant in the earth's crust than uranium, could also be used as a fertile material in breeder reactors.

After the initial development of isotopic separation techniques and nuclear reactors, ^{235}U and ^{239}Pu were obtained in sufficient quantities to construct bombs. When these fissionable materials are assembled into critical masses under properly controlled conditions, an uncontrolled, but of course self-depleting, chain reaction results that releases tremendous quantities of energy. The fissioning of each ^{235}U nucleus releases about 200 Mev of energy. In theory, it is possible for about 5 lb of ^{235}U to release energy with an expansive pressure equal to 20,000 tons of TNT (Behrens, 1969).

Nuclear energy can also be released by fusion of smaller nuclei into larger nuclei if during the process there is a decrease in mass. For fusion to take place, the interacting nuclei must have sufficient kinetic energy to overcome the repulsive force of like electrostatic charges. One method by which a fusion process can be accomplished is at extremely high temperatures ($\sim 10^8$ °K) such as occur following the explosion of fission-type nuclear weapons. These reactions are termed thermonuclear and generally involve isotopes of hydrogen. Thermonuclear or fusion-type weapons have been tested. Fusion reactors for the production of heat and power offer the potential for essentially unlimited power with relatively few pollution problems. There are many technologic problems, however, that must be solved prior to any practical use of fusion for the production of power.

Nuclear Weapons. The first nuclear weapon test explosion took place in 1945 and from then until 1963 large-scale nuclear weapon testing in the atmosphere was conducted by the United States, Russia, and the United Kingdom. In 1963, a ban on atmospheric testing was agreed on by these major powers but limited atmospheric testing has been conducted periodically by France and China. Underground nuclear testing allowed by the treaty has continued and contributes comparatively little to global fallout of radioactive materials (Eisenbud, 1973). After the explosion of atomic weapons, fission products and products of neutron activation from materials used for bomb construction and in the area of the explosion are released as radioactive fallout. The effects of nuclear weapons have recently been reviewed (Glasstone and Dolan, 1977).

Of the many radionuclides produced in nuclear and thermonuclear explosions, the primary contributors to exposure of man are ^{89}Sr, ^{90}Sr, ^{95}Zr, ^{193}Ru, ^{106}Ru, ^{131}I, ^{137}Cs, ^{141}Ce,

and ^{144}Ce. Although ^{239}Pu is present in considerable quantity, its solubility characteristics prevent it from becoming a significant contributor to the dose from fallout. The significance of these and other internally deposited radionuclides is discussed further under Internal Emitters in this chapter. The primary dose from fallout radiation is through external gamma doses, assimilation through the food chain, or beta dose to the skin.

Nuclear Power Production. The production of power by nuclear reactors could increase considerably over the next 50 years. The extent to which this increase occurs will depend largely on technology development, the establishment of the environmental and health costs of nuclear reactors compared to those from conventional sources, and their public and political acceptance. Although dose estimates of potential exposures from the use of nuclear power reactors for power production appear to be reasonable from an environmental standpoint, the impact of catastrophic accidents, however unlikely they are to occur, is more difficult to assess. For the production of power from nuclear reactors, there are a number of areas such as uranium mining, fuel fabrication, the reactor itself, fuel reprocessing, and storage of radioactive wastes that may result in the exposure of man and his environment to radiation. Most of these are discussed below.

Although uranium mining increases the amount of uranium and its decay products accessible to man, the process has not been associated with measurable increases in environmental radioactivity outside the immediate vicinity of the mines. The serious health problems in uranium miners associated with ^{222}Rn and the attachment of its short-lived daughters to dust particles are discussed elsewhere. The same considerations exist for uranium mills and fuel fabrication plants in that proper location and appropriate control of tailings and liquid wastes can prevent significant population exposures from these sources. Previously, failure to control these processes resulted in increased ^{226}Ra in water near plants and its subsequent deposition in crops from irrigation water. Also, the use of tailings in home construction resulted in increased gamma ray and radon exposure of the occupants of the houses (Eisenbud, 1973; NCRP, 1975b).

The quantity and availability of radionuclides for release vary considerably with the type and design of the reactor. The current nuclear power reactors are almost all either boiling-water and pressurized-water types of light water or reactors in which water is utilized as both coolant and moderator. A few gas (helium)-cooled reactors are also in operation, primarily in Great Britain.

As light-water reactors are relatively inefficient and convert only about 1 to 2 percent of the potentially available energy into heat, there is currently a large international research effort under way to produce practical fast-breeder reactors that can use up to about 75 percent of the energy in uranium (Eisenbud, 1973). Of the various possibilities for this reactor type, the so-called liquid metal-cooled fast-breeder reactor (LMFBR) appears to be the first type that will be developed, and commercially used, most likely in Europe.

In the current light-water-cooled reactors, the principal radionuclides present in reactor effluents under normal operations are ^{3}H, ^{58}Co, ^{60}Co, ^{95}Kr, ^{85}Sr, ^{90}Sr, ^{130}I, ^{131}I, ^{131}Xe, ^{133}Xe, ^{134}Cs, ^{137}Cs, and ^{140}Ba (Eisenbud, 1973). Gaseous and volatile radionuclides such as ^{85}Kr, ^{131}Xe, and ^{133}Xe contribute to the external gamma dose while the others contribute to the dose externally by surface deposition and internally by way of the food chain. The average annual dose for the United States population from reactor operations has been estimated to be 0.002 mrem for 1970 and projected to be 0.17 mrem/year for the year 2000, if current estimates of reactor development hold (BEIR Report, 1972).

Under catastrophic accident conditions, radionuclides that may escape from nuclear reactors can be classified as volatile or nonvolatile. The volatile radionuclides of importance include iodine, tritium, and noble gases such as krypton and xenon. The nonvolatile radionuclides include all fission products, many activation products, and fuel components. Under accident situations, the most likely route of exposure is inhalation rather than environment contamination (BEIR Report, 1972). In any accidents involving the LMFBR, there exists the potential for inhalation of particles of plutonium and other transuranic radionuclides as well as ^{22}Na.

Nuclear reactor design has placed considerable emphasis on safeguards against complete failure of containment systems under accident situations. With light-water thermal reactors, the event that could conceivably result in the most catastrophic situation would be a complete failure of the coolant systems including failure of the emergency core cooling systems. This would result in a melting of the core with subsequent rupture of the containment vessel. The subsequent release of volatile and nonvolatile fission products in the form of a cloud would create a potential for exposure of a large number of people downwind from the reactor. For LMFBR, concern for population safety has been expressed because of the use of plutonium, the opportunity for sodium-water reactions, and the risk of accidental changes in core configuration resulting in prompt criticality (Eisenbud, 1973). Catastrophic accidents, however unlikely, probably represent the most difficult risk-versus-benefit judgments concerning the increased use of nuclear reactors for the production of power.

A major study that assessed the accident risks in United States nuclear power plants has recently been completed (WASH-1400, 1975a). The study considered the risks and consequences from accidents involving large nuclear power reactors of the pressurized-water and boiling-water types that are now being used in the United States. The results of this study suggest that the risk to the public from accidents involving nuclear power reactors are relatively small as the consequences of reactor accidents were predicted to be no larger and in many cases smaller than those of nonnuclear accidents and as accidents involving nuclear reactors were predicted to be much less likely than many nonnuclear accidents having similar consequences. They estimated that the likelihood of an individual being killed in any one year in a reactor accident is one chance in 5 billion for each 100 operating reactors. This was in contrast to a chance in 4,000 for being killed in an automobile accident and a chance in 2 million of being killed by lightning. The early somatic effects, the late somatic effects, and the genetic effects in man likely to be associated with a nuclear reactor accident were extensively reviewed in this study (WASH-1400, 1975b).

After reaching the end of its useful life, the reactor core could be reprocessed to convert the fission products to a form suitable for long-term storage and to recover the remaining uranium and the transuranic elements, which could then be used to fuel other reactors. After a period of storage to allow time for decay of the short-lived fission products, the spent cores would then be transported to plants for chemical reprocessing. No reprocessing is now being done in the United States. In fact, the United States is currently actively attempting to discourage reprocessing by other nations due to concerns for nuclear weapon proliferation. Although this temporarily eliminates any problems associated with reprocessing, it creates problems in the storage of unprocessed fuel. If reprocessing plants become operational, the quantities, the types of materials, and the chemical processes used require safety precautions to prevent inhalation and other types of exposures of workers and contamination of the environment by volatile and nonvolatile fission products as well as plutonium.

A very significant problem of the nuclear fuel cycle that has not been adequately resolved is the long-term storage of high-level nuclear wastes. At the present time these wastes are being stored in an aqueous form in large underground tanks ranging in capacity from about 15,000 gallons to 1 million gallons. These tanks have a finite lifetime of about 15 to 40 years. Thus, it will be necessary to store these wastes in some other fashion in the future. The major methods being considered for disposal or long-term storage of these wastes are disposal of solids in salt mines, storage as solids in deep underground caverns, storage as solids in man-made vaults at or near the earth's surface, disposal as solids in the deep ocean, disposal as solids in ice sheet areas, disposal as liquids in deep wells, perpetual storage as liquids in deep wells, perpetual storage as liquids in deep underground caverns, and perpetual storage as liquids in tanks. The disposal of solids in salt mines has received the most study in the United States (Eisenbud, 1973; Schneider, 1974).

Other Radiation Sources

Other miscellaneous sources of radiation exposure such as television, industrial x-ray machines, and air travel have been estimated to result in an average annual dose to the United States population of about 2 mrem (BEIR

Table 19–2. SUMMARY OF ESTIMATES OF ANNUAL WHOLE-BODY DOSE RATES IN THE UNITED STATES (1970)*

SOURCE	AVERAGE DOSE RATE† (mrem/yr)	ANNUAL PERSON-REMS (in millions)
Environmental		
Natural	102	20.91
Global fallout	4	0.82
Nuclear power	0.0003	0.0007
Subtotal	106	21.73
Medical		
Diagnostic	72‡	14.8
Radiopharmaceuticals	1	0.2
Subtotal	73	15.0
Occupational	0.8	0.16
Miscellaneous	2	0.5
Total	182	37.4

* From Biological Effects of Ionizing Radiation (BEIR) Advisory Committee: *Report: The Effects on Populations of Exposure to Low Levels of Ionizing Radiation.* National Academy of Sciences, National Research Council, Washington, DC, 1972.
† The numbers shown are average values only. For given segments of the population, dose rates considerably greater than these may be experienced.
‡ Based on the abdominal dose.

Report, 1972). Other uses of radionuclides such as [238]Pu as a power source for heart pacemakers and electrical power for space flights are also potential sources of exposure to radiation or radioactive materials. The subject of radiation exposure from consumer products and miscellaneous sources has recently been reviewed (NCRP, 1977d). A summary of the estimates of annual whole-body dose rates in the United States for 1970 is given in Table 19–2.

BASIC RADIOBIOLOGIC CONCEPTS

The basic reaction of ionizing radiation with molecules is either ionization or excitation. In ionization, an orbital electron is ejected from the molecule resulting in the formation of an ion pair. In excitation, an electron is raised to a higher energy level. Molecules may receive energy directly from the incident radiation such as when ionization results from interaction of the radiation and an orbital electron. This may be termed a direct effect of radiation. On the other hand, a molecule may receive energy from the molecule originally ionized and become ionized or excited itself, which constitutes an indirect effect of the irradiation. The latter effect is particularly important in aqueous biologic systems. Thus, one of the most fundamental effects of ionizing radiation on biologic systems is the ionization of water with resulting free radical formation, although hydrogen bonds, double bonds, and the sulfhydryl groups of other molecules may be split, also resulting in the formation of free radicals (Karcher and Jentzsch, 1972).

The initial process leading to radiation in a cell is dissipation of the physical energy of the radiation. This occurs within a short time period ($\sim 10^{-6}$ sec) and results in ionization or excitation of molecules within the cell. The process of ionization of water may be written as follows:

$$H_2O \xrightarrow{\text{radiation}} HOH^+ + e^-$$

This results in the production of an ion pair. The energy lost in air by a charged particle is about 34 electron volts for every ion pair produced. The energy gained by tissue per ion pair formed is often assumed to be the same as that observed in air (34 ev). The linear energy transfer or the energy transferred per unit length of tract of the primary ionizing particle in tissue is related to the number of ionizations that may occur within the tissues.

Following energy deposition, ionization, and excitation, there is a period ($\sim 10^{-6}$ sec) in which physicochemical reactions between the ions and other molecules occur. For water this can be written as follows:

$$H_2O + e^- \longrightarrow HOH^-$$

Thus, from the ionization of water both H_2O^+ and H_2O^- result. These then dissociate into free radicals (electrically neutral molecules having an unpaired electron, i.e., $H\cdot$ or $OH\cdot$). For water the process may be written as follows:

$$Radiation \rightsquigarrow HOH \underset{\nearrow e^-}{\longrightarrow} HOH^+$$

$$HOH^+ \longrightarrow H^+ + OH\cdot$$

$$e^- + HOH \longrightarrow HOH^- \longrightarrow H\cdot + OH^-$$

Or the overall reaction as

$$H_2O \xrightarrow{radiation} H\cdot + OH\cdot$$

An alternate theory is

$$Radiation \rightsquigarrow HOH \longrightarrow HOH^+ + e^-$$

$$HOH^* \text{ (excited)}$$

$$H\cdot \qquad OH\cdot$$

In any case, the extremely reactive radicals $H\cdot$ and $OH\cdot$ are formed. These can exist only a minute fraction of a second before undergoing a chemical reaction. A portion of these interact with one another resulting in H_2O, H_2, or H_2O_2 (hydrogen peroxide). The remainder of the free radicals diffuse into solution where they may interact with biologically important molecules.

As oxygen is present in most biologic systems, another free radical HO_2 may be formed by the reaction of the $H\cdot$ radical with oxygen. The HO_2 radical is then reduced to the oxidizing agent H_2O_2. The formation of the HO_2 radical and the increased amounts of H_2O_2 may account for the increased radiosensitivity of cells in the presence of oxygen. The oxygen effect is important for low LET radiations but not for high LET radiations probably because of the high ionization density of high LET radiations.

As was mentioned previously, molecules may be either ionized or excited by radiation. At one time, it was assumed that excited molecules had received energy transfer insufficient for ionization and would lose that energy through such processes as oscillation. However, it is now thought that an excited molecule with energy that exceeds that required for ionization may lose energy through such processes as dissociating into free radicals without passing through the stage of ionization.

The free radicals and other reactive molecules that are formed from the above processes may then react with biologically important molecules within the cell. These reactions (indirect) or the same type of reactions resulting directly from radiation on these biologically important molecules may have a profound effect on the cell when the chemical alterations involve molecules or structures (i.e., chromosomes) of great importance to cell function and viability. Radiation effects have been shown to occur with proteins, enzymes, nucleic acids, lipids, and carbohydrates, all of which may have marked effects on the cell.

The cytopathologic changes observed in cells following radiation are numerous, varied, and complex and are similar to those seen after other types of cellular injury. The response of individual cells and types of cells to radiation is variable depending on such things as the cell cycle and the oxygenation status of the cell. The response of cells and their various components to radiation has recently been reviewed by several authors (Rubin and Casarett, 1968; Berdjis, 1971). Many of these responses may result in cell death, which, if extensive, may result in death of the organism. Other cells may undergo either total or partial repair. These changes may also be expressed at later times by tumors or mutations.

EXTERNAL RADIATION EXPOSURE

General Considerations

The usual exposure of man or animals to external ionizing radiation is to either natural or man-made sources of x-ray or gamma irradiation. Under certain conditions, however, such as in radiotherapy, space flight, and accident situations, other types of radiation such as neutrons, protons, and beta particles may also be sources of external irradiation.

Many factors, both extrinsic and intrinsic, may modify the response of a living organism to a given dose of radiation. The former include external factors such as dose rate, the quality of radiation, the geometry of the exposure, and the portion of the body exposed, and, the latter, biologic factors such as species, age, sex, oxygen tension, and metabolic status of the organism.

Early to Intermediate Effects

Early to intermediate effects can be taken to include the somatic effects of exposure to irradiation excluding life-span shortening and carcinogenesis. These relatively early effects, seen only after exposures to relatively high doses (> 50 rads), include such diverse effects as acute radiation sickness and pulmonary fibrosis.

Probably the most sensitive indicator of

irradiation is the use of the frequency of chromosome aberrations in the lymphocytes of human peripheral blood (Bender and Gooch, 1962; Brewer and Preston, 1975). This method is useful when either the whole body or a substantial part of it has been exposed to a dose of 25 rads or more of penetrating radiation. It should be recognized that many agents are also capable of causing chromosome aberrations in peripheral lymphocytes.

The early effects of exposure to ionizing radiation result primarily from cell death. The radiosensitivity of cells is generally considered to be related to how often they undergo mitosis (Berdjis, 1971). Cells that frequently undergo mitosis are the most radiosensitive, whereas those with no mitosis are the most radioresistant. This principle was recognized as early as 1904 by Bergonie and Tribondeau, who stated in their first "law" of irradiation that the radiosensitivity of cells is related directly to their reproductive capacity and indirectly to their degree of differentiation.

Other investigators (Rubin and Casarett, 1968) have extended the working classification of cells to include five classes of radiosensitivity based on the above principles. The first class is termed vegetative intermitotic cells, which are the most radiosensitive. These cells are characterized as short-lived individual cells, primitive and dividing regularly to produce daughter cells. Included in this class are hematopoietic stem cells, dividing cells in the intestinal glands, type A spermatogonia, granulosa cells of ovarian follicles, germinal cells of the epidermis, gastric and holocrine glands, and large- and medium-sized lymphocytes. Small lymphocytes are also very radiosensitive, but they divide infrequently and are an exception to the relationship.

The second class is termed differentiating intermitotic cells. These cells are not quite as sensitive as vegetative intermitotic cells. This class includes such cells as the differentiating hematopoietic series in the intermediate stages of differentiation in bone marrow, the more differentiated spermatogonia and spermatocytes, and oocytes. The third class is termed multipotential connective tissue cells and is intermediate in radiosensitivity. These cells typically divide irregularly or sporadically and in response to special stimuli. This class includes such cells as endothelial cells, fibroblasts, and mesenchymal cells.

The remaining two classifications include the relatively radioresistant cells. The first of these, reverting postmitotic cells, have long lives and do not divide at a high rate except under conditions of special stimuli. The class includes such cells as epithelial parenchymal cells, duct cells of salivary glands, liver, kidney, and pancreas, cells of the adrenal, thyroid, parathyroid, and pituitary gland, and many other cells. The last class, termed fixed postmitotic cells, includes the most radioresistant cells. These cells, which normally do not divide or have lost completely the ability to divide, are well differentiated and specialized in function. Cells of this type are long-lived neurons, perhaps some muscle cells, neutrophils, erythrocytes, spermatids, spermatozoa, superficial cells of the alimentary tract, and epithelial cells of sebaceous glands.

If the above classification of the relative radiosensitivity of cells is applied to the various organs and systems of the body, the dose-response relationships of radiation injury are more easily understood. For example, if entire populations of essential stem cells are destroyed, such as the hematopoietic stem cells, survival of an individual is virtually impossible, but destruction of the germ cells of the testes would play no role in early lethality even though sterility would result.

Acute Whole-Body Radiation Exposure. Exposure of the whole body or a substantial portion of it to penetrating radiation of various types is likely to occur only under accident situations, nuclear warfare, or possibly during manned space flights (Langham, 1967). Manifestations of early effects occur only after relatively high doses (above about 50 rads) delivered at relatively high dose rates (several rads per hour). Normally these acute early effects, which appear to be threshold phenomena, are dose-rate dependent and their incidence and severity increase nonlinearly with increasing dose.

About one or two hours after an acute whole-body exposure to penetrating ionizing radiation, a combination of gastrointestinal and neuromuscular symptoms, known as the prodromal syndrome, is likely to appear. Anorexia, nausea, vomiting, and diarrhea are the more common symptoms observed, but apathy, tachycardia, fever, and headaches are also likely to occur. Although the time of onset and severity of the symptoms are largely a function of the total absorbed dose, they vary widely among individuals. Langham (1967), from a review of available human data, estimated the following approximate doses required to produce these symptoms in 50 percent of the individuals exposed: anorexia, 120 rads; nausea, 170 rads; vomiting, 210 rads; and diarrhea, 240 rads. At very high doses (~1,000 to ~5,000 rads), the prodromal response merges with the fatal gastroenteric syndrome, whereas at lower doses there is a latent period before the hematologic syndrome. The pathogenesis of the prodromal syndrome is not known.

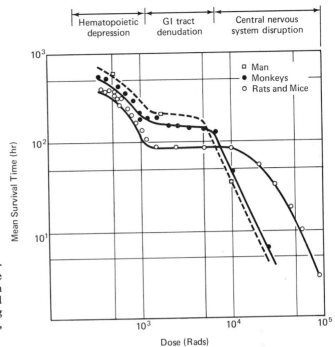

Figure 19–2. Survival time and associated mode of death in relation to dose of acute whole-body irradiation. (From Langham, W. H.; Brooks, P. M.; and Grahn, D.: Biological effects of ionizing radiation. *Aerospace Med.*, **36**:1–55, 1965.)

Depending on the size and distribution of the absorbed dose, the clinical manifestations of the acute radiation syndrome can be divided into three forms: the central nervous system (CNS), the gastrointestinal, and the hematopoietic (Fig. 19–2). At higher doses, however, damage to all tissues and organs may cause the symptoms and effects of one form to blend into the others. With whole-body doses approaching 5,000 rads or more, death apparently results from neurologic and cardiovascular degeneration and usually occurs within minutes to 48 hours, depending on the dose. This has typically been termed the CNS syndrome.

When total-body exposure dose is between 1,000 and 5,000 rads, the survival time may be from five to ten days and death is associated with bloody diarrhea and destruction of the gastrointestinal mucosa, particularly that of the small intestine (gastrointestinal syndrome). The epithelial cells lining the small intestine have a short life and need to be renewed every few days (Patt and Quastler, 1963). Large doses of irradiation cause cell death of the relatively radiosensitive crypt cells, which produce the cells that eventually migrate to replenish the epithelial lining cells. Thus, without continual replacement of the cells, ulceration and hemorrhage develop. These changes develop throughout the gastrointestinal tract but are more pronounced in the small intestine owing to the lack of cell renewal. Gastrointestinal changes are complicated by

changes in many other tissues, particularly the bone marrow where depression also occurs from these doses. At the lower end of the dose range for the gastrointestinal syndrome, animals may be kept alive with the use of large amounts of fluids and antibiotics, and regeneration of intestinal epithelium is quite rapid (Bond *et al.*, 1969). Animals treated in this manner, however, usually die later from the bone marrow syndrome, which is extremely difficult to treat following doses high enough to produce the gastrointestinal syndrome.

Penetrating whole-body doses from about 50 to 1,000 rads cause symptoms related primarily to injury of the bone marrow (hematopoietic syndrome). Damage to the bone marrow cells is reflected by changes in the circulating blood. The severity of bone marrow depression and the latent period between exposure and appearance of the symptoms are related to the magnitude of dose. The changes in the peripheral blood are largely the result of damage to lymphocytes and the precursor stem cells of the bone marrow. The earliest and one of the more dramatic changes in the peripheral blood is a drastic fall in the number of circulating lymphocytes. This is apparent within one to two days after exposure to doses as low as 50 to 100 rads. The circulating lymphocyte count may approach zero at doses in the lethal range. The return to normal of the lymphocyte count is slow and may be depressed months to years after exposure (Langham, 1967).

The total white cell count may be maintained for a few days despite the rapid fall in the lymphocyte count due to a temporary increase in the neutrophil count. However, the neutrophil count soon begins a steady decline followed by a period of leveling off or an "abortive rise." Lack of this abortive rise has been associated with a poor prognosis at doses near the lethal range (Langham, 1967). Following this the neutrophil count again declines, reaching a low at about four to six weeks in man. If death does not occur, the count will increase slowly to normal in a few months. The danger of infection in this stage of the syndrome is closely associated with the level of neutrophils in the peripheral blood.

The platelet count in the peripheral blood decreases similarly to the neutrophil count. When the platelets reach a critical level, hemorrhage is likely to occur and may result in the death of the individual.

Because of the radioresistance and long life-span of mature erythrocytes, red blood cell levels fall slowly if at all in the absence of complicating hemorrhage. Normally, anemia is not an urgently severe consequence of acute exposure to ionizing radiation.

The treatment of acute radiation exposure is very similar to that for any pancytopenia. A complete discussion of the treatment of the acute radiation syndrome has been published (Cronkite et al., 1969).

For acute, high-dose-rate exposure to ionizing radiation, the lethal dose for most species is usually presented as the LD50/30 days. The LD50/30 of various species of animals varies markedly as illustrated in Table 19–3 (Bond et al., 1969). The distribution of deaths at doses near the LD50 as a function of time also varies significantly with species. In rodents most post-exposure deaths occur between 9 and 14 days, in dogs between 10 and 25 days, and in man and most species of monkeys within a range of about 20 to 60 days.

A precise LD50 for acute exposure of man to irradiation is not known. From a review of the data available, Langham (1967) has estimated an LD50/60 days for man of about 300 rads and has proposed a broad basis for relating the dose to survival for man. Survival at doses of 100 to 200 rads is probable and almost certain at doses less than 100 rads, is considered possible at doses from 200 to 500 rads, and is not probable at larger doses. Survivors of the acute radiation syndrome will be at high risk of developing late effects of irradiation such as leukemia.

Acute Partial-Body Radiation Exposure. The effects of acute exposure to penetrating ionizing radiation of a portion of the body are usually seen in patients undergoing radiotherapy for the treatment of cancer. In essence, early to intermediate effects can be produced by irradiation of any tissues and organs of the body. There are several textbooks with complete discussions of the response of various organs and systems to irradiation (Rubin and Casarett, 1968; Berdjis, 1971). The effects usually result in atrophy and fibrosis with a disorder in the architectural pattern of some organs and late necrosis of individual cells in others. Also typical is the presence of foamy, bizarre, or giant cells in some organs and various degrees of cellular proliferation or differentiation, or both, in others. Whether these

Table 19–3. REPRESENTATIVE LD50/30 DAY VALUES FOR VARIOUS MAMMALIAN SPECIES*

SPECIES	TYPE OF RADIATION	Exposure in Air (R)	Absorbed Dose at Midcenter (rads)
Mouse	250 KVP x-ray	443	538
Rat	200 KVP x-ray	640	796
Guinea pig	200 KVP x-ray	337	400
Rabbit	250 KVP x-ray	805	751
Monkey	250 KVP x-ray	760	546
Dog	250 KVP x-ray	281	244
Swine	1000 KVP x-ray	510	247
Sheep	Gamma approx. 0.7 Mev	524	205
Goat	200 KVP x-ray	350	237
Burro	Gamma approx. 1.1 Mev	651	256

* From Bond, V. P.; Cronkite, E. P.; and Conrad, R. A.: Acute whole body radiation injury: Pathogenesis, pre- and post-radiation protection. In Behrens, C. F.; King, E. R.; and Carpender, J. W. J. (eds.): *Atomic Medicine*, 5th ed. Williams & Wilkins Co., Baltimore, © 1969.

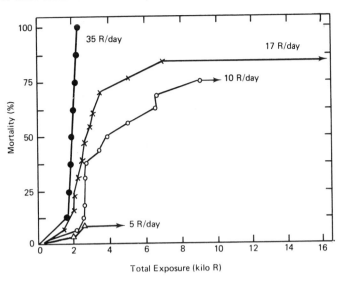

Figure 19–3. Mortality in beagle dogs exposed continuously to either 5, 10, 17, or 35 R/day in a cobalt-60 gamma ray field. The arrows indicate the total exposure reached at the time of early 1971. (From Totter, J. R.: Research programs of the Atomic Energy Commission's Division of Biology and Medicine relevant to problems of health and pollution. In LeCam, L. M.; Neyman, J.; and Scott, E. L. [eds.]: *Effects of Pollution on Health.* Vol. VI, Proceedings of the Sixth Berkeley Symposium on Mathematical Statistics and Probability. Originally published by the University of California Press in 1972; reprinted by permission of The Regents of the University of California.)

changes are related to the eventual development of neoplasia is not known, and many of them are similar to those that develop after other types of injury to the same organ.

With partial-body irradiation at doses less than 500 to 1,000 rads, serious effects are not immediately apparent except in the skin, gonads, or eyes unless a substantial portion of the body is irradiated and significant bone marrow depression occurs. At doses of about 500 rads, many individuals will show skin changes initially as erythema, progressing to dry desquamation and eventually to a dry, hairless skin (McLean, 1973). More dramatic skin changes such as ulceration develop at higher doses.

The germ cells of both males and females are radiosensitive. In males, acute doses of 10 to 100 rads will cause a dose-related depression of the sperm count, which recovers slowly. With doses in the range of 500 rads, permanent sterility is likely. In females, destruction of oocytes results in permanent sterility due to a lack of stem cells in the adult ovary. Also, destruction of germinal epithelium of the ovary involves interruption of the production of the sex hormones (McLean, 1973).

Exposure of the lens of the eye to ionizing radiation such as x-rays, gamma rays, beta particles, and neutrons may cause cataracts. The latent period in man between exposure and cataract formation is dose related and may vary from months to as long as five years or more. Cataracts have not been observed in man from irradiation of gamma or x-rays at doses less than about 600 R, but cataracts have been found in mice exposed to doses as low as 100 rads of x-rays. Neutron doses as low as 1 rad have produced cataracts in mice.

Factors That Modify the Response to Irradiation. Dose rate and dose fractionation both influence the total dose required to produce all of the acute effects of low linear energy transfer (LET) radiation in experimental animals. For example, Figure 19–3 illustrates the effect of dose rate on the survival curves of dogs exposed continuously in a ^{60}Co gamma-ray field. Survival times varied markedly with the different dose rates to which the dogs were exposed and a marked difference existed in the LD50 doses at the various dose rates. For example, at 35 R/day, 50 percent mortality occurred in about 55 days with 2,000 R total dose, while at 10 R/day, 50 percent mortality occurred in about 400 days with 4,000 R total dose. Although the survival times are markedly different, the causes of death for the animals within the groups were related primarily to damage to bone marrow and ranged from septicemia to anemia to leukemia. Similar data on the effect of lowered dose rates on hematologic effects in man are not available, but in one accident case, a man with evidence of severe hematologic depression survived a dose of ^{60}Co gamma irradiation of about 1,000 rads protracted over 119 days (Martinee *et al.*, 1964, *Rev. Med. Inst. Mex. Seguro Social*, 3:14–68, cited in Langham, 1967).

Normally, there is much less dose rate effect from high LET radiation than from low LET radiation. A possible explanation for this is that most cells are incapable of repairing damage caused by high LET radiations (Totter, 1971).

Dose fractionation, where doses are delivered at high dose rates but split into various fractions, is a technique that has been used for many years to alter the therapeutic ratios in tumor therapy. Depending on the schedules used and the tissues irradiated, fractionation can either decrease or increase the effect of a given dose on a given population of cells. Usually, tissues tolerate larger total doses when the dose is fractionated (Rubin and Casarett, 1968).

The age of an animal at the time of exposure may also affect its radiosensitivity. Radiation received by the embryo and fetus during early gestation is likely to cause developmental abnormalities particularly microencephaly or impaired body growth (NCRP, 1977b). In man, abnormalities of this type have only been observed after doses of 100 to 200 rads. Because of the uncertainties over the dose response, therapeutic abortions have been advised by some authors (Rubin and Casarett, 1968) following abdominal exposures of 5 to 10 rads during early pregnancy. Very young animals are also consistently more radiosensitive than adults (Bond et al., 1969). Increased radiosensitivity of aged animals has been observed in only a few of the systems studied (Bond et al., 1969).

Although it is probably of little practical significance except for radiotherapeutic applications, the oxygen tension of cells at the time of irradiation has a marked effect on cellular radiosensitivity. Decreasing the oxygen tension of the cells (hypoxia) decreases their radiosensitivity.

Late Somatic Effects

Within the past few years, there has been increased focus on the potential for even very low doses of irradiation to produce deleterious biologic effects in the human population. Experimental animal data and observations of groups of humans have clearly established that ionizing radiation is carcinogenic and mutagenic at relatively high doses usually delivered at high dose rates. However, owing to uncertainties as to the shape of the dose-response curves, concern exists for the effects of irradiation at doses and dose rates that extend down to doses that may be received from the environment and diagnostic radiography. Furthermore, there is the apparent need for risk-versus-benefit judgments for all of the varied uses and proposed uses of radiation. Animal experiments may provide a sound scientific basis for risk estimates, but the estimation of benefits and the balance between the two remain largely subjective.

For purposes of this discussion, the late somatic effects of ionizing radiation are considered to be carcinogenesis and possibly nonspecific life shortening. The genetic effects of ionizing radiation and the early-to-intermediate effects such as cataract formation and sterility are discussed elsewhere. The scope of this dis-

cussion is necessarily limited; however, comprehensive discussions of the late somatic effects of irradiation have recently been published (BEIR Report, 1972; UNSCEAR, 1972b). Several recent reviews specifically consider the subject of radiation carcinogenesis (Upton, 1973; Storer, 1975; Yuhas et al., 1976).

Laboratory animals, exposed to single or divided doses of radiation in the sublethal range, have demonstrated a shortened life-span (Lindop and Sacher, 1966; Grahn, 1969). Examination of data from many of these experiments has revealed that not all of the excess mortality was due to cancer, but extended over the spectrum of diseases usually observed in the animals. However, analysis of data from various groups of humans exposed to doses of irradiation has not consistently shown any nonspecific life-shortening effects due to exposure (BEIR Report, 1972). The most detailed human study is that of the Japanese atomic bomb survivors in which detailed evaluation through October 1, 1974, of over 14,000 deaths from natural causes other than cancer provided no evidence that diseases other than cancer were involved in the late radiation mortality, the total effect on excess mortality was attributed to neoplasia (Beebe et al., 1978). There has been established, however, a clear relationship between radiation dose and excess risk of cancer in these irradiated human populations and in animal experiments. Thus, carcinogenesis appears to be the primary late somatic effect of ionizing radiation.

A detailed discussion of the dose-response relationship of carcinogenesis following exposure to ionizing radiation is beyond the scope of this discussion. However, the pertinent questions that remain to be resolved along these lines are (1) whether the dose-response curve is linear or nonlinear and/or whether it has a threshold, and (2) the effect of lowering the radiation dose rate or protracting the dose on the dose-response relationship. One set of generalizations that has been made is that high LET radiation is more carcinogenic than low LET radiation and that a dose rate effect exists for low LET radiation (Mole, 1973). There is, however, no general agreement on either of these points, and certain authors contend that applying the maximum permissible dose to the population as recommended in current radiation protection guidelines would result in as many as 100,000 additional cancer deaths per year in the United States (Gofman et al., 1972). Until such questions can be resolved, using results of well-designed animal experiments and human epidemiologic studies, the use of the conservative assumption of a linear, nonthreshold dose response should be continued for risk estimates.

burden measurements of alpha- and beta-emitting radionuclides can be made by radioanalysis of the specific tissues frequently after chemical separation of the radioactive element of interest. Estimation of tissue weight is often uncertain at best. An extensive compilation of data on the mass, dimensions, and elemental composition as well as other key biologic data on man has been published (ICRP, 1975). A discussion of the absorbed fraction of the beta dose has been presented for bone and utilized for other tissues (Parmley et al., 1962). For gamma-emitting radionuclides the situation is considerably more complex since radioactivity deposited in one tissue serves as a source of radiation not only for that tissue but to a varying degree for other tissues dependent upon the spatial relationships of the tissues and the gamma energy of the photons. The subject has been converted in very understandable fashion in the MIRD handbooks (1968; 1969a; 1969b; 1971; 1975a; 1975b).

From this equation it is seen that the radiation dose is a function of (1) the effective retention half-time, (2) the energy released in the tissue, (3) the amount of radioactivity initially introduced, and (4) the mass of the organ. A lower radiation dose will result if the effective retention half-life is shorter, the energy released in the tissue is lower, the amount introduced is smaller, or the mass of the tissue is larger, all other factors being equal. Although these considerations are straightforward, they may be overlooked, for example, in the case of the individual who argues that the effect of 10 μCi of ^{131}I in the rat and man must be similar, neglecting the large difference in the mass of the thyroid in the rat and man and thus differences in radiation dose from identical amounts of radioactivity in the two species.

The dose pattern for radioactive materials in the body may be strongly influenced by the route of entry of the material. For industrial workers, inhalation of radioactive particles with pulmonary deposition and puncture wounds with subcutaneous deposition have been the most frequent (Ross, 1968). The general population has been exposed via ingestion of low levels of naturally occurring radionuclides as well as man-produced radionuclides from nuclear weapons testing and nuclear power operations. Further, the potential exists for catastrophic nuclear accident situations in which members of the general population might be exposed by inhalation.

Routes of Entry

Since there are certain features common to the various modes of entry, irrespective of the radionuclide, the two most important routes of entry, ingestion and inhalation, will be considered in some detail.

Ingestion. Ingestion of radioactive materials is most likely to occur with contaminated foodstuff or water. Ingestion of radioactive material may result in toxic effects as a result of either absorption of the radionuclide or irradiation of the gastrointestinal tract during passage through the tract, or a combination of both. The fraction of a radioactive material absorbed from the gastrointestinal tract is variable, depending on the specific element, the physical and chemical form of the material ingested, and the diet. For example, ^{137}Cs is almost totally absorbed from the gastrointestinal tract (Furchner et al., 1964) whereas ^{144}Ce is very poorly absorbed (McClellan et al., 1965). The absorption of some elements is influenced by age with higher absorption in the very young. Ballou and coworkers (1962) noted this for ^{239}Pu and McClellan (1964) observed this for both ^{45}Ca and ^{90}Sr. The influence of diet is particularly apparent for essential minerals, trace elements, and related elements. For example, ^{90}Sr and ^{45}Ca fractional absorption was decreased in the presence of increased levels of Ca and PO_4 in the diet (Thompson and Palmer, 1960; Palmer and Thompson, 1964).

Eve (1966) has reviewed the physiology of the gastrointestinal tract in relation to radiation doses from radioactive materials. The gastrointestinal tract is viewed as four compartments with the characteristics noted in Table 19–4.

Eve defined the occupancy factor as the fraction of 24 hours during which a section of the gastrointestinal tract is full of food residue. Based on Eve's review, Dolphin and Eve (1966) derived equations for the dosimetry of the gastrointestinal tract following oral intake of radioactive material. Beyond having utility for calculating the radiation dose to the gastrointestinal tract from ingested radionuclides, their work is useful in considering the "dose" to the gastrointestinal tract from ingested nonradioactive toxic materials. Such an approach may be of assistance in relating the pathogenesis of certain diseases of the gastrointestinal tract, such as cancer of the colon, to poorly absorbed toxic materials ingested in small quantities.

Early studies such as those of Quastler (1956) indicated that the damage to crypt cells of the intestine was responsible for early "gastrointestinal" deaths. The critical importance of such information was emphasized by the Rasmussen (WASH-1400, 1975) Study Report on the consequences of reactor accidents, which indicated the importance of ingestion and gastrointestinal tract irradiation in determining early morbidity and mortality following a catastrophic accident with release of massive quantities of

Table 19–4. CHARACTERISTICS OF THE GASTROINTESTINAL TRACT OF
MAN*

PORTION	MASS OF CONTENTS (g)	TIME FOOD REMAINS (hr)	OCCUPANCY FACTOR	EFFECTIVE RADIUS (cm)
Stomach	250	1	6/24	10
Small intestine	400	4	14/24	10
Upper large intestine	220	13	18/24	5
Lower large intestine	135	24	22/24	5

* From Eve, I. S.: A review of the physiology of the gastrointestinal tract in relation to radiation
   doses from radioactive materials. *Health Phys.*, **12**:131–61, 1966.

fission products. Stimulated by the Rasmussen
study, Sullivan *et al.* (1978) critically examined
the dosimetry and effects of ingestion of fission
products, radio-nuclides of varied beta decay
energy, by rats or dogs. Their studies verified
that damage to the crypt cells was responsible
for death. Their work emphasized the importance of estimating the radiation dose to the
crypt cells.

Inhalation. The inhalation mode of exposure
has long been recognized as being of major
importance for both nonradioactive and radioactive materials. This recognition has led to
substantial research on the toxicity of inhaled
radionuclides, research that has already yielded
significant improvement in our general understanding of inhalation toxicology. A report
from a Task Group of the International Commission on Radiological Protection (ICRP,
1966a) provides an excellent overview of our
understanding of the deposition and retention
of inhaled particles in the respiratory tract. An
updated view of this report and other more
recent work in the area is presented in a report
by the International Atomic Energy Agency
Panel on "Inhalation Hazards from Radioactive
Contaminants" (IAEA, 1973). In both reports,
the respiratory tract is viewed as consisting of
three basic compartments: (1) the nasopharynx,
(2) the tracheobronchial compartment, and (3)
the pulmonary compartment (Fig. 19–5). The
nasopharynx (NP) begins with the anterior nares
and extends to the level of the larynx or epiglottis.
The tracheobronchial (TB) compartment consists of the trachea and bronchial tree including
terminal bronchioles. The pulmonary compartment (P) consists of the more distal portions of
the lung, which are involved in functional gas
exchange. To consider the toxicity of inhaled
materials in the context of the total animal, other
compartments should be included: pulmonary
lymph nodes, gastrointestinal tract, blood, and
tissue compartments such as skeleton, liver, and
kidneys.

Using Figure 19–5 as a guide, it is appropriate

to consider in some detail the deposition of
inhaled particles. The Task Group used the
notations D_1 through D_5, where D_1 was the
activity inhaled, D_2 the activity in the exhaled
air, D_3 the activity deposited in NP as a percentage of D_1, D_4 the activity deposited in TB
as a percentage of D_1, and D_5 the activity deposited in P as a percentage of D_1. Deposition,
defined as the process that accounts for the
amount of inhaled or inspired material that remains after expiration, is accomplished by (1)
inertial impaction, (2) gravitational settling, and
(3) diffusion by brownian movement. Inertial
impaction is greatest for particles 5 μm and
larger in diameter and occurs primarily in the
NP and TB compartments. Gravitational settling, involving particles in the range of 0.5 to
5 μm, is of some significance in the NP and TB
compartments but is even more significant in
the P compartment. Diffusion, involving particles smaller than about 0.5 μm, is of great
significance for deposition in the P compartment
and, for very small particles, may be the process
by which large quantities of activity are deposited
in the NP compartment.

In recent years, increased use has been made of
the concept of "equivalent aerodynamic diameter" in considering the deposition of inhaled
particles. This parameter may be defined as the
diameter of a unit density sphere having the same
settling velocity as the particle in question regardless of shape (but crudely spheric) and density
(IAEA, 1973). This approach is realistic when
considering deposition in that it recognizes that
the aerodynamic size of the particle is more
significant than the real size. Adoption of this
concept, in its fullest sense, requires one to use
inertial air-sampling devices such as the cascade
impacter (Mercer *et al.*, 1970) to separate particles according to their aerodynamic size as
contrasted to many sampling devices such as
large filters that collect all of the particles in the
air irrespective of particle size.

Figure 19–5 may again be used in considering
the retention of inhaled material remaining in

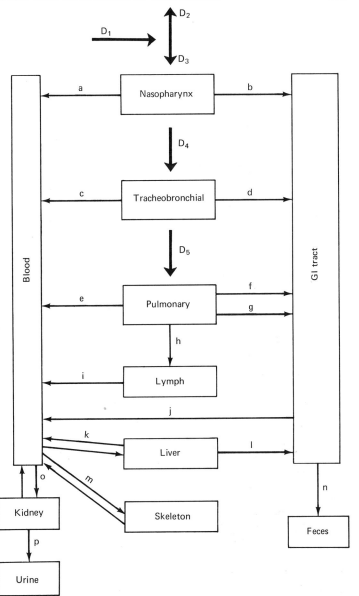

Figure 19–5. Schematic portrayal of deposition sites and clearance processes of the respiratory tract. D_1, total activity inhaled; D_2, the activity in the exhaled air; D_3, activity deposited in nasopharynx as a percentage of D_1; D_4, activity deposited in the tracheobronchial compartment as a percentage of D_1; and D_5, activity deposited in the pulmonary compartment as a percentage of D_1; *a* through *i* represent specific clearance and translocation processes (see text). (From International Commission on Radiological Protection [Task Group on Lung Dynamics]: Deposition and retention models for internal dosimetry of the human respiratory tract. *Health Phys.*, **12**:173–207, 1966.)

the respiratory tract at any time. Retention is a function of clearance and translocation, clearance being the transport of material out of the respiratory tract, and translocation, the absorption and movement of material to other tissues. The letters (a) through (i) in Figure 19–5 represent specific clearance and translocation processes associated with clearance of various compartments as established by the ICRP Task Group. Specifically*

* International Commission on Radiological Protection (Task Group on Lung Dynamics); Deposition and retention models for internal dosimetry of the human respiratory tract. *Health Phys.*, **12**:173–207, 1966.

(a) represents the rapid uptake of material deposited in the nasopharynx directly into the systemic blood:

(b) represents the rapid clearance of all dusts from the nasopharynx by ciliary-mucus transport;

(c) represents the rapid absorption of dust deposited in the TB compartment into the systemic circulation;

(d) is analogous to (b) and represents the rapid ciliary clearance of TB; the dust cleared by (d) goes quantitatively to the GI tract;

(e) represents the direct translocation of dust from the pulmonary region to the blood;

(f) represents the relatively rapid clearance of the pulmonary region, which presumably depends on recruitable macrophages, and this, in turn, is coupled

Table 19–5. AMENDED CONSTANTS FOR USE WITH CLEARANCE MODEL*†

		CLASS (D)	CLASS (W)	CLASS (Y)
N-P	(a)	0.01 d/0.5‡	0.01 d/0.10	0.01 d/0.01
	(b)	0.01 d/0.5	0.40 d/0.90	0.40 d/0.99
T-B	(c)	0.01 d/0.95	0.01 d/0.50	0.01 d/0.01
	(d)	0.20 d/0.05	0.20 d/0.50	0.2 d/0.99
P	(e)	0.5 d/0.80	50 d/0.15	500 d/0.05
	(f)	n.a.	1 d/0.40	1 d/0.40
	(g)	n.a.	50 d/0.40	500 d/0.40
	(h)	0.5 d/0.20	50 d/0.05	500 d/0.15
Lymph	(i)	0.5 d/1.00	50 d/1.00	1000 d/0.90

* From International Commission on Radiological Protection: *The Metabolism of Compounds of Plutonium and Other Actinides.* ICRP Publication No. 19, Pergamon Press, Oxford, 1972, as amended from the International Commission on Radiological Protection (Task Group on Lung Dynamics): Deposition and retention models for internal dosimetry of the human respiratory tract. *Health Phys.*, **12**:173–207, 1966.

† For pulmonary clearance purposes, the radionuclides are classified into three classes: Y for avid retention, W for moderate retention, and D for minimal retention.

‡ The first value is the biologic half-life; the second is the regional fraction. The lymphatic clearance for class Y compounds indicates that a 90 percent regional fraction follows a 1,000-day biologic half-life. The remaining 10 percent is presumed to be permanently retained in the nodes and is subject only to radioactive decay.

to the ciliary-mucus transport process. Therefore, the dust cleared by (f) goes to the GI tract via the tracheobronchial tree;

(g) is a second pulmonary clearance process, which is typically much slower than (f) but still depends on endocytosis and ciliary-mucus transport and the cleared dust goes via TB to the GI tract; the important distinction is that the clearance is apparently rate limited in the pulmonary region by the nature of the deposited dust, per se;

(h) is a process describing the slow removal of dust from the pulmonary compartment via the lymphatic system; we can regard this process as qualitatively similar to (g) with the exception that lymph transport replaces the ciliary-mucus transport;

(i) represents a secondary pathway in which dust cleared by the lymphatic system (h) is introduced into the systemic blood; this pathway obviously depends on the ability of the cleared material to penetrate the lymph tissue, especially the lymph nodes; this implies dissolution of the dust particles, partially or completely, but the turnover of lymphocytes may contribute (Stohlman, 1959);

(j) represents the process by which material in the gastrointestinal tract from processes (b), (d), (f), and (g) reaches the bloodstream. This process is closely related to the gastrointestinal tract considerations of Eve (1966) and Dolphin and Eve (1966) noted earlier.

In considering the clearance of materials from the respiratory tract, the ICRP Task Group found it appropriate to group elements into three categories; class D, expected to exhibit maximal clearance half-times of less than one day; class W, representing material with maximal

clearance half-times of a few days to a few months; and class Y, for materials expected to manifest maximal biologic half-times to six months to several years. The following examples serve to illustrate this classification: class D, cesium chloride; class W, lanthanide carbonates, calcium sulfate; and class Y, lanthanide and actinide oxides. For each class, the Task Group suggested constants for use in the clearance model (Table 19–5).

The Task Group report established the importance of particle solubility in determining long-term pulmonary retention, a concept that was emphasized earlier by Mercer (1967). More recent research (Cuddihy *et al.*, 1974, 1975, 1978; Mewhinney, 1976; Kanapilly, 1977) has indicated the complex nature of particle dissolution phenomena with differences in dissolution rate ascribed to the chemical and physical characteristics of the particles. The surface area of the particles is of special importance.

Specific Radionuclides

Because the toxicity of internally deposited radionuclides is very radionuclide specific, it is appropriate to provide a limited summary on several of the more significant radionuclides. The presentation will be directed toward covering the more important aspects of the radionuclide, element, or group of elements, hopefully providing a base for the interested reader to explore other more detailed references. A recent broad-based review of radionuclide toxicity will be of particular interest (Stannard, 1973).

Alkaline Earth Elements. The metabolic behavior of the alkaline earth elements has recently been reviewed (Marshall *et al.*, 1973). Two alkaline earth elements are of particular interest: radium and strontium. Probably more is known about the late effects in man of ^{226}Ra than any other radionuclide. This large body of knowledge has been and is still being derived from the study of individuals (radium dial painters and chemists) involved in the luminous dial industry that flourished in the early 1900s as well as individuals that received radium as therapeutic nostrums. The radium dial painters were largely young women who used luminous paints containing ^{226}Ra and, as a consequence of an early industrial practice of "tipping" the brush on their lips, ingested significant quantities of ^{226}Ra. Because radium is a metabolic analog of calcium it is deposited in the skeleton. Within the skeleton, a portion is deposited uniformly in the mineral while the remainder is deposited in "hot spots" corresponding to the areas of very active mineral accretion at the time of radium intake. The ^{226}Ra retained in the skeleton serves as a source of alpha radiation of bone and contiguous tissues at a dose rate that decreases slowly with time.

Pioneering studies at Massachusetts Institute of Technology under the leadership of R. D. Evans and at Argonne Cancer Research Hospital and Argonne National Laboratory by A. J. Finkel, R. J. Hasterlik, and C. E. Miller have clearly established that radium induces osteosarcomas of the skeleton and carcinomas of the mastoid and paranasal air sinuses. In general, the lower the burden of radium, the later and less frequent the appearance of a malignant tumor and subsequent death of the subject. In the Argonne series, no malignant tumors had been observed as of 1967 in subjects whose maximum radium burden was estimated to be below 1.2 μCi (Finkel *et al.*, 1969). Generally, similar results were seen in the MIT series and have led Evans and his associates (1969) to suggest the existence of a "practical threshold" of dose, below which the required tumor appearance time generally exceeds the life-span, and hence radiation-induced tumors appear with negligible frequency.

The follow-up of nearly 2000 radium-exposed individuals has now been consolidated at the Argonne National Laboratory and we hope it will be continued through the lifetime of the exposed individuals. Rowland *et al.* (1978) have recently summarized the dose-response information for 759 women who were exposed as "radium dial painters" prior to 1930 and have

been measured for radium content. Through December, 1976, the individuals in the series had manifested 38 bone sarcomas and 17 carcinomas of the head. As in previous analyses, the neoplasms were most prevalent and appeared earliest at the higher levels of radium intake. The dose-response data were fit with a number of mathematical functions. The data for bone sarcoma were best fit with an equation of the form $I = (C + \beta D^2)e^{-\gamma D}$ where C, the natural incidence for this population, was about 10^{-5} per person year, I is the incidence of bone sarcomas, and D is the dose. The data for the carcinomas of the head was best fit with a linear equation of the form $I = C + \alpha D$. The authors viewed their bone sarcoma data as being incompatible with a linear hypothesis. Further, although the bone sarcoma data did not contradict a threshold hypothesis, they felt that since both the bone sarcoma and carcinoma of the head data were fit so well by the continuous functions, they could find no compelling reasons to propose a threshold for either radium-induced neoplasm. The data strongly emphasize the lack of a clear "safe"-versus-"unsafe" dose. A review of all of the data on "radium dial painters" as of 1978 indicates that no bone sarcoma or carcinoma of the head has yet been observed in a dial painter whose exposure started after 1925. This attests to the adequacy of the control procedures instituted once the radiation hazard was recognized. A number of papers on radium toxicity in man and animals may be found in recent symposia proceedings (Jee, 1976).

A second alkaline earth element of major interest, strontium, is related to the abundance of ^{90}Sr in the fission products of nuclear weapon detonations and in the fuel cycle of nuclear power reactors. Because of early concern related to its presence in nuclear weapons fallout, the toxicity of ^{90}Sr has been extensively studied in mice, rats, beagle dogs, and miniature swine with much of the resultant information summarized at several symposia (McClellan and Jones, 1969; Lenihan *et al.*, 1967; Goldman and Bustad, 1972). The basic findings have been that strontium, as a metabolic analog of calcium, is readily absorbed from the gastrointestinal tract or the lung into the bloodstream and is subsequently deposited in bone. A single brief intake orally, intravenously, or by inhalation results in a high incidence of neoplasia of bone and bone-related tissues. The most frequently observed neoplasms have been osteosarcoma, hemangiosarcoma, fibrosarcoma, and epidermoid carcinomas. Chronic ingestion of ^{90}Sr in beagle dogs and miniature swine produced a high incidence of myeloproliferative disease, including frank leukemia, at the highest levels of ^{90}Sr intake, a finding that contrasts sharply with a lack of a similar high incidence with single acute intake of ^{90}Sr. Chronic ^{90}Sr intake resulted in only a few bone tumors in miniature swine while a high incidence was observed in beagle dogs. Mays and Lloyd (1972a) have reviewed ^{90}Sr experimental animal and ^{226}Ra human data and developed estimates of the human bone sarcoma risk from ^{90}Sr. They found that the data did not support a linear dose-response relationship over a wide dose range and that at low levels the data were fit well by practical threshold or sigmoid dose-response relationships. Their best cumulative 50-year risks below 1,000 rads from ^{90}Sr were 1 ± 1 sarcomas/10^6 person rads for a low-dose linear model and 4 ± 4 sarcomas/10^{10} person rads^2 for a dose-squared model.

Iodine. The toxicity of radioiodine, particularly ^{131}I, has received considerable attention related to its widespread use in nuclear medicine applications and its abundance in the inventory of an operating reactor and in nuclear weapons fallout. A 1963 symposium on the *Biology of Radioiodine* provides an excellent summary of our knowledge in this field (Bustad, 1963). More recent publications tend to provide confirmation of the basic information presented in 1963. Radioiodine, irrespective of the route of administration, is rapidly absorbed into the bloodstream and concentrated in the thyroid. High levels of ^{131}I result in virtually complete destruction of the thyroid with an associated decrease in thyroid hormone production. Levels of ^{131}I that damage thyroid but leave some tissue capable of proliferative response lead to hyperplasia, adenomas, and thyroid carcinomas.

The subject of the risk of thyroid neoplasia from radioiodine has recently been reviewed (WASH-1400, 1975b; NCRP, 1977c). The risk of both benign and malignant nodules of the thyroid following ^{131}I exposure appears to be 1/10 to 1/60 on a per rad basis of that from external radiation based on the results of both human epidemiologic studies and animal studies. This difference may be related to the low-energy beta emission of ^{131}I and its nonuniform distribution in the gland. Based on the human epidemiologic data, the estimated absolute risks for children for thyroid nodules is 0.064 and 0.023 per million persons per rem per year for thyroid cancers and total nodules, respectively. Based on the results of the Marshall Islanders exposed to mixed external radiation and radioiodine and on children who received ^{131}I therapy, children appear to be about twice as susceptible as adults to the induction of benign neoplasms, but about equal to adults in the susceptibility to the induction of cancer.

The National Council on Radiation Protection and Measurements has recently provided guidance on the protection of the thyroid gland in the event of release of radioiodine (NCRP, 1977c). For situations that might result in exposures above 10 rad to the thyroid, consideration should be given to the use of potassium iodide as a blocking agent to minimize the dose to the thyroid.

Alkali Metals. Of the alkali metal elements, ^{137}Cs is of greatest interest because of its long physical half-life, 30 years, and its abundance as a fission product in nuclear weapons fallout and in the inventory of a nuclear reactor or a fuel-reprocessing plant. Metabolically, ^{137}Cs behaves as an analog of potassium. Irrespective of the mode of administration, it is rapidly absorbed into the bloodstream and distributes throughout the active tissues of the body. Its distribution throughout the body and the energetic beta and gamma radiation from the decay of ^{137}Cs and its daughter, ^{137}Ba, result in essentially whole-body irradiation (Boecker, 1972). Thus, when large quantities of ^{137}Cs are injected, it is not surprising that acute toxicity with death related primarily to bone marrow destruction is observed, similar to the effects of exposure to high doses of gamma or x-irradiation (Redman *et al.*, 1972). Single acute intakes of lower levels of ^{137}Cs in beagle dogs appear to result in life shortening related to development of neoplasia late in life (Norris *et al.*, 1966). A recent report provides detailed information on the metabolism and dosimetry of ^{137}Cs (NCRP, 1977a).

Lanthanides. A number of lanthanide elements have radionuclides that are produced abundantly in nuclear reactors or in the detonation of nuclear weapons. ^{144}Ce is of particular interest because of its relatively long physical half-life, 285 days, and the energetic beta emissions from it and its daughter, ^{144}Pr. The physical, chemical, and biological properties of radiocerium relative to radiation protection guidelines have recently been summarized (NCRP, 1978d). ^{144}Ce is poorly absorbed from the gastrointestinal tract (McClellan *et al.*, 1965). Its toxicity following inhalation is of special interest since it may be considered as typical of beta-emitting radionuclides. When inhaled as ^{144}CeCl$_3$ by beagle dogs, ^{144}Ce has an effective retention half-time in lung measured in days and weeks with translocation to liver and skeleton such that, by 64 days after a single brief inhalation exposure, liver and skeleton retain 47 and 37 percent, respectively, of the total ^{144}Ce retained in the body (Boecker and Cuddihy, 1974). The morbidity and mortality from ^{144}CeCl$_3$ inhaled in graded activity levels by beagle dogs have been well characterized to over 2,000 days after ^{144}Ce exposure (Benjamin *et al.*, 1973, 1975; Jones *et al.*, 1974). At the highest activity levels, deaths were observed in less than 40 days due to bone marrow aplasia. At slightly lower levels with survival times of less than 1,000 days, the primary causes of death were radiation pneumonitis, hepatic necrosis, and bone marrow aplasia. At generally lower levels and at 799 days or more after ^{144}Ce exposure, deaths were primarily due to myelogenous leukemia or neoplasms of the liver or skeleton.

When ^{144}Ce is inhaled in a more insoluble form, in fused clay particles, it is tenaciously retained in the lung with an effective half-life of approximately 170 days. Small quantities of the cerium, apparently still in particles, are translocated to the tracheobronchial lymph nodes while other ^{144}Ce apparently released from the particles is translocated to liver and skeleton. A long-term study of the effects of single brief exposures to this relatively insoluble form presently provides information to about 1,500 days after ^{144}Ce exposure (Hahn *et al.*, 1970). At the highest exposure levels, deaths have been observed from 5 to 14 months after exposure as a result of radiation pneumonitis and pulmonary fibrosis. At lower levels, deaths have occurred from 25 to 44 months after inhalation exposure related to development of primary lung cancer, the most frequent type being a hemangiosarcoma (Benjamin *et al.*, 1975). The radiation doses to the lung associated with neoplasia were accumulated over long time periods and ranged from 23,000 to 48,000 rads. Primary lung cancers in the form of squamous cell carcinomas have been observed in rats that inhaled ^{144}Ce oxide and received radiation doses to lung as low as 2,500 rads (Thomas *et al.*, 1972). The rat findings contrast sharply with the observations in dogs and may reflect a species-related greater sensitivity in rats or the synergistic effects of radiation exposure and enzootic pneumonia in the rats. Two recent reviews have emphasized the inefficient carcinogenicity of beta-emitting radionuclides in the lung compared to alpha-emitting radionuclides (Bair, 1970; Sanders *et al.*, 1970). Other lanthanide elements have been observed to behave metabolically similar to cerium with deposition primarily in liver and skeleton. Durbin (1962) has reviewed the tissue distribution of the actinide and lanthanide elements and its relationship to the ionic radius of the elements. A good correlation was obtained with decreasing skeletal burden and increasing liver burden with increasing ionic radius.

Actinides. All of the actinide elements are of interest from a radiation toxicity viewpoint because they are all radioactive; however, several are of special interest in view of their abundance. The metabolic properties of the actinides have recently been reviewed (ICRP, 1972; Nenot and Stather, 1979). Natural uranium (^{238}U plus small amounts of ^{235}U and ^{234}U) has been studied extensively because of its importance as the starting point for the uranium fuel cycle for nuclear reactors. In soluble forms, it is largely nephrotoxic with the effects of this very low-specific-activity material thought to be due to chemical rather than radiation effects. Long-term (5 mg U/M^3 for five days per week for five years) inhalation exposures to an insoluble form with subsequent follow-up for 6.5 years resulted in major biologic effects in the lung; in monkeys this was manifest as extensive fibrosis and in beagle dogs with epithelial proliferation, metaplasia, and pulmonary neoplasms (Leach *et al.*, 1970).

Although the toxicity of plutonium has been of interest since its discovery, mostly because of its use in nuclear weapons, there is recent intensified interest in its toxicity as well as that of transplutonium elements such as americium and curium. This intensified interest is multifold and is related to (1) several major incidents involving nuclear weapons or nuclear weapons-related facilities, (2) the use of large quantities of ^{238}Pu as fuel in space electric power systems, and (3) the anticipated development of breeder-reactor systems that will have large inventories of plutonium and transplutonium radionuclides. A number of excellent symposia proceedings and reviews are available on the toxicity of plutonium (Thompson, 1962; Mays *et al.*, 1969; Stover and Jee, 1972; Thompson *et al.*, 1972; Hodge *et al.*, 1973; Bair and Thompson, 1974; Healy, 1975; Jee, 1976).

When inhaled, plutonium is retained in the lung with an effective half-life that varies from hundreds of days for plutonium oxides to tens of days for more soluble forms. A significant portion of the plutonium oxide that leaves the lung is translocated to the tracheobronchial lymph nodes. Plutonium apparently solubilized within the lung is translocated to the liver and skeleton where it is very tenaciously retained (Bair *et al.*, 1973). A classic long-term toxicity study has been performed by Bair and his associates in which the effects of inhaled plutonium oxide were studied in beagle dogs for up to ten years following inhalation exposure. At the highest levels of deposited activity, the dogs died within several hundred days with radiation pneumonitis and pulmonary fibrosis; at later times death was related to severe pulmonary fibrosis, and beyond 1,000 days, although pulmonary fibrosis was still prominent, death was due to primary pulmonary neoplasia. The most common neoplasm was bronchioloalveolar carcinoma. Dogs with 0.6 to 1.2 μCi of initial lung activity died between 1,000 and 3,000 days after inhalation of [239]Pu with an estimated radiation dose to the lung of 3,200 to 5,300 rads.

During the 1970s public interest in the toxicity of inhaled plutonium has been aroused by concern for its continued use in nuclear weapons and the potential for use of large quantities in breeder reactors. Using current standards the present allowable dose for lung from deposited [239]Pu is 15 rem/yr. Tamplin and Cochran (1974) claimed that this was too high by a factor of 115,000 times; later they reduced this to about 1,000. Their contention was based on the hypothesis that a "hot" particle of plutonium in the lung containing just an appropriate amount of radioactivity to intensely irradiate a local volume of lung tissue would be extraordinarily toxic as compared to the same amount of radioactivity distributed more uniformly throughout the lung. The contention of Tamplin and Cochran has been reviewed extensively by a number of groups (NAS, 1976; MRC, 1975; NCRP, 1975b). All have reached the conclusion that there is no unique hazard associated with inhalation of "hot" particles and that standards directed at protection against more uniform irradiation of the lungs are appropriate for use with "hot" particles.

Plutonium citrate injected intravenously deposits primarily in the skeleton and liver resulting in numerous neoplasms of the skeleton and a few bile duct neoplasms. At the lowest level, 0.015 μCi/kg, showing osteosarcomas to date, the mean interval between injection and death was 9.92 years with a dose of 86 rads to the skeleton (Mays and Lloyd, 1972b).

Several publications concerning plutonium in man are of special interest. One by Durbin (1971) critically reviews data collected in 1945 and 1946 on humans who were injected with tracer doses of [239]Pu and compares the results with those obtained in experimental animals. Others by Hempelmann and coworkers (1973) and Voelz (1975) review the follow-up experience on humans who were accidentally exposed in World War II and had estimated burdens of 0.005 to 0.42 μCi, exclusive of lung. To date, there have been no medical findings that can definitely be attributed to the individual's plutonium burdens.

Fewer toxicity data are available on transplutonium radionuclides such as americium and curium; however, the data that are available indicate a qualitative similarity to the toxicity of plutonium (Hodge et al., 1973). McClellan and associates (1972a, 1972b) noted that inhaled americium and curium, even as oxides, appear more soluble than inhaled pluonium and rapidly translocate to liver and skeleton.

Radon and Radon Daughters. An occupational exposure problem of substantial magnitude that has caused problems on two continents involves miners who work underground in uranium mines. This problem was recognized many years ago in the miners in the Erz Mountains of Central Europe who had an excessive incidence of disease of the respiratory system including lung cancer. More recently, the problem has been evident in miners of the Colorado plateau region of the United States. The problem is basically related to the emanation of radon into the mines and decay of the radon with its short-lived radioactive daughters ([216]Po, [214]Pb, [214]Bi, [214]Po) attaching to dust particles, which are inhaled and result in alpha radiation exposure of the respiratory airways. A high incidence of small-cell undifferentiated type of bronchial carcinoma has been observed in the miners. The situation is complicated by recognition that most of the miners are heavy smokers, a factor whose role is uncertain (Lundin et al., 1971; Saccomanno et al., 1971; Archer and Wagoner, 1973).

The BEIR Committee evaluated the risk for the uranium miners and obtained a value of 0.63 excess case per million person-years per rem for white miners (BEIR, 1972). The U.S. population of uranium miners is still being studied very intensively and should yield additional valuable data before the lung disease incidence hopefully returns to normal in association with improved working conditions in the mines.

Although the original concern for radon and its daughters focused on uranium miners, concern has developed in the 1970s for low-level emanations from uranium mine tailings either from tailing piles or when the tailings have been inappropriately used for fill around dwellings. This latter practice has been discontinued and in some cases tailings used as fill around houses have been removed. Increased attention is being given to the maintenance of tailing piles and consideration is being given to remedial treatment of abandoned tailing piles.

Tritium. Tritium, a radioactive isotope of hydrogen (^{3}H), is formed in the upper atmosphere by interactions of cosmic rays with gases. It is also formed in large quantities in both fission and fusion reactions and is present in effluents from nuclear reactors and weapons. Currently, the tritium present in the environment and the relative contribution of the sources have been estimated to be about 0.5 to 1 megacurie from nuclear reactors, 10 to 10^2 megacuries from natural sources, and about 10^3 megacuries from nuclear explosions (BEIR, 1972). Tritium, as tritiated water, is readily absorbed into the bloodstream from the gastrointestinal tract, skin, and lungs and distributes as body water. Any radiation effects are comparable to whole-body irradiation (Osborne, 1972; Stannard, 1973). When tritium enters the body in organic form, particularly as a label for nucleic acids, concern has been expressed over its concentration into vital structures such as DNA. Several recent reviews on the radiotoxicology of tritium have concluded that the use of a quality factor of 1 for tritium is justified, that for chronic environmental exposures to tritium concentration effects and transmutation effects are unimportant, and that the use of body water as the critical organ is conservative since no tissue has a higher proportion of hydrogen (Vennart, 1969; Osborne, 1972). Techniques for measurements of tritium are well developed and documented (NCRP, 1976a). Information on tritium relevant to considering its radiological implications have recently been reviewed (NCRP, 1979).

RADIATION PROTECTION STANDARDS

Biologic injury resulting from exposure to ionizing radiation was observed very soon after the discovery of radiation. Because many of the first applications of radiation were in the medical field, it is not surprising that, in at least qualitative terms, a cause-effect relationship was accepted for radiation and effects such as dermatitis. The establishment of a quantitative relationship, however, was handicapped by a lack of accurate radiation dose measurements. Nonetheless, the observed qualitative cause-effect or dose-response relationship provided a basis for instituting control procedures to limit exposure both to the field of interest of the patient and to the radiologist through the use of protective devices such as gloves and apron and later through protection built into the x-ray machines.

The first organized step toward radiation protection occurred in 1915 at a meeting of the British Roentgen Society when a resolution was introduced calling for stringent rules to assure the personal safety of operators conducting x-ray examinations. Unfortunately, no further organized action was taken until World War I, action that was aided in part by extensive publicity associated with deaths due to aplastic anemia of individuals who had been exposed while working in the military medical corps. The activity that occurred after that war led to the organization of a number of different committees primarily under the aegis of medical and radiologic societies. The work of one of these committees led to publication of the first general set of radiation protection recommendations in the *Journal of the Roentgen Society* in 1921. Later at the First International Congress of

Radiology in London in 1925 and the Second International Congress of Radiology in Stockholm in 1928, there was considerable interest in radiation protection, which led to creation of what is now the International Commission on Radiation Units (ICRU) and the International X-Ray and Radium Protection Committee, the forerunner of the present-day International Commission on Radiological Protection (ICRP). As a prelude to the Second International Congress and organization of the ICRP, the Advisory Committee on X-Ray and Radium Protection, later to become the National Council on Radiation Protection and Measurements (NCRP), was organized in the United States with its "home" to be the National Bureau of Standards.

During the 1920s, the concept of a tolerance dose, the amount of radiation the tissue of concern was able to tolerate, emerged. This concept centered on concern for immediate observable alterations in structure and function of the body, such as erythema of the skin. The importance of dose rate (i.e., variations in units of radiation dose per unit time) and dose fractionation (the delivery of a given radiation dose in several fractions at different times) was recognized and incorporated in the tolerance dose of 0.1 R per day adopted by the NRCP and 0.2 R per day adopted by the ICRP in 1934.

During the late 1930s, several reports were prepared by the NCRP. One of the most significant, NCRP Report No. 5 (1941), concerned the safe handling of radioactive luminous compounds. The impetus for this report derived from the growing body of information on severe or even fatal injury to radium dial painters. This report recommended that any worker who showed a deposit of more than 0.1 μg of radium change his occupation immediately. Later, this recommendation was to be a keystone in the development of standards for other radioactive materials that might be internally deposited. This value and the value of 0.1 R per day for external exposure were to provide the basis for the radiation protection practices used in the World War II Manhattan Project directed toward developing a nuclear weapon.

Within the Manhattan Project, extensive biomedical investigations on the effects of radiation from both external and internal sources were initiated and the body of knowledge on biologic effects of radiation began to increase markedly. After the conclusion of World War II, this extensive research program was continued by the newly created U.S. Atomic Energy Commission. In the years immediately after World War II the ICRP and ICRU were reactivated, their activities having understandably been interrupted by the war. At the same time, the

NCRP activities were expanded and accelerated. In each case this led to a number of reports too numerous for individual citation. One of these on external exposure, NCRP Report No. 17 (1954) issued in preliminary form in 1949 and as a final report in 1954, reduced the basic Maximum Permissible Dose for radiation workers to 0.3 rem per week, a value later adopted by the ICRP (ICRP, 1959).

In the early 1950s, concern over the effects of fallout from nuclear weapons stimulated a wave of concern over radiation effects and radiation protection standards. This concern directed attention to a number of important issues including the adequacy of existing standards, their appropriateness for limiting exposure of the general population, and the adequacy of our knowledge of radiation effects especially as embodied in dose-response relationships. Not surprisingly, one response was the organization of several new committees. One of the new organizations was the United Nations Scientific Committee on the Effects of Atomic Radiation (UNSCEAR) organized in 1956, which has issued five reports (UNSCEAR, 1958, 1962, 1964, 1966, 1972). These reports provide excellent bibliographies to the literature. Within the United States several committees on the Biological Effects of Atomic Radiation (BEAR) were organized under the aegis of the National Academy of Sciences (BEAR, 1956). A recommendation of the latter committees was a further reduction in the basic maximum permissible dose from 15 to 5 rem per year for radiation workers, a reduction stimulated by concern for genetic hazards. To provide latitude for small overdose the concept of age proration was introduced whereby the individual's total exposure was limited to $5 (N - 18)$ rem at a given time where N is the individual's age in years (NCRP, 1957, 1958). At the same time, the principle was enunciated that radiation exposure to persons outside of a controlled area from operations within a controlled area should not exceed one-tenth the value of that for radiation workers.

In 1957, in response to public concern the Joint Committee on Atomic Energy (JCAE) of the U.S. Congress began a series of hearings addressing the question of radiation hazards. These hearings were noteworthy in calling public attention to the problem and emphasizing that radiation standards are inexact: "safe" and "unsafe" have only relative meaning and the meaning may be interpreted differently by different individuals including scientists. A question inherent in this discussion was, and continues to be, the shape of the dose-response curve; i.e., is it linear or curvilinear?

An outgrowth of the JCAE hearing was recognition that the U.S. government had no official standard-setting organization and that in fact it was, by and large, using the standards established by the NCRP and ICRP. Recognizing that there were some desirable features of having a single government agency responsible for establishing radiation standards, an Executive Order was issued in 1959 creating such an agency, the Federal Radiation Council (FRC). Within a short period of time, the FRC arrived at a set of standards essentially identical to those of the NCRP. In 1970, with organization of the Environmental Protection Agency (EPA) the activities and functions of the FRC were transferred to the EPA.

A second outgrowth of the JCAE hearing was the initiation of action to formally sever the relationship between the National Bureau of Standards and NCRP, resulting in establishment of the NCRP as an independent body. This was accomplished in 1964 when the NCRP was issued a federal charter.

During the late 1950s and the 1960s, additional reports of both a general and a specific nature were issued by the ICRP and NCRP. The most significant of these were Reports 1 and 2 of the ICRP (1959, 1960), the first covering both external and internal radiation and the second specifically considering internal radiation. Since ICRP Report No. 2 was prepared under the leadership of individuals also responsible for NCRP activities, a portion of it appeared as NCRP Report No. 22 (1959). ICRP Publication No. 9 (1966c) represents an updated and revised version of ICRP Publication No. 1 and included a discussion of the concept of risk based in large part on ICRP Publication No. 8 (1966b), which specifically addressed the evaluation of risks from radiation. ICRP Publication No. 26 (1977) provides the latest recommendations of the ICRP, recommendations that have not yet been fully adopted within the United States.

The most recent major publication of the NCRP on radiation protection standards is Report No. 39 (1971)—*Basic Radiation Protection Criteria*, which updates the Council's position on basic standards. Because of their importance, the primary recommendations contained in the report are presented in Table 19–6. NCRP Report No. 43 states the position of the NCRP on issues concerning basic standards that were raised by the BEIR report (1972), discussed below, and the 1972 UNSCEAR report. The NCRP has published a number of other reports generally of a more specific nature, some of which have been referenced in this chapter. One additional general report (NCRP, 1976b) providing guidance for personnel working with

Table 19–6. DOSE-LIMITING RECOMMENDATIONS OF THE NCRP*†

Maximum Permissible Dose Equivalent for Occupational Exposure

Combined whole-body occupational exposure	
Prospective annual limit—paragraphs 229, 233	5 rems in any one year
Retrospective annual limit—paragraphs 230, 233	10–15 rems in any one year
Long-term accumulation to age N years—paragraph 231	$(N - 18) \times 5$ rems
Skin—paragraphs 234, 235	15 rems in any one year
Hands—paragraphs 236, 237	75 rems in any one year (25/qtr)
Forearms—paragraphs 236, 237	30 rems in any one year (10 qtr)
Other organs, tissues, and organ systems—paragraphs 238, 239	15 rems in any one year (5 qtr)
Fertile women (with respect to fetus)—paragraphs 240, 241	0.5 rem in gestation period

Dose Limits for the Public or Occasionally Exposed Individuals

Individual or occasional—paragraphs 245, 246, 253, 254	0.5 rem in one year
Students—paragraphs 255, 256	0.1 rem in any one year

Population Dose Limits

Genetic—paragraphs 247, 248	0.17 rem average per year
Somatic—paragraphs 250, 251	0.17 rem average per year

Emergency Dose Limits—Life Saving

Individual (older than 45 years if possible)—paragraph 258	100 rems
Hands and forearms—paragraph 258	200 rems, additional (300 rems, total)

Emergency Dose Limits—Less Urgent

Individual—paragraph 259	25 rems
Hands and forearms—paragraph 259	100 rems, total

Family of Radioactive Patients

Individual (under age 45)—paragraphs 267, 268	0.5 rem in any one year
Individual (over age 45)—paragraphs 267, 268	5 rems in any one year

* From National Council on Radiation Protection and Measurements: *Basic Radiation Protection Criteria*. NCRP Report No. 39. National Council on Radiation Protection and Measurements, Washington, D.C., 1971.

† The paragraph numbers in the table refer to the text of the complete NCRP report. It is important to recognize that many of the recommendations or numbers are qualified by the information in the text, and the reader is referred to the complete report.

radiation or radioactive materials will be of interest to some readers.

Before leaving the subject of radiation standards it is important to note some recent events in the area. In early 1970, a major challenge to existing standards, especially as utilized by the U.S. Atomic Energy Commission, was raised by Gofman and Tamplin who made several calculations of cancer mortality at exposure levels on the order of existing standards. A basic assumption of their calculations was that the dose-response relationship is linear at all dose levels; hence, even at very small doses, if large populations are exposed, a number of deaths may be estimated (Gofman and Tamplin, 1970; Tamplin and Gofman, 1970a, 1970b). Their charges were challenged by U.S. Atomic Energy Commission officials (Thompson and Bibb, 1970) and ultimately provided the major stimulus for an independent evaluation of the question of the effects of low levels of ionizing radiation by a committee of the NAS-NRC. That committee's report (BEIR Report, 1972) provides a valuable and well-documented review of the literature on radiation effects. The committee specifically considered the effects of exposure of the total United States population at 5 rem per 30 years and estimated that such exposures by virtue of genetic risk would lead to an increase of 5 percent in the ill health of the population and that the somatic risk would lead to an increase of about 2 percent in the spontaneous cancer death risk, which is an increase of about 0.3 percent in the overall death rate from all causes. The committee suggested that the current radiation protection guide of 0.17 rem per year was unnecessarily high.

In estimating the risk at low levels of exposure, the committee endorsed the use of a linear dose-response model for standard setting purposes. It should be kept in mind that this endorsement does not represent scientific proof of the linear model; indeed the committee noted that such scientific proof was unlikely: "Some human populations are so large that even very small linear estimates of risk, in the region of dose prescribed by current guidelines, yield finite estimates of induced cancers, i.e., deaths. These estimates of risk are beyond empirical demonstration. It is unlikely that the presence or absence of a true threshold for cancer in human populations can be proved. If the intent of authorities is to minimize the loss of life that radiation exposures may entail, they must indeed, be guided by such estimates, and will not rely on notions of a threshold" (BEIR Report, 1972).

The above quote is worthy of careful consideration relative not only to radiation but to other physical and chemical agents introduced into man's environment. It is obvious that the quantification of societal risks such as those made by the BEIR Committee also demands quantification of societal benefits if critical risk-benefits analyses and judgments are to be made. A recent report specifically addresses considerations in making health benefit-cost analyses for activities involving radiation exposure and alternative activities that may also have associated risks (NAS, 1977). Recognizing the extent to which the basic radiation exposure standards have been successively reduced from time to time in the past, it is not unreasonable to expect that they may be reduced further in the future and that population exposure standards (as contrasted to occupational exposure standards) may be expected to explicitly state the associated risk and approaches to balancing risk versus benefit.

REFERENCES

Altman, K. I.; Gerber, G. B.; and Okada, S.: *Radiation Biochemistry*. Vol. I. Cells. Academic Press, Inc., New York, 1970.
——: *Radiation Biochemistry*. Vol. II. Tissues and Body Fluids. Academic Press, Inc., New York, 1970.
Andrews, H. L.: *Radiation Biophysics*, 2nd ed. Prentice-Hall, Englewood Cliffs, NJ, 1974.
Archer, V. E., and Wagoner, J. K.: Lung cancer among uranium miners in the United States. *Health Phys.*, 25:351–71, 1973.
Attix, F. H., and Roesch, W. C.: *Radiation Dosimetry*, 2nd ed. Vol. I. Fundamentals. Academic Press, Inc., New York, 1968.
——: *Radiation Dosimetry*, 2nd ed. Vol. II. Instrumentation. Academic Press, Inc., New York, 1966.
Attix, F. H., and Tochilin, E.: *Radiation Dosimetry*, 2nd ed. Vol. III. Sources, Fields, Measurements, and Applications. Academic Press, Inc., New York, 1969.
Bair, W. J.: Inhalation of radionuclides and carcinogenesis. In Hanna, M. G., *et al.* (eds.): *Inhalation Carcingoenesis*. AEC Symposium Series 18. U.S. Atomic Energy Commission, Office of Information Services, Springfield, VA, 1970.
Bair, W. J.; Ballou, J. E.; Park, J.; and Sanders, C. L.: Plutonium in soft tissues with emphasis on the respiratory tract. In Hodge, H. C.; Hursch, J. B.; and Stannard, J. N. (eds.): *Uranium, Plutonium and the Transuranic Elements*, Handbook of Experimental Pharmacology, Vol. 36. Springer-Verlag, New York, 1973, chap. 11.

Bair, W. J., and Thompson, R. C.: Plutonium: Biomedical research. *Science*, 183:715–22, 1974.
Ballou, J. E.; George, L. A., II; and Thompson, R. C.: The combined toxic effects of plutonium plus x-ray in rats. *Health Phys.*, 8:581–87, 1962.
Beebe, G. W.; Kato, H.; and Land, C. E.: Studies of the mortality of A-bomb survivors. *Radiat. Res.*, 75:138–201, 1978.
Behrens, C. F.: Nuclear reactors and bombs: some basic considerations. In Behrens, C. F.; King, E. R.; and Carpender, J. W. J. (eds.): *Atomic Medicine*, 5th ed. Williams & Wilkins Co., Baltimore, 1969.
Behrens, C. F.; King, E. R.; and Carpender, J. W. J. (eds.): *Atomic Medicine*, 5th ed. Williams & Wilkins Co., Baltimore, 1969.
Benjamin, S. A.; Hahn, F. F.; Chiffelle, T. L.; Boecker, B. B.; Hobbs, C. H.; Jones, R. K.; McClellan, R. O.; Pickrell, J. A.; and Redman, H. C.: Neoplasia in beagle dogs after inhalation of ^{144}CeCl$_3$. In Sanders, C. L., *et al.* (eds.): *Radionuclide Carcinogenesis*. AEC Symposium Series 29. U.S. Atomic Energy Commission, Office of Information Services, Springfield, VA, 1973.
Benjamin, S. A.; Hahn, F. F.; Chiffelle, T. L.; Boecker, B. B.; Hobbs, C. H.; Jones, R. K.; McClellan, R. O.; and Snipes, M. B.: Occurrence of hemangiosarcomas in beagles with internally deposited radionuclides. *Cancer Res.*, 35:1745–55, 1975.
Bender, M. A., and Gooch, P. C.: Types and rates of x-ray-induced chromosome aberrations in human blood irradiated *in vitro. Proc. Natl. Acad. Sci. U.S.A.*, 48:522–32, 1962.
Berdjis, C. S. (ed.): *Pathology of Irradiation*. Williams & Wilkins Co., Baltimore, 1971, chap. 2, p. 25.
Biological Basis of Radiotherapy. Br. Med. Bull., 29(1): 1–83, January, 1973. British Council, Med. Dept. London, 1973.
Biological Effects of Atomic Radiation (BEAR): *Summary Reports*. National Academy of Sciences, National Research Council, Washington, D.C., 1956.
Biological Effects of Ionizing Radiation (BEIR) Advisory Committee: *Report: The Effects of Populations of Exposure to Low Levels of Ionizing Radiation*. National Academy of Sciences, National Research Council, Washington, D.C., 1972.
Boecker, B. B.: Toxicity of ^{137}CsCl in the beagle: Metabolism and dosimetry. *Radiat. Res.*, 50:556–73, 1972.
Boecker, B. B., and Cuddihy, R. G.: Toxicity of ^{144}Ce inhaled as ^{144}CeCl$_3$ by the beagle dog: Metabolism and dosimetry. *Radiat. Res.*, 60:133–54, 1974.
Bond, V. P.; Cronkite, E. P.; and Conard, R. A.: Acute whole body radiation injury: pathogenesis, pre- and postradiation protection. In Behrens, C. F.; King, E. R.; and Carpender, J. W. J. (eds.): *Atomic Medicine*, 5th ed. Williams & Wilkins Co., Baltimore, 1969.
Brewen, J. G., and Preston, R. J.: The use of chromosome aberrations for predicting genetic hazards to man. In Nygaard, O. F.; Adler, H. I.; and Sinclair, W. K. (eds.): *Radiation Research: Biomedical, Chemical, and Physical Perspectives*. Academic Press, Inc., New York, 1975, pp. 926–36.
Bustad, L. K.: *Biology of Radioiodine*. Pergamon Press, New York, 1964.
Casarett, A. P.: *Radiation Biology*. Prentice-Hall, Inc., Englewood Cliffs, NJ, 1968.
Cronkite, E. P.; Bond, V. P.; and Conard, R. A.: Diagnosis and therapy of acute radiation injury. In *Atomic Medicine*, 5th ed. Williams & Wilkins Co., Baltimore, 1969.
Cuddihy, R. G.; Hall, R. P.; and Griffith, W. C.: Inhalation exposures to barium aerosols; physical, chemical and mathematical analysis. *Health Phys.*, 26:405–16, 1974.

Cuddihy, R. G.; Gomez, S. R.; and Pfleger, R. C.: Inhalation exposures of beagle dogs to cerium aerosols: physical, chemical and mathematical analysis. *Health Phys.*, 29:257–65, 1975.

Cuddihy, R. G.: Deposition and retention of inhaled niobium in beagle dogs. *Health Phys.*, 34:167–76, 1978.

Doll, R.: Cancer following therapeutic external irradiation. In Clark, R. L.; Cumley, R. W.; McCay, J. E.; and Copeland, M. M. (eds.): *Oncology 1970*, Vol. 5. Proceedings on the 10th International Cancer Congress. Year Book Medical Publishers, Chicago, 1971.

Dolphin, G. W., and Eve, I. S.: Dosimetry of the gastrointestinal tract. *Health Phys.*, 12:163–72, 1966.

Durbin, Patricia W.: Distribution of the transuranic elements in mammals. *Health Phys.*, 8:665–71, 1962.

———: Plutonium in man: A twenty-five year review. University of California, Lawrence Radiation Laboratory Report, UCRL-20850, 1971.

Eisenbud, M.: *Environmental Radioactivity*, 2nd ed. Academic Press, Inc., New York and London, 1973.

Elkind, M. M., and Whitmore, G. F. (eds.): *Radiobiology of Cultured Mammalian Cells*. Gordon and Breach, New York, 1967.

Evans, R. D.; Keane, A. T.; KolerKow, R. J.; Neal, W. R.; and Shanahan, M. M.: Radiogenic tumors in the radium and mesothorium cases studied at M.I.T. In Mays, C. W.; Jee, W. S. S.; Lloyd, R. D.; Stover, Betsy J.; Dougherty, Jean H.; and Taylor, G. N. (eds.): *Delayed Effects of Bone-Seeding Radionuclides*. University of Utah Press, Salt Lake City, 1969, pp. 157–94.

Eve, I. S.: A review of the physiology of the gastrointestinal tract in relation to radiation doses from radioactive materials. *Health Phys.*, 12:131–61, 1966.

Fabrikant, J. I.: *Radiobiology*. Year Book Medical Publishers, Chicago, 1972.

Finkel, A. J.; Miller, C. E.; and Hasterlik, R. J.: Radium induced malignant tumors in man. In Mays, C. W.; Jee, W. S. S.; Lloyd, R. D.; Stover, Betsy J.; Dougherty, Jean H.; and Taylor, G. N. (eds.): *Delayed Effects of Bone-Seeking Radionuclides*. University of Utah Press, Salt Lake City, 1969, pp. 195–225.

Furchner, J. E.; Trafton, G. A.; and Richmond, C. R.: Distribution of cesium-137 after chronic exposure in dogs and mice. *Proc. Soc. Exp. Biol. Med.*, 116:375–78, 1964.

Garner, R. J.: *Transfer of Radioactive Materials from the Terrestrial Environment to Animals and Man*. C.R.C. Press, Cleveland, 1972.

Gladstone, S., and Dolan, P. J.: *The Effects of Nuclear Weapons*, 3rd ed. U.S. Department of Defense, U.S. Department of Energy, Washington, D.C., 1977.

Gofman, J. W.; Gofman, J. D.; Tamplin, A. R.; and Kovich, Erma: Radiation as an environmental hazard. In *Environment and Cancer*. Williams & Wilkins Co., Baltimore, 1972.

Gofman, J. W., and Tamplin, A. R.: Low dose radiation and cancer, IEEE (Inst. Elec. Electron Eng.). Transaction on Nuclear Science. Part I, NS-17, 1970, pp. 1–9.

Goldman, M., and Bustad, L. K. (eds.): *Biomedical Implications and Radiostrontium Exposure* AEC Symposium Series 25. U.S. Atomic Energy Commission Office of Information Services, Springfield, VA, 1972.

Grahn, D.: Biological effects of protracted low dose radiation exposure of man and animals. In Fry, R. J. M.; Grahn, D.; Griem, M. L.; and Rust, J. H. (eds.): *Late Effects of Radiation*. Proceedings of a Colloquium held in the Center for Continuing Education, University of Chicago, May 15–17, 1969. Taylor and Francis, Ltd., London, 1970, chap. V.

Haely, J. W. (ed.): *Plutonium; Health Implications for Man*. Proceedings of the Second Los Alamos Life Sciences Symposium held in Los Alamos, New Mexico, May 22–24, 1974. *Health Phys.*, 29(4):489–94, October, 1975. Pergamon Press, New York, 1976.

Hahn, F. F.; Benjamin, S. A.; Boecker, B. B.; Chiffelle, T. L.; Hobbs, C. H.; Jones, R. K.; McClellan, R. O.; and Redman, H. C.: Induction of pulmonary neoplasia in Beagle dogs by inhaled ^{144}Ce fused-clay particles. In Sanders, C. L., *et al.* (eds.): *Radionuclide Carcinogenesis*, AEC Symposium Series 29. U.S. Atomic Energy Commission Office of Information Services, Springfield, VA, 1973.

Health Effects of Alpha-Emitting Particles in the Respiratory Tract. National Academy of Sciences/National Research Council, Washington, D.C., 1976.

Hempelmann, L. H.; Langham, W. H.; Richmond, C. R.; and Voelz, G. L.: Manhattan project plutonium workers: A twenty-seven year follow-up study of selected cases. *Health Phys.*, 25:461–79, 1973.

Hendee, W. R.: *Medical Radiation Physics*. Year Book Medical Publishers, Chicago, 1970.

Hine, G. J., and Brownell, G. L.: *Radiation Dosimetry*. Academic Press, Inc., New York, 1956.

Hodge, H. C.; Hursh, J. B.; and Stannard, J. N. (eds.): *Handbook of Experimental Pharmacology*. Vol. 36, Uranium, Plutonium and the Transplutonic Elements. Springer-Verlag, New York, 1973.

International Atomic Energy Agency: *Inhalation Risks from Radioactive Contaminants*. Technical Report Series No. 142. International Atomic Energy Agency, Vienna, 1973.

———: *Biological and Environmental Effects of Low-Level Radiation*. Proceedings of a Symposium held in Chicago, Nov. 3–7, 1975.

International Commission on Radiation Units and Measurements: *Radiation Quantities and Units*. ICRU Report 19. International Commission on Radiation Units and Measurements, Washington, D.C., 1971.

———: *Dose Equivalents*, ICRU-19 (Suppl.). International Commission on Radiation Units and Measurements, Washington, D.C., 1973.

———: *Conceptual Basis for the Determination of Dose Equivalents*. ICRU Report 25. International Commission on Radiation Units and Measurements, Washington, D.C., 1976.

International Commission on Radiological Protection: *Recommendations of the International Commission on Radiological Protection* (Adopted September 9, 1958). ICRP Publication No. 1. Pergamon Press, Oxford, 1959.

———: *Recommendations of the International Commission on Radiological Protection Report of Committee II on Permissible Dose for Internal Radiation* (1959). ICRP Publication No. 2. *Health Phys.*, 3:1–380, 1960.

———: *Recommendations of the International Commission on Radiological Protection Report of Committee IV on Protection Against Electromagnetic Radiation Above 3 MeV and Electrons, Neutrons and Protons* (Adopted 1962; with revisions adopted 1963). ICRP Publication No. 4. Pergamon Press, Oxford, 1963.

———: (Task Group on Lung Dynamics): *Deposition and Retention Models for Internal Dosimetry of the Human Respiratory Tract*. *Health Phys.*, 12:173–207, 1966a.

———: *Recommendations of the International Commission on Radiological Protection* (Adopted September 17, 1965). ICRP Publication No. 9. Pergamon Press, Oxford, 1966b.

———: (Task Group of Committee 2): *The Metabolism of Compounds of Plutonium and Other Actinides*. ICRP Publication No. 19. Pergamon Press, Oxford, 1972.

———: *Report of the Task Group on Reference Man*. ICRP Publication No. 23. Pergamon Press, Oxford, 1975.

————: *Recommendations of the International Commission on Radiological Protection*. ICRP Publication 26. Annals of the ICRP 1 (3), 1977. International Commission on Radiation Units and Measurements, Washington, D.C., 1977.

Jablon, S., and Kato, H.: Studies of the mortality of A-bomb survivors. 5. Radiation dose and mortality 1950–1970. *Radiat. Res.*, **50**:649–98, 1972.

Jee, W. S. S. (ed.): *The Health Effects Plutonium and Radium*. J. W. Press, Salt Lake City, 1976.

Jones, R. K.; Hahn, F. F.; Hobbs, C. H.; Benjamin, S. A.; Boecker, B. B.; McClellan, R. O.; and Slauson, D. O.: Pulmonary carcinogenesis and chronic beta irradiation of lung. In Karbe, E., and Park, J. F. (eds.): *Experimental Lung Cancer; Carcinogenesis and Bioassays*. Springer-Verlag, Berlin, 1974, pp. 454–67.

Kanapilly, G. M.: Alveolar microenvironment and its relationship to the retention and transport into blood of aerosols deposited in the alveoli. *Health Phys.*, **32**:89–100, 1977.

Karcher, K-H., and Jentzsch, K.: Radiobiology as the basis of radiotherapy. In Ioachim, H. L. (ed.): *Pathobiology Annual*, Vol. 2. Appleton-Century-Crofts, Educational Division, Meredith Corp., New York, 1972.

Langham, W. H. (ed.): *Radiobiological Factors in Manned Space Flight*. National Academy of Sciences, National Research Council, Washington, D.C., 1967.

Leach, L. J.; Maynard, E. A.; Hodge, C. H.; Scott, J. K.; Yuile, C. L.; Sylvester, G. E.; and Wilson, H. B.: A five-year inhalation study with natural uranium dioxide (UO$_2$) dust. I. Retention and biologic effect in the monkey, dog and rat. *Health Phys.*, **18**:599–612, 1970.

Lenihan, J. M. A.; Loutit, J. F.; and Martin, J. H. (eds.): *Strontium Metabolism*. Academic Press, Inc., London and New York, 1967.

Linden, K.: The new special names of SI units in the field of ionizing radiations. *Health Phys.*, **30**:417–18, 1976.

Lindop, P. J., and Sacher, G. A. (eds.): *Radiation and Ageing*. Proceedings of a Colloquium held in Semmering, Austria, June 23–24, 1966. Taylor and Francis, Ltd., London, 1966.

Lundin, F. E.; Wagoner, J. K.; and Archer, V. E.: Radon daughter exposure and respiratory cancer: Quantitative and temporal aspects. NIOSH and MIEHS Joint Monograph No. 1. National Technical Information Service, Springfield, VA, 1971.

McClellan, R. O.: Calcium-strontium discrimination in miniature pigs as related to age. *Nature* (Lond.), **202**:104–106, 1964.

McClellan, R. O.; Barnes, J. E.; Boecker, B. B.; Chiffelle, T. L.; Hobbs, C. H.; Jones, R. K.; Mauderly, J. L.; Pickrell, J. A.; and Redman, H. C.: Toxicity of beta-emitting radionuclides inhaled in fused clay particles—an experimental approach. In Nettesheim, P.; Hanna, M. G., Jr.; and Deatherage, J. W., Jr. (eds.): *Morphology of Experimental Respiratory Carcinogensis*, CONF-700501. U.S. Atomic Energy Commission Office of Information Service, Springfield, VA, 1970.

McClellan, R. O.; Boyd, H. A.; Gallegos, A. F.; and Thomas, R. G.: Retention and distribution of ^{244}Cm following inhalation of ^{244}CmCl$_3$ and ^{244}CmO$_{1.73}$ by beagle dogs. *Health Phys.*, **22**:877–85, 1972b.

McClellan, R. O.; Bustad, L. K.; and Keough, R. F.: Metabolism of some SNAP radionuclides in miniature swine. *Aerospace Med.*, **36**:16–20, 1965.

McClellan, R. O., and Jones, R. K.: ^{90}Sr-induced neoplasia: A selective review. In Mays, C. W., *et al.* (eds.): *Delayed Effects of Bone-Seeking Radionuclides*. University of Utah Press, Salt Lake City, 1969.

McLean, A. S.: Early adverse effects of radiation. *Br. Med. Bull.*, **29**:69–73, 1973.

MacMahon, B.: Prenatal x-ray exposure and childhood cancer. *J. Natl. Cancer Inst.*, **28**:1173–91, 1962.

Mancuso, T. F.; Stewart, A.; and Kneale, G.: Radiation exposures of Hanford workers dying from cancer and other causes. *Health Phys.*, **33**:369–85, 1977.

Margulis, A. R.: The lessons of radiobiology for diagnostic radiology. *Am. J. Roentgenol. Radium Ther. Nucl. Med.*, **117**:741–56, 1973.

Marks, S.; Gilbert, E. S.; and Breitenstein, B. D.: Cancer mortality in Hanford workers. Proceedings of a Symposium "Late Biological Effects of Ionizing Radiation", held March 13–17, 1978, IAEA, Vienna, in press.

Marshall, J. H.; Lloyd, E. L.; Rundo, J.; Liniecki, J.; Marotti, G.; Mays, C. W.; Sissons, H. A.; and Snyder, W. S.: Akaline earth metabolism in adult man. *Health Phys.*, **24**:125–222, 1973 (ICRP Report 20).

Martin, A., and Harbison, S. A.: *An Introduction to Radiation Protection*. Chapman and Hall, Ltd., London, 1972.

Mays, C. W.; Jee, W. S. S.; Lloyd, R. D.; Stover, B. J.; Dougherty, J. H.; and Taylor, G. C. (eds.): *Delayed Effects of Bone-Seeking Radionuclides*. University of Utah Press, Salt Lake City, 1969.

Mays, C. W., and Lloyd, R. D.: Bone sarcoma risk from ^{90}Sr. In Goldman, M., and Bustad, L. K. (eds.): *Biomedical Implications of Radiostrontium Exposure*. AEC Symposium Series 25, CONF-710201, National Technical Information Service, Springfield, VA, 1972a.

————: Bone sarcoma incidence vs. alpha particle dose. In Stover, B. J., and Jee, W. S. S. (eds.): *Radiobiology of Plutonium*. J. W. Press, University of Utah, Salt Lake City, 1972b.

Medical Internal Radiation Dose Committee: MIRD, *Journal of Nuclear Medicine*, Supplement No. 1, Pamphlets 1–3. Society of Nuclear Medicine, Inc., New York, 1968.

————: MIRD, *Journal of Nuclear Medicine*, Supplement No. 2, Pamphlet 4. Society of Nuclear Medicine, Inc., New York, 1969a.

————: MIRD, *Journal of Nuclear Medicine*, Supplement No. 3, Pamphlet 5. Society of Nuclear Medicine, Inc., New York, 1969b.

————: MIRD, *Journal of Nuclear Medicine*, Supplement No. 5, Pamphlet 7–8. Society of Nuclear Medicine, Inc., New York, 1971.

Medical Internal Radiation Dose Committee: *MIRD*, *Journal of Nuclear Medicine*, Supplement, Pamphlet 10. Society of Nuclear Medicine, Inc., New York, 1975.

————: *MIRD*, *Journal of Nuclear Medicine*, Supplement, Pamphlet 11. Society of Nuclear Medicine, Inc., New York, 1975.

Medical Research Council. *The Toxicity of Plutonium*. Her Majesty's Stationery Office, London, 1975.

Mercer, T. T.: On the role of particle size in the dissolution of lung burdens. *Health Phys.*, **13**:1211–21, 1967.

Mercer, T. T.; Tillery, M. I.; and Newton, G. J.: A multi-stage, low flow rate cascade impactor. *Aerosol Sci.*, **1**:9–15, 1970.

Mewhinney, J. A.; Muggenburg, B. A.; McClellan, R. O.; and Miglio, J. J.: The effect of varying physical and chemical characteristics of inhaled plutonium aerosols on metabolism and excretion. In *Diagnosis and Treatment of Incorporated Radionuclides*, IAEA, 1976, pp. 87–97.

Miller, D. G.: *Radioactivity and Radiation Detection*. Gordon and Breach Science Publishers, New York, 1972.

Mole, R. H.: Late effects of radiation: carcinogenesis. *Br. Med. Bull.*, **29**:78–83, 1973.

National Academy of Sciences Advisory Committee on the Biological Effects of Ionizing Radiations (the BEIR Committee): *Considerations of Health Benefit-Cost*

Analysis for Activities Involving Ionizing Radiation Exposure and Alternatives. EPA 5201/4-77-003. National Academy of Sciences, National Research Council, Washington, D.C., 1977.

National Council on Radiation Protection and Measurements: *Safety Handling of Radioactive Luminous Compounds.* NCRP Report No. 5. National Council of Radiation Protection and Measurements, Washington, D.C., 1941.

————: *Permissible Dose from External Sources of Ionizing Radiation.* NCRP Report No. 17. National Council on Radiation Protection and Measurements, Washington, D.C., 1954.

————: Maximum permissible radiation exposure to man: A preliminary statement of the National Commission on Radiation Protection and Measurements (January 8, 1957). *Radiology*, **18**:260, 1957.

————: Maximum permissible radiation exposures to man (April 16, 1958): Addendum to NCRP Report No. 17. *Radiology*, **71**:263, 1958.

————: *Maximum Permissible Body Burdens and Maximum Permissible Concentrations of Radionuclides in Air and Water for Occupational Exposure.* NCRP Report No. 22. National Council on Radiation Protection, Washington, D.C., 1959.

————: *Protection Against Neutron Radiation.* NCRP Report No. 38. National Council on Radiation Protection and Measurements, Washington, D.C., 1971a.

————: *Basic Radiation Protection Criteria.* NCRP Report No. 39. National Council on Radiation Protection and Measurements, Washington, D.C., 1971b.

————: Progress in studies with transuranic elements at the Lovelace Foundation. *Health Phys.*, **22**:815–22, 1972a.

————: *Natural Background Radiation in the United States.* NCRP Report No. 45. National Council on Radiation Protection and Measurements, Washington, D.C., 1975a.

————: *Alpha-Emitting Particles in Lungs.* NCRP Report No. 46. National Council on Radiation Protection and Measurements, Washington, D.C., 1975b.

————: *Tritium Measurement Techniques.* NCRP Report No. 47. National Council on Radiation Protection and Measurements, Washington, D.C., 1976a.

————: *Radiation Protection for Medical and Allied Health Personnel.* NCRP Report No. 48. National Council on Radiation Protection and Measurements, Washington, D.C., 1976b.

————: *Cesium-137 from the Environment to Man: Metabolism and Dose.* NCRP Report No. 52. National Council on Radiation Protection and Measurements, Washington, D.C., 1977a.

————: *Review of NCRP Radiation Dose Limit for Embryo and Fetus in Occupationally-Exposed Women.* NCRP Report No. 53. National Council on Radiation Protection and Measurements, Washington, D.C., 1977b.

————: *Protection of the Thyroid Gland in the Event of Releases of Radioiodine.* NCRP Report No. 55. National Council on Radiation Protection and Measurements, Washington, D.C., 1977c.

————: *Radiation Exposure from Consumer Products and Miscellaneous Sources.* NCRP Report No. 56. National Council on Radiation Protection and Measurements, Washington, D.C., 1977d.

————: *Instrumentation and Monitoring Methods for Radiation Protection.* NCRP Report No. 57. National Council on Radiation Protection and Measurements, Washington, D.C., 1978a.

————: *A Handbook of Radioactivity Measurements Procedures.* NCRP Report No. 58. National Council on Radiation Protection and Measurements, Washington, D.C., 1978b.

————: *Operational Radiation Safety Program.* NCRP Report No. 59. National Council on Radiation Protection and Measurements, Washington, D.C., 1978c.

————: *Physical, Chemical and Biological Properties of Radiocerium Relevant to Radiation Protection guidelines.* NCRP Report No. 60. National Council on Radiation Protection and Measurements, Washington, D.C., 1978d.

Nenot, G. C., and Stather, J. W.: The toxicology of plutonium, americum, and curium. Commission of European Communities, 1979.

Norris, W. P.; Poole, C. M.; and Rehfeld, C. E.: Cesium-137: Current status and late effects. USAEC Report ANL-7278, 1966.

Osborne, R. V.: Permissible levels of tritium in man and the environment. *Radiat. Res.*, **50**:197–211, 1972.

Palmer, R. F., and Thompson, R. C.: Strontium-calcium interrelationships in the growing rat. *Am. J. Physiol.*, **207**:561–66, 1964.

Parmley, W. W.; Jensen, J. B.; and Mays, C. W.: Skeletal self-absorption of beta-particle energy. In Dougherty, T. F., *et al.* (eds.): *Aspects of Internal Irradiation.* Pergamon Press, Oxford, 1962.

Patt, H. M., and Quastler, H.: Radiation effects on cell renewal and related systems. *Physiol. Rev.*, **43**:357–93, 1963.

Redman, H. C.; McClellan, R. O.; Jones, R. K.; Boecker, B. B.; Chiffelle, T. L.; Pickrell, J. A.; and Rypka, E. W.: Toxicity of ^{137}CsCl in the beagle: Early biological effects. *Radiat. Res.*, **50**:629–48, 1972.

Ross, D. M.: A statistical summary of United States Atomic Energy Commission Contractors' internal exposure experience, 1957–1966. In Kornberg, H. A., and Norwood, W. D. (eds.): *Diagnosis and Treatment of Deposited Radionuclides.* Excerpta Medica Foundation, Reidel, Dordrecht, Netherlands, 1968.

Rossi, H. H.: Biophysical implications of radiation quality. In Nygaard, O. F.; Adler, H. I.; and Sinclair, W. K. (eds.): *Radiation Research: Biomedical, Chemical, and Physical Perspectives.* Academic Press, Inc., New York, 1975, pp. 994–97.

Rowland, R. E.; Stehney, A. F.; and Lucas, H. F., Jr.: Dose-response relationships for female radium dial workers. *R diat. Res.*, **76**:368 83, 1978.

Rubin, P., and Casarett, G. W.: *Clinical Radiation Pathology.* W. B. Sanders Co., Philadelphia, 1968, chap. 1, p. 33.

Russell, W. L.: The genetic effects of radiation. In *Peaceful Uses of Atomic Energy.* Proceedings of the Fourth International Conference on the Peaceful Uses of Atomic Energy held jointly by the United Nations and the International Atomic Energy Commission, in Geneva, 6–16 Sept. 1971.

Saccomanno, G.; Archer, V. E.; Auerbach, O.; Kuschner, M.; Saunders, R. P.; and Klein, M. G.: Histologic types of lung cancer among uranium miners. *Cancer*, **27**:515–23, 1971.

Saunders, C. L., Jr.; Thompson, R. C.; and Bair, W. J.: Lung cancer: Dose response studies with radionuclides. In Hanna, M. G., Jr., *et al.* (eds.): *Inhalation Carcinogenesis*, AEC Symposium Series 18. U.S. Atomic Energy Commission Office of Information Services, Springfield, VA, 1970.

Schneider, G. J.; Chone, B.; and Blonnigen, T.: Chromosomal aberrations in a radiation accident. Dosimetric and hematological aspects. *Radiat. Res.*, **40**:613–17, 1969.

Schneider, K. J.: High Level Waste. In Sagan, L. A. (ed.): *Human and Ecologic Effects of Nuclear Power Plants.* Charles C Thomas Publisher, Springfield, IL, 1974, chap. 8.

Schulte, H. F.: Ionizing radiation. In *Industrial Environmental Health*. Academic Press, Inc., New York and London, 1972, pp. 243–69.

Shapiro, J.: *Radiation Protection*. Harvard University Press, Cambridge, Mass., 1972.

Stannard, J. N.: Toxicology of radionuclides. *Annu. Rev. Pharmacol.*, 13:325–57, 1973.

Stewart, A.: Low dose radiation cancers in man. In *Advances in Cancer Researeh*, Vol. 14. Academic Press, Inc., New York and London, 1971, pp. 359–90.

————: The carcinogenic effects of low level radiation. A re-appraisal of epidemiological methods and observations. *Health Phys.*, 24:223–40, 1973.

Stewart, A., and Kneale, G. W.: Radiation dose effects in relation to obstetric x-rays and childhood cancers. *Lancet*, 1:1185–88, 1970a.

————: Age-distribution of cancers caused by obstetric x-rays and their relevance to cancer latent periods. *Lancet*, 2:4–8, 1970b.

Stohlman, F., Jr. (ed.): *The Kinetics of Cellular Proliferation*. Grune & Stratton, Inc., New York, 1959.

Storer, J. B.: Radiation carcinogenesis. In Becker, F. F. (ed.): *Cancer, a Comprehensive Treatise*, Vol. 1. Plenum Press, New York, 1975, chap. 16.

Stover, B. J., and Jee, W. S. S. (eds.): *Radiobiology of Plutonium*. The J. W. Press, University of Utah, Salt Lake City, 1972.

Tamplin, A. R., and Gofman, J. W.: *Population Control Through Nuclear Pollution*. Nelson-Hall Co., Chicago, 1970a.

————: The radiations effects controversy. *Bull. Atomic Scientists*; *Science Public Affairs*, 26(7):2, 1970b.

Tamplin, A. R., and Cochran, T. B.: *Radiation Standards for Hot Particles: A Report on the Inadequacy of Existing Radiation Protection Standards Related to Internal Exposure to Man to Insoluble Particles of Plutonium and Other Alpha-Emitting Hot Particles*. Natural Resources Defense Council, Washington, D.C., 1974.

Thomas, Randi L.; Scott, J. K.; and Chiffelle, T. L.: Metabolism and toxicity of inhaled ^{144}Ce in rats. *Radiat. Res.*, 45:598–610, 1972.

Thompson, R. C. (ed.): Proceedings of the Hanford Symposium on the Biology of the Transuranic Elements held at Richland, Wash., May 28–30, 1962. *Health Phys.*, 8:561–780, 1962.

Thompson, R. C., and Palmer, R. F.: Strontium-calcium interrelationships in the mature rat. *Am. J. Physiol.*, 199:94–102, 1960.

Thompson, R. C.; Park, J. F.; and Bair, W. J.: Some speculative extensions to man of animal risk data on plutonium. In Stover, Betsy J., and Jee, W. S. S. (eds.): *Radiobiology of Plutonium*. J. W. Press, University of Utah, Salt Lake City, 1972.

Thompson, T. J., and Bibb, W. R.: Response to Gofman and Tamplin: The AEC position. *Bull. Atomic Scientists*; *Science Public Affairs*, 26:9–12, 1970.

Totter, J. R.: Research programs of the Atomic Energy Commission's Division of Biology and Medicine relevant to problems of health and pollution. In Le Cam, L. M.; Neyman, J.; and Scott, E. L. (eds.): *Effects of Pollution on Health*. Vol. VI, Proceedings of the Sixth Berkeley Symposium on Mathematical Statistics and Probability held at the University of California, Berkeley, April 9–12, 1971. University of California Press, Berkeley, 1962.

United Nations: Report of the United Nations Scientific Committee on the Effects of Atomic Radiation, 1958, and Supplements thereto for 1962, 1966 and 1972. Official Records of the General Assembly 13th, 17th, 19th, 21st and 24th Sessions. United Nations, New York.

United Nations Scientific Committee on the Effects of Atomic Radiation: *Ionizing Radiation: Levels and Effects*. Vol. I, Levels. Publication No. E.72.IX.17. United Nations, New York, 1972a.

————: *Ionizing Radiation: Levels and Effects*. Vol. II, Effects. Publication No. E.72.IX.18. United Nations, New York, 1972b.

Upton, A. C.: Radiation carcinogenesis. In Busch, H. (ed.): *Methods in Cancer Research*, Vol. 4. Academic Press, Inc., New York, 1968a.

————: The influence of dose rate in mammalian radiation biology. Quality effects. In Brown, D. G., et al. (eds.): *Dose Rate in Mammalian Biology*, CONF-680410, U.S. Atomic Energy Commission, Division of Technical Information, Oak Ridge, TN, 1968b.

————: Radiation. In *Cancer Medicine*. Lea & Febiger, Philadelphia, 1973. chaps. 1–5.

Upton, A. C., and Cosgrove, G. E., Jr.: Radiation-induced leukemia. In Rich, M. (ed.): *Experimental Leukemia*. Appleton-Century-Crofts, New York, 1968.

Upton, A. C.; Randolph, M. L.; and Conklin, J. W.: Late effects of fast neutrons and gamma rays in mice as influenced by the dose rate of irradiation: Induction of neoplasma. *Radiat. Res.*, 41:467–91, 1970.

Vaughan, Janet M.: *The Effects of Irradiation on the Skeleton*. Clarendon Press, Oxford, 1973.

Vennart, J.: Radiotoxicology of tritium and ^{14}C compounds. *Health Phys.*, 16:429–40, 1969.

Voelz, G. L.: What we have learned about plutonium from human data. *Health Phys.*, 29(4):551–61, 1975.

WASH-1400 (NUREG-75/014). United States Nuclear Regulatory Commission: *Reactor Safety Study, An Assessment of Accident Risks in U.S. Commercial Nuclear Power Plants*. United States Nuclear Regulatory Commission, Oct. 1975.

Whitson, G. L. (ed.): *Concepts in Radiation Cell Biology*. Academic Press, Inc., New York, 1972.

Yuhas, J. M.; Tennant, R. W.; and Regan, J. D.: *Biology of Radiation Carcinogenesis*. Raven Press, New York, 1976.

Chapter 20

PLASTICS

John Autian

INTRODUCTION

Polymer science and technology are making it possible to create new man-made materials for numerous human applications. These materials fall into the general categories of plastics, elastomers, and textiles that may compose parts of transportation vehicles, building structures, furniture, clothing, or packaging systems. The same or similar types of materials may be parts of tissue and organs implanted into man to save or prolong life.

In the past, much of the attention given these newer materials was directed at the chemical, physical, and mechanical properties since knowledge in these specific areas is required to develop suitable products for a specific application. More recently, however, attention has been focused on the potential toxic liability of these new man-made materials, particularly when one may be sued for a medical and paramedical application. Since these polymeric materials are prepared from monomers and other chemicals, which of themselves may be toxic, the toxic liability of these various agents in the industrial environment is now receiving considerable attention. The expanding use of all types of man-made materials has also underlined the importance of the toxic potential of thermodegradation and combustion products when these materials are burned or heated deliberately or accidentally.

GENERAL CONSIDERATIONS

Definition of Terms

Plastics are defined in the *Modern Plastics Encyclopedia* (1962) as a "large and varied group of materials which consists of or contain as an essential ingredient, a substance of high molecular weight which while solid in the finished state, at some state in its manufacture is soft enough to be formed into various shapes, usually through the application, either singly or together, of heat and pressure." In the broadest sense, plastics include elastomers (rubbers) and synthetic

textiles. The important feature of plastics is that there is a very long polymer in the material and that this polymer is produced synthetically or semisynthetically.

The smallest unit leading to a polymer is the *mer*. When two mers combine covalently, a dimer is formed, and when many units combine in such a fashion, the polymer chain is formed. For plastic materials the mers may reach into the thousands and even into the hundreds of thousands, depending on the final material that is produced. When two chemically different mers are used to create the final polymer, the term "copolymer" may be used.

Often the term "resin" is used in plastic technology. Here the term signifies the form of the plastic prior to its manufacture into a specific commercial product. The resin may be in the form of a powder, sphere, or pellet. Other ingredients may also be added to the resin to form a specific formulation that when processed will lead to an item having a set of desired physical, chemical, and mechanical properties.

Two other terms are widely used in the plastic field. These are "thermoplastics" and "thermosets." A thermoplastic material is one that can be repeatedly melted and recast into the same form or into a different form, while thermoset materials, once formed, cannot be melted without degradation of the polymer chain. Often it is possible to transform a thermoplastic into a thermoset material by introducing cross-links into the material. Essentially, this means that one polymer chain is tied by a chemical bond to another adjacent chain, either by the use of a chemical agent (cross-linking agent) or by radiation.

For all practical purposes, commercial plastics will have, in addition to the polymer, one or more supplementary agents, collectively referred to as *additives*. These additives may include chemicals to act as plasticizing agents, various types of stabilizing agents, filling agents, colorants, antistatic agents, flame retardants, and other ingredients added to import certain specific

Table 20–1.   NAME AND STRUCTURE OF REPRESENTATIVE PLASTICS

PLASTIC	UNIT CHEMICAL STRUCTURE
1. Polyethylene	$-CH_2-CH_2-$
2. Polypropylene	$-CHCH_3-CH_2-$
3. Polyvinyl chloride	$-CHCl-CH_2-$
4. Polystyrene	$-CHC_6H_5-CH_2-$
5. Nylon-6,6	$-CO-(CH_2)_4-CO-NH-(CH_2)_6-NH-$
6. Delrin	$-O-CH_2-$
7. Polyethylene terephthalate	$-O-CO-C_6H_5-CO-O-CH_2-CH_2-$
8. ABS (acrylonitrilebutadiene styrene)	$-CH_2-CHCN-(CH_2)_4-CHC_6H_5-CH_2-$
9. Polycarbonate	$-O-C_6H_4-C(CH_3)_2-C_6H_4-CO-$
10. Methylpentene polymer (TBX)	$-CCH_2CH(CH_3)_2-C-$
11. Polymonochlorotrifluoroethylene	$-CClF-CF_2-$
12. Polytetrafluoroethylene	$-CF_2-CF_2-$
13. Polymethyl methacrylate	$-CH_2-CCH_3COOCH_3-$
14. Polyurethane	$-CO-NH-R-NH-CO-O-R'-O-$ R = alkyl or aryl group R' = alkyl or aryl group
15. Silicone rubber (dimethyl silicone polymer)	$-Si(CH_3)_2-O-$

properties to the final item. Table 20–1 lists the names and unit structures of a group of plastics.

INDUSTRIAL AND LABORATORY HAZARDS FROM THE MANUFACTURING OF PLASTICS

At one time, it was assumed that harmful effects due to the manufacturing process in the plastic industry have been kept to a minimum because of the generally well-established industrial hygiene and industrial toxicology programs. It is now recognized that injuries to workers due to chemicals are much more prevalent than originally suspected. Particularly in recent years, it has been found that certain chemicals used in the plastic industry have led to incidence of cancer, even though the chemical has been in use for a great number of years. The establishment of the Occupational Safety and Health Administration in 1970 has initiated a very determined effort by both industry and government to search out the most dangerous chemicals in the working environment, in particular those suspected to relate to cancer.

In the early seventies, reports were starting to appear in this country and abroad that several workers in the polyvinyl chloride industry had developed terminal cancer (Selikoff *et al.*, 1975). It was soon found that the causative agent was the monomer vinyl chloride, a chemical that has been used extensively as a major plastic for the past 25 years. More recently, another monomer, acrylonitrile, has also been implicated as a carcinogenic agent. Because of the desire to prevent combustion of synthetic textiles when exposed to heat or flame, chemical agents (flame retardants) have been added. Several of these flame retardants, in particular *tris*-(2,3-dibromopropyl)

phosphate, now appears to be carcinogenic, even though actual human incidence of cancer has not been reported (Blum *et al.*, 1977). Other examples of potentially dangerous chemicals used in the plastic industry that might have mutagenic and carcinogenic properties also exist in the industrial environment but for which no definite information is available establishing the agent or agents as hazardous to the worker. Unfortunately, clinical manifestation of cancer does not occur until the worker is exposed to the agent for a long number of years, and thus it seems appropriate that *in vitro* tests should be found for screening mutagenic or carcinogenic agents. If the chemical is carcinogenic, steps should be taken to reduce the exposure of the worker to that particular agent. The application of the Ames test (Ames *et al.*, 1973) is one *in vitro* method with great promise as a screening test for carcinogenic agents.

In the previous paragraphs, examples of highly dangerous chemicals were cited as causing or possibly causing cancer in workers in the plastic industry. Attention must also be given to less dramatic toxic effects from monomers, catalysts, and various types of additives used in the manufacture of a plastic. These other agents can present from very minor to severe problems if they have contact with the worker's skin or if they are inhaled or ingested. The nearly unlimited number of chemical entities used by the plastic industry precludes a listing of even a small portion of the important chemicals whose toxicity has been studied. Toxicity of a number of these industrial chemicals is discussed in other chapters.

The number of gases and vapors that might be generated or that might be released from an industrial process necessitates the approximation of that level (parts per million) which might be considered harmful when inhaled by industrial workers. These levels, referred to as threshold limit values (TLV), have been compiled for over 400 substances by the American Conference of Government Industrial Hygienists in Cincinnati, Ohio, and can serve as a guide to indicate that a hazard exists to the worker if the concentration of the agent exceeds the TLV. From time to time, threshold values are changed to higher or lower values, depending on new toxicologic information. For example, toluene diisocyanate (TDI), an agent used to manufacture a number of polyurethanes, was assigned a value of 0.1 ppm in 1956, but with additional toxicologic data this figure was changed to 0.02 ppm in 1962. Prior to the discovery that vinyl chloride was a carcinogenic agent, the TLV was 500 ppm and now OSHA has reduced the level to 1.0 ppm.

A great number of chemical agents used in the manufacturing of plastics and rubbers can act as sensitizing agents and do produce a significant number of allergic responses when industrial workers are exposed to these agents. Amine compounds in particular seem to cause numerous allergic responses, and therefore, it is necessary to ensure that proper protection is afforded to workers exposed to these high-potential sensitizing agents. Compounds such as diethylenetriamine and triethylenetetramine are used as curing agents for epoxy polymers and may present considerable sensitizing problems. In the rubber industry, a number of chemical agents used in preparing the rubber can sensitize exposed workers (Wilson *et al.*, 1959). These include accelerators such as mercaptobenzothiazole, tetramethylthiuram monosulfide, diphenylguanidine and antioxidant, monobenzylether of hydroquinone, and phenyl-betanaphthylamine.

In the manufacture of polyurethanes, aromatic isocyanates are used as one of the starting materials. One of the most widely used isocyanates for polyurethanes is toluene-diisocyanate (TDI). Toxicity information on this specific compound has been reported by Zapp (1962). Animal experiments have shown that in general the organic isocyanates of the TDI type are relatively nontoxic following oral ingestion. The LD50 in rats is in the range of 5,800 mg/kg. Skin absorption is poor; concentrations as high as 16,000 mg/kg (rabbits) produce no lethal effects. Inhalation exposure of rats to TDI in a concentration of 600 ppm for six hours is lethal, but when the concentration is reduced to 60 ppm no deaths occur. The primary toxic manifestation of an acute exposure to the aromatic isocyanates is its highly irritant action on skin, mucous membranes, and the eyes.

The danger of the isocyanates in industrial exposure comes from acute and chronic exposures at even low concentrations. Asthmatic attacks have been reported to result from inhalation of the aromatic isocyanates, suggesting that these agents may act as sensitizing agents in certain persons. Subacute and chronic studies in animals suggest that the isocyanates are cumulative toxic agents leading to high morbidity rates in the population exposed. As has been indicated, the present threshold limit value of TDI is 0.02 ppm. Peters and Associates (1970) reported that studies on humans working in a factory manufacturing polyurethanes indicate that the present TLV for TDI is still too high.

Toxicity data in both animals and humans demonstrate the need for utmost care in the use of aromatic diisocyanates in industrial applications, with all provisions being made to keep the chemical from direct contact with the working force.

Long-term exposure to certain types of chemical agents could lead to cancer. Fortunately, modern industrial hygiene and educational programs have helped to reduce the potential cancer problem in those plastics and rubber plants having rigid standards for protecting their employees.

For the most part, the final plastic material will present few hazards to the industrial worker. If a toxic problem does occur, it generally can be associated with one of the additives or other factors not related to the plastic. With at least one plastic, however, a unique industrial hazard has now been established.

Even though polyvinyl chloride has been manufactured in large quantities for over 30 years, it was not until the 1960s that a new occupational disease linked to polyvinyl chloride production was established (Wilson *et al.*, 1967). This occupational entity is now referred to as acroosteolysis (AOL), and the symptoms and signs resemble those of Raynaud's disease but include osteolysis of one or more fingers. At present, the etiology of the disease is not known. Epidemiologic investigations (Dinman *et al.*, 1971) in a number of polyvinyl plants reveal that apparently only those workers who clean the vats where the polyvinyl chloride is made come down with the disease. The total number of workers who have developed AOL is presently very small and may be attributed to the small number of "vat cleaners" in this country.

A growing problem from the point of view of toxicity is the industrial and laboratory use of liquid or dispersed polymer systems, which are then cured *in situ* to form the desired material. This is true for epoxy and polyurethane resins used by workers outside of an industrial setting.

The usual high standards of hygiene practiced in the large manufacturing concerns are not generally observed in the smaller laboratories. Similar types of materials for adhesives and a variety of household applications are used by the layman with little understanding that, if the compounds are not used properly, toxic effects may occur.

MEDICAL AND PARAMEDICAL APPLICATIONS AND TOXIC CONSIDERATIONS

Within the past two decades there has been an increase in the use of a variety of plastic and elastomeric materials in the medical, pharmaceutical, dental, and biochemical engineering fields (Weslowski *et al.*, 1966; Sanders, 1971). In a large number of cases, the same materials that have had success in other fields have found success in the medical fields. In other instances, specific polymers that have had little use in other fields have been synthesized for medical applications.

Man-made materials for a medical or a paramedical application can be classified arbitrarily into five basic groups, as shown in Table 20–2. Items and devices falling into each of these categories will need various levels of toxicity evaluation. It is necessary to consider the effect of any medical material on biologic systems and, for those items in contact with tissues or body fluids, the effect of the biologic environment on the material. It is also necessary to recognize that for items falling in class 4 (collection devices) and class 5 (storage devices) there may be indirect effects to biologic systems, such as an agent being extracted from the plastic and then being administered to the patient (e.g., with transfusion liquids or with drug products). Reviews on toxicity of plastics have been pre-sented by Harris (1959), Wilson and McCormick (1960), Bischoff (1972), and Autian (1964, 1975).

Effects of Materials on Tissue

Short-Term Contact. When a plastic device is placed in contact with tissue, it may release a constituent, causing a local irritation response. For the most part, the response is localized and may vary from a mildly inflammatory response to a highly corrosive reaction. History of use, as well as animal tests, has shown that the final polymerized material has little tendency to cause a tissue response other than a slight foreign-body reaction when implanted into tissue. In the past, tissue responses have been ascribed to the plastic when in reality the response was due to the monomer, catalyst, or unreactive chemicals present in the materials. A great number of plastic and elastomeric materials manufactured today as medical or paramedical devices will produce little or no local irritant response when placed into connective or muscle tissues for short periods of time. For many of these materials, such as polyethylene, polypropylene, Teflon, dacron, polycarbonate, and certain types of silicone rubbers, the propensity for diffusion of an ingredient from the materials is so small that a biologic response cannot be detected. Also many of the materials mentioned have extremely low concentrations of various types of additives, some perhaps having only a stabilizing agent in concentrations of less than 1 part per thousand.

Tissue responses have been noted for certain plastics such as nylon, epoxypolymers, and polyurethanes. With these classes of materials the offending agent can be traced to the monomer, catalyst, or curing agent that has not reacted completely or has not been removed in the manufacturing process.

Table 20–2. CLASSES OF PLASTIC DEVICES ACCORDING TO USE*

CLASS	DEVICE OR ITEM	EXAMPLES
1	Permanent implants	Heart valves, various vascular grafts, orthopedic implants, other artificial organs, etc.
2	Implants having contact with mucosal tissue	Artificial eyes, contact lens, dentures, intrauterine devices, certain types of catheters
3	Corrective, protective, and supportive devices	Splinters, braces, films, protective clothes, etc.
4	Collection and administration devices	Blood transfusion sets, various types of catheters, dialyzing units, hypodermic devices and similar injection devices, etc.
5	Storage devices	Containers, bags for blood, blood products, drug products, nutritional products, diagnostic agents, etc.

* From Autian, J.: Development of standards for plastics to be used in pharmacy and medicine. *J. Dent. Res.*, **45**:1668, 1966. Copyright by the American Dental Association. Reprinted by permission.

Incidence of tissue response increases, however, when the plastic or elastomeric materials require greater concentrations of various types of additives, especially when the additives are dispersed in the polymer system. For plasticized materials such as flexible polyvinyl chloride items the plasticizer enhances the diffusion of a toxic agent from the material to the tissue, bringing about a tissue response. It should be stressed, however, that even though diffusion of an additive may occur, the local irritant response will depend on the intrinsic irritating qualities of the chemical.

Lawrence and associates (1963) demonstrated that a number of tubings (primarily of the polyvinyl chloride type used for administration devices) released a constituent or constituents that were toxic to tissue when implanted into rabbit muscle tissue for one week. Of approximately 50 different tubings examined, one-half were found to elicit a toxic response. Later investigations of these "toxic" tubings revealed that the offending agent was one of the organotin-stabilizing agents. In another study by Autian and coworkers (1965), three different commercially available urinary bags were studied. Two were constructed of flexible polyvinyl chloride while the third was manufactured from polyethylene. Each of the bags was implanted into the rabbit muscle for varying periods of time extending to six weeks. One of the polyvinyl chloride bags was found to be toxic while the remaining two types of bags were not toxic.

Table 20–3. RABBIT MUSCLE TISSUE RESPONSE TO IMPLANTED PVC FORMULATIONS CONTAINING ORGANOTIN COMPOUNDS*

ORGANOTIN IN POLYVINYL CHLORIDE†	TISSUE RESPONSE‡	
	One Week	*One Month*
DBT diisooctyl maleate§	P	N
DBT dilauryl mercaptide	P	N
DBT diisooctyl thioglycolate	N	N
Dioctyltin beta mercapto-propionate	P	N
PVC + 40% plasticizer + 1.5% organotin	P	P
Polyethylene (control)	N	N

* From Guess, W. L.; O'Leary, R. K.; Calley, D.; and Autian, J.: Parenteral toxicity of a series of commercially available dioctyl and dibutyl tin stabilizers used in PVC formulations. *Proceedings, 22nd Annual Technical Conference, Society of Plastic Engineers, Inc.*, Vol. XII, 1966.
† Each of the vinyl plastics contains 100 parts of polyvinyl chloride + 5 parts of the specific organotin compound.
‡ P = tissue response; N = no tissue response.
§ DBT = dibutyltin.

The importance of the intrinsic toxicity of the additive and the further importance of a plasticizer to sustain a tissue response can be seen by examining Table 20–3. In this series of experiments, polyvinyl chloride was prepared with several different types of dibutyltin (DBT) derivatives in the absence of a plasticizer (Guess *et al.*, 1966). One formulation, however, contained 40 percent plasticizer and an organotin compound. As will be noted from the table, each of the vinyl formulations except the one containing DBT diisoctyl thioglycolate elicited a muscle response at the end of the week. At the end of the month none of the originally toxic vinyls showed continued toxicity except the vinyl containing the plasticizer. Here it may be assumed that the plasticizer was helping to prolong the release of the tin compound or in some manner preventing the washing away of the tin in the immediate area of the implant.

As has been emphasized several times, the toxic effects of a material are related to the intrinsic toxicity of the ingredient and its ability to migrate from the material to the tissue in contact with it. It is important to know the toxic potential of each of the ingredients in the final polymerized and formulated material when the material is to be used in an implantable device. Organotin compounds have a high index of irritation and thus when used in plastic formulations may cause tissue necrosis when released to the tissue (Guess *et al.*, 1966).

The plastic materials considered so far have been those that are produced in a polymerized and formulated form by the manufacturer. In certain surgical, medical, and dental applications, however, the final solid material is polymerized and formulated just prior to being used. These items include surgical cements, adhesives, and other items for a variety of medical purposes. In dental practice, similar types of items are also used, such as adhesives, a host of dental filling materials, dentures, implantable plastic teeth, cavity liners, and protective coatings placed on tooth surfaces. In these instances, several components are generally mixed together to form the final material, which, before becoming hard (setting), can be fashioned into the shape desired. In his daily practice, the dentist employs these types of systems primarily as cavity-filling materials. One of the most widely used dental filling materials is that based on esters of methyl acrylic acid. To prepare a final, hard material a liquid component containing the monomer and stabilizers is mixed with a powder containing a polymerized acrylic ester and several different types of additives.

Since these "compounded" plastic or elastomeric systems are placed in contact with tissue immediately after mixing, an unreactive monomer is still present and could migrate to the tissue causing a local irritant or toxic response. In some cases, even after several hours or days this material may still have sufficient residual monomer that can diffuse to tissue.

A few years ago, one manufacturer produced a silicone earplug kit that contained several components that when mixed formed a soft dough. This doughlike material would then be placed into the ears of a worker and would take on the contours of the ear. After about 10 or 15 minutes, the elastic earplugs would be cured and would retain their shape. These tailor-made earplugs could then be used when desired. Biologic tests conducted on this specific material demonstrated that even many days after mixing, the material still contained a toxic unreactive substance (Autian, 1974). A reformulation of the product helped to reduce the toxic liability of the product.

As might be suspected, self-curing plastics or elastomers that are more completely cured (polymerized) will present less toxic liability than those which are less cured. This may be noted by referring to Table 20–4 in which

Table 20–4.   INFLUENCE OF CURING CONDITIONS ON BIOLOGIC RESPONSE*— POLYMETHYL METHACRYLATE

SAMPLE NUMBER	DEGREE OF CURING	TISSUE CULTURE†	HEMO-LYSIS %
9	Lowest	4/3	84
13		2/2	61
11		1/1	1
12		0/0	0
10	Highest	0/0	1

* From Dillingham, E. O.; Webb, N.; Lawrence, W. H.; and Autian, J.: Biological evaluation of polymers. I. Poly(methyl methacrylate). *J. Biomed. Mater. Res.*, 9:569–96, 1975. Reprinted by permission of John Wiley & Sons, Inc.

† Tissue culture-agar overlay test. Numbers indicate degree of cytotoxicity. The higher the number, the greater is the response.

several polymethyl methacrylates having different degrees of curing were prepared. The lowest cured plastic showed the most toxicity in tissue culture and in hemolysis tests, while the highest cured demonstrated no tissue culture toxicity and only a 1 percent hemolysis (this would be considered an insignificant response under the experimental conditions used).

Serious toxic problems have also occurred in orthopedic surgery when methyl methacrylate cement has been used to anchor hip prosthesis. in these cases, an unpolymerized monomer is

released and enters the circulatory system bringing about immediate hypotension and cardiac arrest in elderly patients. In some instances, emboli have also been found due to bone marrow elements and particles of the polymethyl methacrylate. Proper attention to surgery, to mixing ratio of the components, and to proper insertion procedure will generally prevent the toxic responses (Charnley, 1970).

Most dental materials prepared by mixing components show various degrees of local toxicity when tested in rats and other animals (Massler, 1955; Mitchell, 1959; Guttuso, 1962; Rappaport *et al.*, 1964; Matsui *et al.*, 1967). The response may persist for relatively long periods of time or subside within a week or two. Since the materials may have residual monomers or other highly reactive agents that have not been removed, these can be released to tissue causing tissue response. Similar responses, however, may not always be noted in clinical practice when these materials are placed into tooth structure, since the filling material is not generally placed in direct contact with the pulp. It is also possible to prevent access to the pulp by placing a suitable coating on the cavity floor, thereby creating a barrier between the filling material and the tooth below it.

Within the past decade, new adhesive materials have been developed for a number of surgical applications. One of the most promising groups of adhesives for medical purposes is that based on cyanoacrylates. This monomer, when placed in contact with moisture, will polymerize rapidly, creating an extremely tenacious film. It was found that the methyl ester of cyanoacrylic acid was quite irritating to tissue, but that higher-molecular-weight monomers are quite satisfactory and demonstrate a very low order of tissue response. An excellent review on cyanoacrylic adhesives has been presented by Refojo and Associates (1968). In recent years, these cyanoacrylates have fallen out of favor in clinical use.

Perhaps the most commonly used implantable material is silicone rubber. If the material is properly prepared by the manufacturer it will cause no local toxic response (Mullison, 1965). Silicone rubbers may also be prepared *in situ*. In this case the liquid silicone polymer is cured with a suitable agent, producing the rubber.

Various types of epoxy polymers and polyurethane materials also have one or more medical applications. Since the composition of each of these broad groups of polymers can vary greatly, it is impossible to assess the local toxic effects without actually conducting biologic tests on each specific commercial item.

Long-Term Contact: Chronic Toxicity and Cancer. Depending on the specific material and the site of implant, it is possible that man-made materials implanted for long periods of time in animals and humans will degrade, releasing polymer fragments to the body. These compounds may then elicit one or more biologic responses.

Animal experiments, in particular in rodents, have demonstrated that all types of materials can lead to tumor production at the implant sites when these materials have had contact with tissue for longer than six to nine months. As early as 1941, Turner reported that when Bakelite disks were implanted into groups of rats, some animals developed tumors at the implant site after 18 months. Oppenheimer and associates (1948) noted that when kidneys of rats were wrapped with cellophane, tumors were produced after long-term contact. Since then, a number of investigators (Oppenheimer et al., 1952; Laskin et al., 1954; Bering et al., 1955; Russell et al., 1959; Mitchell et al., 1960; Hueper, 1961) have shown that practically all types of materials, when implanted in mice or rats, will result in a higher incidence of tumors at the implantation site than is found in control animals (see Chap. 6).

From the collective data, it is clear that a number of factors will influence tumorigenesis in experimental animals. These include the following: size of implant (Alexander and Horning, 1959), form of implant (Goldhaber, 1961; Oppenheimer et al., 1961), surface (Bates and Klein, 1966), hardness (Shubik et al., 1962), thickness (Roe et al., 1967), and length of implantation (Oppenheimer et al., 1958). Two of the most important factors leading to tumor formation appear to be the size of the implant and an interrupted surface. If these two requirements are met, actual chemical structure of the polymer is unimportant since tumors will result if the polymer is implanted for sufficiently long periods of time. The mechanism for tumor production for rodents is still not clear.

To distinguish "chemical carcinogenesis" from cancer resulting from implanted materials, Bischoff and Bryson (1964) have introduced the term "solid-state carcinogenesis." Perhaps it might be more appropriate to use the term "film or sheet carcinogenesis" since threads and powders are solid but do not cause tumors.

It should be pointed out, however, that the material may act also as a "chemical carcinogen" if the material degrades and releases fragments, which in turn act as the offending agents (Autian et al., 1975, 1976; Heuper, 1960, 1964). With newer polymeric materials entering the medical field, it is important that both "solid-state" and "chemical" carcinogenesis be considered. Up to the present time no well-substantiated evidence has been reported showing that man-made plastics have caused cancer in humans (Harris, 1961; Hoopes et al., 1967) or, in fact, in species of animals besides the rodent. The real answer for humans, however, will not be forthcoming until these materials have been implanted for periods of time exceeding 20 to 30 years.

Allergic Response. Acrylic denture materials (Fisher, 1956) have produced responses in certain patients. Often the cause of the response was the monomer or one of the additives present in the completed denture. Generally, it has been thought that heat-cured resins would not lead to a response, since no active monomer would be present. There have, however, been reports that even the heat-cured acrylic resin dentures can sensitize patients, presumably through the presence in the resin of residual amounts of methyl methacrylate (Crissey, 1965).

The potential sensitizing problems in the dental field will probably increase as newer dentures, restorative materials (such as those used for fillings), and various types of adhesives are introduced into the dental profession. Often these materials come as a two-component system that is then mixed prior to forming the desired polymerized material. Each of the systems can contain a number of ingredients such as monomers, plasticizers, catalysts, inhibitors, dyes, cross-linking agents, and particulate matter, as well as other ingredients included for specific properties or effects.

Self-curing resins are also being used more frequently in surgical procedures where "bone-like" materials or substitutes are needed for restoring a portion of hard tissue. The presence of sensitizing agents in these materials could lead to allergic responses in a small number of patients who are hypersensitive to the offending agent. Unfortunately, the actual ingredients in a formulation are often not revealed, and this potential problem may not be evident until after it has occurred. Fisher (1967) presents a comprehensive accounting of allergic responses to rubbers and plastics in his book.

Systemic Toxicity. When a plastic or elastomer releases a constituent from the material to the tissue, the compound can be absorbed and, if in sufficient concentration, may lead to systemic toxicity. Clinical and experimental evidence of "systemic" effects is extremely sparse. Methyl methacrylate cement used in orthopedic surgery has produced hypotension and cardiac arrest in patients due to the release of an unreacted monomer. Suspicion should be aroused when a plastic or similar type of material contains additives that in themselves could be considered as having a toxic effect if released in sufficient concentration into the circulatory system. Fortunately, up to this time, few reports have appeared that show that released constituents from an implantable plastic have led to serious systemic toxicity. As will be described in another section of this chapter, substances extracted from plastics used for administration devices and for extracorporeal devices may lead to systemic toxicity.

Plastic-Blood Problems

When circulating blood comes into contact with polymeric materials, thrombus formation generally results. Factors causing this blood clot have been attributed to surface charge, zeta potential, surface forces of unspecific nature, surface structure, absorption of certain types of proteins from circulating blood, and the rate of flow of blood (Lyman *et al.*, 1965). The blood-plastic clotting problem, however, has been in certain instances circumvented by treating the material with graphite, followed by benzalkonium chloride and finally by heparin. This method has been developed by Gott and associates (1963) and has had a fair degree of success for certain types of nonflexible plastic prosthetic devices placed into the circulatory system. It has been recognized that the clotting potential for artificial vessels will be reduced if they are knitted or woven into tubes. In these cases, sufficient porosity exists to permit each of the threads to be surrounded with fibrin, which in turn leads to the development of a natural lining facing the blood. In many surgical applications only nonporous materials can be used, and for this reason there is still a great need for the development of nonthrombogenic materials. One approach in this field has been to build into the polymer chain functional groups that will bind heparin. Newer experimental materials are being conceived in which the material has a "heparin"-type functional group.

The plastic-blood problem is perhaps still the most important problem to be solved for the artificial heart program. Experimental work in animals receiving artificial hearts has generally shown that blood clots have formed within the heart during the time period in which the experiments lasted.

Toxicity Due to Treatment of Materials

Up to this point, emphasis has been placed on the toxic potentials of the material due to the additives that are included in the formulation of a material. There are, however, other potential hazards due to treatment of the material for a specific reason. In medical and dental applications it is necessary to have the specific devices

that will have contact with tissue be sterile and be generally pyrogen free. The best way to accomplish this is by the use of an autoclave. Unfortunately, many plastic materials will not withstand autoclaving, and thus other methods of sterilization are used. The most successful alternate method for sterilizing plastics for medical application is through the use of ethylene oxide* or a combination of ethylene oxide with inert carrier gases.

Since ethylene oxide is a strong alkylating agent, it should not be placed in contact with tissue. Residual ethylene oxide, however, has been noted in various types of disposable items and in those devices that are ethylene oxide–sterilized in hospitals for a surgical application. Toxic responses have been observed due to ethylene oxide residues in plastics (Rendell-Baker, 1969). These responses have been seen in clinical practice as well as in experimental studies. Ethylene oxide–sterilized extracorporeal devices, in particular those having polyvinyl chloride tubings, have been found to lead to a higher incidence of hemolysis than nonethylene oxide–sterilized items (Hirose *et al.*, 1963; Clark *et al.*, 1966).

O'Leary and Guess (1968) studied the toxicity of selected medical items sterilized with ethylene oxide. One of the best parameters used by these authors was a hemolysis test. Results of this test indicated that a number of the devices were hemolytic. The authors concluded that the sorption of ethylene oxide by the plastic will be an important factor that in turn will influence the hemolysis. In these tests the presence of plasticizers increased the toxic liability of the device, indicating the sorption of greater quantities of the ethylene oxide, which in turn was released to the blood system.

Gunther (1969) has shown experimentally that if proper degassing procedures are initiated, the level of ethylene oxide in a material can be reduced to zero or to a level where it is not detectable by chemical means.

Since 1968, another problem has been brought to the attention of the medical profession because of ethylene oxide sterilization. Cunliffe and Wesley (1967) reported that polyvinyl chloride tubings contained the toxic agent ethylene chlorohydrin after ethylene oxide sterilization. Since then it has been observed that ethylene chlorohydrin will result from ethylene oxide treatment of materials containing chlorides. Lawrence and associates (1971a, 1971b) conducted acute and subacute toxicity studies on ethylene chlorohydrin in animals and noted that

---

* Recently this chemical has been implicated as a possible carcinogen.

Table 20–5.   LD50 VALUES OF ETHYLENE CHLOROHYDRIN*

SPECIES	SEX	ROUTE OF ADMINISTRATION	ACUTE TOXICITY	
			LD50 mg/kg	*95% Confidence Limits*
Mice	Male	Intraperitoneal	98.3	71.9–134.6
	Male	Oral	81.4	66.4–99.7
Rats	Male	Intraperitoneal	64.0	53.7–76.9
	Male	Oral	71.3	57.8–88.6
Rabbits	Either	Intraperitoneal	84.6	63.7–112.5
	Either	Dermal	67.8	41.2–111.7
Guinea pigs	Female	Intraperitoneal	85.8	—

* From Lawrence, W. H.; Turner, J. E.; and Autian, J.: Toxicity of ethylene chloro-hydrin. I. Acute toxicity studies. *J. Pharm. Sci.*, **60**:568, 1971. Reproduced with permission of the copyright owner.

no significant irritant response was evident when the agent was applied directly to rabbit skin. The compound is, however, readily absorbed from the skin and can lead to death at concentrations equal to oral or intraperitoneal administration.

Table 20–5 summarizes LD50 values for ethylene chlorohydrin in several species of animals. As may be seen from the table, species difference appears to have little effect upon the LD50. Carson and Oser (1969) have indicated that a "no-adverse-effect" level would fall below the range of 45 mg/kg when the compound is taken orally by dogs over a period of time. Subacute toxicity in rats by intraperitoneal administration by Lawrence and coworkers (1971a, 1971b) demonstrated that no adverse effects occurred at a dose of 6.4 mg/kg when the compound was injected daily for 30 days and a dose of 12.8 mg/kg when the compound was injected three times a week for 12 weeks. Systemic toxicity of ethylene chlorohydrin is related to its rate of metabolism to the highly toxic chloroacetaldehyde (Johnson, 1967). Lawrence and associates (1972a) noted that chloroacetaldehyde is inherently more toxic and irritating than ethylene chlorohydrin.

No real information is available on the effects that combinations of ethylene oxide, ethylene chlorohydrin, and other degradation products of ethylene oxide may have on animals.

There are other methods of sterilizing medical devices. Often these include the use of one of the quaternary ammonium salts, such as benzalkonium chloride. Sufficient amounts of one of these agents in certain tissue can be sufficiently irritating to necessitate the removal of the item. Fortunately, in most instances, these quaternary compounds are in concentrations below that which would produce an irritant response, and thus the anticipated problem should not occur. Table 20–6 shows the relationship between concentration of benzalkonium and irritant responses in rabbit skin and eyes.

Dilute solutions of formaldehyde are used as sterilizing agents for medical devices that cannot be autoclaved or that may not be properly

Table 20–6.   RESULTS OF IRRITATION TESTS ON BENZALKONIUM CHLORIDE*†

INTRADERMAL TEST (RABBITS)		EYE TEST (RABBITS)	
Concentration %	*Results*	*Concentration %*	*Results*
5.33	+ + +	0.333	+ + +
2.66	+ + +	0.166	+ +
1.33	+ +	0.0833	+ +
0.333	+	0.0416	+
0.166	+	0.0208	±
0.0833	±		
0.0416	±		

* From Autian, J.: Unpublished data from Materials Science Toxicology Laboratories, University of Tennessee Center for the Health Sciences, Memphis, TN.
† Irritation response scored from 0 (no response) to + + + (marked response).

sterilized by the use of ethylene oxide. For example, certain types of dialysis units can be sterilized by the use of a formaldehyde solution. If the unit is not properly and thoroughly rinsed prior to use, adsorbed formaldehyde can be released to the blood system. Tests on specific dialysis units that were previously sterilized with formaldehyde solution did not indicate that aqueous extracts of the unit could produce a dramatic cardiotoxic effect in isolated rabbit hearts (Autian *et al.*, 1978). In separate experiments, it was found that the response was directly related to the quantity of formaldehyde extracted from the unit.

Fassbinder *et al.* (1976) reported recently that

dialysis units sterilized with formaldehyde led to anti-N-like cold agglutinins in dialysis patients. As indicated in the report, little is known about the possible clinical implications of this antibody but the authors suggest that an alternative to formaldehyde sterilization be sought.

Other toxic problems may occur from plastic items used for medical devices. In these cases, the problem may be due to a chemical substance that was used as an adhesive. For example, it was found that certain lots of polyvinyl chloride infusion containers contained an adulterant that was not part of the plastic formulation (Autian, 1973). Analysis of the substance indicated that the chemical was the solvent cyclohexanone. This solvent is used to affix the tubings to the container. In this specific case, the solvent had migrated into the solution that was stored in the container. This same chemical was also found in tubings used for certain dialyzers, and, when it was extracted from the device and tested in isolated rabbit heart experiments, cardiotoxic responses were noted. Proper manufacturing procedures and good quality control can eliminate this problem.

Radiation of plastic devices has presented few toxic problems. If minor problems have occurred, they have been due to the improper treatment of items, which, in turn, has altered the property of the material. Depending on the specific polymer and the method of radiation treatment, polymer degradation can occur and these substances can be released to tissue or to fluids in contact with the item.

In the early sixties, Lindberg *et al.* (1961) reported a very serious toxic effect when plastic tubings were coated with silicone liquids (which presumably had been bonded to the polymer). As blood flowed through the tubings, the silicone was released and entered the patient, causing embolism and death. Accidents of this type can happen when innovations are made for the purpose of improving a material without recognizing the introduction of a more serious consequence.

Effects of Tissue on Materials

In general, emphasis has been placed on the effect of the specific polymeric material (or its components) on a biologic system. Toxicology of materials, however, must also include consideration of what effect the biologic environment might have on altering the properties of the material, or actually degrading the polymer chain, thereby leading to an immediate or a gradual failure of the prosthetic device. Perhaps not too surprising is the fact that *in vitro* nonbiologic models have often predicted the function and stability of a specific polymer for countless

years, but when the same material has been placed into a biologic environment the failure has often been quite rapid and dramatic. The biologic environment is an extremely complex system with a variety of components, one or more of which may interact with the polymer chain. Unfortunately, this field (degradation of polymers in biologic environments) has not been researched in sufficient depth to permit a clear "cause-effect" relationship, and one must be content to report incidences where failures have occurred. This often is misleading, however, since the same generically named plastic, depending on the stabilizers or other additives, may react quite differently. In other words, one polyethylene may degrade much faster than another because of the presence of a specific additive.

An example of the effects of biologic systems on the properties of a select group of polymers is seen in Table 20–7. It will be noted that each

Table 20–7. CHANGES IN PROPERTIES OF PLASTIC FILMS AFTER IMPLANTATION*

MATERIAL	TENSILE STRENGTH, PSI	ELONGATION %
Polyethylene		
Control	2,700	780
17 months	1,930	420
Teflon		
Control	2,950	320
17 months	3,720	250
Mylar		
Control	18,300	100
17 months	17,400	100
Nylon		
Control	9,300	550
17 months	5,200	140
Silastic		
Control	950	800
17 months	930	890

* From Leininger, R. I.; Mirkovitch, V.; Peters, A.; and Hawks, W. A.: Change in properties of plastics during implantation. *Trans. Am. Soc. Artif. Intern. Org.*, **10**:320, 1964.

of the materials except the silastic material has been altered to some extent after 17 months of implantation in dogs. The importance of the site of implantation must also be recognized. If the material is in a relatively passive site, such as in connective or muscle tissue, the degradation potential most likely would be less than if the material is continually being bathed by body fluids such as blood, stomach contents, or intestinal contents.

Another factor that will influence the rate of alteration and degradation of the material is the actual function of the item. Load-bearing functions or actual motions of the item can introduce other stresses on the material that may help accelerate the failure of the prosthetic device. One of the best examples of prosthetic failures was revealed several years ago; for a very small percent of patients having artificial aortic valves, the ball of the valve had been distorted and even chipped, leading to failure of the valve (Starr *et al.*, 1965). Fortunately, these cases are extremely rare, but they do occur. In another case, it has been noted that a type of heart valve (left type) constructed of Teflon has partially disintegrated, thus negating the value of the valve (Aquino, 1963).

A Japanese worker (Sakurabayashi, 1969) has studied over 3,000 patients utilizing intrauterine devices made from different materials and reported that natural rubber, nylon, and polyethylene underwent varying degrees of degradation leading to a number of clinical effects. In animal experiments, Hueper (1964) has noted that silicone rubber and a specific type of polyurethane degraded after long periods of subdermal and intra-abdominal implantation in rats. Autian *et al.* (1975) have also noted this.

Still another problem with implantable polymeric materials is the possibility that one or more body constituents may be attracted to the material and actually enter the matrix of the item, causing various types of failure. In the late 1950s and early 1960s a very versatile material, Ivalon (a polyvinyl alcohol), when implanted into animals, was noted to become hard and brittle (Adler and Darby, 1960). Clinical experience with Ivalon used for breast plasty has not been good (Hamit, 1957). The implant had to be removed from the patient because of dramatic alterations in the property of the implant. Nylon has also shown failure due to sorption of a constituent followed by degradation of the polymer chains (Creech, 1957).

In a very general way it may be said that as the polarity of the polymer increases, the potential for degradation also increases. It should be remembered, however, that the extremely nonpolar Teflon has been shown to be degraded in a biologic system (Aquino and Skinsnes, 1963), and thus predictions may be extremely hazardous.

The degradation products of the polymer must also be considered. If these substances are sufficiently small and are soluble in the body fluids, they may act as foreign chemical agents and produce one or more biologic responses. Actual documentation of this latter problem has been rare, but could occur with greater use and longer periods of implantation of polymeric materials.

Release of Constituents from Plastics to Solutions and Biologic Products

When plastic and elastomeric administration and extracorporeal devices are used, it is possible for a substance from the synthetic material to be released to blood, infusion solutions, or other products that come in contact with the device. If patients receive acute or chronic doses of these products, even small amounts of the leached constituent could lead to untoward biologic responses. Over long periods of repeated administration, subtle toxic manifestations may develop that may be difficult to detect.

Tubings. Many advantages have been gained by the use of clear, flexible tubings over glass, metal, and rubber. The most successful tubing in medical practice, as well as in a number of laboratory situations, is polyvinyl chloride (PVC), which has been plasticized to give it the desired flexibility. These tubings are used for many applications, such as parts of administration devices, catheters, parts of dialysis devices, and other items requiring clear, flexible tubings.

In the late 1950s, Meyler and coworkers (1960) replaced glass tubings with polyvinyl chloride tubing in their isolated rat heart apparatus. Subsequent experiments in which perfusion solution was passed through the plastic tubing into the isolated heart produced unusual results, such as deterioration of cardiac performance. It soon became clear that the PVC tubing might be responsible for the cardiac response.

A number of separate experiments were conducted using the isolated heart apparatus and the various PVC tubings. In these experiments the cardiotoxic response was recorded if it took place within 15 minutes. Tubing A was highly toxic while tubings B and C showed no cardiotoxic effect within the same time period. The other two tubings (D and E) were cardiotoxic, but to a much lesser extent than A. Chemical analyses of tubing A and tubing B revealed the following:

Tubing A:

Plasticizer (di-2-ethylhexyl phthalate)	43.7 percent
Stabilizer Organotin (extract molecule not identified)	1.0 percent (approximately)
Polyvinyl chloride	Remaining weight of tubing

Tubing B:

Plasticizer (di-2-ethylhexyl phthalate)	34.5 percent of total weight of tubing
Stabilizer (barium-cadmium mixture)	Amount not given
Polyvinyl chloride	Remaining weight of tubing

The authors concluded from these experiments that the cardiotoxic agent was due to the release of the organotin compound to the perfusion solution. As has been stressed in several other sections of this chapter, the name of the plastic can be the same, but two different formulae can give quite different biologic responses, as shown in the table.

In the mid-1960s, Trimble and associates (1966) conducted long-term studies to establish a hormonal basis for the phenomenon of hibernation. Extracts of blood and brown fat of groundhogs were investigated, and it was noted that a constituent in these extracts could prolong the cold tolerance of test animals. Further studies were then conducted to help identify the biologic constituent producing the physiologic effects in the animals. It was only after considerable time had passed that it was finally recognized that the new "biologic agent" was in fact a constituent from the plastic tubings that were being used in the extraction procedure. In this case, the tubings were one of the polyvinyl chlorides and the extracted agent was butyl phthalyl butyl glycolate (a plasticizer).

Duke and Vane (1968) reported that the use of certain types of PVC tubings has an adverse effect on isolated cat lungs due to unidentified contamination from the tubing. This should be a warning to those conducting biologic experiments that they should be alert to possible chemical contamination from specific tubings used in their experiments.

The recent awareness that plastics can release chemical contaminants to various solutions and biologic media has prompted investigators to test tubings and other items in very sensitive biologic systems such as tissue culture. DeHaan (1971) reported that serum-containing solutions passed through polyvinyl chloride tubings used for blood transfusions were extremely toxic to heart cells isolated in tissue culture. Jaeger and Rubin (1970) noted that perfusion solution containing plasma extracted a plasticizer (later identified as butyl glycolybutyl phthalate) from PVC tubing used in isolated rat liver.

Polyvinyl chloride used for catheters can present other problems. With the migration of the plasticizer from the catheter to tissue, the physical property of the plastic changes and the unit becomes more stiff producing physical trauma. The use of PVC catheters in infants has led to problems both from the changes in the properties of the plastic and from the release of the plasticizer, in particular the di-2(ethylhexyl) phthalate. Stetson and Autian (1976) have reviewed the necrotizing enterocolitis resulting from the use of PVC catheters in infants.

As has already been reported in a previous section of this chapter, chemicals that are used as sterilizing agents, if adsorbed to the tubing, can release to fluids in contact with the tubing. Solvents used to seal or to act as an adhesive can also migrate to solutions that pass through the tubings. Since the concentrations of these agents released to solutions are extremely small, the clinical consequences to humans are still unknown even though, as will be reviewed in a later section of the chapter, certain phthalate esters in polyvinyl chloride may have long-term, subtle, toxic effects.

In recent years new flexible, clear tubings resembling polyvinyl chloride without plasticizers have been placed on the market. These types of tubings are generally fashioned from one of the polyurethanes. Depending on the specific polyurethane, some other leachable constituents may be present but in extremely low concentrations. Proper biologic testing of these tubings should, however, ensure the safety of the device when used as intended. Other experimental polymers are also now being considered. These can be prepared without any additives and, if found to be suitable for tubings, could be a great assist to the medical profession.

Blood Bag Assemblies. Today there is widespread use of various types of plastic containers for large volumes of blood and blood products. Recently the same type of plastic containers has been used commercially for the storage and administration of infusion solutions. The term "bags" is often employed instead of containers. There are a number of advantages to using plastic bags for blood and blood products. The plastic bag does not break, is light in comparison to glass, and can be designed in such a way that the container can act as a collecting, storage, and administration device in the same unit. Blood bag assemblies date back to the early 1950s when Walter (1951) introduced them in medical practice. The use of these items has increased until today most of the blood containers are of the plastic type. In this country, the chief material used for the blood bag assemblies is one of the polyvinyl chlorides. In Europe both polyethylene and polypropylene blood containers have been used, although polyvinyl chloride types are also available.

Normal blood bags contain anticoagulant solutions. These bags or containers are generally in a protective packaging system that is opened when the unit is to be filled with blood. A 500-ml-volume bag generally contains 67 ml of anticoagulant solution. Similar bags are used for various blood components such as plasma and platelets. In the United States, practically all the "blood bags and blood component bags" are prepared from a plasticized polyvinyl chloride. The principal plasticizers in these bags are the phthalate esters, primarily the di-(2-ethylhexyl) phthalate (DEHP). During the last five years, several pharmaceutical firms have introduced similar types of PVC containers for a variety of infusion solutions.

Guess and coworkers (1967) reported on a study of blood bag assemblies currently used at the time. The anticoagulant in the bag was ACD solution (anticoagulant citrate dextrose solution, USP). One part of the study included monitoring five PVC blood bags for chemical contaminants when these blood bags were stored at 5° C room temperature and at 50° C over a one-year period. In this particular experiment, representative blood bags (in their original overwrap or container) were pulled from storage and the ACD solutions extracted with carbon tetrachloride to remove the organic compounds released from the PVC. The extracts were then examined spectrophotometrically, by thin-layer chromatography, and tested against several cell lines in tissue culture. In the same experiment, a control ACD solution in glass and a polyethylene container with ACD solution were also included. All of the ACD solutions contained some organic substance. Since all, except one, of the ACD solutions stored in the PVC blood bags were found to have compounds showing cytotoxic effects, they were further examined and the ingredients identified as consisting of di-(2-ethylhexyl) phthalate, 2-ethyl hexanol, phthalic anhydride, phthalic acid, and several unidentified esters. The total concentration of these compounds was small (approximately 15 mg/100 ml).* The authors felt that the presence of even small quantities of contaminants necessitated further work to ensure that there would be no adverse effect on patients, especially if numerous and frequent volumes of blood were to be administered. Chemical contaminants in both the glass and in the polyethylene were found not to be cytotoxic and were assumed to be due in part to the presence of organic compounds as contaminants in the original ingredients used to prepare the solutions. This report was published in 1967 but received little attention.

It was not until the report by Jaeger and Rubin (1970), which documented that several patients having received large volumes of blood stored in PVC blood bags showed the presence of plasticizer (DEHP) in specific organs, that the PVC problem suggested by Guess *et al.* (1967) received serious attention.

Since the report by Jaeger and Rubin, questions have been raised as to the potential problems DEHP or other plasticizers might cause for humans. In another section of this chapter, more detailed information will be presented on the toxicity of phthalate esters, but since it is relevant to the PVC container and tubing problems, some comments will be given here.

It is now well established that DEHP will easily migrate to blood or bloodlike solutions from PVC devices. The extent of migration will depend on the polarity of the solution, the time of contact, and the temperature. Since blood and the various blood fractions are more lipophilic than distilled water, it would be expected that the blood and its products would have a higher content of DEHP than distilled water when these products are placed in PVC containers under identical storage conditions. This, in fact, has been found to be the case. Under various storage conditions in PVC containers, blood and blood products may show concentrations of DEHP ranging from 5 to 20 mg/100 ml. Even though the concentration of DEHP migrating to distilled water is in parts per million, there is the possibility that more can enter the water in colloidal form, in particular when the container is agitated rapidly.

Perhaps the most important evidence suggesting that DEHP might present potential harm to patients has come from the primate research of Jacobson *et al.* (1977) indicating that DEHP does have an effect on the liver and that DEHP can be stored in tissue (liver) many months after the last infusion. Since the specific study by Jacobson was designed to mimic a possible patient experience, it has important implications. A study by Lake *et al.* (1975) appears to support the evidence of Jacobson that liver damage may occur when DEHP enters the body. In the studies by Lake *et al.*, rats were dosed orally with DEHP in corn oil at a concentration of 2,000 mg/kg/day for periods of 4, 7, 14, and 21 days. Biochemical studies were done on liver tissue. Histologic and ultrastructural studies were also performed on the same tissues. Results of the studies indicated that liver size increased to 215 percent; various enzyme levels altered markedly; and ultrastructural changes in the hepatocytes occurred. Daniel and Bratt (1974), however, at doses of 5,000 mg/kg/day (in rats) did not see much evidence of liver alteration but did note an increase in liver size. These investigators alluded to the work of Golberg (1966) who has stated that liver enlargement for many compounds may actually not be a true toxic event but rather a way the body normally handles an exogenous agent. From the work of Jacobson and Lake, however, this may not be the case with DEHP.

It is now well recognized that DEHP is rapidly metabolized and eliminated from the body. In man, it has been estimated that the half-life of DEHP administered i.v. in a solubilized state is approximately 28 minutes. Albero *et al.* (1973) have postulated that DEHP is first hydrolyzed to mono(2-ethylhexyl) phthalate (MEHP), which

---

* Not reported in original paper but obtained from authors.

medical applications have been related to the presence of other chemical agents. Since the number of these chemical agents is so great and so diversified, their toxicity cannot be discussed except in the most sketchy manner. Reference books such as those by Patty (1963) and Lefaux (1968) contain very useful toxicity information on portions of these agents but the information is still inconclusive, and thus a further literature search may be necessary before the desired toxicity data are obtained. Many of these chemical agents are listed under trade names, and the toxicity is obtainable only from the manufacturer or no toxicity information is available at all. Long-term data are still in short supply for many of the chemical agents that are used to manufacture plastics or are included in the plastic for various reasons.

Monomers

Ethylene and Vinyl Chloride. Ethylene is the starting monomer to produce polyethylene. As with all low-molecular-weight hydrocarbon gases, few toxicologic properties exist. In sufficient concentrations, ethylene depletes the oxygen level of the air and through this mechanism acts as an asphyxiant. No long-term toxicologic problems have been attributed directly to the gas. The gas does not have locally toxic effects.

Vinyl chloride is the monomer for the production of polyvinyl chloride. The revelation that this relatively nontoxic agent is a potent carcinogenic agent in man and animals over long exposure periods initiated steps by both government and the plastic industry to reduce drastically the threshold limit value of vinyl chloride in the working environment. Even though this agent has been used in the manufacture of polyvinyl chloride since World War II, it was not until the early seventies that angiosarcomas in workers in PVC plants were related to their exposure to vinyl chloride. Vinyl chloride is considered to have a low order of acute toxicity. Central nervous system depression will occur when animals and man are exposed to moderately high levels of the gas. Guinea pigs exposed to vinyl chloride in air survived in levels of 5 to 7 percent for one hour and in 2½ percent for eight hours. Humans exposed to vinyl chloride in air at a concentration of 6,000 ppm for one-half hour experienced dizziness and drowsiness. This latter property made vinyl chloride at one time a candidate for an anesthetic agent, but other toxicity problems developed at the concentrations necessary for anesthesia. The most serious chronic toxic effect of vinyl chloride, as has already been mentioned, is that it is a potent carcinogenic agent. It is also now considered to be a liver toxicant. A good review on the toxicologic and cancer problems

of vinyl chloride is available for those interested in this specific compound (Selikoff et al., 1975).

Esters of Acrylic Acid. Esters of acrylic and methyl acrylic acids are used to prepare the large class of plastics referred to as the "acrylics." These plastics have a large number of uses outside of medicine in which glass-clear rigid materials are needed. In dentistry and in surgery the monomer is polymerized and prepared into a specific size and shape prior to its use. Charnley (1970) has reviewed the uses of acrylic cement in orthopedic surgery. Many restorative materials in dentistry are formed from one of the acrylic monomers, the most used being the methyl ester of methyl acrylic acid.

The lower-molecular-weight esters of acrylic acids are irritants to skin, eyes, and mucous membranes. Inhalation of these agents can lead to serious toxic events, and thus care must be exercised when these agents are used in an industrial or laboratory setting.

The LD50 in mice for a number of these compounds is shown in Table 20–8. As will be noted

Table 20–8.   LD50 OF A GROUP OF ACRYLIC MONOMERS IN MICE*

NAME OF COMPOUND	ACUTE INTRA-PERITONEAL TOXICITY IN MICE LD50 (ml/kg)
Glacial acrylic acid	0.016
Methyl acrylate	0.265
Ethyl acrylate	0.648
Butyl acrylate	0.926
Isobutyl acrylate	0.854
2-Ethylhexyl acrylate	1.506
Glacial methacrylic acid	0.048
Methyl methacrylate	1.198
Ethyl methacrylate	1.369
Butyl methacrylate	1.663
Isobutyl methacrylate	1.340
Isodecyl methacrylate	3.688
Lauryl methacrylate	24.897
T-Butylaminoethyl methacrylate	0.190
Dimethylaminoethyl methacrylate	0.104
Hydroxyethyl methacrylate	0.497
1,3-Butylene dimethacrylate	3.598
Trimethlyolpropane trimethacrylate	2.727

* From Lawrence, W. H.; Bass, G. E.; Purcell, W. P.; and Autian, J.: Utilization of mathematical models in the study of structure-toxicity relationships of dental compounds. I. Esters of acrylic and methacrylic acids. Presented at the AAAS meeting, Chicago, December 1970.

from the table, all of the esters are less toxic than the parent compound, glacial acrylic acid.

Borzelleca and coworkers (1964) studied the chronic oral toxicity of ethyl acrylate and methyl methacrylate in both rats and dogs. The studies covered a two-year period. Both monomers were added to drinking water of rats in concentrations of 0 to 2,000 ppm (equivalent to about 10, 100, and 3,000 ppm in the food). No mortalities were observed in these animals. In general, except at the highest dose, no adverse effects were noted for either compound in the rats. Dogs received the two compounds in oil that was incorporated into feed. Concentrations in the feed for the dogs ranged from 0 to 1,000 ppm for the ethyl acrylate and up to 1,500 ppm for the methyl methacrylate. No gross toxicity was noted from either compound.

Singh and associates (1972b) studied the embryofetal toxicity and teratogenic effects of a group of methacrylic esters in rats. The esters studied included methyl methacrylate, ethyl methacrylate, butyl methacrylate, isobutyl methacrylate, and isodecyl methacrylate. The esters were administered at 1/10, 1/5, and 1/3 the LD50 dose on the fifth, tenth, and fifteenth days of gestation. At one or more of the dose levels, each ester produced some or all of the following effects: resorptions, gross and skeletal malformations, and fetal death or decreased size. The effects were dose related. Since the chemical was administered IP, it is possible that the toxic effects were due directly to the chemical's passing into the embryo, rather than through systemic absorption.

Cohen and Smith (1971) reported a cardiac arrest in a patient following insertion of acrylic bone cement for anchoring a femoral prosthesis. Autopsy demonstrated that the lungs contained fat and bone marrow emboli. An unidentified foreign material, presumed to be acrylic material, was also noted. Other investigators have also reported toxic effects from the use of acrylic cements as indicated in a previous section of this chapter.

Cyanoacrylates. These monomers have become very useful experimentally and clinically as new tissue adhesives, since they polymerize rapidly when placed on tissue. Initially, methyl cyanoacrylate was used, but this monomer has now fallen out of favor because of its toxic properties. The chief disadvantages of the methyl compound are its irritant properties and its rapid degradation. Kulkarni and associates (1967) implicate the degradation products, formaldehyde and cyanoacetate, in imparting the irritant response.

The butyl and heptyl analogs are less irritating, and their degradation rate is much slower than that of the methyl compound (Ousterhout et al., 1968). The alkyl esters can be absorbed through skin, with the methyl showing the highest rate of urine excretion, 12 percent of compound being excreted in five days when originally applied to rat skin (Ousterhout et al., 1968). When n-butyl 2-cyanoacrylate was implanted subcutaneously in dogs for a period of six months, no adverse effects were noted on liver function, nor was there any apparent pathology of vital organs (Houston et al., 1970). This indicated to the authors that even though the polymerized compound will degrade in a biologic environment, the degradation products released do not present a toxic threat to the host. In more recent years, this group of compounds has come into disfavor in medical practice.

Epichlorohydrin. This monomer is used in the synthesis of a number of epoxy resins. Epichlorohydrin is highly irritating to all types of tissues and is moderately toxic by most routes of administration, such as oral, intravenous, and by inhalation. In mice the intraperitoneal LD50 is 0.1439 ml/kg, for rats 0.0955 ml/kg, for guinea pigs 0.1000 ml/kg, and for rabbits 0.1356 ml/kg (Lawrence et al., 1972b). Dermal LD50 in rabbits is less than 1 ml/kg. Inhalation of the vapors is extremely caustic to the mucous membranes in the respiratory tract. Threshold limit value (TLV) is listed as 5 ppm (19 mg/M^3). However, Formin (1968) recommends that the average daily permissible concentration in air should not exceed 0.2 mg/M^3.

Plasticizers

Esters of Phthalic Acid. Presently the most-used plasticizers from the class of flexible polyvinyl chloride are the esters of phthalic acid. From this group the one that is most widely employed is di-(2-ethylhexyl) phthalate. Other phthalates, however, are used and at times two of the phthalates may be used in the same formulation.

Autian (1973) has reviewed the toxicity and health threats of phthalate esters. Also in a previous section of this chapter, some aspects of the toxicity of di-(2-ethylhexyl) phthalate ester were discussed since this specific plasticizer was used for polyvinyl chloride tubings, blood bags, and infusion containers. In general, the phthalate esters have a very low order of acute toxicity. Table 20-9 summarizes the LD50 values of a group of phthalate esters. In long-term feeding studies in animals in which DEHP was investigated, few toxic problems have been revealed, with the exception that liver involvement was noted at the higher doses. However, in a study involving primates, Jacobson et al. (1977) reported that at even low levels of DEHP administered i.v. liver toxicity was present.

Lawrence et al. (1975) reported that the apparent LD50 in mice receiving IP injections of DEHP five days per week for 12 weeks was reduced from 38.35 ml/kg (single LD50 dose) to 6.40 ml/kg at the end of the first week and 1.37 ml/kg by the end of the twelfth week, indicating the cumulative toxic effect of this agent. A similar pattern was noted for the di-*n*-actyl

phthalate. Other phthalates in the series demonstrated few cumulative effects. It is now well established that for DEHP biotransformation takes place rapidly, first forming the mono-ethylhexyl phthalate, an extremely toxic agent, which

Table 20–9.   ACUTE TOXICITY OF PHTHALATE ESTERS: LD50 IN ANIMALS*

COMPOUND	ANIMAL	ROUTE	LD50 g/kg	REFERENCE
Dimethyl phthalate	Mouse	Oral	7.2	(5c)
	Mouse	IP	3.6	(5c)
	Mouse	IP	1.58	(13)
	Rat	Oral	2.4	(5c)
	Rat	IP	3.38†	(14)
	Guinea pig	Oral	2.4	(5c)
	Rabbit	Dermal	10.0†	(5c)
Diethyl phthalate	Mouse	IP	2.8	(5c)
	Mouse	IP	2.8	(13)
	Rat	IP	5.06†	(14)
	Rabbit	Oral	1.0	(5c)
Dimethoxyethyl phthalate	Mouse	Oral	3.2–6.4	(5c)
	Mouse	IP	2.51	(13)
	Rat	Oral	4.4	(5c)
	Rat	IP	3.7	(13)
	Guinea pig	Oral	1.6–3.2	(5c)
	Guinea pig	Dermal	10.0†	(5c)
Diallyl phthalate	Mouse	IP	0.7	(5c)
	Rat	Oral	1.7	(5c)
	Rabbit	Oral	1.7	(5c)
	Rabbit	Dermal	3.4†	(5c)
Dibutyl phthalate	Mouse	IP	4.0	(13)
	Rat	IP	3.05†	(14)
	Rat	IM	8.0	(5c)
	Rabbit	Dermal	20.0†	(5c)
Diisobutyl phthalate	Mouse	Oral	12.8	(5c)
	Mouse	IP	4.50	(13)
	Rat	IP	3.75†	(14)
	Guinea pig	Dermal	10.0†	(5c)
Butyl carbobutoxymethyl phthalate	Rat	Oral	14.6†	(5c)
	Rat	IP	6.89	(14)
Dihexyl phthalate	Rat	Oral	30.0	(5c)
	Rabbit	Dermal	20.0†	(5c)
Dioctyl phthalate	Mouse	Oral	13.0	(5c)
	Rat	IP	50.0†	(14)
	Guinea pig	Dermal	5.0†	(5c)
Di-2-ethylhexyl phthalate	Mouse	IP	14.2	(13)
	Rat	Oral	26.0	(5c)
	Rat	IP	50.0†	(14)
	Rabbit	Oral	34.0	(5c)
	Guinea pig	Dermal	10.0	(5c)
Butyl benzyl phthalate	Mouse	IP	3.16	(13)
Dicapryl phthalate	Mouse	IP	14.2	(13)
Dinonyl phthalate	Rat	Oral	2.00	(5c)
Dibutyl	Mouse	Oral	11.2	(15)
(diethylene glycol bisphthalate)	Mouse	IP	11.2	(15)
	Rat	Oral	11.2	(15)
	Rat	IP	11.2	(15)
Dialkyl 79 phthalate	Mouse	Oral	20.00	(16)
	Rat	IP	20.00	(16)

* From Autian, J.: Toxicity and health threats of phthalate esters: Review of the literature. *Environ. Health Perspect.*, **4**:(June), 3–26, 1973.
† LD50 in ml/kg.

upon further oxidation leads to other metabolic products.

Singh and coworkers (1972a) studied the teratogenic effects of eight phthalate esters (dimethyl, dimethoxyethyl, diethyl, dibutyl, dimethobutyl, butyl carbobutoxymethyl, dioctyl, and di-[2-ethylhexyl]). For the more toxic esters, 1/10, 1/5, and 1/3 the LD50 dose were administered to rats. The least toxic esters (dioctyl and di-2-ethylhexyl) were administered at dosage levels of 5 and 10 ml/kg. At the doses employed, all of the compounds exerted a deleterious effect on the developing embryo and/or fetus. The lower-molecular-weight esters were generally found to be more teratogenic than the higher-molecular-weight esters, and the effects were dose dependent.

Dominant lethal mutations and antifertility effects in mice have been reported by Singh et al. (1974) for DEHP and for dimethoxyethyl phthalate. In tissue culture, DEHP has been found to be highly cytotoxic to several strains of cells. Studies by Autian and Dillingham (1973) using tissue culture suggest that DEHP has a much greater toxicity to proliferating cells as contrasted to nonproliferating cells.

It should be remembered that even though a number of similarities in toxicity of phthalate esters are evident, unique toxicity to one or more of these esters can also occur. For example, it has been reported that butyl benzyl phthalate may produce central and peripheral neuropathies in animals. A Russian report (Milkov et al., 1973) suggests that certain phthalate esters such as dibutyl phthalate and butyl benzyl phthalate have caused polyneuritis in industrial workers. Similar observations have not been reported in this country.

Esters of Adipic Acid. A number of polyvinyl chloride products utilize one of the higher-molecular-weight diesters of adipic acid. The general toxicity of these esters is similar in many ways to that of the phthalate esters and, in some instances, the toxicity may be less. Toxicity data on the adipates are not quite as extensive as for the phthalate esters, and thus caution should be taken in concluding that the toxic effects of a diester of adipic acid similar to those of a diester of phthalic acid will, in fact, be similar.

Esters of Citric Acid. These esters are used as nontoxic plasticizers for polyvinyl chloride materials as well as for other plastics requiring a plasticizer. Oral LD50 in rats ranged from approximately 8.0 g/kg for triethyl citrate to 31.4 g/kg for acetyl tributyl citrate (Gold et al., 1959). Parenteral toxicity as reflected through intraperitoneal values was much greater in mice, ranging from around 1 g/kg for acetyl triethyl citrate to 4.0 g/kg for acetyl tributyl

citrate (Meyers et al., 1964). Blood pressure experiments in rabbits revealed that triethyl, acetyl triethyl, and tributyl citrates produced complete loss of blood pressure when administered in toxic doses. All four of these compounds were also found to have local anesthetic action in rabbit experiments and to block neural transmission in rats when placed in contact with a nerve trunk (Meyers et al., 1964).

Stabilizers

Organotin Compounds. Organotin compounds are one of the best groups of stabilizers for vinyl materials. In this country, they have been used to stabilize polyvinyl chlorides, but in general their toxicity has decreased their use for medical applications. Guess and coworkers (1966) evaluated a number of dibutyltin compounds used as stabilizers for their toxic potential. A listing of LD50 values for these selected compounds in mice is shown in Table 20–10.

Table 20–10. INTRAPERITONEAL LD50 VALUES OF SOME ORGANOTIN COMPOUNDS*

COMPOUND	LD50 (mg/kg)
Dibutyltin diisoctyl maleate	13.6 ± 1.30
Dibutyltin diisoctyl thioglycolate	13.2 ± 1.50
Dibutyltin dilaurate	13.2 ± 1.40
Dibutyltin dilauryl mercaptide	28.4 ± 1.40
Dioctyltin beta mercaptopropionate	6.6 ± 1.20

* From Guess, W. L.; O'Leary, R. K.; Calley, D., and Autian, J.: Parenteral toxicity of a series of commercially available dioctyl and dibutyltin stabilizers used in PVC formulations. *Proceedings, 22nd Annual Technical Conference, Society of Plastic Engineers, Inc.,* Vol. XII, 1966.

From an acute toxicity point of view, the compounds studied can be considered extremely toxic. The compounds are highly irritating to tissue and, when placed into rabbit eyes, will cause corneal damage leading to blindness if not removed in a relatively short period of time.

Four organotin esters that have been used as stabilizing agents in the formulation of polymeric materials used in medical applications were studied by Calley and coworkers (1967a) in Swiss-Webster albino mice. The compounds included tetrabutyltin, tributyltin acetate, dibutyltin diacetate, and dibutyltin di-(2-ethylhexoate). Oral LD50 of these compounds ranged from 110 mg/kg for dibutyl diacetate to 6,000 mg/kg for tetrabutyltin. These compounds were also found to act as hepatotoxic agents.

In another study, Calley and associates (1967b) studied the effect of dibutyltin diacetate on the ultrastructure of mouse liver. In this study, rats were given orally 1/4 the LD50 dose daily for ten days. One rat was sacrificed each day and the liver tissue removed for both light and electron microscopy. Within a two-to-three-day period, pathologic features were observed, indicating that the agent was acting as a hepatotoxic agent. Changes in ultrastructure of liver cells were evident and early mitochondrial damage was observed. Swelling of granular and agranular endoplasmic reticulum followed soon after the mitochondrial changes were noted. Progressive congestion of bile canaliculi occurred, due in part to cellular and microvilli swelling.

It should be stated that it is extremely difficult to prepare the dialkyltin compounds as pure compounds, there generally being present traces of the corresponding trialkyl derivatives. Commerical organotin compounds used as stabilizers are often not clearly identified about the exact organotin, nor is information given as to the presence of other ingredients, thus making it difficult to predict the toxicity without actually running toxicity studies on the commercial product.

Long-term studies by the parenteral route have not been reported for these compounds, even though it is suspected that some manufacturers may have carried out chronic toxicity studies in animals at least by the oral route.

Other Stabilizers. A large number of other stabilizers are used for plastic materials. Often a synergistic effect can be achieved by combining several of these stabilizers. Toxicity must then be measured by considering the combination rather than each agent alone. Calcium, magnesium, and barium salts (sterate, laurate, and similar types of aliphatic structures) are now used to stabilize a large number of polyvinyl chlorides, but generally they are used in combination with other agents to achieve good polymer stabilization. The acute toxicity of these agents is minimal, and they have not presented any serious hazards as demonstrated by a long history of availability and use.

Various types of epoxy derivatives can also be included in stabilizing systems. The more useful ones are generally of low toxicity, with the toxicity decreasing as the molecular weight increases. In recent years epoxidized oils, such as soybean oil, have been included in stabilizing systems for polyvinyl chloride blood bags and tubings. Most chronic toxicity studies of the epoxy compounds have been of the oral-feeding type, and the toxic effect has generally been considered extremely low. Chronic toxicity studies by a parenteral route in animals have not been reported.

DRUG-PLASTIC PROBLEM

The pharmaceutical industry has made rapid changes in the past several years and is now packaging all types of drug products in plastic systems. Similar innovations have taken place in the packaging of nutritional products, various types of solvents, and a variety of reagent products used for clinical laboratory tests. It has already been mentioned that, depending on the specific plastic and specific product in contact with the material, chemical agents may be released to the contents. Other types of problems can occur when plastic containers and packaging systems are used for drug products. Even though these problems may not appear important, they can change the product composition in a number of ways, negating the value of the item when used. Autian (1963) has discussed these drug-plastic problems.

MIGRATION OF CHEMICALS FROM PLASTICS TO FOODS

With the enactment of the Food Additives Amendment (Public Law 85-929) in 1958, food manufacturers are required to demonstrate the safety of a new ingredient that is added, directly or indirectly, to foods. These substances are defined legally as "food additives." The above act, however, specifically exempted ingredients added to foods that were in common use prior to the amendment. These compounds (in excess of 2,500) became part of the GRAS (generally recognized as safe) substances and by legal definition are not "food additives." The Food and Drug Administration (FDA) can only ban a GRAS ingredient if it has been shown to cause harm in animals or humans.

The Food Additives Amendment includes an extremely important but controversial clause that states that any food additive in any concentration found to cause cancer in animals or humans will be prohibited for food and beverage use.

When chemical agents are placed into food for one or more reasons, the agent can be referred to as a "direct" food additive. The same chemical(s) or other chemical agents might also enter food by contact with articles that come in contact with the food. These can include various types of packaging systems, food-processing apparatus, and household items used to store or serve food. Many of these items are presently prepared from polymeric materials, and thus the possibility exists, depending on the specific plastic, the food, and the conditions of contact, that substances from the plastic will migrate to the food and be consumed. When these substances enter the food, the term "indirect" food additives can be used.

The Food and Drug Administration places limits on the concentration of "indirect" additives that can enter food. In general, the limit is based on the total residue weight that will be extracted from the material under very specific conditions of extraction using selected solvent systems simulating various food systems.* In recent years, questions have been asked as to the toxic potential of "indirect" additives since actual toxicity tests do not need to be conducted on the "extractable" constituents released to foods. With the nearly unlimited number of plastic items that can come in contact with foods, it becomes apparent that an endless list of migrating chemicals could enter foods. Presently, exactly what these chemicals are has not been ascertained even though FDA is giving consideration to this problem. Unfortunately, very little research in this field has been done, and thus there is a knowledge gap concerning the long-term effects of migrating chemicals even though these may be in extremely small concentrations in foods. This problem becomes even more complex when it is realized that most likely there are several migrating chemicals entering foods at the same time. An additional problem is the fact that in food processing or even in preparing the food at home new chemical entities can be produced in the plastic that are quite different from the original chemicals that were present in the material. It seems clear that the use of only physicochemical determinations of the migrating chemical will not answer the problem of the toxic potential presented by a plastic article that will be placed in contact with foods. There is a need for the development of suitable, simple *in vitro* and *in vitro* biologic tests to screen out potentially toxic materials.

TOXICITY OF THERMAL DECOMPOSITION PRODUCTS OF PLASTICS

Perhaps the first awareness of the serious hazards due to thermal decomposition products of plastics was caused by the Cleveland Clinic Fire of 1929 in which 125 people died. Most of the fatalities, it was surmised, were due to the production of carbon monoxide and nitrogen oxide gases from the burning of x-ray films composed of the highly combustible nitrocellulose. Since then other fires throughout the United States have dramatized the fact that degradation products of man-made materials can be dangerous

to the population in the immediate environment of a fire. Periodic warnings are issued that a specific new plastic item should be removed from the market because of its high combustion potential. All fire situations will produce smoke, but other pyrolysis and combustion products will also evolve when polymeric materials are heated and burned. Since most of the polymeric materials contain carbon, carbon monoxide is one of the primary gases generated from the heating and burning of these materials. Depending on the material, the temperature, and the absence or presence of oxygen, other noxious gases can and do develop. These include HCN, HCl, SO_2, and NO_2, various fluorinated gases, and other agents not always well identified.

More recently, a variety of flame retardants has been added to polymeric materials to reduce the combustion properties of the final material. When these materials are heated or subjected to flame, the composition of the degradation products can change, and in turn the inhalation of these agents may produce toxic responses not originally anticipated. Autian (1970) has discussed the toxic problems associated with thermodegradation products of synthetic materials, while Yuill (1972) has emphasized the importance of smoke and its hazards in fire situations.

In the fifties, it was found that when polytetrafluoroethylene (PTFE) was thermodegraded above 300° C, the fumes would lead to symptoms resembling "metal fume" fever in man. The effect was of short duration and generally the worker would recover after 24 or 48 hours from the first signs of the symptoms. In more recent years, workers as meat wrappers using polyvinyl chloride films that were sealed by heating have also developed "asthma"-like symptoms (Vandervort et al., 1977). Proper ventilation and protection of workers have eliminated the toxic effects from both PTFE and PVC. Thermodegradation products of specific polyurethanes have also caused toxic problems to workers. Again, these problems have been eliminated when proper ventilation and health hygiene standards have been initiated. Since research on the toxicology of thermodegradation and combustion products has been very limited, sufficient information is not available to make judgments as to the toxic effects of new man-made polymers that are introduced into commerce.

TOXICITY TESTING

There is a need for the development of suitable toxicity tests for the evaluation of the toxicity of man-made materials that will be used in (1) medical practice and (2) in food packaging or for articles that will have contact with foods. Addi-

---

* It has been proposed that if the migrating agent in food is 0.05 ppm or less, no toxicologic problems would exist for most of the indirect food additives. There would be exceptions, however, as, for example, if the migrating substance has been shown to be a carcinogenic agent or poses some extraordinary toxicity problem.

tional biologic tests are needed for the determination of the toxicity of man-made materials when they are heated or combusted.

The passage of a medical device law, as an amendment to FDA rules and regulations, in 1976 requires manufacturers to show evidence of the safety and efficacy of a new medical device. With certain types of devices, the need for toxicologic evaluation of the materials, as well as the device, will become a necessity for premarket clearance. Even though consideration is being given to evaluation of "indirect" food additives from articles in contact with foods, no definite rule has been promulgated by the FDA as to how these articles should be biologically tested. Neither has legislation been promulgated in regard to toxicity testing of thermodegradation or combustion products of materials. The U.S. Consumer Products and Safety Commission, however, does require certain types of articles such as mattresses and children's clothing to meet certain safety standards in regard to combustion, but no toxicologic tests are required on thermodegradation products. A number of state and local municipalities also have fire codes, but in general, these standards do not include toxicologic studies.

Materials for medical and paramedical applications should be tested or evaluated at three levels: (1) toxicity test on the various ingredients used to manufacture the basic resin, (2) toxicity evaluation of the final plastic or elastomeric material, and (3) evaluation of the final device. Each of these levels would, of course, require a battery of tests. Often toxicity information on individual ingredients may be known and thus lengthy test procedures on these substances would not be required. In other cases, however, with introduction of new chemical compounds, there must be sufficient toxicity testing to establish a broad toxicity profile of the specific ingredient. Special tests may also be needed such as carcinogenic and mutagenic studies on the test substance since these latter two problems are becoming recognized as important health hazards to the public. The information derived from the group of toxicity tests becomes important since it can guide the manufacturer in developing safe-handling and other safety features for the workers who may come in contact with the toxic agent.

In most instances, the final material will not contain the monomer, catalyst, or other reactive ingredients used to manufacture the final resin. There is, however, always the possibility that residues of the reactive chemicals might still be present and these may be adequate to produce one or more types of toxic responses.

One of the first groups in this country to develop a standardized toxicity testing program of items for medical applications was the American Pharmaceutical Manufacturers Association in the early 1960s. Their objective was to develop acceptable testing methods for plastic items to be used with drug products that would be injected into humans. The testing program took on an official status when it became part of the *United States Pharmacopeia* and *National Formulary*. Even though these tests

are for materials that may have contact with drug products, the same test methods are appropriate as an initial test or screening for all types of materials for which acute toxicity information is desired. Details of these tests are available from the official compendia.

Other professional organizations have also directed their attention to the development of toxicity testing procedures. Several of these organizations have now published their programs. Toxicity testing guidelines have now been published by the American Dental Association (1972) for dental materials, and the National Institute of Arthritis, Metabolism, and Digestive Diseases (1977) has issued a report entitled "Evaluation of Hemodialyzers and Dialysis Membranes," which includes a set of toxicity tests.

Organizations such as the Association for the Advancement of Medical Instrumentation (Standards for Anesthesia and Respiratory Apparatus), USA Standard Institute, and the American Society for Testing and Materials (F4 Committee) have developed or are developing toxicity testing programs on materials used for specific medical applications.

Through a joint contract from the Food and Drug Administration and the National Heart, Lung, and Blood Institute to the University of Tennessee, a series of *in vitro* and *in vivo* biologic tests has been developed for the assessment of new biomaterials. The tests are listed in Table 20-11. Each of the tests

Table 20-11. PRIMARY ACUTE TOXICITY SCREENING TESTS FOR MATERIALS*

A. *Tests Directly on Material*

 1. Tissue culture–agar overlay
 2. Rabbit muscle implant (one week)
 3. Hemolysis (rabbit blood)

B. *Tests on Extracts*

 Note: Extracting media: saline, polyethylene glycol 400, and cottonseed oil.
   Extracting conditions: one hour in an autoclave at 121° C.
 1. Tissue culture–agar overlay
 2. Intracutaneous injection in rabbits
 3. Systemic toxicity in mice
 4. Cell growth inhibition on aqueous extract

* From Autian, J.: Toxicological evaluation of biomaterials: Primary acute toxicity screening program. *Artif. Org.*, 1:53–60, 1977.

is given a numerical value depending on the biologic response. From these individual values, a *Cumulative Toxicity Index* may be calculated. The index can range from a "0" (no response in any of the tests) to an index of 1,500 (highest response in each of the individual tests). Table 20–12 includes a number of CTI values for a group of plastics. In general, materials that have a value of 100 or less are considered good candidates for biomedical applications. Autian (1977) has reviewed these tests in a recent publication. The tests alluded to can be considered an "acute toxicity screening program," which can also be applied to food-packaging systems if so

Table 20–12. CUMULATIVE TOXICITY INDEX (CTI) FOR SELECTED PLASTICS AND COMMERCIALLY OBTAINED PLASTICS*

PLASTIC	CTI
Formulated polymethyl methacrylate†	
Sample 13	30
Sample 14	81
Sample 12	128
Sample 19	131
Sample 7	165
Sample 5	249
Sample 3	317
Sample 2	394
Sample 1	508
Formulated silicone rubber†	
Sample 38	93
Sample 39	134
Sample 35	205
Sample 44	251
Sample 30	283
Sample 48	310
Formulated polyurethane A†	
Sample 49	40
Sample 51	65
Sample 66	225
Sample 62	337
Sample 52	471
Sample 53	583
Sample 58	806
Sample 65	1050
Formulated polyurethane B†	
Sample 77	50
Sample 69	98
Sample 84	158
Sample 74	281
Sample 75	646
Sample 80	750
Silicone rubber (#88)	81
Polycarbonate membrane (#89)	30
Polysulfone (#56)	56
Thermoplastic hydrocarbon (#101)	41
Thermoplastic olefin (#102)	516
Polyethylene sample (#107)	65
Ethylcellulose (#108)	56
Epoxy sample (#112)	32
Polyurethane sample (#114)	41
Plastic sample (#117)	383
Polyurethane foam sample (#123)	75
Erythroflex (#130)	40
Polyvinyl chloride (prepared with toxic agents) (#132)	763
Polyethylene sample (#133)	166
Plastic sample (#170)	32
Plastic sample (#182)	126
Plastic sample (#184)	105
Plastic sample (#186)	207
Plastic sample (#187)	216
Plastic sample (#165)	165

* From Autian, J.: Toxicological evaluation of biomaterials: Primary acute toxicity screening program. *Artif. Org.*, 1:53–60, 1977.

† Prepared in MST Laboratories, toxic additives included in a number of these samples. Various curing times were also employed.

desired. The addition of an *in vitro* test such as the Ames test would assist in making a judgment that leachable constituents in the material may have carcinogenic activities. Appropriate "in-use" tests must then be considered to establish the safety of the final item. Depending on the specific device, there may also be the need for long-term animal studies to confirm the safety of the device during the period of actual use.

A large number of biologic tests have been proposed for the determination of the toxicity of thermodegradation and combustion products of man-made materials. Since these tests vary, the toxicity data from the same material may be quite different when different test methods are applied.

REFERENCES

Adler, R. H., and Darby, C.: Use of a porous synthetic sponge (Ivalon) in surgery I. Tissue response after implantation. *U.S. Armed Forces Med. J.*, 11(2):1349–64, 1960.

Albro, P. W.; Thomas, R.; and Fishbein, L.: Metabolism of diethylhexyl phthalate by rats—isolation and characterization of the urinary metabolites. *J. Chromotogr.*, 76:321–30, 1973.

Alexander, P., and Horning, E. S.: Observations on the Oppenheimer method of inducing tumors by subcutaneous implantation of plastic films. *Ciba Foundation Symposium on Carcinogenesis*, 1959, pp. 24–26.

American Dental Association: Recommended standard practices for biological evaluation of dental materials. *J. Am. Dent. Assoc.*, 84:382–87, 1972.

Ames, B. N.; Lee, F. D.; and Durston, W. E.: An improved bacterial test system for the detection and classification of mutagens and carcinogens. *Proc. Natl. Acad. Sci.*, 70:782–86, 1973.

Aquino, T. I., and Skinsnes, P. K.: Teflon embolism of coronary arteries. *Arch. Pathol.*, 80:625–29, 1963.

Aquino, T. I., and Skinsnes, P. K.: Development of standards for plastics to be used in pharmacy and medicine. *J. Dent. Res.*, 45:1668–74, 1966.

Autian, J.: Plastics in pharmaceutical practice and related fields. Part I. *J. Pharm. Sci.*, 52:1–23, 105–22, 1963.

Autian, J.: Toxicity and health threats of phthalate esters: Review of the literature. *Environ. Health Perspect.*, 4:(June) 3–26, 1973.

Autian, J.: Toxicity, untoward reactions and related considerations in the medical use of plastics. *Environ. Health Perspect.*, 53:1289–1301, 1964.

Autian, J.: Toxicologic aspects of flammability and combustion of polymer materials. *J. Fire Flammability*, 1:239–68, 1970.

Autian, J.: Toxicological evaluation of biomaterials: Primary acute toxicity screening program. *Artif. Org.*, 1:53–60, 1977.

Autian, J.: Toxicological problems and untoward effects from plastic devices used in medical applications. In Hayes, W. J., Jr. (ed.): *Essays in Toxicology*, Vol. 6. Academic Press, Inc., New York, 1975, pp. 1–33.

Autian, J.: Unpublished data from Materials Science Toxicology Laboratories, University of Tennessee Center for the Health Sciences, Memphis, TN, 1971, 1972, 1974.

Autian, J., and Dhorda, C. N.: Evaluation of disposable plastic syringes as to physical incompatibilities with parenteral products. *Am. J. Hosp. Pharm.*, 16:1976–79, 1959.

Autian, J.; Lawrence, W. H.; and Dillingham, E. O.: Detection of toxicity of extracted constituents from dialyzers and components, Contract NO1-AM-4-2219, Artificial Kidney-Chronic Uremia Program, National Institutes of Health, Bethesda, Maryland, *Final Report,* Jan. 6, 1978.

Autian, J.; Rosenbluth, S. A.; and Guess, W. L.: An evaluation of two urinary bags as to their biological activity in animals. *Acta Pharm. Succ.,* 2:279–88, 1965.

Autian, J.; Singh, A. R.; Turner, J. E.; Hung, G. W. C.; Nunez, L. J.; and Lawrence, W. H.: Carcinogenic activity of a chlorinated polyether polyurethan. *Cancer Res.,* 36:3973–77, 1976.

Autian, J.; Singh, A. R.; Turner, J. E.; Hung, G. W. C.; Nunez, L. J.; and Lawrence, W. H.: Carcinogenesis from polyurethans. *Cancer Res.,* 35:1591–96, 1975.

Banes, D.: Deterioration of nitroglycerin tablets. *J. Pharm. Sci.,* 57:893–94, 1968.

Bates, R. R., and Klein, M.: Importance of a smooth surface in carcinogenesis by plastic film. *J. Natl. Cancer Inst.,* 37:145–51, 1966.

Bering, E. A., Jr.; McLaurin, R. L.; Lloyd, J. B.; and Ingraham, F. D.: The production of tumors in rats by the implantation of pure polyethylene. *Cancer Res.,* 15:300–301, 1955.

Bischoff, F., and Bryson, G.: Carcinogenesis through solid state surfaces. *Progr. Exp. Tumor Res.,* 5:85–133, 1964.

Bischoff, F.: Organic Polymer biocompatibility and toxicology. *Clin. Chem.,* 18:869–94, 1972.

Blum, A., and Ames, B. N.: Flame-retardant additives as possible cancer hazards, *Science,* 195:17–23, 1977.

Borzelleca, J. F.; Larson, P. S.; Hennigar, G. R., Jr.; Huf, E. G.; Crawford, E. M.; and Smith, R. B., Jr.: Studies on the chronic oral toxicity of monomeric ethyl acrylate and methyl methacrylate. *Toxicol. Appl. Pharmacol.,* 6:29–36, 1964.

Braun, B., and Kummell, H. J.: The use of plastic containers for storing blood and transfusion solutions. *Dtsch. Apoth. Z.,* 103:467–74, 1963.

Calley, D.; Autian, J.; and Guess, W. L.: Toxicology of a series of phthalate esters. *J. Pharm. Sci.,* 55:158–62, 1966.

Calley, D. J.; Guess, W. L.; and Autian, J.: Hepatotoxicity of a series of organotin esters. *J. Pharm. Sci.,* 56:1240–43, 1967a.

Calley, D. J.; Guess, W. L.; and Autian, J.: Ultrastructural hepatotoxicity induced by an organotin ester. *J. Pharm. Sci.,* 56:1267–72, 1967b.

Carpenter, C. P.; Weil, C. S.; and Smyth, H. F., Jr.: Chronic oral toxicity of di-(2-ethylhexyl) phthalate for rats, guinea pigs and dogs. *Arch. Ind. Hyg.,* 8:219–26, 1953.

Carson, S., and Oser, B. L.: Oral toxicity of ethylene chlorohydrin, a potential reaction of ethylene oxide fumigation. Abstract No. 51, Society of Toxicology, 8th Annual Meeting, Williamsburgh, VA, March, 1969.

Charnley, J.: *Acrylic Cement in Orthopedic Surgery.* Williams & Wilkins Co., Baltimore, 1970.

Clarke, C. P.; Davidson, W. L.; and Johnston, J. B.: Hemolysis of blood following exposure to an Australian manufactured plastic tubing sterilized by means of ethylene-oxide gas. *Aust. N.Z.J. Surg.,* 36:53–56, 1966.

Cohen, C. A., and Smith, T. C.: Acrylic bone cement: Report of a case. *Anesthesiology,* 35:547–49, 1971.

Creech, O.: Vascular prosthesis. *Surgery,* 41:62–80, 1957.

Crissey, J.: Stomatitis, dermatitis and denture materials. *Arch. Dermatol.,* 92:45–48, 1965.

Cunliffe, A. C., and Wesley, F.: Hazards from plastics sterilized by ethylene oxide. *Br. Med. J.,* 2:575–76, 1967.

Daniel, J. W., and Bratt, H.: The absorption, metabolism and tissue distribution of di(2-ethylhexyl) phthalate in rats. *Toxicology,* 2:51–65, 1974.

DeHaan, R. L.: Toxicity of tissue culture media exposed to polyvinyl chloride plastic. *Nature* (Lond.), 231:85–86, 1971.

Dillingham, E. O., and Autian, J.: Teratogenicity, mutagenicity and cellular toxicity of phthalate esters. *Environ. Health Perspect.,* 3:(January) 81–89, 1973.

Dinman, B. D.; Cook, W. A.; Whitehouse, W. M.; Magnuson, H. J.; and Ditcheck, T.: Occupational acroosteolysis. I. An epidemiological study. *Arch. Environ. Health,* 22:61–73, 1971.

Duke, H. M., and Vane, J. R.: An adverse effect of polyvinyl chloride tubing used in extracorporeal circulation. *Lancet,* 2:21–23, 1968.

Eubanks, R., and Autian, J.: Evaluation of a polyethylene blood bag. *Am. J. Hosp. Pharm.,* 28:172–77, 1971.

Fassbinder, W.; Pilar, J.; Scheuermann, E.; and Koch, M.: Formaldehyde and occurrence of anti-N-like cold agglutinins in RDT patients. *Proc. Eur. Dialysis Transplant Assoc.,* 13:333–38, 1976.

Fisher, A. A.: Allergic sensitization of the skin and oral mucosa to acrylic resin denture materials. *J. Prosthet. Dent.,* 6:593–602, 1956.

Fisher, A. A.: *Contact Dermatitis.* Lea & Febiger, Philadelphia, 1967.

Fomin, A. P.: Effect of small concentrations of epichlorohydrin vapors on animals. *Vop. Gig. Atmos. Vozdukha Planirovki Naselen Mest.,* 6:50–56, 1968.

Golberg, L.: Liver enlargement produced by drugs: Its significance. *Proc. Eur. Soc. Study Drug Toxicity,* 7:171–84, 1966.

Gold, H.; Modell, W.; and Finkelstein, M.: Toxicology of the citric acid esters: tributyl citrate, acetyl tributyl citrate, triethyl citrate and acetyltriethyl citrate. *Toxicol. Appl. Pharmacol.,* 1:283–98, 1959.

Goldhaber, P.: The influence of pore size on carcinogenicity of subcutaneously implanted millipore filters. *Proc. Am. Assoc. Cancer Res.,* 3:228–330, 1961.

Gott, V. L.; Whiffen, J. D.; and Dutton, R. C.: Heparin bonding on colloidal graphite surfaces. *Science,* 142:1293–94, 1963.

Guess, W. L.; Berg, H. F.; and Autian, J.: Evaluation of a new disposable hypodermic device (the Hypule) by a biological procedure and a compatibility study with parenteral products. *Am. J. Hosp. Pharm.,* 22:181, 1965.

Guess, W. L.; Jacob, J.; and Autian, J.: A study of polyvinyl chloride blood bag assemblies. I. Alteration or contamination of ACD solutions. *Drug Intelligence,* 1:120–27, 1967.

Guess, W. L.; O'Leary, R. K.; Calley, D.; and Autian, J.: Parenteral toxicity of a series of commercially available dioctyl and dibutyltin stabilizers used in PVC formulations. *Proceedings, 22nd Annual Technical Conference, Society of Plastics Engineers, Inc.,* Vol. XXV-4, March 1966, pp. 1–7.

Gunther, D. A.: Absorption and adsorption of ethylene oxide. *Am. J. Hosp. Pharm.,* 26:45–49, 1969.

Guttuso, J.: Histopathologic study of rat connective tissue responses to endodontic materials. *Oral Surg.,* 16:713–27, 1962.

Hamit, H. F.: Implantation of plastics in the breast. *Arch. Surg.,* 75:224–29, 1957.

Harris, D. K.: Some hazards on the manufacture and use of plastics. *Br. J. Ind. Med.,* 16:221–29, 1959.

Harris, H. I.: Research in plastic implants. Their use in augmentation for amastia or hypomastia. *J. Int. Coll. Surgeons,* 35:630–43, 1961.

Harris, R. S.; Hodge, H. C.; Maynard, E. A.; and Blanchet, H. J., Jr.: Chronic oral toxicity of 2-ethylhexyl phthalate in rats and dogs. *Arch. Ind. Health,* 13:259–64, 1956.

Hirose, T.; Goldstein, R.; and Bailey, C. P.: Hemolysis of blood due to exposure to different types of plastic tubing and the influence of ethylene-oxide sterilization. *J. Thorac. Cardiovasc. Surg.*, 45:245–51, 1963.

Hoopes, J. E.; Edgerton, M. T.; and Shelley, W.: Organic synthetics for augmentation mammaplasty: their relation to breast cancer. *Plast. Reconstr. Surg.*, 39:263–70, 1967.

Houston, S.; Ousterhout, D. K.; Sleeman, H.; and Leonard, F.: The effect of n-butyl 2-cyanoacrylate on liver function. *J. Biomed. Mater. Res.*, 4:25–28, 1970.

Hueper, W. C.: Experimental production of cancer by means of implanted polyurethane plastic. *Am. J. Clin. Pathol.*, 34:328–33, 1960.

Hueper, W. C.: Carcinogenic studies on water-insoluble polymers. *Pathol. Microbiol.*, 24:77–106, 1961.

Hueper, W. C.: Cancer induction by polyurethane and polysilicone plastics. *J. Natl. Cancer Inst.*, 33:1005–27, 1964.

Inchiosa, M. A., Jr.: Water-soluble extractives of disposable syringes. Nature and significance. *J. Pharm. Sci.*, 54(2):1379–81, 1965.

Jacobson, M. S.; Kevy, S. V.; and Grand, R. J.: Effects of plasticizer leached from polyvinyl chloride on the subhuman primate: A consequence of chronic transfusion therapy. *J. Lab. Clin. Med.*, 89:1066–78, 1977.

Jaeger, R. J., and Rubin, R. J.: Plasticizers from plastic devices: Extraction, metabolism and accumulation by biological systems. *Science*, 170:460–61, 1970.

Johnson, M. K.: Metabolism of chlorethanol in the rat. *Biochem. Pharmacol.*, 16:185–99, 1967.

Kim, S. W.; Peterson, R. V.; and Lee, E. S.: Effect of phthalate plasticizer on blood compatibility of polyvinyl chloride. *J. Pharm. Sci.*, 65:670–73, 1976.

Kordon, H. A.: Fluorescent contaminants from plastic and rubber laboratory equipment. *Science*, 149:1382–83, 1965.

Kulkarni, R. K.; Hanks, G. A.; Pani, K. C.; and Leonard, R.: The *in vivo* metabolic degradation of poly (methyl cyanocrylate) via thiocyanate. *J. Biomed. Mater. Res.*, 1:11–16, 1967.

Lake, B. G.; Gangolli, S. D.; Grasso, P.; and Lloyd, A. G.: Studies on the hepatic effects of orally administered di-(2-ethylhexyl) phthalate in the rat. *Toxicol. Appl. Pharmacol.*, 32:355–67, 1975.

Laskin, D. M.; Robinson, I. B.; and Weinmann, J. P.: Experimental production of sarcomas by methyl methacrylate implants. *Proc. Soc. Exp. Biol. Med.*, 87:329–32, 1954.

Lawrence, W. H.; Bass, G. E.; Purcell, W. P.; and Autian, J.: Utilization of mathematical models in the study of structure-toxicity relationships of dental compounds. I. Esters of acrylic and methacrylic acids. Presented at the AAAS meeting, Chicago, December 1970.

Lawrence, W. H.; Dillingham, E. O.; Turner, J. E.; and Autian, J.: Toxicity profile of chloroacetaldehyde. *J. Pharm. Sci.*, 61:19–25, 1972a.

Lawrence, W. H.; Itoh, K.; Turner, J. E.; and Autian, J.: Toxicity of ethylene chlorohydrin. II. Subacute toxicity and special tests. *J. Pharm. Sci.*, 60:1163–68, 1971a.

Lawrence, W. H.; Malik, M.; Turner, J. E.; and Autian, J.: Toxicity profile of epichlorohydrin. *J. Pharm. Sci.*, 61:1712–17, 1972b.

Lawrence, W. H.; Malik, M.; Turner, J. E.; Singh, A. R.; and Autian, J.: A toxicological investigation of some acute, short-term and chronic effects of administering di-ethylhexyl phthalate (DEHP) and other phthalate esters. *Environ. Res.*, 9:1–11, 1975.

Lawrence, W. H.; Mitchell, J. L.; Guess, W. L.; and Autian, J.: Toxicity of plastics used in medical practice. I. Investigation of tissue response in animals by certain unit packaged polyvinyl chloride administration devices. *J. Pharm. Sci.*, 52:958–63, 1963.

Lawrence, W. H.; Turner, J. E.; and Autian, J.: Toxicity of ethylene chlorohydrin. I. Acute toxicity studies. *J. Pharm. Sci.*, 60:568–71, 1971b.

Lefaux, R.: *Practical Toxicology of Plastics*. C.R.C. Press, Cleveland, 1968.

Leininger, R. I.; Mirkovitch, V.; Peters, A.; and Hawks, W. A.: Change in properties of plastics during implantation. *Trans. Am. Soc. Artif. Intern. Org.*, 10:320, 1964.

Lindberg, D. A. B.; Lucas, F. V.; Sheargren, J.; and Malm, J. R.: Silicone embolization during clinical and experimental heart surgery employing a bubble oxygenator. *Am. J. Pathol.*, 39:129–44, 1961.

Lyman, D. J.; Muir, W. M.; and Lee, I. J.: The effects of chemical structure and surface properties of polymers on coagulation of blood. I. Surface free energy effects. *Trans. Am. Soc. Artif. Intern. Org.*, 11:301–306, 1965.

Massler, M.: Effects of filling materials on pulp. *J. Tenn. State Dent. Assoc.*, 35:353–74, 1955.

Matsui, A.; Buonocore, M.; Syaegh, F.; and Yamaki, M.: Reactions to implants of conventional and new dental restorative materials. *J. Dent. Child.*, 34:316–22, 1967.

Meyers, D. B.; Autian, J.; and Guess, W. L.: Toxicity of plastics used in medical practice. II. Toxicity of citric acid esters used as plasticizers. *J. Pharm. Sci.*, 53:774–887, 1964.

Meyler, F. L.; Willebrands, A. F.; and Durrer, D.: The influence of polyvinyl chloride (PVC) tubing on the isolated perfused rat's heart. *Circ. Res.*, 8:44–46, 1960.

Milkov, L. E.; Aldyreva, M. V.; Popova, T. B.; Lopukhova, K. A.; Makarenko, Y. L.; Malyar, L. M.; and Shakhova, T. K.: Health status of workers exposed to phthalate plasticizers in the manufacture of artificial leather and films based on PVC resins. *Environ. Health Perspect.*, 3:(January) 175–77, 1973.

Mitchell, D. F.: The irritational qualities of dental materials. *J. Am. Dent. Assoc.*, 59:954–66, 1959.

Mitchell, D. F.; Shankwalker, G. B.; and Shazer, S.: Determining the tumorigenicity of dental materials. *J. Dent. Res.*, 39:1023–28, 1960.

Modern Plastics Encyclopedia. Plastic Products Pub., Inc., New York, 1962, p. 29.

Mullison, E. G.: Silicones and their use in plastic surgery. *Arch. Otalaryngol.*, 81:264–69, 1965.

National Institute of Arthritis and Metabolic Diseases: The evaluation of hemodialysis. Dept. HEW Publ. No. (NIH) 72-103, 1971.

Neergaard, J.; Neilsen, B.; Baurby, V. F.; Christensen, D. H.; and Nielsen, O. F.: Plasticizers in PVC and the occurrence of hepatitis in a hemodialysis unit. *Scand. J. Urol. Nephrol.*, 5:141–45, 1971.

O'Leary, R. K., and Guess, W. L.: Toxicological studies on certain medical grade plastics sterilized by ethylene oxide. *J. Pharm. Sci.*, 57:12–17, 1968.

Oppenheimer, B. S.; Oppenheimer, E. T.; and Stout, A. P.: Sarcomas induced in rats by implanting cellophane. *Proc. Soc. Exp. Biol. Med.*, 67:33–34, 1948.

Oppenheimer, B. S.; Oppenheimer, E. T.; and Stout, A. P.: Sarcomas induced in rodents by imbedding various plastic films. *Proc. Soc. Exp. Biol. Med.*, 79:366–69, 1952.

Oppenheimer, B. S.; Oppenheimer, E. T.; Stout, A. P.; Wilhite, M.; and Danishefsky, I.: The latent period in carcinogenesis by plastics in rats and its relation to the presarcomatous stage. *Cancer*, 11:204–13, 1958.

Oppenheimer, E. T.; Wilhite, M.; Danishefsky, I.; and Stout, A. P.: Observations of the effects of powdered polymer in the carcinogenic process. *Cancer Res.*, 21:132–34, 1961.

Ousterhout, D. C.; Gladieux, G. V.; and Leonard, F.: Cutaneous absorption of N-alkyl cyanoacrylate. *J. Biomed. Mater. Res.*, 2:157–63, 1968.

Patty, F. A. (ed.): *Industrial Hygiene and Toxicology* vol. II, 2nd ed. Interscience, New York, 1963.

Peters, J. M.; Murphy, R. L. H.; Pagnotto, L. D.; and Whittenberger, J. L.: Respiratory impairment in workers exposed to "safe" levels of toluene diisocyanate (TDI). *Arch. Environ. Health*, **20**:364–67, 1970.

Pappaport, H. M.; Lilly, G. E.; and Kapsimalis, P.: Toxicity of endodontic filling materials. *Oral Surg.*, **18**:785–802, 1964.

Refojo, M. F., Dohlman, C. H.; Ahmad, B.; Carroll, J. M.; and Allen, J. C.: Evaluation of adhesives for corneal surgery. *Arch. Ophthalmol.*, **80**:645–56, 1968.

Rendell-Baker, L.: Medical users' views of ethylene oxide sterilization problems. In *Proceedings of the 1969 HIA Technical Symposium*. Sterile disposable devices and sterilizations. Health Industries Association.

Rodkey, F. L.; Collison, H. A.; and Engel, R. R.: Release of carbon monoxide from acrylic and polycarbonate plastics. *J. Appl. Physiol.*, **27**:554–55, 1969.

Roe, F. J.; Dukes, C. E.; and Mitchley, B. C. V.: Sarcomas at the site of implantation of a polyvinyl plastic sponge: incidence reduced by use of thin implants. *Biochem. Pharmacol.*, **16**(1):647–50, 1967.

Rosenbluth, S. A., and Cripps, G. W.: Inhibitory effects of detergents in membrane filters. *J. Pharm. Sci.*, **58**:440–42, 1969.

Rubin, R. J.: Cited in *Chem. & Eng. News*, Feb. 15, 1972, pp. 12–13.

Rubin, R. J.: Transcript of Proceedings, Workshop on Adenine and Red Cell Preservation, October 1, 1976. Department of Health, Education and Welfare, Food and Drug Administration, Bureau of Biologics, pp. 191–205.

Russell, F. E.; Simners, M. H.; Hirst, A. E.; and Pudenz, R. H.: Tumors associated with embedded polymers. *J. Natl. Cancer Inst.*, **23**:305–15, 1959.

Sakurabayashi, M.: Studies on intrauterine contraceptive devices. III. Application of high polymers in cavity of uterus and a new radiopaque Phycon-X ring. *Acta Obstet. Gynaecol. Jap.*, **16**:56–63, 1969.

Sanders, H. J.: Artificial organs—part I. *Chem. & Eng. News*, April 5, 1971, pp. 32–49; and Sanders, H. J.: Artificial organs—part II. *Chem. Eng. News*, April 12, 1971, pp. 68–76.

Selikoff, I. J., and Hammond, E. C. (eds.): Toxicity of vinyl chloride-polyvinyl chloride. *Ann. N.Y. Acad. Sci.*, **246**:1–337, 1975.

Shubik, P.; Saffiottie, W.; Lijinsky, W.; Pietra, G. W.; Rappaport, H.; Toth, B.; Raha, C. R.; Tomatis, L.; Feldman, R.; and Ramahi, H.: Studies on the toxicity of petroleum waxes. *Toxicol. Appl. Pharmacol.*, **4**(suppl.): 1–62, 1962.

Singh, A. R.; Lawrence, W. H.; and Autian, J.: Mutagenic and antifertility sensitivities of mice to di-2-ethylhexyl phthalate (DEHP) and dimethoxyethyl phthalate (DMEP). *Toxicol. Appl. Pharmacol.*, **29**: 35–46, 1974.

Singh, A. R.; Lawrence, W. H.; and Autian, J.: Teratogenicity of phthalate esters in rats. *J. Pharm. Sci.*, **61**:51–55, 1972a.

Singh, A. R.; Lawrence, W. H.; and Autian, J.: Embryofetal toxicity and teratogenic effects of a group of methacrylate esters in rats. *J. Dent. Res.*, **51**:1632–38, 1972b.

Starr, A.; Pierie, W. R.; Raible, D. A.; Edwards, M. L.; Siposs, G. G.; and Hancock, W. D.: Cardiac valve replacement: experience with the durability of silicone rubber. Presented before the American Heart Association Meeting, Bal Harbour, Florida, October, 1965.

Stetson, J. B., and Autian, J.: Necrotizing enterocolitis and plastic catheters. In Stern, L.; Friis-Hansen, B.; and Kildeberg, P. (eds.): *Intensive Care in the Newborn*. Masson Publishing Co., New York, 1976, pp. 79–89.

Trimble, A. S.; Goldman, B. S.; Tao, J. K.; Kovats, L. K.; and Bigelow, W. G.: Plastics—a source of chemical contamination in surgical research. *Surgery*, **59**:857–59, 1966.

Turner, F. C.: Sarcomas at sites of subcutaneously implanted bakelite disks in rats. *J. Natl. Cancer Inst.*, **2**:81–83, 1941.

Vandervort, R., and Brooks, S. M.: Polyvinyl chloride film thermodecomposition products as an occupational illness: I. Environmental exposure and toxicology. *J. Occup. Med.*, **19**:188–96, 1977.

Van Valin, C. C.; Kallman, B. J.; and O'Donnell, J. J., Jr.: Polyethylene as a source of artifacts in the paper chromatography of chlorinated hydrocarbon insecticides. *Chemist-Analyst*, **52**:73, 1963.

Walter, C. M.: A new technique for collection, storage, and administration of unadultered whole blood. *Surg. Forum—1950*. W. B. Saunders Co., Philadelphia, 1951, p. 483.

Wesolowski, S. A.; Martinez, A.; and McMahoh, J. D.: Use of artificial materials in surgery. *Current Problems in Surgery*. Year book Medical Publishers, Inc., Chicago, December 1966, pp. 1–86.

Wilson, R. H., and McCormick, W. E.: Plastics. The toxicology of synthetic resins. *Arch. Ind. Health*, **21**:536–48, 1960.

Wilson, R. H.; McCormick, W. E.; and Tatum, C. F.: Occupational acroosteolysis. Report of 31 cases. *J.A.M.A.*, **201**:577–81, 1967.

Wilson, R. H.; Planek, E. H.; and McCormick, W. E.: Allergy in the rubber industry. *Ind. Med.*, **28**:209–11, 1959.

Yuill, C. H.: Smoke: What's in it? *Fire J.*, **66**:47–55, 1972.

Zapp, J. A., Jr.: Hazards of isocyanates in polyurethane foam plastic production. *Arch. Ind. Health*, **15**:324–30, 1962.

Chapter 21

TOXINS OF ANIMAL ORIGIN

Frederick W. Oehme, John F. Brown, and *Murray E. Fowler*

TOXICOLOGY PROBLEMS OF ANIMAL ORIGIN

A significant part of animal toxicology deals with the toxic chemicals produced by various animal species. The animals that contain or elaborate some of the most violent and toxic chemicals known are scattered throughout various animal phyla, from the single-celled protozoa through the higher animals into mammals, where one species is found that contains venom. Table 21–1 provides a summary of

Table 21–1. DISTRIBUTION OF ZOOTOXINS IN THE ANIMAL KINGDOM

Protozoa—dinoflagellates (shellfish toxicity)
Porifera—sponges
Colenterata—hydroids, Portuguese man-of-war, jellyfish, anemones, coral
Echinodermata—echinoderms, urchins
Mullusca—shellfish, snails, octopus
Annelida—segmented worms
Arthropoda—insects, arachnids
Chordata—fishes, amphibians, reptiles, birds, mammals

the distribution of zootoxins in the animal kingdom. Poisonous spiders, amphibians, and reptiles are important members of this toxic group. Many of the toxic animals are marine and have some unique venom characteristics and methods of releasing the venom into other animals.

The venoms vary greatly, as do the syndromes they produce. Many of these substances are enzymes and provide the biochemist and toxicologist with an array of reactions and metabolic pathways to study. The most significant clinical syndromes are produced by peptides, polypeptides, and amines similar to those produced by mushrooms and toadstools. Glycosides are found in some amphibians, and formic acid is found in other species.

Amid the variety of exposures to these animal toxins possible for man and other animals, it is at once interesting to recognize the existence of this toxic potential and at the same time necessary to understand the hazard due to this widespread and lethal group of toxins. The medical scientist who acknowledges the presence of a poison and has a concept of its toxicity is in a good position to give valuable assistance when needed. It is the purpose of this chapter to explore the different sources for toxicities of animal origin, offer some insight into the characteristics of the poisoning syndromes, and provide some understanding of the therapeutic measures that are helpful in handling clinical cases of intoxication in man and other animals.

CHARACTERISTICS OF VENOMS

Venoms are complex organic substances containing a wide variety of chemical components (Buckley and Porges, 1956; Bücherl *et al.*, 1968–1971; Minton, 1970; Russell and Saunders, 1967), and in fact may be the most complex poisons known (Russell, 1971b). The chief components seem to be proteins, many of them enzymes, and highly toxic polypeptides. The diverse nature of these chemicals is illustrated by the wide variation in chemical components found in venoms.

Perhaps the most commonly known animal toxin is tetrodotoxin, an aminoperhydroquinazoline compound. This poison is toxic in extremely small quantities and produces nervous system involvement when portions of fish containing this chemical are consumed. A lethal fraction of scorpion-fish venom is a complex protein of molecular weight 40,000 to 80,000. Enzymes are especially important components of snake venoms. Phospholipase A is such a component that cleaves lecithin, producing lysolecithin, a hemolytic agent responsible for much of the red cell and tissue damage resulting from snakebites. L-Amino-oxidase converts amino acids to ketonic acids, thereby activating tissue peptidase and furthering tissue destruction from the introduction of venom.

A number of enzymes are present in varying concentrations in venoms from a host of animals. Phosphodiesterase is capable of contributing to hypotension and cardiovascular changes in the victim. The spreading factor of hyaluronidase permits other toxic components of venom to penetrate and distribute themselves away from the site of venom introduction. Proteases produce proteolytic and hemorrhagic actions, further complicating and aggravating the response to the other toxic components present in venom.

A diverse group of peptides, polypeptides, and amines probably does the most damage to the tissues of victims through a direct effect on enzyme systems and cellular structures. Anaphylactic reactions and complex interactions with other biochemical components can produce a vast number of molecular toxic effects.

Some components of venoms act as anticoagulants and prevent normal clotting processes, thereby further permitting the spread and dissemination of the venom's chemical components. Some animals, such as toads, contain glycosides that are rapidly absorbed and affect autonomic nerve endings in addition to producing cardiovascular, central nervous system, or digestive symptoms and signs. Formic acid produced by bees, wasps, and ants will cause tissue irritation upon contact or injection. A choline chloride ester of 3-acetoxyhexadecanoic acid is released from the skin of the boxfish upon stimulation.

A number of other toxic moieties have been isolated from animals, but their characterization is still pending, and their identity is restricted to the use of numbers or letters. The study of such compounds is hindered by the complexity of the animal venoms and by the variations, both qualitatively and quantitatively, that occur from species to species and also among individuals of the same species. Work with "standard" representative venom samples is further confused by alterations that occur in biologic specimens due to the age and sex of the animal, conditions of nutrition and environmental habitat, and the season of the year in which the sample is collected. Despite such fluctuations, venoms within a single phylum in general tend to bear some relationship to each other. Further, venoms liberated from the mouth are generally used for offensive purposes, are high in enzyme activity, and tend to produce pain, while those secreted in other areas of the body are often used as a defensive mechanism, have fewer types and smaller amounts of enzyme action, and do not produce as much pain as those generated from the mouth (Russell, 1971b).

The actions produced by animal venoms are as diversified and complex as their chemical composition (Tu, 1977). Individual venoms cannot be solely considered to affect any single organ or tissue and, in fact, most venoms have effects on several biologic systems. It is thus best to consider venoms as complex mixtures with actions capable of producing toxic changes in several organs simultaneously. The symptoms and signs produced by clinical instances of envenomation may thus involve two or more different toxic reactions.

One of the common body systems affected is the nervous system. A neurotoxic component of venom has been found in almost all examined samples. Coral snakes, the black widow spider, and scorpions produce such symptoms. However, cardiotoxic and hematotoxic activity is also often present with so-called neurotoxic venoms. Alterations in heart function are frequent and are a common toxic action of venoms. The effect of venoms on red blood cells, producing hemolysis and altered red cell functioning, is usually associated with snakebites. Cytotoxic and necrotizing properties of venom result in tissue destruction, which frequently leads to sloughing and loss of varying quantities of skin and deeper structures. Some animal toxins interfere with blood-clotting mechanisms, producing hemorrhagic syndromes with localized or diffuse hemorrhaging. Occasionally such actions are mediated through an effect on blood platelets. This results in a thrombotoxic action and associated clinical syndrome. Proteolytic effects of varying magnitude may result in direct protein precipitation of contacting cells and tissues or more subtle biochemical interactions with specific vital proteins important for enzyme, cell, or organ function.

With the introduction of such diverse foreign chemicals into a victim, it is not at all surprising that allergic and other responses develop in the envenomated individual. The foreign protein injected is an ideal antigen and allergic reactions are common, especially in those individuals with previous exposure to similar proteins. Anaphylactic reactions, and indeed those that have produced fatal results, are common and should be expected in individuals with such sensitivity or history of previous or repeated exposures. The response of the victim may also include the release of biologically active substances, such as bradykinin, histamine, or adenosine. These compounds are sufficiently hazardous in themselves not only to significantly contribute to the clinical manifestations of poisoning, but also to produce effects that may be more serious than that of the actual animal venom. Not only the chemical, but also the emotional effect of venom injection must be considered; cardiac accidents and cerebral strokes may be triggered by the victim's fear reaction upon recognizing the fact that venom injection has occurred. The emotional impact of such realization is often more severe than the actual hazard from the venom. The application of "mind over matter" in this relationship may prove lifesaving.

The variety of animals capable of producing toxic effects in man and other animals suggests that a discussion of these toxins may be accomplished according to biologic classification. Accordingly, the animal toxins potentially poisonous to man and his animals will be presented as marine toxins, arthropod toxins and venoms, amphibian and reptile toxins, and venomous mammals.

MARINE TOXINS

A variety of fishes and other marine animals have toxic components that may produce poisoning in man and animals (Halstead, 1959, 1965–1970; Russell, 1965, 1971a). The chemical composition of the toxins of marine origin varies from one extreme of toxic substances to the other (Martin and Padilla, 1973; Russell, 1971b). Complex organic molecules, often with neurotoxic components, are found in various surface structures of some jellyfish and octopuses and in the livers of some fish. Although contact between marine animals and domestic animals is not common, man often voluntarily exposes himself to marine toxins through his inherent curiosity. He will pick up unusual structures on beaches, explore underwater areas and attempt capture of unusual creatures, and taste exotic foods in an effort to experience new and unusual situations.

Exposure to these marine toxins by topical contact or ingestion of improperly cooked marine products may result in the rapid onset of toxicity with a short clinical course leading either to spontaneous recovery or death. Rarely is sufficient time available to initiate a thorough investigation of the immediate problem, except when recovery permits elucidation of details. Supportive therapy is usually immediately required and indicated. Unfortunately, by the time assistance is available, patients will often have terminated or are on the way to a spontaneous and memorable recovery.

Marine Invertebrates

This interesting group of marine animals includes the jellyfish, coral, univalves, and octopuses, worms, and urchins.

Coelenterates. The coelenterates include the hydroids (which contains the Portuguese man-of-war), the jellyfish, coral, and the sea anemones. These animals are frequently beautiful to observe but present significant hazards associated with their exploration or handling.

The venom apparatus is based in numerous stinging cells called nematocysts. These tiny microscopic organs, used for defensive or food-gathering purposes, number in the thousands on some species of animals. The tentacles of the Portuguese man-of-war (*Physalia*) contain numerous little nematocysts for these purposes. Other marine invertebrates contain nematocysts on various other body structures.

The stinging cell is activated by mechanical or chemical stimulation. Normally it is encased, but upon stimulation is ejected into the victim. Physical damage is instantaneous, with chemical effects following very shortly. It is of interest that some species of fish live within the tentacles of some coelenterates. One species of sea slug will actually consume other coelenterates and concentrate the acquired nematocysts in respiratory organs. These structures are then later used in defense against crustaceans.

The initial effect of contact with nematocysts is the physical stinging sensation of the injected microspears. These are often multiple and produce a burning sensation much like contact with a needle or plant nettle. The toxin associated with the nematocyst is injected at the time of the physical contact through the stinging device. Often within seconds a shooting and throbbing pain is noticed at the site of penetration. The intensity of pain increases rapidly with a dermal reaction producing redness, pruritus, and urticarial-like responses. When several of these nematocysts are injected, the victim often experiences a shocklike effect within minutes and prostration is a frequent result. Persons in water are often unable to reach land and are in great danger of drowning.

Additional clinical signs and symptoms may be observed in milder cases or in individuals with slower onset. Nausea and vomiting are frequent occurrences. Muscle cramps, especially in those areas of the body (often the extremities) nearest the injection sites, produce severe pain and inability to move. Backache may be the result of muscle spasms or neurotoxic effects. Loss of speech and frothing with inability to swallow are prominent signs in some instances. Almost all fatal cases develop paralysis and delirium, with convulsions occurring for several minutes before death.

The treatment of coelenterate-induced toxicity is largely oriented toward relieving pain and controlling the shock reaction that rapidly follows the injection of the toxin. No physiologic or pharmacologic antidote is available to counteract the toxic materials. Symptomatic and supportive care is provided to encourage rapid elimination of the foreign chemicals. Maintenance of vital functions is important. Because of the usual unavailability of medical and supportive assistance at the site of injury, and because of the rapid course of the condition, adequate treatment of such toxicity is infrequent. Most victims are required to rely on their normal detoxication processes and the hope that nonlethal amounts of the venom were injected.

Mollusca. This group consists of the Gastropods or univalves, and the Cephalopods, the octopuses.

The univalves (Gastropods) contain only the cones (*Conus* spp.) that are venomous. However, there are 400 species of this genus that are poisonous. The mollusk, for example, contains a venomous structure in the radular teeth. All the animals in this group appear to have the venom apparatus associated with these radular teeth that are used primarily as a food-securing or feeding structure.

Envenomation produces a sharp stinging pain from the physical act. A localized ischemia rapidly develops at the bite site and numbness in the area of the wound follows. Cyanosis proceeds rapidly with a tingling of the skin followed by a numbness that spreads over the body, including the lips and mouth. Paralysis precedes the coma that then progressively develops.

The octopus (Cephalopods) can inflict a nasty bite that consists of two small but obvious puncture wounds. In certain species a venomous component is present and leads to moderate clinical symptoms and signs. An initial burning or tingling sensation is usually felt at the time that hemorrhage from the wound area is present. Inflammation and swelling of the area are common, but serious consequences or complications are usually not observed.

Of unique and special recent interest is the extremely rapid neurotoxicity that has resulted from the bite of *Octopus maculosus*, the blue-ringed octopus, found in the South Seas. This very attractive species has variously designed blue rings over its natural background color of tan-brown, and it varies in length from 9 to 20 cm or slightly more. Humans may be tempted to handle and play with specimens of this octopus when finding them on seashores or in shallow waters. The toxicity of the salivary venom is potent, and all species must be considered potentially dangerous until further information is available on the nature of the venom. Bites may occur anywhere on the body and result in rapid development of symptoms. Bleeding from the wound is common, together with dryness of the mouth and difficulty in swallowing, vomiting and weakness, ataxia, rapidly progressing respiratory distress, loss of consciousness, and death. Fatalities may occur within five to ten minutes of the bite or two hours may pass before

fatal termination. Attempts at treatment by administration of artificial respiration and positive mechanical respiratory assistance have not been successful (Halstead, 1965–1970).

Annelid Worms. Although only one species of this group produces bites, others have irritating setae or bristles. Persons coming in contact with these structures will develop a local skin inflammation that usually resolves in 36 to 48 hours.

Echinoderms. This group of marine animals is commonly called the sea urchins. They are spiny creatures that skin divers find attractive; however, the spines are vicious and hard to remove. In certain species of urchin the structure is also venomous. These spines on urchins are usually hollow and provide a storage place for venom.

Some species of echinoderm also have small seizing organs, known as pedicellariae, on the shell or surface. These are primarily defense mechanisms, but can produce a mechanical wound on contact. Some of these seizing organs are venomous, while others are not.

Damage from contact with urchins may be due to mechanical puncture wounds or to envenomation. In some species both mechanical trauma and deposition of venom will occur. An immediate and intense burning sensation is felt on contact with these hazardous structures. Inflammation occurs rapidly at the site of wound and numbness follows in a matter of minutes. In severe intoxication muscular weakness and paralysis may set in, but the clinical syndrome is usually not severe or life threatening.

Marine Vertebrates

Toxic vertebrates that live in the seas include the fishes, which generally produce mechanical injury through spines, independently or attached to a venom apparatus, and the sea snakes, whose bite produces a syndrome similar to that of a cobra bite (Halstead, 1959, 1965–1970; Keegan and Mcfarlane, 1963; Russell, 1965, 1971a).

Fishes. Among the approximately 200 species of marine fishes that are known to be venomous via a venom apparatus are the sting rays, scorpion fishes, zebra fishes, stone fishes, weevers, stargazers, and certain of the sharks, ratfishes, catfishes, and surgeonfishes (Russell, 1971b). This approximate number does not include those fishes whose flesh is toxic when eaten.

Fishes do not have venomous bites, but rather have a variety of spines on the body that are either mechanically injurious to contacting individuals or are connected to a venom apparatus, which injects the toxin when the spine contacts or penetrates a surface. The spines are frequently associated with the dorsal or pectoral fins of the fish. Although the toxins of venomous fish have different chemical and pharmacologic properties from the toxins of other venomous animals, a common characteristic of the toxins of venomous fishes is their relative instability at room temperature or even on lyophilization of freshly prepared extracts. This property presents difficulties in study of the toxic properties of venomous fishes, but the heat lability of these chemicals is a helpful tool that may be exploited in the treatment of poisoned individuals. There is sufficient similarity in the toxicologic properties of the toxins of venomous fishes to suggest that their venoms may be similar or at least have some similar chemical components (Russell, 1971b).

A variety of species of fish are hazardous to man and animals through their spines, which may produce mechanical or venomous damage. The horned or spiny sharks are largely hazards because of the mechanical injury produced by their structures. Some of the sting rays are also venomous and have spikes used as protective devices. These fishes are bottom dwellers and are often stepped upon by divers. The traumatic effects of skin puncture produce a sharp shooting pain that develops into persistent throbbing after only a few minutes. Hypotension may also develop. Vomiting, diarrhea, and sweating are less commonly observed symptoms.

Ratfish and elephant fish may also produce such traumatic and toxic signs upon contact with man or animal. Such problems are occasionally observed in domestic animals following exposure to venomous fishes on beaches or other marine areas.

There are a number of different species of catfish that have toxic capabilities. The oriental catfish (*Plotosus lineatus*) is a common species that produces problems in man. Spines are located on the pectoral and dorsal fins and are capable of producing pronounced clinical symptoms. In some catfish the spines are up to 15 cm long. Persons handling such fish may become injured and develop pain instantaneously. Severe stinging and throbbing of the wound are immediately noticed with partial paralysis developing rapidly. Affected individuals usually become incapacitated because of the violent pain and may develop shock following a period of prostration and spasms in response to the injury. The wound often becomes inflamed and gangrene may develop locally. The salt-water catfish are the most toxic; fresh-water catfish also have spines but are not extremely poisonous.

Weever fish are grotesque-appearing creatures that include several venomous species. Dorsal and lateral spines are capable of producing mechanical and venom injury similar to that of all fishes in this group.

The scorpion fish (*Scorpaenidae*) include the zebra fishes or lion fishes (*Pterois*), the scorpion fish proper (*Scorpaena*), and the stone fish (Syranceja). When the spines of these fishes puncture the skin, the venom cells empty their toxin directly into the wounds. Such stings give rise to immediate and intense burning pain, which may develop shooting and throbbing impulses. Inflammation of the wound and swelling of the limb develop rapidly. Weakness, dizziness, and even shock may be present within minutes. The wound site becomes discolored and markedly tender, with paralysis of the limb possible. Systemic signs of hypotension, marked respiratory depression leading to paralysis, and even myocardial ischemia or injury occur (Russell, 1971b). The effect on respiration appears due to cerebral anoxia secondary to a decreased central nervous system blood supply. Although the venom has a direct hemolytic effect, it does not interfere with fibrinogen-thrombin clotting or the generation of plasma thromboplastin or prothrombin (Russell, 1971b). The pain induced by these wounds may persist for several hours and the injured site may be swollen for weeks after the insult. Stings from the stone fishes in this group are especially likely to be fatal. The toadfish, rabbit fish, dragonets, and stargazers are additional marine fishes that produce injury and venom injections due to their spines. The surgeonfishes have sharp knife-like movable spines on the sides of the base of their tail, which may be manipulated by the fish to slash and produce a strictly mechanical, but prominent wound.

Because the venoms of these fishes are extremely heat labile, injuries from these stings respond favorably to placing the injured part of the body in water as hot as the patient can tolerate. This is maintained for up to one hour. If this treatment is delayed, a local anesthetic injection of the injured area or the systemic use of analgesics may be provided. Elevation of the wounded extremity and supportive measures to treat primary or secondary shock, with specific efforts toward maintaining blood pressure, should also be accomplished.

Reptiles. This group includes the wide variety of sea snakes (*Hydrophidae*). Like the cobras (*Elapidae*), these are front-fanged snakes. They are characterized by a tail that is flattened laterally so that it can be used for undulative progress within their aquatic environment. One species of sea snake has adapted to fresh water. All others are marine and are usually found in, but not restricted to, estuary areas.

The clinical syndrome results from a bite, as

opposed to the mechanical injury produced by spines from the previous group of fishes. Venom is injected through the bite wound. Following the insult, initial symptoms may develop within 20 minutes, or may require as long as several hours with bites from certain species of elapids. Pain in the bite site gives way to general aching and anxiety. This is progressively followed by a sensation of thickening of the tongue, muscle stiffness, progressive and ascending generalized paralysis, drooping of the eyelids, difficulty in opening the mouth due to tense jaw muscles (this lockjaw condition is characteristic), dilation of the pupils, pulse rate becoming irregular and weak, and a sensation of thirst and burning of the throat. The syndrome then progresses to shock, with convulsions and respiratory distress preceding death. A 25 percent mortality from sea snake bites is usual.

Shellfish Toxicity

Shellfish filter small organisms called dinoflagellates through their digestive and respiratory systems. These organisms contain toxic substances that may produce poisoning in humans and other animals eating the shellfish. No harm occurs, however, to the host shellfish from the dinoflagellates. Most toxicity is seasonal, primarily in the summer, and is associated with blooms of algal growth. Cockles, mussels, clams especially the Alaskan butter clam (*Saxidomas giganteus*), and oysters are the shellfish species that have proven to be most dangerous.

The toxins from the dinoflagellates are localized in the shellfishes' digestive organs (the dark meat), gills, and siphon. The toxin is water soluble and heat stable; hence cooking the shellfish does not appreciably destroy its poisonous properties, and consumption of the broth from cooked shellfish meals may be equally toxic to consumption of the meat.

The clinical syndromes produced by shellfish poisoning may be classified as allergic, digestive, and paralytic ("paralytic shellfish poisoning"). Each syndrome may be observed separately but it is common to have various degrees of all three types present. Usually, however, one syndrome will predominate.

The allergic syndrome is a typical allergic reaction and anaphylactic signs and symptoms predominate. Previous sensitivity to one or more toxic components is assumed to underlie this reaction.

The digestive signs are probably the result of bacterial or endotoxic contamination of the shellfish. There have been many isolations of *Clostridium botulinum*, types E, F, and even some B, from clams, oysters, crabs, and other fish. In addition to the endotoxin, histadine may

also be released and contribute to the clinical symptoms. Occasional spoilage of shellfish or other marine animals used for food may result in the activation of enzymes, such as thiaminase, with resultant spoilage and poisoning. The gastrointestinal syndrome develops 10 to 12 hours after consumption of the fish materials. Nausea, vomiting, diarrhea, and abdominal pain and colic are common complaints. Except in extreme cases, recovery occurs.

Paralytic shellfish poisoning is caused by a specific dinoflagellate, *Gonyaulaux* sp., that produces a paralytic toxin identified as saxitoxin by K. Meyer in the late 1920s. This particular toxin has been characterized and found to be a poisonous substance not only of shellfish, but also in other fish poisonings, such as red tide. The clinical signs of paralytic shellfish poisoning initially begin with a tingling and burning of the lips, gums, tongue, and face. This rapidly spreads to other parts of the body and is followed by a numbness. Victims frequently complain of difficulty in moving, joint aches, weakness, increased salivation and difficult swallowing, and intense thirst. Progressive and generalized paralysis follows, with death often resulting. Digestive signs are rare, but may occasionally be seen.

Since no direct antidote is available, and the mechanism of action of the toxin's components is ill defined, treatment for any of the forms of shellfish toxicity is symptomatic. Monitoring of vital functions and therapy to reverse the adverse symptoms are provided.

Poisonous Fish

Some food fish may produce toxicity in man and animals when toxic portions of their bodies are consumed. In other instances, toxins may affect the fish, producing toxicity and even death, and consumption by man or animals produces poisoning. The food supply of the fish is often important in determining whether or not the food fish is itself edible. Some fish species are edible when caught in one geographic location, but are extremely toxic when found in other areas. Carnivorous fish may become poisonous by eating herbivorous fish that ate poisonous plant material.

Fish may be toxic to man or other animals if they are poisoned by saxitoxin (red tide) or if the particular fish is a poisonous variety containing unedible organs or toxins such as tetrodotoxin or ciguatoxin.

Red Tide. This toxicity results when fish ingest dinoflagellates that contain saxitoxin. The fish itself may be killed by the toxin or the poisoning may be imparted to other animals, including man, consuming that fish. The dinoflagellate producing red tide is a different species than that which produces shellfish toxicity, but in general the shellfish (clams, oysters) are not damaged by saxitoxin while fish are. Red tide or fish poison is the syndrome that characteristically results in large-scale marine animal losses due to the effect of the toxin on the fish.

Sharks. The livers of some sharks are dangerous. An unknown toxic substance may be found in this organ and upon consumption poisoning occurs in man and animals.

Moray Eels. Tropical forms of this group of poisonous fish should not be eaten. The clinical signs resulting from their consumption are similar to the early signs of shellfish poisoning, but digestive signs are much more prominent. The muscular weakness, joint ache, and salivation and swallowing problems are complicated by the development of vomiting, diarrhea, and abdominal cramps.

Scombroid Fish. For the most part, all portions of tuna, bonito, and mackerel are edible. However, if these are allowed to spoil, there is a change in the histidine present to histamine (sourine), which produces an allergic-type reaction. All fish have some histidine present, but this particular group of fish is most likely to spoil and thereby cause toxicity problems.

Puffer Fish (Tetraodontidae). There are in excess of 90 species of this highly prized food fish. However, unless the fish is specially prepared, toxicity may result from the presence of tetrodotoxin and ichthyocrinotoxin. In Japan puffer fish are sold in restaurants as fugu and belong to the genera *Tetradon* and *Fugu*. The toxins are found in the roe, liver, and skin of the puffer fish. Although specially trained individuals prepare this food fish, in some instances errors are made and human poisoning results. This toxin is also found in the California newt (*Taricha torosa*).

Clinical signs of puffer fish toxicity (tetrodotoxin) include initial tingling of the lips and tongue followed by motor incordination 10 to 45 minutes after ingestion of the toxic fish. Numbness of the skin develops at the same time that salivation and muscle weakness occur. Nausea leads to vomiting and diarrhea. A generalized paralysis occurs with convulsions and death following in terminal cases. Approximately 60 percent of all cases of poisoning due to puffer fish result in death.

Ciguatera. More than 300 species of fish have been found to produce ciguatoxin (ichthyosarcotoxin). This is a serious problem because of the large number of food fish that have this capability. Apparently any fish can acquire the toxicity, which appears to be a result of feeding habits. It is likely that the animals ingest plant material that contains either the toxin or a precursor to the toxin. The large number of fish species that may be involved with ciguatoxin-type toxicity and its sudden appearance in specific marine locations after years of absence make it a great hazard. The red snapper is an example of one species that under certain circumstances accumulates ciguatoxin and will produce toxicity in man.

The clinical signs of ciguatoxin poisoning usually develop with an initial tingling of the lips, tongue, and throat. This is rapidly followed by a numbness of these areas. It is of interest that these signs may not develop for as long as 30 hours after ingestion of the toxic fish. Nausea, vomiting, abdominal pain and intestinal spasms and diarrhea usually follow shortly. A headache that leads to nervousness and even convulsions is a further symptom. Muscle pain, sore teeth, visual disturbances, and dermatitis are additional signs and symptoms that may be seen. Death occurs in only about 7 percent of the clinical cases.

Among the general pharmacologic actions of ciguatoxin is the inhibition of cholinesterase. This results in acetylcholine accumulation at synapses and resulting disruption of nervous function. Respiratory paralysis is the usual mechanism of death.

Due to a lack of specific therapy, treatment for ciguatoxin poisoning is symptomatic. Prevention is the more important control measure. Viscera of tropical marine fish should never be eaten by man or animals. Roe may be especially hazardous. Since ciguatoxin is water soluble and heat stable, it is difficult to remove from the meat of a toxic fish. Soaking the meat in water for up to several days and discarding the toxin-containing water has been advocated as a means of preparing the fish for safe human consumption.

Sea Turtles

Although infrequent, sea turtles have at times been known to be toxic. The livers of sea turtles are thought to be especially hazardous, and marine turtles in the Indo-Pacific regions should be eaten with caution.

The clinical signs of toxicity usually begin with a throbbing or dull headache in the frontal area. Nausea, vomiting, diarrhea, and abdominal pain follow. Dizziness or drowsiness is observed together with irritability and photophobia. Convulsions are seen in patients with severe toxicity.

A quick review of the previous syndromes produced by marine toxins demonstrates that many of the signs and symptoms are similar. Often the toxicities are lethal, although there is some suggestion that the degree of lethality may be exaggerated in some instances. There is no doubt, however, that there is much to be learned about the mechanisms of action, clinical syndromes, and preferred treatments of these interesting marine toxicities.

ARTHROPOD TOXINS AND VENOMS

Many members of the phylum arthropoda secrete substances toxic to other animals and plants. While all classes of *Arthropoda* presumably contain toxin-producing species, discussion will be limited to those insects and arachnids whose toxic secretions are of significant medical importance to man and animals.

Arthropod toxins and venoms produce initial reactions due to their physiopathologic properties as a result of injection through the skin, by bites or stings, or by causing urticaria or blistering. Secondary bacterial infection of the affected site is not uncommon and may be initiated at the time of toxin introduction or as a result of the victim rubbing or scratching the painful or pruritic area. Often, the most serious sequelae of these substances are hypersensitivity reactions of an allergic nature from previous toxin contacts.

Site of Toxin and Venom Production

All arthropod venoms and toxins are produced by exocrine-type glands, which are lined with special secretory epithelium, and are stored in the lumina of the glands, prior to expulsion (Diniz and Corrado, 1971). The venom glands of the mouth and last abdominal segment of arthropods associated with forceful venom injection have a basement membrane underlying the secretory epithelium and a deeper intrinsic muscular sheath in the fibers run in a longitudinal-helical fashion (Snodgrass, 1952). Intracellular organelles associated with venom production seem to be smooth and rough endoplasmic reticulum (Smith and Russell, 1967).

Mechanism of Toxin and Venom Introduction

With the exception of urticarious and blistering arthropod toxins, venoms are usually harmless when they are administered topically or orally. Only when they are injected parenterally or contact broken skin surfaces are their characteristic toxic responses evoked (Diniz and Corrado, 1971). It is therefore necessary for venomous arthropods to be equipped with natural devices for penetrating the unbroken integument to obtain effect with their toxic substances. Probably other glandular secretions of arthropods would be considered toxic were suitable mechanisms available for their introduction into the sensitive tissues of victims.

Intromissions of toxins and venoms by head parts or other anterior structures of arthropods are commonly referred to as bites, even though

the structures and mechanisms employed might be entirely different. Venom is the term applied to the secretions of the highly specialized glandular structures used only for offensive activities. Secretions of other glands, such as salivary and integumentary, that happen to be toxic to sensitive tissues of victims but are not injected as such receive the nominal term of toxin. Envenomations by specialized structures of the posterior region of arthropods are referred to as stings. The stinging apparatus is often closely associated with the ovipositor, accounting for the phenomenon that only the female of some species can sting. Some arthropods may bite and sting independently, whereas others perform the tasks simultaneously. Comparative anatomy and physiology of these mechanisms are well described (Snodgrass, 1944; Herms and James, 1961; Diniz and Corrado, 1971).

The urticaria-producing hairs of various lepidopterous and dermestid coleopterous larvae have a reactive component that evokes toxic reactions on penetration of the skin. Some produce their effect by mechanical irritation, whereas a poison gland has been identified in the hair shaft papilla of the io moth caterpillar (Jones and Miller, 1959). Studies of these structures are in the literature (Weidner, 1936; Kemper, 1958).

Spiders

Spiders are uniformly venomous, but most attack only other arthropods and are generally beneficial to man. Of more than 2,000 genera of spiders known, only a few species have biting mechanisms strong and long enough and venom potent enough to be of significant danger to man. Spiders inject their venom through channeled bilateral hooklets (chelicerae) associated with the head. Since spiders subsist on the body fluids of living animals, their venom is used to subdue or paralyze their prey. The venom of the black widow spider, for example, paralyzes the victim by a yet ill-defined mechanism that appears directed at the peripheral nervous system. The venom may react with the nerve terminal membrane causing release of transmittor substance independently of calcium and depolarization of the terminal (Russell, 1971b).

In the United States, only the female black widow, *Lactrodectus mactans*, and the brown recluse spider, *Loxoscles reclusus*, cause serious envenomation. In Europe, the only dangerous species is the malmignatte, *Lactrodectus mactans tredecimguttatus*. The tarantula, *Eurytelma* sp., is often falsely accused of being extremely poisonous and causing human fatalities. While the tarantula does bite and is mildly venomous, it is for the most part not lethal and produces only mild signs of poisoning, if any. Since spider bites (and for that matter any animal's bite) are anything but sterile, bacterial contamination of the wound may add considerably to the injury produced.

Black Widow (*Lactrodectus mactans*). The toxic fraction of black widow venom is a labile protein (McCrone and Hatala, 1967) that is neurotoxic, causing ascending motor paralysis and destruction of peripheral nerve endings. Initially the bite produces localized pain and paresthesia. A dull, numbing pain is usually present in the affected extremity and leads to muscle rigidity and fasciculations. Neuromuscular dysfunction, evidenced by muscle weakness in the large masses near the injury and even severe muscle spasms, is prominent. Other symptoms include headache, ptosis and occasional eyelid edema, skin rash and conjunctivitis, salivation, inflammation at the site of the bite, and an increase in blood and cerebrospinal fluid pressures (Russell, 1971b). Severe poisonings may cause a lapse into coma, respiratory paralysis, and cardiovascular collapse.

Russell (1971b) suggests that victims of black widow bites under 16 years of age, over 60 years of age, with hypertensive heart disease, or with symptoms and signs of severe envenomation be treated with one ampule of antivenin as early as possible. He recommends that in severe cases the antivenin be given intravenously in 10 to 50 ml of saline solution over a 15-minute period, after appropriate allergic tests. Positive-pressure breathing may be indicated, and monitoring of vital signs should occur frequently during the first ten hours following bites in children. For adults, supportive medications are suggested. Methocarbamol, 10 ml intravenously over a five-minute period with another 5 to 10 ml as a drip in 250 ml of 5 percent dextrose, is given to relieve muscle pains, cramps, and other symptoms. With relief, 500 mg every six hours for 24 hours can then be given orally. Calcium gluconate, meperidine, morphine, atropine, and other drugs may be used to relieve muscle pain and spasms. The patient should be further sedated and, if not hospitalized, advised to rest for at least 12 hours (Russell, 1971b).

Brown Recluse Spider (Violin Spider, *Loxosceles reclusus*). This spider was first recognized in 1950 as a cause of toxicity in the United States. It frequently lived in homes and is found on the floor or behind furniture. It is especially prevalent in the southwestern part of the United States. There are a number of species of *Loxosceles*, which vary in their toxicity. However, bites are always potentially hazardous. The brown recluse spider has a hemolytic and necrotizing venom that produces a long-acting, ulcerating wound, which often leaves an extensive disfiguring scar at the site of the bite. Although the bite itself does not usually produce much pain and individuals often are unaware of the initial wound, the injury commonly does not heal for several weeks and occasionally months. In addition to the localized inflammation and necrosis, systemic signs of fever, muscle weakness, nausea, and vomiting may also occur. In severe cases a hemolytic anemia and thrombocytopenia also develop. Treatment of the wound is symptomatic and aimed at protecting the ulcerating lesion from further bacterial contamination while promoting optimal conditions for healing.

Bees, Wasps, Hornets, and Ants

The important stinging insects belong to the order *Hymenoptera* and inject a hemolyzing venom containing histamine by means of a highly specialized venom gland on the last abdominal segment. The usual reaction to the injected venom in a nonsensitized person is variable local inflammation (pain, swelling, and redness), which usually passes in a few hours. Multiple stings can greatly intensify the severity of reaction; it has been estimated that a total of 500 bee stings within a short time is lethal to man (Martini, 1932).

The site of the sting is of great importance, and if the sting is received in the pharyngeal and buccal areas, asphyxiation from swelling in the glottal area can result. Stings received in highly vascular areas may result in severe systemic symptoms due to rapid venom uptake.

The most severe reactions to hymenopterous stings are hypersensitivity manifestations of an allergic nature. Death resulting from anaphylactic shock due to these stings claims approximately 30 people a year in the United States. Severe circulatory, respiratory, and central nervous system reactions occur in some 250,000 reported nonfatal cases annually.

Insects that are particularly common in producing toxicity are ants (California harvester ant, *Pogonomyrmex californicus*; California fire ant, *Solenopsis xyloni*), wasps and hornets (black hornet, *Vespula maculata*; wasps, *Polistes* spp.), and bees (bumble bee, *Bombus californicus*; honey bee, *Apis mellifera*).

Ants. In addition to the California harvester and fire ants, recent surveys document the increasing health hazard of the imported fire ant, *Solenopsis saevissma var. richeteri*, in the southeastern United States (Triplett, 1971). A hemolytic component of fire ant venom has been reported (Adrouny *et al.*, 1959). The unusually severe immediate and delayed anaphylactic reactions to this venom may be related to its unique alkylated piperidine components (Mac-Connell *et al.*, 1970).

Bees and Wasps. The honey bee probably accounts for more deaths in humans that do all the other venomous terrestrial species. Toxicity has also occurred frequently in domestic animals, such as that seen in horses tied to an old tree and attacked by bees. Multiple stings result and death is ultimately due to shock. An allergic response may be developed to bee venom. Sensitized people should carry adrenaline with them during the summer months in the event of contact with hymenoptera.

Honeybee venom is a complex mixture of carbohydrates, lipids, free amino acids, peptides, proteins, and enzymes (O'Connor *et al.*, 1967). A complex protein named mellitin constitutes approximately 50 percent of dried venom and is suspected to be the major antigen that produces hypersensitivity reactions. A single sting of a bee or wasp will produce a local swelling and may cause severe anaphylaxis if the person or animal has already been sensitized. Multiple stings usually cause severe swelling and an allergic response that may cause death in a few minutes to hours. Routine anaphylactic therapy is indicated.

Mosquitoes, Flies, Fleas, Lice, Bedbugs, and Other Bloodsucking Insects

The above group of insects are most commonly characterized by their bloodsucking activities and only secondarily by the toxic aspect of their feeding activity. Various components of their salivas are introduced during the feeding process, and usually only mild transient tissue reactions are a consequence. Their salivary secretions contain anticoagulant factors that facilitate their bloodsucking activities and also certain antigens that may be of consequence in sensitive individuals (Diniz and Corrado, 1971).

Many members of this group are important vectors of disease, and it is of interest to note that those whose bites produce the most severe tissue reactions are seldom disease vectors. The reverse situation is also true (Herms and James, 1961).

Normally phytophagous *Hemiptera* engaging in bloodsucking activities at times have been reported (Myers, 1929). Certain species of the *Membracidae*, *Cicadellidae*, *Miridae*, *Coreidae*, and *Tingidae* families have exhibted this activity. Several members of the order *Thysanoptera* (thrips), which are normally sapsuckers, have been reported as bloodsuckers (Bailey, 1936).

Assassin Bugs and Other Biting Insects

Assassin bugs, also referred to as kissing bugs, belong to the family *Reduviidae* and produce bites that are scarcely exceeded in severity by any other insect. These bites have been widely compared in intensity to those of snakes. Some species are bloodsuckers, but these usually produce much milder bites and often transmit serious diseases. These painful bites may affect a considerable area of the body, and the effects may last for weeks.

Various water bugs are well known for their painful bites. Those of the family *Belostomatidae* measure up to 6.2 cm or more in length and emit a milky fluid through their beak when biting. The pain produced has been described as a burning sensation that usually lasts only several hours. Other water bugs of the family Notonectidae inflict bites that produce only local tissue reactions similar to bee stings.

Certain flies, lice, bugs, and other insects are not bloodsuckers, yet will bite man and animals on occasion, often as a seemingly defensive or offensive action. The piercing of the skin by the mouthparts may be quite painful, but tissue reactions to the bites are usually mild and transitory unless secondary bacterial infection develops.

Urticarious Insects

Urticarious tissue reactions may be produced by contact with the hairy caterpillars of certain Lepidoptera, especially the saddleback, flannel moth, and io moth caterpillars, and by the hairy larvae of some dermestid coleoptera.

The tissue reaction seems to be caused by a hemolytic toxin that also has the property of liberating histamine (Valette and Huidobro, 1954; Valle *et al.*, 1954). The toxic principle is thought to be a reactive component of the hairs themselves. It is possible that some of the evoked reaction occurs by mechanical irritation, but a poison gland has been identified in the hair shaft papillae of the io moth caterpillar (Jones and Miller, 1959). Studies of these structures are documented (Kemper, 1958; Weidner, 1936).

Vesicating Insects

Insects that produce blistering toxins are from the *Meloidae*, *Oedemeridae*, and *Staphlinidae* families of beetles. Cantharidin, the crystalline anhydride of cantharidic acid, and related substances are the vesicants contained in the blood fluids of these insects.

Generally the vesicant contacts the skin when the beetle is killed by a crushing blow, such as slapping or rubbing. The initial tissue reaction is erythema followed by vesicle formation within 24 hours (Leclercq, 1969).

Millipedes exude a vesicating toxin with an odor resembling cyanide on their body surfaces.

Persons handling them have reported blister formation within a few hours following contact.

Ticks

The wood tick, the eastern dog tick, and the Lone Star tick cause toxic manifestations in man by the injection of a hemorrhagic, neurotoxic saliva during their blood-feeding activities. The toxic principle produces hyperemia and hemorrhage in the central nervous system, which may result in an ascending motor paralysis. The severe symptoms usually appear about six days following attachment of the tick. Tick paralysis most commonly appears in children, cattle, sheep, and dogs.

The tick paralysis syndrome is produced most commonly by tick bites of the genera *Dermacentor* and *Ixodes*. The condition is caused by a neurotoxin produced by the feeding female tick. A clinical syndrome of flaccid, afebrile, ascending motor paralysis is produced. The flaccid paralysis is first evident as incoordination, and the paralysis ascends over 24 to 36 hours from the onset, at which time the victim may be completely immobilized. Death results when the paralysis reaches the respiratory center. Removal of the ticks from the victim results in complete recovery within a few hours with no aftereffects. It is of interest that only one tick is necessary to produce signs, and that recovery will be delayed until all ticks are removed from the patient.

Mites

The mites that cause serious reactions are those which burrow in the skin, producing mange and similar skin conditions. The common chigger or redbug is a six-legged larva of the harvest mite that burrows in hair follicles. It is believed that the skin reaction is due to the hyperemic-hemorrhagic nature of its saliva and possibly its body secretions. It is of interest to note that the demodectic mange mite is a harmless commensal in skin follicles on the oily skin areas of man, yet it is incriminated in the most severe type of canine mange.

Centipedes

Centipedes possess venomous fangs on their first body segments, but their bites are rarely of consequence. The tissue reaction involves local inflammation, erythema, edema, and, rarely, purpura involving an entire limb. The burning, aching, local pain, and other symptoms usually disappear in a few hours.

Scorpions

Scorpions are fearsome arthropods that envenomate their victims by means of a stinging apparatus in the last section of their highly mobile tails. Although they produce much suffering and many deaths in various parts of the world, especially Mexico, the only two dangerous species in the United States (*Centruroides sculpturatus* and *Vejovis spinigerus*) are found in southern Arizona. All of the many other species in this country are relatively harmless to man.

The venoms of scorpions thus far studied appear to have similar toxic activities. The venom of the so-called lethal North American scorpion, *Centruroides sculpturatus*, is the most toxic with an intravenous LD50 in mice of 0.096 mg dried venom per kilogram of body weight (Russell, 1971b). The venom of the other North American scorpion, *Vejovis spinigerus*, appears to contain similar components but is less lethal and has a somewhat different mode of action, with the crude venom having no proteolytic, amylase, or phosphatase activity (Russell, 1971b).

Scorpion venoms are known to have an adverse effect on neuromuscular transmission. The venom stimulates the symptoms of strychnine poisoning by acting chiefly on smooth and striated muscle, causing increased excitability and muscle contraction, trembling, and finally paralysis. The neuromuscular effect is most marked at the presynaptic site and least marked on conduction along the nerve (Russell, 1971b). Any direct effects on central nervous system centers, red blood cells, and coagulation are still unclear.

All scorpion venoms produce pain, perhaps due to the presence of 5-hydroxytryptamine. The clinical signs and symptoms of envenomations are limited to localized pain, minor swelling and edema, redness, and increase in local skin temperature. Stings by the more toxic North American scorpions produce additional symptoms of skin flushing, parasympathetic activity, muscle fasciculations and twitchings, hyperirritability and hyperactivity, hypertension, muscle weakness, and occasional paresthesias of the involved extremity. Severe cases may develop a generalized weakness and paralysis and eventual respiratory distress. Although symptoms usually improve in 15 to 20 hours (Vellard, 1947), fatalities do occur. Mortality is much higher in children than in adults.

Treatment of scorpion stings should include use of appropriate antivenin when the case warrants. Antivenin is usually administered to severely poisoned individuals, the very young, the elderly, or individuals with hypertension (Russell, 1971b). Muscle relaxants and mild sedation are often employed in adults, together with atropine for parasympathetic dysfunction and muscle spasms. Respiratory assistance is necessary when respiratory depression occurs.

AMPHIBIAN AND REPTILE TOXINS

The study of amphibians and reptiles is classified as herpetology. The biology and handling of this group of animals are interesting and unique (VandenBerg, 1972). This class of animals may be the most important and common cause of poisonings of animal origin (Harmon and Pollard, 1948; Rosenfeld and Kelen, 1969). It includes toxicities due to amphibians (toads and salamanders), lizards, and snakes.

Amphibians

Many amphibian species have glandular secretions of the skin that prevent desiccation, control the growth of microorganisms on the skin, and discourage predators. The secretions have cytotoxic effects, and some also have hemolyzing effects on red blood cells.

Toads. All toads secrete substances in skin glands that are repulsive to animals that mouth them. Dogs, especially puppies, are particularly prone to play with toads and thereby come in contact with this repulsive material. Except in the case of children, who accidentally place toads in their mouths or place their fingers in their mouths after handling toads, humans are not particularly affected by toad poisoning.

The more toxic amphibian species are the Colorado River toads (*Bufo alvarius*), marine toads (*Bufo marinus*), and arrow poison frogs of Central America (*Dendrobates* sp.). Most poisonings are observed in dogs and cats that attack and bite or mouth the *Bufo* species of toads. The species mentioned above secrete particularly toxic venom complexes that have a distinct cardioactive digitalis-like action. In the United States the problem of toad poisoning has distinct geographic distribution. Recent imports of toads to the Florida area within the past ten years have resulted in individual veterinarians treating as many as 40 cases of poisoning in dogs and cats annually. The drainage of the Colorado River into Arizona and California has caused the population of toxic toads to present increasing hazards to the small animal population in the southwest. It has been estimated that in excess of 50 dogs a year die from toad poisoning in Hawaii.

The *Bufo* species of toads have parotid glands (skin glands) behind the eyes that secrete a complex venom with an action similar to that of cardiac glycosides. The arrow poison frogs from Central America also contain these cardioactive glycosides in various places on the skin, but they do not have a prominent parotid gland. The other skin glands of *Bufo* spp. also have some of this toxic material, although concentrations are not as great as those secreted by the parotid glands. Other species of toads also contain substances that are objectionable to animals when they are mouthed. Particularly sensitive are young puppies and kittens, since the toxic glycosides are sufficiently potent to cause death within 10 to 15 minutes in these small, immature animals.

The clinical syndrome is developed within a few minutes after the dog or cat mouths the toad or the child places fingers coated with the glandular secretion in its mouth. Initial signs are those of a profuse salivation with pulmonary edema, cardiac arrhythmia, hypertension, and prostration developing within minutes. Convulsions develop rapidly, and death due to cardiac arrest may be observed as early as 15 minutes after initial contact with the toxic secretions.

Treatment is largely aimed at removing as much as possible of the unabsorbed secretions from the mouth and controlling the clinical signs. Washing of the victim's mouth with abundant water, frequently from a garden hose, and administering atropine to control salivation are early treatments that should promptly be implemented. Barbiturates should be additionally administered to control convulsions, and calcium gluconate may be useful in combating some of the physiologic effects (Knowles, 1968). Artificial respiration to maintain respiratory function may also be useful in prolonging the life of acutely exposed animals. Because of the cardioactive effect of the toxins, Otani *et al.* (1969) have found that adrenergic-blocking agents are useful in toad poisoning. Phenoxybenzamine is recommended to block alpha-adrenergic receptors, and propranolol is used to block the beta-adrenergic receptors. The latter compound also has an antifibrillatory action against the cardiac glycosides. This therapy has proven very effective in experimental cases, apparently because the cardiac syndrome produced by the *Bufo* toxin is similar to synergistic effects of cardioactive glycosides and ephedrine. Supportive care in maintaining vital functions contributes to a satisfactory and rapid clinical recovery.

Salamanders. This group of amphibians with potential toxic capabilities includes the California newt (*Taricha torosa*), the European newt (*Tariturus* sp.), and the unk (*Bombia variegota*).

Tetrodotoxin, the same toxin found in puffer fish, and additional toxic components are found associated with the salamander group. The roe or eggs from these animals, and the skin, contain quantities of this potent poison that is toxic at levels of 10 μg/kg of body weight. Ingestion of the toxin results in tingling of the oral cavity with salivation, muscle weakness and motor incoordination, skin numbness, vomiting and diarrhea, and a generalized paralysis with convulsions and death in severe cases.

Salamander poisoning is rare and when it occurs is most often observed in small, young domestic animals.

Lizards

The only genus of poisonous lizard, *Heloderma*, contains the two species of poisonous lizards *Heloderma suspectum* (gila monster) and *Heloderma horridum* (the Mexican beaded lizard).

Toxicity due to lizards is a result of envenomation during bites from the grooved upper teeth. All the teeth are dangerous, not just the rear fangs as is occasionally incorrectly cited in the literature. There are four venom glands on each side that bathe the teeth from the top and provide the venom to produce toxicity. Lizards usually bite and then hang on to their victims. The resulting chewing may help to increase the degree of envenomation, but even a simple bite is sufficiently dangerous to produce poisoning. Fortunately, lizards are quite lethargic and are not aggressive. Humans and animals are usually not bitten.

However, in instances of lizard bites, the clinical syndrome initiates with pain and swelling at the wound site. Since the bite is usually on an extremity, the clinical reaction then progresses toward the body. Vomiting may occur and is followed by shock and central nervous system depression. Only rarely do fatalities occur, and then usually it is in debilitated or very young individuals. Treatment is aimed at supporting vital functions and reducing the clinical effects of the toxicity.

Poisonous Snakes

Snakes are the most widely distributed of all reptiles; both poisonous and harmless species are found on all continents (Dowling *et al.*, 1968; Moore, 1965; Russell and Scharffenberg, 1964). In the United States, some 2,500 species of snakes are found. Poisonous species occur in all the states except Maine, Alaska, and Hawaii. Texas, Georgia, Florida, Alabama, and southern California are areas that tend to have higher-than-normal incidences of snakebite (Wadsworth, 1973). The most common intoxication of animal origin is probably that produced by snakes.

Classification of Poisonous Snakes. A great variety of venomous snakes are in existence (Brown, 1973; Dowling *et al.*, 1968; Moore, 1965). All are in the Class *Reptilia*, Order *Squamata*, and Suborder *Ophidia*. The poisonous species all fall into one of the following families:

Elapidae, the elapids, which include the cobras and coral snakes; *Hydrophidae*, the sea snakes; *Viperidae*, including the true vipers such as the Russell's viper and puff adder; *Crotalidae*, the pit vipers such as the rattlesnakes; and Colubridae, containing the boomslang and mangrove snake.

The elapids (Family *Elapidae*) include the most poisonous snakes in the world. The cobras, kraits, coral snakes, and tiger snake fall into this family. They may not, however, account for the most deaths in either animals or humans. They are characterized by having a fixed front fang that is rather short but still very effective. It does not rotate as it does in the vipers. The venom gland is located superficially behind the eye of the snake. Injury produced by bites may be prevented by sewing the snake's mouth shut, as is done by exotic dancers, or by performing a vasectomy to eliminate the channeling of the venom of the gland to the fang. This group is extremely dangerous. The king cobra, which is 5.4 to 6 m in length, is capable of killing a man in just a few minutes. The most toxic species, however, is the small (0.9 to 1.2 m long) Australian tiger snake. Although it is a cobra type, it does not hood up. There are two different types of coral snakes in the United States—the Eastern and the Arizonan—both of which have a cobra-like venom. They are small species with characteristic red and black bands separated by white or yellow bands. The tip of the nose is black. Some species may not be much larger than a pencil. The coral snakes are nonaggressive and are usually not seen because they are under cover. Inquisitive small domestic animals or children may be bitten when traveling through underbrush.

The sea snakes (*Hydrophidae*) are strictly marine and usually live in brackish water. All the sea snakes are poisonous and have a cobra-like appearance with fixed front fangs. Toxicity does not occur, due to lack of contact between these snakes and potential victims.

The Family *Viperidae* are the true vipers and include species that account for more human and animal deaths than any other group of snakes. They are characterized by having long, movable fangs on the upper jaw that rotate back up into the mouth when not in use. The fang is attached to a venom gland. The Russell viper is a pretty snake that has good concealment in undergrowth. It kills more people in Asia than does the cobra. The African puff adder kills more people in Africa than do all the other animals put together. Another African species, the gaboon viper, is closely related to the puff adder, is extremely pugnacious, and is capable of lethal effects.

The pit vipers of the Family *Crotalidae* are

snake venoms. More likely, phospholipase A may facilitate the penetration of other neuro-pharmacologically active venom components into nerve tissue (Russell, 1971b). The specific pharmacologic effects of phospholipase B and phospholipase C are not currently known, but their activity has been found in a number of snake venoms.

Several phosphatases involved in the hydrolysis of phosphate bonds in nucleotides are found in snake venoms. In most instances 5′-nucleotidase is the most active phosphatase in the venom. It catalyzes the hydrolysis of 5′-mononucleotides and yields the ribonucleoside and orthophosphate. Phosphodiesterase has also been found in almost all snake venoms tested and causes the release of 5′-nucleotides from polynucleotides. Several phosphodiesterases with similar enzymatic properties may also be in some venoms.

Acetylcholine is found in large amounts in venom from mambas (*Dendroaspis* sp.) and is present in smaller amounts in other elapid and crotalid venoms. It may act directly on the heart or at the neuromuscular junction of the victim. It may also facilitate the distribution of more toxic components of the venom (Brown, 1973; Russell, 1971b).

Pit Viper Bites. The eastern or Florida diamondback rattlesnake and the western or Texas diamondback rattlesnake are the most dangerous and powerful poisonous snakes in the United States. The Texas diamondback probably causes more deaths than any other rattlesnake. The copperhead is the least poisonous of the pit vipers, while the water moccasin (or cottonmouth) is the meanest tempered of the pit vipers. It has been known to attack unprovoked, which most snakes seldom do (Wadsworth, 1973).

Most pit vipers have fangs long enough to penetrate the muscle of their victim. They strike in less than a second and can accurately strike a distance of one-half their body length. Although diamondback rattlesnakes may eject 75 percent of their venom per strike, most snakes rarely empty their venom glands at one ejection. Even though a snake's head is severed from the body, the bite reflex may persist for nearly an hour (Wadsworth, 1973).

Pit vipers produce one or two large puncture marks with rapid swelling and discoloration developing at the bite site. This reaction develops into a marked edema and erythema that may extend over the entire portion of the body. Immediate excruciating pain is characteristic. The swelling is extremely sensitive to touch and, if on a leg, produces painful and stiff locomotion. If swelling at the bite site does not occur within

30 minutes, the bite was probably not produced by a pit viper.

Although most bites occur on one of the extremities, strikes may also occur on the head or neck. This is especially common in domestic animals where curiosity results in their probing the snake with their nose. Such bites may result in respiratory distress due to rapid swelling of facial or throat tissues. Difficult respiration, cyanosis, and suffocation may result if individuals so bitten are not promptly treated to provide an unobstructed air passageway.

The victim of pit viper bite usually becomes excited, apprehensive, and anxious. Nausea, vomiting, and diarrhea may result. Victims often complain of excessive thirst. Shock is an important clinical result in infants, elderly persons, and small animals. Anaphylactic reactions to the proteins in the snake venom occur, but are rare. Cardiac effects are observed as a rapid, weak pulse and a profound fall in systemic arterial blood pressure. A fall in circulating blood volume appears to be due to pooling in abdominal organs. Central nervous system signs of incoordination may lead to respiratory paralysis in severe cases.

With increasing survival time, the necrotizing and hemolytic properties of the venom will be demonstrated. A hemolytic anemia and hemoglobinuria will be seen if the patient survives for several hours. By that time the tissue reaction to bites of the head or neck may have produced sufficient swelling to seal the eyes shut and interfere with eating. A blood-stained frothy exudate may be discharged from the nose and reflects the tissue destruction from the bite. Additional changes that occur with increasing survival time are thrombosis and hemorrhage into peripheral tissues, changes in resistance and permeability of blood vessels, alterations in the integrity of blood cells, changes in heart dynamics and nerve conduction, and the development of cerebral anoxia, pulmonary edema, and heart failure (Arena, 1970; Russell, 1971b). The clinical effects are usually more severe in young persons and in small domestic animals and humans.

The necrotizing effect of the pit viper venom on the injected tissues is manifested as painful, localized necrosis and tissue sloughing of the bite area several days after the bite. This is often complicated with wound infections produced by organisms introduced at the time of the bite or during the subsequent sloughing process. These local necrotic areas may persist for several weeks. Healing is usually slow due to the continual drainage from the wound. Granulation and scar formation ultimately reestablish tissue continuity.

Since the swelling of the bite area frequently

reduces the opportunity for observing the fang wounds, the diagnosis of snakebite may be easily confused with other conditions causing swelling of an extremity. Fractures of the limbs or head, bruises, hematomas, infections of the head or subcutaneous tissue (cellulitis), allergic reactions, arthritis, and even photosensitization may all resemble snakebite and must be included in a differential diagnosis.

The *therapy* of snakebite should be handled as an emergency, since it requires immediate attention and considerable judgment. The attending doctor is faced with a patient who may die from the effects of one or several of the venom components. Since several organ systems may be involved and death may result within several minutes or several days, multiple modes of action must be considered (Arena, 1970; Kaye, 1970; Russell, 1971b).

The first 30 to 45 minutes are most important, and it is important to retard venom absorption, to remove as much of it as possible, or to neutralize or reduce its effects. The physician must give careful attention to the patient's electrocardiogram and respiration, to the location and extent of local tissue involvement, and to electrolyte and blood studies. The patient should be kept quiet and calm, and he should be encouraged not to move the affected part of the body. The affected limb should be lowered below the level of the heart and for body bites the individual should remain seated or lie down. Since the snake producing the bite will usually remain in the immediate area, it should be found and killed, if possible. It should not, however, be handled (Wadsworth, 1973).

Occasionally patients may develop allergic reactions and may die in minutes following the bite. The administration of corticosteroids or epinephrine will be of lifesaving value in such instances. Antihistamines are not uniformly recommended since they are of questionable value and have been shown experimentally to compound snakebite toxicity in some instances.

Prevention of spread of the toxin may be accomplished by applying a light constrictive band or tourniquet 2.5 to 10 cm above the bite. Since the venom travels via the lymphatics and not the bloodstream, the application of a tight tourniquet is not necessary. The band should be released every 10 to 15 minutes for one to two minutes. This tourniquet should be removed as soon as antivenin is given. Cold packs to the area may also be employed to reduce circulation. Freezing of the treated wound, however, must be avoided. Incision of the fang marks and the application of suction for approximately one hour after the bite may also be employed to remove the injected venom. Since a large portion of the venom will be injected subcutaneously, the incision does not have to penetrate very deeply. If more than one hour has elapsed since the bite, local incision and suction may not be of much benefit. Oral suction should be avoided, if possible, since absorption of the venom from the oral mucosa and through mucosal wounds is possible. The surgical excision of the bitten area (removing a disk of skin and subcutaneous tissue around the fang marks) has also been recommended. Its use is controversial, since in many patients the venom may already have been distributed well beyond the bitten area before treatment is instituted. Although 20 percent or more of the venom may be removed by such a procedure if performed shortly after the bite, the traumatic effect of the surgery and the usual slow healing that follows suggest that surgical intervention during the acute phase of the toxicity is contraindicated except in rare cases (Russell, 1971b).

The most beneficial single action for snakebite therapy is probably the early and vigorous use of antivenin, and preferably species-specific antivenin. When the snake producing the bite is identified or a reasonable estimate can be made of its identity, antivenin may be secured from large hospitals, from poison control centers, or directly from suppliers such as Wyeth Laboratories or Merck Sharp & Dohme. Polyvalent antivenin is available for various species; 5 to 50 ml is administered depending on the victim's size and the location and severity of the bite.

In individuals with wounds around the head, nose, or neck, the maintenance of a patent airway is often lifesaving. Small animals and horses are frequently bitten in the head region, and the swelling often necessitates a tracheotomy or the passage of a nasal tube to assure adequate ventilation. The administration of oxygen may be necessary in some animals that are already exhibiting signs of anoxia due to respiratory embarrassment prior to the establishment of a patent air passage.

Symptomatic therapy should then be instituted to reduce some of the more severe signs and symptoms associated with snakebite. Shock must be avoided and precautions taken for its treatment if initial signs develop. Muscle spasms are treated with calcium gluconate, convulsions with sedatives, and any impending coma with appropriate stimulants (Arena, 1970). Evidences of hemolysis and/or hemorrhage should be combated by blood transfusions, fluid and electrolyte therapy, or the administration of calcium gluconate solutions. Pain may be relieved by the administration of analgesics. However, except in certain cases, such supportive measures should not be considered substitutes for antianaphylactic therapy, procedures to reduce the spread of the toxin, and the administration of antivenin (Russell, 1971b).

Additional therapy that may be useful to reduce tissue damage and complications includes the treatment of tissue necrosis by the application of cold packs and proteolytic enzymes, and routine open-wound therapy. Because bacterial infections frequently complicate snakebite wounds, the administration of tetanus antitoxin and the prolonged applications of broad-spectrum antibiotics are useful additional measures. Scarring and bacterial complications are significantly reduced by these efforts. The use of ligatures and cryotherapy are of questionable value because of the large amount of tissue destruction that results. The application of potassium permanganate to the wound is of additional dubious benefit. While potassium permanganate may inactivate venom *in vitro*, such is not its action *in vivo*.

Humans bitten by pit vipers often undergo good recovery with prompt and thorough therapy. Individuals who receive delayed and limited treatment develop toxicity that is largely dependent upon the species of snake involved, the amount of venom injected, and the victim's own physical and biologic characteristics. Recovery is usual in most domestic animals, although persistent treatment is required for small pets and horses, and especially for those receiving bite wounds that result in respiratory distress. In the majority of cases, tissue necrosis of the bite area is the only common persistent lesion.

Coral Snakebites. Although coral snakes have bitten humans and dogs in the area of the United States in which they are found naturally, this elapid snake is not aggressive and usually produces injury only if disturbed. In some large metropolitan areas, certain individuals keep poisonous snakes and are potential victims for elapid (coral snake or cobra) bite toxicity. It is estimated that there are approximately 3,000 pet cobras within the Los Angeles city limits.

Coral snakes have permanent, immovable fangs. In order to inject its venom the snake must bite and hang on to the area attacked. Because it must gain leverage to bite, it cannot bite a flat surface. Hence, few deaths are produced by coral snakes, even though it is one of the most poisonous snakes in the United States. Although its venom is highly toxic, many of its bites are ineffective in injecting sufficient venom to produce poisoning (Wadsworth, 1973).

Coral snake venom is predominantly neurotoxic in effect and produces little to no local reaction or swelling at the bite site. No local pain is felt. However, within minutes (often indicated as a 20-minute period) the victim will begin showing signs of the neurotoxic effect of the venom. Depression, inability to swallow, paralytic signs, recumbency and paresis, evidence of pain that is associated with the paresis, and finally vital center paralysis and death may occur within a few hours (Arena, 1970; Brown, 1973; Wadsworth, 1973). These central nervous system effects also include numbness of limbs, disorientation, and skeletal paralysis. Death is due to respiratory paralysis (Simpson, 1971).

The *therapy* of elapid snakebites is more specific than that of pit viper bites. The rapidity of the neurotoxic action limits the effectiveness of the general and symptomatic measures previously suggested. Such efforts, however, should be attempted while more specific antivenin treatment is being secured. The only effective therapy for elapid poisoning is the specific antivenin. Although more general or polyvalent elapid antivenins are available from commercial institutions, the nearest and often most specific antivenin may be available from the closest large zoologic collection having a reptile collection. Most such zoos maintain a reasonably complete line of antivenins for the snake species they are housing. Communication with such facilities will usually result in rapid delivery of the necessary antivenin and a great strengthening of the victim's prognosis for recovery.

Pharmacologic Uses of Snake Venoms. Facilities are now functioning to collect the venom of various snakes for use in research and for therapeutic purposes. The production of antivenin is an important public and animal health function that requires diligence and specific techniques. The availability of this lifesaving product is a priceless commodity for the victim of a severe snakebite. Research activities utilizing snake venoms have included studies of enzyme activity, investigations into the mechanisms of blood coagulation, and extensive studies of the factors governing nerve activity. Venoms or fractions of venoms have also been used therapeutically to control intractable pain. The future will no doubt see further uses of snake venom. These ongoing investigations will continue to contribute significantly to man's understanding of the factors governing his biologic functions.

A Word to the Wise. A few precautions to assist in avoiding snakebites may be well spent if they are taken and applied conscientiously. In order to avoid snakes, and their bites, potential victims should stay away from them. Since snakes are fearful of animals and humans, deliberate attempts to handle or capture snakes should be recognized as hazardous. Since snakes swim, waters known to contain snakes should be avoided. Snake-den areas should be left alone so as not to disturb possible snake nests. Individuals should not go barefooted or alone into country known to contain poisonous snakes. Hands should never be placed on rock ledges, under boards, or into hollow logs, and camping should be avoided near brush piles, rocks, or dead logs. Playing with a live or dead snake, or going out of one's way to kill a snake, merely increases the danger of becoming snakebitten (Wadsworth, 1973).

VENOMOUS MAMMALS

Even within the group of mammals, known venomous species exist. These include the platypus, the spiny anteater, and shrews (Bücherl et al., 1968–1971). The biology, physiology, general husbandry, and medicine of the marine mammals have been documented by Ridgway (1972).

Platypus

The venom apparatus of the duckbill platypus (Ornithorhynchos anatinus) is found only in the male. It is a movable horny spur found on the inside of each hind leg near the heel. The venomous spur is enfolded into the skin, but is extended when required. Each spur is connected to a crural or poison gland. While usually used against other members of the species, it has also been used against man occasionally.

Attacks on man have been few and, since the venom is not highly lethal, have usually not been fatal. Following an attack by the platypus, the clinical signs include immediate intense pain at the site of the injury, swelling that extends some distance from the wound, and a feeling of numbness around the injury. Varying degrees of shock, such as weakness, may also occur. The edema of the injured tissue usually subsides in a few days. No specific treatment is recommended except for rest, sedatives, and routine treatment of the injured area. Animals other than man have also been attacked and similar signs are described (Bücherl et al., 1968–1971).

Spiny Anteaters

The spiny anteaters (Tachyglossus sp. and Zaglossus sp.) belong to the order Echidna. The anatomy of their venom apparatus and the action of their venom are similar to those of the platypus. Injuries inflicted by the spur produce immediate pain and subsequent swelling of the injured area. The degree of toxicity and the recovery are similar to those of the platypus.

Insectivora

The Order Insectivora has venom-bearing species in only two families, the Solenodontidae

and the Soricidae (Bücherl et al., 1968–1971). The toxin is carried in the saliva of the submaxillary glands and is transmitted to the victim by bite wounds.

Solenodon paradoxus. These squirrel-sized mammals are found only on the island of Haiti. Their submaxillary glands are quite large and have ducts that open near the base of the large, deeply channeled second incisor. The toxin-bearing saliva is carried from the gland duct along the channels of the second incisors and is drawn upward into the bite wound by capillary action (Bücherl et al., 1968–1971). Pain and inflammation around the bite punctures of the lower incisors result, but little if any inflammation occurs at the wounds produced by the upper incisors. Recovery from clinical signs usually occurs within one to three days. Experimental animals injected with extracts of the submaxillary glands have developed systemic toxicity terminating in paralysis and convulsions. This syndrome has not been described in field cases of bites.

Sorex, sp. The European water shrew and the short-tailed shrew both have abundant cells in the submaxillary salivary glands that produce toxins secreted into the saliva and transmitted to the victim by bite wounds. Large amounts of saliva are excreted by the shrews, and the concavity of the first incisors serves to collect and transmit the copious amounts of poison-bearing secretion to the bite-wound area from the submaxillary ducts that open near the base of the incisors. Shrew bites produce immediate burning sensations at the site of the punctures, followed by shooting pains that reach maximum intensity in about one hour. Pain is present for several days and subsequent discomfort often lasts more than a week (Bücherl et al., 1968–1971). Deaths have not been reported in humans, although investigations of the insectivore toxin indicate that it pharmacologically resembles that of the elapid snakes. Neurotoxic signs have been experimentally produced in animals, with convulsions and death occurring.

MAMMALS WITH HIGH HEPATIC VITAMIN A

Polar Bear

This white mammal of the polar regions has induced toxicity when its liver has been consumed as human or animal food. The polar bear's liver is extremely high in vitamin A, and toxicity from hypervitaminosis A has resulted.

Other Marine Mammals

The bearded seal and the walrus also have livers that are high in vitamin A content. Use of

Chapter 22

PHYTOTOXICOLOGY

John M. Kingsbury

INTRODUCTION

At the subcellular level, plants and animals display more similarities than differences. Consider the processes of replication of information, genetic recombination, development of subcellular structures, and respiration. Attention should be focused on the fact that, although plants and animals are different, they are evolving branches of a common origin. The study of phytotoxicology, then, is an examination of those products characteristic of one major part of the biota that produce or evoke a specific deleterious reaction when they interact with systems characteristic of the other. This view emphasizes the differences that have evolved between plants and animals despite their common beginnings. In every plant poisoning case it should be possible to identify precisely the plant product and the animal system involved, the route by which they are brought together, and the specific subsequent events that occur until the animal either dies or recovers. However, according to a recent authoritative statement on this subject, "Probably no field of scientific endeavor exists in which it is more difficult to separate fact from fiction than in the study of poisonous plants. Examination of the pertinent literature will reveal considerable confusion tending to mask an even greater amount of ignorance. . . . Unbelievable chaos reigns in the area of plant identification and nomenclature as applied by the nonspecialist" (Claus *et al.*, 1970).

This chapter is directed toward three main topics: (1) the importance of poisonous plants to man and animals, (2) an assessment of current knowledge of poisonous plants, and (3) a discussion of the effects of toxic principles elaborated by plants.

IMPORTANCE OF POISONOUS PLANTS TO MAN AND ANIMALS

Although incomplete, the best figures on incidence of human poisoning by plants are those collected from individual poison control centers and analyzed by the National Clearinghouse for Poison Control Centers (National Clearinghouse for Poison Control Centers, 1972). Ingestions are grouped by categories in the annual summaries. Plants as a category have consistently ranked in the top seven, accounting for about 4 percent of the reported ingestions until the 1970s. In 1970, plants (excluding mushrooms and toadstools) accounted for 4,059 reported ingestions, representing 4.8 percent of all reported ingestions for that year. This was greater than the number of disinfectant, tranquilizer, insecticide, hormone, acid and alkali, antiseptic, polish, or paint ingestions and was exceeded only by the incidence of ingestion of aspirin and soap-detergents-cleaners. Since then, however, plants as a category has come to the top of the list of "products" most frequently implicated in poisoning of children under 5 years of age. Now, about one out of every ten cases reported by poison control centers is related to plants. This conspicuous rise in importance of plants since 1965 is related to the equally dramatic decrease in cases of poisoning from aspirin. These have fallen from greater than 25 percent of reported incidents in 1965 to just 4.1 percent in 1976. Safety packaging, limited quantities per package, and increased public awareness of hazards—the result of governmental and private compaigns—have been the main contributing factors in reducing the importance of aspirin. Only the latter method of decreasing incidents is easily applicable to the unnecessarily high volume (O'Leary, 1964; Subcommittee on Weeds, 1968) of ingestions involving plants now being experienced at poison control centers. According to reported figures (O'Leary, 1964) there are approximately 75,000 human ingestions of poisonous plants in the United States each year (Subcommittee on Weeds, 1968). According to Canadian figures (MacEachen *et al.*, 1968), ingestions of nonfood plants are more than ten times greater than the number of reported incidents involving venomous bites or stings.

The above figures need to be viewed with a certain amount of caution. First, the majority of the ingestions were of materials, or in amounts,

The foregoing discussion presents reasons why current practices make it difficult to deal with poisonous plants. There are historic reasons as well. At the risk of oversimplification, they may be summarized as follows (for a detailed discussion, see Kingsbury, 1964).

The Greeks and Romans were astute and recorded, in some detail and with commendable accuracy, their conclusions concerning the useful, medicinal, or toxic characteristics of the natural world. For most areas of knowledge, these collected observations went into eclipse during the Dark Ages, surviving largely as manuscripts copied from generation to generation without significant addition or modification. This was not the case with poisonous materials, for the practice of poisoning to obtain succession of royalty or ecclesiastical authority, inheritance of wealth, or defeat of armies became a highly developed art (Lewin, 1920). Persons able to get results commanded high fees. In order to protect their hard-won trade secrets, these artisans compounded recipes with many esoteric ingredients, thereby obscuring the identity of the actual active principle. A perhaps overdrawn, but nonetheless illuminating example is the several-stanza list of ingredients that went into the witches' cauldron in Shakespeare's *Macbeth*; only two (yew and hemlock) could be expected to do the job.

With the Renaissance, it became necessary to separate fact from fiction, something that was only imperfectly accomplished. Further confusion resulted from an innocent attempt to relate the reports of the classic authors, who dealt mainly with Mediterranean plants, to the flora of central and northern Europe. Keep in mind that the science of naming plants originated with Linneaus' *Species Plantarum* of 1753; before that time all names applied to plants had no more authority than the common names used today.

Herbals supplanted classic manuscripts around 1470; floras and tomes on materia medica supplanted herbals around 1670; all contained frequent reference to toxic capacities of plants. Monographs devoted solely to poisonous plants began to appear shortly before 1700. All of these works were European, and interested educated persons were expected to know the literature of their subject well enough so that citation of authority for particular statements was not deemed necessary. Hence, for the most part, the first books dealing with poisonous plants do not say where the information came from. Most later writers on poisonous plants have apparently been reluctant to eliminate anything that sounds reasonable, in spite of their inability to verify the information. Some patently unreasonable things are also perpetuated. Even today, books may appear in which medieval error is repeated unconsciously (Baskin, 1967) but with devastating effect (Dress, 1967) if taken as scientifically accurate documents.

In 1814 M. J. B. Orfila published the first edition of his substantial work on toxicology, to which the use of an experimental approach in toxicology is generally traced. Orfila experimented with a number of plants, describing their effects and attempting to trace the distribution of the poisonous principle in

that would not have proved capable of eliciting a toxic response, or else treatment, usually emesis, intervened before such a response occurred. These, strictly speaking, are better defined as ingestions than as poisonings, without implying whether a toxic reaction was or was not possible. Second, many incidents (possibly a majority) are treated by private physicians who do not report to a poison control center. In addition, some poison control centers fail to report to the National Clearinghouse. Thus, the precise number of toxic responses that occur from plants annually in the human population cannot be determined from these data.

Poisoning of pets and livestock is even more extensive than is poisoning of man. No reliable figures exist, but estimates as to loss of range livestock in western states consistently place the annual figure at more than one million dollars per state or region. Certainly, well-documented instances in which more than 1,500 animals have been killed at a single time, such as losses of sheep to *Halogeton glomeratus*, represent considerable economic impact and do not need to be multiplied by many such events or by many similar plants to assume major importance to the livestock industry. The resulting economic loss includes not only the value of the animals but also the diminution in real value of the range acreage following its infestation with a poisonous weed. Losses of pets (Kingsbury, 1974) and wild animals are so poorly documented that no useful generalizations are possible.

CURRENT KNOWLEDGE OF POISONOUS PLANTS

Effective consideration of phytotoxicology requires a synthesis across wide academic boundaries and is thus difficult. This, and the diversity of natural phenomena dealt with, perhaps more than other factors, have inhibited a more rapid, rigorous, development of the subject. Comparison of the principal current references (Kingsbury, 1964; Radeleff, 1964; Food Protection Committee, 1966; Lampe and Fagerström, 1968, Liener, 1969; Morton, 1971; Hardin and Arena, 1974) dealing with North American poisonous plants shows immediately that fundamental input and analysis are required from botany, physiology, and pathology. In all cases, full development of a particular topic also requires the attention of one or more academic or practical specialists, such as physician, veterinarian, toxicologist, clinician, organic chemist or biochemist, plant physiologist, pharmacologist, pharmacognocist, agronomist, horticulturist, geneticist, and animal husbandman. Consideration must be given to identification and description of a toxic reaction; practical understanding of the history, to aid in diagnosis and in formulating control; secure determination of the etiology (species of plant involved); identification and perhaps isola-

tion of a toxic principle; specific description of its action; the seasonal, ecologic, and genetic control of production of the toxic principle by the plant; and the way in which man or animals were or may be exposed. The latter involves agricultural practices in the case of livestock. In man, a plethora of possibilities exist, from overuse of plant-derived drugs by adults to accidental or experimental ingestions of drugs or whole plant parts by children.

Approximately 700 species of North American plants are considered to be poisonous on the basis of case histories, experimental investigations, or other specific reasons (Kingsbury, 1964). More will be discovered. This is only a small fraction of the perhaps 30,000 species of plants in the wild and cultivated floras of North America. Nevertheless, it is a large number, and no generalization emerges from a review of their botany, ecology, or management by man to allow systematizing them for easier comprehension. Poisonous species are scattered throughout the plant kingdom from algae, to ferns, to gymnosperms, to angiosperms, and in the latter large groups they appear almost randomly among the plant families. One sometimes hears that certain groups such as the nightshade or potato family (Solanaceae) are particularly dangerous, but such statements are not entirely valid. Such families are the larger ones, and contain poisonous species more or less in relation to their size.

Toxicity usually exists at the level of the genus. If one species of a genus is toxic, some or all others in that genus usually display similar toxicity. This is why species names are sometimes omitted in general discussions of toxicity. This is a mistake. First, exceptions to the generalization are numerous and important. Second, even when similar species display similar toxicity, they may have other important differences. For example, most species of the genus *Asclepias* (milkweeds) are toxic, but the most toxic species (*A. labriformis*) is found only in a limited area of Utah. However, the most troublesome milkweeds (*A. subverticillata*, *A. eriocarpa*) differ in appearance from the former and have significantly less toxicity on a weight basis, but are much more widely distributed geographically. Important distinctions such as these are lost when species names are not used.

In some cases, groups of genera within a single family display similar toxicity. This is true, for example, of the laurel group of the heath family (Ericaceae). At the other extreme, however, are those instances in which closely related species differ in toxicity. *Eupatorium rugosum* is closely related to the numerous other species of *Eupatorium*, but *only* the former is known to be toxic. Occasionally the same toxic principle is found in plants of great botanical or habitat difference.

For example, the only other plant known to contain the same poisonous principle as *Eupatorium rugosum* is *Aplopappus heterophyllus*. These two are in the same plant family (Compositae), but the former is found in woodlands of eastern North America while the latter is limited to the dry ranges of the Southwest. Nicotine, as another example, can be isolated from plants as botanically distant as tobacco (*Nicotiana tabacum*) of the nightshade or potato family of angiosperms, and from club moss (*Lycopodium* spp.) of the primitive, spore-bearing lycopods.

The content of a given poisonous principle, and even to some extent its molecular structure, can vary widely in some species with the environmental conditions under which the plant grew. This is particularly true of many glycosides. In other cases, certain alkaloids for instance, elaboration of the poisonous principle in a given species in under reasonably tight genetic control and varies little with growing conditions. Even when under strict genetic control, the content of a poisonous principle in a given plant may vary with stage of growth; it may concentrate in particular parts of the plant, or it may vary with the particular variety or strain of plant.

Exemplifying the last point, one of the nightshades exists in two distinct populations, which fortunately do not normally interbreed. The botanic distinctions between them are so small that the two populations were originally recognized as a single species (*Solanum nigrum*). One kind, however, is quite toxic. The other, now set off taxonomically as *Solanum intrusum*, is not known to be toxic. In fact, *S. intrusum* has entered trade as "garden huckleberry" or "wonderberry" and is sometimes recommended to home gardeners for its edible fruits. Poinsettia (*Euphorbia pulcherrima*) may represent a similar example. Its listing as toxic was founded originally on a reported case of human mortality in Hawaii in 1919. Recent feeding experiments (Stone and Collins, 1971), prompted by the belief of horticulturists that the poinsettia is really not poisonous, showed no toxic effect in rodents fed large quantities of the red bracts. However, poison control centers continue to report instances of gastric distress in children after ingestion of poinsettia. A possible explanation for the apparent conflict in these several observations is the very great horticultural manipulation that has in recent years been devoted to breeding showier, longer-lasting, and differently colored poinsettias. It is reasonable to suppose that the ability to form a toxic principle may have been consciously selected against at the same time that desirable floral characteristics were sought. If this is the case, older varieties of poinsettia, or ones dis-

The National Clearinghouse for Poison Control Centers published a detailed review of the collected reports of plant ingestions for 1965 that were treated as poisoning emergencies (Verhulst and Crotty, 1966). Their list of the "top ten" is shown in Table 22–1. If reporting were accurate,

Table 22–1. PLANTS RESPONSIBLE FOR INGESTIONS REPORTED MOST FREQUENTLY BY POISON CONTROL CENTERS IN 1965*

Pokeweed	Holly
Yew	Honeysuckle
Philodendron	Pyracantha
Bittersweet	Castor bean
Nightshade	Jerusalem cherry

* Data from Verhulst and Crotty (1966).

this list should contain the most troublesome plants of the United States. It is not difficult, however, to show (Kingsbury, 1969) that the clearinghouse list is actually of little value for this purpose. Assuming that the personnel of most poison control centers are competent, concerned, conscientious, and medically trained, this list represents a summation of their frustrations in obtaining useful histories, identifying plants, finding or interpreting appropriate literature, discovering that useful or recent experimental results do not exist for the plant in question, or finding that no tested treatments have been recommended for particular circumstances, as was suggested earlier in this chapter.

Taking the plants in order as named:

Standard botanical manuals for the United States list at least three different genera to which the name "pokeweed" or "pokeroot" is commonly applied. All three (*Phytolacca americana* [= *P. decandra*], *Veratrum viride*, and *Symplocarpus foetidus*) have histories of toxicity, but the syndromes differ greatly, as would appropriate treatments. All three are discussed later in this chapter. (*Symplocarpus foetidus*, also called skunk cabbage, is an aroid or member of the plant family Araceae.)

"Yew" is another common name that can cause trouble. It normally refers to a species of *Taxus*. One of these species, *T. canadensis*, is more commonly called "ground hemlock" in some areas. Thus, it is easy for the uninitiated to trans-

fer inadvertently in the literature from "yew" to "hemlock," especially since the latter is a well-known name associated with toxic plants. However, "hemlock" is applied as a common name to at least four genera of plants (Table 22–2, Fig. 22–1), only one of which is not lethal. Again the syndromes and appropriate treatments vary.

"Philodendron" is both a scientific name and a common name. As the latter, it is applied by the public, and nearly as loosely by many florists, to almost any viny, leafy, nondeciduous (not shedding) potted plant, with or without holes in the leaf blade. A survey of plants with these characteristics, made with the help of the staff at Cornell's Hortorium, resulted in a tally of several score species of plants in nine genera. Only a plant specialist could accurately identify the plant involved when a call comes to a poison control center that a child has eaten "philodendron," and then probably only by seeing the actual plant.

The name "bittersweet" is commonly applied to two entirely different plant genera, one of which has only an ancient European record of putative toxicity. The other is a species of *Solanum* (*dulcamara*), thus a "nightshade." "Nightshade" is perhaps the worst possible designation for a poisonous plant. Usually it refers to one of the multitude of species of *Solanum*. However, it can apply to more than one genus (for example, *Atropa belladonna* is commonly called "nightshade") and is also regularly used to designate the family that contains these plants, the Solanaceae. This is one of the larger plant families and contains such useful plants as potato (*Solanum tuberosum*) and tomato (*Lycopersicon esculentum*). Any member of the family can be called a "nightshade" in a general way, and many are poisonous ("deadly nightshade") under some circumstances including potato and tomato, despite their widespread daily use as food. The last plant named in Table 22–1 is also a nightshade (Jerusalem cherry = *Solanum pseudocapsicum*), but is at worst only mildly poisonous according to the available information. In conclusion, "nightshade" and "deadly nightshade" are words many parents know. They are likely to come up when a child has eaten a wild plant whose identity is not known by the distraught mother. Under these circumstances, the usefulness of "night-

Table 22–2. "HEMLOCKS"

Ground hemlock	*Taxus canadensis*	Woody shrub	Lethal
Poison hemlock	*Conium maculatum*	Herb	Lethal
Water hemlock	*Cicuta maculata* and others	Herb	Lethal
Common hemlock	*Tsuga canadensis*	Tree	Harmless

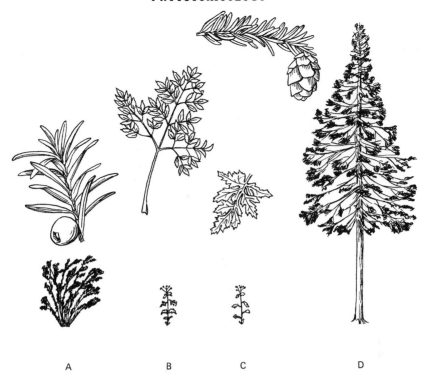

Figure 22–1. Plants commonly called "hemlock," approximately to scale. *A.* Ground hemlock (*Taxus canadensis*): habit sketch of a particularly erect specimen, below; detail of leafy twig with "berry," above. *B.* Water hemlock (*Ciruta maculata*): habit sketch, below; detail of leaf, above. *C.* Poison hemlock (*Conium maculatum*): habit sketch, below; portion of leaf, above. *D.* Hemlock tree (*Tsuga canadensis*): habit sketch, with detail of leafy twig and cone, above left. (Drawn by Elfriede Abbe.)

shade" for indicating the identity of a species of plant is virtually nil.

"Holly" is applied to a dozen species of the genus *Ilex*. Many are native American plants and have no record of toxicity. English holly (*I. opaca*) figures in a wealth of Middle Ages mythology. The only definite published reference to the toxicity of *Ilex* is in a second-hand French report from 1889, with authority not stated. Although this has been carried forward in texts to the present, and may even have some validity to it, the present-day physician would be unwise to base his treatment on this kind of information.

"Honeysuckle" refers to more than a score of species of plants in eight genera belonging to four different plant families. The plant commonly referred to in the East as "honeysuckle" is not known to be toxic.

"Pyracantha" is a scientific name and, although several common names are available for this shrub, it is the only plant to be designated by scientific name in Table 22–1. Without a species name this particular plant is identified only partially, although probably better than with only a common name. The berries of *Pyracantha*, however, have been shown by experiments to be nontoxic in four species of laboratory animals. At present there is no reason to assume that *Pyracantha* berries are poisonous to man.

"Castor bean" is a satisfactory (i.e., unambiguous) common name designation for a single plant species, *Ricinus communis*. The seeds of this plant are well known to be lethal if ingested in small to moderate amount. However, the plant has been subjected to horticultural manipulation so that two main commercial selections now exist. One is grown for production of oil; the other, as a showy, ornamental hedge or garden plant. The unselected native type grows wild in Florida. Whether these three types have equivalent toxicity is not known.

Greater impetus for detailed experimentation with poisonous plants might develop if more investigators realized the important discoveries that have come from such research in the past. Some, such as ergot, digitalis, belladonna, and morphine, are classic. The discovery of dicoumarol as an anticoagulant and the development of warfarin as a rodenticide came directly from an experiment station investigation of why cattle fed moldy sweetclover hay (*Melilotus* spp.) bled to death. More recently, investigation of the toxicity of cyads (*Cycas* spp.) has yielded important information about carcinogenesis (see Chapter 6); of bracken fern (*Pteridium aquilinum*), about avitaminosis B_1 in nonruminants; of pokeweed (*Phytolacca americana*), about mitogenesis in leukocytes (Farnes *et al.*, 1964); of hellebore (*Veratrum californicum*) and lupine (*Lupinus sericeus*) (Shupe *et al.*, 1967), about teratogenesis; and of groundsels (*Senecio* spp.) (Schoental, 1960), about liver function.

Other sources of sophisticated information on the effects of plants on animals are the pharmaceutical industry and feed manufacturers, or academic laboratories functioning in these areas. The pertinence of investigations of natural drug products is obvious. Less obvious, perhaps, is the work that has been done to analyze and determine nutritional insufficiencies or minor toxicities associated with utilizing large amounts of particular crops for feedstuffs. A good example is the detailed analysis of gossypol, the toxic component of cottonseed (*Gossypium* spp.) that makes cottonseed meal potentially poisonous to livestock.

EFFECTS OF TOXIC PRINCIPLES ELABORATED BY PLANTS

Poisonous principles of plants range from single elements or simple salts accumulated by some species under certain circumstances (e.g., selenium in cereal crops or oxalates in *Halogeton glomeratus*) to the elaboration of complex molecules of high toxicity (the phytotoxin abrin, a protein, in *Abrus precatorius*, the infamous Rosary pea or Jequirity bean). Table 22–3 presents a summary of major categories. The specific action of a toxic principle in an animal as presently understood may range from simple irritation of mucous tissues to disruption of an enzymatic process at the microsomal or mitochondrial level. Thus, it is difficult to organize the available information along lines of either molecular structure or fundamental physiology. This difficulty is compounded by the fact that precise knowledge of the toxicity of the 700 species of plants known to be toxic is lacking for more than half. Different authors use various more or less successful schemes based on physiology, pathology (signs and lesions), chemistry, or some combination. Any attempt to categorize poisonous principles of plants on chemical grounds suffers not only from the fact that the exact chemistry is rarely known but also that the common categories employed for such purposes

Table 22–3. MAJOR CATEGORIES OF POISONOUS PRINCIPLES*

Alcohols
Alkaloids
Polypeptides
Amines
Glycosides-glucosides
    Cyanogenetic (nitrile) glycosides
    Goitrogenic substances
    Irritant oils
    Coumarin glycosides
    Steroid and triterpenoid glycosides
        Cardiac glycosides
        Saponins
Oxalates
Resins or resinoids
Phytotoxins (toxalbumins)
Mineral poisonings
    Copper, lead, cadmium, fluorine, manganese
Nitrogen
    Nitrites-nitrates
    Nitrosos
    Gaseous oxides of nitrogen
    Selenium
    Molybdenum
Compounds causing photosensitivity
    Primary photosensitization
    Hepatogenic photosensitization

* Modified from Kingsbury, J. M.: *Poisonous Plants of the United States and Canada.* Prentice-Hall, Inc., Englewood Cliffs, N.J., 1964.

(alkaloids, glycosides, saponins, etc.) are not parallel and therefore not mutually exclusive.

Information on poisonous principles and actions is organized below according to observed responses to average toxicologic exposures, and this in turn is considered in sequence of major target organ or tissue as the poison passes through the body, assuming initial exposure by ingestion. Poisons and responses they elicit are so numerous and varied that what follows is more of a summary than a discussion. Only one example is given for each situation, although numerous examples may exist, and subsidiary effects or consequences in additional organs or tissues are ignored, although they are often clinically important. The discussion is also limited to effects of plants ingested as such, not to overdoses of drugs of plant origin, and does not include consideration of differential diagnosis, clinical signs, pathology, or treatment, except as specifically important to the point singled out for attention. Specific references have not been included for each point, for this would have burdened the chapter with an unwieldy bibliography, and these references are readily available in general texts on poisonous plants (Hardin and Arena, 1974; Kingsbury, 1964; Lampe and Fagerström, 1968).

External Structure and Mouth

The sap of some plants is acrid and irritating to skin and mucous membranes. The mown stubble of a field of spurge (*Euphorbia esula*) has caused inflammation and loss of hair on the legs of horses used to mow it. Some plants taken into the mouth cause intense stomatitis by direct irritation. The foliage or berries of the ornamental shrub daphne (*Daphne mezereum*), for example, cause corrosive lesions of the mouth, if chewed or eaten (Stout *et al.*, 1970). Animals will take such distasteful materials into the mouth out of curiosity, and most poisonings occur when prunings or clippings are thrown into a pasture or stall. Children exhibit similar curiosity and will swallow distasteful material as readily as they spit it out, just to get it out of the mouth. Either of these plants, and many others of course, will produce intense irritation of the esophagus and, if swallowed, the gut. The exact nature of the irritant is usually unknown. Many aroids (members of the plant family Araceae) cause a similar intense burning sensation in the mouth. Perhaps the most notorious is dumbcane (*Dieffenbachia* spp.). These plants contain needle-like crystals of calcium oxalate that may cause some mechanical as well as chemical irritation. The severity of the reaction has been traced (Walter, 1967), however, to the presence of a proteolytic enzyme in the plant that attacks the oral tissues. This reaction is often accompanied by swelling and glottic edema and has been fatal in man when the breathing passages have been blocked as a consequence.

Degree of mastication of seeds and fleshy or thick plant parts may determine the severity of the subsequent reaction, or whether it takes place at all. Seeds of precatory bean (*Abrus precatorius*), for example, are highly toxic if chewed, but will pass through the gut undigested if the seed coat is left intact.

Rumen, or Foregut

Ruminants may react to plant poisons quite differently from nonruminants due to differences in digestive structure and function between these two major groups of animals. Ability to vomit effectively is one difference. Some plants stimulate a strong vomit reflex. The vomiting disease of swine, for example, requires ingestion of only a very small amount of barley grain parasitized by a mold fungus (*Gibberella* sp.). Cardioactive glycosides such as those in foxglove (*Digitalis purpurea*) similarly provoke vomiting in most species of animals, even when administered parenterally. Many simple-stomached animals (e.g., man and dog) vomit easily. Ruminants can vomit, but the reflex is not as easily stimulated and the degree to which vomiting is effective in removing poisonous material from the gut is much less than in nonruminants. Vomiting in ruminants is not equivalent to normal eructation. Horses can vomit, but the structure of the oral cavity leads to complications if vomiting occurs. In horses, vomitus is directed into the trachea. Pneumonitis is a common result, and this can develop into pneumonia and result in death. In severe cases, death may result directly from asphyxiation after vomiting.

Many glycosides, as they exist in plants, are not toxic to animals. Toxicity comes from breakdown of the glycoside to release a toxic component. Breakdown often occurs more readily or more rapidly in the rumen than in the digestive tract of monogastric animals. Also, small molecules can be absorbed at the rumen and thus enter the circulation rapidly. Breakdown of cyanogenic glycosides, such as amygdalin, from members of the rose family (Rosaceae) is an example. The ruminant is more likely to achieve toxic levels of cyanide in the blood in the balance between breakdown of the glycoside, absorption of cyanide, and its detoxification and excretion, than is the nonruminant. Occasionally, unexpected events occur. Sheep on dry range pasture may die of cyanide poisoning shortly after drinking water. The loss of life from ingestion of poison suckleya (*Suckleyea suckleyana*) is an example. It is hypothesized that the ruminal contents are too dry for effective breakdown of the glycoside until the animal drinks, whereupon the reaction is intense. Sometimes such instances are erroneously diagnosed as poisoning from the water itself. Many of the symptoms are similar to those of nitrate poisoning.

Ingestion of abnormally large amounts of various forages or grains, or sudden massive change in diet, can provoke unusual reactions in the rumen that have toxicologic consequences. These can range from a simple pH shift to the elaboration of specific highly toxic molecules. For example, it has been suggested that, under unusual circumstances, silage of high nitrate content can undergo a reaction in the rumen that yields nitrogen oxide gases. Taken into the lungs, small amounts of nitrogen oxides cause severe, irreversible pulmonary emphysema. The same thing happens when nitrogen oxides are formed in silage made from forage (usually corn, *Zea mays*) of high nitrate concentration. Being heavier than air, the nitrogen oxides accumulate around the base of the silo. Breathed by man, they cause a similar syndrome, which is called "silo-filler's disease."

A syndrome of cattle, associated clinically with reduced levels of magnesium in the blood, is characterized by staggering that develops shortly after they are placed on lush pasturage. It has been postulated that, under these pasturage conditions, sufficient ammonia is formed in the rumen to react with, and tie up enough, magnesium (as hydroxide) to produce dietary insufficiency.

Some plants cause ruminal stasis. When this happens, a low-grade toxemia commences that becomes more severe with time. Also, signs of starvation appear. Mesquite bean (*Prosopis juliflora*) poisoning, recognized on southwestern ranges in cattle, is an example. Stasis is complete or nearly so. Mesquite beans have been found in the rumen on postmortem examination of animals that had not had access to this plant for as long as nine months. Under these conditions, the seeds have sometimes sprouted and begun to grow in the rumen.

Ruminants are more susceptible to bloat (the foamy entrapment of gases) than are monogastric animals. Bloat, if unrelieved, can have lethal consequences. Some plants promote bloat. These include some common leguminous forage crops and certain wild plants. Among the latter is the wild larkspur (*Delphinium* spp.) of western ranges. Under range conditions bloat may not be observed in time to be treated effectively.

Just as the rumen can promote the release of a toxic compound from an innocuous precursor, so can it sometimes aid in the detoxification of an initially poisonous compound. Sheep fed high-calcium alfalfa hay, for example, are protected to some degree against the toxic effects of halogeton (*Halogeton glomeratus*), which contains soluble oxalates. It is postulated that calcium is precipitated by the oxalate ions in the rumen, thus making the oxalate unavailable for absorption from the gut.

Another situation in which the ruminant has the advantage over the nonruminant occurs in the case of ingestion of plants containing a thiaminase, such as field horsetail (*Equisetum arvense*). In the horse, continued exposure to such plants causes destruction of the thiamine in the diet and the development of a definite and eventually lethal B_1 deficiency with classic signs of polyneuritis. This is one of the few instances where the ultimate biochemical lesion, disruption of carboxylation in the Krebs cycle, is known. In a ruminant, the microflora of the rumen manufacture copious quantities of thiamine, which apparently is carried intact in the bacterial cell to a point in the gut beyond which the thiaminase is inactivated or destroyed. There it is released by digestion of the bacterial cell and absorbed by the ruminant. In any event, ruminants do not suffer from thiamine deficiency despite having a level of thiaminase in the diet that would kill a horse.

The initial distribution of ingested materials in the ruminant is determined partly by density.

Seeds tend to pass quickly through the rumen and to concentrate in the abomasum. Here irritant substances may be released from seeds in concentrated form and promote irritation and hemorrhage of the abomasal wall. Seeds of members of the mustard family (Cruciferae) are examples.

Lower Gut

Two important actions, irritation and absorption, may occur in the stomach and intestines. Many plants cause irritation, varying in severity from mild to ulcerative, and the principal signs or symptoms in many cases of poisoning are simply those of gastroenteritis. Pokeroot (*Phytolacca americana*), for example, experimentally produces hemorrhagic gastritis, and ulcers are found in postmortem examination at locations where pieces of root lie against the mucosa of the gut. Pokeweed poisoning in cattle results in copious, almost explosive diarrhea that may contain signs of hemorrhage. In contrast, although blood-tinged feces are characteristic of oak (*Quercus* spp.) poisoning of cattle, the gastroenteritis is usually accompanied by constipation.

Absorption of toxins into the bloodstream normally takes place in the lower gut. Some toxic principles are large molecules, not readily absorbed. Saponins, such as those of the cockles (*Saponaria* spp.), are examples. As irritants, however, they promote their own absorption. Cardioactive glycosides are saponic in physical properties. It has been shown that the nature of the sugar portion of the intact glycoside is important in determining the solubility of these molecules and, therefore, their physiologic availability.

Liver

Poisonous principles absorbed into the circulatory system pass first to the liver. Here many different things can happen. A number of plant substances are severely poisonous to hepatic tissue, causing rapid destruction and necrosis where contact is made. A common finding on necropsy is a pathologic liver, but the exact pathology varies considerably. In many cases, the assault is somewhat chronic, and the appearance and function of the liver represent whatever current balance exists between destructive and regenerative changes.

A great deal of recent work has gone into elucidation of the exact hepatoxic effects of pyrrolizidine alkaloids (Clarke and Clark, 1967). Alkaloids of this configuration are found in a number of genera of higher plants (such as *Senecio* spp.). The primary lesion is a characteristic megalocytosis accompanied by venous obstruction or occlusion. Some plants (e.g., *Tri-*

folium subterraneum, subterranean clover) accumulate copper from soils of high copper content. Copper then accumulates in and produces degenerative changes of the liver. In akee (*Blighia sapida*) poisoning of man, a hypoglycemic poisonous principle in the plant reduces the glycogen content of the liver to nearly zero (Tanaka *et al.,* 1972).

One of the types of liver dysfunction that commonly occurs in plant poisonings is the reduced ability to eliminate certain pigmented molecules in the bile. These, instead, enter general circulation. When they reach the capillaries of the skin, they react with light and cause the capillaries to leak serum. This reaction and its consequences constitute the syndrome of photosensitization. If edematous swelling is severe, the involved tissues die and are sloughed off. Thus, in range sheep, the disease known as bighead is characterized initially by erythema, then by edematous swelling, and ultimately by necrosis of portions of the ears, cheeks, and lips, if severe. Animals that have lost the lips are unable to forage effectively and die of starvation. The identity of all pigments involved in photosensitization is not yet known, but several have been established. One or more are breakdown products of chlorophyll and are normally present in the hepatic portal circulation. In other cases, the photosensitizing pigment is contained in the plant itself and passes unchanged through digestion, absorption, and the normal liver. Photosensitization caused by the first type of pigment, always accompanied by signs of liver damage, and usually by icterus, is termed secondary. Photosensitization involving a normal liver and lacking any signs of liver dysfunction is termed primary. A range plant commonly provoking secondary photosensitization (bighead) is horsebrush (*Tetradymia* spp.). Primary photosensitization is less common, but can be caused by ingestion of St. Johnswort (*Hypericum perforatum*).

Circulatory System

The discussion of photosensitization has taken us from the liver to the general circulation. A number of other disease syndromes may occur in the circulatory system or involve the blood itself. The toxic principle of sweet pea (*Lathyrus odoratus*), β-aminopropionitrile, causes dissecting aneurysm of the aorta in small animals. A number of plants contain toxins that provoke lysis of red blood cells and consequent hemolytic anemia. Among them are cultivated onion (*Allium cepa*) and rape forage (*Brassica napus*). Saponins and phytotoxins cause lysis of red blood cells *in vitro*. Their role *in vivo* is less clear.

Coumarin, contained in sweetclover hay (*Melilotus* spp.), is converted to dicoumarin by molds under certain conditions. This compound interferes with prothrombin synthesis and results in a hemorrhagic disease when molded sweetclover hay is ingested over a period of time. Animals bleed to death from minor injuries or, in advanced cases, bleed to death internally. Large subdermal hemorrhages are usually found in these cases. Soluble oxalates in the diet can result in the precipitation of calcium ions in the circulating blood. The resulting ionic imbalance has neurologic consequences. Hypomagnesemia and its consequences have already been mentioned.

Kidney

Once a toxin is in the blood, all organs are exposed to its effect unless a membrane barrier intervenes. Many plant toxins are destructive to parenchymatous organs in general. Degenerative effects are seen primarily in liver and kidneys on postmortem examination. In some cases described above, the liver is the primary target organ. In a few others, the kidney shows the major pathology. The latter includes the effects of tannins in oak (*Quercus* spp.) poisoning, and the crystallization of oxalates in kidney tubules in oxalate poisoning as by halogeton (*Halogeton glomeratus*).

Heart

In many lethal poisonings, the immediate cause of death is heart failure. Heart dysfunction can be brought about by malfunction of innervation or of the heart's conducting tissues, or it may be a result of a more direct effect on the heart musculature. Ingestion of foxglove (*Digitalis purpurea*) is similar to an overdose of the drug digitalis, which acts by stimulating the vagus center. At toxic levels, cardioactive glycosides produce cardiac irregularities and heart block. The alkaloid of yew (*Taxus cuspidata*) depresses the conducting tissue of the heart and stops it, often very quickly, in diastole. Hypotensive alkaloids, such as in false hellebore (*Veratrum viride*), cause a marked slowing of the heart rate.

Bone

Bracken fern (*Pteridium aquilinum*) contains two toxins. One is a thiaminase. The other, more slowly acting, has as its target the bone marrow. Thus, ruminants exposed to a steady diet of bracken for many weeks develop a blood dyscrasia, characterized particularly by diminished counts of leukocytes and platelets, which may be traced in origin to severe destruction of bone marrow. Clinical signs of this disease are unusual for a poisoning and consist chiefly of hemorrhaging throughout the body due to thrombocytopenia, and invasion of the body by ordinarily nonpathogenic bacteria due to leukocytopenia, and the concomitant development of an elevated temperature. This disease is basically indistinguishable from radiation poisoning.

Pokeweed (*Phytolacca americana*), in contrast, contains an active principle that promotes the division of white blood cells. The pokeweed mitogen is also associated with the stimulation of production of interferon (Friedman and Cooper, 1967).

Some unusual plant toxins act on the skeletal structure itself. Sweet pea (*Lathyrus odoratus*) poisoning in laboratory animals consists primarily of disturbance of the normal deposition and resorption of bone in such a way that cartilage proliferates. The gross effect includes a twisting of the vertebral column. The poisonous principle is the same as that causing dissecting aneurysms in other animals. "Crooked-calf disease" is associated with lupines (*Lupinus sericeus*) (Shupe *et al.*, 1967).

Lung

Under some circumstances, ingestion of rape (*Brassica napus*) forage results in lesions of the lung. Edematous swelling and emphysema are followed by rupture of the alveoli and passage of air from the lungs to collect subdermally on either side of the backbone, where it may be palpated. Somewhat similar lesions are produced by nitrogen gases, as described before.

Thyroid

Many members of the cabbage family (Cruciferae) contain glycosides that release goitrogenic factors (thiocyanates and thiooxazolidone) when digested. The thyroid responds to these compounds by enlarging, and other signs of goiter appear. These goitrogens are iodine responsive.

Eye

The eyes are sometimes involved in signs of poisoning. Severe mydriasis that may provoke visual disturbance is a common sign of poisoning by alkaloids of the tropane configuration, such as atropine found in jimsonweed (*Datura stramonium*). Blindness accompanies a number of poisonings in which other signs may be primary. Often the eye appears normal in structure and function, and blindness may be ascribed to malfunction in the central nervous system. An example of a plant that causes functional blindness is tansy mustard (*Descurainia pinnata*). In man, ingestion of poppy (isoquinoline) alkaloids as from prickly poppy (*Argemone mexicana*) often causes generalized edema and has been held responsible for producing glaucoma.

Nervous System

Nervous signs are perhaps second in frequency only to gastroenteric signs in cases of plant poisoning. Nervous involvement and the consequent specific signs are extremely varied and may depend as much on species of animal as on the poisonous principle itself. When nervous tissue is the principal target, lesions are usually absent. There are exceptions. Cerebral demyelination has been reported in lambs born to ewes fed heavily on seaweeds. Liquefactive necrosis of cerebellar areas has been associated with molded forage and with ingestion of sensitive fern (*Onoclea sensibilis*) by horses. More recently, focal necrosis in the anterior globus pallidus of the cerebrum and substantia nigra of the mesencephalon has been described as the primary lesion in "chewing disease" of horses fed on yellow star thistle (*Centaurea solstitialis*). Pigs born to sows that have fed heavily on white clover (*Trifolium repens*) may under some circumstances display demyelination of the spinal cord and be unable to suckle (McClymont, 1954). The exact signs associated with lesions of cranial and spinal nervous tissue vary widely and depend on exactly what areas are involved. An example of a type of poisoning in which obvious lesions of the nervous tissue do not occur is the convulsive syndrome characteristic of water hemlock (*Cicuta maculata*) poisoning.

In many cases a nervous syndrome may be characterized grossly as excitatory or depressive. An example of the former is the hyperexcitable condition produced in animals after ingestion of Dallis grass (*Paspalum dilatatum*) parasitized by an ergot (*Claviceps paspali*). In contrast, weakness and paralysis are characteristic of the effect of poisons that interfere with the normal action of the voluntary musculature through its innervation. For example, guajillo (*Acacia berlandieri*) provokes a classic syndrome of ascending posterior paralysis. In this case, the identity of the poisonous principle, N-methyl-β-phenylalanine, has been worked out (Camp *et al.*, 1963). Coniine, the alkaloid of poison hemlock (*Conium maculatum*), the first alkaloid to be synthesized, has an action that is essentially similar in gross effect. Sleepy grass (*Stipa robusta*), found in a limited area of the American Southwest, provokes drowsiness in horses in small amounts and deep sleep in larger doses. The active principle is unknown.

Additional nervous symptoms can be described in man. Paresthesias and hallucinations are associated with particular types of poisoning. The alkaloid aconitine (e.g., from monkshood, *Aconitum napellus*) causes the former, and jimsonweed (*Datura stramonium*) in moderate amount gives rise to the latter.

In gangrenous ergotism, chronic ingestion of ergot (usually *Claviceps purpurea* on rye—*Secale cereale*) causes constriction of the musculature of arterioles. This results in a predisposition to thromboses or other occlusions of the circulation, particularly in the extremities where blood pressure is minimal. The tissue distal to the occlusion dies, becomes septic, and eventually is lost.

Respiratory System

Respiration can be inhibited or prevented at any level, from the mouth to the respiring cells themselves. Cases involving the oral cavity, the lungs, and the cardiovascular system have already been mentioned. In addition to these, respiration can be blocked by the inability of blood to carry oxygen, as in nitrate poisoning, or of the cells to use it, as in cyanide poisoning. Many plants can take up dangerously high levels of nitrogen under conditions of heavy fertilization; a few (such as corn—*Zea mays*) are predisposed to do so. Treatment of crops with 2,4-D can upset nitrogen metabolism with similar results. Nitrate in plants is largely converted to nitrite in the gut. This reacts with hemoglobin to form methemoglobin. The ability of the blood to carry oxygen is impaired in proportion to conversion. Cyanide, released from cyanogenetic glycosides of various kinds elaborated in a large number of plants (e.g., wild cherries—*Prunus* spp.), blocks the action of cytochrome oxidase and thereby interferes with the uptake of oxygen into cellular respiration. In both cases the general signs are those associated with asphyxiation.

Reproductive System

Some plants can elaborate estrogenic factors under certain conditions. Certain forage legumes are known to do so. Corn (*Zea mays*) molded by an unknown fungus has provoked a similar syndrome. Poisoning is characterized by vaginal swelling and prolapse in female animals. Some effects may also be observed in male animals.

Some plants, ingested by pregnant animals, have a pronounced teratogenic effect on the developing embryo. Perhaps the best example is the cycloptic lambs born to ewes that have been exposed to ingestion of hellebore (*Veratrum californicum*) on the fourteenth day of gestation. At that time the embryo is sensitive in development of facial structure. A massive exposure to the plant results in severely inhibited facial development. While the lower jaw remains more or less normal, the upper jaw disappears nearly entirely, and both eyes occupy a single orbit in the center of the forehead, or there may be but one central eye.

Some poisonous principles (fortunately few) are readily excreted in milk. These include especially those of high fat solubility, which may be concentrated in the butterfat. While excretion of toxic principles is beneficial to the animal doing so, the consumption of milk from poisoned animals can induce poisoning in man or nursing animals. The secondary poisoning can be more severe than that in the lactating animal because of the concentration of the poison and the lesser ability of the nonlactating consumer to eliminate it. Perhaps the best example is given by white snakeroot (*Eupatorium rugosum*). The poisonous principle (tremetol) it contains provokes a disease in cattle called trembles. Ingestion of milk from poisoned cattle causes a serious debilitating disease, "milksickness," in man.

Farmers commonly associate abortion in livestock with ingestion of weeds. The actual causes of abortion are many. Some plants in toxic amounts (e.g., broomweed—*Gutierrezia microcephala*) undoubtedly can lead to abortion in pregnant animals, but the mechanism is undetermined.

Hair and Skin

The effect of photosensitization on the skin has been mentioned above. Thickening of the skin (hyperkeratosis), usually accompanied by loss of hair, can result from a variety of causes but is often related to a deficiency of vitamin A. It has been shown that some isolates of the imperfect fungus *Aspergillus* can induce the formation of a factor in the substrate that produces well-developed cases of hyperkeratosis in experimental animals.

Some forage plants, particularly legumes, grown on high molybdenum soils accumulate enough molybdenum to become toxic to grazing animals. One of the chief signs of poisoning is depigmentation of the hair. The incidence of this disease in cattle at pasture can be mapped by airplane. Depigmentation, which develops slowly, is ascribed to the inability of tyrosinase to mediate the formation of melanin in the absence of copper, the availability of which in the body is reciprocally related to the bodily concentration of molybdenum.

Loss of long hair and hoof deformity accompany one type of selenium poisoning. On certain seleniferous soils, grain crops may develop concentrations of selenium, in organic combination, of 5 ppm or more. At this level, continued ingestion of grain or forage produces the syndrome known as "alkali disease." It appears that selenium substitutes for sulfur in amino acids. Hoof deformity and sloughing will become severe enough in time that affected animals will graze from a kneeling position and eventually starve to death. The amino acid mimosine (as in koa haole, *Leucaena glauca*) is held responsible for causing a similar syndrome when ingested.

CONCLUSIONS

Poisonous plants are numerous, ubiquitous, troublesome, and poorly studied. No general botanic, ecologic, or geographic relationship exists among them to bring order to an understanding of the diversity. Similar diversity exists in the variety of toxic principles contained in plants, viewed either chemically or physiologically, and in the syndromes provoked by them in man and animals. Syndromes in which a plant poison is the prime etiologic factor may involve the integument and hair, the mouth and any portion of the digestive system (with a major distinction possible between ruminant and simple-stomached animals), the parenchymatous organs (especially the liver and kidney), the circulatory system (including the heart, vascularization, and blood itself), the skeletal system, the lungs and respiratory system (including cellular respiration), various glands (especially the thyroid), the central and autonomic nervous systems, the eye, and the reproductive system. Full elucidation of a poisonous plant syndrome usually requires the efforts of a team of research specialists. Some past investigations have yielded results of great medical or economic importance. Results are needed even more urgently so that reaction to poisoning by plants, its treatment, and prevention can be more intelligently founded than at present.

REFERENCES

Baskin, E.: *The Poppy and Other Deadly Plants.* Delacorte Press, New York, 1967.

Camp, B. J.; Adams, R.; and Dollahite, J. W.: The chemistry of the toxic constituents of *Acacia berlandieri. Ann. N. Y. Acad. Sci.*, 111:744–50, 1963.

Clarke, E. G. C., and Clark, M. L.: *Garner's Veterinary Toxicology*, 3rd ed. Williams & Wilkins Co., Baltimore, 1967.

Claus, E. P.; Tyler, V. E.; and Brady, L. R.: *Pharmacognosy*, 6th ed. Lea & Febiger, Philadelphia, 1970.

Dress, W. J.: Review of Baskin, E., The Poppy and Other Deadly Plants. *Baileya*, 15:165–66, 1967.

Farnes, P.; Barker, B. E.; Brownhill, L. E.; and Fanger, H.: Mitogenic activity in *Phytolacca americana* (pokeweed). *Lancet*, 2:1100–1101, 1964.

Food Protection Committee: *Toxicants Occurring Naturally in Foods.* National Academy of Sciences, Publ. 1354, National Research Council, Washington, D.C., 1966.

Friedman, R. M., and Cooper, H. L.: Stimulation of interferon production in human lymphocytes by mitogens. *Proc. Soc. Exp. Biol. Med.*, 125:901–905, 1967.

Hardin, J. W., and Arena, J. M.: *Human Poisoning from Native and Cultivated Plants*, 2nd ed. Duke University Press, Durham, N.C., 1974.

Kingsbury, J. M.: Poisonous plants of particular interest to animal nutritionists. In *Proceedings, Cornell Nutrition Conference of Feed Manufacturers*, 1960, pp. 14–23.

——: *Poisonous Plants of the United States and Canada.* Prentice-Hall, Inc., Englewood Cliffs, N.J., 1964.

——: Phytotoxicology. I. Major problems associated with poisonous plants. *Clin. Pharmacol. Ther.*, 10:163–69, 1969.

——: Poisoning by plants. In Kirk, R. W. (ed.): *Current Veterinary Therapy V.* W. B. Saunders Co., Philadelphia, 1974.

Lampe, K. F., and Fagerström, R.: *Plant Toxicity and Dermatitis: A Manual for Physicians.* Williams & Wilkins Co., Baltimore, 1968.

Lewin, L.: *Die Gifte in der Weltgeschichte.* Springer, Berlin, 1920.

Liener, I. E. (ed.): *Toxic Constituents of Plant Foodstuffs.* Academic Press, Inc., New York, 1969.

McClymont, G. L.: Paresis associated with spinal cord myelin sheath degeneration in new born pigs. *Aust. Vet. J.*, 30:345–46, 1954.

MacEachen, A. J.; Crawford, J. N.; Willard, J. W.; Napke, E.; Adams, D. M.; and Fournier, L. deG: Canadian poison control program statistics, 1965. *Clin. Toxicol.*, 1:91–131, 1968.

Morton, J.: *Plants Poisonous to People in Florida and Other Warm Areas.* Hurricane House, Miami, 1971.

National Clearinghouse for Poison Control Centers: Tabulations of 1971 reports. *Bull. Natl. Clearinghouse Pois. Cont. Centers*, Sept.–Oct., 1972.

O'Leary, S. B.: Poisoning in man from eating poisonous plants. *Arch. Environ. Health*, 9:216–42, 1964.

Radeleff, R. D.: *Veterinary Toxicology.* Lea & Febiger, Philadelphia, 1964.

Schoental, R.: The chemical aspects of seneciosis. *Proc. Roy. Soc. Med.*, 52:284–88, 1960.

Shupe, J. L.; Binns, W.; James, L. F.; and Keeler, R. F.: Lupine, a cause of crooked calf disease. *J. Am. Vet. Med. Assoc.*, 151:198–203, 1967.

Stone, R. P., and Collins, W. J.: *Euphorbia pulcherrima*: toxicity to rats. *Toxicon*, 9:301–302, 1971.

Stout, G. H.; Balkenhol, W. G.; Poling, M.; and Hickenell, G. L.: The isolation and structure of daphnetoxin, the poisonous principle of *Daphne* species. *J. Am. Chem. Soc.*, 92:1070–71, 1970.

Subcommittee on Weeds: Weeds injurious to the health of man and animals. *Weed Control*, National Academy of Sciences, Publ. 1597, Washington, D. C., 1968.

Tanaka, K.; Isselbacher, K. J.; and Shih, V.: Isovaleric and α-methylbutyric acidemias induced by hypoglycin A: mechanism of Jamaican vomiting sickness. *Science*, 175:69–71, 1972.

Verhulst, H. L., and Crotty, J. J.: Survey of products most frequently named in ingestion accidents—1965. *Bull. Natl. Clearinghouse Pois. Contr. Centers*, July–Aug., 1966, pp. 1–12.

Walter, W. C.: Dieffenbachia toxicity, *J.A.M.A.*, 201:154–55, 1967.

UNIT IV
ENVIRONMENTAL TOXICOLOGY

insanitary conditions in meat-packing plants, the use of poisonous preservatives and dyes in foods, and cure-all claims for worthless and dangerous patent medicines. This act prohibited interstate commerce of misbranded and adulterated foods, drinks, and drugs. In addition, the Meat Inspection Act was also passed at the same time.

Most manufacturers observed the law of 1906, and adulteration with known harmful substances was rare. Finally, in 1938, the U.S. Congress passed the Food, Drug and Cosmetic Act, which contained certain new provisions relating to foods:

Provided for tolerances for unavoidable poisonous substances.

Authorized standards of identity, quality, and fill of containers for foods.

Authorized factory inspection.

Added the remedy of court injunction to previous remedies of seizure and prosecution.

The problem of how to protect the consumer from inadequately tested food additives was studied intensively by Congressional committees from 1950 to 1958. In 1951 the "Delaney Committee" started to investigate the safety of chemicals in foods and cosmetics, laying the foundation for effective controls for the use of pesticides, food additives, and colors. In 1954 the passage of the Miller Pesticides Amendment by Congress streamlined procedures for setting safety limits for pesticide residues on raw agricultural commodities and greatly strengthened consumer protection. The Food Additive Amendment, Public Law 85-929, also known as the Delaney Amendment, became law September 6, 1958, to prohibit the use of new food additives until the sponsor establishes safety and the U.S. Food and Drug Administration (FDA) issues regulations specifying conditions of use.

Under the Food Additive Amendment of 1958, a substance newly proposed for addition to food must undergo strict testing designed to establish the safety of the intended use *before* it is marketed. Information must be presented to the FDA in the form of a petition as to the identity of the new additive, its chemical composition, how it is manufactured, and analytic methods to be used to detect and measure its presence in the food supply at the levels of expected use. Data must establish that the proposed analytic method is of sufficient sensitivity to adequately determine compliance with the regulations. There must also be data establishing that the additive will accomplish the intended effect in the food and that the level sought for approval is no higher than that reasonably necessary to accomplish the intended effect. Finally, data must be provided establishing that the additive is safe for its intended use. This requires experimental evidence ordinarily derived from extensive feeding studies and other tests using the proposed additive at various levels in the diets of two or more species of animals. Results of these tests must be submitted to the Food and Drug Administration. If FDA scientists are satisfied that the additive may be used safely, a regulation—called an "order"—will be issued permitting its use. This regulation may place a limit, or "tolerance," on the amount that may be used and will specify any other conditions necessary to protect the public health. If the evidence submitted is not convincing as to safety, the additive will not be permitted. This applies equally to substances added directly to foods, including animal feeds, and to substances likely to contaminate food as a result of some incidental use in food processing. Food-packing materials that may be absorbed by the food itself are covered. The law also applies specifically to processes for irradiating foods for preservation, and it covers any residues that may carry over into meat, milk, or eggs as a result of use in animal feeds.

The 1958 Amendment specifically states that no additive may be permitted in any amount if the tests show that it produces cancer when ingested by man or animals, or by other appropriate test. And it specifies that only the smallest amount necessary to produce the intended effect may be permitted. It prohibits the use of any chemical that would result in consumer deception.

The Color Additives Amendment was enacted in 1960 to allow the FDA to establish by regulations the conditions of safe use for color additives in foods, drugs, and cosmetics, and to require manufacturers to perform the necessary scientific investigations to establish safety.

The Food, Drug, and Cosmetic Act with its various amendments is administered by the FDA, which was organized in 1938 under the U.S. Department of Agriculture, but in 1940 was transferred to the Federal Security Agency. These regulations affect about 60 percent of the food produced in the United States. The remaining 40 percent is under state regulations, which in many cases parallel federal legislation. For public protection food safety is under constant review by the Food and Drug Administration. It is important to note that, as our knowledge of toxicology advances and better diagnostic and analytic methods become available, a formerly permissible additive can be declared unacceptable.

In the United Kingdom, food regulations are incorporated in the Revised Food and Drug Act of 1955 and supplemental regulations. Authority is vested in the Ministry of Agriculture, Fisheries, and Food, which works closely with several committees, including the Food Standards Committee and Food Additives and Contaminants Committee (Kent-Jones, 1971). Most nations now have laws regulating some aspects of food additives and sanitation. Early laws were often modeled on the British Statute of 1875. More recently, some of the emerging nations have followed the concepts of food regulations adopted in the United States. With increasing control of food additives within national borders and increasing international redistributions of food supplies, a serious new problem has arisen. An additive legal in one country may be illegal in another.

Several international agencies are attempting to solve the problems of international trade and set up criteria to evaluate the safety of food additives. Under the United Nations, FAO (Food and Agriculture Organization) and WHO (World Health Organization) formed the FAO/WHO Joint Expert Committee on Food Additives. It has issued a series of monographs and technical reports, which cover the principles for the use of food additives, methods of evaluating the safety of food additives (including evaluation of carcinogenic hazards and specifications for the use of antimicrobial preservatives), antioxidants, food colors, emulsifiers, stabilizers, and bleaching and maturing agents. Pesticide residues and radioactive contaminants are covered by separate programs under Joint FAO/IAEA/WHO Expert Committees. The FAO/WHO recommendations are based on the acceptable daily intake (ADI) of the additive. Three classes of acceptance have been defined (Joint FAO/WHO Expert Committee on Food Additives, 1968):

1. An unconditional ADI is given only to those substances for which full and adequate biologic data are available.

2. A conditional ADI is given to those substances used for specific purposes arising from special dietary requirements.

3. A temporary ADI is granted when the available data are judged not fully adequate to establish the safety of the substance and it is considered necessary that additional evidence should be provided within a stated period of time.

No ADI would be allocated to substances for which the available biologic data were grossly inadequate to establish their safety.

The FAO/WHO Codex Alimentarus Commission and its subcommittees are also concerned with what additives are used and in what quantity and in establishing acceptable international food standards (Koenig, 1965). Through study of national dietary surveys, it attempts to determine whether the total diet load approaches the ADI in the various diets. The first list of recommended international standards proposed by the Commission was published by the FDA in the Federal Register of October 5, 1972. Each member country has three options: to accept the standards, to accept with change, or to reject the recommendations. Hopefully, the major food-producing countries will eventually accept the regulations. Waters (1972) has analyzed the importance and impact of acceptance of the proposed standards.

The Council of Europe has among its aims the harmonization of legislation in the public health area. The Sub-committee on the Health Control of Foodstuffs and the Working Party on Flavoring Substances have prepared an acceptable list of flavorings (Council of Europe, 1970). Action by the Council of Europe is not binding on the member nations but is presented for national legislation of the member nations (Elias, 1972).

On the other hand, actions of the European Economic Community (EEC) are binding on the member countries. One of the aims of the EEC also is harmonization of national food laws of the member states through directives drafted by the EEC commission. Enforcement, however, is a matter for national authorities. Several authors have discussed in more detail the international aspects of regulation of food additives (Luckey, 1968; Egan and Hubbard, 1971; Kent-Jones, 1971; Elias, 1972).

PRESENT STATUS OF FOOD ADDITIVES

Additives Generally Considered as Safe

The 1958 Food Additives Amendment to the Food, Drug, and Cosmetic Act of 1938 called for prior approval by the FDA of new commercially added food ingredients. Petitioners for food additives were required to present evidence of the usefulness and harmlessness of the ingredients when used as proposed. However, at that time, a number of substances, including many that had been used in food for a considerable number of years, were exempted from the requirements of the food additives amendment because they were generally recognized as safe (GRAS). These substances, collectively known as the GRAS list, numbered better than 600. For regulatory purposes, GRAS substances are not considered as food additives. Substances legally classified as food additives are more tightly regulated than GRAS ingedients. The first GRAS list was published in the U.S. Federal Register in 1958

(CFR 121.101). The substances covered are as follows:

CODE OF FEDERAL REGULATION (CFR)	NUMBER OF ITEMS
Section 121.101	
(d) (1) Anticaking agents	7
(d) (2) Chemical preservatives	31
(d) (3) Emulsifying agents	9
(d) (4) Nonnutritive sweeteners	4
(d) (5) Nutrients and/or dietary supplements	86
(d) (6) Sequestrants	31
(d) (7) Stabilizers	12
(d) (8) Miscellaneous and/or general purpose	81
(e) (1) Spices and other natural seasonings and flavorings	89
(e) (2) Essential oils, oleoresins, and natural extractives	172
(e) (3) Natural substances used in conjunction with spices and other Natural seasonings and flavors	3
(e) (4) Natural extractives used in conjunction with spices, seasonings, and flavors	9
(e) (5) Miscellaneous (used in flavors, etc.)	5
(f) Trace minerals added to animal feeds (46 items not included in this count)	
(g) Synthetic flavorings, substances, and adjuvants	27
(h) Substances migrating to food from paper and paper board products used in food packaging	67
(i) Substances migrating to food from cotton and cotton fabrics used in dry food packaging	41
Total	674

These lists were compiled largely from lists of substances already recognized in 1958 as suitable for food by publication in FDA Food Standards or by publication in certain state regulations and from lists of substances known to have been used in food for some years without reported adverse effects. As provided for by the law, some substances could be considered generally recognized as safe merely because of a history of use in food. Thus there are certain GRAS substances permitted in food for which no recent tests have been made that are comparable to the rigorous laboratory test required for approval of a new food additive.

The Flavor and Extract Manufacturers Association (FEMA) also published a list of substances that they recognized as having GRAS status through evaluation by the expert Panel of FEMA and other accepted authorities (Hall and Oser, 1965). This first list contains some 1,100 flavoring substances and their use levels, and FDA adopted virtually the entire list in the form of two regulations (21 CFR 121.1163 and .1164). The Panel has evaluated the safety of flavoring substances, the vast majority of which have been in wide use for many years and generally regarded as normal components of food. The results of these studies have been reported in a series of papers in *Food Technology* (Hall and Oser, 1965, 1970; Oser and Ford, 1973a, 1973b, 1974, 1977, 1978; Oser and Hall, 1972, 1977). Recently, the Food and Drug Administration solicited submission of safety data on 933 flavoring substances as part of the GRAS review. Included in the list of flavors on which data is being sought were 533 substances on which Scientific Literature Reviews (SLR) are being prepared by the FEMA and 460 substances for which FEMA previously prepared SLRs. Additionally, FDA also solicited submission of unpublished data on 27 GRAS or prior sanctioned substances added to food for which SLRs are being prepared.

Substances on the GRAS list are subject to review and removal or transfer to the food additives category as additional toxicologic information and usage data are available. The FDA in 1970 began a comprehsnsive GRAS evaluation program in response to the President's directive to the federal government to evaluate the substances on the GRAS list. This action came amid public concern that arose in the 1960s as a few GRAS ingredients came under the suspicion of scientists who had been subjecting some of them to the comprehensive testing with experimental animals that the FDA requires for modern food additives before permitting their use. One GRAS substance, cyclamate, was banned from use in food as a consequence of findings that it produced bladder cancer in rats. The wide concern over substances that had been thought to be safe figured in the decision to give the entire GRAS list a thorough reappraisal under modern safety standards for food ingredients. It was apparent that there was a need for the revision of the food additive law with more stringent control in general and clarifications of the cancer clause in particular. Hall (1971) lists as reasons

1. The information on which the original GRAS determinations were made might now be outdated.

2. Conditions of use have changed.

3. New data on toxicology and metabolism are available.

4. Nearly 300 substances have dropped from use and others have been shifted to replace them.

5. Some new materials are in use.

The first step was taken with the announcement in the *Federal Register* (April 9, 1970) of revocation of prior sanctions and setting up of a survey under the National Research Council, National Academy of Sciences, Food Protection

Committee to collect information on additives being used in the food industry along with published data supporting their safety as used. The FEMA has conducted a separate survey on flavoring ingredients that will also be used by the FDA in review of GRAS substances. The FDA in the *Federal Register* of March 23, 1972 (37 FR 6207), announced proposed procedures for affirmation and determination of GRAS and food additive status. Important features are that the commission after studying the data can affirm the GRAS status of substances found to meet GRAS criteria. Food ingredients that do not meet GRAS criteria may be eliminated completely or may be permitted to remain in food subject to food additive regulation or may be given interim food additive status pending further study. In each case, the ruling is subject to a further hearing of interested parties after filing of notice in the *Federal Register*.

In the *Federal Register* of July 26, 1973 (38[143]FR,PtII), the FDA published a report on the status of the project, listing those substances that had been reaffirmed to be permissible food additives or to be GRAS substances. The announcement included a proposed classification of foods and ingredients and a partial listing of banned substances.

On December 7, 1976, the FDA issued regulations defining the criteria for determining whether food ingredients are generally recognized as safe (GRAS) or subject to prior sanctions. These regulations also implemented certain procedures related to the Agency's review of the safety of food ingredients; they became effective January 6, 1977 (Federal Register 41:53599-53623).

In approaching the evaluation of the GRAS substances, the FDA contracted, through the Life Sciences Research Office (LSRO) of the Federation of American Sciences for Experimental Biology (FASEB), a group of nongovernmental scientific experts, to review the available information and make evaluations. This group, known as the Select Committee on GRAS Substances, began its evaluation in 1972.

In a 1977 "white paper" on "lessons learned and questions unanswered" during the first five years of the GRAS review, under contract to the FDA, the Select Committee has recommended the eventual scrapping of the GRAS concept. The Committee said:

We envision this exercise as making a transition of a new phase of regulatory procedures. We expect that GRAS substances will eventually be brought into the mainstream of food additives. Gradually, the special treatment of being evaluated for the lack of evidence of hazard will give way to being evaluated for the evidence of safety, as is the practice with other commerically added ingredients

(Federation of American Societies for Experimental Biology, 1977).

By February 1, 1978, the Committee had made 84 final reports covering 232 substances and eight tentative reports covering an additional 40 substances. The Committee expects to issue a total of 140 reports covering well over 400 GRAS substances by June 1979. Although the Committee's recommendations are not binding, the FDA gives them careful consideration in deciding what action to take on each GRAS substance under review. After evaluating the Committee's recommendations and other information available to it, the FDA publishes its proposed final action in the *Federal Register* for comments.

The FDA now expects to have all its regulations resulting from the GRAS review completed or at least in proposal stage by the end of 1983 (Hopkins, 1978). The Agency also has committed itself to conduct cyclic reviews of all food ingredients and currently has undertaken review of direct and indirect food additives, GRAS and non-GRAS flavors, and color additives in a long-range plan to assure that all food ingredients are without hazard as judged by the existing state of scientific knowledge.

Delaney Amendment

The Food Additive Amendment of 1958 also included the cancer or Delaney clause, which states: "That no additive shall be deemed to be safe if it is found to induce cancer when ingested by man or animal, or if it is found, after tests which are appropriate for the evaluation of the safety of food additives, to induce cancer in man or animal . . ." (Federal Food, Drug, and Cosmetic Act, Section 409 [c] [3] [A]). Although the aim of the Delaney clause is excellent, serious problems exist in the evaluation of data, protocols for testing for carcinogenicity, and the extrapolation of the data to man (U.S. Department of Health, Education, and Welfare, 1969; Kilgore and Li, 1973). These problems have polarized scientific and legislative authorities as well as the consuming public into proponents and opponents of the measure (Wade, 1972).

The controversy was brought to a head but not solved when cyclamates and saccharin were banned under the Delaney clause in 1969 and 1977, respectively. In the case of saccharin, the FDA proposed to ban the use of saccharin as a food additive in prepackaged foods, such as soft drinks, and as tabletop nonnutritive sweeteners. (Federal Register 42:19995-20010, April 15, 1977). The document said:

The Commissioner's determination that saccharin must be banned as a food additive is based on a series of scientific studies conducted in accordance with currently accepted methods for determining whether compounds can cause cancer. The most recent of these studies, conducted by Canadian scientists under the auspices of the Canadian Government, confirms what earlier American studies have suggested: that saccharin poses a significant risk of cancer for humans. Under these circumstances, conscientious concern for the public health requires that FDA prohibit the continued general use of saccharin in foods.

This conclusion is also dictated by the so-called Delaney clause of the Food, Drug, and Cosmetic Act (21 U.S.C. 348(c)(3)), which prohibits the use in food of any food additive which has been shown, by ingestion or other appropriate tests, to cause cancer in laboratory animals.

A loud public outcry followed because saccharin is the only general-use artificial sweetener approved for use in this country. A debate ensued over the wisdom of the Delaney clause in light of the need for an artificial sweetener, not just by casual dieters but by diabetics and others for whom obesity is a health problem. The FDA received more than 100,000 comments, most opposing the ban.

In response to this unprecedented public outcry, the U.S. Congress in November 1977 passed the Saccharin Study and Labeling Act (Public Law 95-203). The primary purpose of the law was to impose an 18-month moratorium on the FDA's proposed ban of saccharin, which provides time to study existing evidence, to gather new information, and to consider the impact that a ban would have (Anonymous, 1978a). The law also requires certain warning labels and notices for foods containing saccharin, which has been determined to cause cancer in laboratory animals (Anonymous, 1978b).

The 18-month moratorium imposed on the FDA's proposed ban on saccharin provides time to gather and study new evidence but it does not solve the problem. Saccharin's ultimate fate depends on a number of factors, among them additional information that may be developed on the substance's safety and possible congressional action on how food additives should be regulated.

The U.S. National Academy of Sciences, conducting a federally funded study of the nation's food safety policy and saccharin in particular, is reviewing present available research findings and other data. The Academy's saccharin findings were sent to the FDA in November 1978 and the complete study was finished by February 1979.

In Europe, the adoption of restrictions on the use of saccharin has been recommended by the Commission of the European Communities to all its member states. Recommended actions include banning of the use of saccharin in baby foods; regulating the use of saccharin in food and requiring food labels to note the presence of saccharin; setting an acceptable daily level; and reducing to a minimum the consumption of saccharin by children.

INTENTIONAL FOOD ADDITIVES

Intentional food additives are natural or synthetic substances added to the original food or mixture of foods for specific purposes. Generally, they are classified according to use, rather than chemical structure. The most commonly used categories are

1. Anticaking agents
2. Chemical preservatives
3. Emulsifying agents
4. Nutrients and dietary supplements
5. Sequestrants
6. Stabilizers
7. Synthetic flavoring substances
8. Miscellaneous additives

On occasion substances are removed from the list by the FDA in the light of new evidence. Cyclamate sweeteners were removed because of reports that large doses cause the development of tumors in laboratory test animals (Anonymous, 1969). Similarly, the FDA has proposed the banning of saccharin; a final order has not yet been issued. A partial list of typical food additives is given in Table 23–1.

A more complete listing can be obtained from the U.S. Food and Drug Administration.

The word "chemical" is not ordinarily used to describe intentional food additives because both additives and foods are made up of chemicals, although "food chemical" is the term preferred by some authors. Perhaps the major reason for its use is that "food additive" has a definite legal meaning under the Food Additive Amendment.

Certain natural foods are also used as food additives (Table 23–1). A fact not widely recognized is that some essential dietary compounds can be toxic when consumed in excessive amounts.

Although the margin of safety for most nutrients is many times the normal intake, it is possible in some instances to exceed the toxic threshold when the diet is too restricted or unlimited use of the additive is permitted. An interesting example is vitamin A (retinol). This vitamin is present in foods in the form of vitamin A itself or of several carotenes that are precursors of vitamin A. The recommended daily allowance (RDA) has been set at 5,000 International Units (IU), or 1,000 retinol equivalents, for adults and 2,000 IU (400 retinol equivalents) for infants six months to one year of age (National Research Council, 1974). Carotenes are not known to cause any acute toxic problems, although ingestion of large quantities will cause a distinct

Table 23–1.

SELECTED FOOD ADDITIVES

Anticaking Agents
Aluminum calcium silicate
Calcium silicate
Sodium aluminosilicate
Sodium calcium aluminosilicate

Chemical Preservatives
Ascorbic acid
Ascorbyl palmitate
Butylated hydroxyanisole
Butylated hydroxytoluene
Calcium propionate
Calcium sorbate
Dilauryl thiodipropionate
Erythorbic acid
Methylparaben
Potassium bisulfite
Potassium sorbate
Propionic acid
Propylparaben
Sodium ascorbate
Sodium bisulfite
Sodium metabisulfite
Sodium sorbate
Sodium sulfite
Stannous chloride
Sulfur dioxide
Tocopherols

Emulsifying Agents
Cholic acid
Desoxycholic acid
Glycocholic acid
Mono- and diglycerides
Propylene glycol
Ox bile extract

Nutrients and Dietary Supplements
Alanine
Arginine
Aspartic acid
Biotin
Calcium citrate
Calcium glycerophosphate
Calcium pantothenate
Calcium phosphate
Calcium sulfate
Carotene
Choline chloride
Copper gluconate
Cysteine
Cystine
Ferric pyrophosphate
Ferric sodium pyrophosphate
Ferrous lactate
Ferrous sulfate
Histidine
Inositol
Isoleucine
Leucine
Lysine
Magnesium oxide
Magnesium sulfate
Manganese chloride
Manganese gluconate
Manganese glycerophosphate
Manganese sulfate

Manganous oxide
Methionine
Methionine hydroxy analogue
Niacinamide
D-Pantothenyl alcohol
Potassium chloride
Potassium glycerophosphate
Proline
Pyridoxine hydrochloride
Riboflavin-5-phosphate
Serine
Sodium phosphate
Sorbitol
Thiamine mononitrate
Threonine
Tocopherol acetate
Tryptophane
Valine
Vitamin A
Vitamin A palmitate
Vitamin B_{12}
Vitamin D_3
Zinc sulfate
Zinc chloride
Zinc oxide

Sequestrants
Calcium acetate
Calcium chloride
Calcium diacetate
Calcium gluconate
Calcium phosphate, monobasic
Calcium phytate
Dipotassium phosphate
Disodium phosphate
Monoisopyropyl citrate
Potassium citrate
Sodium citrate
Sodium diacetate
Sodium hexametaphosphate
Sodium metaphosphate
Sodium potassium tartrate
Sodium pyrophosphate
Sodium tartrate
Sodium thiosulfate
Stearyl citrate
Tartaric acid

Stabilizers
Acacia (gum arabic)
Agar-agar
Calcium alginate
Carob bean gum
Ghatti gum
Guar gum
Sodium alginate
Sterculia (or karaya) gum

Miscellaneous Additives
Acetic acid
Adipic acid
Aluminum potassium sulfate
Aluminum sodium sulfate
Ammonium bicarbonate
Ammonium carbonate
Ammonium phosphate
Ammonium sulfate

Bentonite
Butane
Calcium carbonate
Calcium chloride
Calcium gluconate
Calcium hydroxide
Calcium oxide
Calcium phosphate
Carbon dioxide
Carnauba wax
Dextrans
Ethyl formate
Glutamic acid hydrochloride
Glycerin
Helium
Hydrochloric acid
Lactic acid
Lecithin
Magnesium hydroxide
Magnesium oxide
Malic acid
Methylcellulose
Monopotassium glutamate
Nitrogen
Papain
Phosphoric acid
Potassium bicarbonate
Potassium carbonate
Potassium hydroxide
Potassium sulfate
Propylene glycol
Rennet
Sosium acetate
Sodium acid pyrophosphate
Sodium bicarbonate
Sodium carbonate
Sodium carboxymethylcellulose
Sodium caseinate
Sodium hydroxide
Sodium pectinate
Sodium potassium tartrate
Sodium sesquicarbonate
Succinic acid
Sulfuric acid
Triacetine
Triethyl citrate

Synthetic Flavoring Substances
Acetaldehyde
Acetoin
Anethole
Benzaldehyde
d- or *l*-carvone
Cinnamaldehyde
Decanal
Diacetyl
Ethyl butyrate
Ethyl vanillin
Geraniol
Geranyl acetate
Limonene
Linalool
1-malic acid
Methyl anthranilate
Piperonal
Vanillin

yellowing of the skin. This condition, known as carotenemia, developed in a woman who drank 2 quarts of tomato juice daily for several years (Beckman, 1961). On the other hand, doses as low as 18,500 IU vitamin A have been toxic to infants when the mother inadvertently or over-zealously gave the infant excess doses of the vitamin supplement. The severe illness that Eskimos and Arctic explorers suffered after eating polar bear liver has been traced to the extremely high vitamin A content of the bear liver (Moore, 1957). Since vitamins A and D can be toxic when

consumed at excessive levels, on August 3, 1973, they were removed from the GRAS list by the FDA regulated for use as a permitted nutrient additive under specified conditions. The problem has been compounded because of the extra-high-potency vitamin tablets that have been available.

In countries that have adequate legislation, financial resources, and facilities for testing and enforcement of regulations, acute toxicologic problems caused by intentional additives are rare. However, in some areas of the world, food adulteration and indiscriminate addition of in-

Table 23–2. IMPORTANT FOOD ADDITIVE FUNCTIONAL CLASSES, SIGNIFICANT EXAMPLES, AND TYPICAL LEVELS OF USE

CLASS	EXAMPLES	LEVEL OF USE	FAO/WHO ACCEPTABLE DAILY INTAKE, mg/kg BODY WEIGHT
Acids, alkalies, buffers, and neutralizing agents	Acetic acid		Unlimited
	Citric acid	1%	Unlimited
	Phosphoric acid	1%	0–70 (as total phosphorus)
	Alkali hydroxides and carbonates		Unlimited
Anticaking	Magnesium carbonate		Unlimited
Bleaching and maturing agents, bread improvers	Benzoly peroxide	0.001%	0–40
Flavorings	Synthetic (esters, aldehydes, ketones)	1–300 ppm	0–2.5
	Spice extracts		
	Essential oils		
Enhancers	Monosodium glutamate (MSG)		0–120
Food colors	Synthetic	0.005%	0–12.5
	Natural: annatto, carotene	0.01%	0–1.25
		5 ppm	0–5
Humectants	Propylene glycol	0.05%	0–125
Miscellaneous	Nitrates	0.02%	0–5
Nutrient supplements	Amino acids		
	Iodide (in salt)	0.01%	
	Vitamins		
Nonnutritive sweeteners	Saccharin	0.001%	0–5
			5–15 (dietetic purposes)
Preservatives	Sodium benzoate	0.1%	0–5
	Sulfur dioxide	0.005%	0–0.7
	Sorbic acid	0.1%	0–25
	Propionates	0.15%	0–10
Antioxidants	Butylated hydroxyanisole	0.005%	0–0.5
	Butylated hydroxytoluene	0.005%	0–0.5
	Propyl gallate	0.003%	0–0.2
Propellants	Nitrogen, nitrous oxide, carbon dioxide		
Sequestering agents	Ethylenediaminetetraacetic acid	0.01%	0–2.5
Surface-active agents	Mono- and diglycerides	0.1%	Unlimited
	Polyoxyethylene sorbitan fatty esters	0.4%	0–25
	Vegetable gums	0.5%	
	Acacia, guar		Unlimited
	Carrageenan		0–75

tentional additives, sometimes toxic, continue to be problems.

The questions currently being raised about intentional food additives fall into three general categories. They are

1. What additives are really necessary to produce acceptable, safe, and nutritious products?

2. Should all additives, including GRAS substances, be listed on the label?

3. What additives may be carcinogens, mutagens, and teratogens capable of slowly causing biologic injury to present and future generations?

The first two points are not toxicologic problems within the range of this discussion, although the second may be of great importance to allergic individuals. The third is of major importance both to the food industry and to the consumer.

Teratogenic and mutagenic compounds are not specifically banned at present, but efforts are being made to include them in any revision of the Delaney clause. Some authorities believe all three classes should be banned completely; others believe that such substances should be accepted under the "no-effect" or, better, "no-ill-effect" clause (Golberg, 1971; Wade, 1972). Again, one problem is the positive identification of carcinogenic, teratogenic, and mutagenic compounds in man and determination of a "no-ill-effect" level. The protocols for testing continue to be debated by recognized authorities within the fields (Wade, 1972). Progress has been made for testing for carcinogens with the publication by the Food and Drug Administration Advisory Committee on Protocols for Safety Evaluation of the "Panel on Carcinogenesis Report on Cancer Testing in the Safety Evaluation of Food Additives and Pesticides" (1971). This report recommends that at least two species, preferably two rodent species, be used for tests for carcinogenicity. The test usually runs for two years—the average life-span of rats. For mutagens the problems of testing are even greater as several generations may be required (Sanders, 1969). After all the testing is completed, the next question is how to extrapolate the data to man and what margin of safety is adequate. The widely used rule of thumb of 10×10 or 100 times the "no-effect" level may not be adequate in some cases (Oser, 1969) based on analyses of the slope of dose-response curves.

A related problem is the possibility of toxic compounds being formed through interaction of nontoxic materials or through metabolism of a nontoxic additive either during food processing of after ingestion (Golberg, 1971; Conney and Burns, 1972). The possible metabolism of nitrites and nitrates to carcinogenic nitrosoamines is currently being extensively studied (Institute of Food Technologists' Expert Panel on Food Safety and Nutrition and the Committee on Public Information, 1972b; Wolff and Wasserman, 1972), and the long-accepted use of nitrites and nitrates in the curing of meats is being reevaluated.

Some important intentional food additives, with levels of use and the FAO/WHO acceptable daily intake, are listed in Table 23-2.

NONINTENTIONAL ADDITIVES

Nonintentional additives include substances that are not present in the food as produced and that have not been added to serve a stated desirable purpose in the finished product. Some authors have further divided them into unintentional additives and incidental additives. Unintentional additives are considered to be those coming from the environment in which the foods are produced, and incidental additives are those resulting from some production or processing treatment but which do not serve any purpose in the finished product. Since some substances can become additives under either condition, they will all be classified here as nonintentional additives. These substances run the gamut from sand to pesticides and radioactive fallout, with a corresponding range in toxicity from harmless to acutely toxic compounds. Therefore, it was necessary to select from the wide variety of substances a few examples that illustrate toxicologic problems that may be encountered with nonintentional additives.

The aim of good production practices and food regulations is to prevent the inclusion of harmful additives or at least to keep their inclusion below the toxic level. Definite standards are possible for known toxic agents, but once again much of the current discussion and concern reflect the problems in assessing the potential for biologic damage caused by low levels of suspected teratogens, mutagens, and carcinogens from residues remaining after treatment with pesticides, growth-promoting agents, and so forth. Table 23-3 lists some types of nonintentional additives considered to be of toxicologic significance today.

TOXICOLOGIC PROBLEMS

Carcinogenicity, Mutagenicity, and Teratogenicity of Food Additives

The possible carcinogenicity, mutagenicity, and teratogenicity of a wide variety of food additive compounds are major problems in the field of toxicology for which there are no quick or easy answers. Some of the compounds are or have been widely used as intentional additives, e.g., cyclamates, saccharin, nitrates, and some natural and synthetic food colorings and flavorings; others are incidental residues from production practices, e.g., growth hormones, pesticides, and fertilizers. Many food additives, including some

Table 23–3. SOURCES OF NONINTENTIONAL ADDITIVES OF POSSIBLE TOXICOLOGIC SIGNIFICANCE

During Production

1. Animal and insect filth (including insects and insect parts)
2. Antibiotics and other agents used for prevention and control of disease
3. Growth-promoting substances
4. Microorganisms of toxicologic significance
5. Parasitic organisms
6. Pesticides residues (insecticides, fungicides, herbicides, etc.)
7. Toxic metals and metallic compounds
8. Radioactive compounds

During Processing

1. Animal and insect filth (including insects and insect parts)
2. Microorganisms and their toxic metabolites
3. Processing residues and miscellaneous foreign objects
4. Radionuclides

During Packaging and Storage

1. Animal and insect filth
2. Labeling and stamping materials
3. Microorganisms and their toxic metabolites
4. Migrants from packaging materials
5. Toxic chemicals from external sources (including vapors and solvents)

generally recognized as safe (GRAS), have not been tested for mutagenicity or teratogenicity. There is no question that proven carcinogens, mutagens, and teratogens should be prohibited from use as food additives in any quantity that would be toxicologically significant. The problems are how to determine if a compound is carcinogenic, mutagenic, or teratogenic at extremely low levels of intake and if there is a permissible level of intake below which there would be no significant risk to the consumer.

The criteria for determining carcinogenicity of orally consumed substances are still in the formative stages. The Food and Drug Administration Advisory Committee on Protocols for Safety Evaluation has issued a Carcinogenesis Report on Cancer Testing in the Safety Evaluation of Food Additives and Pesticides (1971). However, not all laboratories have used the methods suggested. Therefore, the evaluation and comparison of data from different sources are difficult. There is also disagreement among experts as to whether certain tumors are malignant or non-malignant (U.S. Department of Health, Education, and Welfare, 1969; Kilgore and Li, 1973). The evaluation of data for mutagenicity and teratogenicity is even more difficult. The National Center for Toxicological Research (National Center for Toxicological Research, 1973) has set as one of its primary goals carcinogenic, teratogenic, and mutagenic studies for the safety evaluation of chronic (long-term, low-level) exposure to chemicals and to enable better extrapolation of data from laboratory animals to man.

The conclusion of Bonser (1967) in discussing the factors concerned in the location of human and experimental cancer is especially pertinent in the consideration of the carcinogenic, mutagenic, and teratogenic risks in food additives:

1. A return to a "natural" way of living would not eliminate carcinogenic risks; it might even increase them.

2. We can expect that further carcinogenic chemicals will be introduced into man's environment, but as safeguards we can observe such restrictions in their use as are called for in the light of present and future knowledge.

3. No strict relation has yet been formulated between chemical structure and carcinogenic potency. For this reason there is justification for continuing the search for new classes of chemical carcinogens in the hope that such a relation will eventually be found.

Metals and the Mercury Problem

In foods, the problem of toxicity of metals and metallic compounds is very complex because of several factors. A number of the metals are dietary essentials and all food contains at least trace quantities of many metals. Some that are dietary essentials are toxic when ingested in excessive quantities. Iron, copper, magnesium, cobalt, manganese, and zinc are recognized as dietary essentials, and there are indications that trace amounts of molybdenum, selenium, and several others are also required by man (National Research Council, 1968, 1971). A normal, varied diet of plant and animal food will usually supply an individual's needs except perhaps that for iron. Metallic compounds used as intentional food additives include nutrients (iron salts), anti-caking agents (magnesium silicate), and buffers and neutralizing agents (aluminum ammonium sulfate, magnesium carbonate). They may also be present as contaminants from packaging materials or the result of processing procedures. Small amounts of tin and zinc compounds may be present from stabilizers as well as from the container in which the food is packed. Some of the permitted compounds have been on the GRAS list (ferric phosphate, ferrous sulfate, magnesium carbonate), but most of them are additives with stated tolerances and/or restrictions (Manufacturing Chemists' Association, 1961).

The uptake, utilization, metabolism, and toxicity of metals vary greatly for both plants and animals, depending on the chemical forms of the metallic compounds available in the environment of that species. Selenium is an interesting example. Some species of plants known as "selenium indicators" require and selectively accumulate selenium when grown on seleniferous soils. These accumulators, which can contain as much as 1,000 ppm selenium, are not normally consumed by grazing animals unless there is a shortage of other feeds. However, food and forage crops can accumulate potentially toxic levels (> 5 ppm) when grown on soils containing soluble organic selenium compounds or selenates (Rosenfield and Beath, 1964). The critical level of dietary selenium below which chronic deficiency symptoms are observed in animals is apparently about 0.02 ppm for ruminants and 0.03 to 0.05 ppm for poultry. A level of 1 ppm appears to be completely safe. Chronic selenium toxicity occurs in animals when plants containing 3 to 20 ppm selenium are consumed over a prolonged period. Plants containing 400 to 800 ppm of selenium have been lethal to sheep, hogs, and calves (National Research Council, 1971). Symptoms of chronic selenium poisoning in man have been reported but are not common, probably because of the diversity of his diet (Rosenfield and Beath, 1964).

Metals that are introduced into foods through the equipment in which the food is prepared or served are an old but continuing toxicologic problem. The decline in vitality and fertility of the Romans has been attributed to the lead in the pewter dishes they used (Gilfillan, 1965). Although many countries have regulations for the control of toxic metals in dishes and cooking ware, the problem still exists. Glazes on some earthenware dishes (Harris and Elsea, 1967) and even decals on the inside of cocktail glasses (Dickinson et al., 1972) have been found to be sources of lead poisoning. Chronic lead poisoning in alcoholics has been traced to the contamina-tion of moonshine whiskey from homemade stills (Whitfield et al., 1972).

A potentially more serious source of heavy metals in foods is the result of environmental pollution whereby increased quantities of the metals are incorporated into the foods during production. Air pollution, fertilizer and pesticide residues, and industrial waste products have all contributed to the problem. Lagewerff and Specht (1970) have reported that the concentration of cadmium, nickel, lead, and zinc in roadside soil and vegetation was significant near heavily traveled roads and decreased with distance from traffic. The contamination was related to the composition of gasoline, motor oils, and tires and to roadside deposition of their waste products. Some plants and some parts of plants are known to be able to selectively accumulate lead (Jones and Clement, 1972) and cadmium (Nilsson, 1970), which metabolize them so that they are more toxic to animals and man than when deposited as environmental pollutants.

The possible hazards from mercury in fish are presently of great concern. The problem is more accurately stated as the organic or methyl mercury problem. Inorganic mercury industrial waste products have been discharged into waterways for many years but were of little concern because they are not considered to be hazards. Inorganic mercury is only minimally absorbed by plants and animals (Lisk, 1971). Organic mercury compounds, especially dimethyl mercury, are readily absorbed and accumulated through the food chain. Previously all organic mercurials were considered to be man-made compounds, but is is now known that inorganic mercury can be converted to methyl- and dimethylmercury primarily by microorganisms present in silt of river and lake beds (Jensen and Jernelov, 1969).

Realization that toxic levels of heavy metals such as mercury can be present in foods by accumulation through the food chain has been an important factor in recognition of the complexity and magnitude of environmental pollution problems. Outbreaks of mercury poisoning in Minimata and Niigata, Japan, have been traced to the methyl mercury content of fish from nearby heavily polluted water. These fish, which contained mercury up to 1 mg/kg, were eaten daily or several times a week by many of the villagers (Kutsuna, 1968; Study Group on Mercury Hazards, 1971).

Mercury can also enter the food chain at other points. Abnormally high levels of mercury have been found in seed-eating birds from Scandinavia and North America. The source of the mercury was seeds treated with mercurial fungicides (Study Group on Mercury Hazards, 1971). The unfortunate poisoning of members of a New

Mexico family who consumed pork from hogs fed mill sweepings of mercury-treated grain is another example of mercury accumulation through the food chain (Study Group on Mercury Hazards, 1971).

The identification of methyl mercury accumulation has resulted in curtailment of the use of methyl mercury seed dressings and the establishment of an interim tolerance limit of 0.5 ppm mercury for fish. Several reports (Expert Group, Stockholm, 1971; Study Group on Mercury Hazards, 1971; Wallace *et al.*, 1971) have reviewed the mercury problem and made recommendations for future studies. The Expert Group, Stockholm (1971), has recommended an acceptable daily exposure or average daily intake (ADI) of about 0.03 mg or about 0.04 μg of mercury per kilogram of body weight. Probably these levels would only be approached by individuals who consume 500 g of fish containing 0.6 mg of mercury per kilogram daily.

Foodborne Pathogens and Their Toxic Metabolites

Microbial Infections and Intoxications. Problems arising from pathogenic microorganisms and their toxic metabolites in food are many and varied. They range in severity from relatively mild intestinal disturbances caused by *Clostridium perfrigens* or *Staphylococcus* organisms to the highly lethal intoxication caused by ingestion of the toxins produced by *Clostridium botulinum*. Modern methods of food processing and distribution have influenced the pattern of foodborne infections and intoxications. Poor hygiene control of a widely distributed product can result in infection of consumers over an extended period of time and many miles from the source of contamination. Unpasteurized or inadequately pasteurized batch-processed eggs (frozen liquid or dried), used in the baking industry, have been found to be sources of *Salmonella* infections over wide areas (Taylor and McCoy, 1969).

Although *Escherichia coli* has traditionally been considered to be an indicator of fecal contamination in food and is the leading cause of seizure of foodstuffs by the FDA, it has not been considered to be a major problem in foodborne illnesses in the United States. However, in 1971, enteropathogenic *E. coli* in imported cheese was identified as the source of 96 gastroenteritis outbreaks in eight states (U.S. Public Health Sercice, 1971). It appears that either pathogenic strains themselves or enterotoxins produced by the organisms can produce illness. The food industry ·has been alerted to enteropathogenic *E. coli* as a potential food problem (Insalata, 1973).

Taylor and McCoy (1969) in their discussion of *Salmonella* and related "Arizona infections" have emphasized that the intestinal tracts of poultry, cattle, and swine form permanent reservoirs from which human foodborne *Salmonella* infections are derived, and that mass rearing and slaughtering have contributed to the problem. They believe that the greatest reduction in human infections will result from "the application of proven simple hygienic principles from the birth of the food to the final appearance on the plate of the consumer." This would include pasteurization of all egg and milk products.

The principles stated above apply also to many other forms of foodborne infections and intoxications. However, since pathogenic organisms cannot be completely eliminated by these practices, one must add proper heating, cooling, and storage practices during final food preparation to minimize further growth of organisms. Ideally food should be consumed promptly after final preparation. When this is not feasible, cooked foods, especially those containing meat and dairy products, should be cooled rapidly and stored below 5° C (41° F). *Clostridium perfrigens* and *Bacillus cereus* infections and staphylococcal food intoxication are frequently the result of improper heating and cooling practices (Angelotti, 1969; Hobbs, 1969). Another factor in controlling pathogenic microorganisms in processed food may be competition from certain nonpathogenic bacteria such as lacti cocci (Spittstoesser, 1973). In studying the microbiology of frozen vegetables, Spittstoesser concludes that in frozen food processing "the reduction of microbial contamination is a virtue—up to a point."

Botulism, the intoxication resulting from the ingestion of the highly lethal toxins produced by *Clostridium botulinum* organisms, is the most widely known and feared of the foodborne intoxications. The actual incidence is surprisingly low in humans, but large-scale outbreaks have been reported in animal populations. Six different antigenic types of toxins have been identified (Reimann, 1969; Institute of Food Technologists' Expert Panel on Food Safety and Nutrition, 1972). All members of *C. botulinum* are anaerobic organisms, but large numbers of cells can be produced under suitable growth conditions. The spores are quite heat resistant, but the toxins are readily destroyed by normal cooking. The Institute of Food Technologists' Expert Panel on Food Safety and Nutrition (1972a) has issued a summary report on botulism, in which they state that "botulism is usually associated with foods that have been given an inadequate or minimal preservation treatment, [that were] held for some time unrefrigerated, and [that were] consumed without appropriate heating."

In commercially canned foods there is minimal chance of spore survival. From the estimated 775 billion cans of food commercially produced between 1925 and 1972 in the United States, only three outbreaks of botulism were recorded. During the same period of time, an average of 10 to 20 outbreaks of botulism were reported annually, the majority being traced to improperly heated, home-canned, nonacid foods (Institute of Food Technologists' Expert Panel on Food Safety and Nutrition, 1972a). The food habits and preservation practices of a region largely determine the types of food involved in outbreaks. Almost any type of food with a pH above 4.5 can, under suitable conditions, support the growth of *C. botulinum* and consequent toxin production (Riemann, 1969). Smoked and fermented fish, liver paste, and even beef jerky have been identified as causing botulism outbreaks. Home-canned vegetables, especially green beans, have frequently been identified as sources of outbreaks. Vacuum-packed, moist, low-acid goods, such as uncured meat and smoked fish in plastic packages, have been found to be potential sources of botulism toxins. Such products should always be kept under refrigeration (preferably below 3° C) or frozen until used.

Antitoxin (a combination of type A, B, and E antitoxins) is available through the U.S. Public Health Service. It appears to be particularly effective against type E botulism (Sakaguchi, 1969). Probably because of the availability of the antitoxin, the mortality rate for botulism has dropped from 60 to 25 percent in recent years (Institute of Food Technologists' Expert Panel on Food Safety and Nutrition, 1972a). Toxoids have also been produced that can be used for vaccination. Because of the low incidence of the disease, only workers regularly exposed by *C. botulinum* have so far been vaccinated (Riemann, 1969).

Mycotoxins. Fungi, which contaminate a wide variety of foodstuffs, especially cereal grains, also produce toxic metabolites, frequently termed mycotoxins. Molds are capable of producing a wide variety of complex organic molecules, most of which are nontoxic. Ergotism from rye infected with *Claviceps purpurea* was probably the first mycotoxicosis to be recognized, but it has largely been eliminated as a human food problem (Wogan, 1969).

Aflatoxins, the toxic metabolites produced by some strains of the fungus *Aspergillus flavus*, have been widely studied in recent years because of their known toxicity and carcinogenicity in many species of animals and because of the wide distribution of the fungus in foodstuffs, especially peanut meals (Wogan, 1969). Aflatoxicosis was first recognized in 1960 in England when serious outbreaks of the intoxication occurred in turkeys. Since then outbreaks have been reported in ducks, swine, and young cattle. Aflatoxins have been found in samples of oilseeds, pulses, and other food staples from various parts of the world. Although they are not as acutely toxic to humans as to some other species, the chronic ingestion of aflatoxins has been implicated as a contributing factor in the high incidence of human liver cancer in certain areas of southeast Asia and Africa where the inhabitants consume cereals, peanuts, and other foodstuffs frequently infested with molds (Shank *et al.*, 1972).

Viral Infections. Recognition of food as an agent for the transmission of viral infections is of relatively recent origin (Cliver, 1969). The literature on foodborne viral infections is not extensive, but it documents how viral infections may be spread by food. Cliver (1969) suggests that recent developments in food technology enabling more efficient and widespread distribution of food may accentuate the problem. Infectious hepatitis is a common food-associated viral disease. The organism is ordinarily destroyed by thorough cooking, but foods can easily be contaminated by infected handlers during final preparation. Some foods, such as shellfish that are consumed raw, can be sources of this viral disease. Cliver (1969) has identified ten outbreaks of infectious hepatitis caused by the ingestion of raw shellfish. In most instances, the shellfish were found to be from water polluted with raw sewage.

Some cases of poliomyelitis have been traced to virus-infected foods. In most instances, raw milk was the vehicle in transmission (Cliver, 1969). With the development of poliomyelitis vaccine and the decline in the use of raw milk, the incidence of such outbreaks has largely ceased. The relationship of animal influenza viruses to man and vice versa is being extensively studied at the present time. There is considerable support for the theory that animals, particularly swine, are reservoirs of influenza viruses and that they are potential contributors to new pandemic strains of influenza viruses that periodically appear (Kaplan and Beveridge, 1972).

Migrants from Packaging Materials

With increased urbanization and growth of the food industry, more and more foodstuffs are prepackaged before reaching the retailer's shelves. Many problems are involved in packaging because almost any packaging material is subject to slow chemical or physical attack from the food or storage conditions. When some of the packaging material becomes a part of the food as consumed, it is termed a migrant and is classed as an incidental or unintentional additive. Therefore, it is subject to control under the various food additive regulations.

The traditional metal containers that came into use in the nineteenth century have been improved over the years so that the contents are minimally exposed to lead solder. The one exception appears to be canned milk, which is still packaged in a can with a flat-soldered seam and the filling hole closed by solder flux. The lead content of canned evaporated milk has been found to be higher than that present in either fresh or powdered milk. Although no cases of lead poisoning in infants have been traced to the use of canned milk, there is concern that the lead content of canned milk could increase the body burden at the age when children are particularly susceptible to lead poisoning (Shea, 1973).

The packaging of foodstuffs in plastic materials presents very complex problems that are being studied at the present time. Although the plastic itself may be relatively insoluble, partially reacted polymers, plasticizers, and contaminants can be dissolved and migrate into the food or become environmental problems. Phthalic acid esters (PAES), which are extensively used as plasticizers in food wrap films, have been found in whole blood stored in plastic bags (Jaeger and Rubin, 1970). PAES are now widely dispersed throughout the environment, but their significance as environmental pollutants is not fully known. The use of polyvinyl chloride (PVC) plastic bottles for packaging of liquors was banned by the FDA and the U.S. Treasury Department in 1973 because of possible toxic interaction between the alcohol and PVC. (See Chapter 20).

CONCLUSIONS

The points made by Bonser (1967) for carcinogenic risks can well apply to the whole field of toxicologic problems of food additives. There are inherent risks in eating that we must take in order to live. By ingesting a wide variety of foodstuffs chosen from carefully selected, produced, processed, and prepared foods, we can greatly reduce the calculated risks while ensuring ourselves of an adequate diet. Continuing research in many areas will also reduce the inherent risks from both added and natural toxins that may be present in foodstuffs.

REFERENCES

Anonymous: Cyclamates barred as "food additives" under Delaney clause. *Food Chem. News* (Washington, D.C.), special suppl., Oct. 20, 1969.

Anonymous: Saccharin: Where do we go from here? *FDA Consumer*, **12**(3):16–21, 1978a.

Anonymous: Saccharin warning notice required in stores. *FDA Consumer*, **12**(5):4, 1978b.

Angelotti, R.: Staphylococcal infections. In Riemann, H. (ed.): *Food-Borne Infections and Intoxications*. Academic Press, Inc., New York, 1969.

Beckman, H.: *Pharmacology. The Nature, Action and Use of Drugs*, 2nd ed. W. B. Saunders Co., Philadelphia, 1961.

Bonser, G. M.: Factors concerned in the location of human and experimental tumors. *Br. Med. J.*, **2**:655–60, 1967.

Cliver, D. O.: Viral infections. In Riemann, H. (ed.): *Food-Borne Infections and Intoxications*. Academic Press, Inc., New York, 1969.

Conney, A. H., and Burns, J. J.: Metabolic interactions among environmental chemicals and drugs. *Science*, **178**:576–86, 1972.

Council of Europe (Partial Agreement) Natural and Artificial Flavoring Substances. Strasbourg, 1 July, 1970 (as noted in Elias, 1972).

Davis, J. G.: Food additives: An introductory paper on general problems. In Goodwin, R. W. L. (ed.): *Chemical Additives in Foods*. Little, Brown & Co., Boston, 1967.

Egan, H., and Hubbard, A. W.: Food additives specifications. *Chem. Ind.*, 1971:1181–86, 1971.

Elias, P. S.: Food additives, toxicology and the EEC. *Chem. Ind.*, 1972:139–44, 1972.

Expert Group, Stockholm: Methylmercury in fish. A toxicologic-epidemiologic evaluation of risks. *Nodisk Hygienski Tidskrift*, suppl. 4, Stockholm, Sweden, 1971 (English translation).

Federation of American Societies for Experimental Biology. Select Committee on GRAS Substances: Evaluation of Health Aspects of GRAS Food Ingredients: Lessons learned and questions unanswered. *Fed. Proc.*, **36**:2519–62, 1977.

Food and Drug Administration Advisory Committee on Protocols for Safety Evaluation: Panel on carcinogenesis report on cancer testing in the safety evaluation of food additives and pesticides. *Toxicol. Appl. Pharmacol.*, **20**:419–38, 1971.

Gilfillan, S. C.: Lead poisoning and the fall of Rome. *J. Occup. Med.*, **7**:53–60, 1965.

Golberg, L.: Trace chemical contaminants in food: Potential for harm. *Food Cosmet. Toxicol.*, **9**:65–80, 1971.

Hall, R. L.: GRAS review and food additive legislation. *Food Technol.*, **25**:466–70, 1971.

Hall, R. L., and Oser, B. L.: Recent progress in the consideration of flavoring ingredients under the Food Additives Amendment. 4. GRAS substances. *Food Technol.*, **24**:25–34, 1970.

Harris, R. W., and Elsea, W. R.: Ceramic glaze as a source of lead poisoning. *J.A.M.A.*, **202**:544–46, 1967.

Hobbs, B. C.: *Clostridium perfrigens* and *Bacillus cereus* infections. In Riemann, H. (ed.): *Food-Borne Infections and Intoxications*. Academic Press, Inc., New York, 1969.

Hopkins, H.: The GRAS list revisited. *FDA Consumer*, **12**(4):13–15, 1978.

Insalata, N. F.: Enteropathogenic *E. coli*—A new problem for the food industry. *Food Technol.*, **27**(3):56, 58, 1973.

Institute of Food Technologists' Expert Panel on Food Safety and Nutrition: Botulism. A scientific status summary. *J. Food Sci.*, **37**:985–88, 1972a.

———: Nitrites, nitrates, and nitrosamines in food—A dilemma. *J. Food. Sci.*, **37**:989–92, 1972b.

Jaeger, R. J., and Rubin, R. J.: Plasticizers from plastic devices: Extraction, metabolism, and accumulation by biological systems. *Science*, **170**:460–62, 1970.

Jensen, S., and Jernelov, A.: Biological methylation of mercury in aquatic organisms. *Nature* (Lond.), **223**:753, 1969.

Joint FAO/WHO Expert Committee on Food Additives: Specifications for the identity and purity of food additives and their toxicological evaluation. Seventh Report. FAO Nutrition Meetings, Report Series No. 35, 1964.

Jones, L. H. P., and Clement, C. R.: Lead in the environment: Possible health effect on adults. In Hepple, P. (ed.): *Lead in the Environment*. Institute of Petroleum, London, 1972.

Kaplan, M., and Beveridge, W. I. B.: Influenza in animals. Introduction. *Bull. WHO*, **47**:439–43, 1972.

Katsuna, M. (ed.): Minamata report, Minamata disease. Kumamoto University, Kumamoto, Japan, 1968.

Kent-Jones, D. S.: Modern food and food additives. *Chem. Ind.*, 1971:1275–83, 1971.

Kilgore, W. W., and Li, M. Y.: The carcinogenicity of pesticides. In Gunther, F. A. (ed.): *Residue Reviews*, vol. 48. Springer-Verlag, New York, 1973, pp. 141–61.

Koenig, N.: A new vital influence international standards. *Food Technol.*, **48**:148–50, 1965.

Lagerwerff, J. V., and Specht, A. W.: Contamination of road side soil and vegetation with cadmium, nickel, lead, and zinc. *Environ. Sci. Technol.*, **4**:583–86, 1970.

Lisk, D. G.: Ecological aspects of metals. *N. Y. State J. Med.*, **71**:2541–55, 1971.

Luckey, T. D.: Introduction to food additives. In Furia, T. E. (ed.): *Handbook of Food Additives*. The Chemical Rubber Co., Cleveland, 1968.

Manufacturing Chemists' Association: *Food Additives: What They Are, How They Are Used*. Manufacturing Chemists' Association, Inc., Washington, D.C., 1961.

Moore, T.: *Vitamin A*. Elsevier Publishing Co., Amsterdam, 1957.

National Center For Toxicological Research: Report prepared for Society of Toxicology, Jefferson, AR, 1973.

National Research Council: *Recommended Dietary Allowances. A Report of the Food and Nutrition Board*, 7th rev. ed. National Academy of Sciences, Washington, D.C., 1968.

———: *Recommended Dietary Allowances. A Report of the Food and Nutrition Board*, 8th rev. ed. National Academy of Sciences, Washington, D.C., 1974.

———: *Selenium in Nutrition, Report of Committee on Animal Nutrition, Subcommittee on Selenium*. National Academy of Sciences, Washington, D.C., 1971.

———: *Food Chemical Codex*, 2nd ed. National Academy of Sciences, Washington, D.C., 1972.

National Research Council, Food Protection Committee: *Toxicants Occurring Naturally in Foods*. National Academy of Sciences Publication 1354. Washington, D.C., 1966.

———: *Evaluating the Safety of Food Chemicals*. National Academy of Sciences, Washington, D.C., 1970.

Nilsson, R.: *Aspects on the Toxicity of Cadmium and Its Compounds*. Ecological Research Committee Bull. No. 7. Swedish Natural Science Research Council, Stockholm, Sweden, 1970.

Oser, B. L.: Much ado about safety. *Food Cosmet. Toxicol.*, **7**:415–24, 1969.

Oser, B. L., and Ford, R. A.: Recent progress in the consideration of flavoring ingredients under the Food Additives Amendment. 6. GRAS substances. *Food Technol.*, **27**(1):64–67, 1973a.

———: Recent progress in the consideration of flavoring ingredients under the Food Additives Amendment. 7. GRAS substances. *Food Technol.*, **27**(11):56–57, 1973b.

———: Recent progress in the consideration of flavoring ingredients under the Food Additives Amendment. 8. GRAS substances. *Food Technol.*, **28**(9):76–77, 80, 1974.

———: Recent progress in the consideration of flavoring ingredients under the Food Additives Amendment. 9. GRAS substances. *Food Technol.*, **29**(8):70–72, 1975.

———: Recent progress in the consideration of flavoring ingredients under the Food Additives Amendment. 10. GRAS substances. *Food Technol.*, **31**(1):65–67, 70, 72, 74, 1977.

———: Recent progress in the consideration of flavoring ingredients under the Food Additives Amendment. 11. GRAS substances. *Food Technol.*, **32**(2):60–62, 64–66, 68–70, 1978.

Oser, B. L., and Hall, R. L.: Recent progress in the consideration of flavoring ingredients under the Food Additives Amendment. 5. GRAS substances. *Food Technol.*, **26**(5): 35–37, 40–42, 1972.

Riemann, H. (ed.): *Food-Borne Infections and Intoxications*. Academic Press, Inc., New York, 1969.

Rosenfield, I., and Beath, O. A.: *Selenium: Geobotany, Biochemistry, Toxicity and Nutrition*. Academic Press, Inc., New York, 1964.

Sakaguchi, G.: Botulism—type E. In Riemann, H. (ed.): *Food-Borne Infections and Intoxications*. Academic Press, Inc., New York, 1969.

Sanders, H. J.: Chemical mutagens. An exploding roster of suspects. *Chem. Engin. News*, **47**(23):54–68, 1969.

Shank, R. C.; Bhamarapravati, N.; Gordon, J. E.; and Wogan, G. N.: Dietary aflatoxins and human liver cancer. IV. Incidence of primary liver cancer in two municipal populations in Thailand. *Food Cosmet. Toxicol.*, **10**:171–79, 1972.

Shea, K. P.: Canned milk. *Environment*, **15**:6–11, 1973.

Spittstoesser, D. F.: The microbiology of frozen vegetables. *Food Technol.*, **27**(1):54–60, 1973.

Study Group on Mercury Hazards, Nelson, N. (Chairman): Hazards of mercury. *Environ. Res.*, **4**:1–69, 1971.

Taylor, J., and McCoy, J. H.: Salmonella and Arizona infections. In Riemann, H. (ed.): *Food-Borne Infections and Intoxications*. Academic Press, Inc., New York, 1969.

U.S. Department of Health, Education, and Welfare: *Report of the Secretary's Commission on Pesticides and Their Relationship to Environmental Health*, Parts I and II. Superintendent of Documents, Washington, D.C., 1969.

U.S. Public Health Service: *Morbidity and Mortality Weekly Report*, vol. 20. Center for Disease Control, Atlanta, GA, 1971, p. 445.

Wade, N.: Delaney anti-cancer clause: Scientists debate on article of faith. *Science*, **177**:588–91, 1972.

Wallace, R. A.; Fulkerson, W.; Shutts, W. D.; and Lyons, W. S.: *Mercury in the Environment, the Human Element*. Oakridge National Laboratory, Oakridge, TN, 1971.

sulfur dioxide reach values of 0.75 mg/m³ for smoke and 0.25 ppm for sulfur dioxide, excess mortality is observed.

There is also clear-cut evidence that more ordinary day-by-day fluctuations in pollution levels have adverse effects on sick people. By giving chronic bronchitic patients a very simple diary in which they recorded whether they felt better or worse than usual, and then relating these entries to daily air pollution data in London, a striking correlation was obtained (Lawther, 1958). It was plain the patients felt worse on days of greater pollution. These studies were continued after the British Clean Air Act had reduced the levels of both pollutants. It was then possible to conclude that when the 24-hour mean concentrations for smoke and sulfur dioxide were respectively below 0.25 mg/m³ and 0.19 ppm, the patients showed no response (Lawther, 1975).

The acute effects discussed have been associated with the reducing type of pollution. There is less clear-cut evidence to associate the photochemical oxidant type of pollution with acute effects on human health. There is of course no question of the ability of this type of pollution to produce severe eye irritation that can be correlated with the concentration of pollution present. Studies made of daily mortality among persons 65 and over in Los Angeles County indicated that this was strongly influenced by a heat wave but was not altered consistently by variations in oxidant concentrations. There has been no adequately demonstrated relationship between daily hospital admissions and variations in concentrations of photochemical oxidants. Admissions for conditions considered "highly relevant" (allergic disorders, inflammatory disease of the eye, acute upper respiratory infections, influenza, and bronchitis) were, however, found to show significant correlations with oxidant levels, carbon monoxide, and ozone. It is possible to show a high degree of correlation between diminished performance of high-school cross-country track runners and increased oxidant levels occurring in the hour before the meet.

CHRONIC HEALTH EFFECTS OF AIR POLLUTION

Ambient air pollution concentrations occurring in many cities of the world contribute to the occurrence and/or aggravation of disease in urban populations. The diseases that fall into this category are the following: acute nonspecific upper respiratory disease (i.e., the "common cold"), chronic bronchitis, chronic obstructive ventilatory disease, pulmonary emphysema, bronchial asthma, and lung cancer.

Chronic bronchitis is characterized by exces-

sive mucus secretion in the bronchial tree. A chronic or recurrent productive cough is present. In order for the condition to be officially defined as "chronic" these symptoms should have been present on most days for a minimum of three months in the year and for not less than two consecutive years. There appears to be little question that there is a relationship between chronic bronchitis and both cigarette smoking and air pollution. The effect of smoking is by far the greater of the two as a contributing factor to respiratory disease. Unless careful data are included on smoking histories it is impossible to assess the contribution made by air pollution. This does not mean, however, that air pollution makes no contribution. The following indices have been shown to be associated with chronic bronchitis mortality: population size of the community, amounts of fuel burned in large cities, levels of annual sulfur dioxide, levels of dust fall as well as airborne dust levels, decreased visibility. The following have been shown to be associated with aggravation of symptoms of chronic bronchitis: decreased visibility, outdoor ambient air as contrasted with less polluted indoor air, temporal changes in concentrations of smoke and sulfur dioxide.

In chronic obstructive ventilatory disease the movement of air in and out of the lungs is impeded by partial closure of the airways. After eliminating the smoking factor, it was found that residents of a polluted area showed lower values for one-second forced expiratory volume (FEV_1) than did residents of an area of low pollution. The difference was small but measurable and was attributed to air pollution. Japanese studies have shown that the airway resistance of school-children living in polluted areas is greater than that of similar children living in nonpolluted areas.

The fact that pulmonary emphysema seems to be increasing, especially in urban areas, points toward air pollution as a possible etiologic factor. If patients with emphysema are placed in a room in which the smog typical of Los Angeles can be removed from the air, after 24 hours they have both subjective relief and objective improvement, which can be measured by pulmonary function tests. Such patients have a decreased oxygen need when they are breathing cleansed air than when they are breathing untreated community air.

Bronchial asthma is produced by many aeroallergens of natural origin, which are dispersed by natural forces rather than from man's activities. Sometimes these natural allergens can be introduced by man as air pollutants, for example, castor bean dust from factories processing the material, or material from grain handling and milling. Various studies have suggested that asthmatic attacks are associated with higher levels of pollution.

The cause of cancer is, as far as we know, a multiplicity of factors. Among the compounds known to occur as urban air pollutants are some, such as benzopyrene, that have known carcinogenic potency. The adsorption of carcinogenic substances on inert particulate material could prolong residence time at sensitive sites in the respiratory tract. Many air pollutants have an irritant action on the mucous membranes of the respiratory tract. There is experimental evidence that when benzopyrene is inhaled by rats whose respiratory tracts have chronic irritation (produced by chronic sulfur dioxide inhalation), bronchogenic carcinoma results (Kuschner, 1968). Experimental evidence also exists that when ozonized gasoline was inhaled by mice that had been infected with influenza virus, epidermoid carcinomas were produced (Kotin and Falk, 1963). There is an urban-rural gradient in incidence of lung cancer, which is real when corrected for the effects of cigarette smoking. Kotin and Falk say, "Chemical, physical and biologic data unite to form a constellation that strongly implicates the atmosphere as one dominant factor in the pathogenesis of lung cancer."

GENERAL CONSIDERATIONS OF REDUCING TYPE POLLUTION

The acute air pollution incidents made plain that under certain meteorologic conditions the reducing type pollution characterized by sulfur dioxide and smoke was capable of producing disastrous effects. This stimulated toxicologic research on experimental animals and human subjects. Special emphasis, perhaps too much for too long, was given to studies of sulfur dioxide alone.

Recognition of the critical importance of atmospheric interactions among components of the sulfurous pollution complex was long overdue when it finally found general acceptance. Sulfur dioxide does not remain unaltered in the atmosphere. Instead, a portion of it is converted to sulfuric acid, ammonium sulfate, and other sulfates. The conversion to sulfuric acid can be brought about by soot or by trace metals such as vanadium or manganese. Recent evidence indicates that stable sulfite complexes may be formed in the presence of metals such as copper or iron. Gas-particle interactions are complicated and on the whole incompletely understood. Toxicologic studies suggest that some, but not all, of the sulfur-containing particulate materials are more irritant than sulfur dioxide. Research to permit definitive identification of the sulfur aerosols in the atmosphere has lagged behind our

needs. Until this gap is closed it will be very difficult, if not impossible, to do definitive epidemiology.

In 1969 the National Air Pollution Control Administration (now under the Environmental Protection Agency) issued two documents: *Air Quality Criteria for Sulfur Oxides* (USDHEW, 1969a) and *Air Quality Criteria for Particulate Matter* (USDHEW, 1969b). These reviewed the state of knowledge as of that time and were intended to relate observed effects to concentrations of the pollutants. Criteria Documents were the legal prerequisites for Air Quality Standards and formed the data base for the standards that were promulgated. Currently all of the criteria documents are scheduled for revision and updating by the EPA.

Millions of dollars are involved in control measures designed to meet these air quality standards. Thus, it is indeed valid to inquire as to the adequacy of the data base upon which current standards rest. The proposed increase in the use of coal further emphasizes this question. In the decade since the criteria for sulfur oxides and for particulate matter were issued, an almost unbelievable amount of time has been spent in reviewing and rereviewing the literature and in identifying and reidentifying gaps in our knowledge. A cynic might wish more effort had been spent in filling in the major gaps. The report of a committee chaired by Dr. David Rall provides an excellent and balanced summary (Rall, 1974). It has thoughtfulness, brevity, and complete lack of bias to commend it. Another well-balanced, more detailed review was issued by the Electric Power Research Institute (1976).

TOXICOLOGY OF SULFUR DIOXIDE

Studies of Mortality and Lung Pathology

Early studies of the mortality produced by sulfur dioxide utilized mice, rats, guinea pigs, and insects. The concentrations required to kill animals are so high that these studies have little relevance to air pollution problems.

Chronic exposure of animals to sulfur dioxide produces a thickening of the mucous layer in the trachea and a hypertrophy of goblet cells and mucous glands that resembles the pathology of chronic bronchitis. The important point is that such changes can be produced by irritant exposure alone without the intermediary of infection. Infection is of unquestioned importance in the etiology of chronic bronchitis, but experimental evidence indicates that it is not an essential factor in the development of the excessive mucous cells characteristic of this disease. An excellent discussion of the respiratory mucous membrane and its response to irritant agents by Jeffrey and Reid (1977) is recommended reading for students interested in pulmonary toxicology.

In experiments done by Dalhamn (1956), daily exposures of rats to 10 ppm sulfur dioxide for 18 to 67 days produced a thickening of the mucous layer in the trachea of rats. This layer, normally about 5 μm, increased in the exposed animals to about 25 μm. The rate of transport of the mucous layer was decreased and remained so for a month after the end of the exposure. In acute *in vivo* exposures of the trachea of rats to sulfur dioxide, 12 ppm caused cessation of the ciliary beat in four to six minutes. The cilia regained mobility a few minutes after the exposure ceased. In the chronic exposures, however, the frequency of the beat of the cilia was normal. They were unable to move the thickened mucous layer efficiently, thus slowing clearance mechanisms. Normally beating cilia under a mucous blanket too thick for them to move almost suggests the end result of a self-defeating protective mechanism.

Reid (1963) exposed rats five hours a day, five days a week for three months, to 300 to 400 ppm sulfur dioxide. Mucus-secreting cells increased in number in the main bronchi, where they are normally frequent, and appeared in the peripheral airways, from which they are normally absent. Cessation of exposure arrested the increase in cells but the excess persisted for at least three months after the termination of exposure. One group of rats obtained from a supplier who had attempted to breed a strain less susceptible to bronchiectasis showed a lesser response to sulfur dioxide exposure.

Mawdesley-Thomas *et al.* (1971) exposed rats for ten periods of six hours to 50, 100, 200, and 300 ppm and examined them 72 hours post-exposure. In the trachea the highest dose produced considerable epithelial damage and almost complete destruction of goblet cells. A dose-related increase in goblet cells, however, occurred at lower concentrations in the trachea and at all concentrations in the bronchiolus. Excess mucus that reaches the alveolar spaces must be removed by the alveolar macrophages. Exposure to sulfur dioxide did not increase the number of macrophages but did increase their metabolic activity, as indicated by a dose-related increase in acid phosphatase. This increase could be detected at a concentration of 25 ppm.

Dogs exposed for four to five months to 500 to 600 ppm, for two hours, twice a week showed similar alterations in histochemistry and histology of the respiratory mucous membranes (Spicer *et al.*, 1974). The magnitude of the pathology suggests that the very high concentrations were probably not necessary to produce critical alterations, the more so as other workers found that daily exposures of dogs to 1 ppm for a year produced detectable effects indicating a slowing of tracheal mucous transport (Hirsch *et al.*, 1975). In rats, daily exposures to a total of 70 to 170 hours to 0.1, 1.0, and 20 ppm interfered with the clearance of inert particles. The most marked effects were seen with lower doses administered over a longer period of time (Ferin and Leach, 1973).

Following continuous exposure of guinea pigs or monkeys for periods of up to a year or more to concentrations of 0.1 to 5 ppm, no evidence of pulmonary pathology was detected (Alarie *et al.*, 1972, 1975). Unfortunately the more sensitive techniques discussed above for evaluation of alterations in respiratory mucous membranes were not included in the protocol of these studies.

Studies on Absorption and Distribution of Inhaled Sulfur Dioxide

On the basis of its solubility in water, one would predict that sulfur dioxide would be readily removed during passage through the upper respiratory tract. This prediction can be tested experimentally by making measurements of the drop in sulfur dioxide concentration when an airstream passes through the upper respiratory tract of larger animals, such as dogs or rabbits, or in human subjects. Indirect assessment of this factor may be made by comparison of the response to given sulfur dioxide concentrations inhaled through the nose or through a tracheal cannula in animals or by comparison of the response to nose and mouth breathing in human subjects.

By the use of $S^{35}O_2$, Strandberg (1964) was able to examine the absorption by the upper respiratory tract of rabbits over a concentration range of 0.05 to 700 ppm. At higher concentrations removal was 90 percent or greater; this is in agreement with the findings of other workers on dogs and human subjects. At concentrations below 1 ppm, however, only 5 percent or less was removed by the upper respiratory tract. These data fit with the observation that guinea pigs breathing through a tracheal cannula to bypass removal by the upper respiratory tract showed an increased response to concentrations of 2, 20, or 100 ppm but no difference at a concentration of 0.4 ppm (Amdur, 1966). This fitting together of data obtained by different methods on different species makes a strong case for the fact that at levels pertinent to air pollution, sulfur dioxide is not efficiently removed by the upper respiratory tract.

The penetration of sulfur dioxide to the lungs is greater during mouth breathing than during nose breathing. An increase in flow rate markedly increases the penetration. In dogs breathing orally, 99 percent of 1 ppm was removed orally at a flow rate of 3.5 liters/minute. Increasing the flow rate tenfold decreased the removal efficiency to 33 percent (Frank *et al.*, 1969). These data are of significance in connection with increased uptake in persons exercising and/or mouth breathing during incidents of heavy pollution.

Studies using $S^{35}O_2$ have shown that inhaled sulfur dioxide is readily distributed throughout the body. This also occurs when only an isolated segment of the trachea or the upper airways is exposed. Systemic absorption occurs from these sites, although to a lesser extent than when the lungs are exposed. It is possible that the lungs release some of the gas absorbed in this manner, since radioactivity could be detected in exhaled air samples collected at the carina or below when the lungs had had no sulfur dioxide exposure (Frank *et al.*, 1967). The gas was presumably carried to the lungs from the pulmonary capillaries.

Inhaled sulfur dioxide is only slowly removed from the respiratory tract. Radioactivity can be detected in the respiratory system for a week or more following exposure. Some of the S^{35} appears to be attached to protein.

Studies of Pulmonary Function

A basic physiologic response to the inhalation of sulfur dioxide is a mild degree of bronchial constriction, which is reflected in a measurable increase in flow resistance. This increase in resistance has been demonstrated in guinea pigs, dogs, cats, and human subjects. A method for studying the response of guinea pigs (Amdur and Mead, 1958) provides a biologic assay for examining such factors as dose-response relationships, comparison of irritant potency of pollutants, and the effect of aerosols on the response to irritant gases. The method is sufficiently simple that data on many animals exposed only once can be readily obtained. This eliminates the need for reexposure following "recovery," which is an understandable part of the protocol of experiments that use complicated physiologic preparations of larger animals. Unless repeated exposure is the factor being tested, reuse of an experimental animal is not sound toxicologic practice. Studies on larger animals permit the use of more elaborate methods of respiratory physiology that shed light on the mechanisms that underlie the changes.

Exposure of guinea pigs to sulfur dioxide produces a dose-related increase in flow resistance. The lower curve in Figure 24–1 shows a dose-response curve relating increase in resistance to sulfur dioxide concentration. Because the figure is designed primarily to demonstrate comparative irritant potency of sulfuric acid and sulfur dioxide, the concentrations are plotted as mg of sulfur per m^3 (1 ppm sulfur dioxide = 1.31 mg S/m^3). In exposures to 100 ppm or less of sulfur dioxide alone the resistance returns to control values by the end of a one-hour postexposure period.

The increase in flow resistance is accompanied by a decrease in compliance of the lungs. The units of resistance are cm $H_2O/ml/sec$. The units of compliance are ml/cm H_2O. The product of resistance times compliance has the unit of time and is referred to as the time constant of the lungs. An increase in the time constant is associated with a decrease in

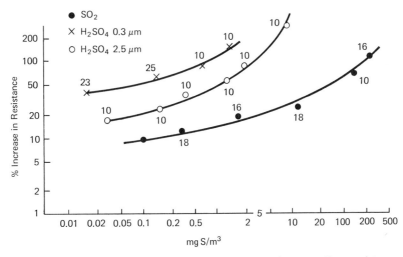

Figure 24–1. Dose-response curves of increase in pulmonary flow resistance produced in guinea pigs exposed for one hour to sulfur dioxide or sulfuric acid. The number beside each point represents the number of animals exposed.

frequency of breathing. In sulfur dioxide exposures, the increase in resistance is proportionately greater than the decrease in compliance, resulting in an elevated time constant. A decrease in respiratory frequency is observed that becomes statistically significant at concentrations above 25 ppm. Tidal volume increases, but not enough to compensate for the decrease in frequency. The end result is a decrease in the minute volume.

This pattern of respiratory response, characterized by increased flow resistance and decreased frequency of breathing, is typical of a variety of irritants. Among them are sulfur dioxide, sulfuric acid, formaldehyde, formic acid, acetic acid, acrolein, zinc ammonium sulfate, zinc sulfate, ammonium sulfate, ferric sulfate, and iodine. For this group of irritants, increase in flow resistance is the most sensitive criterion of response. For another group of irritants the pattern of respiratory response is different. There is a major decrease in compliance with minimal change in resistance and an increase in the frequency of breathing. This second pattern of response is typical of deep lung irritants.

Dogs also respond to inhalation of sulfur dioxide with an increase in resistance (Frank and Speizer, 1965). The gas was given to anesthetized dogs by nose, by tracheal cannula, and by exposing an isolated segment of the trachea to sulfur dioxide while the lungs were ventilated with air. The response was greatest when the gas was introduced directly into the lungs via a tracheal cannula and least when only a segment of trachea was exposed. The fact that resistance increased by exposure of only the tracheal segment suggests a referred reflex constriction of the bronchi. Nasal resistance also increased in a manner roughly proportional to sulfur dioxide concentration over a range of 7 to 61 ppm for 15 minutes. At concentrations above 23 ppm the nasal resistance became progressively greater throughout the exposure period. These changes probably reflect mucosal swelling and/or increased secretion of mucus.

The mechanism of bronchoconstriction produced by sulfur dioxide has been studied in cats (Nadel et al., 1965). Anesthetized cats were ventilated with a pump via a tracheal cannula. Sulfur dioxide gas was delivered either to the lungs or to the upper airways. Total pulmonary resistance increased during the first breath when sulfur dioxide was delivered to the lower airways and lungs during a single inflation cycle. It had returned to control values within one minute. Exposing only the upper airways also produced an increase in resistance. An IV injection of atropine or cooling of the cervical vagosympathetic nerves abolished these effects; rewarming of the nerve reestablished the response. The rapidity of the response and its reversal suggests that changes in smooth muscle tone are the cause of the bronchoconstriction. The response depends on intact parasympathetic pathways.

The cough reflex in cats is elicited when sulfur dioxide is given through an endobronchial catheter to the lungs and smaller bronchi without coming in contact with the trachea (Widdicombe, 1954). The cough reflex produced in this way was stronger than that produced when sulfur dioxide contacted only the trachea and main bronchi. After several inhalations, the cats became completely refractory to sulfur dioxide but still gave normal response to mechanical stimulation of the trachea. Procaine solution sprayed into the trachea blocked the mechanical cough reflex but failed to affect the response to sulfur dioxide. These data suggest that the receptors for the mechanical stimulus and the sulfur dioxide stimulus are distinct.

This was further confirmed in elegant experiments in which single vagal fibers that were excited by inflation of the lungs were dissected for study (Widdicombe, 1954). One group of these fibers, distributed throughout the lower trachea and main bronchi, was sensitized and then inhibited by sulfur dioxide. These fibers were not inhibited by procaine. Another group of fibers was sensitive to mechanical stimulation but not to sulfur dioxide. Vagal temperatures of $7°$ to $10° C$ blocked the fibers sensitive to sulfur dioxide. Sulfur dioxide acts via the sympathetic nervous system as well as via the vagus nerve. The group of fibers sensitive to sulfur dioxide sends fibers to the sympathetic trunk.

Human subjects exposed for brief periods to sulfur dioxide also show alterations in pulmonary mechanics. Sensitive physiologic methods that yield essentially the same respiratory data as discussed above can be made without interrupting exposure to sulfur dioxide. Frank et al. (1962) exposed 11 subjects to 1, 5, and 13 ppm sulfur dioxide for periods of ten minutes. At 1 ppm only one individual showed an increase in flow resistance. It is of interest to note that this was the individual with the highest control resistance of the group. At a concentration of 5 ppm the average increase in resistance for the group was 39 percent above control values. Nine out of the group showed a statistically significant increase in resistance. At 13 ppm the resistance of all subjects increased, with an average increase for the group of 72 percent. It is thus possible by meticulous attention to experimental protocol and by the use of sensitive physiologic methods to demonstrate a dose-response relationship in human subjects. Extension of some of the exposures to 30 minutes showed that the resistance remained elevated but decreased slightly compared with the ten-minute response. Extension of the exposures to 1 ppm to 30 minutes did not produce an increase in resistance. These data suggest that the response is related to concentration of sulfur dioxide and not to a $C \times T$ relationship. There was a slight decrease in functional residual capacity at 13 ppm, but the two lower concentrations produced no effect.

Speizer and Frank (1966) compared the effects of breathing sulfur dioxide by nose and by mouth in ten-minute exposures to 15 or 28 ppm. In mouth breathing the pulmonary flow resistance increased in 9 out of 12 experiments. When the same concentrations were breathed through the nose, pulmonary flow resistance increased in only 3 out of 12 experiments and decreased in one experiment. When the gas was breathed by nose, the pulmonary flow resistance was often higher during the postexposure period than during the exposure itself. In 8 of the 12 experiments nasal resistance increased, in three it decreased, and in one it decreased and then increased during the same exposure.

Lawther et al. (1975) found that airway resistance increased when subjects inhaled 1 to 3 ppm deeply by mouth. There was a dose-response relationship between the number of breaths taken (up to 32) and the observed increase in resistance. Airway resistance was increased when concentrations of 5 to 30 ppm were inhaled normally. Although concentrations as high as 3 ppm are unlikely as daily or hourly averages, they could be encountered briefly as pockets of pollution from local sources. The fact that as few as eight deep breaths will produce increased airway resistance could be of significance to individuals with diseased lungs. The relationship between ventilation and perfusion could be further disturbed with undesirable clinical consequences. Although the subjects used in these studies were normal, healthy individuals, 3 out of 25 showed a greater change that persisted for a longer period after exposure was discontinued.

Almost all of the studies of human subjects mention some individual who was more sensitive than the rest of the subjects. Upon occasion, exposures to 5 to 10 ppm have been reported to cause severe bronchospasm. These individuals who were more sensitive have been "normal, healthy subjects," not individuals with respiratory disease. Unfortunately there are no studies of how these individuals would react to even lower concentrations of sulfur dioxide, nor do we have data that would indicate in any way what percentage of an urban population might be expected to show a greater-than-average sensitivity to sulfur dioxide.

The changes we have been discussing have been observed when animals or human subjects have been exposed for short periods of an hour or less to sulfur dioxide. Alarie et al. (1970) exposed guinea pigs to 0.13, 1.01, and 5.72 ppm sulfur dioxide continuously for a year. When the guinea pigs were compared with a comparable control group breathing clean air, no evidence was found of adverse effects on the mechanical properties of the lung. Measurements included tidal volume, respiratory rate, minute volume, flow resistance, and work of breathing. Monkeys (groups of nine animals) were exposed continuously for 78 weeks to 0.14, 0.64, and 1.28 ppm sulfur dioxide (Alarie et al., 1972). No detrimental alterations in pulmonary function were detected. A fourth group had been started at a level of about 5 ppm. After 30 weeks on experiment, there was an accidental high exposure for an hour to somewhere between 200 and 1,000 ppm. These animals were continued for the functional measurements but shifted to room air instead of continuing the exposure. Following the overexposure, these animals showed a definite deterioration in pulmonary function, which was shown clearly by the change in the distribution of ventilation.

Lewis et al. (1969) exposed dogs to levels of 5 ppm sulfur dioxide about 21 hours a day for 225 days. One group of dogs was normal and the other had had lung impairment produced by prior exposure to nitrogen dioxide (191 days at 26 ppm). The exposure to sulfur dioxide produced about a 50 percent increase in resistance and about a 16 percent decrease in compliance. In general, the adverse effects were less in the dogs with impaired function from previous nitrogen dioxide exposure, which might suggest that a lung previously remodeled by a toxicant may be more difficult to alter physiologically than one that had never been exposed to toxic concentrations of irritant. Vaughan et al. (1969) exposed dogs for 16 hours a day for 18 months to a combination of 0.5 ppm sulfur dioxide and 0.1 mg/m^3 sulfuric acid and concluded there was no impairment in pulmonary function.

Well-planned and carefully executed studies of the effect of sulfur dioxide on human subjects exposed continuously for periods of 120 hours were reported by Weir et al. (1972). Their subjects lived throughout the exposure period in a 30-m^3 dynamic flow chamber. Daily pulmonary function measurements included airway resistance at varying lung volumes, functional residual capacity, dynamic lung compliance, and total lung volume. In the initial series, 0, 3, 6, and 8 ppm sulfur dioxide were used. Dose-related changes were observed in subjective complaints, clinical evaluations, blood gases, airway resistance, and dynamic lung compliance. The second group of experiments used concentrations of 0.3, 1, and 3 ppm sulfur dioxide. No dose-related changes were observed in subjective complaints, clinical evaluations, or most pulmonary function measurements at these lower concentrations. Significant but minimal reversible increases were noted in airway resistance accompanied by a decrease in compliance at high frequencies of breathing at the 3-ppm concentration. Unfortunately a detailed report of these studies has never been published.

Biochemical Studies

Information on biochemical aspects of the toxicology of sulfur dioxide is very limited. Some early studies indicated that radioactive sulfur persisted in the lung incorporated into protein, but no evidence was presented on the nature of this complex. Work by Gunnison and Palmes (1974) has indicated the presence in plasma of S-sulfonate formed by the reaction of sulfite with the disulfide bond inproteins. This has been found in rabbits and in human subjects. They examined the plasma from subjects exposed in Weir's experiments and found a positive correlation of plasma S-sulfonate levels with exposure concentrations of sulfur dioxide. Most recently they have found S-sulfonate present in the plasma and aorta of rabbits infused with sulfite. While the biologic significance is not at present understood, this finding represents the first biochemical alteration observed in target organs.

TOXICOLOGY OF SULFURIC ACID AND PARTICULATE SULFATES

Sulfuric Acid

The guinea pig is the small mammal most sensitive to sulfuric acid inhalation. Rabbits, rats, and mice are much less sensitive (Treon et al., 1950). Two early studies (Amdur et al., 1952; Pattle et al., 1956) used guinea pigs to examine the lethal effects of eight-hour exposures to sulfuric acid. The concentration required to kill the animals ranged from 18 to 60 mg/m^3. Animals were more sensitive at one to two months of age than at 18 months. Particles of 2.7 μm were more toxic than 0.8-μm particles when mortality was the criterion of response. This is probably because the larger particles deposited in areas of the respiratory tract where major spasm of the airways would be rapidly lethal. Dropping the temperature to 0° C significantly increased the toxicity of the sulfuric acid, probably due to the cold stress on a tropical animal. Sufficient ammonium carbonate in the chamber to provide an excess of ammonia protected against the effects of sulfuric acid.

The pathologic findings in the lungs were similar in the two investigations. The cause of death in animals that succumbed rapidly appeared to be bronchoconstriction and laryngeal spasm. Animals dying after a longer exposure showed gross pulmonary pathology, including hemor-

rhage, capillary engorgement, and some edema. The animals surviving the exposure showed spotty areas of old hemorrhage and areas of consolidation, especially around the hilar regions. Such damage is repaired only slowly.

Extending the exposure time to 72 hours did not increase the mortality beyond that observed for eight-hour exposures, but did increase the lung pathology (Amdur et al., 1952). The mortality was related to concentration of sulfuric acid, and the degree of lung pathology was related to the total dose (concentration × time). This suggests that sulfuric acid has two actions. First, it promotes laryngeal spasm and bronchospasm, which are the causes of death. These actions are related primarily to concentration and individual sensitivity. Sulfuric acid can also cause parenchymal lung damage and this action is related to the total dosage.

Sulfuric acid produces an increase in flow resistance in guinea pigs, the magnitude of which is related to both concentration and particle size (Amdur, 1958; Amdur et al., 1978a). In the following discussion, particle size is expressed as mass median diameter (MMD). Particles of 7 μm produced only a slight increase in resistance even at very high concentration (30 mg/m^3). Since these particles would not penetrate beyond the upper respiratory tract, this response was probably a referred reflex or an increase in nasal resistance. Particles of 2.5 μm gave a response that was slow in onset and accompanied by a major decrease in compliance. These mechanical changes were suggestive of closure of large areas of the lung due to constriction or obstruction with mucous secretions. Particles of 1 μm or below produced a swift response similar to that observed with irritant gases. Irritant potency increased with decreasing particle size. At concentrations below 1 mg/m^3 the response was greater for 0.3-μm than for 1-μm particles (Amdur et al., 1978a). Elevated flow resistance produced by sulfuric acid is much slower to return to control values than is the increase produced by sulfur dioxide. The action of irritant particles deposited on the lung surface is more prolonged than that of a gas, which is rapidly cleared from the lungs when exposure ceases.

Dose-response curves shown in Figure 24–1 indicate that at a given concentration of sulfur, sulfuric acid produces a greater response than sulfur dioxide. Even the less irritant 2.5-μm particles produce a two- to threefold greater response than the equivalent amount of sulfur dioxide.

There is evidence that on a chronic basis as well, sulfuric acid is a more potent irritant than sulfur dioxide (Alarie et al., 1972, 1975). These studies involved the exposure of monkeys to either sulfur dioxide or sulfuric acid for periods

Table 24-1. COMPARATIVE TOXICITY OF SO_2 AND H_2SO_4: PULMONARY FUNCTION OF MONKEYS EXPOSED TWO YEARS

COMPOUND	CONCENTRATION	mg S/M³	ALTERATIONS		
SO_2	1 ppm	1.31	None		
			Histopathology	Distribution of Ventilation	Arterial O_2
H_2SO_4 (2.15 μm)	0.38 mg/m³	0.12	Slight	0	0
H_2SO_4 (3.60 μm)	2.43 mg/m³	0.80	Moderate	Moderate	Slight
H_2SO_4 (0.73 μm)	4.79 mg/m³	1.57	—	Slight	0
H_2SO_4 (0.54 μm)	0.48 mg/m³	0.16	Moderate to severe	Moderate	Moderate

of 78 weeks. Table 24-1 indicates some of the changes observed. When compared on the basis of mg S/m³, it is evident that far higher levels of sulfur administered as sulfur dioxide had no effect on the animals.

The effect of sulfuric acid (0.3 to 0.6 μm) on tracheobronchial mucociliary clearance of radioactively tagged ferric oxide particles has been studied in the donkey (Schlesinger et al., 1978). Previous studies have shown that the donkey is a good experimental model, as clearance changes are consistent with and quantitatively comparable to similar data obtained in human subjects. Three out of four animals demonstrated short-term slowing of clearance as a result of single, one-hour exposures to 194 to 1,364 μg/m³. Two of the four animals showed a more persistent slowing of control clearance values as the series of weekly exposures progressed. Pulmonary flow resistance, compliance, and regional deposition of aerosol were unchanged. Concentrations of ammonium sulfate up to 2 mg/m³ had no effect on clearance or on pulmonary mechanics. Sulfur dioxide affected clearance only at concentrations of 300 ppm or greater. This is another piece of evidence indicating the greater toxicity of sulfuric acid as compared to sulfur dioxide.

Particulate Sulfates

The irritant potency of zinc ammonium sulfate, which was reported as a constituent of the Donora fog, was studied at four particle sizes, from 0.29 to 1.4 μm, at concentrations from 0.25 to 3.6 mg/m³ (Amdur and Corn, 1963). The lowest concentration is of the order of magnitude of what might have occurred during the fog incident. All concentrations tested produced an increase in flow resistance in guinea pigs. The irritant potency increased as the particle size decreased. The slope of the dose-response curves also steepened as the particle size decreased, so that a smaller increment in concentration produced a larger increment in response. This paper points out the utter inadequacy of relying on information on mass concentration alone when attempting to assess the irritant potency of particulate matter. Information on particle size can be equally critical.

Nadel et al. (1967) found that zinc ammonium sulfate produced a response similar to, but lesser in degree than, that produced by histamine. The experiments were made on anesthetized cats artificially ventilated with a pump. The aerosol was submicron in size and the concentration was 40 to 50 mg/m³. The response to a three-minute inhalation included increased pulmonary resistance, decreased compliance, and increased end-expiratory transpulmonary pressure. Isoproteronol prevented the changes, suggesting that they were due to smooth muscle contraction. Cardiac arrest during histamine inhalation did not prevent the changes. This suggests that the action was directly on the airway smooth muscle and was not dependent on circulation. To correlate with the physiologic responses, anatomic studies were made after rapid deep freezing of the lungs in the open thorax. The principal sites of constriction were the alveolar ducts and terminal bronchioles. Bronchi and bronchioles larger than 400 μm were not constricted. Physiologic response and anatomic data combine to indicate the locus of action of the submicron particles.

The sulfate ion per se is not irritant; therefore, sulfates vary widely in irritant potency. For comparison, the increase in flow resistance can be calculated per μg of sulfate. Data were obtained with 0.3-μm aerosols (Amdur et al., 1978b). Table 24-2 expresses the response to the sulfate salts as a percentage of the corresponding response to sulfuric acid. Pharmacologic studies also indicate differences among sulfates. Ammonium sulfate causes histamine release by guinea pig lungs, whereas sodium sulfate does not. The removal of intratracheally injected sulfate from the lung is markedly influenced by the cation present (Charles et al., 1977). These data suggest that "suspended sulfate" without further characterization is unlikely to be a definitive atmos-

Table 24–2. RELATIVE IRRITANT POTENCY OF SULFATES

Sulfuric acid	100
Zinc ammonium sulfate*	33
Ferric sulfate†	26
Zinc sulfate*	19
Ammonium sulfate	10
Ammonium bisulfate	3
Cupric sulfate	2
Ferrous sulfate	0.7
Sodium sulfate‡	0.7
Manganous sulfate†	−0.9§

* Data of Amdur and Corn, 1963.
† Data of Amdur and Underhill, 1968.
‡ Particle size: 0.1 μm.
§ Resistance decreased; change N.S.

pheric measurement for the assessment of health effects. Certainly it is toxicologically meaningless.

EFFECT OF AEROSOLS ON THE RESPONSE TO SULFUR DIOXIDE

Measurement of flow resistance in the guinea pig is a bioassay of sufficient sensitivity to detect quantitatively the potentiation of irritant gases by aerosols. The aerosols are "inert," in that they do not affect resistance when used alone. The dose-response curve for sulfur dioxide plus the aerosol can be compared with the dose-response curve for sulfur dioxide alone.

Early studies with sodium chloride delineate several factors affecting the potentiation (Amdur, 1961). Particle size of the aerosol is important. Submicron particles potentiate but 2.5-μm particles do not. Concentration of the aerosol is important. At a relative humidity of 50 percent, 10 mg/m^3 potentiates but 4 mg/m^3 does not. Postexposure resistance values remain elevated (typical of irritant aerosols) and can be related directly to total aerosol dose. The potentiation is relatively slow to develop; at ten minutes the response is the same as that to sulfur dioxide alone (Amdur, 1961; Amdur and Underhill, 1968). Relative humidity is important (McJilton et al., 1973). At 80 percent RH 1 mg/m^3 is as effective as 10 mg/m^3 at 50 percent RH. At high humidities the potentiation occurs rapidly.

The aerosols that have produced a major potentiation of the response to sulfur dioxide are soluble salts of such metals as manganese, ferrous iron, and vanadium (Amdur and Underhill, 1968). These materials form droplets that can dissolve sulfur dioxide, and the metal ions promote oxidation to sulfuric acid. These aerosols potentiate the response about threefold when present at a concentration of 1 mg/m^3 at 50 percent RH. This is far greater than the potentiation produced by sodium chloride except at a high relative humidity. At a sulfur dioxide concentration of 0.2 ppm, about 10 percent of the sulfur was converted to sulfuric acid. When this amount of sulfuric acid was added to 0.2 ppm of sulfur dioxide, the response to the gas plus metal aerosol could be duplicated (Amdur, 1974).

The response to sulfur dioxide was not altered by the presence of solid aerosols of carbon, iron oxide, open hearth dust, fly ash, or manganese dioxide. The response was attenuated by aerosols of triphenyl phosphate or motor oil (Costa and Amdur, 1979).

Results of studies of flow resistance in human subjects exposed to sulfur dioxide alone and in combination with sodium chloride aerosol are conflicting. Frank et al. (1964) exposed human subjects to 1, 5, and 15 ppm of sulfur dioxide alone and with the addition of sodium chloride aerosol. In an initial series of experiments the exposures were given in sequence with a 15-to-20-minute recovery period between them. Whether the gas alone or the combination was given first was randomized. The only consistent finding was that the resistance increase in response to the second exposure was less than that evoked by the first exposure. The series was repeated, allowing the lapse of a month between exposures. No difference could be detected between the response to the sulfur dioxide alone and the response to sulfur dioxide plus the aerosol. Although the paper does not so indicate in the discussion, the variability of the response of the same individual on different occasions to the same concentration of sulfur dioxide alone is greater than the potentiating effect of sodium chloride observed in guinea pigs. Burton et al. (1969) tested the effect of about 2 mg/m^3 sodium chloride aerosol on the response of ten subjects to 1 to 3 ppm sulfur dioxide. As would have been predicted on the basis of experiments with guinea pigs, at this gas concentration and 4 mg/m^3 sodium chloride, no potentiation was observed.

Toyama (1962) reported that sodium chloride did potentiate the response of human subjects to sulfur dioxide. The dose-response curves for sulfur dioxide alone and plus aerosol resemble strikingly data on guinea pigs. The major toxicologic problem in accepting these results is the fact that the exposures were given in sequence and the second exposure was always to the sulfur dioxide plus aerosol. If data were given on responses of a similar number of subjects to sequential exposures to sulfur dioxide alone, the results could be properly interpreted. As was indicated above, Frank et al. (1964) found a lesser response to a second exposure given in sequence, which is the reverse of these findings. Sequential exposures are a toxicologic trap into which unwary physiologists fall.

Toyama and Nakamura (1964) observed potentiation by an aerosol of hydrogen peroxide, which would be a liquid droplet and also oxidize sulfur dioxide to sulfuric acid. Again, there is the problem of sequential exposures. No published data exist on the effect of the soluble metal salts on the response of human subjects to sulfur dioxide.

The techniques of the experimental toxicologist who can use many animals, exposed only once, may be more suitable for the elucidation of potentiation responses than are the techniques of the physiologist who can expose only a few human subjects.

COMPONENTS AND FORMATION OF PHOTOCHEMICAL AIR POLLUTION

Photochemical air pollution arises from a series of atmospheric reactions. The main components are ozone, oxides of nitrogen, aldehydes, peroxyacetyl nitrates, and hydrocarbons. From the point of view of a discussion of the toxicology of air pollutants, the hydrocarbons as such do not concern us. The concentrations of hydrocarbons in ambient air do not reach levels high enough to produce any toxic effect. They are important because they enter into the chemical reactions that lead to the formation of photochemical smog.

The chemical reactions that lead to the formation of this particular complex of pollutants in the atmosphere are extremely complex. A detailed discussion and review of this subject, as well as the toxicology of ozone, was recently released by the National Academy of Sciences Committee on Medical and Biological Effects of Environmental Pollutants (1977).

The oxidant found in the largest amounts in polluted atmospheres is ozone (O_3). Several miles above the earth's surface there is sufficient short-wave ultraviolet light to convert O_2 to O_3 by direct absorption, but these wavelengths do not reach the earth's surface. Of the major atmospheric pollutants, nitrogen dioxide is the most efficient absorber of the UV light that does reach the earth's surface. This absorption of UV light by NO_2 leads to a complex series of reactions, which may be simplified as follows:

$$NO_2 \xrightarrow{UV} NO + O \tag{1}$$
$$O + O_2 \longrightarrow O_3 \tag{2}$$
$$O_3 + NO \longrightarrow NO_2 + O_2 \tag{3}$$

Since NO_2 is regenerated by the reaction of the NO and O_3 formed, the overall result is a cyclic reaction that can be perpetuated.

This NO_2 photolytic cycle serves to explain the initial formation of O_3 in polluted atmospheres, but cannot explain the development of concentrations of O_3 as great as those that have been measured. If no additional mechanisms were involved, most of the O_3 would be broken down by reaction with the NO formed, and in steady-state conditions O_3 and NO would be formed and destroyed in equal quantities. The hydrocarbons, especially olefins and substituted aromatics, become important by providing the necessary added reactants. Oxygen atoms attack the hydrocarbons. The resulting oxidized compounds and free radicals react with NO to produce more NO_2. Thus the balance of the reactions shown in equations 1 to 3 is upset so that NO_2 and O_3 levels build up while NO levels are depleted. These reactions are very complex and involve the formation of intermediate free radicals that are very reactive and undergo a series of changes.

Aldehydes are major products in the photo-oxidation of hydrocarbons, and in the reactions of hydrocarbons with ozone, oxygen atoms, or free radicals. Formaldehyde and acrolein have been specifically identified in urban atmospheres. About 50 percent of the total aldehyde is present as formaldehyde and about 5 percent as acrolein.

Peroxyacetyl nitrate, often referred to as PAN, is most likely formed in the atmosphere from the reaction of the peroxyacetyl radical with NO_2. Its chemical formula is CH_3COONO_2. Higher homologs are probably also present, but PAN is the one that has been positively identified as present in urban atmospheres.

TOXICOLOGY OF OZONE

Studies of Mortality and Lung Pathology

Ozone is a deep lung irritant capable of causing death from pulmonary edema. The early studies, many of them from his own research group, have been well reviewed by Stokinger (1965). The LC50 following three-hour exposures varies from about 50 ppm for guinea pigs to about 20 ppm for mice. The lethality of ozone is influenced by factors other than concentration and length of exposure. Young mice are more susceptible. Elevated ambient temperature or exercise increases the toxicity. Intermittent exposures are much less toxic than the same total dose administered continuously.

Early studies reported gross pulmonary edema in mice exposed four hours to 3.2 ppm. Exposures to 1 ppm produced engorged blood vessels and excess leukocytes in lung capillaries. Rats exposed to 2 ppm for three hours showed an increased water content of the lung. More sensitive techniques, which utilize recovery of radio-labeled blood albumin in lung lavage fluid, indicate that the threshold for edema formation in rats is 0.25 to 0.5 ppm for six hours (Alpert *et al.*, 1971).

Boatman *et al.* (1974) reported desquamation of the ciliated epithelium throughout the ciliated airways of cats exposed four to six hours to 0.25, 0.5, and 1.0 ppm. The degree of damage was dose related. Alveolar damage included swelling and denudation of the cytoplasm of type I cells, swelling or rupture of the capillary endothelium, and lysis of erythrocytes. In rats, Stephens *et al.* (1974) observed degenerative changes in type I alveolar cells after three-hour exposure to concentrations as low as 0.2 ppm. These are replaced by type II cells beginning a day after exposure.

Rats and monkeys exposed for eight hours a day on seven consecutive days to 0.2, 0.5, or 0.8 ppm showed mild but significant morphologic lesions at the lowest concentrations. When an exposure of rats was extended continuously, lesions reached a peak in three to five days and then diminished. After 90 days at 0.8 ppm there was obvious damage but this was less severe than at seven days. The biochemical and morphologic changes associated with this adaptation are currently under active investigation (Dungworth, 1976).

It is important to note that in the case of ozone, pulmonary pathology has been observed in experimental animals following relatively short exposures to concentrations that can occasionally be attained for short periods in polluted urban areas.

Early studies suggested that long-term exposure to ozone results in effects on morphology and function of the lung and acceleration of lung-tumor formation and of aging. Chronic bronchitis, bronchiolitis, fibrosis, and emphysematous changes were observed in a variety of species exposed to ozone concentrations slightly above 1 ppm.

Electron microscopy has been used to document morphologic changes in the lungs of dogs exposed to 1 to 3 ppm ozone for up to 18 months (Stephens *et al.*, 1973). Daily exposure times were 8, 16, or 24 hours. The effects increased in severity in a manner related more to concentration than to duration of exposure. A thickening of the terminal and respiratory bronchioles was accompanied at the highest concentration by an infiltration of cells that reduced the caliber of the small airways. Young rats exposed for up to three weeks to 0.5 to 0.9 ppm showed morphologic lesions in respiratory bronchioles, distal portions of the terminal bronchiolar epithelium, the alveolar duct, and alveoli (Stephens *et al.*, 1974). It is thus evident that damage from ozone occurs in peripheral areas of the lung.

Tolerance Development

Early studies (Stokinger, 1965) indicated that a single brief (one-hour) exposure to low concentrations of ozone (0.3 ppm) would protect against subsequent exposure to otherwise lethal concentrations. Tolerance lasted four to six weeks in rats and up to 14 weeks in mice. Water content of the lungs remained normal and there was less histopathologic damage. Lung alkaline phosphatase and glutathione levels remained normal in tolerant animals. Cross-tolerance was found between ozone and other edema-producing irritants such as nitrogen dioxide and phosgene.

The tolerance protects against pulmonary edema but not against alterations in pulmonary function. More recent evidence indicates that the antibacterial defense mechanisms of the lung are not protected (Gardner *et al.*, 1972). Other investigations showed that repeated exposures to low levels of nitrogen dioxide conferred less protection against subsequent exposures than did a single exposure. It is thus unlikely that tolerance development plays a significant role in protecting human populations exposed to low concentrations of oxidant pollutants.

Studies of Pulmonary Function

Exposure to ozone produces alterations in respiration, the most characteristic of which are shallow, rapid breathing and a decrease in pulmonary compliance. Alterations in resistance occur only at high concentrations. This pattern is typical of materials that have their site of action in the smaller airways and peripheral portions of the lung.

In two-hour exposures of guinea pigs to 0.34 to 1.35 ppm (Murphy *et al.*, 1964b), the earliest effects detected were an increase in frequency and a decrease in tidal volume that were observed at all concentrations. Higher concentrations produced a greater change that was present earlier in the exposure period. Higher concentrations also produced an increase in flow resistance. These changes were reversible during a 90-minute recovery period. More recent work from Amdur's laboratory has shown that concentrations of 1.3 to 1.8 ppm will reduce pulmonary compliance by about 50 percent. A lesser change in compliance was detected as low as 0.4 ppm, but not at 0.2 ppm.

Ozone exposure increases the sensitivity of the lung to bronchoconstrictive agents such as histamine, acetylcholine, and allergens. Easton and Murphy (1967) found an increased respiratory response to histamine injected s.c. in guinea pigs two hours after a two-hour exposure to 1 to 5 ppm ozone. Increased mortality from higher levels of histamine could be produced by as little as 0.5 to

1 ppm ozone. The increased susceptibility persisted up to 12 hours after a two-hour exposure to 5 ppm ozone. More recent studies on dogs (Lee *et al.*, 1977) have shown an increased respiratory response to an aerosol of histamine following exposure to 1 ppm ozone. This sensitivity can persist for 7 to 28 days. Compared to air controls, guinea pigs exposed one hour to 0.1 ppm O_3 showed a more marked decrease in compliance in response to s.c. injection of histamine two hours after exposure (Gordon and Amdur, 1980). These studies raise important questions in regard to the possibility of ozone sensitizing to subsequent exposure to other pollutants.

Alterations in pulmonary function have also been observed in human subjects, especially when intermittent light exercise is superimposed on exposure. This entire area, including emphasis of points that are critical to appropriate experimental design, is discussed at length in the 1977 National Academy of Sciences monograph referenced earlier. Hazucha *et al.* (1973) exposed human subjects for two hours to 0.37 and 0.75 ppm with alternate periods of rest and exercise. These exposures produced alterations in several pulmonary function tests, including a decrease in forced vital capacity, forced expiratory volume at one second (FEV_1), maximal flow rate at 50 percent of vital capacity, and maximal midexpiratory flow rate. Closing volume and residual volume increased. The subjects in these studies were Canadians. A group of southern Californians studied by Hackney *et al.* (1975) did not respond to a four-to-five-hour exposure to 0.5 ppm ozone alone or combined with 0.3 ppm nitrogen dioxide or 0.3 ppm nitrogen dioxide and 30 ppm carbon monoxide. Another group of subjects, each with either a history of developing symptoms during light activity in smog or a history of asthma, developed clinical discomfort and were unable to complete a similar protocol. These experiments indicate the wide variation in sensitivity and indicate that sensitive people develop significant symptoms under exposure conditions similar to those occurring during pollution episodes. In further exploration of the difference between Canadians and Californians, it was found that Canadians also showed a larger increase in red cell fragility after exposure. These differences, if real, might suggest an adaptation by the Californians. Studies done by Kerr *et al.* (1975) on 20 healthy adults showed alterations in pulmonary function from exposure for six hours to 0.5 ppm ozone. Ten were smokers and ten were nonsmokers. When the smokers were considered separately as a group, no significant alterations in pulmonary function were seen. Cough and chest discomfort were more frequent in nonsmokers.

Experiments in the chamber in Montreal suggested that if 0.37 ppm sulfur dioxide, which had a negligible effect on pulmonary function, was combined with 0.37 ppm ozone, observed effects were much greater than with ozone alone. This effect was not observed in the California chamber at Rancho Los Amigos. A major joint endeavor (Bell *et al.*, 1977) has finally resolved this conflict. Conditions in the Montreal chamber led to the formation of about 200 μg of sulfate, most likely sulfuric acid, which was not present in the Rancho chamber. There is evidence from air pollution incidents in Japan and in Holland that when both ozone and sulfur dioxide are present at about 0.3 ppm, symptoms of respiratory distress are greater than would be expected, especially among persons exercising. Although there is no direct evidence, experimental data would suggest that perhaps this increased response was the result of the formation of sulfuric acid aerosol.

Increased Susceptibility to Bacterial Infection

Exposure to ozone prior to challenge with aerosols of infectious agents produces a higher incidence of infection than seen in control animals (Coffin and Blommer, 1967). It is assumed that this results from inhibition of clearance mechanisms, either mucociliary streaming or phagocytosis. Exposure of mice to concentrations as low as 0.08 ppm ozone for three hours enhanced the mortality from subsequent exposure to a bacterial aerosol of *Streptococcus* (group C). The susceptibility of mice and hamsters to *Klebsiella pneumoniae* aerosol was increased by prior exposure to ozone, as indicated by a higher mortality, shorter survival time, and lower LD50 for *K. pneumoniae* in ozone-exposed animals as compared with controls.

It has been shown that exposure to ozone reduced the number as well as the *in vitro* phagocytic ability of pulmonary macrophages in rabbits. This could help to explain the increased survival time of bacteria observed in the lungs of animals preexposed to ozone.

Biochemical Studies

The similarity of some of the effects of ozone to those of radiation suggested that ozone toxicity might result from the formation of reactive free-radical intermediates. Stokinger (1965) and Menzel (1970) have reviewed the evidence on this subject. Ozone and x-irradiation are nearly additive in producing chromosomal aberrations in plants and animals. Antioxidant and radical trapping agents such as quinones, ascorbic acid, and α-tocopherol protect against ozone toxicity. Ozone-induced free radicals may be derived from interaction with sulfhydryls and/or from oxidative decomposition of unsaturated fatty acids. It is likely that more than one radical is formed either directly from ozone or from its interaction with normal cellular constituents. Further research is needed to determine the exact radicals produced by ozone *in vivo*.

Various investigators have noted protection from ozone by sulfhydryl compounds. Decreases in lung glutathione and succinic dehydrogenase occur following ozone exposure. Exposure of rats to 2 ppm for four to eight hours produced a decrease in both protein and nonprotein lung sulfhydryl groups. The bulk of the glutathione oxidized in rat lung was in the form of mixed disulfides with lung protein sulfhydryl groups. Peak oxidation of nonprotein sulfhydryl groups did not occur until 24 hours after exposure and recovery was evident by 48 hours (DeLucia *et al.*, 1975).

Chow and Tappel (1973) have examined the effect of ozone on enzymes active in the defense against intracellular oxidation and oxidant stress. Rats were exposed to ozone at 0.2, 0.5, or 0.8 ppm continuously for eight days. Increases in glucose-6-phosphate dehydrogenase, glutathione peroxidase, and glutathione reductase were linearly related to dose. Histochemical studies have demonstrated an alteration in NADPH- and NADH-diaphorase activity in the lungs of rats exposed to 0.8 ppm ozone for seven days (Castleman *et al.*, 1973).

Several lines of evidence indicate that one of the biologic actions of ozone is reaction with unsaturated fatty acids. The biologic implications and resulting products of ozonization of these fatty acids are essentially equivalent to lipid peroxidation. This subject has been reviewed by Menzel (1970).

Incubation of human red cells *in vitro* with ozone or ozonides provides evidence for a role of lipid peroxidation in cellular damage from ozone. Incubation with ozonized liposomes (Tiege *et al.*, 1974) or with ozonized serum (Menzel *et al.*, 1975) was more damaging than incubation with ozone itself. Lung toxicity similar to that seen after ozone exposure was produced in rats by IV injection of fatty acid hydroperoxidases or ozonides (Cortesi and Privett, 1972). Conjugated diene bonds were found in extracts of lungs of mice exposed to 0.4 to 0.7 ppm ozone for four hours (Goldstein *et al.*, 1969).

One piece of indirect evidence for a role of lipid peroxidation is the finding that animals deficient in vitamin E were more susceptible to ozone (Goldstein *et al.*, 1970). Data on the protective effect of added supplements of vitamin E are conflicting. Menzel *et al.* (1975) found that oral administration of vitamin E did protect against Heinz body formation in cells incubated *in vitro* with ozonides.

Alterations in the protein fraction of lung tissue have been observed in rabbits following one-hour exposure to 1 ppm ozone (Buell *et al.*, 1965). A variety of aldehydes and ketones were identified. The aldehydes formed may bring about an intra- or intermolecular cross-linking of proteins that would alter normal lung structure. There was also evidence of oxidative degradation of hyaluronic acid, which would suggest alterations in the ground substance of the lungs. Since the ground substance serves as a lubricant and matrix for the fibers of the lung, a decreased slippage and flexibility of elastic protein molecules could result. This could be enhanced by cross-linking of aldehydes with fibers of elastic protein molecules. The authors suggest these alterations may help explain the increased sensitivity of ozone-exposed animals to bacterial infection because a breakdown of ground substance by ozone exposure would facilitate penetration of bacteria into the lung tissue.

Extrapulmonary Effects

Various studies have reported effects other than those directly related to the lung in laboratory animals exposed to ozone at a concentration as low as 0.2 ppm. Included are reduction of voluntary activity in mice, chromosomal aberrations in circulating lymphocytes of hamsters, and increased neonatal mortality as well as incidence of jaw abnormalities in offspring of mice exposed to ozone. The National Academy of Sciences monograph reviews and documents these and other studies.

TOXICOLOGY OF NITROGEN DIOXIDE

Studies of Mortality and Lung Pathology

Nitrogen dioxide, like ozone, is a deep lung irritant capable of producing pulmonary edema if inhaled in sufficient concentrations. This is a practical problem to farmers, as sufficient amounts can be liberated from ensilage to produce the symptoms of pulmonary damage known as silo-filler's disease.

Even over short time intervals, Haber's law does not hold for nitrogen dioxide. This law states that $C \times T = K$, where C is the concentration of the toxic material, T is time, and K is a constant. For example, for a 15-minute exposure, 420 ppm nitrogen dioxide kills 50 percent of the animals (Gray *et al.*, 1954). Applying Haber's law, one would predict 105 ppm for one hour or 26 ppm for four hours would kill 50 percent of the animals so exposed. Experimental results indicate, however, that the rats exposed for longer times can withstand higher concentrations than predicted. The LC50 values found for one-hour and four-hour exposures were 166 and 88 ppm, respectively. Even short exposure to the higher concentration was sufficient to produce overwhelming pulmonary edema and death.

Some earlier work in which animals were allowed to remain in an atmosphere of nitrogen dioxide until they died suggested a low toxicity. Because death from pulmonary edema is delayed, not immediate, the animals unquestionably received multilethal doses of nitrogen dioxide. In the case of irritant agents that produce delayed edema, the experimental design that measures survival time under continuous exposure will underestimate the lethal dose.

Damage to mast cells in the lungs of rats was produced by exposure to as little as 0.5 ppm for four hours or 1 ppm for one hour. The damage, which was repaired within 24 hours, was interpreted as the potential onset of an acute inflammatory reaction. More prolonged alterations in lung collagen were produced in rabbits by exposure to 0.25 ppm four hours a day for six days. Damage was still evident seven days after the final exposure (Mueller and Hitchcock, 1969).

In rats exposed to 17 or 2 ppm nitrogen dioxide, changes in cell proliferation in the lung were estimated by determining the proportion of cells that could be labeled with tritiated thymidine. A dose-related increase was found that peaked on the second day of exposure and had returned to control levels by the fifth day. This occurred in terminal bronchioles and alveoli and represented an increased turnover rate of type II alveolar cells. Type I cells are damaged, slough off, and are replaced by cuboidal cells that have some of the characteristics of type II cells.

Exposure of squirrel monkeys for two hours to 10 to 50 ppm nitrogen dioxide produced primary lesions in the alveoli (Henry et al., 1969). The degree of damage was related to the concentration of nitrogen dioxide. At 10 ppm, there were many septal breaks and the alveoli were markedly expanded. In some areas there were large air vesicles with very thin septal walls. At 15 ppm, the alveolar tissue was expanded with minimal wall thinning and patchy interstitial infiltration with lymphocytes. The bronchioles were normal. At 35 ppm, some lung areas were collapsed and alveolar septa had become very basophilic. In other areas the alveoli were expanded and had thin septal walls. The bronchi were moderately inflamed with some showing epithelial proliferation. Frank edema was produced by 50 ppm. The lungs of these monkeys showed extreme vesicular dilatation or total collapse of alveoli with lymphocyte infiltration. The bronchi showed epithelial surface erosion and the absence of cilia.

Over the past 15 years the pathologic effects of chronic exposure of rats to nitrogen dioxide have received extensive and meticulous study with both light and electron microscopy (Freeman et al., 1972). The emphysematous nature of the changes observed makes these studies extremely pertinent to cigarette smoking as well as to air pollution. Cigarette smoke contains nitrogen dioxide and increases the incidence of emphysema.

Rats grew normally and survived their natural lifespans in atmospheres containing 0.8 or 2 ppm nitrogen dioxide. They showed moderate tachypnea without apparent distress. The lungs were grossly normal except for slight bloating. They were able to contract on exposure to the atmosphere, although lungs from the rats exposed to 2 ppm retained some air and weighed about 20 percent more than control lungs. The lungs of the rats exposed to 2 ppm showed histologic alterations in the bronchiolar epithelium. The cells were broader and more uniform than controls. The cilia were either reduced or absent. The possibility exists that such a deficiency in ciliary cleansing mechanisms could lead to increased residence time of materials such as carcinogenic hydrocarbons. The group exposed to 0.8 ppm occasionally showed similar cellular alterations that were not seen in controls of the same age. A 16-week exposure to 4 ppm produced no gross changes in lung volume. The terminal bronchiolar epithelium was tall and hypertrophied. Exposure to 10 and 25 ppm produced large, air-filled heavy lungs without edema or increased blood volume. The animals died of respiratory failure. The development of emphysema-like lungs was accompanied by enlargement of the thoracic cage with dorsal kyphosis.

The terminal bronchiolar lumen of the "emphysematous" lungs was narrowed due to hypertropy of the epithelium and to amorphous proteinaceous material, fibrin strands, and alveolar macrophages accumulated at the junctions with alveolar ducts. Such obstructive lesions may have led to the distention of the lungs and to the broken alveolar septa.

Lungs from rats exposed for 20 weeks to 18 ppm nitrogen dioxide were stained appropriately for detection of collagen and elastic tissue. In the exposed lungs both materials stained more prominently and were thicker and more prevalent, especially at the level of the alveolar ducts. The lengthwise elastic tissue fibers were often replicated and fractured into straighter and shorter pieces than could be found in control lungs. Such changes very likely contributed to the increased lung weight and to the reduction observed in pulmonary compliance.

Rats exposed for a lifetime to 15 ppm had voluminous, dry lungs with a large functional residual capacity. At maximal standard pressure the lung volume was greater than in control animals. Terminal bronchioles and alveolar ducts showed loss of cilia, epithelial hypertrophy, and narrowing. Alveoli were distended and exposed animals had approximately one-third the number of alveoli of control animals with a resultant reduction in ventilatory surface. Arterial oxygen tension was reduced and secondary polycythemia was evident. The disease state resembled human emphysema.

Emphysema-like lesions were also produced in the lungs of beagle dogs exposed for six months to 25 ppm nitrogen dioxide (Riddick *et al.*, 1968). The lungs of one of six exposed dogs showed bullous emphysema. The lungs of the other five exposed dogs showed increased firmness with scattered small bullae. The lungs of all dogs exposed showed a diffuse increase in collagen.

Effects on Pulmonary Function

Experimental exposure of animals or human subjects to nitrogen dioxide can cause measurable alterations in pulmonary function. The pattern of changes produced is in general similar to the pattern produced by ozone. This is an increase in respiratory frequency, with a decrease in compliance as the predominant alteration in mechanical behavior of the lungs. Pulmonary flow resistance is minimally altered.

Exposure of guinea pigs for periods of two to four hours at nitrogen dioxide concentrations of 5 to 13 ppm caused an increase in respiratory frequency and a decrease in tidal volume (Murphy *et al.*, 1964b). The overall minute volume remained the same. The magnitude of the changes in frequency and tidal volume was related to the concentration of nitrogen dioxide. In addition, the time at which the maximum response was reached was shorter at higher concentrations. At 5 ppm the respiratory frequency continued to increase and the tidal volume continued to decrease for three hours. After this no further change was produced by an additional hour of exposure. At a concentration of 13 ppm, the maximum change was reached in one hour and no further alteration was noted during a second hour of exposure. The values for respiratory frequency and tidal volume had returned to pre-exposure values by four hours after the end of exposure. The method used for studying pulmonary mechanics in this investigation did not measure compliance. There is, however, little doubt that there was an accompanying decrease in compliance.

In the long-term studies of rats by Freeman's group, an increase in frequency and a decrease in compliance were observed as chronic effects. In the studies of squirrel monkeys discussed earlier, exposure for two hours to 10 or 15 ppm caused a decrease in tidal volume and minute volume, but no increase in respiratory frequency. Recovery was complete within 24 to 48 hours after exposure. Concentrations of 35 to 50 ppm for two hours caused an increase in respiratory frequency and a decrease in tidal volume that was completely reversible in 72 hours. Similar changes were produced by two-months' exposure to 5 ppm.

Abe (1967) exposed five human subjects for ten minutes to 5 ppm nitrogen dioxide. He observed a mean increase in airway resistance of 92 percent. This response was delayed and did not become apparent until 30 minutes after the exposure ended. The mean value of pulmonary compliance was 40 percent below control levels by 30 minutes after the exposure. There was a marked reduction in three subjects and no change in the other two. No indication is given of the time interval over which these delayed effects would be reversed.

In the late 1970s a number of investigators examined the response of human subjects to nitrogen dioxide. The results on the whole are more conflicting and less definitive than those obtained in similar studies of sulfur dioxide or ozone. There seems little doubt that alterations of pulmonary function can be produced in normal, healthy subjects by exposure to 2 to 3 ppm and above. There is also the suggestion in these data that a concentration of 5 ppm may render normal subjects more sensitive to bronchoconstrictive agents and that similar effects may occur at far lower (0.1-ppm) concentrations in some asthmatic subjects (Orehek *et al.*, 1976).

Effects on Susceptibility to Respiratory Infection

Data obtained on a variety of species of experimental animals (mice, hamsters, rabbits, squirrel monkeys) suggest that either short-term or long-term exposures to nitrogen dioxide can increase susceptibility to respiratory infection by bacterial pneumonia or influenza virus. The evidence for this effect falls into three categories: (1) increased mortality rates; (2) reduced survival time; and (3) reduced ability to clear pathogenic organisms from the lung, as indicated by the number of viable organisms that can be cultured.

Coffin *et al.* (1976) tested the effect of varying both concentration and time of exposure on the mortality of mice exposed to *Streptococcus pyrogenes*. A $C \times T$ value of 7 ppm-hours was used with exposures from 14 ppm for 0.5 hour to 1 ppm for seven hours. The concentration was more critical than time in increasing the mortality from infection. In other experiments, 1.5 ppm for 18 hours increased mortality by 25 percent but a two-hour exposure to 14.5 ppm caused a 65 percent increase.

Exposure of two hours to 5 ppm nitrogen dioxide reduced the rate of clearance of *K. pneumoniae* from the lungs of mice and hamsters. The bacterial challenge took place one hour after the irritant exposure. The number of bacteria in the lungs was measured one, three, five, six, seven, and eight hours after infection. In control animals the bacterial population was markedly reduced during the six hours postinfection. The bacterial count then increased, reaching its initial concentration in about eight hours. In the exposed animals the initial period of clearance was reduced to 4.5 (mice) or 5 hours (hamsters) and the original concentration was reestablished in less than seven hours. In rabbits there is evidence that short-term exposure (three hours) to nitrogen dioxide will inhibit phagocytic activity (Gardner *et al.*, 1969).

Both increased mortality and reduced clearance rates of *K. pneumoniae* from the lungs were observed in mice exposed chronically to 0.5 ppm nitrogen dioxide (Ehrlich and Henry, 1968). Statistically significant increases in mortality following infection were observed in mice exposed continuously for three months and after six months of daily 6- or 18-hour exposures. The clearance rate of bacteria from the lung was reduced by exposure for 6 or 18 hours a day for nine months. These effects were more pronounced after 12 months of exposure. When exposure was continuous, a reduced capacity to clear bacteria from the lung was observed after six months of exposure as well as at 9 and 12 months.

Increased mortality was seen in squirrel monkeys exposed for short periods of two hours to 50 ppm nitrogen dioxide or for periods of one or two months to 10 or 5 ppm when they were infected with *K. pneumoniae* (Henry *et al.*, 1970). Monkeys exposed to 10 ppm nitrogen dioxide for two hours and then infected had viable bacteria present in their lungs up to 50 days after challenge. Squirrel monkeys were infected with nonlethal levels of A/PR-8 influenza virus and then exposed continuously to 5 or 10 ppm nitrogen dioxide. All six monkeys exposed to 10 ppm died within three days and one out of three exposed to 5 ppm died. Other experiments suggested that exposure of squirrel monkeys for five months to 5 ppm nitrogen dioxide depressed the formation of protective antibody against this influenza virus.

Biochemical Effects

Both acute and chronic exposure to nitrogen dioxide can cause biochemical alterations as well as histologically demonstrable lung damage. Short exposures of one hour to as little as 1 ppm nitrogen dioxide caused alterations in the configuration of collagen and elastin in the lungs of rabbits (Buell *et al.*, 1966). Differential ultraviolet spectrophotometry showed molecular alterations in both collagen and elastin in animals killed immediately after exposure. The changes were not observed in an animal killed 24 hours after exposure, which demonstrates the reversibility of the change. It may be remembered that the structural changes in collagen produced by repeated exposure were not reversible up to at least seven days after the final exposure. One might speculate that repeated denaturation of the sort observed here can lead on to irreversible structural change.

It is interesting to note that hydroxylysine glycosides, probably originating from the degradation of collagen, were found in the urine of the Apollo crew of the Apollo-Soyuz mission. They had been exposed to an average of 250 ppm nitrogen dioxide for four to five minutes. Pulmonary damage was evident on roetgenograms.

Nitrogen dioxide, like ozone, can cause lipid peroxidation. Four-hour exposures to 1 ppm produced evidence of lipid peroxidation in extracts of lipids from rat lung (Thomas *et al.*, 1968). Peroxidation was maximum 24 hours after exposure and lasted for at least 24 hours longer. When six daily exposures were given, lipid peroxidation increased. This suggests a cumulative effect. Rats fed a diet deficient in vitamin E showed more peroxidation in surfactant and tissue lipids than rats fed a diet normal in vitamin E content.

ALDEHYDES

Various aldehydes in polluted air are formed as reaction products in the photo-oxidation of hydrocarbons. The two aldehydes of major interest are formaldehyde and acrolein. The irritant nature of these materials probably contributes to the odor and eye irritation of photochemical smog. Formaldehyde accounts for about 50 percent of the estimated total aldehydes in polluted air. Acrolein, the more irritant of the two, may account for about 5 percent of the total aldehydes. A recent study by Kane and Alarie (1978) indicates that these aldehydes act as competitive agonists. Irritation would not be related to "total aldehyde" but to specific concentrations of acrolein and formaldehyde.

Formaldehyde

Formaldehyde is a primary irritant. Because of its high water solubility, it produces signs of irritation of mucous membranes of the nose, upper respiratory tract, and eyes. Concentrations of 0.5 to 1 ppm are detectable by odor, 2 to 3 ppm produce mild irritation, and 4 to 5 ppm are intolerable to most people.

The effect of low concentrations of formaldehyde on the respiration of guinea pigs has been studied (Amdur, 1960). A one-hour exposure to concentrations of 0.3 ppm and above produced an increase in pulmonary flow resistance accompanied by a lesser decrease in compliance. The respiratory frequency and minute volume decreased, but changes in these factors did not become statistically significant until concentrations of 10 ppm and above were used. The overall pattern of respiratory response produced by formaldehyde is similar to that produced by sulfur dioxide. A concentration of 0.05 ppm produced no alterations in any of the respiratory criteria used. Below concentrations of 50 ppm the alterations were reversible within an hour after the exposure.

The response to a given concentration of formaldehyde was greater when the gas was inhaled through a tracheal cannula that bypassed the scrubbing effect of the upper respiratory tract and permitted a greater concentration of the irritant to reach the lungs. The response in these animals was also readily reversible and the flow resistance values had returned to preexposure levels by one hour after the end of exposure.

The response to formaldehyde was potentiated by the simultaneous administration of an aerosol of submicron particles of sodium chloride. The values for pulmonary resistance remained above preexposure levels for one hour after the end of exposure when the gas-aerosol combination was used. This prolonged response, which is typical of the response of irritant aerosols, suggests that the potentiation is brought about by the attachment of formaldehyde to the particles to form an irritant aerosol. This hypothesis is further supported by the fact that when 3, 10, and 30 mg/m³ concentrations of sodium chloride were used, the potentiation increased with the increasing concentration of particles. The response to a given concentration of formaldehyde plus aerosol breathed by nose was greater than the response to the gas alone breathed through a tracheal cannula. This indicates that the increment added by the aerosol is not due to the transfer of an additional amount of formaldehyde gas as such to the lungs, since it was greater than could be accounted for by the transfer of the full concentration of formaldehyde to the lungs.

The particles of Los Angeles type smog are capable of carrying a considerable amount of formaldehyde. This would suggest that the biologic data obtained may have some practical significance.

Acrolein

The fact that it is an unsaturated aldehyde makes acrolein much more irritant than formaldehyde. Concentrations of below 1 ppm cause irritation of the eyes and mucous membranes of the respiratory tract.

The effect of acrolein on the respiratory function of guinea pigs has been studied (Murphy et al., 1963a). Exposure to 0.6 ppm and above increased pulmonary flow resistance, increased tidal volume, and decreased respiratory frequency. The effects were reversible when the animals were returned to clean air. In the case of irritants of this type, flow resistance is increased by concentrations below those which cause a decrease in frequency. This would suggest that flow resistance increases would be produced by far lower concentrations of acrolein than were tested. Atropine, aminophylline, isoproterenol, and epinephrine partially or completely reversed the changes. Pyrilamine and tripelennamine were without effect. The mechanism of increased resistance appears to be bronchoconstriction mediated through reflex cholinergic stimulation.

Inhalation of acrolein also has effects on various rat liver enzymes (Murphy, 1965). Elevated alkaline phosphatase activity occurred in the liver following 40 hours' continuous exposure to acrolein at concentrations as low as 2.1 ppm. Exposure to higher concentrations for shorter times also increased the enzyme activity, but the effect was not constant with a constant CT. Continuous exposure to 4 ppm acrolein for 4, 8, and 20 hours resulted in liver AP values that were 135, 222, and 253 percent of their respective controls. When a constant CT of 80 ppm-hours was given as 4 ppm for 20 hours, 2 ppm for 40 hours, and 1 pp. for 80 hours, the increases in alkaline phosphatase were 233, 146, and 103 percent of respective control values. This suggests that a threshold level of irritation must be reached to initiate processes that result in elevated enzyme activity. Liver alkaline phosphatase and tyrosine-ketoglutarate transaminase activities were markedly increased in rats 5 to 12 hours after injection or inhalation of acrolein. These effects could be prevented or substantially reduced by prior adrenalectomy or hypophysectomy or by pretreatment of the animals with chemicals that inhibit protein synthesis. The data suggest that the irritant action of acrolein stimulates the pituitary-adrenal system, leading to hypersecretion of glucocorticoids, which act to induce or stimulate the synthesis of increased amounts of the enzyme proteins by the liver.

CARBON MONOXIDE

Carbon monoxide would be classed toxicologically as a chemical asphyxiant and its toxic action stems from its formation of carboxyhemoglobin (COHb). The fundamental factors of the toxicology of carbon monoxide and the physiologic factors that determine the level of carboxyhemoglobin reached in the blood at various atmospheric concentrations of carbon monoxide are dealt with in Chapter 14. A monograph from the New York Academy of Sciences (Coburn, 1970) gives an excellent discussion of all aspects of the toxicology of carbon monoxide.

The literature is also extensively reviewed in the *Air Quality Criteria for Carbon Monoxide* (USDHEW, 1970).

The normal concentration of COHb in the blood of nonsmokers is about 0.5 percent. This is attributed to endogenous production of CO from such sources as heme catabolism. Uptake of exogenous CO increases blood COHb in proportion to the concentration in the air as well as the length of exposure and the ventilation rate of the person. Continuous exposure of human subjects to 30 ppm CO leads to an equilibrium value of 5 percent COHb. About 80 percent of this value is approached in four hours and the remaining 20 percent is approached slowly over the next eight hours. It can be calculated that continuous exposure to 20 ppm CO gives an equilibrium COHb value of about 3.7 percent and 10 ppm CO gives an equilibrium value of 2 percent COHb. The equilibrium values are generally reached after eight or more hours of exposure. The time required to reach equilibrium can be shortened by physical activity.

Analysis of data from air-monitoring programs in California indicates that eight-hour average values, which may be exceeded for 0.1 percent of the time, ranged from 10 to 40 ppm CO. Depending on location within a community, CO concentrations can vary widely. Concentrations predicted inside the passenger compartments of motor vehicles in downtown traffic were almost three times those for central urban areas and five times those expected in residential areas. Occupants of vehicles traveling on expressways had CO exposures somewhere between those in central urban areas and in downtown traffic. Concentrations above 87 ppm have been measured in underground garages, in tunnels, and in buildings over highways.

No human health effects have been demonstrated for COHb levels below 2 percent. Above 2 percent COHb in nonsmokers (the median value for smokers is of the order of 5 percent COHb) it has been possible to demonstrate effects on the central nervous system. At COHb levels of 2.5 percent resulting from about 90-minutes exposure to about 50 ppm CO, there is an impairment of time-interval discrimination; at approximately 5 percent COHb, there is an impairment of other psychomotor faculties. Cardiovascular changes may be produced by exposure sufficient to produce over 5 percent COHb. These include increased cardiac output, AV oxygen difference, and coronary blood flow in patients without coronary disease. Decreased coronary sinus blood P_{O_2} occurs in patients with coronary heart disease. Impaired oxidative metabolism of the myocardium may occur. These changes could produce an added burden on patients with heart disease. Some adaptation to chronic low levels of CO may occur through such mechanisms as increased hematocrit, increased hemoglobin, and increased blood volume.

AUTO EXHAUST AND SYNTHETIC SMOG

Many investigators have studied the effect of atmospheres designed to simulate photochemical smog. These have included irradiated and non-irradiated auto exhaust or ozonized gasoline. In such experiments the observed effects are those of a mixture of components, some of which are known, others of which are unknown. Such experiments have the advantage of being a step closer to actual urban air pollution than studies of individual specific chemicals and the disadvantage that it is difficult to determine which of the many substances present are critical for the observed effects.

Short-Term Exposures

Exposure of two to three hours to heavy Los Angeles smog containing 0.4 ppm total oxidant or synthetic smog containing 0.5 ppm total oxidant was capable of producing ultrastructural changes in alveolar tissue of mice ranging in age from 5 to 21 months (Bils and Romanovsky, 1967). The severity of the damage increased with increasing age. No change was detectable in the youngest animals. In eight-to-nine-month-old animals there were definite alterations, but by 14 to 18 hours after exposure there was no detectable difference from control animals. In animals 15 months of age alterations were still present 24 hours after exposure. The endothelial cells were seriously affected but the lining epithelium and basement membrane were intact. In the oldest animals changes that could be interpreted as edema-like occurred in the lining epithelium. The alterations were still present 18 hours after exposure. The implication is clear that loss of regenerative capacity of alveolar tissue following damage is one result of aging.

Exposure of A-strain and C_{57} black mice to 1 to 3.8 ppm ozonized gasoline produced an increased incidence of lung tumors (Kotin and Falk, 1956; Kotin et al., 1958). True carcinomas have been produced in C_{57} black mice by combined exposure to ozonized gasoline and influenza virus.

Mice were exposed for four hours to auto exhaust containing 0.08 to 0.67 ppm oxidant and 12 to 100 ppm CO for four hours (Coffin and Blommer, 1967). Immediately following this exposure the mice were exposed to a bacterial aerosol of *Streptococcus* (group C) at the rate of 100,000 organisms per mouse. When the exhaust contained 0.35 to 0.67 ppm oxidant and 100 ppm

CO, there was enhanced mortality from streptococcal pneumonia: 53 percent among the exposed and 11 percent among the controls. The mortality was not enhanced by exhaust containing 0.12 ppm oxidant and 25 ppm CO. The increased mortality was probably related to the oxidant content. The levels involved are well below peak concentrations reported for heavy pollution.

The respiratory function of guinea pigs exposed to irradiated and nonirradiated auto exhaust has been measured (Murphy et al., 1963a). Increases in flow resistance were produced by 150:1 dilutions of irradiated exhaust but not by similar dilution of nonirradiated exhaust. This was attributed to the formation of aldehydes, nitrogen dioxide, and total oxidant by irradiation. The nature of the response would suggest aldehyde as the most likely component responsible for the observed change.

Chronic Exposures

In an extensive experiment designed to assess the long-term effects of auto exhaust, beagle dogs were exposed daily for 16 hours for a total of 68 months (Lewis et al., 1974). A variety of pulmonary function studies were made at intervals throughout the exposure years. At the end of the exposure period the dogs were moved from the EPA laboratory in Cincinnati to the College of Veterinary Medicine at Davis, California. There a series of physiologic measurements were made both on arrival and two years after the exposure had terminated. The dogs were then sacrificed and extensive morphologic examination by light and electron microscopy was made of the lungs. These experiments thus provided an opportunity to correlate physiologic and morphologic observations.

One hundred and four dogs were divided into eight groups. One group included 20 dogs that served as controls and were exposed in similar chambers to clean air. The seven experimental groups each contained 12 dogs. The exposures were to (1) nonirradiated auto exhaust; (2) irradiated auto exhaust; (3) sulfur dioxide plus sulfuric acid; (4) and (5) the two types of exhaust plus the sulfur mixture; and (6) and (7) a high and a low level of nitrogen oxides. The irradiated exhaust contained oxidant (measured as ozone) at about 0.2 ppm and nitrogen dioxide at about 0.9 ppm. The raw exhaust contained minimal concentrations of these materials and about 1.5 ppm nitric oxide. Both forms of exhaust contained close to 100 ppm carbon monoxide.

The values for physiologic tests done on the control dogs showed no change between the end of exposure and two years after. All other exposure groups had pulmonary function values different from controls and had more functional abnormalities at the end of the two-year post-exposure period. Pulmonary function tests suggested that auto exhaust exposure injured the airways and parenchyma while oxides of sulfur or nitrogen injured the parenchyma.

Two important exposure-related pulmonary lesions were observed. Enlargement of air spaces and loss of interalveolar septa in proximal acinar regions were most severe in dogs exposed to oxides of nitrogen, oxides of sulfur, or the latter with irradiated exhaust. Hyperplasia of nonciliated bronchiolar cells was most severe in dogs exposed to raw auto exhaust alone or with oxides of sulfur.

These studies indicate that alterations in function that are reflected by morphologic injury are persistent in nature following exposure to quite realistic levels of mixed pollution.

CONCLUSIONS

Since it was written for a textbook of toxicology, this chapter has discussed mainly the results of experimental studies related to specific compounds that occur as pollutants of urban air. Data of this kind are among the factors considered in the practical deliberations on the development of air quality criteria and standards.

The Clean Air Act sets forth the legal steps leading to the establishment of air quality standards. The initial step in this process is the preparation of an air quality criteria document, which sets forth the state of knowledge in regard to the effects of the substance on animals, man, plants, and materials. It is in this step that the availability of pertinent toxicologic data is of prime importance. This has been and should continue to be an incentive to toxicologists to develop sensitive methods capable of assaying the response to low concentrations of materials that occur as air pollutants.

REFERENCES

Abe, M.: Effects of mixed NO_2-SO_2 gas on human pulmonary functions. Effects of air pollution on the human body. *Bull. Tokyo Med. Dental Univ.*, **14**:415–33, 1967.

Alarie, Y. C.; Ulrich, C. E.; Busey, W. M.; Swann, H. E., Jr.; and MacFarland, H. N.: Long-term continuous exposure of guinea pigs to sulfur dioxide. *Arch. Environ. Health*, **21**:769–77, 1970.

Alarie, Y. C.; Ulrich, C. E.; Busey, W. M.; Krumm, A. A.; and MacFarland, H. N.: Long-term continuous exposure to sulfur dioxide in cynomolgus monkeys. *Arch. Environ. Health*, **24**:115–28, 1972.

Alarie, Y. C.; Krumm, A. A.; Busey, W. M.; Ulrich, C. E.; and Kantz, R. J., Jr.: Long-term exposure to sulfur dioxide, sulfuric acid mist, fly ash, and their mixtures. Results of studies in monkeys and guinea pigs. *Arch. Environ. Health*, **30**:254–62, 1975.

Alpert, S. M.; Schwartz, B. B.; Lee, S. D.; and Lewis, T. R.: Alveolar protein accumulation. A sensitive indicator of low level oxidant toxicity. *Arch. Intern. Med.*, **128**:69–73, 1971.

Amdur, M. O.: The respiratory response of guinea pigs to sulfuric acid mist. *Arch. Ind. Health*, **18**:407–14, 1958.

————: The response of guinea pigs to inhalation of formaldehyde and formic acid alone and with a sodium chloride aerosol. *Int. J. Air Pollut.*, **3**:201–20, 1960.

————: The effect of aerosols on the response to irritant gases. In Davies, C. N. (ed.): *Inhaled Particles and Vapours.* Pergamon Press, Oxford, 1961, pp. 281–92.

————: Respiratory absorption data and SO_2 dose-response curves. *Arch. Environ. Health*, **12**:729–32, 1966.

————: 1974 Cummings Memorial Lecture: The long road from Donora. *Am. Ind. Hyg. Assoc. J.*, **35**:589–97, 1974.

Amdur, M. O., and Corn, M.: The irritant potency of zinc ammonium sulfate of different particle sizes. *Am. Ind. Hyg. Assoc. J.*, **24**:326–33, 1963.

Amdur, M. O., and Mead, J.: Mechanics of respiration in unanesthetized guinea pigs. *Am. J. Physiol.*, **192**:364–68, 1958.

Amdur, M. O., and Underhill, D. W.: The effect of various aerosols on the response of guinea pigs to sulfur dioxide. *Arch. Environ. Health*, **16**:460–68, 1968.

Amdur, M. O.; Schultz, R. Z.; and Drinker, P.: Toxicity of sulfuric acid mist to guinea pigs. *Arch. Ind. Hyg. Occup. Med.*, **5**:318–29, 1952.

Amdur, M. O.; Dubriel, M.; and Creasia, D. A.: Respiratory response of guinea pigs to low levels of sulfuric acid. *Environ. Res.*, **15**:418–23, 1978a.

Amdur, M. O.; Bayles, J.; Ugro, V.; and Underhill, D. W.: Comparative irritant potency of sulfate salts. *Environ. Res.*, **16**:1–8, 1978b.

Bell, K. A.; Linn, W. S.; Hazucha, M.; Hackney, J. D.; and Bates, D. V.: Respiratory effects of exposure to ozone plus sulfur dioxide in Southern Californians and Eastern Canadians. *Am. Ind. Hyg. Assoc. J.*, **38**:696–706, 1977.

Bils, R. F.: Ultrastructural alterations of alveolar tissue of mice. I. Due to heavy Los Angeles smog. *Arch. Environ. Health*, **12**:689–97, 1966.

Bils, R. F., and Romanovsky, J. C.: Ultrastructural alterations of alveolar tissue of mice. II. Synthetic photochemical smog. *Arch. Environ. Health*, **14**:844–58, 1967.

Boatman, E. S.; Sato, S.; and Frank, R.: Acute effects o ozone on cat lungs. II. Structural. *Am. Rev. Resp. Dis.*, **110**:157–69, 1974.

Buell, G. C.; Tokiwa, Y.; and Mueller, P. K.: Potential cross-linking agents in lung tissue. Formation and isolation after *in vivo* exposure to ozone. *Arch. Environ. Health*, **10**:213–19, 1965.

————: Lung collagen and elastin denaturation *in vivo* following inhalation of nitrogen dioxide. Paper No. 66-7, *59th Air Pollution Control Association Meeting*, San Francisco, June, 1966.

Burton, G. G.; Corn, M.; Gee, J. B. L.; Vasallo, C.; and Thomas, A. P.: Response of healthy men to inhaled low concentrations of gas-aerosol mixtures. *Arch. Environ. Health*, **18**:681–92, 1969.

Castleman, W. L.; Dungworth, D. L.; and Tyler, W. S.: Histochemically detected enzymic alterations in rat lung exposed to ozone. *Exp. Mol. Pathol.*, **19**:402–21, 1973.

Charles, J. M.; Gardiner, D. E.; Coffin, D. L.; and Menzel, D. B.: Augmentation of sulfate ion absorption from the rat lung by heavy metals. *Toxicol. Appl. Pharmacol.*, **42**:531–38, 1977.

Chow, C. K., and Tappel, A. L.: Activities of pentose shunt and glycolytic enzymes in lungs of ozone-exposed rats. *Arch. Environ. Health*, **26**:205–208, 1973.

Coburn, R. F. (ed.): Biological effects of carbon monoxide. *Ann. N.Y. Acad. Sci.*, **174** (Art. 1):1–430, 1970.

Coffin, D. L., and Blommer, E. J.: Acute toxicity of irradiated auto exhaust. Its indication by enhancement of mortality from streptococcal pneumonia. *Arch. Environ. Health*, **15**:36–8, 1967.

Coffin, D. L.; Gardiner, D. E.; and Blommer, E. J.: Time-dose response for nitrogen dioxide exposure in an infectivity model system. *Environ. Health Perspect.*, **13**:11–15, 1976.

Cortesi, R., and Privett, O. S.: Toxicity of fatty ozonides and peroxides. *Lipids*, **7**:715–21, 1972.

Costa, D. L., and Amdur, M. O. Effects of oil mist on the irritancy of sulfur dioxide: II motor oil. *Am. Ind. Hyg. Assoc. J.*, **40**:809–15, 1979.

Dalhamn, T.: Mucous flow and ciliary activity in the trachea of healthy rats and rats exposed to respiratory irritant gases (SO_2, H_3N, HCHO). A functional and morphologic (light microscopic and electron microscopic) study, with special reference to technique. *Acta Physiol. Scand.*, **36** (suppl. 123):1–161, 1956.

DeLucia, A. J.; Mustafa, M. G.; Hussain, M. Z.; and Cross, C. E.: Ozone interaction with rodent lung. III. Oxidation of reduced glutathione and formation of mixed disulfides between protein and nonprotein sulfhydryls. *J. Clin. Invest.*, **55**:794–802, 1975.

Dungworth, D. L.: Short-term effects of ozone on lungs of rats, mice, and monkeys. (Abstract) *Environ. Health Perspect.*, **16**:179, 1976.

Easton, R. E., and Murphy, S. D.: Experimental ozone preexposure and histamine. Effect on the acute toxicity and respiratory function effects of histamine in guinea pigs. *Arch. Environ. Health*, **15**:160–66, 1967.

Ehrlich, R., and Henry, M. C.: Chronic toxicity of nitrogen dioxide. I. Effect on resistance to bacterial pneumonia. *Arch. Environ. Health*, **17**:860–65, 1968.

Electric Power Research Institute: *Sulfur Oxides: Current Status of Knowledge.* EPRI Document EA-316, Electric Power Research Institute, Palo Alto, CA, 1976.

Evans, M. J.; Stephens, R. J.; Cabral, L. J.; and Freeman, G.: Cell renewal in the lungs of rats exposed to low levels of NO_2. *Arch. Environ. Health*, **24**:180–88, 1972.

Ferin, J., and Leach, L. J.: The effect of SO_2 on lung clearance of TiO_2 particles in rats. *Am. Ind. Hyg. Assoc. J.*, **34**:260–63, 1973.

Frank, N. R., and Speizer, F. E.: SO_2 effects on the respiratory system in dogs. Changes in mechanical behavior at different levels of the respiratory system during acute exposure to the gas. *Arch. Environ. Health*, **11**:624–34, 1965.

Frank, N. R.; Amdur, M. O.; Worchester, J.; and Whittenberger, J. L.: Effects of acute controlled exposure to SO_2 on respiratory mechanics in healthy male adults. *J. Appl. Physiol.*, **17**:252–58, 1962.

Frank, N. R.; Amdur, M. O.; and Whittenberger, J. L.: A comparison of the acute effects of SO_2 administered alone or in combination with NaCl particles on the respiratory mechanics of healthy adults. *Int. J. Air Water Pollut.*, **8**:125–33, 1964.

Frank, N. R.; Yoder, R. E.; Yokoyama, E.; and Speizer, F. E.: The diffusion of $^{35}SO_2$ from tissue fluids into the lungs following exposure of dogs to $^{35}SO_2$. *Health Phys.*, **13**:31–38, 1967.

Frank, N. R.; Yoder, R. E.; Brain, J. D.; and Yokoyama, E.: SO_2 (^{35}S labeled) absorption by the nose and mouth under conditions of varying concentration and flow. *Arch. Environ. Health*, **13**:315–22, 1969.

Freeman, G.; Crane, S. C.; Furiosi, N. J.; Stephens, R. J.; Evans, M. J.; and Moore, W. D.: Covert reduction in ventilatory surface in rats during prolonged exposure to subacute nitrogen dioxide. *Am. Rev. Resp. Dis.*, **106**:563–79, 1972.

Gardner, D. E.; Holzman, R. S.; and Coffin, D. L.: Effects of nitrogen dioxide on pulmonary cell population. *J. Bacteriol.*, **98**:1041–43, 1969.

Gardner, D. E.; Lewis, T. R.; Alpert, S. M.; Hurst, D. J.; and Coffin, D. L.: The role of tolerance in pulmonary defense mechanisms. *Arch. Environ. Health*, 25:432–38, 1972.

Goldstein, B. D.; Lodi, C., Collinson, C.; and Balchum, O. J.: Ozone and lipid peroxidation. *Arch. Environ. Health*, 18:631–35, 1969.

Goldstein, B. D.; Buckley, R. D.; Cardenas, R.; and Balchum, O. J.: Ozone and vitamin E. *Science*, 169:605–606, 1970.

Gordon, T., and Amdur, M. O.: Effect of ozone on the response of guinea pigs to histamine. *J. Environ. Sci. Toxicol.* (in press).

Gray, E. L.; Patton, F. M.; Goldberg, S. B.; and Kaplan, E.: Toxicity of the oxides of nitrogen. II. Acute inhalation toxicity of nitrogen dioxide, red fuming nitric acid, and white fuming nitric acid. *Arch. Ind. Hyg. Occup. Med.*, 10:418–22, 1954.

Gunnison, A. F., and Palmes, E. D.: *S*-Sulfonates in human plasma following inhalation of sulfur dioxide. *Am. Ind. Hyg. Assoc. J.*, 35:288–91, 1974.

Hackney, J. D.; Linn, W. S.; Mohler, J. G.; Pederson, E. E.; Breisacher, P.; and Russo, A.: Experimental studies on human health effects of air pollutants. II. Four-hour exposure to ozone alone and in combination with other pollutant gases. *Arch. Environ. Health*, 30:379–84, 1975.

Hazucha, M.; Silverman, F.; Parent, C.; Field, S.; and Bates, D. V.: Pulmonary function in man after short-term exposure to ozone. *Arch. Environ. Health*, 27:183–88, 1973.

Henry, M. C.; Ehrlich, R.; and Blair, W. H.: Effect of nitrogen dioxide on resistance of squirrel monkeys to *Klebsiella pneumoniae* infection. *Arch. Environ. Health*, 18:580–87, 1969.

Henry, M. C.; Findlay, J.; Spangler, J.; and Ehrlich, R.: Chronic toxicity of NO_2 in squirrel monkeys. III. Effect on resistance to bacterial and viral infection. *Arch. Environ. Health*, 20:566–70, 1970.

Hirsch, J. A.; Swenson, E. W.; and Wanner, A.: Tracheal mucous transport in beagles after long-term exposure to 1 ppm sulfur dioxide. *Arch. Environ. Health*, 30:249–53, 1975.

Jeffery, P. K., and Reid, L. M.: The respiratory mucous membrane. In Brain, J. D.; Proctor, D. F.; and Reid, L. M. (eds.): *Respiratory Defense Mechanisms*, Part I. Marcel Dekker, New York and Basel, 1977.

Kane, L. E., and Alarie, Y.: Evaluation of sensory irritation from acrolein-formaldehyde mixtures. *Am. Ind. Hyg. Assoc. J.*, 39:270–74, 1978.

Kerr, H. D.; Kulle, T. J.; McIlhany, M. L.; and Swidersky, P.: Effects of ozone on pulmonary function in normal subjects. An environmental-chamber study. *Am. Rev. Resp. Dis.*, 111:763–73, 1975.

Kotin, P., and Falk, H. L.: The experimental induction of pulmonary tumors in strain-A mice after their exposure to an atmosphere of ozonized gasoline. *Cancer (Philadelphia)*, 9:910–17, 1956.

———: Atmospheric factors in pathogenesis of lung cancer. *Adv. Cancer Res.*, 7:475–514, 1963.

Kotin, P.; Falk, H. L.; and McCammon, C. J.: The experimental induction of pulmonary tumors and changes in the respiratory epithelium of C57BL mice following their exposure to an atmosphere of ozonized gasoline. *Cancer (Philadelphia)*, 11:473–81, 1958.

Kuschner, M.: The J. Burns Amberson Lecture: The causes of lung cancer. *Am. Rev. Resp. Dis.*, 98:573–90, 1968.

Lawther, P. J.: Climate, air pollution and chronic bronchitis. *Proc. R. Soc. Med.*, 51:262–64, 1958.

———: Compliance with the clean air act: Medical aspects. *J. Inst. Fuel*, 36:341–44, 1963.

———: Air pollution and public health—a personal appraisal. *Edwin Stevens Lectures for the Laity*, Royal Society of Medicine, 1975.

Lawther, P. J.; MacFarlane, A. J.; Waller, R. E.; and Brooks, A. G. F.: Pulmonary function and sulphur dioxide, some preliminary findings. *Environ. Res.*, 10:355–67, 1975.

Lee, L. Y.; Bleeker, E.; and Nadel, J. A.: Ozone-induced airway hyperirritability in dogs. *Fed. Proc.*, 36:616, 1977.

Lewis, T. R.; Campbell, K. I.; and Vaughan, T. R., Jr.: Effects on canine pulmonary function. Via induced NO_2 impairment, particulate interaction, and subsequent SO_x. *Arch. Environ. Health*, 18:596–601, 1969.

Lewis, T. R.; Moorman, W. J.; Yang, Y. Y.; and Stara, J. F.: Long-term exposure to auto exhaust and other pollutant mixtures. *Arch. Environ. Health*, 21:102–106, 1974.

Mawdesley-Thomas, L. E.; Healey, P.; and Barry, D. H.: Experimental bronchitis in animals due to sulphur dioxide and cigarette smoke. An automated quantitative study. In Walton, W. H. (ed.): *Inhaled Particles and Vapours, III*. Unwin Brothers Ltd., Old Woking, Surrey, England, 1971.

McJilton, C.; Frank, N. R.; and Charlson, R. E.: Role of relative humidity in the synergistic effect of a sulfur dioxide–aerosol mixture on the lung. *Science*, 182:503–504, 1973.

Mead, J.: The control of respiratory frequency. *Ann. N.Y. Acad. Sci.*, 109:724–29, 1963.

Menzel, D. B.: Toxicity of ozone, oxygen, and radiation. *Annu. Rev. Pharmacol.*, 10:379–94, 1970.

Menzel, D. B.; Slaughter, R. J.; Bryant, A. M.; and Jauregui, H. O.: Heinz bodies formed in erythrocytes by fatty acid ozonides and ozone. *Arch. Environ. Health*, 30:296–301, 1975.

Mueller, P. K., and Hitchcock, M.: Air quality criteria—toxicological appraisal for oxidants, nitrogen oxides, and hydrocarbons. *J. Air Pollut. Control Assoc.*, 19:670–76, 1969.

Murphy, S. D.: Mechanism of the effect of acrolein on rat liver enzymes. *Toxicol. Appl. Pharmacol.*, 7:833–43, 1965.

Murphy, S. D.; Klingshirn, D. A.; and Ulrich, C. E.: Respiratory response of guinea pigs during acrolein inhalation and its modification by drugs. *J. Pharmacol. Exp. Ther.*, 141:79–83, 1963a.

Murphy, S. D.; Leng, J. K.; Ulrich, C. E.; and Davis, H. V.: Effects on animals of exposure to auto exhaust. *Arch. Environ. Health*, 7:60–70, 1963b.

Murphy, S. D.; Davis, H. V.; and Zaratzian, V. L.: Biochemical effects in rats from irritating air contaminants. *Toxicol. Appl. Pharmacol.*, 6:520–28, 1964a.

Murphy, S. D.; Ulrich, C. E.; Frankowitz, S. H.; and Xintaras, C.: Altered function in animals inhaling low concentrations of ozone and nitrogen dioxide. *Am. Ind. Hyg. Assoc. J.*, 25:246–53, 1964b.

Nadel, J. A.; Salem, H.; Tamplin, B.; and Tokiwa, Y.: Mechanism of bronchoconstriction during inhalation of sulfur dioxide. *J. Appl. Physiol.*, 20:164–67, 1965.

Nadel, J. A.; Corn, M.; Zwi, S.; Flesch, J.; and Graf, P.: Location and mechanism of airway constriction after inhalation of histamine aerosol and inorganic sulfate aerosol. In Davies, C. N. (ed.): *Inhaled Particles and Vapours, II*. Pergamon Press, Oxford, 1967, pp. 55–66.

National Academy of Sciences, Committee on Medical and Biologic Effects of Environmental Pollutants: *Ozone and Other Photochemical Oxidants*. National Academy of Sciences, Washington, D.C., 1977.

Orehek, J.; Massari, J. P.; Gayrard, P.; Grimaud, C.; and Charpin, J.: Effect of short-term, low-level nitrogen dioxide exposure on bronchial sensitivity of asthmatic patients. *J. Clin. Invest.*, 57:301–307, 1976.

Pattle, R. E.; Burgess, F.; and Cullumbine, H.: The effects of a cold environment and of ammonia on the toxicity of sulphuric acid mist to guinea pigs. *J. Pathol. Bacteriol.*, **72**:219–32, 1956.

Purvis, M. R., and Ehrlich, R.: Effect of atmospheric pollutants on susceptibility to respiratory infection. II. Effect of nitrogen dioxide. *J. Infect. Dis.*, **113**:72–76, 1963.

Rall, D. P.: Review of the health effects of sulfur oxides. *Environ. Health Perspect.*, **8**:97–121, 1974.

Reid, L.: An experimental study of hypersecretion of mucus in the bronchial tree. *Br. J. Exp. Pathol.*, **44**: 437–45, 1963.

Riddick, J. H., Jr.; Campbell, K. I.; and Coffin, D. L.: Histopathologic changes secondary to nitrogen dioxide exposure in dog lungs. *Am. J. Clin. Pathol.*, **49**:239, 1968.

Schlesinger, R. B.; Lippmann, M.; and Albert, R. E.: Effects of short-term exposures to sulfuric acid and ammonium sulfate aerosols upon bronchial airway function in the donkey. *Am. Ind. Hyg. Assoc. J.*, **39**: 275–86, 1978.

Speizer, F. E., and Frank, N. R.: The uptake and release of SO_2 by the human nose. *Arch. Environ. Health*, **12**: 725–28, 1966.

———: A comparison of changes in pulmonary flow resistance in healthy volunteers acutely exposed to SO_2 by mouth and by nose. *Br. J. Ind. Med.*, **23**:75–79, 1966.

Spicer, S. S.; Chakrin, L. W.; and Wardell, J. R., Jr.: Effect of chronic sulfur dioxide inhalation on the carbohydrate histochemistry and histology of the canine respiratory tract. *Am. Rev. Resp. Dis.*, **110**:13–24, 1974.

Stephens, R. J.; Freeman, G.; Stara, J. F.; and Coffin, D. L.: Cytologic changes in dog lungs induced by chronic exposure to ozone. *Am. J. Pathol.*, **73**:711–18, 1973.

Stephens, R. J.; Sloan, M. F.; Evans, M. J.; and Freeman, G.: Early response of lung to low levels of ozone. *Am. J. Pathol.*, **74**:31–57, 1974.

Stokinger, H. E.: Ozone toxicology. A review of research and industrial experience: 1954–1964. *Arch. Environ. Health*, **10**:719–31, 1965.

Strandberg, L. G.: SO_2 absorption in the respiratory tract. Studies on the absorption in rabbits, its dependence on concentration and breathing pace. *Arch. Environ. Health*, **9**:160–66, 1964.

Thomas, H. V.; Mueller, P. K.; and Lyman, R. L.: Lipoperoxidation of lung lipids in rats exposed to nitrogen dioxide. *Science*, **159**:532–34, 1968.

Tiege, B.; McManus, T. T.; and Mudd, J. B.: Reaction of ozone with phosphatidylcholine liposomes and the lytic effect of products on red blood cells. *Chem. Phys. Lipids*, **12**:153–71, 1974.

Toyama, T.: Studies on aerosols. 1. Synergistic response of the pumonary airway resistance on inhaling sodium chloride aerosols and SO_2 in man. *Jpn. J. Ind. Health*, **4**:86–92, 1962.

Toyama, T., and Nakamura, K.: Synergistic response of hydrogen peroxide aerosols and sulfur dioxide to pulmonary airway resistance. *Ind. Health*, **2**:34–45, 1964.

Treon, J. F.; Dutra, F. R.; Cappel, J.; Sigmon, H.; and Younker, W.: Toxicity of sulfuric acid mist. *Arch. Ind. Hyg. Occup. Med.*, **2**:716–34, 1950.

U.S. Dept. of Health, Education, and Welfare: *Air Quality Criteria for Particulate Matter.* National Air Pollution Control Administration, Publication AP-49, Washington, D.C., January, 1969a.

———: *Air Quality Criteria for Sulfur Oxides.* National Air Pollution Control Administration, Publication AP-50, Washington, D.C., January, 1969b.

———: *Air Quality Criteria for Carbon Monoxide.* National Air Pollution Control Administration, Publication AP-62, Washington, D.C., March, 1970.

Vaughan, T. R., Jr.; Jennelle, L. F.; and Lewis, T. R.: Long-term exposure to low levels of air pollutants. Effects on pulmonary function in the beagle. *Arch. Environ. Health*, **19**:45–50, 1969.

Weir, F. W.; Stevens, D. H.; and Bromberg, P. A.: Pulmonary function studies of men exposed for 120 hours to sulfur dioxide. *Toxicol. Appl. Pharmacol.*, **22**: 319, 1972.

Widdicombe, J. G.: Respiratory reflexes from the trachea and bronchi of the cat. *J. Physiol.*, **123**:55–70, 1954.

———: Receptors in the trachea and bronchi of the cat. *J. Physiol.*, **123**:71–104, 1954.

Chapter 25

WATER AND SOIL POLLUTANTS

Robert E. Menzer and *Judd O. Nelson*

INTRODUCTION

The ultimate sinks for most chemicals produced and used by man are water and soil. Three-quarters of the earth's surface is covered by water, and the remainder that is not covered by asphalt or concrete is covered by soil. Although water and soil are usually considered as separate ecologic systems, one needs to realize that suspended soil particles in water represent an interface between the two systems and serve as a mechanism for contamination of the one by the other. In reality it is impossible to consider any component of the real world in isolation from any other, as illustrated in Figure 25–1. For our purposes, however, we shall consider the presence, fate, and effects of chemicals in water and in soil as separate systems, as far as that is possible.

Systems of water may be compartmentalized based on their natural occurrence and the use made of them. One may consider separately the naturally occurring bodies of water: marine systems, fresh water systems, and the interface between them, the estuarine systems. One may also consider these systems on the basis of the use made of water removed from them for drinking purposes or other domestic consumption. Water systems are also the recipients of the products of domestic and industrial sewage systems. Bodies of water, including rivers, lakes, ponds, and the ground water, are also the recipients of runoff from agricultural and urban areas, which greatly modifies their capability to support life and their usefulness for other purposes.

Although water can be ultimately purified to a specific, definite chemical entity, soil has no commonly accepted compositional definition. Soils are composed of inorganic and organic constituents. The inorganic are silt, sand, and clay in varying ratios. These inorganic particles are coated and admixed with organic constituents, living and dead. The behavior of soil to a major degree is determined by the size and shape of the particles of which it is composed. Soil particles range in size from less than 0.002 mm to about 2.0 mm in diameter. Soils are classified according to particle size ranges as follows: clay, < 0.002 mm; silt, 0.002 to 0.02 mm; fine sand, 0.02 to 0.20 mm; and coarse sand, 0.2 to 2.0 mm. The most important use of soil is for agriculture. Soil is the ultimate support of man's sources of most food and much fiber. In addition, the soil has been the final disposal site for much of the industrial and urban waste generated by man's societies.

The interface between soil and water is an intimate one. Virtually all water systems contain suspended soil particles, and virtually all soil contains at least a small amount of water. The sediment that is the end product of soil erosion is by volume the greatest single pollutant of surface waters and is the principal carrier of most pollutants found in water. In a joint study the United States Department of Agriculture and the Environmental Protection Agency have estimated that potential annual water erosion losses range from negligible to more than 100 tons of soil per acre. About 20 percent of the 438 million acres of crop land in the United States averages more than 8 tons of soil loss per acre per year; 30 percent averages less than 3 tons; and the other 50 percent between 3 and 8 tons (Stewart *et al.*, 1975). In fact, the sedimentary materials in water resulting from soil erosion accumulate more than 700 times more than those derived from sewage discharges (Weber, 1972). Thus, any treatment of the environmental toxicology of soil and water must consider each as a two-phase system, each containing the other and interacting through the water-sediment system.

Sources of Chemicals in the Environment

Chemicals in the environment may be classified in a variety of ways. In this chapter we have chosen to consider chemicals primarily according to their use; secondarily, by chemical properties. Thus, we will consider chemicals by their source as follows: (1) industrial, (2) agricultural, (3) domestic and urban, and (4) naturally occurring. No matter what use is made of chemicals, contamination of the environment may be either

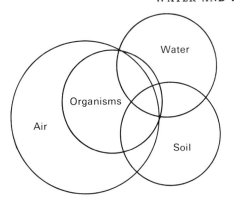

Figure 25–1. Overlapping relationships of environmental compartments.

from point sources or from nonpoint sources. The results of point source pollution are generally easy to identify and the remedies are frequently more attainable. Nonpoint source pollution, on the other hand, is generally less dramatic in its initial effects, but is more difficult to contain or correct.

The production, use, and disposal of industrial chemicals all lead to contamination of soil and water. Production activities lead to soil and water contamination when by-product chemicals are not properly conserved during manufacturing processes. For example, in various smelting operations toxic chemicals present in ores may not be properly controlled. Naturally occurring arsenic in copper ores, for example, frequently finds its way into soil and water. Accidental spillage of industrial chemicals may also result in contamination, sometimes dramatically, of soil and water. Careless manufacturing practices in a small chemical firm in Hopewell, Virginia, led to serious contamination of the James River and Chesapeake Bay by the pesticide Kepone. Even though these practices have now ceased, the contamination of the estuarine system will be present for many decades. Another example is the contamination of the Ohio River with carbon tetrachloride resulting from an accidental dumping of the material from a chemical plant. Such incidents of point source contamination of water can generally be prevented or controlled by the appropriate use of technology. The result, however, of not controlling such point source pollution is frequently a very high cost for decontamination, where that is even possible, and frequently both acute and chronic detrimental effects on organisms.

The use of chemicals for their intended purpose often leads to contamination, sometimes undesirably, of soil and water. Lead contamination of soils and occasionally water near highways results from the use of tetraethyl lead as an anti-knock component of gasoline for automobiles. Although a commitment has been made to reduce the use of this compound in gasoline, the many years during which it was used and the nonpoint source nature of the contamination have resulted in concentrations of lead that will remain for many years in soils and water. A chemical that is intentionally added to water for therapeutic purposes is fluorine. The use of water fluoridation to prevent tooth decay is well known and has been practised in the United States for many years. Excessive concentrations of fluorine, however, can result in undesirable effects in teeth, manifested primarily by their mottling and discoloration. Careful attention must be paid to the use of fluorine to prevent overfluoridation with its undesirable side effects.

The disposal of industrial chemicals following their use presents a major problem in several industries. Detergents used in clothes laundering are discharged into sewage systems and ultimately into rivers, lakes, and streams. Phosphate detergents then serve as nutrients for algae and other organisms that can cause major difficulties in these bodies of water. The green scum resulting from algal blooms is a familiar sight in some areas. The contamination of rivers resulting from discharge of water containing organic mercurials used in paper manufacturing presents a problem in some local situations. Other chemicals resulting from paper making can also present serious water pollution problems. Asbestos tailings resulting from mining operations have also contaminated water systems in some parts of the United States, and this has resulted in concern over the potential health effects of the material that then finds its way into drinking-water systems.

The use of chemicals in agriculture results in contamination of soil and water through the direct use of pesticides and fertilizers. Pesticides are, of course, applied directly to the soil in some cases to control insects, weeds, and plant diseases. Some of these chemicals can persist for many years and thereby cause concern about their potential movement from soil into water systems and from both soil and water into organisms that live in and on water and soil. The effects of pesticides in the food chain are now generally familiar. Likewise, fertilizers applied to the soil to promote plant growth and productivity can leach or run off from soil and find their way into natural water systems, causing an upset in the ecologic balance to the degree that organisms living in those systems can be either enhanced or otherwise affected.

The domestic and urban use and disposal of chemicals also result in the contamination of soil and water. Domestic wastes are concentrated in sewage systems and landfill operations. Frequently, large buildups of heavy metals occur as a result. Pesticides and fertilizers used in suburban and some urban situations for lawn and home garden purposes or pest control in other situations also are serious problems when improperly used. Detergents may also cause difficulties as referred to above. Recently, the discovery that the process of purifying water can result in the chlorination of certain small organic chemicals to produce chlorinated hydrocarbons that are potential carcinogens has generated concern. In some parts of the country concentrations of such chemicals above levels considered to be safe have been found in drinking-water systems.

Finally, metals, minerals, and plant or animal toxins are found in the environment as natural components of water and soil systems. Although they have always been there and always will be, man's activities frequently result in excessive production or movement of such chemicals found naturally occurring in the environment and can result in concentrations detrimental to man or other organisms. Furthermore, the possibility of interaction of synthetic chemicals and pollutants with naturally occurring metals, minerals, and toxins must be considered.

Transport, Mobility, and Disposition

The fate and distribution of chemicals in the environment are determined by several variables that can interact in numerous ways. An analogy between pharmacodynamics and chemodynamics can be drawn to illustrate some basic similarities in each approach. First, one must appreciate the physicochemical properties of a chemical, such as water solubility, lipid solubility, partitioning behavior, vapor pressure, pKa

for ionic species, chemical stability, etc., if one is to predict the behavior of a chemical in a system—be it man or an ecosystem. Second, the processes that act within the system must be considered. Transport, via serum proteins versus suspended sediments; circulation, via the circulatory system versus the hydrologic cycle; degradation, in liver versus soil microorganisms; and excretion, via urine, feces, and expired air versus dilution in water and air to nondetectable levels or deposition in ultimate sinks such as deep ocean sediments, are all processes that act on chemicals to determine the mobility and final disposition of a chemical in a system. The analogy can be carried one step further to include target organs or tissues affected by the chemical in comparison with the susceptible species of an ecosystem. The fundamental difference in this consideration is one of scale, in both time and dimension, which then requires models of varying scale. Mathematical transport models for predicting the fate of chemicals remain primitive and approximate at best; the reader is referred to a National Academy of Sciences (1975) report on the subject for further information and references.

Water Solubility. The water solubility and latent heat of solution are critical properties of a chemical that affect its environmental fate. Many environmental toxicants are hydrophobic, having solubilities in the parts-per-million (ppm, mg/l) to parts-per-billion (ppb, μg/l) range. Reported solubility values vary with the method used for determination (Gunther et al., 1968). Water solubilities are affected by pH (for ionizable chemicals), presence of dissolved salts and organics, and temperature.

Soil Adsorption. Adsorption to particulate matter is a major mechanism by which chemicals

---

Table 25–1. CLASSES OF MATERIALS RELATED TO THE EFFECT OF pH ON ADSORPTION*

CLASS	EXAMPLE	pK_a	MOLECULAR FORM Low pH	MOLECULAR FORM High pH	pH Effect
Strong acid	Linear alkylsulfonates		Anion	Anion	Small
Weak acid	Picloram	3.7	Free acid	Anion	Large adsorption; pH approx. pK_a
Strong base	Diquat		Cation	Cation	Decrease at very low pH (18 N H_2SO_4)
Weak base	Ametryne		Cation	Free base	Increasing adsorption to pH approx. pK_a and then decrease
Polar molecules	Diuron		Nonionized	Un-ionized	Small
Neutral molecules	DDT	Nil	Nonionized	Un-ionized	Probably none

* From Hamaker, J. W., and Thompson, J. M.: Adsorption. In Goring, C. A. I., and Hamaker, J. W. (eds.): *Organic Chemicals in the Soil Environment*, Vol. 1. Marcel Dekker, Inc., New York, 1972. Reprinted by courtesy of Marcel Dekker, Inc.

are removed from solution. Adsorbent materials in soils and sediments can be divided into clay minerals and soil organic matter. Clay minerals include various hydrous silicates, oxides, and layer silicates. The clay minerals have been extensively studied and are characterized by physical structure or layering type, either 1:1 or 2:1, swelling ability, cation exchange capacity, and specific surface (m^2/g) (Weber, 1972). These parameters are important considerations in the behavior of organic cations, polar organic molecules, and metal ions in soils. High specific surface is associated with small particle size; therefore, the colloidal fraction of the soil is a dominant factor in chemical-soil interactions. Cation exchange capacity of the inorganic fraction is a function of the magnitude and distribution of the structural charge. Exchangeability is dependent on the adsorbed cations, usually sodium, potassium, or calcium, and the nature of the replacing cations.

The water associated with clay plays an important role in defining its characteristics. Adsorbed water on clay surfaces is more ordered than free water. Water on the clay surface may also be more ionized than otherwise. Thus, the hydrogen ion concentration of the clay surface is high. The effect of pH on the adsorption of classes

pletely decomposed plant and animal material, and (2) humic substances, which are more or less completely altered or resynthesized materials. The former serve as a source for the latter. Nonhumic materials include well-known organic chemical groups with definite characteristics: proteins, carbohydrates, organic acids, sugars, fats, waxes, resins, lignins, pigments, and low-molecular-weight compounds. These materials comprise 10 to 15 percent of the soil organic matter. Their composition and residence times are quite variable. Humic substances account for 85 to 90 percent of soil organic matter and their nature is not well understood. Humic substances are fractionated to give fulvic acid, which is soluble in both alkali and acid; humic acid, which is soluble in alkali but not in acid; and the humin fraction, which cannot be readily extracted with cold alkali. Humic acid and fulvic acid are aromatic polymers with molecular weights that range from 5,000 to 100,000 and from 2,000 to 9,000, respectively. Functional groups that have been identified on humic substances are carboxyl, phenolic hydroxyl, alcoholic hydroxyl, carbonyl, and methoxy. Heterocyclic rings with oxygen and nitrogen atoms are also present. A hypothetic structure for humic acid has been proposed by Kononova (1966) as follows:

of chemicals has been summarized by Hamaker and Thompson (1972) (Table 25-1).

Adsorption data for chemicals in soils is usually expressed by the Freundlich isotherm, $x/m = KC^n$; x/m is the amount of chemical sorbed per weight of the adsorbent, C is the equilibrium concentration of the chemical, and K and n are constants. The constant K represents the extent of adsorption while the value n sheds light on the nature of the adsorption mechanism and the role of the solvent, water.

Soil organic matter usually ranges from 0.1 to 7.0 percent and serves as the most important sorptive surface for nonionic chemicals. Above a few percent organic matter, all the soil mineral surfaces are effectively blocked and thus no longer function as adsorbents. Soil organic matter can be divided into two main groups: (1) nonhumic substances, which are fresh or incom-

Vaporization. Vaporization from soil, water, or plant surfaces is a major transport process for many chemicals. The volatility of a chemical is a function of its vapor pressure, but the rate of vaporization also depends on environmental conditions such as temperature, degree of adsorption, soil properties, and soil water content. Airflow over the evaporating surface affects vaporization rate since air movement continuously replaces and mixes air around the evaporating surface. Many chemicals evaporate simultaneously with water, which leads some researchers to believe that chemicals such as DDT "codistill" with water. This phenomenon can be demonstrated in laboratory distillations at 100° C, but does not occur at normal environmental temperatures. Instead, water evaporation and DDT volatilization occur independently. Higher vapor loss from most soil surfaces correlates with pesticide volatilization, but is due to desorption of chemicals from soil adsorption sites by water molecules and the mass flow of chemical to the soil surface by the "wick effect." This phenomenon has been noted with chemicals such as 2,4-D esters, thiolcarbamates, triazines, organochlorine insecticides, and N-methyl-carbamates. Volatility of organic chemicals from water increases with decreasing water solubility. As a result, a chemical with both low vapor pressure in the solid phase and very low water solubility would be much more volatile from aqueous solution than might be expected. DDT is again the example.

Partitioning. Many chemicals have low water solubility but high solubility in nonpolar solvents (lipophilicity). The partition coefficient as a measure of these properties is often determined in a system of n-octanol/water. The relationship between water solubility and partition coefficient is illustrated in Figure 25–2. The importance of partitioning behavior of chemicals lies primarily in the phenomenon of bioaccumulation (biomagnification or bioconcentration). Organisms in contact with a solution of chemical that has a high partition coefficient will act as the nonpolar phase of the binary system and accumulate it through a partitioning process.

Bioaccumulation. Bioaccumulation is different from other environmental transport processes because it concentrates rather than diffuses the chemical in question. This concentration effect is expressed as the ratio of the concentration of a chemical in the organism to that in the medium (usually water). The two properties of a chemical that are responsible for high bioaccumulation ratio values are (1) high partition coefficient, i.e., lipophilic, and (2) recalcitrance toward all types of degradation. Bioaccumulation ratios have been determined for a variety of environmental chemicals in laboratory model ecosystems and correlate well with the n-octanol/water partition coefficients (Fig. 25–2).

Degradation. Transformations of chemicals in soil and water occur by chemical, photochemical, and biochemical reactions. Degradation results in the true "disappearance" of a chemical's molecular form, as opposed to transport processes, which merely move chemicals from one environmental compartment to another. However, it must be recognized that transport processes that move chemicals to ultimate sinks, such as deep ocean sediments, for all practical purposes do remove chemicals from the environment.

Chemical transformations are classified as hydrolyses, oxidations, reductions, nucleophilic substitutions involving water, and free radical reactions. These reactions may be catalyzed by the presence of metal ions, metal oxides, clay

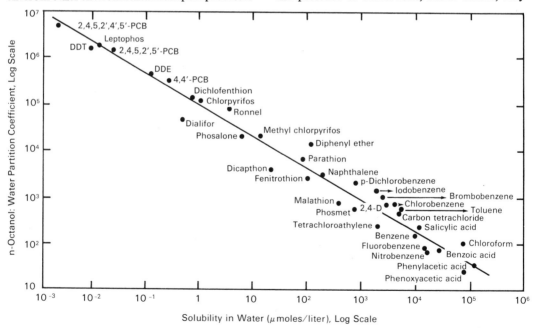

Figure 25–2. Relationship between water solubility and n-octanol/water partition coefficient. (From Freed, V. H.; Chiou, C. T.; and Hague, R.: Chemodynamics: transport and behavior of chemicals in the environment—a problem in environmental health. *Environ. Health Perspect.*, **20:**55–70, 1977.)

surfaces, organic compounds, and organic surfaces. The pH of solutions and the effective pH of clay surfaces, which may be quite different from the surrounding aqueous environment, can significantly influence rates of degradation. Other obvious conditions that affect degradation rates are temperature, moisture content in soils, and other environmental processes that alter chemical concentrations. The kinetics of degradation rates are dependent on the mechanism of degradation. Some degradative processes follow first-order kinetics, while others are best described by a "hyperbolic rate model" (Hamaker, 1972).

Photochemical reactions of chemicals occur in air and water but are probably of little or no significance in soils. For a chemical to undergo a photochemical reaction, it must absorb light energy from an appropriate portion of the spectrum or have the light energy transferred through an intermediate substance known as a sensitizer. Ultraviolet light (4- to 400-nm wavelengths) has sufficient energy to break existing chemical bonds, but light above 450 nm, which represents an energy of 65 kcal/mole, is usually not sufficient to initiate reactions. Light of wavelengths shorter than 295 nm does not reach the earth's surface in appreciable amounts. The principal reactions are photo-oxidations and photoreductions which proceed through light-formed free radicals and which then react with molecular oxygen or abstract hydrogen from organic compounds, respectively.

Biologic reactions of chemicals in soil and water are mediated primarily by microorganisms. Microorganisms are quite versatile when confronted with foreign chemicals. The major reactions involved are dehalogenation, hydrolysis, oxidations, reductions, conjugations, and methylations. They are also very important in the natural cycles of many elements, such as mercury and arsenic. These natural cycles can be disturbed by introduction of various forms of metals and can increase formation of toxic species, e.g., methylmercury. The types and rates of microbiologic reactions are determined by the microbial ecology of any given system. Thus, pH, temperature, redox potential, nutrient availability and microbial interactions will affect the microbial degradation of a chemical.

Chemodynamics. As we have seen above, there are numerous routes by which chemicals enter the environment and many factors to consider in understanding their behavior once they are there. Much of what is known about chemodynamics is derived from studies of pesticides and, to a lesser extent, industrial chemicals and heavy metals. Certainly, pesticide applications, sewage sludge disposal, and industrial waste effluents each present different starting points for a consideration of chemodynamics. We shall deal with environmental processes in the following sections and attempt to relate the (1) physicochemical properties of a chemical and (2) the environmental conditions that serve as modifiers of the processes. Each process has a rate that describes the transport from one component to the next and a rate that describes the degradation of the chemical in question. A complete analysis of all of the rates for entry, transport, and degradation of a chemical will describe its ultimate fate in the water and soil.

PESTICIDES

The major classes of pesticides have been grouped as "nonpersistent" or "slightly residual," "moderately persistent" or "moderately residual," or "persistent" or "highly residual" (Harris, 1969; Kearney et al., 1969). Persistence times reflect the time required for 75 to 100 percent disappearance of pesticide residues from the site of application. Nonpersistent pesticides have persistence values of 1 to 12 weeks; moderately persistent pesticides, 1 to 18 months; and persistent pesticides, two to five years. Persistence times vary with environmental conditions and the generalizations about the classes are subject to several exceptions by individual pesticides within the class (Fig. 25–3).

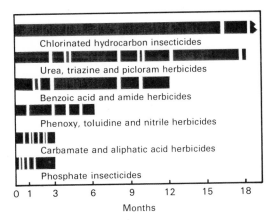

Figure 25–3. Persistence in soils of several classes of insecticides and herbicides. (From Kearney, P. C.; Nash, R. G.; and Isensee, A. R.: Persistence of pesticide residues in soils. In Miller, M. W., and Berg, G. G. [eds.]: *Chemical Fallout.* Charles C Thomas Publisher, Springfield, IL, 1969.)

Persistent Pesticides

Chlorinated Hydrocarbon Insecticides. This group of chemicals includes DDT, TDE (a major metabolite of DDT), methoxychlor, and related chemicals; the cyclodiene insecticides, aldrin, dieldrin, endrin, heptachlor, chlordane, mirex, and Kepone; the hexachlorocyclohexanes (commonly referred to as BHC) and the purified gamma isomer, lindane; and the polychloroterpenes, toxaphene and Strobane. The technology, application, and biologic and environmental aspects of this class of insecticides have been authoritatively reviewed in a two-volume treatise by Brooks (1974). The persistence of pesticides in the environment has been the subject of numerous books and reviews.

DDT, its major metabolites, DDD (TDE) and DDE (which are collectively referred to as DDT-R), and dieldrin, which is both an insecticide and the major metabolite of the insecticide aldrin, are ubiquitous residues and the prime examples of persistent pesticides. Studies with DDT and dieldrin have elucidated several important concepts in environmental toxicology. First, persistence is not a desirable attribute as originally believed. Second, the transport and disposition of persistent pesticides is affected by physical and biologic processes, which occur from the micro to the global scale. Third, high lipid solubility combined with chemical and biologic stability can lead to biologic magnification of pesticide residues.

Persistence is primarily a function of physicochemical properties of substances. In addition, the sorption/desorption process is one of the important factors controlling the fate of pesticides in soils. Sorption of pesticides in soils has been reviewed by numerous authors (Goring, 1967; Bailey and White, 1970; Weber, 1972). Chlorinated hydrocarbon insecticides are highly soluble in lipids and most organic solvents, but have low water solubilities and relatively low vapor pressures. Studies of the adsorption of chlorinated hydrocarbons on various soils are difficult because of their low water solubility. However, studies with PCBs, which have many similar physicochemical properties to the chlorinated hydrocarbons, show that adsorption of the hydrophobic chlorinated hydrocarbons depends strongly on the presence of soil organic matter. Once adsorbed, these chemicals do not readily desorb. Two implications are readily apparent: (1) such compounds will not leach or diffuse in soils and (2) transport into the hydrosphere from contaminated soils will be through erosion of soil particles or sediment, not by desorption and dissolution. When chlorinated hydrocarbons are poorly adsorbed, as in sandy soils, the vaporization loss will be significant as compared to that in soils with higher organic matter.

Volatilization of pesticides into the atmosphere from water and soils is also a transport route. The volatility of a chemical from soil or water is a function of its vapor pressure, but the actual vaporization rate depends on several environmental parameters. Temperature, soil properties, soil water content, and other physicochemical properties such as water solubility and degree of adsorption affect the vaporization rate of pesticides from soil. Soil properties such as high organic matter that cause the pesticide to be strongly adsorbed reduce volatility greatly. The importance of soil moisture in volatilization of chlorinated hydrocarbons led to the use of the term "codistillation." DDT codistills with water in the laboratory (Acree et al., 1963). However, the effect observed in soils is more adequately described as displacement of the sorbed pesticide by water molecules, plus a carrier action by water to the soil-air interface. The distribution of a pesticide between water and air is dependent on both water solubility and vapor pressure. As a result, compounds like DDT with very low water solubilities are quite volatile from water.

Degradation of the chlorinated hydrocarbons is quite slow as compared to the other classes of insecticides, and in soil and water is due mainly to the action of microorganisms. To a lesser extent, chemical reactions and photochemical reactions degrade the chlorinated hydrocarbons under certain conditions. A summary of the pathways for DDT (Fig. 25–4) emphasizes the importance of dechlorination and dehydrochlorination reactions. Oxidative reactions are only moderately important in this scheme. The formation of DDCN in sewage sludge and lake sediment is an example of the unique reactions carried out by microorganisms. Epoxidations and rearrangement reactions are common among the cyclodiene insecticides. The most thoroughly studied of these reactions is the epoxidation of aldrin to dieldrin and heptachlor to heptachlor epoxide (Lichtenstein and Schulze, 1960). The rearrangement products are mainly complicated "caged" structures that are still toxic. The caged compounds mirex and Kepone undergo very little detectable degradation. Toxaphene and BHC are degraded initially by dechlorinations and dehydrochlorinations.

The bioaccumulation of the chlorinated hydrocarbons DDT and dieldrin is well documented by environmental residue data (Edwards, 1970). Bioaccumulation ratios relate organism residues to environmental residue levels and are higher in aquatic ecosystems as opposed to terrestrial ecosystems (Table 25–2). The processes involved in bioaccumulation are quite complex due to population fluctuations, food web relationships, metabolic capabilities of various species and numerous other ecologic considerations. However, the physicochemical parameters of lipid solubility, low water solubility, and chemical stability, which characterize the chlorinated

tion by hydrolysis of the urea. The various
, acidic metabolites formed by oxidation
ions react further to yield various conjugates.
e combination of low mammalian toxicity
biodegradability of the phenylurea herbi-
leads to the conclusion that these com-
ds are not significant factors in the
mination of soil and water systems, and
significance as environmental pollutants
s to be minimal.

bstituted Dinitroanilines. The substituted
oanilines are an important group of herbi-
. Included are trifluralin, benefin, nitralin,
elated materials. These compounds are only
ly soluble in water, have generally low
r pressures, and are relatively immobile in
systems, remaining essentially where they
pplied. They have been classed among the
mobile of the herbicides. Like many of the
cides they appear to be readily adsorbed by
organic matter. Compounds that were the
highly adsorbed were also the least available
owing plants and hence the least effective as
icides. The dinitroanilines are considered to
oderately persistent herbicides in the soil.
are generally considered to have a very low
ee of toxicity to mammals and are degraded
e environment to products without signifi-
adverse effects on organisms.

onpersistent Pesticides

enoxy and Related Acidic Herbicides. A
group of compounds may be designated as
ic herbicides, since they are chemicals that
ess carboxyl or phenolic functional groups
which ionize in aqueous systems yielding
s of < 4. The behavior of these chemicals is
ely correlated with their acid character. The
significant factor with respect to mobility of
compounds is the organic matter content of
soil. Various adsorption studies have shown
the compounds are readily adsorbed by soil
nic matter. Furthermore, in acidic systems
compounds are also adsorbed by clay
icles. A number of these compounds are
mercially available in either the acid form or
sters. The behavior of the esters might be
cted to be considerably different from that
e acid forms.
ncluded within this group of herbicides are
ral important herbicide classes. The phenoxy-
ic acids, including 2,4-D and its esters, were
oduced following World War II for their
activity against many broad-leaved weeds.
chlorinated aliphatic acids include dalapon
trichloroacetic acid, compounds used against
nnial weeds. The benzoic acid herbicides
ude chloramben, dicamba, diclobenil, and
ral other compounds. This is a very hetero-

genous group of herbicides used for a variety
of purposes. The dinitrophenols are a group of
broad-spectrum herbicides, the most common of
which is dinitro-*o*-cresol (DNOC).

Phenylcarbamate and Carbanilate Herbicides.
The phenylcarbamate herbicides are much more
water soluble than the substituted anilines. In
spite of this, however, they are very immobile in
soil systems. Again, these compounds have been
shown to be inactivated by adsorption to soil
organic matter. Compounds in this group include
propham, chlorpropham, barban, terbutol, and
dichlormate. The mechanism of adsorption to
soil organic matter is thought to involve hydrogen
bonding between the carboxyl groups of the
organic matter and the nitrogen and carbonyl
oxygen of the carbamate.

Ethylenebisdithiocarbamate Fungicides. The
metal derivatives of the ethylenebisdithiocarbamates are one of the most important groups of
fungicides currently used in agriculture. The
principal compounds in this group are the manganese and zinc derivatives, maneb and zineb,
and the disodium derivative, nabam. A closely
related group is dithiocarbamates, represented
by ferbam, ferric dimethyldithiocarbamate, and
ziram, zinc dimethyldithiocarbamate. From a
toxicologic standpoint these compounds have
caused concern because of their degradation to
ethylene thiourea, a known carcinogen. This
group is thoroughly considered in a two-volume
treatise on antifungal compounds (Siegel and
Sisler, 1977).

These compounds may be used as seed protectants and foliar fungicides. Only small quantities
find their way into the soil, and once there, are
rapidly degraded. In soil ethylene thiourea, ethyl-
enethiuram monosulfide, CS₂, and H₂S result
from treatment with nabam, zineb, and maneb.
Ethylene thiourea is further degraded to ethylene-
urea. These fungicides appear to have some
systemic activity, and plants growing on treated
soil will take up residues of the compounds, as
well as ethylene thiourea.

Because of the carcinogenic activity of ethylene thiourea, the significance of residues of this
compound found in soils, plants, and food is of
concern. Although the residues of ethylene
thiourea itself may be small, it has been shown
that cooking vegetables containing residues of
ethylenebisdithiocarbamates releases ethylene
thiourea. Hence, the toxicologic significance of
residues of these chemicals in soil, once thought
to be of little consequence, is now a matter of
considerable attention.

Organophosphorus and Carbamate Insecticides.
In contrast to the persistent insecticides, particularly the chlorinated hydrocarbons, the organophosphorus and carbamate insecticides are

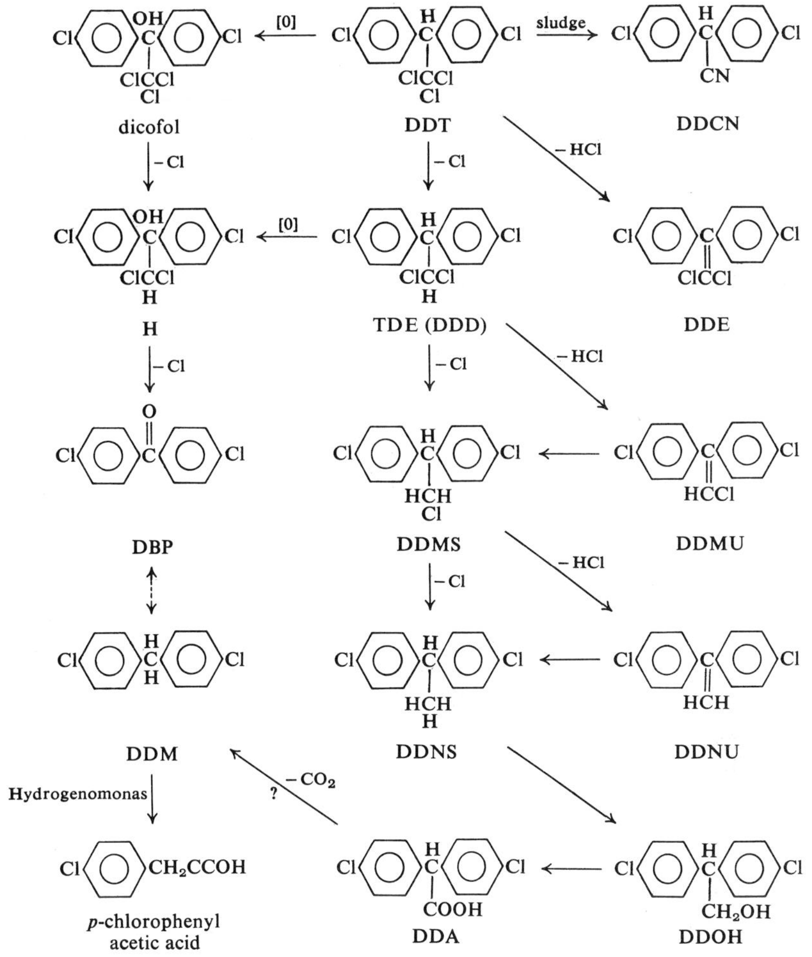

Figure 25–4. Microbiologic and environmental degradation of DDT, illustrating the importance of dechlorination and dehydrochlorination reactions. (Modified from Matsumura, F.: *Toxicology of Insecticides*. Plenum Press, New York, 1975.)

hydrocarbons, appear to be most important in
bioaccumulation of organic pesticides.

DDT was used extensively in the three decades
between 1942 and 1972 for a variety of agricultural
pest control purposes and in many public health
disease control programs worldwide. High levels of
the compound were applied over wide areas. The
result of this heavy usage was the widespread contamination of many components of the environment with
residues of DDT that are likely to persist for many
years. Figure 25–5 illustrates the complicated relationships that have now been shown to exist as a result.
Very low levels of the insecticide, only marginally
detectable in many cases, exist in the air, atmospheric
dust, and rainwater. From there the compound is
transported to soil and water ecosystems where it
becomes available to a variety of organisms. These
residues are then bioaccumulated, with man, of
course, sitting atop the food chain as the ultimate

consumer. Although direct toxicity to man has not
been documented as a result of the accumulation of
DDT, the thin eggshells and reproductive failures of
birds and chronic toxic effects on fish served as the
warning signs that led to restriction of the use of this
chemical.

It may be observed that the effects of bioaccumulation of DDT-R and dieldrin are manifest primarily at the tops of food chains.
Predatory fish and birds suffer from acute toxicity, chronic toxicity, and reproductive failures.
Behavioral changes in DDT-treated fish have
also been demonstrated. Thus, the effects can
range from obvious toxicity to subtle behavioral
changes, the ecologic consequences of which are
unknown.

Cationic Herbicides. The two chemicals of
importance in this group are diquat and para-

Table 25–2. BIOCONCENTRATION OF DDT-R RESIDUES IN PLANTS OR ANIMALS FROM ITS ENVIRONMENT*

ENVIRONMENT	PLANT OR ANIMAL ORGANISM	(DDT-R RESIDUE IN ORGANISM DIVIDED BY RESIDUE IN ENVIRONMENT)	
		Maximum Value Observed	*Minimum Value Observed*
Soil	Earthworm	73	0.67
	Beetles	2.81	0.31
	Slugs	3.70	2.33
	Crop roots	0.13	0.04
	Crop foliage	0.08	—
Water	Sea squirt	1,000,000 †	200 †
	Sea hare	178,000 †	—
	Eastern oyster, clam	70,000 †	60
	Shrimp	2,800 †	280
	Crabs	144	—
	Crayfish	97	17
	Snails	1,480 †	—
	Plankton	16,666 †	250
	Fish	829,300 †	5–(1,450) †
	Fish (DDD)	9,214 †	417
	Algae	33	0.34
	Aquatic plants	100,000 †	0.45
Diet	Pheasant	2.91	—
	Woodcock	4.5	2.6
	Bald eagle		
	Brain	0.1	—
	Liver	1.9	—
	Fat	35.7	—

* Modified from Edwards, C. A.: *Persistent Pesticides in the Environment.* CRC Press, Cleveland, 1970.
† DDT may be present in excess of solubility in water.

quat, which are used in "no-till" methods of farming. These compounds readily dissolve and dissociate in aqueous solution. As cations, they are strongly adsorbed to soil particles by cation exchange reactions (Weber, 1972):

$$\text{Paraquat}^{2+} + 2\text{Na-clay} \rightleftharpoons \text{paraquat-clay} + 2\text{Na}^+$$

X-ray studies show that these planar molecules interlayer between the parallel silicate sheets of various clays. The adsorption behavior is also related to surface charge densities on various clays. Adsorption isotherms for these cationic compounds indicate a high affinity of the solute for the adsorbent until the cation exchange capacity is reached.

Paraquat and diquat as soil-bound residues are resistant to microbial degradation and photodecomposition. Tightly adsorbed residues are not biologically available and therefore persist indefinitely. Both diquat and paraquat are nonvolatile and are not transported in the vapor phase. Environmental transport is thus tied to sediment transport processes.

Moderately Persistent Pesticides

Triazine Herbicides. The triazines behave as weak bases in aqueous solution with pK_a values

that range from 1.1 to 4.3. Water solubilities are therefore determined by the pH level, with the triazines being more soluble at low pH levels. The behavior and fate of triazines in soils has been extensively studied and reviewed (Gunther, 1970). Adsorption of triazines through an exchange process to organic matter and clay minerals is dependent on the pH of the solution and the acidity of the adsorbent surface. Hydrogen bonding and hydrophobic bonding are other mechanisms by which soil organic matter adsorbs triazine herbicides, especially at higher pH levels.

Hydrolysis and oxidation are the general routes of soil metabolism for triazine herbicides. Photodecomposition appears to be minimal on soils. Vapor transport losses of triazines are dependent on vapor pressure and pH of the evaporating surface, since ionized compounds are less volatile. Transport from soil to water occurs in solution and in sediments.

Phenylurea Herbicides. Between 20 and 25 different substituted phenylurea compounds are presently commercially available as herbicides for the control of annual and perennial grasses in alfalfa, cotton, sugar cane, pineapple, grapes, apples, and citrus. The phenylureas can be divided into three categories based on their water

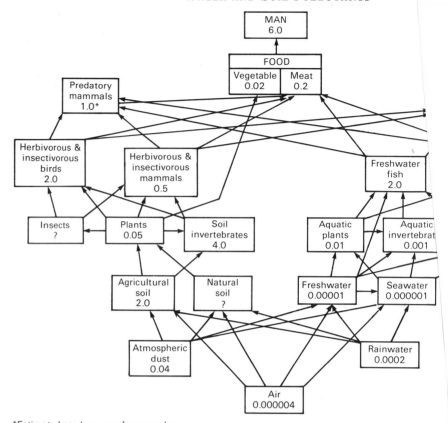

*Estimate based on very few samples
? Insufficient data available

Figure 25–5. Typical levels of DDT (ppm) in environmental compartments, media, and aquatic organisms, and man and the relationships between them. (Reprinted with p from Edwards, C. A.: *Persistent Pesticides in the Environment.* Copyright 1970 The Rubber Co., CRC Press, Inc.)

solubilities, which in turn seem to be related to a number of other properties that each group holds in common (Weber, 1972). Fenuron, the most water soluble of the phenylureas at approximately 2,900 to 3,850 ppm, is in a category by itself. This compound is also the most mobile in soil systems of all the phenylureas. Fenuron has been shown to move substantially in a lateral direction over the soil surface and in a vertical direction into the subsoil. Its movement is also related to soil texture and organic matter content. Movement was greater in coarse-textured soils and was decreased at higher organic contents.

The middle group of phenylureas in terms of water solubility includes monuron, diuron, linuron, monolinuron, fluometuron, metobromuron, norea, and siduron, in which water solubilities range from 18 to 580 ppm. Compounds in this category are moderately mobile in the soil; their relative movement decreases as the water solubilities decrease. Movement of the com-

pounds also decreases as organic of the soil increases, and in turn activity of the phenylureas decrease pounds are bound to the soil organi

The least soluble of the phe neburon and chloroxuron, where bilities range from 2.0 to 4.8 ppm. pounds are rather immobile in the s

Most of the phenylurea compoun tively low vapor pressures and a volatile from the soil. Soil pH does n significantly affect adsorption, m herbicidal activity of the phenylurea persistence of these compounds is with residues remaining following app several months at the longest.

The phenylurea herbicides are readi lized by most biologic systems. D reactions involve *N*-dealkylation an koxylation, ring hydroxylation, oxidati substituents, and a small amount c relatively nonpersistent in the environment. They are typically applied to crops, sometimes directly to the soil as systemic insecticides, for the control of phytophagous pests. These chemicals generally persist from only a few hours through several weeks to months. Only in rare instances are organophosphorus or carbamate residues found in crops beyond the growing season during which they were applied. These chemicals are rapidly replacing the chlorinated hydrocarbon insecticides as the principal weapons in the arsenal of American agriculture against the invasion of the pests that compete with man for food and fiber. More than half (57 percent in 1971) of the total volume of insecticides applied in the United States is made up of members of this group of chemicals. These compounds have been the subject of two recent monographs (Eto, 1974; Kuhr and Dorough, 1976).

The organophosphates and carbamates used as insecticides are neutral esters of phosphoric and carbamic acids. A large number of these compounds representing a variety of chemical, physical, and biologic properties are presently in commercial use, allowing their specific application to be tailored to particular needs. They act as anticholinesterase agents by phosphorylating or carbamylating acetylcholinesterase, freeing in the process a leaving group that is generally easily further degraded. This reaction may take place as well in the environment by chemical or photochemical mechanisms. Thus, these compounds do not represent a serious problem as contaminants of soil and water. Their breakdown products are generally nontoxic, being composed of low-molecular-weight, volatile molecules that are easily degraded and utilized by organisms.

The specific rate of chemical and biochemical transformation of the organophosphorus and carbamate insecticides depends on the specific properties of the individual compounds. Some of these compounds are relatively soluble in water. Being esters, they are also susceptible to hydrolysis. The half-lives of a number of common organophosphorus insecticides at various temperatures and pH values are given in Table 25-3. Most organophosphorus and carbamate compounds are stable at acid pH values. However, under alkaline conditions hydrolysis is rapid, the breakdown rate increasing approximately tenfold for each pH unit above 7. An increase of $10°$ of temperature will increase the hydrolysis rate approximately fourfold (Mühlmann and Schrader, 1957).

Organophosphorus and carbamate insecticides may contaminate soils by either direct application or through runoff from applications to crops. When these compounds are present in the soil, their disappearance is influenced by their interaction with the physical characteristics of the soil, the water content of the soil, and the microflora present. They may be tightly bound in certain types of soils, even to the point where they are unavailable for biologic decomposition. Under such conditions very little movement takes place even though water may be running through the soil or over its surface. The combination of interaction with soil components and rapid

Table 25-3. EFFECT OF TEMPERATURE AND pH ON THE HYDROLYSIS IN WATER OF SOME ORGANOPHOSPHORUS INSECTICIDES*

TEMP. (°C)†	HALF-LIFE						
	Parathion	Paraoxon	Methyl Parathion	Disulfoton	Trichlorofon	Dichlorvos	Azinphos-methyl
Days							
10	3,000	1,200	760	4,830	2,400	240	1,070
20	690	320	175	1,110	526	61.5	240
30	180	93	45	290	140	17.3	61.5
40	50	29	12.5	78	41	5.8	18
50	15	9.6	4.0	24	10.7	1.66	5.46
60	4.75	3.2	1.34	7.8	3.2	0.58	1.9
70	1.65	1.2	0.47	2.7	1.13	0.164	0.61
Hours							
70							
pH 1	34	18.5	15.4	62	32	2.3	24
3	21	23	11.2	62	33	3.4	9
5	19.5	24.4	10.7	60	15.3	2.8	8.9
7	7.8	11.5	6.9	27.6	0.7	0.45	4.8
9	2.7	2.1	1.5		0.1		

* Data from Mühlmann, R., and Schrader, G.: Hydrolyse der insektiziden Phosphorsäureester. *Z. Naturforsch.*, **12b**:196–208, 1957.
† At pH 1 to 5.

chemical and biochemical degradation in the soil results in minimal contamination of water supplies and soil to which compounds have not been applied.

The detection of organophosphorus and carbamate insecticides in soil can be difficult. Their interaction with soil components renders them unavailable to exert their toxic action on organisms and makes them difficult to remove by conventional solvent extraction techniques. Hence, methods that depend on removal of residues from soil particles often underestimate the presence of these compounds. The analysis of organophosphorus and carbamate residues in water, on the other hand, is relatively uncomplicated and easily done. Extraction of large quantities of water with organic solvents and subsequent analysis provides a very sensitive assay for small quantities of organophosphorus and carbamate insecticides in water, although other water pollutants may complicate the analyses when they are coextracted with the insecticide.

When organophosphates or carbamates reach the soil, their subsequent disposition is influenced by interaction with the mineral components of the soil, soil organic matter, soil pH, and soil moisture. In addition, the flora and fauna present in the soil are responsible for the degradation of these insecticides into innocuous breakdown products. A number of workers have found that after treatment of soil in laboratory or controlled field studies, extraction of the material from the soil was increasingly difficult as time progressed. For example, in a comparative study with ^{14}C-dimethoate applied to three different soil types at two different times of the year, recovery of dimethoate-^{14}C-equivalents from the soil with organic solvent extraction decreased from nearly 100 percent immediately after application to between 60 and 80 percent by 37 days after application, depending on the soil type and moisture content (Duff and Menzer, 1973). In greenhouse experiments where Mocap was applied to the soil in pots, very little of the applied ^{14}C-Mocap was taken up by bean or corn plants, and again the extractability of the compound from soil was increasingly difficult with the passage of time. In these experiments, Mocap was labeled either at the ^{14}C-propyl position or the ^{14}C-ethyl position, and it was noted that more radioactivity was recovered from the ethyl-labeled compound than the propyl-labeled compound (Menzer et al., 1971).

The persistence of these compounds is, at least in part, a function of interactions with the mineral components of soil. Metallic ions in soils interact with organophosphorus insecticides. Malathion, for example, is quickly incor-

porated into the montmorillonite clay interlayer region where it is adsorbed as a double layer. The mechanism was shown to be hydrogen binding between carbonyl oxygen atoms and the hydration water shells of cations. In this case adsorption was so strong that no degradation of the malathion was observed. In these studies sodium, calcium, copper, iron, and aluminum montmorillonite were used (Bowman et al., 1970). Similarly, Saltzman and Yaron (1972) have shown a strong affinity of parathion for sodium montmorillonite. On the other hand, diazinon and chloropyrifos were decomposed rapidly upon contact with copper (II)-montmorillonite (Mortland and Raman, 1967). Calcium and magnesium montmorillonites were relatively ineffective in degrading these compounds.

Binding of organophosphorus and carbamate insecticides correlates well with the organic matter content of soils (Edwards, 1966). It has been shown, for example, that the amount of mevinphos bound by soils increased with increasing organic matter content. Furthermore, the absorption of phorate from the soil by plants appeared to be in competition with the binding of the compound with the organic matter content of the soil.

In a kinetic study of the adsorption of carbaryl to soil organic matter surfaces, Leenheer and Ahlrichs (1971) found that carbaryl was more readily adsorbed to acid soils than to neutral or alkaline soils. This may be due to decreased displacement of the carbamate from the active sites by water at lower pH values.

Soil moisture has a major influence on the availability and extractability of residues of organophosphorus and carbamate insecticides, apparently because of competition between the insecticides and water for the adsorption sites on the soil particles. Harris (1964) has shown, for example, that diazinon, parathion, trichlorfon, and mevinphos are 135-fold, 28-fold, 20-fold, and 1.4-fold, respectively, more active in moist soils than in dry soils. Analytic procedures for the recovery of residues from soils generally recommend the addition of water for the desorption of the residues from soil particles before extraction with an organic solvent. However, even though there is a major interaction between these insecticides and water, they do not appear to move freely in soils with water, and loss by leaching does not appear to be a major factor in the disappearance of these compounds from soils. In studies designed to test the behavior of phorate in soils, Getzin and Chapman (1960) applied the radiolabeled compound on the surface of various soil types and applied 10 to 30 mm of water every two days for a total of 250 mm over 24 days. More than 80 percent of the radiolabeled phorate-equivalents remained near the surface with silt loam and muck soils, although only 50 percent remained in sandy soil and 76 percent in quartz sand.

The fact that microorganisms exert a major influence on the behavior of pesticide residues in soil has been demonstrated by observing the effect of soil sterilization on the breakdown of a number of compounds. Getzin (1968) showed that zinophos degraded faster in nonautoclaved soil, although the decomposition of diazinon was unaffected by autoclaving. Getzin and Rosefield (1968) showed that malathion, Ciodrin, dichlorvos, mevinphos, parathion, methyl parathion, Supracide, dimethoate, and chloropyrifos were all degraded faster in nonsterile soils. Lichtenstein et al. (1968) showed that both sodium azide treatment and autoclaving reduced soil bacteria and resulted in an increased persistence of parathion. It was also shown in these studies that sodium azide affected diazinon residues in the soil directly, but the studies were unable to assess the effect of soil sterilization on this compound. Bro-Rasmussen et al. (1968) reported that sterilization extensively affected diazinon degradation in loam and sandy loam soils. The effect of sterilization of soil on pesticide degradation may appear to be somewhat ambiguous because of changes other than the destruction of soil microorganisms that would have an effect on the degradation of compounds applied. Autoclaving, for example, is known to change the physicochemical properties of soil and to destroy heat-sensitive soil components other than microorganisms that participate in the degradation of organophosphorus insecticides. As in the case of diazinon, chemical sterilization may result in direct reactions between the insecticide and the soil sterilant. In general, however, there is at least strong evidence that microorganisms exert a major influence on the degradation of pesticides in soils.

Harris has proposed a classification scheme in which all pesticides are ordered into three groups. Group I is defined as "highly residual" compounds; group II, "moderately residual"; and group III, "slightly residual" (Harris, 1969). Various studies by many workers allow the classification of the organophosphorus and carbamate insecticides in groups II and III. In group II are dazanit, carbofuran, dimethoate, methomyl, Mocap, and Mobam, and in group III, parathion, diazinon, phorate, chloropyrifos, bromophos, and disulfoton (Harris, 1969; Harris and Hitchon, 1970). Group II compounds persist between 4 and 16 weeks, and group III compounds persist between two and four weeks in soils.

There is little information on the effects of organophosphates and carbamates on organisms living in water and soil. In general, only minute amounts of residues of the insecticides and their toxic degradation products are found in natural water systems. Thus, their biologic effect seems to be minimal. In soil, however, there is greater likelihood of the presence and buildup of toxic residues. Several studies have shown that some compounds can cause reduction in bacterial populations. Garretson and San Clemente (1968) showed that parathion inhibited nitrifying chemolithotrophic bacteria, although malathion did not. Sommer (1971) showed that organophosphates had little effect, while carbamates markedly inhibited nitrification. In studies to assess the effect of diazinon on soil microorganisms Gunner and coworkers (Gunner et al., 1966; Gunner, 1970) have shown that the compound exerts a selective effect on both soil and rhizosphere microflora expressed as selective enrichment of coccidioidal rods. Although the numbers of fungi were unaffected, a large number of the genus *Streptomyces* appeared as a climax population. In another instance the microflora that arose in response to diazinon belonged primarily to one species of *Arthrobacter*. Similar results were obtained by Stojanovic et al. (1972) with carbaryl as the test insecticide. The various studies show that these insecticides may cause a variety of effects on the soil flora and fauna not always expressed as directly toxic effects.

NONPESTICIDAL ORGANIC CHEMICALS

Data gathered by the United States Environmental Protection Agency through November, 1975, indicate that 253 different organic chemicals have been detected in drinking water in the United States. There is every reason to believe that an additional number, yet unidentified, may also be present, and the total number of chemicals could be considerably larger. The list of chemicals includes both aliphatic and aromatic hydrocarbons, pesticides, industrial chemicals, plasticizers, and solvents. Many of these materials are halogenated and some are produced by chlorination of the water during the purification process. Others appear through industrial and municipal discharges, urban and rural runoff, natural sources, and sewage purification practices.

The principal objective of the nationwide survey of organic chemicals in drinking water made by the Environmental Protection Agency was to determine the extent and significance of the occurrence of suspected carcinogens in water (Environmental Protection Agency, 1975). These data were considered in a report of the potential health effects of chemicals in drinking

Table 25–4. ORGANICS DETECTED IN WATER IN THE EPA NATIONAL ORGANICS RECONNAISANCE SURVEY*

| | RAW WATER ANALYSIS | | FINISHED WATER ANALYSIS | | |
| | | | | Concentration | |
COMPOUND	No. of Locations Where Detected	Concentration Range (μg/1)	No. of Locations Where Detected	Range (μg/1)	Median
Chloroform	49	<0.1–0.9	80	<0.1–311	21
Bromodichloromethane	7	<0.2–0.8	78	0.3–116	6
Dibromochloromethane	1	3	72	<0.4–110	1.2
Bromoform	0	—	26	<0.8–92	5
Carbon tetrachloride	4	<2–4	10	<2–3	—
1,2-Dichloroethane	11	<0.2–3	26	<0.2–6	—

* Data derived from *Preliminary Assessment of Suspected Carcinogens in Drinking Water, Report to Congress*. U.S. Environmental Protection Agency, Washington, D.C., 1975.

water that was produced by the National Academy of Sciences (National Research Council, 1977) under mandate of the Safe Drinking Water Act of 1974.

Low-Molecular-Weight Halogenated Hydrocarbons

Of particular concern is the possibility of the production of low-molecular-weight chlorinated hydrocarbons through the use of chlorination for water purification. This concern focuses principally on the four trihalomethanes, chloroform, bromodichloromethane, dibromochloromethane, and bromoform; and carbon tetrachloride and 1,2-dichloroethane. A two-part study was conducted by the Environmental Protection Agency to ascertain the presence of these chemicals in water, and whether they were produced by chlorination. A National Organics Reconnaissance Survey was initiated in November, 1974, for this purpose. The results are summarized in Table 25–4. It was noted that all of these materials were found in drinking water and most were found in the raw water before chlorination. The second part of the study, an intensive study of the situation in midwestern United States, led to several conclusions:

1. Raw water with low turbidity resulted in finished water that was relatively free of chloroform and related halogenated compounds.
2. Chloroform, bromodichloromethane, dibromochloromethane, and bromoform do result from chlorination of precursors in the raw water. On the other hand, carbon tetrachloride, methylene chloride, and 1,2-dichloroethane do not appear to be produced chemically during the treatment process.
3. There appears to be a correlation between chloroform, dibromochloromethane, bromodichloromethane, and bromoform concentrations. The ratio between the four chemicals appears to

be relatively constant in all water examined, indicating the probability of a common precursor or group of precursors for these halogenated hydrocarbons.
4. The use of granular activated carbon treatment was not effective in removing volatile organic compounds during the water treatment process.

The four halogenated hydrocarbons produced by chlorination seem to result from naturally occurring humic substances as precursors (Bellar et al., 1974; Bunn et al., 1975; Rook, 1974). The maximum concentrations of these materials found were chloroform, 54 μg/l; bromodichloromethane, 20 μg/l; dibromochloromethane, 13 μg/l; and bromoform, 10 μg/l.

Studies were conducted to compare the rate and extent of chloroform formation when chlorine was added to raw river water, filtered water, and activated-carbon-treated water (Environmental Protection Agency, 1975). These experiments were carried out at constant pH and 25° C. When sufficient chlorine was added to satisfy the chlorine demand, chlorination of raw river water yielded approximately seven times as much chloroform as did chlorination of the filtered water and approximately 80 times as much as chlorination of activated-carbon-treated water. Similar results were obtained when the same experiments were conducted with realistic concentrations of humic acid. Concentrations of humic materials are probably reduced during coagulation, settling, and filtration, thereby reducing the rate and extent of chloroform formation by chlorination. Thus, it may be possible to reduce the quantity of chlorinated hydrocarbons formed during chlorination by altering the water purification process so that chlorination is performed following the removal of humic materials through filtration and coagulation steps.

As yet, there is no generally accepted substitute for the use of chlorine as a disinfectant in water purification. However, the confirmation that chlorination produces a number of halogenated hydrocarbons has stimulated an extensive investigation of other chemicals that could be used for this purpose, such as chloramines, chlorine dioxide, ozone, bromine, and iodine.

The seriousness of the concern about low-molecular-weight halogenated hydrocarbons in drinking water is illustrated by the situation that developed in mid-1970s with respect to the water supply of the city of New Orleans, Louisiana. In 1975 Dowty *et al.* (1975) reported that the tap water in New Orleans contained more chlorinated hydrocarbons than untreated Mississippi River water. In addition, these workers reported the presence of chlorinated hydrocarbons, including carbon tetrachloride, in blood plasma collected from human volunteers in New Orleans. Following that report Page *et al.* (1976) reported a statistical correlation between the incidence of cancer among the New Orleans population and the source of the water supply. They noted that the cancer mortality rate was 15 percent higher among white males who drank water from the Mississippi River than among those who obtained their water from wells. They compared the percentage of the individual parish populations drinking water from the Mississippi River or its distributaries with total cancer incidence, cancer of the urinary organs, and cancer of the gastrointestinal organs, for four subgroups of the population—white males, nonwhite males, white females, and nonwhite females. The regression coefficients on mortality rates were significantly higher for all groups of the population with respect to cancer of the gastrointestinal organs, with all groups except white females for total cancer, and for white males and nonwhite females for cancer of the urinary organs. The analysis also included consideration of the effects that degree of urbanization, income, and certain occupational exposures could have had on cancer mortality; no relationship could be established for these variables. Other variables such as smoking, diet, alcohol consumption, and air pollution were not considered because the necessary data were unavailable.

While statistical studies cannot by themselves establish causality, the authors concluded that they support the hypothesis that there is a link between chlorinated hydrocarbons in drinking water in New Orleans and cancer mortality. These data coincided with the consideration in the United States Congress of the Safe Drinking Water Act of 1974 and provided a dramatic backdrop to the passage of this legislation.

Aromatic Halogenated Hydrocarbons

In recent years a number of halogenated aromatic compounds have engendered increasing concern about their effects as environmental pollutants. The polychlorinated biphenyls (PCB) have appeared as ubiquitous contaminants of soil and water. Chlorophenols used for a variety of purposes have been detected in surface waters and drinking water. The extremely toxic 2,3,7,8-tetrachlorodibenzo-*p*-dioxin (TCDD) has contaminated large areas of both water and soil through industrial accidents and through widescale application of herbicides containing small quantities of the chemical as a contaminant.

Polychlorinated Biphenyls. PCBs are very stable materials of low flammability, which contain from 12 to 68 percent chlorine. They are exceptionally persistent in the environment, even more persistent than the chlorinated hydrocarbon insecticides, with which they often have been confused in analytic studies of environmental samples. They have been used as insulating materials in electrical capacitors and transformers, plasticizers in waxes, in paper manufacturing, and for a variety of other industrial purposes. The diversity of their use patterns, the large quantities used, and their stability have led to widespread occurrence of these compounds in soil and water. Fish from the upper Hudson River and Lake Ontario have been found to contain PCB concentrations from 5 to 20 ppm. Fish from a number of other rivers throughout the United States have also been found to contain comparable quantities of PCBs. Waterfowl have also accumulated high concentrations of PCBs. These examples of PCB pollution have occurred in spite of efforts to restrict and eventually eliminate the release of such compounds into the environment.

The health effects of PCBs are well established. Investigations have shown that PCBs interfere with reproduction in phytoplankters (Mosser *et al.*, 1972). Other observed effects in mammals and birds include microsomal enzyme induction, porphyrogenic action, estrogenic activity, and immunosuppression (Bitman, 1972; Vos, 1972). Other adverse effects are possible since the PCBs are lipophilic, a property, along with their stability, that leads to bioaccumulation and the possibility of long-term effects that have not been completely identified.

Chlorophenols. Pentachlorophenol has been used in significant quantities since 1936 as a wood preservative. As a result of this use surface water and treated drinking water have been found to contain as much as 0.70 and 0.06 ppb, respectively, of pentachlorophenol (Buhler *et al.*, 1973). Hexachlorophene (2,2'-methylene-*bis*-[3,4,6-trichlorophenol]) has been widely used as an antibacterial agent in a number of consumer products, including soaps and deodorants. It has been detected in surface waters as high as 48 ppb and in drinking water at 0.01 ppb (Buhler *et al.*, 1973). Hexachlorophene is resistant to metabolic attack and tends to persist in the environment and bioaccumulates in food chains (Sims and Pfaender, 1975).

Pentachlorophenol has a fairly high acute toxicity and has been shown to cause reproductive failures in rats. However, the full extent of its health effects has not been completely evaluated (National Research Council, 1977). The acute toxicity of hexachlorophene is also quite high. The compound has exhibited neurotoxicity in dogs, sheep, and rats. The presence of these chemicals in water needs to be closely monitored because of their high toxicity and the possibility of adverse health effects in man.

2,3,7,8-Tetrachlorodibenzo-*p*-dioxin. What was probably the most dramatic and catastrophic occurrence of environmental pollution by a toxic chemical occurred in Seveso, Italy, July 10, 1976. On that date a safety disk in a reaction vessel being used to manufacture 2,4,5-trichlorophenol, an intermediate in the production of hexachlorophene and 2,4,5-trichlorophenoxyacetic acid (2,4,5-T), ruptured, releasing a chemical cloud over the region. The cloud contained predominantly 2,4,5-trichlorophenol. However, an estimated 3 to 16 kg of 2,3,7,8-tetrachlorodibenzo-*p*-dioxin (TCDD), a potent teratogen, was also released. The area was thus contaminated with the greatest concentration of TCDD ever found in the environment, up to 51.3 ppm in some samples.

When the safety disk of the reaction vessel ruptured, the chemicals blew up into a plume 30 to 50 m high above the factory, then cooled and came down over a cone-shaped area about 2 km long and 700 m wide, all over a matter of minutes. The result was that some people become ill immediately, while others began to show symptoms ranging from skin burns to stomach pains and internal bleeding a few days later. Animals and vegetation within the area began to die. Shortly after the incident the entire area was evacuated and cordoned off. It was expected that a 123-acre area, which became a wasteland of shriveled and dying plants and evacuated homes, would have to remain entirely closed for ten years or longer before the levels of TCDD would degrade sufficiently for the area to be safe for habitation (Rawls and O'Sullivan, 1976).

TCDD is extremely toxic, as indicated by its acute oral LD50, reported to be between 0.6 and 115 μg/kg for several animal species (National Research Council, 1977). The compound causes degenerative changes in liver and thymus, porphyria, altered serum enzyme concentrations, and loss in body weight. Thymic atrophy is a very sensitive index of TCDD exposure. TCDD is also a potent fetotoxic agent in various animal species.

The significance of TCDD as an environmental pollutant lies primarily in the fact that it is a trace by-product in the synthesis of 2,4,5-T, an important herbicide that has been widely used in agricultural and other weed control programs. It was extensively used as a defoliant in Vietnam by the United States Army. Fortunately, water transport of TCDD is limited since its solubility in water is only 0.2 ppb. Its only accumulation, therefore, will likely be in soils to which heavy applications of 2,4,5-T have been made. TCDD is firmly bound to soil where it tends to persist for more than one year (Crosby *et al.*, 1971, 1973). Degradation of the chemical in the soil will be largely by photochemical mechanisms.

Phthalate Ester Plasticizers

The phthalate ester plasticizers are used in virtually every major product category, including construction, automotive, household products, apparel, toys, packaging, and medical products, resulting in the widest possible distribution of these materials. The industry today comprises 13 major suppliers who produced in 1972 approximately 1 billion pounds of 20 different compounds (Graham, 1973). The two most abundantly produced phthalate ester plasticizers are di-2-ethylhexylphthalate (DEHP) and di-*n*-butylphthalate (DBP).

The phthalate esters are now known to be ubiquitously distributed in the environment. They have been found complexed with the fulvic acid components of humic substances in soil (Ogner and Schnitzer, 1970) and in both marine and estuarine waters. Fulvic acid apparently functions as a solubilizer for the rather insoluble phthalate esters and thus serves to mediate the mobilization, transport, and immobilization of these materials in soil and water. Hites (1973) reports the presence of phthalate esters in the Charles and Merrimack Rivers in Massachusetts. In the Charles River it was shown that the phthalate concentration increased as one moved upstream to about river mile 7 where apparently the phthalate esters were added to the river. The concentration decreased as the contaminated water flowed downstream, diluting the phthalates present. Concentration at river mile 7 of phthalate esters was approximately 1.9 ppb, while at the mouth of the river concentrations had decreased to 0.97 ppb. In another study (Giam *et al.*, 1978) phthalate ester plasticizers were detected in the open ocean environment of the Gulf of Mexico and the North Atlantic. DEHP and DBP were found in almost all samples analyzed, including a deep sea jellyfish, *Atolla*, from 1,000-M depths in the North Atlantic (Morris, 1970). Concentrations of DEHP in surface water ranged from 4.9 to 130 ng/l. DBP ranged from a nondetectable level to 95 ng/l. Lower levels of both compounds were found in sediment. It has become clear that the phthalate ester plasticizers are general contaminants of virtually all soil and water ecosystems; it has become very difficult to analyze any soil or water sample without detecting the presence of phthalate esters.

Because of the widespread occurrence of these compounds, their toxicity is of concern. In general, the phthalate esters have a low order of acute toxicity. For example, the intraperitoneal LD50 dose in mice ranges from 1.5 to 14.2 g/kg (Rubin and Jaeger, 1973). Furthermore, 90-day and two-year feeding studies of DEHP in rats and one-year feeding studies in guinea pigs and dogs indicated a low order of chronic toxicity. On the basis of these results the Food and Drug Administration approved DEHP for use in plastic wrapping of food. Although these studies indicated a low order of toxicity, they emphasized evaluation of gross overt effects, not taking into account subtle toxicologic effects. Rubin and Jaeger (1973) investigated a number of more subtle effects of DEHP on a variety of biologic systems. They found of particular note a sensitivity of cultured beating chick embryo heart cells to DEHP. As little as 4 μg/ml in the culture medium was lethal to 97 to 98 percent of the cells. This concentration could be reached in human blood stored in vinyl plastic bags for a period of one to two days. These results indicated the need for caution in assuming the safety of low concentrations of phthalate esters. Other studies on the toxicity of phthalates have been summarized in Chapter 20 and by Krauskopf (1973), Gesler (1973), Dillingham and Autian (1973), and Peters and Cook (1973).

Data reported by Mayer and Sanders (1973) indicate that DEHP and DBP may also be detrimental to the reproduction of some aquatic organisms at low concentrations. *Daphnia magna* reproduction was decreased by approximately 80 percent by continuous exposure of 30 μg/l DEHP for up to 21 days. Reproduction in zebra fish and guppies was also decreased by low concentrations of DEHP.

Although the concentrations of phthalate esters in soil and water are quite low and the toxicity of the compounds is also quite low, some concern is evident because of the ubiquitous nature of environmental contamination by these compounds. They have been shown to occur in drinking water in the United States (Environmental Protection Agency, 1975), are undoubtedly present in food, and may reach man through other mechanisms as well.

METALS

The toxicology of metals, including their use, occurrence, and effects, has already been presented in Chapter 17. In this section we will deal only with some aspects of the natural cycles of elements and conditions that alter the process involved. It is necessary to limit this treatment to the best-studied examples of environmentally important elements: mercury, cadmium, lead, arsenic, and selenium. (Note: arsenic and selenium are not metals, but the term will be used to include these metalloids.)

Mercury. Methyl mercury pollution of Minimata Bay and the subsequent human poisoning from consumption of contaminated seafood has stimulated much research on the origin and fate of methyl mercury. An important theme throughout the discussion of metals is the question of chemical species. Mercury, for example, exists in the inorganic form as free mercury, $Hg°$, mercury ion in salts and complexes, Hg^{2+}; or as organic mercury compounds, such as phenylmercuric salts, which have been used as fungicides and herbicides, and the alkyl-mercury compounds including methyl mercury. In natural systems, a dynamic equilibrium that is determined by the physiochemical and biologic conditions of the soil-water system exists between the various chemical species. Some organic forms of mercury are man-made, such as the phenylmercuric compounds, while methyl mercury is produced by man, sediment microorganisms, nonbiologically in sediments, and possibly by some fish. As expected, each species of mercury has its own set of physical, chemical, and toxicologic properties.

Mercury is transported to aquatic ecosystems via surface runoff and through the atmosphere. It is complexed or tightly bound to both organic and inorganic particles. Sediments with high sulfur content will strongly bind mercury. Organic acids such as fulvic and humic acid are usually associated with the mercury that is not bound to particles.

Methylation of mercury by microorganisms is a detoxication response that allows the organism to dispose of heavy metal ions as small organometallic complexes. Conditions for methylation by sediment microorganisms are strict and occur only within a narrow pH range. The rate of synthesis of methyl mercury also depends on the redox potential, composition of the microbial population, availability of Hg^{2+}, and temperature. Vitamin B_{12} derivatives are believed to be the methylating agents, since mechanistically they are the only methyl carbanion and methyl radical donating coenzymes known (Ridley *et al.*, 1977). An understanding of the biomethylation reaction mechanisms together with oxidation-reduction chemistry of elements allows predictions of the environmental conditions necessary for the biomethylation of mercury and several other metals. However, the best conversion rate for inorganic mercury to methyl mercury under ideal conditions is less than 1.5 percent per month (Jensen and Jernelov, 1969).

Little or no methyl mercury is found in sediments. Conversion of inorganic mercury to methyl mercury results in its desorption from sediment particles at a relatively fast rate. Demethylation by sediment microorganisms also occurs at a rapid rate when compared to methylation. Methyl mercury released in surface waters can undergo photodecomposition to inorganic mercury. However, methyl mercury can also be bioaccumulated by plankton algae and fish. In fish, the rate of absorption of methyl mercury is faster than that for inorganic mercury, and the clearance rate is slower with a net result of high methyl mercury concentrations in the muscle tissue. Selenium, which is present in seawater and seafood, readily complexes with methyl mercury and is believed to have an important protective action against the toxic effects of methyl mercury. In summary, the danger of methyl mercury poisoning, as occurred in Minimata, arises from direct methyl mercury contamination rather than methylation of environmental sources of inorganic mercury.

Cadmium. Cadmium has long been recognized as a toxic element. Its importance as an environmental contaminant was demonstrated in the outbreak of *itai-itai* disease caused by smelter wastes that contaminate rice paddies (see Chap. 17). Cadmium deposits are found as sulfides with zinc, copper, and lead deposits, and cadmium is recovered as a by-product of smelting processes for those metals. A major environmental source of cadmium is vapor emissions that contaminate surrounding soil and water through fallout during smelting. Natural soil concentrations of cadmium are less than 1 ppm and average about 0.4 ppm. Sewage sludge is often contaminated with cadmium, which can then concentrate in plants grown on contaminated soils. The problem of heavy metal contamination, especially cadmium, has been one of the most serious concerns impeding the use and disposal of domestic sewage sludge on agricultural lands. Cadmium also enters agricultural soils as a contaminant of phosphate fertilizers. There is some evidence for the leaching of cadmium in soils.

Cadmium concentrations in fresh waters are usually less than 1 ppb while sea water ranges from 0.05 to 0.2 ppb and averages about 0.15 ppb (Fleischer *et al.*, 1974). Higher concentrations of cadmium in surface water are usually due to metallurgic plants, plating operations, cadmium pigments, batteries, plastics manufacture, or from sewage effluent. Mine drainage and mineralized areas also contribute significantly to cadmium fluxes in the Mississippi River in the Missouri-Tennessee-Kentucky area.

Drinking water in soft water areas can serve as a source of cadmium through corrosion of plumbing. However, this source is estimated to be small in relation to food intake. As in the association of selenium and mercury, there appears to be a protective effect with zinc and calcium against cadmium toxicity.

Lead. The use of lead, its mining, and its processing date back several centuries. Changing usage patterns rather than increased consumption determine present environmental inputs from man's use of lead. Batteries, gasoline additives, and paint pigments are major uses, but combustion of gasoline additives is the major source of environmental pollution by lead. Thus, lead is primarily an atmospheric pollutant that enters soil and water as fallout, a process determined by physical form and particle size. The net result is a buildup of lead near heavily traveled roads.

Lead enters aquatic systems from runoff or as fallout of insoluble precipitates and is found in sediments. Typical fresh water concentrations lie between 1 and 10 $\mu g/l$ while natural lead concentration in soil range from 2 to 200 ppm and average 10 to 15 ppm. Deep ocean waters, below 1,000 m, contain lead at 0.02- to 0.04-$\mu g/kg$ concentrations, but surface waters of the Mediterranean Sea and Pacific Ocean contain 0.20- and 0.35-$\mu g/kg$ levels (National Academy of Sciences, 1972). Drinking water concentrations of lead may be greatly increased in soft water areas through corrosion of lead-lined piping and connections. However, average drinking water intake is considerably less than food sources.

The biologic methylation of inorganic lead to tetramethyl lead by lake sediment microorganisms has been demonstrated (Wong *et al.*, 1975). However, the fate of this volatile, water-insoluble form of lead is unknown.

Arsenic. Arsenic is widely distributed in the environment. Man's input of arsenic into the global cycle occurs through smelting, coal burning, and the use of arsenical pesticides. Speciation of arsenic is an important consideration in the fate, movement, and action of this element. The chemical and biochemical transformations of arsenic include oxidation, reduction, and methylation, which affect the volatilization, adsorption, dissolution, and biologic disposition of the arsenic species involved.

Arsenic contamination of soils from point sources such as copper smelters or coal-burning power plants is easier to control than the dispersive use of arsenical pesticides, resulting in nonpoint source pollution. Various forms of

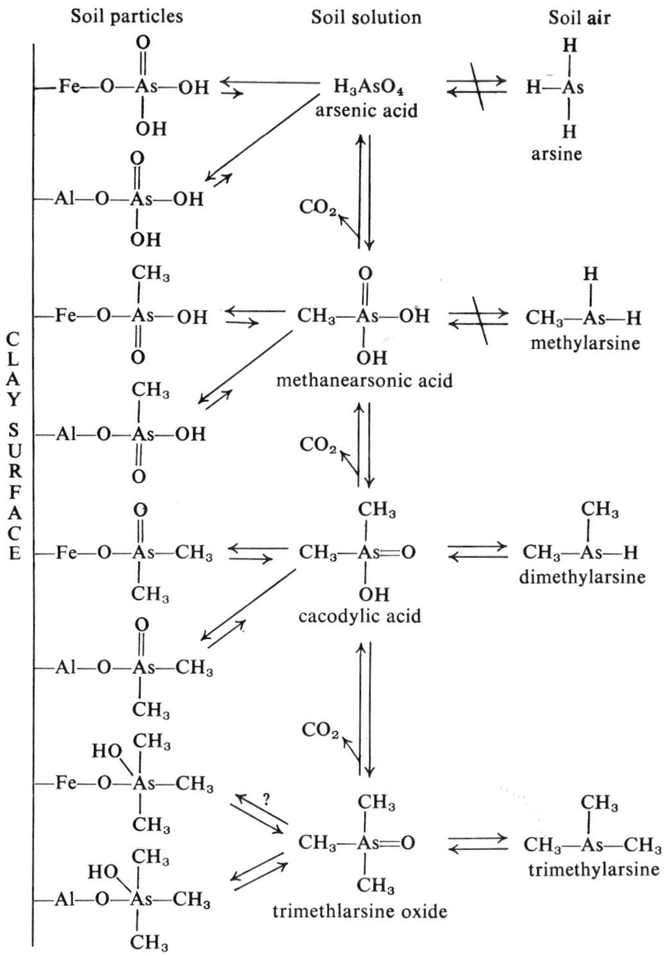

Soil particles Soil solution Soil air

CLAY SURFACE

$$-Fe-O-\underset{\underset{OH}{|}}{\overset{\overset{O}{||}}{As}}-OH \rightleftharpoons H_3AsO_4 \rightleftharpoons H-\underset{\underset{H}{|}}{\overset{\overset{H}{|}}{As}}$$

arsenic acid arsine

$$-Al-O-\underset{\underset{OH}{|}}{\overset{\overset{O}{||}}{As}}-OH$$

CO_2

$$-Fe-O-\underset{\underset{O}{||}}{\overset{\overset{CH_3}{|}}{As}}-OH \rightleftharpoons CH_3-\underset{\underset{OH}{|}}{\overset{\overset{O}{||}}{As}}-OH \rightleftharpoons CH_3-\underset{\underset{H}{|}}{\overset{\overset{H}{|}}{As}}$$

methanearsonic acid methylarsine

$$-Al-O-\underset{\underset{O}{|}}{\overset{\overset{CH_3}{|}}{As}}-OH$$

CO_2

$$-Fe-O-\underset{\underset{CH_3}{|}}{\overset{\overset{O}{||}}{As}}-CH_3 \rightleftharpoons CH_3-\underset{\underset{OH}{|}}{\overset{\overset{CH_3}{|}}{As}}=O \rightleftharpoons CH_3-\underset{\underset{H}{|}}{\overset{\overset{CH_3}{|}}{As}}-H$$

cacodylic acid dimethylarsine

$$-Al-O-\underset{\underset{CH_3}{|}}{\overset{\overset{O}{||}}{As}}-CH_3$$

CO_2

$$-Fe-O-\underset{\underset{CH_3}{|}}{\overset{\overset{HO \quad CH_3}{|}}{As}}-CH_3 \overset{?}{\rightleftharpoons} CH_3-\underset{\underset{CH_3}{|}}{\overset{\overset{CH_3}{|}}{As}}=O \rightleftharpoons CH_3-\underset{\underset{CH_3}{|}}{\overset{\overset{CH_3}{|}}{As}}-CH_3$$

trimethlarsine oxide trimethylarsine

$$-Al-O-\underset{\underset{CH_3}{|}}{\overset{\overset{HO \quad CH_3}{|}}{As}}-CH_3$$

Figure 25–6. Dissolution and reactions of arsenicals within the soil environment. (From Woolson, E. A.: Fate of arsenicals in different environmental substrates. *Environ. Health Perspect.*, 19:73–81, 1977.)

arsenic are used as pesticides. Arsenic acid (H_3AsO_4) is a leaf desiccant used in cotton production, lead and calcium arsenates are insecticides, and organic arsenicals, which include methanearsonic acid and its sodium salts as well as dimethylarsinic acid (cacodylic acid), are used as postemergence herbicides. The transport of arsenic in the environment is largely controlled by adsorption/desorption processes in soil and sediments. Therefore, sediment movement is responsible for transfer of arsenic soil residues to their ultimate sinks in deep ocean sediments. The clay fraction, plus ferrous and aluminum oxides that coat clay particles, adsorbs arsenicals as depicted in Figure 25–6. The reactions of arsenicals in soil include oxidation, reduction, methylation, and demethylation. Conversion of arsenic to volatile alkylarsines leads to air transport loss from soils. The transformation processes of arsenic and its transport processes are intimately linked.

Arsenic concentrations in water are generally much lower than in sediments. In Lake Michigan, the concentrations in water range from 0.5 to 2.3 $\mu g/l$ while sediment concentrations range from 7.2 to 28.8 mg/kg (Seydel, 1972). Inorganic arsenic exists in water in different oxidation states, depending on the pH and E_h of the water. Arsenate is apparently reduced by bacteria to arsenite in marine environments since the ratio of arsenate to total arsenic is much lower than is predicted thermodynamically. Methylation of arsenic occurs in both freshwater and marine systems and where arsenic is detected as arsenate, arsenite, methanearsonic acid, and dimethylarsinic acid (Braman and Foreback, 1973).

Bioaccumulation of arsenic species occurs readily in some aquatic organisms. Some seaweeds, fresh water algae, and crustaceans accumulate significant amounts of arsenic. Some arsenic in *Daphnia magna* and algae occurs as arseno analogs of phospholipids, indicating the mistaken accumulation and utilization of arsenate in place of phosphate. Crabs, lobsters, and other marine organisms accumulate organo-arsenicals along the food chain.

Selenium. Selenium concentrations in natural waters depend largely on the occurrence of seleniferous soils. Average concentrations for selenium in natural waters are less than 10 μg/l, but can reach several hundred micrograms per liter in certain areas of some Western states. Dietary sources of selenium are usually more important than drinking-water sources.

Environmental redistribution of selenium through man's activities is due to copper smelting; lead, zinc, phosphate, and uranium mining and processing; manufacturing of glass ceramics and pigments; and burning of fuels.

Selenium can be methylated as also demonstrated for mercury, arsenic, lead, and tin. Sediment microorganisms are responsible for the production of dimethyl selenide and dimethyl diselenide from both inorganic and organic selenium compounds (Chau, 1976). The importance of volatile methyl selenide compounds in the biogeochemical cycling of this element is still uncertain.

INORGANIC IONS

Nitrate, phosphate, and fluoride are inorganic ions that have caused considerable concern over their environmental effects. With nitrates and fluorides the concern is principally human health, but nitrates and particularly phosphates also cause eutrophication of lakes and ponds, a process that is considered environmentally undesirable. Midsummer algal blooms are familiar sights in some parts of the United States.

Nitrates. Man has altered the nitrogen cycle through his agricultural and technologic practices; changing patterns in agriculture, food processing, urbanization, and industrialization have had an impact on the accumulation of nitrate in the environment. Intensive agricultural production has consumed an increasing amount of nitrogen-based fertilizers, particularly with corn, vegetables, other row crops, and forages. Nitrogenous wastes from livestock and poultry production as well as urban sewage treatment have contributed nitrogenous wastes to the soil and water environments. Nitrate and nitrite are used extensively for color enhancement and preservation of processed meat products. These practices inevitably lead to increased exposure of man and animals to significant nitrate levels in food, feed, and water (National Academy of Sciences, 1972).

The nitrate form of nitrogen is of concern because of the high water solubility of this ion and consequent leaching, diffusion, and environmental mobility in soil and water. Nitrate can contaminate ground water to unacceptable levels.

The current recommended limit for nitrate nitrogen in drinking water is 10 mg/l (45 ppm nitrate). In the Community Water Supply survey of the Bureau of Water Hygiene in 1969, the range of nitrate concentrations found was 0 to 127 mg/l. Nineteen systems, about 3 percent of those examined for nitrate, had concentrations in excess of the recommended limit (National Research Council, 1977). Nitrite is formed from nitrate or ammonium ion by certain microorganisms in soil, water, sewage, and the alimentary tract. Thus, the concern with nitrate in the environment relates to its conversion by biologic systems to nitrite.

Methemoglobinemia is caused by high levels of nitrite or indirectly from nitrate in humans. It results in difficulties in the oxygen transport system of the blood. Poisoning of infants from nitrate in well water was first reported in the United States in 1944. Cases numbering in the thousands have now been reported, mostly in rural areas, mostly involving poisonings in infants.

Of more recent concern is the production of nitrosamines in food by the reaction of nitrite with secondary amines. Other nitroso compounds can result from the analogous reactions of nitrites with amides, ureas, carbamates, and other nitrogenous compounds. Various dialkyl and related nitrosamines have been shown to produce liver damage, hemorrhagic lung lesions, and convulsions and coma in rats (Heath and McGee, 1962). *N*-Nitroso compounds represent a major class of important chemical carcinogens and mutagens. The various forms of cancer for which the environmental *N*-nitroso compounds are suspected to play a causative role occur after long latency periods and at relatively low absolute frequency in the general population. These factors make it difficult to establish cause-and-effect relationships between specific carcinogens and disease incidence (Wogan and Tannenbaum, 1975).

Phosphates. Although the principal problem of phosphates in the environment is not directly related to human health, there is considerable concern about the effects of phosphorus from various sources on water quality. There remains considerable disagreement and controversy about the principal source of phosphate found in water ecosystems. Some maintain that phosphate fertilizers are a major contribution to the levels of phosphates found in water while others claim that phosphate detergents are the major contribution (Griffith, 1973).

Phosphorus applied to the soil as fertilizer moves primarily by erosion because phosphate adsorbs strongly on soil particles. However, some soluble phosphorus compounds do move in runoff water. The total phosphorus content of soils ranges from 0.01 to 0.13 percent (Stewart *et al.*, 1975). The phosphorus fertilizers applied as soluble orthophosphate soon revert to insoluble forms in soil. This conversion limits leaching and leads to a higher phosphorus concentration in sediments than in the original soil since phosphorus seems to be associated with finer particles. Control of phosphate pollution from agriculture will result from efforts to reduce erosion and sediment loss by modified agricultural practices.

The contribution of phosphorus to water from detergents is likely to be associated with the degree of urbanization. Efforts to control phosphates in water have concentrated on the detergent problem. Some states and local areas have restricted or banned the use of phosphate detergents completely. In some areas secondary treatment of sewage waste results in the precipitation and removal of phosphates from the effluent before discharge.

Phosphate is a major contributor to the eutrophication process in lakes and ponds (Thomas, 1973). The observer of a lake undergoing eutrophication notices first an extraordinarily rapid growth of algae in the surface water. Planktonic algae cause turbidity and flotation films. Shore algae cause ugly muddying, films, and damage to reeds. Decay of these algae causes oxygen depletion in the deep water and in shallow water near the shore. This rapid growth of algae gives rise to a number of undesirable effects on treatment of the water for consumption, on fisheries, and on the use of lakes for recreational purposes.

Fluorides. The beneficial effect of low levels of fluorides in preventing dental caries has led to the extensive use of fluoride in drinking water. The Safe Drinking Water Committee of the National Academy of Sciences has evaluated this practice as follows:*

Fluoride is found widely in water supplies, but the concentration is usually not great enough to be undesirable. The maximum concentration found for the 969 supplies studied in the 1969 Community Water Supply Survey was 4.4 mg/liter. Most supplies that were not intentionally fluoridated had fluoride concentrations less than 0.3 mg/liter.

A more extensive survey by the Dental Health Division of the U.S. Public Health Service showed more than 2,600 communities with a population of 8 million people had water supplies with more than 0.7 mg/liter of naturally occurring fluoride. Most of these communities are in Arizona, Colorado, Illinois, Iowa, New Mexico, Ohio, Oklahoma, South Dakota, and Texas. Of these, 524

communities representing 1 million people had supplies with fluoride concentrations greater than 2 mg/liter.

Small amounts of fluoride, on the order of 1 mg/liter, depending on the environmental temperature, in ingested water and beverages, are generally conceded to have a beneficial effect on the rate of occurrence of dental caries, particularly among children.

Two forms of chronic toxic effects are recognized generally as being caused by excess in intake of fluoride over long periods of time. These are mottling of teeth enamel or dental fluorosis, and skeletal fluorosis. In both cases, it is necessary to consider the severity since the very mild forms are considered beneficial by some. The most sensitive of these effects is the mottling of tooth enamel, which, depending on the temperature, may occur to an objectionable degree with fluoride concentrations in drinking water of only 0.8–1.6 mg/liter. (These observations were made a number of years ago and there have been no recent studies to determine if these levels still cause mottling.) Apparently there has been little systematic investigation of the degree to which consumers of drinking water with several mg/liter of fluoride regard the resultant mottling as an adverse health effect.

Skeletal fluorosis has been observed with use of water containing more than 3 mg/liter. It now appears that there is some probability that objectionable dental mottling and increased bone density may occur in those with long-standing renal disease or polydipsia who consume water containing more than 1 mg/liter of fluoride for long periods of time. Increased bone density, however, has often been regarded as a beneficial rather than an adverse effect. (This therefore makes the implications of such changes unclear.) Intake of fluoride for long periods in amounts greater than 20–40 mg/day may result in crippling skeletal fluorosis.

Epidemiological studies where water is naturally high in fluoride have shown no adverse effects other than dental mottling except in rare cases. Controlled studies with fluoridation at the 1 mg/liter level have reported no instances of adverse effects. Available evidence does not suggest that fluoridation has increased or decreased cancer mortality rates.

ASBESTOS

Asbestos is a general term applied to a family of silicate minerals that have a number of properties in common that render them useful for several commercial purposes. These minerals are fibrous in structure and have electrical and thermal insulating properties as well as being sufficiently flexible that they can be woven into fabrics. The production and use of such materials has been described by Rosato (1959). Approximately 88 percent of asbestos use is in the construction industry, including cement products, floor tile, paper products, and paint and caulking,

---

* Reproduced from *Drinking Water and Health*, pp. 433–34, with the permission of the National Academy of Sciences, Washington, D.C.

with the remainder being used in transportation, textiles, and plastics industries (May and Lewis, 1970).

The definition of asbestos listed in the Glossary of Geology is as follows:*

(a) a commercial term applied to a group of highly fibrous silicate minerals that readily separate into long, thin, strong fibers of sufficient flexibility to be woven, are heat resistant and chemically inert, and possess a high electric insulation, and therefore are suitable for uses (as in yarn, cloth, paper, paint, brake linings, tiles, insulation cement, fillers, and filters), where incombustible, nonconducting, or chemically resistant material is required.

(b) a mineral of the asbestos group, principally chrysotile (best adapted for spinning) and certain fibrous varieties of amphibole (example: tremolite, actinolite, and crocidolite).

The mineral fibers that comprise the asbestos group are the serpentine: chrysotile; and the amphiboles: actinolite, amosite (a cunningtonite-grunerite mineral), anthophyllite, crocidolite, and tremolite. Asbestos minerals are mined in Canada and the United States, where chrysotile accounts for about 95 percent of the production. Amosite and crocidolite make up most of the remainder. The largest chrysotile deposit in the world is found between Danville and Chaudiere, Quebec, Canada. Other deposits are found in northern Ontario, northern British Columbia, and Newfoundland in Canada, and in California, Vermont, Arizona, and North Carolina in the United States.

Asbestos is made up of fibrils of individual tubes of single crystals that bind together to produce a fiber. The size of the individual fibers varies greatly for the various minerals making up the asbestos group. Minimum fiber widths range between 0.06 μm for crocidolite to 0.25 μm for anthophylite. Fiber lengths in general range between 0.2 and 2.0 μm. Occasional longer fibers up to 100 μm are found, although these are much rarer in the general environment than in occuptational situations (Rendall, 1970).

Solubility is an important consideration in assessing the presence and impact of chemicals in soil and water. Asbestos minerals are soluble in acid solution to varying degrees (Choi and Smith, 1971). The isoelectric point of the various minerals differs widely; chrysotile has an isoelectric point of 11.8 while the amosite isoelectric point falls between 5.2 and 6.0 (Parks, 1967). As the pH of an aqueous medium falls below the isoelectric point, the charge of suspended asbestos particles will become more positive, thereby

---

* From American Geological Institute: *Glossary of Geology*. The Institute, Washington, D.C., p. 41, 1972.

attracting other dissolved minerals that can interact with them. Therefore, the mobility, transport, disposition, and biologic properties of asbestos will vary widely depending on the mineral involved, the pH of the medium, and the presence of other materials with which the asbestos may interact.

A major difficulty in assessing the environmental impact of asbestos is the difficulty in detecting and analyzing it. Since asbestos is a very heterogeneous material, its detection is also difficult. A number of methods have been proposed for the identification and quantitation of asbestos in air, water, and biologic materials. Optical and electron microscopy, x-ray diffraction, and differential thermal analysis have all been proposed. Analytic problems are complicated by the difficulty of distinguishing between asbestos fibers and other fibers and particles of minerals that may be present in the same sample with them. The quantities present in environmental samples, furthermore, are generally quite small, and the particles present may exist in a wide range of sizes, making identification difficult and greatly complicating the quantitation of the mineral present. It is generally felt that transmission electron microscopy is the most satisfactory method for the detection of asbestos. A useful summary of the advantages, disadvantages, possibilities, and difficulties of various analytic techniques that have been investigated is given by Langer (1974) and Langer et al. (1974).

Asbestos is found ubiquitously in the environment. Chrysotile asbestos is a common air pollutant in most large urban areas in the United States (Selikoff et al., 1972). In fact, because of the industrial use of asbestos, the highest concentrations found in air and water are generally in metropolitan areas (Cunningham and Pontefract, 1971; Kay, 1973). Asbestos fibers have been detected as contaminants of domestic water supplies derived from Lake Superior, generally thought to result from mine waste discharges.

An example of the contamination of a domestic water supply by asbestos minerals is illustrated by the case of Duluth, Minnesota. An iron ore mining company located at Silver Bay, Minnesota, discharges tailings into Lake Superior to the extent of approximately 70,000 tons per day. These tailings are the residue from the processing of taconite ore into pellets and are predominantly of the amosite type of asbestos. Bottom currents in Lake Superior carry some of this discharged tailing material to Duluth, approximately 70 miles southwest. Duluth draws its water directly from Lake Superior and distributes and uses it unfiltered. The water in the Duluth domestic supply had been shown to contain numerous amphibole fibers and pieces as well as other crystalline material. The concentration of verified asbestos mineral fibers in the Duluth water supply ranges from approximately 20×10^6 to 75×10^6 fibers per liter of water. These concentrations correspond to approximately 5 to 30 μg of asbestos fibers per liter of water (Nicholson, 1974). An analysis of the water system of Superior, Wisconsin, the neighbor city of Duluth, which draws only a portion of its water from Lake Superior, shows considerably fewer fibers. An analysis of the water from Grand Marais, Minnesota, which is upstream from Silver Bay, detected no asbestos fibers.

The health effects of asbestos in water have so far been incompletely ascertained. Asbestos is known to lead to asbestosis characterized primarily by pulmonary fibrosis, the formation of plural plaques, a greatly increased risk of bronchogenic carcinoma, plural mesothelioma, and peritoneal mesothelioma after occupational exposure to inhaled asbestos dust, as discussed elsewhere in this book. It is not clear, however, whether the ingestion of asbestos-contaminated water will lead to the same or similar diseases in man. Epidemiologic studies of cancer death rates in Duluth, Minnesota, have not yet revealed any increase in such conditions as compared with other areas in relation to the contamination of the water with mineral fibers. However, the contamination of the Duluth water supply began about 20 years ago, and it is not certain whether such conditions might show an increase within the next 5 to 15 years because of characteristic long latency periods. The assessment of the carcinogenicity of inhaled asbestos is complicated by the fact that synergism has been demonstrated by cigarette smoking. Whether some sort of synergistic effect may also occur with asbestos in drinking water is entirely unknown.

IMPACT OF CHEMICALS ON SOIL AND WATER SYSTEMS

The traditional view of the environment embodied in the phrase "balance of nature" represents an outmoded conceptualization of the forces that control environmental processes. There is, in fact, no simple balance of nature. The environment is composed of many systems and subsystems, each internally balanced in a dynamic way and influenced by many external processes that tend to interact and influence the structure and function of the whole system. The thrust of nature's "balance" is an evolutionary movement toward greater diversity, greater speciation, and more complex structure.

Man has been altering the course of evolution through technologic advances in agricultural and industrial practices. A side effect of a number of these advances is the introduction of chemicals resulting from agricultural and industrial practices to the soil and water ecosystems and the resulting impact of these chemicals on organisms residing there. The effects of chemical pollution are threefold (Woodwell, 1970; Stickel, 1974): (1) a tendency toward simplification of communities through the elimination of more sensitive species and their replacement by larger populations of tolerant species, (2) the change in species relationships within communities, whereby the species that earlier might have enjoyed only a minor niche dominated by other species are allowed to expand into a dominant role in the ecosystem by the disappearance of the control species, and (3) alterations in nutrient cycles, which may have a long-lasting effect on the basic composition of the ecosystem. Alteration of nutrient cycles may lead in turn to permanent changes in an ecosystem through erosion and leaching, which in turn change the basic physical structure.

Effects of pollutants are seen primarily at the tops of food chains and are observed by man usually as changes in population levels of predator species. The chlorinated hydrocarbon pesticides and industrial chemicals, for example, may cause reproductive difficulties in birds, such as the peregrine falcon. Mink are highly sensitive to methyl mercury, while apparently other mammals are not so sensitive. Contamination with methyl mercury can thus alter the diversity and dominance characteristics of the ecosystem. Disturbances in the ecosystem can be detected in nutrient cycling even though no effects are measured in the diversity or population of the community. Several studies have now shown that changes in nutrients, such as nitrates, are more sensitive than biologic parameters to chemical stress (O'Neill et al., 1977; Jackson et al., 1977). This results from the fact that changes in nutrient pools must eventually directly affect the productivity of the entire ecosystem, even though the effects may not be measurable in biologic terms until a number of years later.

The net effect of decreased diversity in an ecosystem is a more unstable system. Such communities are subject to wide fluctuations in populations of organisms and are more easily influenced by outside pressures such as chemical pollutants. This leads in turn to the necessity for man's further intervention in an attempt to stabilize the system, a process that historically has sometimes been self-defeating.

In terms of human ecology we are just beginning our efforts to understand the impact of chemicals in the environment. The full range of effects of the loss of species diversity in the ecosystem on man is yet to be understood. Changes in the dominance characteristics of ecosystems will have a major effect on man's activities as they cause him to change strategies of pest control, alter his use of water systems for consumption

Seydel, I. S.: Distribution and circulation of arsenic through water, organisms and sediments of Lake Michigan. *Arch. Hydrobiol.*, **71**:17–30, 1972.

Siegel, M. R., and Sisler, H. D.: *Antifungal Compounds*, 2 Vols. Marcel Dekker, Inc., New York, 1977.

Sims, J. L., and Pfaender, F. K.: Distribution and bio-magnification of hexachlorophene in urban drainage areas. *Bull. Environ. Contam. Toxicol.*, **14**:214–20, 1975.

Sommer, K.: Effect of various pesticides on nitrification and nitrogen transformation in soils. *Landwirtsch. Forsch. Sonderh.*, **25**:22–30, 1970.

Stewart, B. A.; Woolhiser, D. A.; Wischmeier, W. H.; Caro, J. H.; and Frere, M. H.: Control of Water Pollution from Cropland. USDA/EPA, Report No. ARS-H-5-1/EPA-600/2-75-026a, 1975.

Stickel, W. H.: Some Effects of Pollutants in Terrestrial Ecosystems. In McIntyre, A. D., and Mills, C. F. (eds.): *Ecological Toxicology Research: Effects of Heavy Metal and Organohalogen Compounds*. Plenum Press, New York, 1975, pp. 25–74.

Stojanovic, B. J.; Kennedy, M. V.; and Shuman, F. L., Jr.: Edaphic aspects of the disposal of unused pesticides, pesticide wastes, and pesticide containers. *J. Environ. Qual.*, **1**:54, 1972.

Thomas, E. A.: Phosphorus and Eutrophication. In Griffith, E. J.; Beeton, A.; Spencer, J. M.; and Mitchell, D. T. (eds.): *Environmental Phosphorus Handbook.* John Wiley & Sons, New York, 1973, pp. 585–611.

Vos, J. G.: Toxicology of PCBs for mammals and for birds. *Environ. Health Perspect.*, **1**:105–17, 1972.

Weber, J. B.: Interaction of organic pesticides with particulate matter in aquatic and soil systems. In Gold, R. F. (ed.): *Fate of Organic Pesticides in the Aquatic Environment*. American Chemical Society, Washington, D.C., 1972, pp. 55–120.

Wogan, G. N., and Tannenbaum, S. R.: Environmental N-nitroso compounds: Implications for public health. *Toxicol. Appl. Pharmacol.*, **31**:375–83, 1975.

Wollast, R.; Billen, G., and Mackenzie, F. T.: Behavior of mercury in natural systems and its global cycle. In McIntyre, A. D., and Mills, C. F. (eds.): *Ecological Toxicology Research: Effects of Heavy Metal and Organohalogen Compounds*. Plenum Press, New York, 1975, pp. 145–66.

Wong, P. T. S.; Chau, Y. K.; and Luxon, P. L.: Methylation of lead in the environment. *Nature*, **253**:263–64, 1975.

Woodwell, G. M.: Effects of pollution on the structure and physiology of ecosystems. *Science*, **168**:429–33, 1970.

Woolson, E. A.: Fate of arsenicals in different environmental substrates. *Environ. Health Perspect.*, **19**:73–81, 1977.

UNIT V
APPLICATIONS OF TOXICOLOGY

Chapter 26

FORENSIC TOXICOLOGY

Randall C. Baselt and *Robert H. Cravey*

INTRODUCTION

The science of forensic toxicology is a hybrid of analytic chemistry and fundamental toxicologic principles. It is concerned with the medicolegal aspects of the harmful effects of chemicals upon humans and animals. Although the techniques for the isolation, detection, and estimation of toxic substances in biologic materials are primarily invoked for the purpose of aiding in establishing the cause or in elucidating the circumstances of death in a postmortem investigation, they are applicable as well to certain aspects of clinical toxicology, forensic determinations made on living subjects, and drug abuse monitoring programs.

GENERAL CONSIDERATIONS

Role of Chemicals in Fatalities

The harmful effects of exposure to chemicals have been well established in the United States. Poisoning fatalities now approximate 10,000 annually; in 1968 about 3 percent of all accidental deaths and 26 percent of suicides involved poisons (Table 26–1). In addition, it is estimated

Table 26–1. THE ROLE OF POISONS IN ACCIDENTAL AND SUICIDAL DEATHS IN THE UNITED STATES IN 1968*

	ACCIDENTS	SUICIDES
Poisoning by gases and vapors	1,526	2,408
Poisoning by solids and liquids	2,583	3,276
Total all poisonings	4,109	5,684
Total all causes	114,864	21,372

* Data from U.S. Department of Health, Education, and Welfare, National Center for Health Statistics.

that for every successful suicide, there are 15 to 20 cases of attempted suicide, and that the total number of nonfatal poisonings exceeds 1 million per year (Goldstein *et al.*, 1974).

A particular class of chemicals, the barbituric acid derivatives, were implicated in 75 percent of the suicides by drugs in the United States in 1968. Table 26–2 illustrates the frequency with

Table 26–2. SELECTED DATA IN FATAL ACCIDENTAL AND SUICIDAL POISONINGS IN CALIFORNIA IN 1976*

CAUSATIVE AGENT	SUICIDES	ACCIDENTS
Barbiturates	374	109
Vehicle exhaust	185	21
Opiates and opioids	†	505
Salicylates	12	12
Arsenic	5	†
Strychnine	4	†
Total all poisonings	1233	1025

* Data from State of California Department of Public Health, Bureau of Health Intelligence.
† Data not tabulated for this classification.

which some selected toxicants were involved in fatal poisonings in California in a recent year. There, as nationwide, barbiturates are statistically prominent, accounting for 30 percent of all suicides resulting from chemicals. Carbon monoxide, present in motor vehicle exhaust gas, represents an auxiliary means of suicide and additionally contributes to another sizable classification, death by conflagration, which is not generally categorized as a chemical means. Salicylates, although they are the principal agents in accidental poisoning in the United States (U.S. Public Health Service, 1970), do not represent a major cause of death. Toxicants such as arsenic, strychnine, and other classic poisons, of considerable historic significance in toxicology, are now rarely encountered in forensic analysis.

Ethyl alcohol, while not prominent as a primary lethal agent, is a truly ubiquitous chemical in the viewpoint of the analytic toxicologist. It has been held indirectly responsible for up to 50 percent of the more than

50,000 annual nationwide motor vehicle traffic accident fatalities (Smith, 1965) and is commonly detected in the bodies of many victims of homicide, suicide, and accidents.

Most forensic laboratories today routinely analyze for alcohol in all the samples they receive. Of 25,000 coroner's cases investigated over a ten-year period in San Francisco, alcohol was found present in 16.7 percent (Committee on Medicolegal Problems, 1968). If one includes tests performed on intoxicated drivers, the analytic determination of alcohol has been the forensic chemical examination most frequently executed over the past 50 years.

The Forensic Analyst

It is the primary responsibility of the forensic toxicologist, as a member of the medicolegal team, to elucidate the nature and extent of chemical involvement in human fatalities. Inaugurated in this country by a handful of chemists performing crude chemical assays for arsenic and strychnine from the gastric contents of poisoning victims, the profession currently includes several hundred toxicologists skilled in analytic chemistry, who utilize sophisticated instrumentation for the identification of potentially thousands of toxicants, which must be isolated from virtually every organ and body fluid.

Table 26–3 exemplifies the variety and frequency of substances encompassed in the domain of a coroner's toxicologist. While alcohol, carbon monoxide, the barbiturates, and morphine remain the substances most commonly encountered by the forensic toxicologist, it is the uncommon substances that constitute the greatest analytic challenge and probably require more of the toxicologist's time. These compounds are, for the most part, representative of the ever-increasing therapeutic arsenal of the physician, each new drug contributing to the complexity of the analyst's task. For instance, several years ago the antianxiety agents diazepam and chlordiazepoxide were the only benzodiazepine derivatives available therapeutically. The toxicologist, armed with the knowledge that these two drugs were among the most frequently prescribed to persons over the age of 65 (Task Force on Prescription Drugs, 1968), would have equipped himself with a scheme for the isolation and detection of the compounds and their metabolites, and in certain areas of the country may have included this scheme in his initial or secondary search for poisons. Within the past few years, however, the number of benzodiazepine drugs on the world market has risen to 13, all close chemical relatives. To further complicate the situation,

seven of the compounds—chlordiazepoxide, clorazepate, medazepam, diazepam, prazepam, temazepam, and oxazepam—have a common metabolic pathway (DiCarlo et al., 1970; Randall et al., 1970; Dixon et al., 1976; Brooks et al., 1977). Thus, the chore of isolating and identifying a benzodiazepine derivative has been multiplied manyfold.

The example of the benzodiazepines has been and is being paralleled by other classes of drugs, such as the barbiturates, 25 of which are now prescribable in this country, and the phenothiazines, numbering approximately 16 (Goodman and Gilman, 1975). The continued emergence of new drugs and chemicals that are made available to the public calls for perseverance on the part of the forensic toxicologist in the constant modernization of his analytic methodology.

While chemically very similar, the drugs within a class may vary widely in terms of pharmacologic activity, toxicity, and pharmacokinetic properties. Thus, the goal of absolute qualitative identification of a compound isolated from a tissue sample becomes increasingly important with the continued availability of new and closely related chemical entities. Simply determining that a compound is a barbiturate, for example, does not justify interpretation of its blood concentration in terms of clinical symptoms. And often-requested estimates of the amount ingested, time of administration, and time of death are unattainable without explicit knowledge regarding the rate of absorption, pattern of body distribution, and extent of metabolism and excretion of a compound.

Obviously, the forensic toxicologist must be a first rate chemical analyst, intimately acquainted with the modern equipment and techniques that can furnish him with the qualities of speed, sensitivity, and specificity he requires. Further, he must be equally skilled in the application of toxicologic principles and pharmacologic facts to the interpretation and assessment of his findings in order to form conclusions regarding the circumstances of death.

Objectives of Toxicologic Analysis

Besides playing a major role in postmortem medicolegal investigations, the forensic toxicologist serves another equally important, although not so apparent, purpose. The data on human toxicology accumulated by him and his colleagues are often lifesaving to others, in that they lead to recognition of particular hazards in regard to drugs or chemicals either accidentally contacted or intentionally abused.

A dramatic example involves the recent epidemic of halogenated hydrocarbon inhalation

Table 26–3. DRUGS AND CHEMICALS DETECTED IN CORONER'S CASES IN ORANGE COUNTY, CALIFORNIA, 1967–1976

AGENT	FREQUENCY	AGENT	FREQUENCY
Acetone	30	Meprobamate	126
Acetaminophen	20	Mesoridazine	2
Amitriptyline	44	Methadone	8
Amphetamine	28	Methamphetamine	9
Arsenic	4	Methane	4
Barbiturates	1,165	Methanol	5
Brompheniramine	2	Methapyrilene	27
Carbamazepine	3	Methaqualone	57
Carbon Monoxide	354	Methocarbamol	8
Carbromal	9	Methyl bromide	2
Carisoprodal	4	Methylenedioxyamphetamine	1
Chlordiazepoxide	61	Methylphenidate	2
Chloroquine	2	Methyprylon	15
Chlorpheniramine	2	Morphine	416
Chlorpromazine	35	Nitrous Oxide	1
Chlorprothixene	2	Nortriptyline	11
Clorazepate	5	Oxazepam	4
Cocaine	11	Oxycodone	2
Codeine	92	Oxyphenbutazone	21
Cyanide	18	Papaverine	2
Desipramine	10	Paraquat	3
Diazepam	328	Pentazocine	13
Dichlorodifluoromethane	9	Perphenazine	13
Diethyl ether	1	Phenacetin	69
Diethylpropion	1	Phencyclidine	13
Digoxin	18	Phentermine	1
Diphenhydramine	5	Phenylbutazone	4
Diphenoxylate	1	Phenytoin	60
Doxepin	16	Procainamide	5
Ergonovine	2	Procaine	11
Ethanol	2,444	Prochlorperazine	10
Ethchlorvynol	63	Promazine	6
Ethinamate	2	Promethazine	6
Ethoheptazine	5	Proparacaine	1
Fluphenazine	1	Propoxyphene	112
Flurazepam	17	Propranolol	5
Furosemide	11	Pyrilamine	1
Glutethimide	31	Quinidine	11
Halothane	2	Quinine	2
Hydromorphone	1	Salicyclic acid	263
Hydroxyzine	7	Scopolamine	1
Hydrochlorthiazide	4	Strychnine	3
Imipramine	23	Theophylline	16
Isopropanol	3	Thioridazine	47
Levallorphan	1	Trifluoperazine	18
Levorphanol	1	Trichloroethane	3
Lidocaine	7	Trichloroethylene	3
Malathion	3	Trichloromonofluoromethane	8
Meperidine	10		

by youths. Some early reports by toxicologists of fatalities resulting from this abuse (Hall and Hine, 1966; Baselt and Cravey, 1968) gave rise to a nationwide epidemiologic study that turned up 110 similar deaths over a seven-year period (Bass, 1970). The predominantly sudden deaths, which generally lack conclusive autopsy findings, have recently been attributed to ventricular fibrillation due to cardiac sensitization to

epinephrine (Reinhardt et al., 1971). It is hoped that education of the public through continued publication of the potential dangers of these chemicals will lead to a decrease in the incidence of abuse.

Recognition of the heroin epidemic that has plagued the metropolitan areas of the United States may be partly ascribable to the work of forensic toxicologists. The geometric progression in the incidence of death due to heroin overdose in large cities over the ten years from 1960 to 1970 was a major indicator of the impending heroin crisis. Heroin fatalities in Philadelphia rose from five in 1962 to over 170 in 1970, while narcotic overdosage was the leading cause of death for those between 15 and 35 years of age in New York City, which reported over 1,200 such deaths in 1970 (Spelman, 1970). The Baden formula (after Dr. Michael Baden, New York City Deputy Chief Medical Examiner), which is now used by many cities in calculating their total addict population, is based on a city's annual heroin fatality rate. Through the application of this formula and increased surveillance on the part of the district coroner's toxicologist, the District of Columbia adjusted its estimated addict population upward to 16,800 (representing 2.2 percent of the District's population) from a previous figure of 4,200 (DuPont, 1971).

Although the avenues of relief of this and related situations have yet to be fully charted, the appreciation of a problem is the first step in its solution. To this end the living are able to profit from knowledge the dead can provide through the expedient application of forensic toxicology.

RISE OF FORENSIC TOXICOLOGY

Any attempt at tracing the early foundations of forensic toxicology must necessarily focus on the Spanish chemist and physician Mathieu J. B. Orfila (1787–1853), whose extensive influence on the development of this discipline is undeniable. An interest in forensic medicine and knowledge of analytic chemistry led Orfila to devote several years to experimentation with the poisons of that period, culminating in his textbook of general toxicology, *Traité des Poisons*, in 1814. As professor of legal medicine at the University of Paris, he devised analytic methods for the detection of poisons in human viscera, investigated the reliability of antidotes to poisons, and authored numerous other monographs on various phases of forensic medicine and toxicology. Orfila served as expert witness in the courts of Europe for many years, espousing his firm belief that only through the use of chemical analysis could a case of criminal poisoning be properly adjudicated.

Undoubtedly his most noteworthy contribution to modern forensic toxicology was his discovery that poisons, after administration via the oral route, were absorbed from the gastrointestinal tract and distributed to the various organs, in which they could be detected by chemical analysis. Fundamental as this concept seems today, the chemists of Orfila's time, having failed to find a poison in the contents of victim's stomach or intestines, would have concluded that poisoning was not responsible for the death (Bodin and Cheinisse, 1970).

Orfila also served to arouse popular interest in the infant science of toxicology, notably through his role as expert witness in the murder trial of the infamous Marie Lafarge in 1840. Utilizing a technique developed by the English chemist James Marsh several years earlier, Orfila demonstrated the presence of arsenic in the tissues of a victim of poisoning and for the first time toxicologic data was used as evidence in a medicolegal trial. His testimony resulted in the conviction and life imprisonment of Madame Lafarge and stimulated a furor of worldwide disputes over the validity of toxicologic premises. The aftermath of this trial saw the arrival in Paris of numerous young chemists eager to study under Orfila and other French toxicologists (Thorwald, 1966).

Orfila's influence was extended to England by Robert Cristison (1797–1882), a physician who had studied toxicology under the master in Paris. Returning to the University of Edinburgh, Cristison was appointed professor of forensic medicine and thus became the first British toxicologist. His excellent *Treatise on Poisons*, incorporating many of the toxicologic concepts of Orfila, was published in 1829 and survived a number of revisions, the fourth of which became the first American edition in 1845 (Camps, 1968).

The next 60 years witnessed the further development of qualitative and quantitative assays for the detection and estimation of small amounts of poisonous chemicals. One of the most noteworthy advances is attributed to Jean Servais Stas, professor of chemistry at Brussels and former student of Orfila, who in 1850 was requested by a Belgian magistrate to perform an analysis for poison in a case of suspected murder. Stas succeeded in isolating the alkaloid nicotine from the dead man's tissues. In so doing he developed a means of extraction and purification, which, after numerous refinements and modifications, forms the basis for the method of solvent extraction used universally by toxicologists today in isolating a wide variety of toxicants from biologic samples (Thorwald, 1966).

While the methodology was fast becoming available, toxicologic analysis for medicolegal purposes was not to become an accepted and routine procedure in the United States until well into the twentieth century. In 1918 the coroner system in New York City was replaced by a medical examiner system. Simultaneously, a laboratory of forensic toxicology was established, the first in the United States, under the supervision of A. O. Gettler. Over the years the numerous associates of Dr. Gettler have radiated out to establish many of the laboratories presently operating within coroners' and medical examiners' offices in the urban centers of this country (Gettler, 1956).

The American Academy of Forensic Sciences was established in 1949 to uphold and further the practice of all phases of legal medicine in the United States; the present 300 members of the toxicology section represent the majority of the analytic toxicologists in the country, including a number of hospital and private clinical laboratory analysts. The annual meetings of the Academy and its quarterly publication, the *Journal of Forensic Sciences*, serve an important role as forum for all matters of professional interest to forensic toxicologists. This Academy, together with the Society of Forensic Toxicologists and the California Association of Toxicologists, sponsors the American Board of Forensic Toxicologists, which certifies properly trained and qualified forensic toxicologists in their chosen speciality.

Forensic science organizations such as this have evolved concurrently in other countries such as Great Britain and Australia, and in order to bridge these gaps the International Association of Forensic Toxicologists was formed in 1963. With more than 500 members from 45 countries, the Association publishes an informal bulletin that presents analytic techniques and scientific data on cases involving new or infrequently encountered drugs and other chemicals.

The number and variety of poisons met with in the practice of forensic toxicology today provide a formidable obstacle to any one person attempting to master the art. With a view toward alleviating this problem by providing an opportunity for promulgation of pertinent professional information on an interpersonal basis, several informal organizations have been formed throughout the country. The California Association of Toxicologists, for example, whose meetings are open to any person demonstrating an interest, holds quarterly workshops involving lively discussions on timely topics.

The current situation regarding the training of novitiate forensic toxicologists is somewhat less than satisfactory. Customarily a person entering the field undergoes a form of apprenticeship in one of the practicing laboratories, often sidestepping theory and principle in favor of basic laboratory technical skills. This tends to produce an individual inadequately prepared for interpreting the results he has obtained, for acting as an expert witness, or for adapting existing laboratory techniques to new situations, all of which are requisite abilities for a true forensic toxicologist. The future holds promise of relief of this situation, however for there now exist a number of postgraduate training programs in toxicology that emphasize the forensic and analytic aspects of the discipline, including those at Indiana University, University of Maryland, Medical College of Virginia, and the University of Puerto Rico. Development of additional programs such as these should be heartily encouraged and supported by all practicing forensic scientists.

FROM THE DEATH SCENE TO THE LABORATORY

Approximately 20 percent of the population die under circumstances entailing an official inquiry into the cause of death (Snyder, 1967). Deaths that warrant investigation under the laws of most states are those unattended by a physician, or occurring under violent, unusual, or sudden circumstances. Determining the cause of death in these cases becomes the responsibility of the medical examiner or coroner and much depends on the accuracy of his determination. The innocence or guilt of the accused in many cases may depend solely on the proper postmortem diagnosis of the cause of death of the victim. Other legal problems hinging on the final classification of a death include insurance benefits, workmen's compensation benefits, and civil accident liability. Aside from the legal aspects, there is to be considered the emotions of the living. Interpretation of a case due to drug poisoning as accidental or suicidal, for example, should not be taken lightly. The forensic toxicologist plays a paramount role in the evaluation of a significant proportion of unclassified deaths. Prerequisite to the comprehension of this role is a basic understanding of the mechanics of a medicolegal investigation.

The Medicolegal Investigative Team

In order to properly evaluate a case, the coroner, who may or may not be a physician, or the medical examiner, who is trained in anatomic and clinical pathology as well as forensic pathology, must depend not only on his expertise but on the help of the best-qualified team available. This team consists of a homicide investigator, a medical examiner's investigator, a forensic pathologist, a forensic toxicologist, and, in certain cases, specialists trained in hematology, microbiology, sociology, odontology, anthropology, or criminalistics.

The Homicide Investigator

In cases of sudden and unexplained death, the first investigator called and consequently the first to arrive on the scene is the police homicide investigator. The rule of preservation of the death scene must be enforced until all details can be photographed and any witnesses interrogated. The homicide investigator will fingerprint the victim and collect such evidence as firearms, knives, and other articles relevant to the case that will later be examined by appropriate specialists. Other experts will be called to assist as needed, including identification technicians, police photographers, and criminalists.

The Medical Examiner-Coroner's Investigator

Two types of investigators are found in medical examiner and coroner systems in the United States. The first is the medical investigator or deputy medical examiner, a physician who has been trained in forensic medicine. The second is the lay investigator who has a suitable academic background and has gained experience through on-the-job training while serving an apprenticeship under a senior investigator. The increasing complexity of present-day cases makes it imperative that the investigator possess highly specialized skills and expertise not found in other areas of medicolegal investigation. In cases of sudden and unexplained death, he is frequently the only member of the medicolegal team to actually view the scene and collect the evidence that other members of the team will need to assist them in their investigation.

The medical examiner-coroner's investigator is responsible for the identification of the decedent, the documentation of circumstances surrounding the death, the collection and preservation of evidence including medications and other toxic substances in the area, photographs of the body and the total scene, interviews with witnesses, family, and friends as indicated by the nature of the case, and a complete medical history. All information is incorporated into a formal report, which becomes a part of the case record.

The information given the pathologist must also be given orally or in formal report to the toxicologist at the time the tissues and the preliminary pathology report are submitted to the laboratory. The investigator will also make the photographs available to the toxicologist and will submit all medications and other toxic substances directly to him.

The Forensic Pathologist

The forensic pathologist differs from the clinical pathologist in that the latter specializes in death due to natural causes while the former specializes in sudden and unexplained deaths.

The forensic pathologist can make dead men tell tales by being cognizant of the pathology associated with various injuries or poisons. For example, a murderer might smother his victim and then burn the building to disguise the death. A forensic pathologist, with proper laboratory support would be alerted to this ruse by the lack of carbon particles in the lungs and the absence of carbon monoxide in the blood.

The possibility of death due to a poisonous substance arises whenever the cause of death is not readily apparent from the gross examination of the body at autopsy. Any unmarked body without stab wounds, gunshot wounds, or crushing injuries is potentially a case of poisoning. Although the majority of cases referred to the medical examiner-coroner are finally resolved as natural deaths, many of these do not exhibit characteristic and recognizable morbid anatomic changes and may be difficult or sometimes impossible for the pathologist to ascertain unaided. Among these are metabolic diseases such as "thyroid storm," porphyria, addisonian crisis, and diabetes mellitus and functional disorders such as epilepsy and cardiac irregularities, including sudden ventricular fibrillation in the presence of only moderate arteriosclerotic heart disease.

The autopsy report prepared by the pathologist consists of the gross findings, negative as well as positive, describing the body both externally and internally in great detail, followed by the results of the histochemical or microscopic studies. On the basis of the gross and microscopic examinations the pathologist will give his opinion as to the cause of death. In those cases in which the cause of death is not evident and in those cases in which there is pathologic and/or historic evidence of poisoning, the pathologist will submit tissues for toxicologic examination. Chemical determinations are both expensive and time-consuming, and the toxicologist should not be expected to begin his task until all preliminary investigation has been completed. If an adequate history has been obtained and a thoroughly complete necropsy has been performed, the toxicologist need not be faced with a "general unknown."

The complete autopsy report often provides information pinpointing a toxic substance or class of substances. If multiple needle marks are found, for instance, the toxicologist will suspect the use of opiates and direct his initial efforts toward the disclosure of this group of compounds. The report will also allow the toxicologist to omit the search for poisons obviously not suspect. If the gastrointestinal tract is normal, one does not analyze for corrosives. If the liver and kidneys show no gross or microscopic damage, one omits the search for heavy metals.

Collection and Preservation of Postmortem Specimens

The forensic pathologist additionally is experienced in the practice of the rule of evidence, thereby ensuring that specimens for toxicologic analysis are properly obtained, placed in appropriate containers, sealed, signed, and dated. These specimens are taken immediately to the laboratory, where the toxicologist will sign or initial the seal on each container and record the hour and date received. The chain of possession, in all cases, must be intact, guaranteeing complete chronologic accountability of the samples in the expectation of judicial proceedings.

Tissues Required for Analysis

Inasmuch as it is usually impossible to determine at autopsy what tissues the toxicologist will need in his analysis, adequate samples of all tissues should be taken. These can be disposed of later if not required, whereas the possibility for disinterment of a body is remote (Curran, 1971). The pathologist should confer with his toxicologist to establish the quantity of tissue needed, since this will largely depend on the methods and instrumentation used for analysis.

Blood.   Great care should be exercised in the collection of the blood sample to ensure freedom from contamination. Heart blood is preferred and peripheral blood is acceptable. Under no circumstances should the sample be "scooped up" from the body cavity since this blood may be contaminated with fluids from the viscera and/or the stomach contents. A 100-ml sample will usually suffice for routine studies. Alcohol, cyanide, carbon monoxide, barbiturates and other depressants, and tranquilizers are among the poisons easily and readily detected from the blood.

Brain.   At least 50 g should be collected. This tissue is especially useful in the demonstration of alcohol and other volatile poisons.

Kidney.   The equivalent of one kidney should be taken. This is the tissue of choice for most metals and sulfonamides.

Liver.   A sample of 100 g is a minimal requirement. The liver is the site of biotransformation for the majority of toxicants, and the levels found in this tissue may be up to several hundred times higher than found in the blood. In many instances, the liver may be the only tissue in which the toxic substance will be found in sufficiently high concentration for absolute identification and quantitation.

Lung.   At least 100 g of lung should be obtained. This tissue will be especially useful in fatalities due to substance inhalation. It may likewise be a strategic tissue in certain instances of injection or ingestion of a poison. It has been the experience of the authors that in acute deaths resulting from the intravenous injection of heroin, morphine, the principal biotransformation product, is found in significant concentrations in the blood and lungs and may not be present at detectable levels in other tissues.

Bone.   Bone should be collected if there is any indication that a pesticide or metal is suspected. A total of 100 g should prove adequate.

Hair and Fingernails.   These specimens should be taken if chronic metal poisoning is suspected.

Adipose.   A minimum sample of 50 g should be taken routinely. In cases in which the victim has survived some days following ingestion of an unknown poison, or if pesticides or insecticides are suspected, adipose tissue should be analyzed. Among the drugs that will accumulate in the fat are thiopental, glutethimide, and ethchlorvynol.

Urine.   All available urine should be collected, and if the bladder appears empty the bladder should be submitted intact. A small amount of urine will be present in the empty bladder and this can be utilized for a micro sugar and acetone determination. Postmortem blood sugar levels are of little or no value, but the urine analysis may give evidence of diabetes. Urine often provides a concentrated, relatively unadulterated form of a poison and its metabolites and is applicable to a variety of preliminary screening tests.

Bile.   The gallbladder should not be opened at the time of autopsy but, rather, should be removed intact and placed into a separate container. Biliary excretion is an important route of elimination for a number of foreign compounds, including drugs such as morphine, methadone, and glutethimide.

Stomach and Contents.   The stomach should be ligated at both ends and disturbed as little as possible en route to the laboratory. The pathologist may wish to be present when it is opened and emptied so that he may take it back to his laboratory for closer inspection. Tablets and capsules are frequently found intact in cases of overdosage and may be easily and quickly identified. The volume of the stomach contents should be recorded so that the total quantity of drug(s) present may be calculated. This value, together with the tissue concentrations, is necessary for an estimate of the amount of a compound actually ingested.

FROM THE LABORATORY TO THE COURTROOM AND BEYOND

Analysis

As previously stated, on the basis of a good investigation and autopsy the toxicologist may be able to proceed directly to the tissue of choice and expeditiously elucidate the nature of the poison in question. The cherry red color of blood taken from the victim of a fire would suggest that a carbon monoxide determination should be performed first. Other obvious (but rare) examples are toxicants with characteristic odors, such as cyanide and organic solvents, or materials producing distinctive pathology, such as the corrosives.

In those cases in which the medical history is sparse and the autopsy shows little other than visceral edema and congestion, a number of toxic substances must be searched for as a matter of routine. The techniques involved in this search often necessarily compromise sensitivity or specificity in favor of speed, reliability, and comprehensiveness. While it is not the purpose of this chapter to provide a detailed modus operandi for toxicologic screening, a brief presentation of a general approach to the problem is in order.

Analysis of the Stomach Contents. The intact stomach should be emptied into a large flat container for careful inspection of the gastric contents. If death has been rather rapid, the dosage forms of ingested drugs may be discrete and readily identified. The contents should be checked for odor, color, and gross appearance and the pH measured. Sodium salts of weakly acidic drugs may give an alkaline pH. Description of the contents should include any recognizable food as well as foreign materials.

The contents are then weighed and a portion taken for analysis. The stomach contents may be examined for heavy-metal compounds using the Reinsch test, which consists of boiling a short spiral of copper wire in the acidified contents. Any metals depositing on the wire must be confirmed by further testing (Kaye, 1970; Clarke, 1969).

A weighed sample of stomach contents can be extracted for acid, basic, and neutral drugs by direct extraction with organic solvents. Ultraviolet spectroscopy and thin-layer or gas-liquid chromatography offer a means of rapid screen for the majority of drugs (Stewart and Stolman, 1961; Stolman, 1963, 1965, 1967, 1969, 1974; Curry, 1976; Sunshine, 1969, 1971, 1975; Finkle et al., 1971).

Analysis of the Urine. A battery of screening tests can be rapidly accomplished directly from the urine (Curry, 1976; Kaye, 1970; Sunshine, 1971):

1. Sugar and acetone determinations using Clinistix and Ketostix
2. Tumeric paper test for borates
3. Furfural spot test for meprobamate and other carbamates
4. FPN spot test for phenothiazines and related compounds
5. Five percent ferric chloride reagent for salicylates
6. Fujiwara test for chloral and other halogenated hydrocarbons
7. Reinsch test for heavy metals

A sample of urine is also extracted for acidic, neutral, basic, and amphoteric drugs and analyzed utilizing methods corresponding to those for the gastric contents.

The information gained from the analysis of the stomach contents and the urine will often provide all the information necessary to determine what procedures to follow with respect to the viscera. As a general rule the toxicologist should analyze the blood, brain, lung, liver, kidney, and bile for the purpose of establishing toxicant concentrations. It may be effectively argued that complete body distribution studies are not necessary in all cases. Certainly in the case of death due to acute alcoholism the blood, brain, and stomach contents offer all information of relevance and no other tissues are really satisfactory. Likewise, in the case of death due to the intravenous injection of heroin it may be impossible to demonstrate its metabolite, morphine, in many of the tissues. However, following overdosage of the majority of drugs, concentrations in the specimens mentioned are substantive to valid estimation of the amount administered.

Curry (1976) states that three questions will be asked of the toxicologist upon completion of his analyses. These are (1) Did you find any poison, and if so, what was it? (2) When and how was the poison taken into the system? (3) How much did you find? To these queries should be added: (4) Are the levels found consistent with death? To answer these questions the authors feel that the analysis of blood, liver, urine, and stomach contents will be minimally required.

Report of Findings

The format of toxicology reports will vary from laboratory to laboratory, but authorities appear to be in agreement as to the information the report should contain (Stewart and Stolman, 1961; Curry, 1976). A representative example is shown in Figure 26-1. The case number, name of decedent, tissues taken at autopsy, drugs, and other physical evidence found at the

```
                                        CASE  # 71-0873

                      TOXICOLOGY REPORT

NAME OF DECEDENT____Doe, Jane____SEX__F__AGE__21__WEIGHT 110 lb

TISSUES SUBMITTED Blood, bile, brain, liver, adipose,

              stomach contents, kidney

CHAIN OF POSSESSION           Smith, Jones, Baselt


*************************************************************************
```

A 1-ml sample of blood was screened for alcohol and other common volatiles employing the gas chromatographic method developed in this laboratory. None were found.

A 10-g portion of homogenized stomach contents was screened for acid, basic and neutral drugs by ultraviolet spectroscopy, thin-layer chromatography, and chemical tests. Ethchlorvynol was found present. Employing the method of Wallace *et al.* (*J. For. Sci.*, 9:342–51, 1964), it is estimated that the total stomach contents submitted contain 1.2–g.

A 5-ml sample of blood and a 10-g section of liver were screened for acidic drugs by gas chromatography. None were found.

A 50-g section of liver was screened for basic drugs by gas chromatography. None were found.

A 5-ml sample of blood, a 10-g section of brain, a 10-g section of kidney, a 10-g section of liver, a 10-g section of adipose, and the total contents of the gallbladder were analyzed for ethchlorvynol by the method of Wallace *et al.* The following levels were found: blood 8.5 mg%; kidney 5.4 mg%; liver 7.0 mg%; bile 12.5 mg%; adipose 104.0 mg%.

CONCLUSIONS:

The high levels of ethchlorvynol found in the tissue analyzed would have produced coma and may have proved fatal. Peak blood levels following the ingestion of 500 mg of ethchlorvynol usually range from 0.2 to 0.5 mg%. The levels found in this case are indicative of the ingestion of a large overdose.

Figure 26–1. Organization of toxicologist's case report.

scene and the chain of possession of these samples must be clearly stated. The body of the report must list the concentrations of any toxicants found present in the tissues as well as toxicants analyzed for but not present in levels above the limits of detection for the methods used. Methods applied in the analyses should be briefly described or a reference given if the method has been published. This information will enable medical examiners, forensic pathologists, and other toxicologists to form an opinion concerning the validity and reliability of the analyses performed.

Since many persons who are not forensic medical specialists or forensic toxicologists may be concerned with the report, an interpretation of the findings is essential. This is a most difficult task for the toxicologist since he is reasoning from data collected from other fatal cases from his case files as well as data collected by other workers that have been published in the literature. Therefore, the interpretation given

by the toxicologist is his "opinion" based on these data. This opinion must be an honest one. If all data lead to one conclusion, it should be so stated. The majority of cases, however, are not that simple, and in cases liable to more than one interpretation the toxicologist should state the arguments both for and against each and, if possible, weigh the relative probabilities. A statement on the toxicity of the chemical compound found may be included with an opinion as to whether this represents a therapeutic level, or a moderate or large overdose. If the case involves a new toxicant, the interpretation may have to be deferred until more data are available.

Interpretation of Findings

One of the most difficult problems facing the forensic toxicologist is that of interpreting his analytic findings. While the task of isolating, identifying, and estimating the level of a toxic substance from biologic specimens is not to be considered commonplace, with present-day instrumentation and the toxicologist's chemical expertise this aspect is not insurmountable.

An approach to the problem of interpretation usually begins with a review of data abstracted from the literature or culled from previous cases investigated by the toxicologist and his colleagues. The former often supplies information concerning blood levels resulting from therapeutic administration of a drug or from overdosage in which the patient survived (Baselt and Cravey, 1977). The latter concerns statistical data on body distribution studies from fatalities known to have arisen from a particular compound. An experienced analyst will usually have available a substantial body of information that greatly enhances his ability to evaluate toxicologic findings. Information from well-documented and well-investigated cases that the toxicologist personally obtains is of the foremost value in understanding toxic and fatal levels. In evaluating data received from outside sources, one must bear in mind that there is no uniformity or standardization of toxicologic procedures among clinical and forensic laboratories. Methods for isolating, identifying, and quantitating toxic substances from tissues often differ greatly in their degree of specificity, sensitivity, and accuracy.

Recovery alone poses a problem since drug-protein complexes formed in plasma and other tissues may be difficult to break down without substantial loss of the drug. Thus, the values reported are indicative only of the amount of a compound recovered and do not necessarily reflect the amount actually present in the tissue.

Since for the majority of drugs and chemicals the blood or plasma level most clearly reflects the clinical state of the patient, it is this level that is most often cited in the toxicologist's report as the deciding factor in a case of possible overdosage. It is certainly true that in clinical studies involving naïve subjects, individuals do not vary significantly with respect to the pharmacologic effects produced by certain well-defined blood concentrations of most drugs (Vesell and Passananti, 1971). However, in interpreting levels exceeding these therapeutic concentrations the toxicologist should be aware of modifying factors likely to be encountered.

Factors Affecting the Clinical State at a Given Blood Concentration of a Drug. Tolerance, a state of decreased responsiveness to a drug, is a result of prior exposure, usually long term, to a given drug or its congener. Cellular adaptation is one type of tolerance in which ever-increasing blood concentrations of a drug are required in order to maintain a certain pharmacologic response. This situation is exemplified by the methadone maintenance patient who may be receiving a daily oral dose of 100 mg of methadone hydrochloride. This same dose, although it produces no noticeable narcotic effects in the tolerant patient, could easily prove fatal if ingested by a nontolerant individual. While it is tempting, the toxicologist should refrain from classifying a blood level as consistent with death according to literature values until the decedent's history of drug usage has been determined.

The problem of drugs in combination is a frequent obstacle to interpretation of toxicologic findings. The possibility of antagonism of one

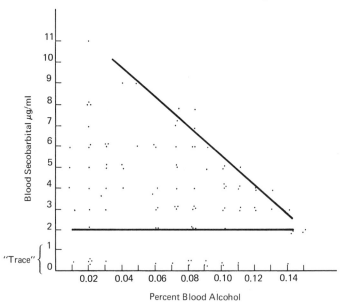

Figure 26–2. Blood concentrations of secobarbital and alcohol in 102 drug abusers ranging in age from 12 to 25 years. All subjects exhibited overt signs of intoxication. (From Finkle, B. S.: Ubiquitous reds: a local perspective on secobarbital abuse. *Clin. Toxicol.*, 4:253–64, 1971. Courtesy of Marcel Dekker, Inc.)

drug by another, although rare, should not be overlooked. More often the additive or synergistic effects produced by the interaction of two or more depressant drugs may result in coma or death, although none of the drugs is present in toxic levels. The combination of alcohol and secobarbital is commonly employed for purposes of intoxication or as a means of suicide and has been well investigated (Finkle, 1971). Figure 26–2 illustrates the simultaneous blood alcohol-secobarbital concentrations attained by young living drug abusers; the heavy lines indicate the apparent limitations for blood values that result in overt intoxication without producing coma.

Unfortunately, the effects of many other drug combinations are not known. A significant number of coroner's cases are those revealing no pathologic changes, in which the toxicologist has isolated several drugs, each in relatively low levels. In these cases only previous reports can help elaborate on whether the effect created is that of addition, synergism, untoward reaction to one or more of the drugs, or some other mechanism. However, if the chemical findings constitute the only positive findings in a case in which a complete autopsy and investigation have been performed, it may be reasonable to conclude that the terminal episode was produced by the chemicals found. However, this conclusion may occasionally assume a degree of competency on the part of the toxicologist and pathologist that is not justified.

A further, possibly obvious, factor in the interpretation of blood levels is the likelihood of the analyst mistaking a pharmacologically inactive metabolite for a parent drug and thus recording an inordinately high test result. While this problem is usually avoided with the newer chromatographic techniques used in toxicologic analysis, many of the traditional visible and ultraviolet spectrophotometric methods are less specific and will yield positive results with certain products of drug metabolism, such as the hydroxylated barbiturates (Stewart and Stolman, 1961).

Factors Affecting Blood Concentrations of Drugs. Quite often the forensic toxicologist is requested by the coroner or the court to estimate the amount of a drug ingested by a decedent strictly on the basis of a given blood concentration. This information could be invaluable in classifying a death as either suicide or accidental. Or assuming that the dosage and blood level are known, the toxicologist may be asked to predict the elapsed time between drug administration and death.

There are many variations of this theme, but in essence it requires an assumption on the part of the toxicologist that there exist for this drug both a well-defined dose-blood concentration relationship and pharmacokinetic constants for its rates of metabolism and excretion. Any estimate of dosage or of time until death on this basis is at best a gross approximation, and the toxicologist should approach this field of speculation with great caution.

The primary factor determining blood concentration produced by a given amount of most drugs (assuming standardization as to weight of the subject and route of administration) is the rate of drug metabolism. This is largely

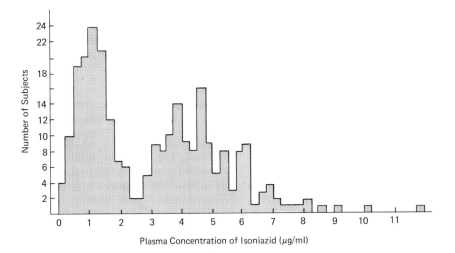

Figure 26–3. Plasma concentrations of isoniazid in 267 human subjects six hours after oral administration of the drug at a dose of 9.8 mg/kg. (From Evans, D. A. P.; Manley, K. A.; and McKusick, V. C.: Genetic control of isoniazid metabolism in man. *Br. Med. J.*, 2:485–91, 1960.)

DuPont, R. L.: Profile of a heroin-addiction epidemic. *N. Engl. J. Med.*, **285**:320–24, 1971.

Evans, D. A. P.; Manley, K. A.; and McKusick, V. C.: Genetic control of isoniazid metabolism in man. *Br. Med. J.*, **2**:485–91, 1960.

Finkle, B. S.: A progress report on a statewide computer program for analytical and case toxicology data. *Forensic Sci. Gaz.*, **1**:2–4, 1970.

———: Ubiquitous reds: a local perspective on secobarbital abuse. *Clin. Toxicol.*, **4**:253–64, 1971.

Finkle, B. S.; Cherry, E. J.; and Taylor, D. M.: A GLC based system for the detection of poisons, drugs, and human metabolites encountered in forensic toxicology. *J. Chromatogr. Sci.*, **9**:393–419, 1971.

Gerber, S.: Expert medical testimony and the medical expert. In Schroeder, O. (ed.): *Medical Facts for Legal Truth.* W. H. Anderson Co., Cincinnati, 1961, pp. 195–212.

Gettler, A. O.: The historical development of toxicology. *J. Forensic Sci.*, **1**:3–25, 1956.

Gochman, M., and Bowie, L. J.: Automated systems for radioimmunoassay. *Anal. Chem.*, **49**:1183A–90A, 1977.

Goldstein, A.; Aronow, L.; and Kalman, S. M.: *Principles of Drug Action*, 2nd ed. Harper & Row, New York, 1974.

Gonzales, T. A.; Helpern, M.; and Umberger, C.: *Legal Medicine, Pathology and Toxicology.* Appleton-Century-Crofts, New York, 1954.

Goodman, L. S., and Gilman, A. (eds.): The *Pharmacological Basis of Therapeutics*, 5th ed. Macmillan Publishing Co., Inc., New York, 1975.

Hall, F. B., and Hine, C. H.: Trichloroethane intoxication: a report of two cases. *J. Forensic Sci.*, **11**:404–13, 1966.

Kaye, S.: *Handbook of Emergency Toxicology*, 3rd ed. Charles C Thomas, Publisher, Springfield, Ill., 1970.

Law, N. C.; Aandahl, V.; Fales, H. M.; and Milne, G. W. A.: Identification of dangerous drugs by mass spectrometry. *Clin. Chim. Acta*, **32**:221–28, 1971.

Mannering, G. J.: Significance of stimulation and inhibition of drug metabolism. In Burger, A. (ed.): *Selected Pharmacological Testing Methods.* Marcel Dekker, Inc., New York, 1968, pp. 51–119.

Mendelson, J. H.; Stein, S.; and Mello, N. K.: Effects of experimentally induced intoxication on metabolism of ethanol-1-^{14}C in alcoholic subjects. *Metabolism*, **14**:1255–66, 1965.

Milne, M. D.: Drugs, poisons, and the kidney. In Black, D. (ed.): *Renal Disease.* Blackwell Scientific Publications, Oxford, 1967, pp. 546–60.

Newman, H. W.: Acquired tolerance to ethyl alcohol. *Q. J. Stud. Alcohol*, **2**:453–63, 1941.

Orfila, M. J. B.: *Traits des poisons tires des regnes mineral, vegetal et animal ou toxilogie general consideree sous les rapports de la pathologie et des la medicine legale.* Crochard, Paris, 1814.

Randall, L. O.; Scheckel, C. L.; and Pool, W.: Pharmacology of medazepam and metabolites. *Arch. Int. Pharmacodyn.*, **185**:135–48, 1970.

Reinhardt, C. F.; Azar, A.; Maxfield, M. E.; Smith, P. E.; and Mullin, L. S.: Cardiac arrhythmias and aerosol "sniffing." *Arch. Environ. Health*, **22**:265–79, 1971.

Rubin, E., and Lieber, C. S.: Alcoholism, alcohol, and drugs. *Science*, **172**:1097–1102, 1971.

Smith, S. D. (ed.): *Traffic Accident Facts.* National Safety Council, Chicago, 1965.

Snyder, L.: *Homicide Investigation*, 2nd ed. Charles C Thomas, Publisher, Springfield, Ill., 1967.

Spelman, J. W.: Heroin addiction: the epidemic of the 70's. *Arch. Environ. Health*, **21**:589–90, 1970.

Starrs, J. E.: The ethical obligations of the forensic scientist in the criminal justice system. *J. Asso. Off. Anal. Chem.*, **54**:906–14, 1971.

Stewart, C. P., and Stolman, A. (eds.): *Toxicology, Mechanisms and Analytical Methods*, 2 vols. Academic Press, Inc., New York, 1961.

Stolman, A. (ed.): *Progress in Chemical Toxicology*, vol. 1. Academic Press, Inc., New York, 1963; vol. 2, 1965; vol. 3, 1967; vol. 4, 1969; vol. 5, 1974.

Sunshine, I. (ed.): *Handbook of Analytical Toxicology.* Chemical Rubber Co., Cleveland, 1969.

———: *Manual of Analytical Toxicology.* Chemical Rubber Co., Cleveland, 1971.

———: *Methodology for Analytical Toxicology.* CRC Press, Cleveland, 1975.

Task Force on Prescription Drugs: *The Drug Users.* U.S. Dept. of Health, Education, and Welfare, Washington, D.C., 1968.

Thorwald, J.: *Proof of Poison.* Thames and Hudson, Ltd., London, 1966.

U.S. Public Health Service: *Bulletin of the National Clearinghouse for Poison Control Centers.* Dept. of Health, Education, and Welfare, Washington, D.C., Sept.-Oct., 1970.

Vesell, E. S., and Passananti, G. T.: Utility of clinical chemical determinations of drug concentrations in biological fluids. *Clin. Chem.*, **17**:851–66, 1971.

Wallace, J. E.; Wilson, W. J., Jr.; and Dahl, E. V.: A rapid and specific method for determining ethchlorvynol. *J. Forensic Sci.*, **9**:342–52, 1964.

Wright, J. T.: The value of barbiturate estimations in the diagnosis and treatment of barbiturate intoxication. *Q. J. Med.*, **24**:95–108, 1955.

Chapter 27

CLINICAL TOXICOLOGY

Barry H. Rumack and Robert G. Peterson

INTRODUCTION

Treatment of the poisoned patient based on pharmacologic principles promotes the institution of rational methods most beneficial to recovery. Unfortunately the communication of these principles and methods has not always been appropriate, and some current reference sources still recommend procedures that are antiquated and should be contraindicated. For example, the eighth edition of *Harrison's Principles of Internal Medicine* still recommends in the treatment of acute barbiturate intoxication, "analeptics such as coffee or parenteral caffeine sodium benzoate may be used" (Victor and Adams, 1977). This statement appears despite the acceptance of the Scandinavian method introduced before 1951 utilizing only conservative, supportive care (Clemmesen, Nilsson, 1961).

The material presented in this book provides a framework for the approach to the poisoned patient exposed to drugs, chemicals, plants, or other situations that confront the clinical toxicologist. This chapter reviews some of the principles of clinical management, as well as specific current theory and treatment of frequently encountered toxic situations.

TOXICOKINETICS

The basic application of pharmacokinetics to the toxic substance exposure is often useful in monitoring the course of the poisoning and determining therapeutic manipulations. The ability to calculate a body burden of a drug, its half-life, route of excretion, and other physical characteristics will aid in decisions such as use of diuresis, dialysis, or hemoperfusion. However, it must be be recognized that most pharmacokinetic data are based on the therapeutic evaluation of drugs, and significant changes in kinetic parameters may occur in overdoses. For example, it is well known that salicylate peak blood levels are prolonged up to six hours from the normal values of one or two hours and that its half-life increases from two to four hours to 25 to 30 hours in significantly overdosed patients (Done, 1960).

Conversely, digoxin half-life may be shortened to one-third its expected value in overdose (Rumack *et al.*, 1974), and paradoxically hyperkalemia is a hallmark of acute overdose rather than the hypokalemia frequently seen with chronic digitalis toxicity. Thus, it is critical for the clinician to determine that the data on which decisions are to be based are related to overdose rather than therapeutic information.

LD50 and MLD

The LD50 and MLD values are considered important to many clinicians in formulating a plan for dealing with the poisoned patient. Unfortunately they are rarely of practical value clinically.

First, these values are obtained from various animal trials that establish a dose that will statistically kill half of a group or some other predetermined number. Differences in metabolism between humans and animal species are remarkable, and linear correlation or extrapolation of animal metabolism data to humans is rarely possible.

Second, the clinician obtains a *history* of overdose and attempts to relate the amount ingested by history with the LD50. This disregards factors such as the accuracy of history (which is often accurate less than 50 percent of the time), rate and extent of absorption of agent, metabolism/disposition of the agent, and the clinical response of the patient.

Consequently, the generally accepted recommendation is to disregard LD50 and MLD data on a particular poison and to determine the expected toxicology of the drug followed by appropriate monitoring to determine if the patient demonstrates the predicted clinical findings. The adage "Treat the patient not the *poison*" represents the most basic and important principle in clinical toxicology.

Half-Life

The half-life is a measure of rate for the time required to eliminate one half of a quantity of an

Table 27–1. TOXICOKINETIC DATA OF DRUGS AND TOXINS (NUMBERS EXPRESSED AS A MEAN OR AS A RANGE)

AGENT	pK_a	Vd l/kg	THER. $t_{1/2}$ hrs	O.D. $t_{1/2}$ hrs	DIURESIS	DIALYSIS	SPECIFIC THERAPY
Acetaminophen	9.5	0.75	2	4	No	No	N-Acetylcysteine
Amitriptyline	9.4	40+	36	72	No	No	Physostigmine
Amobarbital	7.9	2.4	16	36+	No	No	
Amphetamine	9.8	0.60	8–12	18–24	Acid	Yes	Chlorpromazine
Bromide	—	40+	300	300	Yes	Yes	
Caffeine	13	0.75	3.5	4–120	No	No	
Chloral hydrate	—	0.75	8	10–18	No	No	
Chlorpromazine	9.3	40+	16–24	24–36	No	No	
Codeine	8.2	3	2	2	No	No	Naloxone
Coumadin	5.7	0.1	36–48	36–48	No	No	Vitamin K
Desipramine	10.2	50+	18	72	No	No	Physostigmine
Diazepam	3.3	1–2	36–72	48–144	No	No	
Digoxin	—	7–10	36	13	No	No	
Diphenhydramine	8.3	—	4–6	4–8	No	No	Physostigmine
Ethanol	—	0.6	2–4	—	Yes (?)	No	
Ethchlorvynol	8.7	3–4	1–2	36–48	No	No	
Glutethimide	4.5	20–25	8–12	24+	No	No	
Isoniazid	3.5	0.60	2–4	6+	Alkaline	Yes	
Methadone	8.3	6–10	12–18	12–18	No	No	Naloxone
Methicillin	2.8	0.60	2–4	2–4	Yes	Yes	
Pentobarbital	8.11	2.0	10–20	50+	No	No	
Phencyclidine	8.5	—	—	12–48	Acid	Yes	
Phenobarbital	7.4	0.75	36–48	72–120	Alkaline	Yes	
Phenytoin	8.3	0.60	24–30	36–72	No	No	
Quinidine	4.3, 8.4	3	7–8	10	No	No	
Salicylate	3.2	0.1–0.3	2–4	25–30	Alkaline	Yes	
Tetracycline	7.7	3	6–10	6–10	No	No	
Theophylline	0.7	0.46	4.5	6+	No	Yes	

agent in the body. For drugs exhibiting first-order kinetics the half-life can be calculated with the use of the following equation where Kel is the elimination rate constant.

$$t_{1/2} = \frac{0.693}{Kel}$$

Clinically it is estimated simply by plotting several concentration values of the agent against time on semilogarithmic paper. Once several values have been plotted, a straight line should be evident, and the amount of time that it takes for the drug concentration to decrease by half from any point on the line can be determined.

The clinical value of determining a patient's half-life during the course of a poisoning is to see the rate at which a patient is approaching therapeutic levels of a drug and whether methods of therapy being employed are effective. For some drugs, half-life values in the overdose situation are prolonged over values seen in normal dose. Therefore, measures to enhance elimination to shorten drug half-life are desirable. With digoxin, however, the $t_{1/2}$ has been reported to be shorter in overdose than in therapeutic situations. In such cases supportive rather than elimination-enhancing measures are more practical.

Kinetic Relationships

The volume of distribution is the apparent space in which an agent is distributed following absorption and subsequent distribution in the body. Salicylate is distributed in total body water or about 60 percent of body mass. Digoxin, on the other hand, has an enormous volume of distribution of 500 liters or more in a 70-kg man (approximately 7 liters/kg). Since this is impossible practically, the term *apparent* volume of distribution is utilized to denote that while this is the apparent volume based on the measured value of the drug in the blood, the drug is concentrated or sequestered somewhere out of the blood, i.e., tissue compartments (see Chap. 3).

Some useful mathematic relationships are

$$Vd = \frac{D}{Cp} \qquad Cp = \frac{D}{Vd} \qquad D = Cp \cdot Vd$$

Where Vd = value of distribution
D = dose administered
Cp = plasma concentration

$$Cl = Kel \cdot Vd$$

Where Cl = clearance of drug
Kel = elimination rate constant

$$Kel = \frac{0.693}{t_{1/2}}$$

Thus, if the history is that of a 25-kg child who was estimated to have consumed 500 mg of phenobarbital and the Vd for phenobarbital is approximately 60 percent body weight, then the estimated blood level would be 33.3 μg/ml. This approximates phenobarbital's high therapeutic range.

Example calculations:

25 kg $\times$ 0.60 l/kg = 15 l = Vd
500 mg/15 l = 33.3 mg/l or 33.3 μg/ml

In this case, the decision would be made clinically that the maximum possible dose by history assuming total absorption could produce toxicity, and, therefore, the child probably needs to be seen and observed by medical personnel.

MEASURES TO ENHANCE ELIMINATION

Once a patient has been observed clinically to be in a seriously toxic state, then it must be determined whether or not the agent can be eliminated more rapidly, thereby shortening the duration of coma or other toxic manifestations. Procedures to enhance elimination are indicated in severely poisoned patients.

Diuresis

The basic principles of diuresis are ion trapping and increasing urine flow. The ion-trapping phenomenon occurs when the pK_a of the agent is such that, after filtering into the renal tubular fluid, alteration of the pH of the urine can ionize and "trap" the agent. Once the toxin is ionized, then reabsorption from the renal tubules is impaired and the result is that more of the drug is excreted in the urine. Salicylates and phenobarbital elimination is significantly enhanced by forced alkaline diuresis, while strychnine, phencyclidine, and amphetamine elimination is hastened in an acid urine. Even though a drug's pK_a may indicate that the drug might be successfully eliminated by this method, other factors, such as lipid solubility and volume of distribution, may render this method ineffective (see Table 27–1).

For some drugs urine flow rate is important. Normal urine output is 1 to 2 ml/kg/hour. Forced diuresis results in a urine flow rate of 3 to 6 ml/kg/hour. In theory, for drugs whose renal elimination is flow dependent, increasing urine output by the use of fluids or diuretics may enhance drug or toxin elimination.

Dialysis

The dialysis technique, either peritoneal or hemodialysis, relies on the dialysis membrane permeability of the toxic agent so it can equilibrate with the dialysate and subsequently be removed. This is in part dependent on the molecular weight of the compound. Some drugs

Table 27–2. **DRUG TOXIN REMOVAL BY DIALYSIS, INTENSIVE SUPPORTIVE CARE, AND USE OF ACTIVATED CHARCOAL**

Dialysis Indicated on Basis of Condition of Patient

Alcohol	Iodides
Ammonia	Isoniazid
Amphetamines	Meprobamate (Equanil,
Anilines	Miltown)
Antibiotics	Paraldehyde
Barbiturates (long)	Potassium
Boric acid	Quinidine
Bromides	Quinine
Calcium	Salicylates
Chloral hydrate	Strychnine
Fluorides	Thiocynates

Dialysis Not Indicated Except for Support in the Following Poisons; Therapy Is Intensive Supportive Care

Antidepressants (tricyclic and MAO inhibitors also)
Antihistamines
Chlordiazepoxide (Librium)
Digitalis and related
Diphenoxylate (Lomotil)
Ethchlorvynol (Placidyl)
Glutethimide (Doriden)
Hallucinogens
Heroin and other opiates
Methaqualone (Quaalude)
Noludar (Methyprylon)
Oxazepam (Serax)
Phenothiazines
Synthetic anticholinergics and belladonna compounds

Well Adsorbed by Activated Charcoal

Alcohol	Muscarine
Amphetamines	Nicotine
Antimony	Opium
Antipyrene	Oxalates
Atropine	Parathion
Arsenic	Penicillin
Barbiturates	Phenol
Camphor	Phenolphthalein
Cantharides	Phenothiazine
Cocaine	Phosphorus
Digitalis	Potassium permanganate
Glutethimide	Quinine
Iodine	Salicylates
Ipecac	Selenium
Malathion	Silver
Mercuric chloride	Stramonium
Methylene blue	Strychnine
Morphine	Sulfonamides

such as phenobarbital can readily cross these membranes and go from high concentrations in plasma to that in the dialysate. Since the volume of distribution of phenobarbital is 75 percent of the body weight, there is a reasonable opporninty for enough drug to be removed from total body burden that the technique is valuable in serious cases. Conversely, drugs with large volumes of distribution would be expected to be poorly dialyzable. Similarly, drugs that are highly serum protein bound are not expected to be well removed by dialysis (see Watanabe, 1977).

Lipid dialysis has been suggested for lipid-soluble drugs (like glutethimide) that do not readily concentrate in aqueous dialysate. Unfortunately, most lipophilic drugs have extremely large volumes of distribution, and consequently even with four to six hours of dialysis only a small percentage may be removed (see Table 27–2).

Hemoperfusion

Passing blood through a column of charcoal or adsorbent resin is the newest technique of extracorporeal drug/toxin removal. While some agents are better removed by this technique because of the adsorptive capacity of the column, the volume of distribution of an agent may limit removal in a similar manner as with dialysis. If the drug is highly tissue bound such as in fat stores and only a small proportion is presented via the blood compartment to a device, then only the proportion that is in blood is available for removal. To date there is no known agent that is able to significantly displace toxins from either fat stores or protein binding. At the present time the literature in this area contains no controlled studies demonstrating conclusive results, and the available optimistic results must be viewed skeptically (see Table 27–1).

APPROACH TO THE POISONED PATIENT

Telephone management of the pediatric patient, especially under the age of five, is responsible for 85 percent of this patient population's treatment. Epidemiologic data clearly demonstrate that the peak age of ingestion is two years of age, which is consistent with the ambulatory growth and development of children. Most children suffer *ingestion* rather than poisoning with fewer than 1 percent becoming symptomatic. In fact, the major traumatic event associated with a pediatric ingestion is the emesis that results from the therapeutic administration of syrup of ipecac. Poison centers, therefore, have adopted standard protocols for dealing with these childhood accidents so as to preclude missing those that actually become symptomatic (Rumack *et al.*, 1978). In addition, it is prudent

for the clinician to become familiar with the local and regional poison control centers for consultative toxicology services.

Key Steps in Telephone Management

When dealing with a potential ingestion, the history represents the first step in determining the necessity for instituting therapeutic measures. The following represent critical history points and subsequent measures.

1. Telephone number, name, address, age, weight
2. Time of ingestion, route, agent
3. Assessment of severity
4. Assessment of reliability of history
5. Determination of safety of home therapy
6. Instructions in home therapy—emesis, catharsis, charcoal, decontamination
7. Follow-up

1 hour—Determine success of therapy, usually emesis, and assess patient

4 hours—Determine condition of patient

24 hours—Determine condition of patient, suggest psychotic services, social services, or visiting nurses service if appropriate. Basically, if the status changes or if it seems that more than these calls need to be made, then the patient should be seen. A rule of thumb in most poison centers is that children under six months of age should be seen or referred to a physician regardless of history. Child abuse should be considered in any repeat poisoning case (Rumack, 1978).

Evaluation of the Patient

The decision that determines whether or not the patient should be hospitalized is based on an evaluation of the severity of the potential poisoning. If it is apparent that the patient is in no danger, hospital referral in most cases is unlikely, and poison control center experience indicates that a vast majority of these situations can be appropriately handled at home. However, if it is judged that the patient's life is in immediate or potential danger, the patient should be brought or taken by ambulance to the nearest hospital or emergency room. Initial emergency room contact requires determining if the patient is breathing and/or is in shock with immediate life support instituted as necessary. Clinical evaluation, in addition to the usual physical examination of the poisoned patient, includes several widely used scoring systems for coma, hyperactivity, and withdrawal. They are not only useful to assess the condition of the patient but also as a reminder to check certain key points. They also serve as a useful monitoring parameter to follow and to determine if the patient's condition is improving or deteriorating. Table 27–3 identifies these scoring methods and criteria.

Table 27–3. SCORING SYSTEMS FOR COMA, HYPERACTIVITY, AND WITHDRAWAL

Classification of Coma

0	Asleep, but can be aroused and can answer questions.
1	Comatose, does withdraw from painful stimuli, reflexes intact.
2	Comatose, does not withdraw from painful stimuli, most reflexes intact, no respiratory or circulatory depression.
3	Comatose, most or all reflexes are absent but without depression of respiration or circulation
4	Comatose, reflexes absent, respiratory depression with cyanosis, circulatory failure or shock.

Classification of Hyperactivity

1+	Restlessness, irritability, insomnia, tremor, hyperreflexia, sweating, mydriasis, flushing.
2+	Confusion, hyperactivity, hypertension, tachypnea, tachycardia, extrasystoles, sweating, mydriasis, flushing, mild hyperpyrexia.
3+	Dilirium, mania, self-injury, marked hypertension, tachycardia, arrhythmias, hyperpyrexia.
4+	Above plus: convulsions, coma, circulatory collapse.

Classification of Withdrawal

Score the following finding on a 0-, 1-, 2-point basis:

Diarrhea	Hypertension	Restlessness
Dilated pupils	Insomnia	Tachycardia
Gooseflesh	Lacrimation	Yawning
Hyperactive bowel sounds	Muscle cramps	

       1–5, mild
       6–10, moderate
       11–15, severe

Seizures indicate severe withdrawal regardless of the rest of the score.

Emesis

Syrup of ipecac in appropriate doses (30 ml, adult; 10 to 15 ml, pediatric) has been shown to be a safe and effective means of producing emesis. While apomorphine has a more rapid onset of action than ipecac syrup, the average percent recovery is the same. Apomorphine is notoriously toxic in children with its narcotic depressant effects, which may persist past the reversal effects of naloxone administered to counteract the toxicity of this emetic. In addition, apomorphine may result in protracted vomiting, which is often unresponsive to narcotic antagonist intervention. Emesis 60 minutes after ingestion produces recovery of 30 percent of gastric contents.

Emesis is generally contraindicated when the patient is comatose, convulsing, or without the gag reflex. Strong acid or base ingestion is another reason for not inducing emesis since this will reexpose the patient's esophagus to these agents, thus contributing to further damage. While hydrocarbons have been a contraindication in the past, they are no longer considered a contraindication for emesis in many cases (Subcommittee on Accidental Poisoning, 1976).

Lavage

Gastric lavage with a large-bore tube is a rapid and effective way to empty the stomach. While there has been criticism in the past of this technique, most comparative studies were performed with ipecac emesis and small-bore (16-French) lavage tube. Proper lavage with large (36- to 40-French) tubes utilizing 10 to 20 liters of warm saline in an adult or 5 to 10 liters of warm tap water in a child is the method of choice to empty the stomach if a contraindication to emesis exists, if the patient is symptomatic, or if an adult has ingested an unusually large or toxic amount of agent (Matthew and Lawson, 1975).

Cathartics

The rationale for the administration of cathartics in the poisoned patient is to hasten the toxin through the gastrointestinal tract to minimize its absorption. Although no controlled data are available for the use of cathartic agents, they are indicated in several situations: ingestion of enteric-coated tablets, when the lag time since ingestion is greater than one hour, and with hydrocarbons. Preferred agents are the saline cathartics (sodium sulfate, magnesium sulfate, citrate, or phosphates), which have a relatively prompt onset of action and lower toxicity than the oil-based cathartics, which have attendant aspiration risks.

Charcoal

The classic paper of Corby and Decker (1970) demonstrates the value of administration of sufficient quantities of charcoal to bind toxin that has not been removed by emesis or lavage.

Although concern has been raised that charcoal cannot "catch up" with drugs and other agents once they have passed through the pylorus, there is ample evidence to show that administration of charcoal-following methods to empty the stomach will result in lower plasma levels than if emesis or lavage alone is used. Concomitant administration of activated charcoal with syrup of ipecac often renders the ipecac ineffective.

Laboratory

Measurement of plasma, urine, or gastric levels of drugs or toxins when done in appropriate relationship to time and clinical status can have a significant impact in the clinical management of the poisoned patient. When a toxic screen is requested, the clinician must be aware of which drugs are actually being examined. Too often the clinician interprets a negative toxic screen to mean that there are no toxic agents on board. Interpretation of a patient's levels should be related to the therapeutic levels from the same laboratory. Statements such as "lethal level" are not relevant since toxicologists assume that most patients arriving alive in the emergency department will eventually recover. Specific relationships of blood levels will be presented with each drug discussed in the next sections of this chapter (Curry, 1974).

ACETAMINOPHEN

Acetaminophen has been utilized as an analgesic and antipyretic since the mid-1950's and has become more prominently recognized as a potential hepatotoxin in the overdose situation since the original British reports in the late 1960s (Proudfoot and Wright, 1970). Recent work on the mechanism of liver toxicity of the drug has provided a theoretic basis for therapy (Mitchell et al., 1973).

Acetaminophen in normal individuals is inactivated by sulfation (approximately 52 percent) and by glucuronide conjugation (42 percent). About 2 percent of the drug is excreted unchanged. The remaining 4 percent is detoxified by the cytochrome P-450 mixed-function oxidase system. This P-450 metabolic process results in a potentially toxic metabolite that is detoxified by conjugation with glutathione and excreted as the mercapturate. Evidence extrapolated from animals indicates that when 70 percent of endogenous hepatic glutathione is consumed, the toxic metabolite becomes available for covalent binding to hepatic cellular components. The ensuing hepatic necrosis would be expected to take place after absorption of 15.8 g of acetaminophen, the amount needed to deplete glutathione in a normal 70-kg man. Other factors may alter this figure. Ingestion of 15.8 g may not produce toxicity if all of the dose is not absorbed, if the history is inaccurate, if the patient has a metabolic inhibitor on board such as piperonyl butoxide, or if he suffers from anorexia nervosa.

On the other hand, patients on long-term metabolic enhancers (microsomal enzyme inducers) such as phenobarbital may produce more than 4 percent of the toxic metabolite. The range of metabolic response and the difficulty of estimating accurately the amount ingested and absorbed precludes making therapeutic decisions on a historic predictive basis alone (Peterson and Rumack, 1978).

The clinical presentation of these patients is also sufficiently confusing in some cases to make waiting for appearance of symptoms inadequate for diagnosis. The usual patient presents in the following stages:

Stage I—2 to 24 hours
   Anorexia, nausea, vomiting
   A general feeling of malaise not unlike the common cold or flu.
Stage II—Improvement; the patient begins to feel better—may become hungry and willing to get out of bed. At this same time the SGOT, SGPT, bilirubin, and prothrombin time become abnormal. Right upper quadrant pain may occur.
Stage III—3 to 5 days
   Hepatic necrosis with peak abnormalities of hepatic function.
Stage IV—7 to 8 days
   Return to normal of hepatic functions and general clinical improvement.

Follow-up liver biopsy studies of patients who have recovered three months to a year after hepatotoxicity have demonstrated no long-term sequelae or chronic toxicity (Clark et al., 1973). A very small percentage (0.25 percent) of patients in the national multiclinic study conducted in Denver may progress to hepatic encephalopathy with subsequent death. The clinical nature of the overdose is one of a sharp peak of SGOT by day 3 and with recovery to less than 100 IU/l by day 7 or 8. Patients with SGOT levels as high as 20,000 IU/l have shown complete recovery and no sequelae one week after ingestion (Arena et al., 1978).

Laboratory evaluation of the potentially poisoned patient is crucial in terms of both hepatic measures of toxicity and plasma levels of acetaminophen. Accurate estimation of acetaminophen in the plasma, preferably by high-pressure liquid chromatography or gas chromatography, should be done on samples drawn three to four hours after ingestion when peak plasma levels can be expected. While p-aminophenol was once considered an adequate urine screening test, it is no longer indicated for this purpose since acetaminophen does not produce this metabolite in significant measurable quantities.

Once an accurate plasma level is obtained, it

SEMILOGARITHMIC PLOT
OF PLASMA ACETAMINOPHEN LEVELS VS. TIME

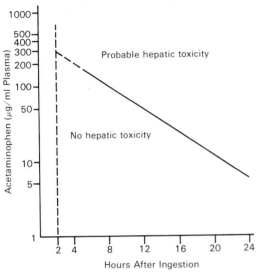

Figure 27–1. Rumack-Matthew nomogram for acetaminophen poisoning. Cautions for use of chart: (*1*) The time coordinates refer to time of ingestion. (*2*) Serum levels drawn before four hours may not represent peak levels. (*3*) The graph should be used only in relation to a single acute ingestion. (*4*) A half-life of greater than four hours indicates a high likelihood of significant hepatic injury. (From Rumack, B. H., and Matthew, H.: Acetaminophen poisoning and toxicity. *Pediatrics*, 55:871, 1975. Copyright American Academy of Pediatrics 1975.)

should be plotted on the Rumack-Matthew nomogram to determine whether therapy is or is not indicated (see Fig. 27–1). This nomogram is based on a series of patients with and without hepatotoxicity and their corresponding blood levels. While half-life was once considered an accurate way to determine potential acetaminophen hepatotoxicity, it is no longer considered adequate since the toxic metabolite comprises only about 4 percent of the total metabolism. Similarly, back extrapolation of data to the zero-hour axis may not accurately reflect initial levels since the slope of excretion curve does not necessarily reflect hepatic toxicity.

Treatment should be instituted in any patient with a plasma level in the potentially toxic range. Standard support with gastric lavage should be followed by oral administration of N-acetylcysteine (Mucomyst), currently the subject of a major national multiclinic open study. Activated charcoal, unless administered within a few minutes of ingestion, should be avoided because

of its potential adsorptive capacity for N-acetylcysteine (NAC). Because NAC is most effective if given prior to 16 hours, postingestion patients in whom blood levels cannot be obtained should have NAC treatment instituted and therapy terminated only if levels are nontoxic. The dosing regimen for NAC is a loading dose of 140 mg/kg orally, followed by 70 mg/kg orally for 17 additional doses (Peterson and Rumack, 1977). Cysteamine has been used effectively in Great Britain but is generally unavailable in the United States. Methionine has been shown to be less effective than NAC or cysteamine (Prescott *et al.*, 1976).

Daily SGOT, SGPT, bilirubin, and prothrombin time should be monitored, as well as constructional dyspraxia.

Chronic toxicity is unlikely with acetaminophen because of its lack of accumulative kinetics (Peterson and Rumack, 1978).

ACIDS

Acids such as hydrochloric acid, nitric acid, sulfuric acid, and sodium bisulfate are commonly found around the home in products such as toilet bowl cleaners, automobile batteries, swimming pool cleaning agents, and other such products. Despite the fact that these agents have various degrees of toxicity, even a very small amount (milliliters) can result in serious sequelae that can occasionally progress to death, for example, if the caustic acid agent is aspirated. Clinically, the patient may present with irritation and crying, in association with inability to swallow or pain upon swallowing, mucous membrane burns, circumoral burns, hematemesis, abdominal pain, respiratory distress (secondary to epiglottal edema), shock, and renal failure. Once the patient has been treated through the initial stages of the ingestion, residual sequelae may occur with lesions of the esophagus and gastrointestinal tract that may progress to scarring and strictures.

The use of emetics and lavage are absolutely contraindicated. Dilution or therapy with water or milk immediately following ingestion represents the treatment of choice since these substances do not result in an exothermic chemical reaction. Despite labeling of many acid-containing products, alkaline substances or carbonate preparations are contraindicated since, when administered, they may produce tremendous amounts of heat and carbonates may form carbon dioxide gas, which presents an unacceptable risk of gastric perforation. In addition, immediate irrigation with copious amounts of water should be instituted to the exposed areas of skin, mucous membranes, and other affected areas. Olive oil is not indicated and may interfere with further therapy. Analgesics, administered by the parenteral route, may be indicated. Development of shock requires appropriate treatment with fluid therapy and pressor agents as indicated. Development of laryngoedema may require placement of an endotracheal tube, and esophagoscopy should be considered in all patients with significant symptoms indicating extensive burn involvement. Acids are more likely to produce gastric burns than esophageal burns, and the institution of corticosteroid therapy may be of some value in preventing stricture and scarring development.

ALKALIES

Strong alkaline substances are found in such products as Drano, Liquid Plum'r, and Clinitest Tablets, all of which contain compounds such as sodium hypochlorite, sodium hydroxide, or potassium hydroxide. Experience has shown that strongly basic substances such as these are more likely to produce more severe injuries than are seen with acidic caustic ingestions. Recent experience has determined that the chlorinated bleaches, which contain a 3 to 6 percent concentration of sodium hypochlorite, are not as toxic as formerly thought. Following an ingestion of sodium hypochlorite, this compound interacts with the acidic milieu of the stomach, producing hypochlorous acid, which has irritant properties to the mucous membranes and skin. More serious problems are presented following ingestions of compounds such as Drano, which can cause burns of the skin, mucous membranes, and eyes almost immediately on contact. However, the absence of any evidence of burns, irritation, erythema, or other such signs in the oral or circumoral area does not necessarily indicate that esophageal or other involvement does not exist. There have been cases demonstrating the absence of oral involvement with subsequent esophagoscopy proving esophageal burns. Edema of the epiglottis may result in respiratory distress, and inhalation of fumes may result in pulmonary edema or pneumonitis. Shock may occur.

Alkaline caustic exposures require immediate irrigation of the affected areas with large amounts of water. Exposures to the eyes require irrigation for a minimum of 20 to 30 minutes and may require instillation of a local anesthetic to treat the blepharospasm. Oral ingestions require immediate dilution therapy with water or milk. Antiquated antidotes such as vinegar or lemon juice are absolutely contraindicated. Ingestion of chlorinated bleaches does not necessarily require esophagoscopy unless a large amount has been ingested or the patient is symptomatic. Institution of a three-week course of corticosteroids such as dexamethasone, in a dose of 10 mg

initially followed by 1 mg every four hours, is indicated when esophageal burns are demonstrated. Bougienage has been reported to be of some therapeutic benefit, and antibiotic therapy should be instituted if mediastinitis occurs. Further information on the treatment of alkaline poisoning can be found in the following publications: Leape et al., 1971; Haller et al., 1971; Burrington, 1974; Rumack et al., 1977.

AMPHETAMINE AND RELATED DRUGS

Stimulant drugs such as amphetamine, methylphenidate, and others can produce anxiety, hyperpyrexia, hypertension, and severe CNS stimulation. A toxic psychosis of a paranoid nature is not uncommon, especially as the patient begins to come off the "high." These tablets and capsules are used as "diet" pills even though they are clearly not effective as anorexic agents after two weeks of therapy. Street "speed" or "crystal" may contain in addition to or in lieu of amphetamine such compounds as caffeine, strychnine, or phencyclidine (PCP).

Therapy of the severely agitated patient should be directed toward tranquilization with chlorpromazine and acid diuresis to ion-trap and promote excretion (Espelin and Done, 1968). The dose of chlorpromazine should be 1 mg/kg in pure amphetamine overdose and 0.5 mg/kg if the amphetamine has been mixed with a barbiturate. A major problem with this therapy is the interaction of chlorpromazine with several street drugs such as STP, MDA, or DMT, which may produce dramatic hypotension. If the history is not definitive for amphetamine, then diazepam at 0.1 to 0.3 mg/kg as a starting intravenous dose should be administered.

Acid diuresis may be instituted with sufficient intravenous fluids to produce a urine flow of 3 to 6 ml/kg/hour. Ammonium chloride, at 75 mg/kg/dose administered intravenously four times per day, to a maximum of 6 g total dose per day, may be used. This will produce a urine with a pH range of 4.5 to 5.5.

ANTICHOLINERGICS

A number of agents may produce anticholinergic toxicity following acute overdose, and these agents include drugs such as antihistamines (e.g., Benadryl, Dramamine, Chlortrimeton), atropine, homatropine, over-the-counter sleeping medications (which contain both antihistamines and belladonna-like agents), and certain plants (e.g., jimsonweed, deadly nightshade) (Mikolich et al., 1975; Rumack et al., 1974; Bryson et al., 1978). Antihistamines are readily available in many common nonprescription products as well as prescription medications. Plants containing belladonna alkaloids such as jimsonweed are frequently used in folk medicine cures for the common cold or as an hallucinogen by thrill seekers. Patients with anticholinergic toxicity may present with atropinic symptoms including dry mouth; thirst; fixed, dilated pupils; flushed face; fever; hot, dry, red skin; and tachycardia. Speech and swallowing may be impaired in association with blurred vision. In infants, particularly those ingesting antihistamines, paradoxic excitement may occur subsequently followed by a more characteristic central nervous depression. Severe overdoses can present with hallucination-like delirium, tremors, convulsions, coma, respiratory failure, or cardiovascular collapse. Potentially fatal doses of most antihistamines have been estimated to be approximately 25 to 30 mg/kg.

Immediate treatment should include instituting emesis with syrup of ipecac or lavage followed by administration of activated charcoal and saline cathartics. In ingestions of antihistamines related to the phenothiazines or in massive ingestions, induced emesis may be ineffective. Development of severe symptoms such as convulsions, coma, or hypotension presents an immediate indication for physostigmine therapy in a dose of 0.5 to 2 mg, administered intravenously which can be repeated every 30 minutes as needed (Rumack, 1973). Physostigmine dramatically reverses the central and peripheral signs of anticholinergic toxicity, which are usually not seen with other cholinergic antagonists such as neostigmine since they do not cross the blood-brain barrier and enter the central nervous system (Rumack, 1973). Measures such as forced diuresis and dialysis have not yet been shown to be effective in treating severe anticholinergic poisonings.

BENZODIAZEPINES

Benzodiazepine agents are widely prescribed in the treatment of anxiety and nervousness. In fact, in 1976 and 1977, the no. 1 prescribed drug in the United States was Valium. A large number of congeners have been marketed by the pharmaceutical industry with little, if any, significant differences between the agents. Available products include chlordiazepoxide (Librium), clonazepam (Clonopin), flurazepam (Dalmane), lorapezam (Atvian), and oxazepam (Serax). Although their pharmacologic effects do not differ greatly in terms of their clinical application, there are some minor differences with respect to their pharmacokinetics. Chlordiazepoxide and oxazepam have shorter half-life values than the other agents such as diazepam and flurazepam. Following acute overdose, clinical symptoms or manifestations may include sleepiness, which,

following larger overdoses, can progress or range from stage-zero to stage-one coma. Initially, excitement may be seen as a result of the disinhibition effects of these drugs, which then progresses to central nervous system depression, hypotension, respiratory depression, and coma (Welch et al., 1977). On occasion, anticholinergic symptoms such as dry mouth, tachycardia, dilated pupils, and absent bowel sounds may be seen. Patients who have been receiving or ingesting benzodiazepines on a chronic basis (40 to 80 mg or more per day for one to two months or more) may exhibit mild to moderate symptoms of withdrawal, with severe withdrawal symptoms seen in patients taking the drug for many months to years. Symptoms may include jitteriness, nervousness, anxiety, agitation, confusion, hallucinations, and seizures. Patients exhibiting withdrawal symptoms should be reinstituted on benzodiazepine and slowly withdrawn over a period of several months (Rifkin and Floyd, 1976). In most cases, ingestions of a benzodiazepine agent alone of up to 1.5 g results in only minor toxicity, i.e., CNS depression. Fatality, following oral ingestion, is rare unless a combination of drugs is taken with benzodiazepine (Greenblatt et al., 1978). Therapeutic levels of diazepam or chlordiazepoxide are reported to be about 0.5 mg/100 ml.

Treatment of benzodiazepam overdose is primarily supportive. Establishment of respiration with assisted ventilation if necessary should be instituted immediately. Emesis should be considered unless the patient is comatose, convulsing, or has lost his gag reflex. If these contraindications exist, the patient may be intubated and lavaged followed by administration of activated charcoal and a saline cathartic such as sodium or magnesium sulfate. Hypotension, if it occurs, should be treated initially with fluid. Institution of vasopressor agents should be used only if the patient is unresponsive to other measures. Physostigmine has been reported to be effective in treating diazepam overdose; however, since this type of drug overdose has been associated with morbidity and essentially no mortality, there is no clinical indication for the use of physostigmine unless the patient has also ingested anticholinergic substances and is demonstrating cardiac arrhythmias, hypertension, and/or convulsions. Forced diuresis and dialysis are of no value in the treatment of benzodiazepine overdoses.

CYANIDE

Cyanide is commonly found in certain rat and pest poisons, silver and metal polishes, photographic solutions, and fumigating products. Compounds such as potassium cyanide can also be readily purchased from chemical stores. Cyanide is readily absorbed from all routes, including the skin, mucous membranes, and by inhalation, although alkali salts of cyanide are toxic only when ingested. Death may occur with ingestion of even small amounts of sodium or potassium cyanide and can occur within minutes or hours depending on route of exposure. Inhalation of toxic fumes represents a potentially rapidly fatal type of exposure. Sodium nitroprusside (Smith and Kruszyna, 1974) and apricot seeds (Sayre and Kaymakcalan, 1964) have also caused cyanide poisoning. A blood cyanide level of greater than 0.2 μg/ml is considered toxic. Lethal cases have usually had levels above 1 μg/ml. Clinically, cyanide poisoning is reported to produce a bitter, almond odor on the breath of the patient; however, only a small proportion of the population is genetically able to discern this characteristic odor. Typically, cyanide has a bitter, burning taste, and following poisoning, symptons of salivation, nausea without vomiting anxiety, confusion, vertigo, giddiness, lower jaw stiffness, convulsions, opisthotonos, paralysis, coma, cardiac arrhythmias, and transient respiratory stimulation followed by respiratory failure may occur. Bradycardia is a common finding, but in most cases heartbeat usually outlasts respirations (Wexler et al., 1947). A prolonged expiratory phase is considered to be characteristic of cyanide poisoning.

Artificial respiration should be started immediately in patients with respiratory difficulty or apnea. Administration of 1 to 2 ampules of amyl nitrite by inhalation to the patient for 15 to 30 seconds every minute should be instituted concurrently while preparing sodium nitrite for intravenous administration (Chen and Rose, 1952). Amyl nitrite has the ability to induce methemoglobin, which has a higher affinity for cyanide than hemoglobin; however, amyl nitrite alone is not adequate to maintain or attain desirable methemoglobin levels (Stewart, 1974). The Lilly cyanide kit (Lilly stock no. M76) contains ampules of amyl nitrite, sodium nitrite, and sodium thiosulfate with appropriate instructions. Sodium nitrite, 300 mg intravenously, should be administered to adults. However, doses this high should not be administered to children, as potentially fatal methemoglobinemia may result (Berlin, 1970). Children weighing less than 25 kg must be dosed on the basis of their hemoglobin levels. In the absence of immediate serum hemoglobin levels, a dose of 10 mg/kg is considered safe (Berlin, 1970). Once intravenous sodium nitrite is administered, sodium thiosulfate should be immediately given. Thiosulfate combines with available cyanide to form thiocyanate, which is then readily excreted

(Stewart, 1974; Chen and Rose, 1952). Oxygen should also be given since it increases the effects of the nitrites and the thiosulfate. Oxygen therapy should be maintained during and after thiosulfate therapy to ensure adequate oxygenation of the blood. A hemoglobin level of greater than 50 percent is an indication for exchange transfusion or administration of blood. Since cyanide toxicity may reoccur, the patient should be observed for no less than 24 to 48 hours, and reoccurrence is an indication for retreatment with sodium nitrite and sodium thiosulfate in one-half the recommended doses. Some data indicate that the use of cobalt compounds such as hydroxocobalamin or dicobalt edetate (Kelocyanor) may be of value in the treatment of cyanide poisoning (Hillman et al., 1974; Bain and Knowles, 1967; Paulet, 1965). However, experience in the United States with these compounds is limited and most of the data available are in the foreign literature. Further clinical experience is required to evaluate the role of these agents in the treatment of cyanide poisoning.

DIGITALIS GLYCOSIDES

Digitalis glycosides are available in prescription medications as digoxin (Lanoxin) and digitoxin as well as through a number of plant sources (oleander, foxglove). Many ingestions of digitalis occur in infants who inadvertently get into a grandparent's heart medication, although the drug has been used on occasion by persons with suicidal intent. Acute toxic manifestations of the digitalis glycosides represent extensions of the compound's vagal effects. Clinical manifestations seen in the acute overdose include nausea, vomiting, bradycardia, heart block, cardiac arrhythmia, and cardiac arrest. Younger individuals without significant heart disease tend to present with bradycardia and heart block, while other patients may present with ventricular arrhythmias, with or without heart block (Ekins and Watanabe, 1978). While hypokalemia is a frequent hallmark associated with chronic digitalis poisoning, in the acute-overdose situation hyperkalemia is more frequently found. Serum digoxin levels in excess of 5 mcg/liter (ng/ml) are often seen.

Emesis or lavage is indicated followed by administration of activated charcoal with saline cathartics. Potassium administration is contraindicated unless there is documented hypokalemia since potassium administration with unsuspected concurrent digitalis-induced hyperkalemia in the overdose situation may result in heart block progressing to sinus arrest. Patients should be monitored by ECG and antiarrhythmics instituted for the treatment of arrhythmias. Phenytoin (Dilantin) is considered to be the antiarrhythmic

the contaminated environment. Decontamination may be achieved by using soap washings followed by alcohol-soap washings using tincture of green soap. Rescuers and medical personnel should also be protected from contamination by use of rubber gloves and aprons.

Maintaining adequate respiratory function should be the first treatment measure taken. In cases of ingestion, emesis is indicated unless the patient is comatose, convulsing, or has lost the gag reflex. This should be followed by administration of activated charcoal and sodium or magnesium sulfate as a cathartic. Atropine is the drug of first choice (especially in patients with respiratory problems) and should be administered until signs of atropinism occur, i.e., dry mouth, tachycardia. In some cases, large doses (up to 2 g of atropine) may be required in order to reverse cholinergic excess. The presence of significant cholinesterase depression in red blood cells requires treatment with 2-PAM in conjunction with atropine. In an adult a dose of 1 g intravenously administered at a rate of 500 mg/minute should be given and repeated every 8 to 12 hours. After administration of three doses of 2-PAM, the drug is not likely to be of any additional benefit. The pediatric dose is 250 mg/dose administered slowly by the intravenous route and repeated every 8 to 12 hours. The use of aminophylline/theophylline, succinylcholine, physostigmine, and morphine is contraindicated.

Carbamates

Carbamate insecticides include agents such as aminocarb, carbaryl (Sevin), and landrin. These insecticides are reversible inhibitors of cholinesterase, whose actions are often enhanced by formulating them with pyrethrin or piperonyl butoxide. Clinical manifestations are those seen with cholinesterase inhibition but may not be identical to the signs and symptoms seen with organophosphate poisoning. However, with carbamate exposure the degree of toxicity is considered less severe due to the rapid reversal of the cholinesterase inhibition. Symptoms such as headache, blurred vision, weakness, sweating, myosis, chest pain or tightness, salivation, lacrimation, nausea, vomiting, urination, abdominal cramps, and diarrhea may occur. More severe exposure may result in muscle cramps, fasciculations, pulmonary edema, areflexia, and convulsions. Blood cholinesterase activity can be measured but may not show significant depression unless blood samples are drawn and assayed immediately due to rapid cholinesterase regeneration. Atropine in large doses for maintenance of airway and respiration is the treatment of choice, dosed initially at 2 mg intravenously in an adult and 0.05 mg/kg intravenously in a child, with the

drug repeated at five- to ten-minute intervals if needed. The patient should be thoroughly decontaminated and other measures instituted to prevent absorption. Again care must be exercised to protect rescuers and medical personnel from exposure. 2-PAM is usually not needed due to the rapid regeneration of cholinesterase and is considered to be contraindicated in certain carbamate poisonings, e.g., carbaryl. Data for this contraindication are questionable.

IRON

Iron is available in a wide variety of preparations including iron supplement tablets (ferrous sulfate, ferrous gluconate, ferrous fumarate), multiple-vitamin preparations, and prenatal vitamin preparations. As described on the labels of these preparations, iron may be given in terms of a milligram amount of the salt form (e.g., ferrous sulfate 300 mg or ferrous gluconate 320 mg) or by the actual amount of elemental iron. It is important to note that iron toxicity relates to the amount of *elemental* iron and, therefore, for the salt forms the actual elemental iron content must be calculated.

SALT FORM	% ELEMENTAL IRON
Ferrous fumarate	33
Ferrous gluconate	12
Ferrous sulfate (exsiccated)	30
Ferrous sulfate	20

Clinically, there are generally five phases of toxicity subsequent to ingestion of iron. The first phase lasts from 30 minutes to two hours after ingestion and may be characterized by symptoms of lethargy, restlessness, hematemesis, abdominal pain, and bloody diarrhea. Necrosis of the gastrointestinal mucosa is a result of the direct corrosive effect of iron to the tissue and may result in severe hemorrhagic necrosis with development of shock. Iron absorbed through intact mucosa may also cause shock. The second phase presents as an apparent recovery period, which then progresses into the third phase. This third phase occurs 2 to 12 hours after the first phase and is characterized by the onset of shock, acidosis, cyanosis, and fever. Acidosis results from the release of hydrogen ion from the conversion of ferric (Fe + 3) to ferrous (Fe + 2) ion forms and accumulation of lactic and citric acids. The fourth phase occurs two to four days after ingestion and is sometimes characterized by the development of hepatic necrosis, which is thought to be due to a direct toxic action of iron on mitochondia. The fifth phase occurs from two to four weeks after ingestion and is characterized by gastrointestinal obstruction, which is secondary to gastric or pyloric scarring and healed tissue. Oral ingestion of iron is a potentially fatal occurrence, and ingestions of over 30 mg/kg body weight should be considered for hospital admission for observation depending on clinical symptoms and findings (Stein *et al.*, 1976).

Emesis or lavage with a large-bore tube is indicated. Abdominal x-rays may reveal full tablets or tablet fragments in the gastrointestinal fract since they are radiopaque. Fleet phosphate enema solution is the preferred lavage solution since when given orally and diluted in a 1:4 concentration this will result in the formation of a nonabsorbable iron phosphate complex. However, excessive use (more than 60 ml) of the enema solution may result in hypernatremia, hyperphosatemia, and hypokalemia. The use of deferoxamine is considered somewhat controversial since this drug may induce severe hypotension following oral doses. When used, the dose is 2 to 10 g of deferoxamine dissolved in 25 ml of lavage fluid followed by a second dose of 50 percent of the initial dose in four hours and a similar third dose in 8 to 12 hours. If free iron is present in serum and the patient is exhibiting shock, or coma, or if the serum iron is greater than 350 mcg/ml intravenously, deferoxamine should be administered at a rate not to exceed 15 mg/kg/hour for eight hours followed by 5 mg/kg/hour if needed (Stein *et al.*, 1976). If the patient is not in shock, deferoxamine may be administered intramuscularly (20 mg/kg every four to six hours), depending on the clinical condition. Shock and dehydration should be treated with appropriate fluid therapy (Robertson, 1971).

LOMOTIL

Lomotil is a frequently prescribed antidiarrheal preparation that contains 2.5 mg of the narcotic diphenoxylate and 0.025 mg of atropine per tablet or 5 ml of liquid. The atropine is allegedly included in the dosage form to discourage abuse since the dose per tablet or teaspoon is essentially homeopathic. However, in the overdose situation, the clinical picture is often a mixture of that seen for narcotics and atropine overdosage, with early findings primarily due to atropine toxicity. The atropinic symptoms seen may include flushing, lethargy, hyperpyrexia, tachycardia, urinary retention, reduced bowel motility, and hallucinations. Mydriasis, although expected, is often not seen due to the narcotic effects of diphenoxylate, and pinpoint pupils may be noted. Cyclic coma has been seen in some cases and is probably due to changes in gastrointestinal motility with subsequent absorption of the drug (Snyder *et al.*, 1973). In many cases, there may be a delay in the onset

of toxicity and/or coma of up to 6 to 12 hours even in the face of appropriate therapy such as emesis. Patients, particularly pediatric patients, should be monitored for a minimum of 12 to 24 hours, depending on the history of the ingestion (Rumack and Temple, 1974; Rosenstein *et al.*, 1973).

Establishment of respiratory support as necessary and measures to prevent absorption should be instituted immediately. If the patient is comatose or convulsing, endotracheal intubation should be instituted followed by gastric lavage and administration of activated charcoal and saline cathartics. Forced diuresis does not appear to enhance the elimination of diphenoxalate (Rumack and Temple, 1974) and fluid should be administered cautiously to avoid cerebral edema, which is particularly frequent in patients with anoxic episodes (Ginsberg, 1973). Naloxone in a dose of 0.005 mg/kg administered intravenously is the drug of choice, and it should be administered at frequent intervals in order to maintain a therapeutic effect since the duration of naloxone's effect is less than that of the opiate. In some cases, up to 11 to 13 doses of Narcan have been administered in order to reverse opiate effects (Rumack and Temple, 1974). Physostigmine should be considered in the face of severe anticholinergic toxicity.

MERCURY

Mercury in its various forms is available widely in the forms of metallic mercury (thermometers, Miller-Abbott tubes), fungicides, paints, mercurial drugs, and antiquated cathartics and ointments. Poisoning may occur from either chronic or acute exposure to such agents or through the food chain (Eyl, 1971; Teitelbaum and Ott, 1969). Toxicity of the mercury is primarily related to its form since metallic mercury is relatively nontoxic unless it is converted to an ionized form, such as occurs on exposure to acids or strong oxidants. In general, the mercuric salts are more soluble and produce more serious poisoning than do the mercurous salts (Goldwater, 1957; Shoemaker, 1957). Inorganic forms of mercury are corrosive and produce symptoms of metallic taste, burning, irritation, salivation, vomiting, diarrhea, upper gastrointestinal tract edema, abdominal pain, and hemorrhage. These effects are seen acutely and may subside with subsequent lower gastrointestinal ulceration (Goldwater, 1957). Large ingestions of the mercurial salts may produce kidney damage, which may present with nephrosis, oliguria, and anuria. Ingestion of organic mercurials such as ethylmercury may produce symptoms of nausea, vomiting, abdominal pain, and diarrhea, but in most cases the main toxicity is neurologic involvement presenting with paresthesias, visual disturbances, mental disturbances, hallucinations, ataxia, hearing defects, stupor, coma, and death. Symptoms may occur for several weeks after exposure. Exposure and poisoning can occur following ingestion of mercury-contaminated seafood, grains, or inhalation of vaporized organomercurials. Chronic inorganic mercury poisoning may occur following repeated environmental exposure and may present with a neurologic syndrome often described as the "mad hatter syndrome."

Therapy should be initiated with emesis or lavage followed by administration of activated charcoal and a saline cathartic. Milk may be administered to help precipitate the mercury compound. Blood and urine levels of mercury may be of value in determining the indication of administration of chelating agents such as D-pencillamine or dimercaprol (BAL) (Kark, 1971). D-Penicillamine is administered in a dose of 250 mg orally four times a day in adults, 100 mg/kg/day in children, to a maximum recommended dose of 1 g per day for three to ten days with continuous monitoring of mercury urinary excretion. In patients who cannot tolerate penicillamine, BAL can be administered in a dose of 3 to 5 mg/kg/dose every four hours by deep intramuscular injection for the first two days followed by 2.5 to 3 mg/kg/dose intramuscularly every six hours for two days followed by 2.5 to 3 mg/kg/dose every 12 hours intramuscularly for one week. Adverse reactions associated with BAL administration such as urticaria can often be controlled with antihistamines such as diphenhydramine. The development of renal failure contraindicates penicillamine therapy since the kidney is the main route of renal excretion for penicillin. BAL therapy can be used cautiously in spite of renal failure since BAL is excreted in the bile; however, BAL toxicity, which consists of fever, rash, hypertension, and CNS stimulation, must be closely monitored. Dialysis does not remove either chelated or free mercury metal (Robillard et al., 1976).

NARCOTIC OPIATES

Narcotic overdose may occur in a number of different situations in addition to drug addiction such as in the newborn infant. Accidental or intentional overdoses frequently involve Lomotil, Darvon, Talwin, morphine, or dextromethorphan. Acute overdoses of any narcotic drug may result in respiratory arrest and coma with an initial clinical presentation of pinpoint pupils, hypertension, bradycardia, and respiratory depression, urinary retention, muscle spasm, and itching. Propoxyphene overdose has been associated with convulsions (Lovejoy et al., 1974). Other symptoms such as leukocytosis, hyperpyrexia, and pulmonary edema may occur, particularly in drug abusers injecting street drugs intravenously. Ingestions of methadone or propoxyphene may have a prolonged or protracted clinical course lasting 24 to 48 hours or more. Chronic narcotic use is often associated with skin abscesses, cellulitis, endocarditis, myoglobinuria, cardiac arrhythmias, tetanus, and thrombophlebitis. Lomotil ingestion is frequently complicated by the presence of atropine in the proprietary dosage forms with a resultant mixed picture of narcotic and anticholinergic symptoms (Rumack and Temple, 1974).

Emesis or lavage should always be performed since delayed gastric emptying is common following narcotic ingestions (Rumack and Temple, 1974). Emesis can be induced in the alert patient; however, if seizures or coma exist, intubation and gastric lavage with a large-bore (28-French or larger) Ewald tube should be carried out. Activated charcoal, five or ten times the estimated weight of ingested drug (minimum of 10 g), as well as a nonabsorbable saline cathartic (sodium sulfate or magnesium sulfate, 250 mg/kg of body weight) should be instilled following emesis or lavage. The cathartic should be repeated every three to four hours until stooling has occurred. Other basic supportive measures should be provided as needed. Naloxone at a dose of 0.005 mg/kg intravenously is a drug of choice for all narcotic ingestions including pentazocine and propoxyphene as well as methadone, morphine, and codeine (Martin, 1976). In some cases doses of naloxone as high as 24 mg may be required, and there is little evidence that such doses of naloxone are associated with any ill effects. Due to the short duration of action of naloxone (60 to 90 minutes) (Evans et al., 1974), repeated doses of naloxone may be necessary until the narcotic is metabolized, particularly in the treatment of methadone overdoses (Aranol et al., 1972; Frand et al., 1972). In some cases of narcotic overdose, up to 20 mg of naloxone may be required (Moore et al., 1978). Other narcotic antagonists such as nalorphine (Nalline) and levallorphan (Lorfan) possess narcotic antagonistic effects, i.e., respiratory depressant effects (Foldes et al., 1969), and are no longer recommended.

PHENCYCLIDINE (PCP)

Phencyclidine, which is commonly called PCP, was originally developed as an anesthetic for humans but was abandoned due to its postoperative side effects, i.e., hallucinations and agitation. It is now legally available as a veterinary medication for use as an animal tranquilizer. It is also known by various street names: angel dust, dust, embalming fluid, elephant or horse tranquilizer, killer weed, super weed, monkey dust, peace pill, rocket fuel, and hog. It is frequently sold as THC (tetrahydrocannabinol), but may appear also as mescaline, psilocybin, LSD, amphetamine, and cocaine. It is closely related to the anesthetic ketamine (Ketalar), and both agents produce what has been called disassociative anesthesia. Due to the availability and ease of manufacture, there has been an increased use of PCP, particularly in the teenage population where it is ingested orally, smoked, or snorted. Intravenous use is less common but on occasion has been reported. Clinical manifestations from phencyclidine use include symptoms of excitation with marked paranoid or aggressive behavior, which is frequently characterized as self-destructive. Characteristically, nystagmus, both horizontal and vertical, is noted in association with ataxia, impaired speech, bizarre behavior, tachycardia, hypertension that may progress to later stages of hypotension, increased reflexes, seizures, respiratory depression, and coma (Bolter, 1970; Tong et al., 1975). The sensations that the user may feel subsequent to PCP ingestion are feelings of depersonalization, distortion of body image, a sense of distance and estrangement from the environment in association with time expansion, and slowed body movements. Phencyclidine can be analyzed in serum, urine, and gastric contents.

Initial management of phencyclidine ingestion requires isolation of the patient from all sensory stimuli such as noise, lights, and touch (Stein, 1973). Provision of a quiet, supportive, and non-threatening environment may help reduction of psychotomimetic effects from bad trips. Therapy by talking the patient down with continual verbal reassurance in many cases may be all that is required. Extremely agitated or convulsing patients should be protected from self-inflicted harm and given diazepam intravenously in 2- to 3-mg increments. In severe cases with hypotension this should be treated with use of plasma expanders before vasopressors are attempted. Diazoxide has been used with good success in hypertensive crisis secondary to phencyclidine (Eastman and Cohen, 1975). Gastric lavage or gastric dialysis has been suggested to be of benefit in capturing PCP excreted into the stomach. Acidification of the urine in association with forced diuresis may hasten renal elimination of phencyclidine (Done et al., 1977).

PHENOTHIAZINES

The phenothiazine class of antipsychotic agents includes a broad class of drugs with similar therapeutic effects. Individual agents depending on the class of phenothiazine (aliphatic, piperidine, or piperazine) differ primarily in their milligram potencies and their tendencies to produce extrapyramidal symptoms, sedation, and hypotension. Agents such as fluphenazine (Prolixin) and trifluoperazine (Stelazine) have a high tendency to produce extrapyramidal effects, while chlorpromazine (Thorazine) and thioridazine (Mellaril) have a lesser tendency to produce extrapyramidal effects but a higher tendency to produce sedation and hypotension. Two other classes of antipsychotic drugs that are non-phenothiazine-related include butyrophenones such as haloperidol (Haldol) and the thioxanthine class such as chlorprothixene (Taractane) and thiothexene (Navane). These non-phenothiazine-class drugs have a higher tendency to produce extrapyramidal symptoms over sedation and hypotension. These drugs possess significant anticholinergic, alpha-adrenergic blocking, quinidine-like, and extrapyramidal effects. In addition, phenothiazines also lower the seizure threshold (Logothetis, 1967). Overdose with these drugs may result in CNS depression, which can present initially with reduced activity, emotional quieting, and affective indifference, although such patients may also exhibit a period of agitation, hyperactivity, or convulsions prior to the depressed state (Hollister, 1966). Hyperthermia or hypothermia may develop due to phenothiazine's effects on the temperature-regulating mechanisms at the hypothalamus. Tachycardia with hypotension as a result of anticholinergic and alpha-blocking effects may occur. In addition, widening of the QRS complex due to the "quinidine-like" effect of these drugs can occur and may result in ventricular tachycardia. Extrapyramidal symptoms, present as torticollis, stiffening of the body, spasticity, impaired speech, and opisthotonos, may occur. These symptoms may frequently occur in children who have been administered prochlorperazine (Compazine) in the treatment of nausea and vomiting.

Emesis or lavage is indicated, followed by administration of activated charcoal and a saline cathartic. Phenothiazines are radiopaque, and unabsorbed drug in the form of full or partial tablets may be visualized in the gastrointestinal tract by abdominal x-ray (Barry et al., 1973). Development of convulsions should be treated with intravenous diazepam in a dose of 0.1 to 3 mg/kg in pediatric patients and 5 to 10 mg in an adult. Hypotension requires the use of a pure alpha agonist such as norepinephrine (levarternol or Levophed) since administration of epinephrine may cause hypotension. Dialysis is ineffective in removing phenothiazine since these drugs are highly tissue bound. Cardiac arrhythmias may respond to the use of phenytoin (Dilantin) or lidocaine in patients with refractory arrhythmias; a cardiac pacemaker may be required. Extrapyramidal reactions are usually adequately treated by the use of intravenous diphenhydramine (Benadryl) in a dose of 1 to 5 mg/kg (Davies, 1970). Hypothermia or hyperthermia should be treated appropriately. Drugs that can potentiate the depressant effect on phenothiazine, such as barbiturates, sedatives, alcohol, narcotics, and anesthetics, are best avoided.

SALICYLATES

Accidental or intentional ingestion of salicylates by children and adults continues to represent a major poisoning problem due to the high incidence of use of these compounds, their widespread availability, their numerous proprietary and nonproprietary products and preparations, and their mass promotion through advertising media. Most salicylate poisonings involve the use of aspirin or acetylsalicylic acid, although other serious salicylate exposures may result from such compounds as oil of wintergreen (methylsalicylate). Generally, ingestion of doses larger than 150 mg/kg (or 1.0 gr/lb) can produce toxic symptoms such as tinnitus, deafness, nausea, and vomiting. Serious toxicity can be seen with ingestions greater than 400 mg/kg (approximately 3 gr/lb), with symptoms of severe vomiting, hyperventilation, hyperthermia, convulsions, coma, hyper- or hypoglycemia, and acid-base disturbances such as respiratory alkalosis or metabolic acidosis (Gabow et al., 1978; Pierce, 1974). In severe cases, the clinical course may progress to pulmonary edema, hemorrhage, acute renal failure, oliguria, or death (Anderson et al., 1976). It is important to note that the salicylate-overdosed patient can progress to a more serious condition with time as additional drug is absorbed from the gastrointestinal tract. Chronic salicylism presents clinically in a similar fashion to the acute situation, although it is often associated with a higher morbidity and mortality as well as a more pronounced acidosis, hypokalemia, dehydration or fluid retention, and hyperpyrexia. Although acute overdoses may be associated with salicylate levels of 25 to 35 mg/100 ml or more, chronic salicylism can result in death at lower salicylate levels, i.e., 10 to 15 mg/100 ml or less. It is important to remember that the kinetics of salicylates are dose dependent, and at higher serum concentrations of salicylate the drug's half-life may be prolonged, i.e., 15 to 30 hours. The Done nomogram (Fig. 27–2) can be utilized as an aid in interpreting a given salicylate level as

long as the blood sample was not drawn prior to six hours after ingestion. In addition, the Done nomogram is not useful in cases of chronic salicylism. Salicylates are exceptionally sensitive to pH changes, with resulting ionization changes having a pronounced effect on disposition in the body. Acidosis, which is a common finding in acute salicylate overdose, can result in a larger percentage of the drug distributing into the central nervous system. Similarly, alkalinization of the urine results in ion trapping of salicylate in the kidney tubule, causing greater urinary excretion (Hill, 1973).

Emesis should be initiated unless the patient is comatose, convulsing, or has lost the gag reflex. If these contraindications exist, intubation should proceed with gastric lavage, using a large-bore tube such as a 36 French. Subsequently, activated charcoal should be administered followed by saline cathartics to hasten the elimination of any unabsorbed drugs through the gastrointestinal tract. Alkalinization of the urine can result in a

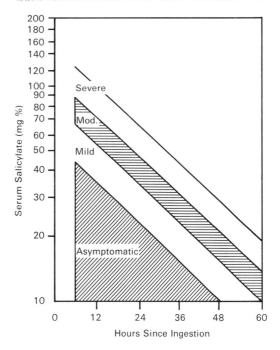

Figure 27–2. Done nomogram for salicylate poisoning. Cautions for use of chart: (1) The patient has taken a single acute ingestion and is not suffering from chronic toxicity. (2) The blood level to be plotted on the nomogram was drawn six hours after ingestion. (3) Levels in the toxic range drawn before six hours should be treated. (4) Levels in the nontoxic range drawn before six hours should be repeated to see if the level is increasing. (From Done, A. K.: Pediatrics, 26:805, 1960. Copyright American Academy of Pediatrics, 1960.)

Table 27-4. SEDATIVE HYPNOTICS

DRUG	Vd (% BODY WEIGHT)	PROTEIN BINDING, (%)	pKa	PEAK CONCERN TIME, (hr)	T1/2, (hr)	THERAPEUTIC BLOOD LEVEL	MAJOR ROUTE OF ELIMINATION	DIURESIS	DIALYSIS	HEMOPERFUSION
Long-acting barbiturates										
Phenobarbital	75	20	7.41	1–6	48–96 (overdose)	10–20 μg/ml	20–40% excreted unchanged; remainder metabolized	Alkaline	Yes	Yes
Short-acting barbiturates										
Pentobarbital	200–300	30	8.1	0.5–2	36	50 μg/ml	Metabolism	No	No	No
Secobarbital	200–300	45	7.9	0.5–2	24					
Benzodiazepines										
Diazepam	100–200	90			25–30	<0.5 mg/100 ml	Metabolism	No	No	Yes
Chlordiazepoxide	25	90			7–15					
Chloral hydrate	25	40–80 for trichlor-ethanol	6.8		6–9	10–15 μg/ml	Metabolism to active metabolite	Yes	No	Yes
Ethclorvynol	600	50	8.7	1	100 (overdose)	<100 μg	Metabolism	No	No	No
Glutethimide	—	—	4.52	—	40 (overdose)	—	Metabolism to active metabolite	No	No	?
Meprobamate	75	10–20	9.2	1–2	8	<4 mg/100 ml	Metabolism with 25–50% excreted unchanged	Yes	Yes	Yes
Methyprylon	>100	?	7.1	1/2–1	3–6	<1 mg/100 ml	Metabolism	No	No	?
Methaqualone	100–200	?	—	1–4	2–3	<2 mg/100 ml	Metabolism	No	?	Yes

tenfold increase in a drug's excretion by increasing urinary pH from 6.5 to 7.5. Hypokalemia secondary to respiratory alkalosis induced by salicylate poisoning should be corrected, since this condition may make alkalinization of urine difficult.

Acetazolamide (Diamox) is not indicated for urine alkalization since this drug may contribute to metabolic acidosis. Hemodialysis, peritoneal dialysis, exchange transfusion, and hemoperfusion can be effective in removing salicylate from blood compartments but are indicated in only severe cases. Adequate fluid therapy should be instituted to prevent dehydration and to correct electrolyte imbalances. Should hemorrhagic complications in association with a prolonged prothrombin time occur, vitamin K_1 or phytonadione is indicated. It is important to note that salicylate may cause coagulation defects due to platelet effects that will not be responsive to vitamin K administration (Pierce, 1974). The patient's serum electrolytes, renal function, and cardiac status should be monitored. If hyperpyrexia occurs, appropriate treatment measures should be instituted (Hill, 1973).

SEDATIVE-HYPNOTICS

Sedative hypnotics include a wide range of pharmacologic agents used in the treatment of anxiety, nervousness, and sleep disorders. The most widely known agents are the barbiturates (short acting and long acting), benzodiazopines, chloral hydrate, ethchlorvynol (Placidyl), meprobamate (Miltown), methyprylon (Noludar), glutethimide (Doriden), and methaqualone (Quaalude). These agents have the propensity following chronic overuse or abuse to cause physical addiction, and the possibility of physical withdrawal symptoms should be considered in the treatment of patients overdosed on sedative-hypnotics. Table 27–4 compares some of the different pharmacokinetic properties of the more commonly used agents. Patients presenting with sedative-hypnotic overdose may manifest symptoms of confusion, poor coordination, ataxia, respiratory distress, apnea, and coma. Barbiturate overdose cases may present characteristically with "barb burns" or clear vesicular bullous skin lesions appearing on the hands, buttocks, and between the knees (Groschel et al., 1970). Glutethimide may present with a clinical course characterized by an unusually prolonged coma or cyclic coma with periods of alternating unconsciousness and wakefulness (Decker et al., 1970). Much of the severity of this drug's toxicity is related to its metabolism to and accumulation of a metabolite that has a long half-life and is twice as potent as the present agent, 4-hydroxyglutethimide (Hansen et al., 1975). Gastric drug mass or drug bezoar formation has been reported, particularly in association with sedative-hypnotic agents that are poorly soluble in water (Schwartz, 1976). In such cases, gastrotomy has been required to surgically remove drug bezoars.

In the vast majority of sedative-hypnotic overdoses, conservative treatment represents the most successful approach to managing such patients. If the patient is conscious, vomiting may be indicated, although in many cases gastric lavage followed by administration of activated charcoal and saline cathartics is required to terminate the exposure. Maintaining a patent airway, providing adequate ventilation, and control of hypotension and other supportive measures are the mainstays of therapy. In some cases, such as with phenobarbital, forced alkaline diuresis has been shown to be of benefit to hasten elimination of the drug. For lipid-soluble drugs such as glutethimide, methaqualone, and ethchlorvynol, dialysis procedures have not been shown to be effective. Results from lipid dialysis of these agents are equivocal. Some data suggest that meprobamate may be adequately treated in severe cases with the use of diuresis and/or dialysis, while chloral hydrate may be significantly removed by hemodialysis (Stalker et al., 1978). Analeptics or other stimulants (e.g., caffeine) have never been shown to be of any value and are therefore contraindicated. In sedative-hypnotic overdose, patients may develop pulmonary edema or shock that should be treated appropriately.

TRICYCLIC ANTIDEPRESSANTS

The tricyclic antidepressants are available in a wide variety of brands, including amitriptyline (Elavil), doxepin (Sinequan), and imipramine (Tofranil), and in combination with phenothiazine drugs in Triavil and Etrafon. Tricyclic antidepressants have three primary pharmacologic actions, including anticholinergic effects, reuptake blockade of catecholamines at the adrenergic neuronal site, and quinidine-like effects on the cardiac tissue. Tricyclic antidepressant overdose represents a life-threatening episode. Initial symptoms seen are those of central nervous system depression with manifestations of lethargy, disorientation, ataxia, respiratory depression, hypothermia, and agitation. Severe toxicity may be associated with hallucinations, deep tendon reflex loss, muscle twitching, coma, and convulsions. Anticholinergic or atropinic effects of these drugs include dry mouth, pyrexia, dilated pupils, urinary retention, tachycardia, and reduced gastrointestinal motility, which may result in marked delay of the onset of symptoms but also allows for the institution of emesis and lavage long after ingestion to still be effective. Life-threatening sequelae of the tricyclic antidepressants are the cardiovascular effects, resulting in cardiac arrhythmias such as supraventricular tachycardia, premature ventricular contractions, ventricular tachycardia, ventricular flutter, and ventricular fibrillation that progresses to hypotension and shock. The electrocardiogram characteristically demonstrates prolonged PR interval, widening of the QRS complex, QT prolongation, T-wave flattening or inversion, ST segment depression, and varying degrees of heart block progressing to cardiac standstill (Tobis and Das, 1976). In pediatric patients, toxic effects of a tricyclic antidepressant can occur after ingestion of only one tablet. Widening of the QRS complex has been reported to correlate well with the severity of the toxicity following acute overdose ingestions (Biggs et al., 1977). Widening of the QRS complex past 100 milliseconds or greater within the first 24 hours is an indication of severe toxicity.

Emesis and lavage are indicated as appropriate, followed by administration of activated charcoal and a saline cathartic such as sodium or magnesium sulfate. Patients admitted with tricyclic antidepressant overdose but without symptoms should be monitored for a minimum of six hours to detect any possible delayed symptom onset. Vital signs and the electrocardiogram should be monitored for 48 hours in symptomatic patients since fatal cardiac arrhythmias have occurred late in the course. Hypotension should be treated with fluids and a vasopressor such as levarterenol (Levophed) administered as needed. The development of convulsions, severe hallucinations, hypotension, and cardiac arrhythmias is an indication for physostigmine use and it should be administered intravenously in adults in a therapeutic trial of 2 mg slowly followed by 1 to 2 mg. For pediatric patients the trial dose is 0.5 mg, administered slowly by the intravenous route, followed by the lowest total effective trial (Rumack, 1973). Physostigmine should be administered with caution in the presence of asthma, gangrene, cardiovascular disease, and mechanical obstructions of the gastrointestinal or urogenital tract. Cardiac arrhythmias refractory to physostigmine may be treated with phenytoin (Bigger et al., 1977). Convulsions not responding to physostigmine may be treated with intravenous diazepam.

REFERENCES

Anderson, R. J.; Potts, D. E.; Gabow, P. A.; Rumack, B. H.; and Schrier, R. W.: Unrecognized adult salicylate intoxication. Ann. Intern. Med., 85:745–48, 1976.

Aronow, R.; Shashi, D. P.; and Wooley, P. V.: Childhood poisoning and unfortunate consequences of methadone availability. J.A.M.A., 219:321–24, 1972.

Arena, J. M.; Rourke, M. H.; and Sibrach, C. D.: Acetaminophen: Report of an unusual poisoning. Pediatrics, 61:68–72, 1978.

Bain, J. T. B., and Knowles, E. L.: Successful treatment of cyanide poisoning. Br. Med. J., 2:763, 1967.

Baldochin, B. J., and Melmed, R. N.: Clinical and therapeutic aspects of kerosene poisoning: A series of 200 cases. Br. Med. J., 2:28–30, 1964.

Barry, D.; Meyskens, F. L., Jr.; and Becker, C. E.: Phenothiazine poisoning: A review of 48 cases. Cal. Med., 118:1, 1973.

Beamon, R.; Seigel, C.; and Landers, G.: Hydrocarbon ingestion in children: A six year retrospective study. J.A.C.E.P., 5:771–75, 1976.

Bergson, F.: Pneumatocoeles following hydrocarbon ingestion. Am. J. Dis. Child, 129:49–54, 1975.

Berlin, C. M., Jr.: The treatment of cyanide poisoning in Children. Pediatrics, 46:793, 1970.

Bigger, J. T.: Is physostigmine effective for cardiac toxicity of tricyclic antidepressant drugs? J.A.M.A., 273:1311, 1977.

Biggs, J. T.: Tricyclic antidepressant overdose: Incidence of symptoms. J.A.M.A., 238:135–38, 1977.

Bolter, A.: Phencyclidine (PCP) abuse. West. J. Med., 127:80, 1970.

Boylan, J. L.; Egle, J. L.; and Guzelian, P. S.: Cholestyramine: Use as a new therapeutic approach for chlordecone (Kepone) poisoning. Science, 199:893–95, 1978.

Bratton, L., and Haddow, J. E.: Ingestion of charcoal lighter fluid. J. Pediatr., 87:633–36, 1975.

Brown, J.; Burke, B.; and DaJanias, C.: Experimental kerosene pneumonia: Evaluation of some therapeutic regimens. J. Pediatr. 84:396–401, 1974.

Bryson, P. D.; Watanabe, A. S.; Rumack, B. H.; and Murphy, R. C.: Burdock root tea poisoning: Case report involving a commercial preparation. J.A.M.A., 239:2157, 1978.

Burrington, J. P.: Clinitest burns of the esophagus. Ann. Thorac. Surg., 20:400, 1974.

Chen, K. K., and Rose, C. L.: Nitrile and thiosulfate therapy in cyanide poisoning. J.A.M.A., 149:113, 1952.

Clark, R.; Borirakchanyavat, V.; Davidson, A. R.; Thompson, R. P. H.; Widdop, B.; Goulding, R.; and Williams, R.: Hepatic damage and death from overdose of paracetamal. Lancet, 1:66, 1973.

Clemmesen, C., and Nilsson, E.: Therapeutic trends in the treatment of barbiturate poisoning: The Scandinavian method. Clin. Pharmacol. Ther., 2:220–29, 1961.

Corby, D. G., and Decker, W. J.: Activated charcoal for sedative overdosage. Pediatr. Clin. North Am., 17:620, August 1970.

Curry, A. S.: The Poisoned Patient: The Role of the Laboratory. Elsevier, Amsterdam, 1974.

Davies, D. M.: Treatment of drug-induced dyskinesias. Lancet, 1:567, 1970.

Decker, W. J.: Gluthethimide rebound. Lancet, 1:778, 1970.

Done, A. K.; Aronow, R.; and Miceli, J. N.: Pharmacokinetic observation in the treatment of phencyclidine poisoning. In Rumack, B. H., and Temple, A. R. (eds.): Management of the Poisoned Patient. Science Press, Princeton, NJ, 1977.

Eastman, J. W., and Cohen, S. N.: Hypertensive crisis and death associated with phencyclidine poisoning. J.A.M.A., 231:1270–71, 1975.

Ekins, B. R., and Watanabe, A. S.: Acute digoxin poisoning: Review of therapy. Am. J. Hosp. Pharm., 35:268–77, 1978.

Elbel, H., and Schleyer, F.: In Blutalkatal: Die Wissenschaftlichen Grudlagen der Beurteilung von

Blutalkoholbefunden bei Strassenverke-Msdelkten Stutt-gart. Georg Thiene, Heidelberg, 1956, p. 226.

Espelin, D. E., and Done, A. K.: Amphetamine poisoning: Effectiveness of chlorpromazine. *N. Engl. J. Med.*, **278**:1361–65, 1968.

Evans, J. M.; Hogg, M. I. J.; Lynn, J. N.; and Rosen, M.: Degree and duration of reversal by naloxone of effects of morphine in conscious subjects. *Br. Med. J.*, **2**:589–91, 1974.

Eyl, T. B.: Organic-mercury food poisoning. *N. Engl. J. Med.*, **284**:706, 1971.

Fischer, D. S.; Parkman, R.; and Finch, S. C.: Acute iron poisoning in children. *J.A.M.A.*, **218**:1179–84, 1971.

Foldes, F. F.; Duncalf, D.; and Kuwabara, S.: The respiratory, circulatory, and narcotic antagonistic effects of nalorphine, levallorphan, and naloxone in anesthetized subjects. *Can. Anaesth. Soc. J.*, **16**:151–61, 1969.

Frand, U. I.; Chang, S. S.; and Williams, M. H., Jr.: Methadone induced pulmonary edema. *Ann. Intern. Med.*, **76**:975–79, 1972.

Gabow, P. A.; Anderson, R. J.; and Potts, D. E.: Acid-based disturbances in the salicylate-intoxicated adult. *Arch. Intern. Med.*, **138**:1481–84, 1978.

Ginsburg, C. M.: Lomotil intoxication. *Am. J. Dis. Child.*, **925**:241–42, 1973.

Greenblatt, D. J.: Rapid recovery from massive diazepam overdose. *J.A.M.A.*, **240**:872–74, 1978.

Groschel, D.; Gerstein, A. R.; and Rosenbaum, J. M.: Skin lesions as a diagnostic aid in barbiturate poisoning. *N. Engl. J. Med.*, **283**:409–10, 1970.

Haller, J. A., Jr.: Pathophysiology and management of acute corrosive burns of the esophagus. *J. Pediatr. Surg.*, **6**:578, 1971.

Hammond, R. B.; Rumack, B. H.; and Rodgerson, D. O.: Blood ethanol: A report of unusually high levels in a living patient. *J.A.M.A.*, **226**:63–64, 1973.

Hansen, A. R.; Kennedy, K. A.; Ambre, J. J.; and Fischer, L. J.: Glutethimide poisoning—a metabolite contributes to morbidity and mortality. *N. Engl. J. Med.*, **292**:250–52, 1975.

Hill, J. B.: Salicylate intoxication. *N. Engl. J. Med.*, **2–8**:1110, 1113, 1973.

Hillman, B.; Bardham, K. D.; and Bain, J. T. B.: The use of dicobalt edetate (Kelocyanor) in cyanide poisoning. *Postgrad. Med. J.*, **50**:171–74, 1974.

Hollaster, L. E.: Overdoses of psychotherapeutic drugs. *Clin. Pharmacol. Ther.*, **7**:142–46, 1966.

Kark, R. A. P.: Mercury poisoning and its treatment with N-acetyl-D, L-penicillamine. *N. Engl. J. Med.*, **285**:1, 1971.

Lambecier, M. R., and DuPan, R. M.: L'intoxication alcoolique aigue' et les accidents d'automobile. *Schweiz Med. Wochenschr.*, **76**:395–98, 421–28, 1968.

Leape, L. L.; Ashcraft, K. W.; Scarpelli, D. G.; and Holder, T. M.: Hazards to your health, liquid lye. *N. Engl. J. Med.*, **284**:578–81, 1971.

Lloyd, B. L., and Smith, T. W.: Contrasting rates of reversal of digoxin toxicity by digoxin specific IgG and Fab fragments. *Circulation*, **58**:280–83, 1978.

Logothetis, J.: Spontaneous epileptic seizures and EEG changes in the course of phenothiazine therapy. *Neurology*, **17**:869–77, 1967.

Lovejoy, F. H.; Mitchel, A. A.; and Goldman, P.: Management of propoxyphene poisoning. *J. Pediatr.*, **85**:98–100, 1974.

Mann, J. B.: Diagnostic aids in organophosphate poisoning. *Ann. Intern. Med.*, **67**:905–906, 1967.

Marks, M. I.; Chicoine, L.; and Legere, G.: Adreno-corticosteroid treatment of hydrocarbon pneumonia in children—a cooperative study. *J. Pediatr.*, **81**:366–69, 1972.

Martin, W. R.: Naloxone. *Ann. Intern. Med.*, **85**:765, 1976.

Matthew, H., and Lawson, A. A.: *Treatment of Common Acute Poisoning*, 3rd ed. Livingston, London, 1975.

Mitchell, J. R.; Jollow, D. J.; Potter, W. Z.; Davis, D. C.; Gillette, J. R.; and Brodie, B. B.: Acetaminophen induced hepatic necrosis. *J. Pharmacol. Exp. Ther.*, **187**:185, 1973.

Mikolich, J. R.; Paulson, G. W.; and Cross, C. J.: Acute anticholinergic syndromes due to jimson weed ingestion. *Ann. Intern. Med.*, **83**:321, 1975.

Moore, R. A.; Rumack, B. H.; and Conner, C. S.: Naloxone: underdosage after narcotic poisoning. *Am. J. Dis. Child.* 1979 (in press).

Namba, T.: Poisoning due to organophosphate insecticides: Acute and chronic manifestations. *Am. J. Med.*, **50**:475–92, 1971.

Paulet, G.: Intoxication cyanhydrique et chelater de cobalt. *J. Physiol. Path. Gen.*, **50**:438, 1958.

Peterson, R. G., and Rumack, B. H.: Treating acute acetaminophen poisoning with acetylcysteine. *J.A.M.A.*, **237**:2406–2407, 1977.

Pierce, A. W.: Salicylate poisoning. *Pediatrics*, **54**:342–47, 1974.

Prescott, L. E.; Sutherland, G. R.; and Park, J.: Cysteamine, methionine and penicillamine in the treatment of paracetamal poisoning. *Lancet*, **2**:109–13, 1976.

Proudfoot, A. T., and Wright, N.: Acute paracetamal poisoning. *Br. Med. J.*, **2**:557, 1970.

Rifkin, A.; Quitkin, F.; and Klein, D. F.: Withdrawal reaction to diazepam. *J.A.M.A.*, **236**:2172–73, 2976.

Robertson, W. O.: Treatment of acute iron poisoning. *Mod. Treat.*, **8**:552–60, 1971.

Robillard, J. E.; Rames, L. K.; Jensen, R. L.; and Roberts, R. J.: Peritoneal dialysis in mercurial-diuretic intoxication. *J. Pediatr.*, **88**:79–81, 1976.

Rosenstein, G.; Freeman, M.; Standard, A. L.; and Westen, N.: Warning: The use of Lomotil in children. *Pediatrics*, **51**:132–34, 1973.

Rumack, B. H.: Anticholinergic poisonings: Treatment with physostigmine. *Pediatrics*, **52**:449, 1973.

Rumack, B. H.: Anticholinergic poisoning: Treatment with physostigmine. *Pediatrics*, **2**:449, 1973.

Rumack, B. H.: Hydrocarbon ingestions in perspective. *J.A.C.E.P.*, **6**:4, 1977.

Rumack, B. H.; Anderson, R. H.; Wolfe, R.; Fletcher, E. C.; and Vestal, B.: Ornade and anticholinergic toxicity: Hypertension, hallucination and arrhythmias. *Clin. Toxicol.*, **7**:573–81, 1974.

Rumack, B. H.; Wolfe, R. R.; and Gilfrich, H.: Diphenylhydantoin treatment of massive digoxin overdose. *Br. Heart J.*, **36**:405–408, 1974.

Rumack, B. H.: *Poisindex.* Micromedex, Inc. Denver, 1978.

Rumack, B. H.: Management of acute poisoning and overdose. In Cozzetto, E. J., and Brettell, H. R.: *Topics in Family Practice.* Symposia Specialists Medical Books, New York, 1976.

Rumack, B. H., and Burrington, J. P.: Antidotal therapy of caustic reactions. *Clin. Toxicol.*, **11**:27, 1977.

Rumack, B. H.; Ford, P.; Sbarbaro, J.; Bryson, P.; and Winokur, M.: Regionalization of poison centers—a rational role model. *Clin. Toxicol.*, **12(3)**:367–75, 1978.

Rumack, B. H., and Matthew, H.: Acetaminophen poisoning and toxicity. *Pediatrics*, **55**:871, 1975.

Rumack, B. H., and Temple, A. R.: Lomotil poisoning. *Pediatrics*, **53**:495–500, 1974.

Rumack, B. H., and Temple, A. (eds.): *Management of the Poisoned Patient.* Science Press, Princeton, NJ, 1977.

Rumack, B. H.; Wolfe, R. R.; and Gilfrich, H.: Phenytoin treatment of massive digoxin overdose. *Br. Heart J.*, **36**:405–408, 1974.

Sayre, J. W., and Kaymakcalen, S.: Cyanide poisoning from apricot seeds among children in central Turkey. *N. Engl. J. Med.*, **270**:1113, 1964.

Schwartz, H. S.: Acute meprobamate poisoning with gastrotomy and removal of a drug-contained mass. *N. Engl. J. Med.*, **295**:1177, 1976.

Smith, R. P., and Kruszyna, H.: Nitroprusside produces cyanide poisoning via a reaction with hemoglobin. *J. Pediatr.*, **191**:557, 1974.

Smith, T. W.; Haber, E.; Yeatman, L.; and Butler, V. P., Jr.: Reversal of advanced digoxin intoxication with Fab fragments of digoxin—specific antibodies. *N. Engl. J. Med.*, **294**:797–800, 1976.

Snyder, R.; Mofenson, H.; and Greensher, J.: Toxicity from Lomotil. *Clin. Pediatr.*, **12**:47, 1973.

Stalker, N. E.; Gambertoglio, J. G.; Fukumitsu, C. J.; *et al.*: Acute massive chloral hydrate intoxication treated with hemodialysis: A clinical pharmacokinetic analysis. *J. Clin. Pharmacol.*, **18**: 136–42, 1978.

Steele, R. W.; Conklin, R. H.; and March, H. M.: Corticosteroids and antibiotics for the treatment of fulminant hydrocarbon aspiration. *J.A.M.A.*, **219**:1434–37, 1972.

Stein, J. L.: Phencyclidine induced psychosis: The need to avoid unnecessary sensory influx. *Milit. Med.*, **138**:590, 1973.

Stein, M.; Blayney, D.; Feit, T.; Goergen, T. G.; Micik, S.; and Nyhan, W. L.: Acute iron poisoning in children. *West. J. Med.*, **125**:289–97, 1976.

Stewart, R.: Cyanide poisoning. *Clin. Toxicol.*, **7**:561, 1974.

Subcommittee on Accidental Poisoning: Kerosene and related petroleum distillates. In *Handbook of Common Poisonings in Children*. U.S. Department of HEW, Rockville, MD, 1976 (FDA-76-7004).

Tobis, J., and Das, B. N.: Cardiac complications in amitriptyline poisoning—successful treatment with physostigmine. *J.A.M.A.*, **234**:1474–76, 1976.

Tong, T. G.; Benowitz, N. L.; Becker, C. E.; Forni, P. J.; and Boerner, U.: Phencyclidine poisoning. *J.A.M.A.*, **234**:512–13, 1975.

Victor, M., and Adams, R. D.: Barbiturate. In *Harrison's Principles of Internal Medicine*. McGraw-Hill Book Co., New York, 1977, Chap. 120.

Watanabe, A. S.: Pharmacokinetic aspects of the dialysis of drugs. *Drug. Intall. Clin. Pharmacol.*, **11**:407–16, 1977.

Welch, T. R.; Rumack, B. H.; and Hammond, K.: Clonazepam overdose in resulting cyclic coma. *Clin. Toxicol.*, **10**:433–34, 1977.

Wexler, J.; Whittenberger, J. L.; and Dumke, P. R.: The effect of cyanide on the electrocardiogram of man. *Am. Heart, J.*, **34**:163–73, 1947.

Wilkinson, P. K.: Blood ethanol concentrations during and following constant rate IV infusion of alcohol. *Clin. Pharmacol. Ther.*, **19**:213, 1976.

Chapter 28

OCCUPATIONAL TOXICOLOGY

Robert R. Lauwerys

INTRODUCTION

The main objective of industrial toxicology is the prevention of health impairments in workers handling or exposed to industrial chemicals. This objective can only be reached if conditions of exposure or work practices are defined that do not entail an unacceptable health risk. With the possible exception of carcinogenic substances, for which it is still debatable whether "safe" conditions of exposure can presently be defined, this implies in practice the definition of permissible levels of exposure to industrial chemicals. These levels can be expressed either in terms of allowable atmospheric concentrations (maximum allowable concentrations—MAC; threshold limit values—TLV; time-weighted averages —TWA; short-term exposure limits—STEL; emergency exposure limits—EEL) or in terms of permissible biologic levels for the chemicals or their metabolites (biologic TLV). To evaluate with some degree of confidence the level of exposure at which the risk of health impairment is negligible, a body of toxicologic information is required that derives from two main sources, experimental investigations on animals and clinical surveillance of exposed workers (including retrospective studies on previously exposed workers). In some circumstances, limited investigations on volunteers can also be considered.

The large-scale use of any chemical in industry should be preceded by certain types of toxicologic investigations on animals in order to establish a tentative "no-adverse-effect" level. Other important information that may also be derived from these investigations concerns methods of biologic monitoring and preexisting pathologic states that may increase the susceptibility to the chemical. Animal testing can provide only an estimate of the toxicity of a chemical for man. For example, there is a great risk of missing allergic reactions in testing new materials in animals. Thus when the compound is actually handled in industry, monitoring of the work places and careful clinical surveillance of the

workers are essential. The design of these clinical surveys will to a large extent depend on the information collected during the first experimental phase of the investigations. The main objectives of the clinical work are (1) to test the validity of the provisional permissible level of exposure based on animal experiments; (2) to detect as early as possible hypersensitive reactions unpredictable from animal investigations; and (3) to confirm the usefulness of biologic methods of monitoring workers. One must, however, recognize that for many chemicals toxicologic investigations on animals have not been performed before the chemicals' use in industry. In that case clinical work (retrospective epidemiologic studies; historic prospective studies) is aimed at defining the no-adverse-effect level directly in man.

In some circumstances exposure of volunteers can be considered when the information, e.g., threshold for upper respiratory tract irritation, is not easily obtainable by other means and when the experiments entail no risk for the volunteers (which means that extensive biologic information should already be available before any experiments on volunteers are undertaken). Experimental investigations on animals and clinical studies on workers or volunteers are closely related, and I will illustrate below how collaboration between disciplines or approaches helps accomplish more rapid progress in the field of industrial toxicology.

PRELIMINARY TESTING ON ANIMALS

It is evident that certainty as to the complete safety of a chemical can never be obtained, whatever the extent of toxicologic investigations performed on animals. Nevertheless, some basic requirements can be suggested to estimate with some degree of confidence the level of exposure at which the risk of health impairment is negligible and thus acceptable. We are excluding from the following considerations chemicals that have only very limited use, as in a research laboratory, and can be handled by a limited number of skilled persons in a way that prevents any exposure.

General guidelines for assessing experimentally the toxicologic hazards of industrial chemicals have been recommended (Lauwerys, 1976). Their principles do not differ much from the investigations presently required for evaluating the toxicity of substances to which the general public can be exposed (drugs, food additives, pesticides residues, etc.) (NAS, 1975). I do not propose to review these tests (local and systemic acute toxicity tests; skin sensitization tests; toxicity following repeated exposure; short-term tests for detecting potential mutagens and carcinogens; studies of effect on reproduction and of teratogenic activity; investigations of metabolism and mechanism of action; interaction studies; etc.), which have been extensively described in previous chapters. I wish only to stress a few points that are important or more relevant to the field of industrial toxicology.

The need for performing some (or all) of those investigations should be carefully evaluated for any industrial chemical to which workers will be exposed. The toxicologist is guided in selecting the studies most relevant for safety evaluation by an understanding of the physicochemical properties of the chemical; the conditions of use and degree of exposure, including the possibility of generating toxic derivatives when the chemical is submitted to various chemical and physical factors (heat, pH change, etc.); the type of exposure, which may be continuous or accidental; and possibly toxicologic information already available on other chemicals with similar chemical structure and reactive chemical groups. It should be stressed that conclusions drawn from any toxicologic investigation are valid only if the exact composition (e.g., nature and concentration of impurities or degradation products) of the tested preparation is known precisely. The assessment of the toxicity of 2,4,5,-T illustrates this point. Its teratogenic hazard is estimated differently depending on the content of the highly toxic impurity 2,3,7,8-tetrachlorodibenzodioxin in the preparation tested (Courtney and Moore, 1971; Emerson et al., 1971). Accurate methods of analysis of the chemical in air and in biologic material should also be available. Flexibility of approach is essential in deciding the duration of tests necessary to establish a reasonable no-effect level for occupational exposure. This depends mainly on the type of toxic action that is suspected, but it is generally recognized that subacute and short-term toxicity studies are usually unsatisfactory for proposing permissible exposure levels. Subacute and short-term toxicity tests are usually performed to find out whether the compound exhibits some cumulative toxic properties and to select the doses for long-term exposure and the kind of tests that may be most informative when applied during long-term exposures. Several studies have recently drawn attention to the fact that the reproductive system may also be the target organ of industrial chemicals (e.g., anesthetic gases, monochlorodibromopropane, vinyl chloride). Studies designed to evaluate reproductive performance and teratogenic action should therefore also be considered during routine toxicologic testing of industrial chemicals.

Information derived from similar exposure routes (skin, lung) to those sustained by workers is clearly most relevant. For airborne pollutants, inhalation exposure studies provide the basic data on which provisional permissible levels are based. Experimental methodology is certainly much more complicated for inhalation studies than for oral administration experiments. For example, in the case of exposure to aerosol, particle size distribution should be estimated and the approximate degree of retention in the respiratory tract of the animal species selected should be known. Ideally, particle size should be selected according to the deposition pattern of solid or liquid aerosols in the particular animal species used. It should also be kept in mind that the concentration of the material in the air and the duration of exposure do not give a direct estimate of the dose, which is also dependent on the minute volume and percent retention. The appropriateness of other routes of administration (usually oral) in combination with limited data from tests by inhalation or skin application must be scientifically evaluated for each chemical (depending on its main site of action, metabolism, etc.). The morphologic, physiologic, and biologic parameters that are usually evaluated, either at regular intervals in the course of the exposure period or at its termination, have been reviewed (Lauwerys, 1976; NAS, 1975; Shibko and Flamm, 1975). It is evident that investigations that can make use of specific physiologic or biochemical tests based on the knowledge of the "critical" organ or function produce highly valuable information and hence increase confidence in the TLV derived from them. In the field of industrial toxicology, knowledge of the metabolic handling (absorption, distribution, biotransformation, excretion) of the chemical and/or its mechanism of action is of major interest. Indeed, as indicated in the introduction, the main objective of occupational toxicology is to prevent the development of occupational diseases. In this respect the biologic monitoring of workers exposed to various industrial chemicals may play an important role, by detecting excessive exposures as early as possible, before the occurrence of significant biologic disturbances, or at least when they are still reversible or have not yet caused any health impairment. A rational biologic monitoring is possible only when sufficient toxicologic information has been gathered on the mechanism of action and/or the metabolism of xenobiotics to which workers may be exposed. These studies must be performed first on animals.

OBSERVATIONS ON WORKERS

When a new chemical is being used on a large scale, careful clinical survey of the workers and monitoring of the work places should be planned. In addition to the specific actions immediately taken if any adverse effect on the health of the workers is discovered, a clinical survey may have two main general objectives: to evaluate the validity of the "no-adverse-effect" level derived from animal experiments, and to test the validity of a biologic method of monitoring.

Evaluation of the Validity of Animal Experiments

Evaluation of the validity of the "no-adverse-effect" level derived from animal experiments is certainly the prime objective since, as stated by Barnes (1963), "studies and observations on man will always be the final basis for deciding whether or not a MAC set originally on the basis of tests on animals is, in fact, truly acceptable as one that will not produce any signs of intoxication." This means that behavioral, clinical, biochemical, physiologic, or morphologic tests that are considered to be the most sensitive for detecting an adverse effect of the chemical should be regularly applied to the workers at the same time their overall exposure is evaluated to provide personal monitoring of airborne contaminants.

Since the adverse effects under scrutiny for the early detection of health impairment are subtle, and since individual variations exist in the response to a chemical insult, results can only be evaluated on a statistical basis. This means that the dose-response curves found among exposed workers should always be compared to similar responses in a group of unexposed workers matched for other variables such as age, sex, socioeconomic status, and smoking habits. The importance of selecting a control group that is well matched with the exposed group and that undergoes exactly the same standardized clinical, biologic, or physiologic evaluation at the same time as the exposed group must be emphasized. Since an employed population is a group selected to a certain degree for health, comparison with the general population is not valid. Since such a survey lasts for several years

(prospective survey or observational cohort study), the importance of good standardization of all methods of investigation, such as questionnaires related to subjective complaints, instrumentation, and analytic techniques, must be stressed before the start of the survey.

If labor turnover is too high to allow a typical cohort study (i.e., regular examination of the same exposed and control workers), repeated cross-sectional studies of exposed and matched controls should be undertaken. If exposure is above the threshold level of response, these studies may permit (1) establishment of the relationship between integrated exposure (intensity × time) and frequently of abnormal responses, and consequently (2) a redefinition of the "no-adverse-effect" level.

When this surveillance program has not been planned before the introduction of a new chemical, it is more difficult to obtain the desired information through investigations designed after the fact. Indeed, in this case, evaluation depends on retrospective cohort studies or, more usually, simple cross-sectional studies. Since the information regarding the past exposure of the workers is often incomplete, a correct evaluation of the no-effect level is much more difficult. Whether or not clinical investigations are planned from the introduction of a new chemical or process, it is essential to keep standardized records of workers' occupational histories and exposures. The need may arise for mortality or case history studies in order to answer an urgent question on a suspected risk. The evaluation of the "no-effect" level of vinyl chloride in man illustrates this point.

In addition to these clinical surveys, it is useful to report in case studies any particular observations resulting from exposure to the chemicals (e.g., accidental acute intoxications). Although such isolated observations are not helpful for determining the "no-effect" level in man, they are of interest, mainly for new chemicals. They may indicate whether human symptomatology is similar to that found in animals, and hence may suggest the functional or biologic tests that might prove useful for the routine control of exposed workers.

Testing the Validity of a Biologic Method of Monitoring

Experimental work may have suggested a biologic method for monitoring of workers (e.g., evaluation of current exposure, internal load, or early biologic response by measuring a metabolite or the compound itself in urine or blood, or by determining blood enzyme activity). Clinical investigations must then be made to test the applicability of such methods in industrial situations. A brief review of the main biologic monitoring methods presently available for evaluating exposure to some industrial toxicologic hazards is presented at the end of this chapter.

EXPERIMENTAL STUDIES ON VOLUNTEERS

Experimental studies on volunteers are usually designed to answer very specific questions, e.g., time course of metabolite excretion during and after exposure; threshold doses for blood cholinesterase inhibition; evaluation of the threshold concentration for sensory responses (odor, irritation of the nasal mucosa, etc.); effect of solvent exposure on perception, vigilance, and the like. For evident ethical reasons, such studies can only be undertaken when the same results cannot be obtained through other means and under circumstances where the risk for the volunteers can reasonably be estimated as nonexistent. The experimentation should comply with the Declaration of Helsinki (1964), i.e., it should be carried out under proper medical supervision on duly-informed volunteers.

INTEREST OF CLOSE COLLABORATION BETWEEN EXPERIMENTAL INVESTIGATIONS ON ANIMALS AND CLINICAL STUDIES ON WORKERS (OR VOLUNTEERS)

Perhaps in the field of industrial toxicology more than in other areas of toxicology, close collaboration between experimental investigations on animals and clinical studies on workers plays an important role in explaining the potential risk linked with overexposure to chemicals, and hence in suggesting preventive measures to protect the health of the workers. A few examples will illustrate the complementarity of both disciplines in occupational toxicology.

The firm identification of an occupational carcinogen requires both epidemiologic and experimental evidence; an excess of cancer is found in a group exposed to a known chemical and tumors can be produced in experimental animals by the same chemical (Higginson and Muir, 1976). The carcinogenicity of vinyl chloride was first demonstrated in rats (Viola, 1971) and a few years later epidemiologic studies confirmed the same carcinogenic risk for man (Creech and Johnson, 1974; Monson et al., 1974). This observation stimulated several investigations on its metabolism in animals and on its mutagenic activity in various in vitro systems. Identification of vinyl chloride metabolites led to the conclusion that an epoxy derivative is first formed that is suspected to be the proximate

carcinogen. This report triggered a number of investigations on the biotransformation of structurally related chemicals extensively used in industry, such as trichloroethylene, vinylidene chloride, vinyl benzene, and chlorobutadiene. It is likely that all give rise to reactive epoxy intermediates (Bonse et al., 1975; Leibman, 1975; Uehleke et al., 1977). Retrospective epidemiologic studies on persons who are or have been occupationally exposed to these chemicals are therefore indicated. Furthermore, several of these chemicals or their metabolites exhibit mutagenic activity in vitro. This observation stimulated the search for chromosomal aberrations in workers. Such anomalies were indeed found in workers exposed to vinyl chloride (Heath et al., 1977), and an epidemiologic study suggests that vinyl chloride can induce genetic damage in man. Again, in view of the results of the experimental studies cited above, extension of these clinical studies to chemically related compounds is highly desirable.

Dioxane is an industrial solvent with a variety of industrial applications. When it is administered at high doses, the principal toxic effects in rats are centrilobular hepatocellular and renal tubular epithelial degeneration and necrosis and induction of hepatic and nasal carcinoma (Kociba et al., 1974). The major metabolite in rats was identified as either β-hydroxyethoxyacetic acid (HEAA) or p-dioxane-2-one, depending on the acidity and the alkalinity of the solution. It was found, however, that the biotransformation of dioxane to HEAA may be saturated at high doses of dioxane. This observation led Young to suggest that the toxicity of dioxane occurs when doses are given sufficient to saturate the metabolic pathway for its detoxification (Young et al., 1976a). On the premise that similarity of the metabolic pathway of dioxane in rats and humans would greatly facilitate the extrapolation of toxicologic data from rats to man (Young et al., 1976b), the same authors examined the urine of plant personnel exposed to dioxane vapor. In urine of workers exposed to a time-weighted average concentration of 1.6 ppm dioxane for 7.5 hours, they found the same product (HEAA) as found previously in the rat. Furthermore, the high ratio of HEAA to dioxane, 118 to 1, suggests that at a low-exposure concentration dioxane is rapidly metabolized to HEAA. The authors concluded that since saturation of the metabolism of dioxane in rats was correlated with toxicity, their results on man support the hypothesis that low levels of dioxane vapor in the workplace pose a negligible hazard. This conclusion is debatable, however, since dioxane is a carcinogen and the existence of a threshold level for such chemicals is still controversial

(Claus *et al.*, 1974; Dinman, 1972; Henschler, 1974).

Furthermore, Woo *et al.* (1977) have reported that *p*-dioxane-2-one is more toxic than dioxane and its production *in vivo* may be related to dioxane toxicity and/or carcinogenicity, in view of the fact that a number of lactones with similar structure are known to be carcinogenic. If it can be shown that *p*-dioxane-2-one is really a proximate carcinogen, workers found to excrete the metabolite will have to be considered at risk.

Dimethylformamide (DMF) is an hepatotoxic solvent extensively used in laboratories and in the production of acrylic resins. Exposure of workers occurs mainly by inhalation of vapor and through skin contact. Its metabolism was first investigated in rats and in dogs *in vitro* and *in vivo* (Barnes and Ranta, 1972; Kimmerle and Eben, 1975a). These investigations demonstrated that DMF is rapidly metabolized *in vivo*. The biotransformation consists of a progressive demethylation, possibly followed by the hydrolysis of the amide bond. The main urinary metabolite is the monomethyl derivative, N-methylformamide (NMF). The animal studies stimulated human studies to evaluate whether *in vivo* biotransformation could lead to the proposal of a biologic method for monitoring workers exposed to DMF. First, two groups of workers investigated the metabolism of DMF on volunteers (Kimmerle and Eben, 1975b; Maxfield *et al.*, 1975). They both found that the majority of the absorbed substance is eliminated within 24 hours and that the main urinary metabolite is NMF. Its concentration was related to the intensity of exposure. The next logical test was to evaluate the practicability of this biologic monitoring method on workers. A preliminary investigation in an acrylic fiber factory confirmed that NMF in urine is a sensitive biologic indicator of exposure since its presence could be easily detected, even when the average airborne DMF concentration was below the current ACGIH-TLV (30 mg/m^3). Furthermore, in a group of workers, the amount of DMF excreted at the end of the shift seems to reflect the intensity of exposure of the same day (Lauwerys *et al.*, 1975).

These examples (vinyl chloride, dioxane, dimethylformamide) demonstrate that the study of the metabolic handling of an industrial chemical in animals is very important because it may lead to the characterization of reactive intermediates, suggesting yet-unsuspected risks, or it may indicate new methods of biologic monitoring, which must first be validated by a field study.

Conversely, clinical observations on workers may stimulate the study of the metabolism or the mechanism of toxicity of an industrial chemical in animals. This may help in predicting the human response to structurally related compounds or in evaluating the health significance of a biologic disturbance. In 1973 an outbreak of peripheral neuropathy occurred in workers exposed to the solvent methyl butyl ketone (MBK) (Allen *et al.*, 1975; Billmaier *et al.*, 1974; McDonough, 1974). The same lesion was reproduced in animals (Duckett *et al.*, 1974; Mendell *et al.*, 1974; Spencer *et al.*, 1975). Metabolic studies were then undertaken in rats and guinea pigs (Abdel-Rahman *et al.*, 1976; DiVincenzo *et al.*, 1976, 1977), and some MBK metabolites (2,5-hexanedione, 5-hydroxy-2-hexanone) were also found to possess neurotoxic activity (DiVincenzo *et al.*, 1977; Spencer and Schaumburg, 1975).

Similar oxidation products are formed from *n*-hexane, the neurotoxicity of which is probably due to the same active metabolite as that produced from MBK. According to DiVincenzo *et al.* (1977), the most probable active intermediate is 2,5-hexanedione. Since methyl isobutyl ketone and methyl ethyl ketone cannot give rise to 2,5-hexanedione (DiVincenzo *et al.*, 1976), they should preferably replace MBK as solvents. *n*-Hexane derivatives that are oxidized to 2,5-hexanedione are probably also neurotoxic for man (DiVincenzo *et al.*, 1977).

Investigations on volunteers and on workers have shown that for the same level of exposure to lead the accumulation of free erythrocyte porphyrin (FEP) is more important in women than in men (Roels *et al.*, 1975; Stuik, 1974). Whether this finding justifies the proposal of different permissible levels of exposure to lead for women and for men is debatable, since its health significance is still unknown. A study on the mechanism of the sex difference could clarify its health significance. A joint experimental and clinical approach seems very promising in being able to yield an understanding of the mechanism of this sex-lead interaction. A difference in the level of the iron pool between men and women was first proposed as the main mechanism of the different susceptibility to lead. A relative iron deficiency in women could synergize the action of lead on the enzyme chelatase in the bone marrow. Two arguments, one clinical and one experimental, suggest that the lead-sex interaction may also involve other biologic factors. In women moderately exposed to lead who did not suffer from iron-deficiency anemia, no correlation was found between FEP and plasma iron, nor between concentration of lead in blood and plasma iron (Lauwerys, unpublished results). Furthermore, it was possible to reproduce the sex difference in FEP response to lead in rats (Buchet *et al.*, 1978). In this species under normal feeding conditions the action of lead on FEP accumulation is apparently independent of the

Table 28–1   (*continued*)

CHEMICAL AGENT	ANALYSIS	TENTATIVE BIOLOGIC TLV*	REMARKS
$(C_2H_5)_4Pb$	Pb in urine	110 μg/l	
Se	Se in urine	100 μg/l	
Tl	Tl in urine		
Ur	Ur in urine	50 μg/l	
V	V in urine	50 μg/l	
Zn	Zn in urine	800–1,200 μg/l	

B. *Organic Substances*

1. Nonsubstituted Aliphatic Hydrocarbons

Hexane, heptane, octane	Substance in blood		
	Substance in expired air		

2. Nonsubstituted Aromatic Hydrocarbons

Benzene	Phenol in urine	50 mg/l	
		20 mg/l	If TLV is 1 ppm
	Benzene in expired air	0.12 ppm	16 hr after exposure to 10 ppm for 8 hr
	Benzene in blood		
Toluene	Hippuric acid in urine	2.0 g/l	
	Toluene in expired air		
	Toluene in blood		
Xylene	Methylhippuric acid in urine	2.5 g/l	
	Xylene in expired air		
	Xylene in blood		
Cumene	2-Phenylpropanol in urine	200 mg/l	
	Cumene in expired air		
	Cumene in blood		
Mesitylene	3,5-Dimethylhippuric acid in urine		
Styrene	Mandelic acid in urine	2 g/l	
	Phenylglyoxylic acid in urine	250 mg/l	
	Styrene in blood		
	Styrene in expired air		
Biphenyl	4-Hydroxybiphenyl in urine		

3. Halogenated Hydrocarbons

Dichloromethane	HbCO in blood	3%	Nonsmokers
	Dichloromethane in blood		
	Dichloromethane in expired air		
Trichloroethylene	Trichloroethanol and trichloroacetic acid in urine	250 mg/l	
	Trichloroethanol in blood	2–3 mg/l	
	Trichloroethylene in expired air	0.3–0.8 ppm	18 hr after exposure
1,1,1-Trichloroethane	Trichloroethanol and trichloroacetic acid in urine	30–50 mg/l	
	Trichloroethane in blood		
	Trichloroethane in expired air		
Tetrachloroethylene	Tetrachloroethylene in expired air	8 ppm	18 hr after exposure
Other halogenated hydrocarbons			

(*continued*)

Table 28-1 *(continued)*

CHEMICAL AGENT	ANALYSIS	TENTATIVE BIOLOGIC TLV*	REMARKS
(CCl$_4$, CHCl$_3$, vinyl chloride, halogenated anaesthetics)	Substances in expired air		
4. Amides			
Dimethylformamide	N-Methylformamide in urine	100 mg/l	
Dimethylacetamide	N-Methylacetamine in urine		
5. Alcohols, Glycols, Phenol, and derivatives (see also pesticides)			
Methanol	Methanol in urine	5 mg/l	
Ethylene glycol	Oxalic acid in urine		
Methycellosolve	Oxalic acid in urine		
Phenol	Phenol in urine	250 mg/l	
p-Tert-butylphenol	*p*-Tert-butylphenol in urine	2 mg/l	
Dioxane	*p*-Dioxane-2-one in urine		
6. Amino- and Nitroderivatives			
Nitrobenzene	*p*-Nitrophenol in urine	5 mg/l	
	Methemoglobin in blood	5%	
Aniline	*p*-Aminophenol in urine	10 mg/l	
	Methemoglobin in blood	5%	
7. Pesticides			
Organophosphorus esters	Cholinesterase in RBC or in plasma	− 50%	
Parathion	*p*-Nitrophenol in urine	100 μg/l	
Carbamate insecticides	Cholinesterase in RBC or in plasma		
Carbaryl	Naphthol in urine		
Baygon	2-Isopropoxyphenol in urine		
8. Organochlorine Pesticides			
DDT	DDT in serum	20–50 μg/100 ml	
	DDT and DDE in blood		
	DDA in urine		
Dieldrin	Dieldrin in blood	15 μg/100 ml	
Lindane	Lindane in blood	2 μg/100 ml	
Endrin	Endrin in blood	5 μg/100 ml	
Hexachlorobenzene	2,4,5-Trichlorophenol in urine		
Pentachlorophenol	Pentachlorophenol in urine	3 mg/l	
Phenoxyacetic acid derivatives (2,4-D; 2,4,5-T; MCPA)	2,4-D in urine 2,4,5-T in urine MCPA in urine		
Dinitro-*o*-cresol	Dinitro-*o*-cresol in blood Amino-4-nitro-*o*-cresol in urine	20 mg/100 ml	
9. Carbon disulfide			
	Sodium azide test in urine	> 6.5	

*The values apply to biologic samples collected at the end of the workshift unless otherwise indicated.

CONCLUSION

The working environment will always present the risk of workers' overexposure to various chemicals. It is self-evident that the control of these risks cannot wait until epidemiologic studies have defined the no-adverse-effect level directly in man. However, extrapolation from animal data has its limitations. A combined experimental and clinical approach is certainly the most effective for evaluating the potential risks of industrial chemicals, hence for recommending adequate preventive measures and for applying the most valid screening procedures on workers.

Thus the field of industrial toxicology provides many opportunities for scientists with different backgrounds (physicians, chemists, biologists, hygienists) who are convinced of the usefulness of working in close collaboration to understand and prevent the adverse effects of industrial chemicals on workers' health.

REFERENCES

Abdel-Rahman, M. S.; Hetland, L. B.; and Couri, D.: Toxicity and metabolism of methyl n-butyl ketone. *Am. Ind. Hyg. Assoc. J.*, 37:95–102, 1976.

Allen, N.; Mendell, J. R.; Billmaier, D. J.; Fontaine, R. E.; and O'Neill, J.: Toxic polyneuropathy due to methyl n-butyl ketone. *Arch. Neurol.*, 32:209–18, 1975.

Barnes, J. M.: The basis for establishing and fixing maximum allowable concentrations. *Trans. Assoc. Ind. Med. Off.*, 13:74–76, 1963.

Barnes, J. R., and Ranta, K. E.: The metabolism of dimethylformamide and dimethylacetamide. *Toxicol. Appl. Pharmacol.*, 23:271–76, 1972.

Billmaier, D.; Yee, H. T.; Allen, N.; Craft, R.; Williams, N.; Epstein, S.; and Fontaine, R.: Peripheral neuropathy in a coated fabrics plant. *J. Occup. Med.*, 16:665–71, 1974.

Bonse, G.; Urban, T.; Reichert, D.; and Henschler, D.: Chemical reactivity, metabolic oxirane formation and biological reactivity of chlorinated ethylenes in the isolated perfused rat liver preparation. *Biochem. Pharmacol.*, 24:1829–1834, 1975.

Buchet, J. P.; Roels, H.; and Lauwerys, R.: Influence of sex hormones on free erythrocyte protoporphyrin response to lead in rats. *Toxicol.*, 9:249–53, 1978.

Claus, G.; Krisko, I.; and Bolander, K.: Chemical carcinogens in the environment and in the human diet: Can a threshold be established? *Food Cosmet. Toxicol.*, 12:737–46, 1974.

Courtney, K. D., and Moore, J. A.: Teratology studies with 2,4,5-trichlorophenoxyacetic acid and 2,3,7,8-tetrachlorodibenzo-P-dioxin. *Toxicol. Appl. Pharmacol.*, 20:396–403, 1971.

Creech, J. L., and Johnson, H. M.: Angiosarcoma of the liver in the manufacture of polyvinylchloride. *J. Occup. Med.*, 16:150–51, 1974.

Dinman, B. D.: "Non-concept" of "no-threshold" chemicals in the environment. *Science*, 175:495–97, 1972.

DiVincenzo, G. D.; Kaplan, C. J.; and Dedinas, J.: Characterization of the metabolites of methyl-n-butyl ketone, methyl iso-butyl ketone, and methyl ethyl ketone in guinea pig serum and their clearance. *Toxicol. Appl. Pharmacol.*, 36:511–22, 1976.

DiVincenzo, G. D.; Hamilton, M. L.; Kaplan, C. J.; and Dedinas, J.: Metabolic fate and disposition of ¹⁴C-labeled methyl n-butyl ketone in the rat. *Toxicol. Appl. Pharmacol.*, 41:547–60, 1977.

Duckett, S.; Williams, N.; and Francis, S.: Peripheral neuropathy associated with inhalation of methyl n-butyl ketone. *Experientia*, 30(11):1283–84, 1974.

Emerson, J. L.; Thompson, D. J.; Strebing, R. J.; Gerbig, C. G.; and Robinson, V. B.: Teratogenic studies on 2,4,5-trichlorophenoxyacetic acid in the rat and rabbit. *Food Cosmet. Toxicol.*, 9:395–404, 1971.

Heath, C. W.; Dumont, C. R.; Gamble, J.; and Waxweiler, R. J.: Chromosomal damage in men occupationally exposed to vinyl chloride monomer and other chemicals. *Environ. Res.*, 14:68–72, 1977.

Henschler, D.: New approaches to a definition of threshold values for "irreversible" toxic effects? *Arch. Toxicol.*, 32:63–67, 1974.

Higginson, J., and Muir, C. S.: The role of epidemiology in elucidating the importance of environmental factors in human cancer. *Cancer Detection Prevention*, 1:79–105, 1976.

Kimmerle, G., and Eben, A.: Metabolism studies of N,N-dimethylformamide. I. Studies in rats and dogs. *Int. Arch. Arbeitsmed.*, 34:109–26, 1975(a).

Kimmerle, G., and Eben, A.: Metabolism studies of N,N-dimethylformamide. II. Studies in persons. *Int. Arch. Arbeitsmed.*, 14:127–36, 1975(b).

Kociba, R. J.; McCollister, S. B.; Park, C.; Torkelson, T. R.; and Gehring, P. J.: 1,4-Dioxane. I. Results of a 2-year ingestion study in rats. *Toxicol. Appl. Pharmacol.*, 30:275–86, 1974.

Lauwerys, R.; Buchet, J. P.; Roels, H.; Berlin, A.; and Smeets, J.: Intercomparison program of lead, mercury, and cadmium analysis in blood, urine, and aqueous solutions. *Clin. Chem.*, 21:551–57, 1975.

Lauwerys, R.: Biological criteria for selected industrial toxic chemicals: A review. *Scand. J. Work Environ. Health*, 1:139–72, 1975.

Lauwerys, R.: Experimental and clinical investigations for assessing the toxicological hazards of industrial chemicals. *Proceedings of the Meeting of the Scientific Committee, Carlo Erba Foundation, Occupational and Environmental Health Section*, Milan, 1976, pp. 9–48.

Lauwerys, R.; Buchet, J. P.; Roels, H.; and Bernard, A.: Industrial toxicology: a collaborative approach to laboratory animal research and clinical field studies. In Duncan, W., and Plaa, G. (eds.): *Proceedings First International Congress in Toxicology*. Academic Press. Inc., Toronto, 1977, pp. 311–26.

Leibman, K. C.: Metabolism and toxicity of styrene. *Environ. Health Perspect.*, 11:115–19, 1975.

Linch, A. L.: *Biological Monitoring for Industrial Chemical Exposure Control*. CRC Press, Cleveland, 1974.

Maxfield, M. E.; Barnes, J. R.; Azar, A.; and Trochimowicz, H. T.: Urinary excretion of metabolite following experimental human exposures to DMF or to DMAC. *J. Occup. Med.*, 17:506–11, 1975.

McDonough, J. R.: Possible neuropathy from methyl n-butyl ketone. *N. Engl. J. Med.*, 290:695, 1974.

Mendell, J. R.; Saida, K.; Ganasia, M. F.; Jackson, D. B.; Weiss, H.; Gardier, R. W.; Chrisman, C.; Allen, N.; Couri, D.; O'Neill, J.; Marks, B.; and Hetland, L.: Toxic polyneuropathy produced by methyl N-butyl ketone. *Science*, 185:787–89, 1974.

Monson, R. R.; Peters, J. M.; and Johnson, M. N.: Proportional mortality among vinyl-chloride workers. *Lancet*, 2(7877):397–98, 1974.

N.A.S. (National Academy of Sciences): *Principles for Evaluating Chemicals in the Environment*. Washington, D.C., 1975.

Roels, H. A.; Lauwerys, R. R.; Buchet, J. P.; and Vrelust,

M. T.: Response of free erythrocyte porphyrin and urinary δ-aminolevulinic acid in men and women moderately exposed to lead. *Int. Arch. Arbeitsmed.*, **34**:97–108, 1975.

Shibko, S. I., and Flamm, W. G. (eds.): Symposium on safety evaluation and toxicological tests and procedures. Jointly sponsored by the AOAC and the Society of Toxicology. *J. Assoc. Off. Anal. Chem.*, **58**:633–93, 1975.

Spencer, P. S.; Schaumburg, H. H.; Raleigh, R. L.; and Terhaar, C. J.: Nervous system degeneration produced by the industrial solvent methyl *n*-butyl ketone. *Arch. Neurol.*, **32**:219–22, 1975.

Spencer, P. S., and Schaumburg, H. H.: Experimental neuropathy produced by 2,5-hexanedione—a major metabolite of the neurotoxic industrial solvent methyl *n*-butyl ketone. *J. Neurol. Neurosurg. Psychiatry*, **38**:771–75, 1975.

Stuik, E. J.: Biological response of male and female volunteers to inorganic lead. *Int. Arch. Arbeitsmed.*, **33**:83–97, 1974.

Uehleke, H.; Tabarelli-Poplawski, S.; Bonse, G.; and Henschler, D.: Spectral evidence for 2,2,3-trichlorooxirane formation during microsomal trichloroethylene oxidation. *Arch. Toxicol.* **37**:95–105, 1977.

Viola, P. L.; Bigotti, A.; and Caputo, A.: Oncogenic response of rat skin, lungs, and bones to vinyl chloride. *Cancer Res.*, **31**:516–22, 1971.

Woo, Y. T.; Arcos, J. C.; and Argus, M. F.: Metabolism *in vivo* of dioxane: identification of *p*-dioxane-2-one as the major urinary metabolite. *Biochem. Pharmacol.*, **26**:1535–38, 1977.

Young, J. D.; Braun, W. H.; LeBeau, J. E.; and Gehring, P. J.: Saturated metabolism as the mechanism for the dose dependent fate of 1,4-dioxane in rats. *Toxicol. Appl. Pharmacol.*, **37**:138, 1976(a).

Young, J. D.; Braun, W. H.; Gehring, P. J.; Horvath, B. S.; and Daniel, R. L.: 1,4-Dioxane and β-hydroxyethoxyacetic acid excretion in urine of humans exposed to dioxane vapors. *Toxicol. Appl. Pharmacol.*, **38**:643–46, 1976(b).

Chapter 29

REGULATORY TOXICOLOGY

Morton Corn

INTRODUCTION

The term "regulatory toxicology" is herein used to cover those situations in which the public has transferred authority to a governmental body for overseeing restrictions imposed on citizens or organizations of citizens in their utilization of chemicals. In these cases the chemicals are judged, by some societal mechanism, to pose sufficient risk to those exposed to require regulatory measures.

The history of regulatory toxicology dates to antiquity. Regulation of public water quality and supplies of food, albeit qualitative in nature, is documented from as early as 33 B.C. (Corn and Corn, 1976; Rosen, 1958). The pace of regulatory toxicology quickened in the eighteenth and early nineteenth centuries, culminating in what is now referred to as the sanitary movement (Sand, 1952). The sanitary movement was based on the conviction that the physical and social environment of citizens has a direct effect on their health. It laid the groundwork for organized municipal effort to provide regulations of water supply, improved sewage, and removal of refuse. Most of the provisions of regulation during these periods were what we today call work practices, procedures that individuals follow to ensure the desired protective result. It remained for the scientific advances of the late nineteenth century and the understanding by health professionals of the germ theory of disease to establish quantitative measures of the effectiveness of work practices to control bacteriologic contamination.

In the United States, the Public Health Service was formed in 1902; the U.S. Bureau of Mines was formed in the Department of the Interior in 1910. In 1914, the predecessor of the Occupational Health Division of the United States Public Health Service was started. Government intervention in regulation of industry was concomitant with Labor Department formation and activity during the 1930s. The pace of federal regulation in the United States quickened after World War II. In retrospect, the period 1955 through 1977 will be remembered for the large number of federal regulatory standards that are applicable to our environment, both at work and in the community. Some of the U.S. statutes which regulate our chemical environment and which have come into existence since 1959 are the following: the Clean Air Act; the Clean Water Act; the Occupational Safety and Health Act; the Mine Safety and Health Act; the Coastal Zone Management Act; the Endangered Species Act; the Energy Supply and Environmental Coordination Act; the Federal Environmental Pesticide Control Act; the Federal Insecticide, Fungicide and Rodenticide Act; the Fish and Wildlife Coordination Act; the Hazardous Materials Transportation Act; the Marine Protection, Research and Sanctuaries Act; the Resources Conservation Recovery Act; the Solid Waste Disposal Act; the Transportation Safety Act; the Consumer Product Safety Act; and most recently, in December 1976, the Toxic Substances Control Act, an umbrella act covering the handling and elimination of chemicals in the United States. Each of these statutes has implications for professional practitioners in the fields of medicine, environment, and toxicology. There are aspects of these statutes that legally and ethically obligate professionals, or specifically assign duties to professionals in responsible charge (Corn, 1978).

One might ask, "Is all this governmental regulation of chemicals a response to a real problem?" Table 29–1 indicates the production of synthetic organic chemicals in the United States between 1949 and 1969. Table 29–2 lists the production and sales of organic pesticides in the United States during 1960–1975. The increased production of chemicals results in increased exposure of the population to chemical risks, be it in the occupational environment where the product is manufactured, in the outdoor environment where effluents to air, water, or solid wastes are encountered by the public, or at the commercial product user stage. Tables and graphs depicting the increase in effluents to air

Table 29-1. PRODUCTION OF SYNTHETIC ORGANIC CHEMICALS IN THE U.S. BETWEEN 1949 AND 1969*

	1949 (lb)	1969 (lb)	% INCREASE
Raw materials and intermediates†	8×10^9	1×10^{11}	1,150
Consumer products Grand total:	1.6×10^{10}	1.1×10^{11}	581
Pesticides and related products	1.4×10^8	1.1×10^9	686
Medicinal chemicals	4.2×10^7	2×10^8	376
Flavors and perfumes	2.4×10^7	1.2×10^8	400
Plastics and resins	1.5×10^9	1.9×10^{10}	1,167
Elastomers	9.5×10^8	4.5×10^9	374
Surfactants	4.3×10^8	3.9×10^9	807
Plasticizers	1.7×10^8	1.4×10^9	724
Rubber chemicals	8×10^7	3×10^8	275
Dyes	1.4×10^8	2.4×10^8	71
Organic pigments	3.7×10^7	6.1×10^7	65
Miscellaneous	1.2×10^{10}	7.6×10^{10}	533

* From *Chemicals and Health*. National Science Foundation, Washington, D.C., 1973. † Includes crude products from petroleum and natural gas, and intermediates derived therefrom.

and water and increased occupational usage of chemicals are available. The best sources of these data are the Congressional hearings preceding adoption of regulations or the continuing oversight hearings of the regulatory agency by the Congress, or audits by the General Accounting Office (GAO). One example of Congressional probing into chemical hazards is the report

Table 29-2. THE PRODUCTION AND SALES OF ORGANIC PESTICIDES PRODUCED IN THE UNITED STATES 1960-1975*

YEAR	QUANTITY, MILLION POUNDS	VALUE, MILLION DOLLARS
1960	648	307
1965	877	577
1970	1,034	1,058
1971	1,136	1,283
1972	1,158	1,345
1973	1,289	1,493
1974	1,417	1,985
1975	1,609	2,918

* From *1977 Statistical Abstract of the U.S.* Government Printing Office, Washington, D.C., 1977.

Chemical Dangers in the Workplace (1976). The reader is referred to the ongoing Congressional literature for perhaps the most up-to-date information on chemicals and their regulation. An example of the complexity of the chemical "mix" in any definable area of production or effluent media is revealed by Table 29-3, which lists drugs and other promoting chemicals added to animal feeds in the United States.

Table 29-3. EXAMPLES OF DRUGS AND OTHER PROMOTING CHEMICALS ADDED TO ANIMAL FEEDS IN THE UNITED STATES*

GROWTH PROMOTANTS

Hormonal	*Arsenicals*	*Antibiotics*
Diethylstilbestrol	Roxarsone	Chlortetracycline
Aeralanol		Bacitracin
Dinestrol diacetate		Oleandromycin
		Tylosin
		Sulfamethazine

USED FOR DISEASE PROPHYLAXIS

Antibacterials	*Antiprotozoals*	*Pesticides*
Chlortetracycline	Aklomide	Ronnel
Furazolidone	Buquinolate	Coumaphos
Racephenicol	Amprolium	Famphur
Bacitracin	Zoalene	
	Ipronidazole	
	Monensin	

Antimycotics	*Anthelmintics*
Copper sulfate	Coumaphos
Griseofulvin	Hygromycin

Physiologic Disease Prevention
Antibloat—poloxalene
Ketosis—propylene glycol
Aortic rupture—reserpine

USED FOR DISEASE TREATMENT

Bacterial	*Antimycotics*
Novobiocin	Griseofulvin
Sulfaethoxypyridazine	Nystatin
Oxytetracycline	
Furazolidone	
Streptomycin	

Antiprotozoals	*Anthelmintics*
Sulfadimethoxine	Dichlorvos
Amprolium	Levamisole
	Thiabenzadole

* From *Chemicals and Health*. National Science Foundation, Washington, D.C., 1973.

The impact on the population of increased chemical usage is difficult to unravel. There are positive and negative impacts to evaluate. Suffice it to say that with the exception of the startling revelations of a chemical tragedy such as the misuse of Kepone in Virginia during 1975–1976, or the exposed population associated with excess cancer from asbestos, there is limited quantitative information on the impact of increased chemical usage in our economy. It must be concluded that the sheer magnitude of the growth in chemical usage and indicators of impact led to the surge in regulatory toxicology during the 1955–1977 period, but particularly during the 1960s.

It is not the purpose of this chapter to delineate the details of one or another of the regulations cited above. Rather, it is my purpose to discuss the related philosophic and scientific principles that either have been accepted or are evolving, and that dictate the form of final regulations and administrative procedures associated with regulation of chemicals. It is the purpose of this chapter to look at the general structure of these regulations and to examine the basis for their passage, construction, and implementation. In so doing, illustrations will be drawn from selected regulations. Before embarking on this examination it should be noted that the approach utilized in the United States is not that adopted by other industrialized nations.

In general, other nations approach regulatory toxicology with less specific regulations than the United States. The Health and Safety Executive in England is delegated sweeping authority to regulate the workplace (Health and Safety at Work Act, 1974). The Executive transmits to the person having control of any premises the "general duty" to "use the best practical means for preventing the emission into the atmosphere from the premises of noxious or offensive substances and for rendering harmless and inoffensive such substances as may be emitted." The Executive only in the case of very highly toxic compounds elaborates on this duty in the form of specific standards. Inspectors employed by the Executive to enforce the regulation are, in general, less familiar with specific technical aspects of the work environment or toxic chemicals than their United States counterparts, who enforce highly specific regulatory standards administratively promulgated by the agency created in the enabling regulatory statute.

The Swedish Act, in effect since January 1974, is part of a broader act entitled "The Act on Co-Determination at Work" (Workers Protection Act, 1974). The approach in Sweden is to focus responsibility on joint labor-management committees to resolve dangers in the workplace.

There are few specific standards. Professional physicians, environmentalists, and toxicologists are employed by the government, industry, or the university and together they resolve the nature of the problem. It is only when the negotiations encouraged by establishment of specific organizational components fail that the regulatory agency is called on the scene to resolve the problem. As an example, paragraph 40B of the Workers Protection Act reads as follows: "If a work involves immediate and serious danger to the life or health of an employee and if no immediate remedy can be obtained through representations to the employer, the safety delegate may order the suspension of the work pending a decision by the labor inspectorate . . . the safety delegate cannot be held liable for any damage resulting from a measure referred to in the first paragraph." The Norwegians, on the other hand, have chosen to spell out in the law the demands that may be put upon the working conditions. The Swedes have left the specifics of regulation open, to be finally decided by the people in the particular working situation or, if necessary, by the labor inspectorate and its board.

The rationale for the Swedish approach is that technology changes and so do social values and norms. Such changes shall be incorporated in the demands on the work environment without cumbersome procedures required to change the law. The Swedes believe that the working conditions should be adapted to workers' physical and mental prerequisites—that is, needs and capacities. The same philosophy extends to their approach to regulation of toxic materials in the environment. The Swedish approach has been extended, for the most part, by the Danes in their Working Environment Act (The Working Environment Act, 1975). Thus, we should be aware that the approach that will be elaborated upon in this chapter is unique to the United States, to its historic tradition, and to its human resources. It would probably be a mistake for another nation to adopt verbatim the approach embodied in United States statutes or standards without carefully considering their relevance to the historic tradition, population, and current societal problems of that nation.

ASSESSMENT OF RISK

The level of exposure to a toxic substance may be free of risk under one set of circumstances but not under another. Permissible levels of exposure must be considered against the backdrop of the specific conditions in which they will be used. For example, it is not suprising to find lower permissible exposures to a toxic substance for the general population where there are susceptible individuals present, i.e., infants, senior citizens, those suffering from disease, than among the working population. The decision making for regulating chemicals in the environment is evolving (Committee on Principles of Decision Making for Regulating Chemicals in the Environment, 1975). A critical concept in the evolution of considerations for decision making is that of risk (Lowrance, 1976; Rowe, 1977). Lowrance differentiates between the evaluation or estimate of risk, which is a scientific endeavor, and the acceptance of levels of risk, which involves sociopolitical decision making. For example, Table 29–4 indicates the estimated comparative risks of selected activities in the United Kingdom.

Table 29–4. ESTIMATED RISKS FOR SELECTED ACTIVITIES*†

RISKS	ACTIVITY
1/400	Smoking (10 cigarettes/day)
1/2,000	All accidents
1/8,000	Traffic accidents
1/30,000	Work in industry
1/50,000	Natural disasters
1/1,000,000	Driving 80.5 kilometers‡
1/1,000,000	Being struck by lightning

* From Flowers, B. D. (chairman): *Royal Commission on the Environment, Sixth Report: Nuclear Power and the Environment*. Her Majesty's Stationery Office, London, 1976.
† Risk is expressed as probability of death for an individual for a year of exposure and orders of magnitude only are given.
‡ This risk is conveniently expressed in the form indicated rather than in terms of a year of exposure.

The comparative risks tabulated in Table 29–4 reflect perception of risk, which is not absolute; it is arrived at in relation to an individual's personal experience and his or her environment. A society arrives at the acceptance of these risks by a very complex interaction of individual perceptions and societal procedures. Until recently, risk-benefit analyses have been made without explicit consideration of how risks and benefits are distributed among various societal sectors. Those who accept risk and those who benefit from the acceptance of risk are not always the same individuals.

Recent focus on the topic of risk has categorized risk as follows (Science Council of Canada, 1977):

1. Voluntary risks.
2. Risks that can be modified by the risk-taker's behavior.
3. Risks that are taken involuntarily.
4. Risks taken in ignorance of the hazard.
5. Risks in which there can be no direct awareness of the level of risk although there is a general awareness of the existence of a hazard, for example, in a low-level radiation exposure.

6. Short-term hazards, as opposed to long-term risks, where the consequences of exposure may only be seen years after the exposure is ended, as in the case of asbestos or vinyl chloride exposure.

7. A category of special hazards where the individual involved may not be in a position to assess the benefit of the damage of the procedure, for example, in psychosurgery and medicinal use of drugs.

Inherent in consideration of risk is the acceptance of the statistical basis for assigning risk to any hazard. As Alvin Weinberg has noted, there is a category of problems with which society deals that he designates as "trans-science." These problems do not have objective proof or certainty and such proof or certainty is unattainable (Weinberg, 1972). The public perception of what constitutes an acceptable risk can be viewed as an exercise in "trans-science" problem solving.

A current controversy involves the so-called exportation of high-risk industries by highly industrialized Western nations. Thus, Brazil has indicated it is anxious to import industries with large pollution potential because it has extensive tracts of remote land where such industries can be located. Air and water pollutants can be discharged with little risk to the public. The perception of Brazilians vis-à-vis pollutant effluents is obviously different from the perception of the public in technologically advanced, high-population-density nations such as the United States, Germany, and England, for example.

The measurement of risk is a scientific activity. Existing information must be summarized and carefully considered before a regulatory body takes action on the data at hand. Those opposed to regulatory decisions often attempt to place the risk associated with the decision in perspective with other risks. Thus, Wilson (1978) questioned the decision of the Occupational Safety and Health Administration to regulate benzene to an airborne concentration of 1 part per million (ppm). He calculated that the cost of saving one life attributable to benzene exposure would be approximately 300×10^6. Wilson considers risks in everyday life that increase the change of death 1 part in a million, or expressed differently, risks that reduce one's life expectancy by eight minutes. Table 29–5 is a summary of activities with this level of risk.

Clearly, Table 29–5 represents estimates rather than firm calculations of risk. It illustrates current probing to develop comparisons for the purpose of decision making.

The perception of hazards is continuously

Table 29–5. EXPOSURES THAT INCREASE THE CHANCE OF DEATH BY 1 PART IN A MILLION, OR REDUCE LIFE EXPECTANCY BY EIGHT MINUTES*

Smoking 1.4 cigarettes
Living two months with a cigarette smoker
One x-ray (in a good hospital)
Eating 100 charcoal-broiled steaks
Eating 40 tablespoons of peanut butter
Drinking 10,000 24-ounce soft drinks from recently banned plastic bottles
Drinking 30 12-ounce cans of diet soda containing saccharin
Living 20 years near a polyvinyl chloride plant
Living 15 years within 30 miles of a nuclear-powered plant

---

* From Wilson, R.: A rational approach to reducing cancer risk. *New York Times*, July 7, 1978.

altering. The changing attitude of society toward lead as a toxic agent is illustrative of this process of change (Corn, 1975). The significance of the history of plumbism up to this point is that an ancient disease once considered acceptable has been reevaluated; it is now perceived as a serious medical, human, and social problem. This change of focus is based on new scientific data that have changed our perceptions of the earlier manifestations of lead poisoning and created new attitudes toward the effect of lead poisoning on the health of industrial workers and the general population exposed to lead. The new uses of lead, the new ability to make more accurate measurements, advances in biochemical science, and new attitudes toward the public health have all meshed to challenge the traditional concept of lead poisoning. In the dialogue that has been initiated between those who see a threat and those who do not, the concept of health risk and even the concept of disease itself are undergoing redefinition.

There are numerous examples of the altering perceptions of risk. Asbestos has been known to cause asbestosis, a fibrosis of the lung, since the 1920s. In the 1950s it was associated with increased incidence of lung cancer and in the 1960s it was specifically associated with a very rare form of lung cancer, mesothelioma. In general, as more specific and more readily identifiable effects of the hazard came to the forefront, the time frame for public response and regulatory action shortened. Chronic toxic agents with long periods of latency are the most difficult to treat within a regulatory framework, because the arguments advanced for regulation can be refuted on the basis of lack of data on human populations. Because the regulatory measures are often extreme, the public is reluctant to accept these measures in the absence of "real data."

In the real world, risk is seldom encountered by exposure to single chemical agents. Members of society are exposed to multiple chemical agents on the job and in the community. The biologic action of these agents in complex mixtures cannot, in general, be assessed. It is known that certain chemical agents acting together have an effect greater than that of either acting alone, i.e., synergism, and that some acting together have an effect that is less than the summation of the effects of each acting alone, i.e., antagonism. In the complex interactions of air pollutants, for example, the combined effect of sulfur dioxide suspended particulate matter, nitrogen oxides, polynuclear aromatic hydrocarbons, oxidants, etc., are not clearly understood.

The nature of the evidence contributing to the assessment of risk and the problems of inference stemming from incomplete data or data based on animals and extrapolated to man are discussed by Lowrance (1976). Lowrance also lays the groundwork for discussion of factors entering into the judgment of the level of acceptance of risk. These topics will increasingly enter into rule making in the United States and elsewhere for regulation of toxic agents in the environment. The process of rule making is becoming increasingly analytic, with the demands for benefit-risk analysis increasing in direct proportion to the cost borne by the community as a result of regulatory action.

The remainder of this chapter is devoted to the implementation of regulation after a risk has been judged to be unacceptable. In the United States, a host of regulatory agencies have been created on the basis of statutes promulgated, as noted above. One or more agencies have responsibility for regulating the hazardous substance or condition. The Occupational Safety and Health Administration will be frequently utilized as illustrative of the problems encountered by regulatory agencies in implementing enabling legislation passed by the Congress to protect the public from unacceptable risks associated with toxic substances. OSHA is not unrepresentative of other agencies, such as the Environmental Protection Agency, the Food and Drug Administration, and the Mine Safety and Health Agency. Where OSHA does differ from these regulatory bodies it will be noted.

SKELETON OF ENABLING LEGISLATION FOR CONTROL OF TOXIC SUBSTANCES

Enabling regulatory legislation consists, in general, of the following major categories of descriptive material. For purposes of illustration, the Occupational Safety and Health Act of 1970 (Commerce Clearing House, 1978) is utilized.

Each piece of enabling legislation is associated with a documented legislative history, which includes verbatim transcripts of Congressional debates, supplementary materials, etc. (Legislative History of the Occupational Safety and Health Act of 1970, 1971).

1. Coverage
2. Duties of employers and employees
3. Safety and health standards
4. National Advisory Committee
5. Inspections
6. Citations
7. Enforcement
8. Occupational Safety and Health Review Commission
9. Imminent danger
10. Penalties
11. State-federal arrangements
12. Records to be maintained
13. National Institute for Occupational Safety and Health (NIOSH)
14. Research
15. Training
16. Statistics
17. Federal agency programs

Some of these areas are specific to the Occupational Safety and Health Act (OSHA); others are not. The specific OSHA sections will have their counterparts in other statutes. The regulatory act establishes the responsibilities and creates an agency or agencies to fulfill the needs to be met by the enabling legislation. Each of the areas noted above will be briefly discussed in terms of the Occupational Safety and Health Act.

Coverage

The Act is applicable to all employers whose business affects commerce except the U.S. Government, or any state or political subdivision of a state, mining, railroads, or those employers under regulations of the Atomic Energy Commission. Special provisions are included prescribing the responsibility of the federal government. State employees are covered by the Act, when the state's plan for an occupational safety and health program is approved by the Secretary of Labor.

Duties of Employers and Employees

Employers are to furnish to their employees employment and a place of employment free of recognized hazards that are causing or likely to cause death or serious physical harm to employees, and are required to comply with the occupational safety and health standards promulgated under the Act.

Thus, the employer's responsibility is not only to comply with standards but also to mitigate or eliminate "recognized hazards" even if there are no standards promulgated concerning that hazard.

Employees are also required to comply with all standards, rules, and regulations issued pursuant to the Act that are applicable to their actions and conduct.

Safety and Health Standards

The initial standards package that was published was adopted by the Secretary of Labor from the so-called consensus standards of the American National Standards Institute (ANSI), the National Fire Protection Agency (NFPA), and certain established federal standards. Consensus standards could be adopted until April 28, 1973. The rules of procedure call for public review of any new standards before they are adopted.

Any standards that deal with toxic materials should prove that "no employee will suffer material impairment of health or functional capacity even if such employee has regular exposure to the hazard dealt with by such standard for the period of his working life," on the basis of the best available evidence.

The Secretary is required to issue emergency temporary standards that take effect immediately if he determines that employees are exposed "to grave danger" from exposure to substances determined to be toxic or from new hazards, and if such emergency standard is necessary to protect employees. The emergency standard then stays in effect until a permanent standard is promulgated, which must be done within six months. Procedures are established for judicial review of these actions.

National Advisory Committee

A National Advisory Committee on Occupational Safety and Health representing labor, management, safety and health professions, and the public is created. There are provisions for other advisory committees, as well.

Inspections

Inspections may be made by representatives of the Secretary of Labor (compliance officers) at reasonable times and during working hours. The Secretary of HEW also has the right of entry to determine the adequacy of records of injuries, illnesses, and exposures to potentially toxic and harmful materials. Both employer and employee representatives may accompany the Department of Labor representatives on inspection tours. Provisions are made for employees or their representatives to request inspections from the Secretary.

Citations

When a violation of the standards or a recognized hazard is found, the Secretary issues a citation in writing describing the violation or hazard and specifying the amount of time allowed to abate the violation. The Secretary is authorized to establish procedures for the issuance of "*de minimis*" notices where no direct relationship to safety or health is involved. Citations are to be posted in the workplace at or near the location of the violation.

Enforcement

When a citation is issued, the Secretary notifies the employer of any penalty. The employer has 15 days to contest either the citation, the penalty, or the abatement period. If the employer does not respond within 15 days, the citation shall be considered a final order of the Occupational Safety and Health Review Commission. If the employer contests the citation or any penalty within the time limits specified, the Commission holds hearings giving all parties an opportunity to be heard. The Commission issues a decision based on the record at the hearings.

Occupational Safety and Health Review Commission

The Commission consists of three members appointed by the President for six-year terms. Appointments are confirmed by the Senate. The Act authorizes the appointment of hearing examiners (called judges), whose decisions will become the order of the Commission unless a Commission member requests within 30 days that the report be reviewed by the Commission.

Imminent Danger

The Secretary may petition the U.S. Court to shut down an operation where a "danger exists which could reasonably be expected to cause death or serious physical harm immediately or before the imminence of such danger can be eliminated through enforcement procedures otherwise provided by this Act."

Penalties

Civil penalties are provided up to $1,000 (1) for each violation (where they are not of a serious nature, such penalty is discretionary) and (2) for each day in which a final order is violated. A penalty of up to $10,000 is provided for each willful or repeated violation of employer duties. Criminal penalties are set for willful violations resulting in death.

State-Federal Arrangements

The Act places all jurisdiction regarding occupational safety and health under its terms in the federal government, except for those occupational safety and health issues for which no federal standards are in effect. A state can assume jurisdiction by submitting a state plan that is approved by the Secretary of Labor.

Records to Be Maintained

Each employer is required to maintain and make available such records as the Secretary, in cooperation with the Secretary of HEW, may prescribe as appropriate for the enforcement of the Act or for developing information regarding the causes and prevention of occupational accidents and illnesses. Such rules may include provisions requiring employers to conduct periodic inspections (but not to determine or report their own state of compliance). The Secretary must prescribe regulations requiring employers to (1) maintain accurate records of work-related deaths, injuries, and illnesses other than minor injuries requiring only first-aid treatment and which do not involve medical treatment, loss of consciousness, restriction of work or motion, or transfer to another job; and (2) maintain records of employee exposure to potentially toxic materials or harmful physical agents. Certain information must be provided to the employee in the latter instance. Records must be kept for periods of time specified by the Secretary.

National Institute for Occupational Safety and Health (NIOSH)

A National Institute is created within the Department of HEW and it is authorized, among other things, "to develop and establish recommended safety and health standards."

Research

The Act provides for research by HEW relating to occupational safety and health including, but not limited to, (1) psychologic factors involved, (2) criteria dealing with toxic materials and harmful agents, and (3) effects of chronic or low-level exposure to materials and processes on the potential for illness.

Training

The Secretary of HEW is to conduct, directly or by grants or contracts, (1) education programs to provide an adequate supply of qualified personnel to carry out the purpose of the Act, and (2) informational programs on the importance of the proper use of safety and health equipment.

Statistics

The Secretary, in consultation with the Secretary of HEW, is required to develop and maintain a system for collecting and analyzing occupational safety and health statistics. Included are work injuries and illnesses that are serious or significant even if they do not cause loss of time. Those injuries and illnesses specifically excluded are minor injuries requiring only first-aid treatment, or that do not involve medical treatment, loss of consciousness, restriction of work or motion, or transfer to another job.

JUDGMENT OF RISK: THE CONCEPT OF A TOXIC SUBSTANCE STANDARD

The word standard is here used in the sense of a legally enforceable body of requirements that must be met by those in responsible charge of the environment, the workplace, or a commercial product. Because of the legal ramifications of standards, the standard-setting process must result in goals that are achievable by those legally charged with meeting them. Failure to do this results in lack of confidence in the standards and in those drafting them, and resistance to the enforcement process. Where guidelines, which are not legally binding, are involved, an entirely different set of circumstances apply. The usual result of unrealistic guidelines is that they are ignored by all concerned. They remain a scholarly ideal having little relationship to reality. Apparently, from all eyewitness accounts, U.S.S.R. guidelines for the concentrations of substances in workplace air fall into this category.

If we use control of chemicals in the workplace as an example, the control of occupational hazards is an exercise in sorting out the risk associated with a particular agent or situation in relation to all the other risks we must accept as a part of our daily lives. Lowrance (1976) made a major contribution by differentiating between risk assessment, which is an empiric, scientific endeavor, and judgment of risk, which is a normative political exercise. In the United States, it is the latter exercise that now leads to the proposal for, and promulgation of, an occupational safety or health standard under the provisions of the Occupational Safety and Health Act.

Lowrance stresses that "safety is not measured; risks are measured. Only when those risks are weighed on the balance of social values can safety be judged: a thing is safe if its attendant risks are judged to be acceptable."

The mixing of these two activities, the assessment of risk and the judgment of risk, in U.S. occupational health standards–setting processes since 1971 has been the cause of much of the bitterness engendered in politically identifiable groups associated with occupational standards setting in the United States. The confusion of these two activities by those charged with straightforward administration of the regulatory machinery, as well as by those intent on achieving often parochial results related to a single standard, has confused the public and jeopardized the entire regulatory process. Because there are often insufficient scientific data to assess risk, the final recommendations of each individual concerned are a judgment of the acceptability of the risk and not a contribution to the assessment of the risk. However, it has not been couched in those terms in the formative steps of standards setting, such as the hearing. The Occupational Safety and Health Agency has, in contrast, taken pains on many occasions to separate risk assessment from judgment of the acceptability of risk. The following quotation from the Coke Oven Emissions Standard (Exposure to Coke Oven Emissions, 1976) illustrates the explicit nature of judgment of risk acceptability, which was made by OSHA. The judgment was sustained as reasonable and valid by the Third Circuit Court of Appeals after the standard was challenged by the American Iron and Steel Institute.

> Then from the point of view of choosing a safe level of exposure, the permissible exposure limit should be set at zero. However, based on the evidence in the record, OSHA does not believe that a zero standard for exposure to coke oven emissions is technologically feasible. In fact, it is clear that for any of the indicator substances considered, certain quantities of each substance are present in the ambient environment as a result of natural phenomena and as artifacts of human activity . . . . OSHA has determined that 150 μg/m³ is the level which most adequately assures, to the extent feasible, the protection of coke oven workers. Several factors have been considered in making this determination and are discussed below.*

The judgment of risk acceptability will be challenged in the U.S. framework of government. The judgment of acceptability of risks is a controversial exercise in regulatory government with often very expensive ramifications following from the final judgments. In the case of the Coke Oven Emissions Standard, the cost to the coking industry was estimated to be $275 × 10⁶ per year. Of course, these costs will be passed on to U.S. citizens, but the differential impacts of these costs to individual employers within an industry and to the industry in its international conduct of business cannot be ignored; the impacts are real and they stimulate intensive, sustained involvement of these sectors in the rule making. When faced with judgments that differ from those they

---

* Exposure to Coke Oven Emissions: Department of Labor, Occupational Safety and Health Administration, Occupational Safety and Health Standards. *Federal Register*, **41**(no. 206):46742–90, Oct. 22, 1976.

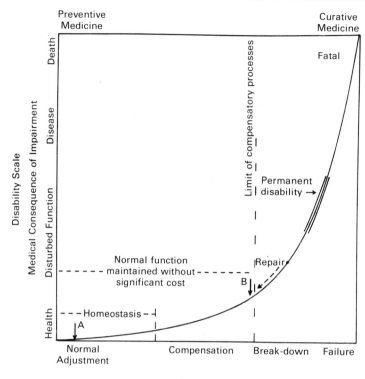

Figure 29–1. Suggested relationship between impairment and disability. Considerable movement along the scale of impairment accompanied by relatively little disability. Basic man-environment relationships are between environmental stress and impairment, the precursor of disease. (From Hatch, T. F.: Changing objectives in occupational health. *Am. Ind. Hyg. Assoc. J.*, **23**:1–7, 1962.)

would make if they were the regulators, the private sector, or organized labor, becomes the aggrieved party and presses for the judgment of risk by a third, objective party, i.e., the courts. OSHA operates on the assumption that *every* standard will be challenged in the courts.

In the case of occupational standards, Congress in its wisdom intended to separate risk assessment and risk judgment in the OSHA of 1970. NIOSH was to assess risk, and OSHA in the standards-setting process was to reflect the wishes of the body politic in judging the risk. The process was to be an open one with the widest possible participation of all of our society. The judgment of risk process has been open, and, although hectic, has adhered to the aims of the Act. In the cases of clean air, clean water, and toxic substances control regulation by the Environmental Protection Agency, assessment and judgment of risk are vested in one agency of government.

The question raised by the concept of standards for toxic chemicals is how do we place and monitor individuals in environments so that a risk judged to be unacceptable to that individual is not encountered. Can our standards act as a template for such management through medical and environmental surveillance, administrative

and engineering controls, etc.? Can we establish surveillance methods to identify those at high risk and can we devise acceptable administrative procedures to reduce this risk?

Figure 29–1 illustrates some guiding principles, both in the assessment of risk and in the judgment of risk procedures.

In Figure 2 [Fig. 29–1] a distinction is made between impairment and disability, the two scales representing, respectively, the underlying disturbance of the system and the consequence of such disturbance in terms of identifiable disease. Starting with normal health, the individual progresses, for one reason or another, along the scale of impairment and of disability, ultimately to death. Early departures from health (impairment) are accompanied by little disability. In the beginning, normal homeostatic processes insure adequate adjustment to offset stress and for a distance beyond this early zone of change, compensatory processes similarly maintain the overall function of the system without serious disability. Further increments in impairment beyond the limits of compensatory processes, however, are accompanied by rapidly increasing increments in disability and the individual moves into the region of sickness and disability, terminating in death. A healthy individual, functioning at point A on the curve and subjected to a given kind

processes reasonably necessary or appropriate to provide safe and healthful employment and places of employment. Thus, a standard for a toxic chemical is not merely the limiting concentration of the material in air below which those dealing with the agent may be exposed. It has a much broader interpretation. It applies to the way in which the chemical is handled, to work practices to reduce exposure, etc. This interpretation extends to statutes other than the Occupational Safety and Health Act. There are workplace standards (OSHA), ambient air quality standards (Clean Air Act), emissions standards governing the amount of material that can be released into the atmosphere or into waterways (Clean Air Act and Clean Water Act), and standards for maximum content of specific chemicals (Consumer Product Safety Act). Under OSHA, standards in the sense defined above have been passed for regulation of coke emissions, acrylonitrile, and 14 carcinogens, for examples. Under the Mine Safety and Health Act (MSHA), standards in the above sense are in effect for respirable coal mine dust, methane, noise, and visible light in underground mines.

In order to clarify the ingredients of a typical standard, including the extent of the detail contained therein, the OSHA Coke Oven Emissions Standard is used here as an example.

Typical Ingredients of OSHA Coke Oven Emission Standard

1. Scope and Application. This section indicates extent of coverage of the Standard.

2. Definitions. The technical terms relevant to the Standard are defined.

3. Permissible Exposure Limit. The maximum-time-weighted average concentration (mg/m^3) to which an employee can be exposed is defined.

4. Regulated Areas. Defines areas of limited employee access on coke batteries.

5. Exposure Monitoring and Measurement. Defines the obligations of the employer to measure the exposure of employees to the agent and indicates required frequency, type, and required accuracy of sampling, among other sampling aspects.

6. Methods of Compliance. Indicates specific, required engineering controls and work practices, including employee training programs in these areas.

7. Regulatory Protection. Indicates requirements for respirators where other control methods are in progress. Respirators are regarded as an interim control.

8. Protective Clothing and Equipment. Indicates the minimum protective gear required.

9. Hygiene Facilities and Practices. Change rooms, showers, lunchroom, and lavatory requirements are presented.

10. Medical Surveillance. Indicates in detail the frequency and types of examinations to be conducted with the employee's consent. Also indicates the period during which records must be retained.

11. Employee Information and Training. Discusses the requirements for institution and maintenance of an employee training program related to provisions of the standard.

12. Precautionary Signs and Labels. Cites specific employer obligations for designation of plant areas affected by the standard, including specific legend of signs for posting.

All of the above requirements represent the standard; employers are subject to citation for failure to comply with any of the above sections of the standard.

PROCEDURES FOR RULE MAKING IN REGULATORY TOXICOLOGY

The procedures for promulgating a rule regulating the substance or mixture against unreasonable health or environmental risks under the Toxic Substances Control Act (TOSCA) are no different than the procedures specified in the Occupational Safety and Health Act or the Mine Safety and Health Act of 1977. Therefore, TOSCA procedures are here cited as illustrative.

The Administrator must publish a statement concerning the following:

1. The effects of the substance or mixture on health and the environment.

2. The magnitude of the exposure of human beings in the environment to the substance or mixture.

3. The benefits of the substance or mixture for various uses and the availability of substitutes for such uses.

4. The reasonably ascertainable economic consequences of the rule after consideration of the effect on the national economy, small business, technologic innovation, the environment, and public health.

The EPA Administrator also must make determinations regarding the adequacy of actions under other federal laws administered by EPA to eliminate or reduce the risks. If the risks may be regulated by another federal law administered by EPA, the Administrator may not promulgate a regulation under TOSCA unless he determines that it is in the public interest to resort to the Act rather than the other law in question.

The Toxic Substances Control Act has some significant modifications and additions to the administrative procedures act, which in general is followed by OSHA and MSHA. Under TOSCA there must be an opportunity for an informal hearing, the requirements of which are prescribed. In an informal hearing, any interested person can present his/her position both orally and in writing. An interested person also has a limited conditional right to cross-examine at an informal hearing. Cross-examination is conditioned on the Administrator's determination that there are disputed issues. The Administrator has discretion on what may be covered in the cross-examination. There must be a verbatim transcript of any oral presentation and cross-examination in an informal hearing. This requirement also covers formal hearings.

The concept of standards embodied in many of the Acts discussed, namely complete protection of all those exposed, is well intentioned, but tends to ignore some of the basic toxicologic insights that are currently available to us and that make fulfillment of the Congressional mandate in many of these Acts virtually impossible. The first difficulty encountered is that of the highly susceptible individual exposed to a chemical agent. High-risk groups are a reality in all populations convered by standards (Calabrese, 1978). Can the standard be protective of the most susceptible individual(s)? In certain cases, e.g., lead and its effect on the human fetus, there is evidence that such a policy may not be technologically feasible. This is a particularly difficult regulatory issue (Workshop on the Assessment of Reproductive Hazards in the Workplace, 1978). The administrative procedures for standards development are designed to provide extensive examination of these difficult issues before promulgation of the final standard by an agency. In making final judgments on controversial issues, the agency must rely on the record of the hearing(s) and submitted comments. The evidence must support the final rule promulgation or it will not withstand challenge in the courts. Therefore, it is desirable to document all aspects of a standard in the official record.

ADDITIONAL SELECTED ASPECTS OF REGULATORY TOXICOLOGY

Temporary Emergency Standard

The due process of law followed under the Administrative Procedures Act or a modified Administrative Procedures Act need not be followed in most regulatory enabling acts if the Administrator declares that an emergency temporary standard is appropriate. Under TOSCA this is referred to as an imminent hazard. Under the Occupational Safety and Health Act

of 1970, an emergency temporary standard can take immediate effect upon publication in the *Federal Register*. It can be promulgated if the Administrator determines (1) that employees are exposed to grave danger from exposure to substances or agents determined to be toxic or physically harmful or from new hazards and (2) that such emergency standard is necessary to protect employees from such danger. The emergency temporary standard remains in effect for six months; it must then be replaced by a permanent standard, one promulgated after due process is followed. The concept of imminent danger or imminent hazard implies that the individual agent or the environment will cause injury to health or unreasonable risk. The Administrator, with the backing of a court order, can take immediate action under these conditions. Under TOSCA, in addition to civil actions against a person or persons, a civil action is authorized for seizure of an imminently hazardous chemical substance or mixture.

General Duty Clause

Most regulatory enabling acts include a general duty clause. In the Occupational Safety and Health Act it is Section V of the Act: "Each employer 1) shall furnish to each of his employees employment and a place of employment which are free from recognized hazards that are causing or are likely to cause death or serious physical harm to his employees, and 2) shall comply with occupational safety and health standards promulgated under this Act." In general, the courts have recognized the appropriateness of the general duty clause when a standard does not cover the particular hazard at issue. The general duty clause cannot be used where a standard for that hazard is active.

The heart of a regulatory agency's activities are the standards. The Occupational Safety and Health Act permitted the Assistant Secretary of Labor to adopt consensus safety standards and standards that existed in preexisting federal statutes, these adoptions to occur within the first two years of the Act. Many standards were adopted that were never meant to be legally enforceable, particularly in the areas of safety hazards. However, the very presence of these standards rules out citation of violations in areas covered, however inadequately, by adopted consensus standards. In retrospect, one can conclude that the adoption of many of these consensus standards led to many of the problems that the Occupational Safety and Health Administration encountered during its early years. The Agency has taken steps to revoke many of these standards. The lesson to all regulatory agencies is that standards tuned to the goals of the enabling legislation must be carefully developed. Existing standards, originally developed for other purposes, cannot be adopted *en masse* and be expected to lend themselves to the procedures authorized by the Congress for enforcement.

Enforcement

Each regulatory agency must ensure that it fairly and without bias extends the adopted standards to all regulatees. Most agencies work out of regional and area offices in the United States. U.S. federal jurisdiction is divided into ten regional areas. Policy from the central offices of the agency must be transmitted by the regional administrator to each of the area offices in his/her jurisdiction and then to inspectors in the field. This represents a vast network of regulatory personnel, all of whom must deal with the public in a consistent, equitable manner. Extensive communications are essential between central offices, usually in Washington, DC, where policy is established, and field offices that interface with the public. Figure 29–2 shows the organization of the Occupational Safety and Health Administration. It is representative of regulatory agency organization where inspection is part of agency function.

The major tool of the regulatory force in the field is the on-site inspection. The inspector must be qualified in the subject area that he/she is enforcing and must determine if the regulatee is in compliance with all existing standards. The inspector can observe work practices, check monitoring records to determine exposures of personnel, determine quantities of materials handled, labeling practices, test emissions from sources by obtaining samples for laboratory analyses, etc. Records, including photographic documentation of procedures, can be obtained.

If the compliance officer or inspector finds a violation of standards, a citation is recommended. The recommended citations are usually reviewed at the area office and in some agencies at the regional office before issuance. The citation must be specific and must reference the standard violated. There are civil penalties associated with citations; in some regulatory acts there are also criminal penalties, usually for willful violation of the standard when grave harm or death has resulted.

Review of Citations

There is usually a provision in the enforcement procedure for the regulatee to obtain review of the citation. Under OSHA a quasi-judiciary three-member review commission was created for this purpose. A similar five-member board functions under the Mine Safety and Health Act.

If the regulatee disagrees with the conclusions of the review commission, the appeal can be carried to the Federal Circuit Court of Appeals and, if necessary, to the Supreme Court. There are cases on record where the regulatee has gone the full route for judicial review, including seeking a Supreme Court ruling. Thus, due process provides for administrative review of citations followed by judicial review.

Records, Statistics, Reports

The paucity of data relating to the effects on exposed population of potentially toxic chemicals has led to a record-keeping requirement in most regulatory statutes. This, in turn, has stimulated the private sector to establish computer-based health statistics information systems, or health service data systems.

Under the Toxic Substances Control Act, reports submitted to the EPA may be required to include the common or trade name, the chemical identity, and the molecular structure of chemicals produced; proposed categories of use of the chemicals; total amount manufactured, estimates of future promotion, the amount manufactured for each category use and estimates of future production, description of by-products resulting from use; all existing data concerning the environmental and health effects of the chemicals; occupational exposures, including the number of people exposed and the workplace estimates of the number of people to be exposed in the future and the duration of such exposures; and the methods of disposal of the chemicals. TOSCA does not require the reporting of changes in the proportions of mixtures unless the Administrator finds it necessary for efficient enforcement of the Act. The information so received, together with premarket notification information, will be used by EPA to compile an inventory list of chemicals manufactured or processed in the United States. For purposes of the Act, importing is considered to be the same as manufacturing. The reporting provisions of the Act do not apply to small manufacturers, as defined by the EPA, except that small manufacturers may be required to submit data for use in compiling an initial inventory list. Manufacturers are required to keep records of significant adverse reactions to health or the environment alleged to have been caused by a chemical substance. This information may have come to the manufacturer from any source, including consumer complaint of injury, occupational injury reports, and complaints of injury to the environment. The seriousness, duration, and frequency of reaction should be taken into account in establishing what constitutes a significant adverse reaction. An individual

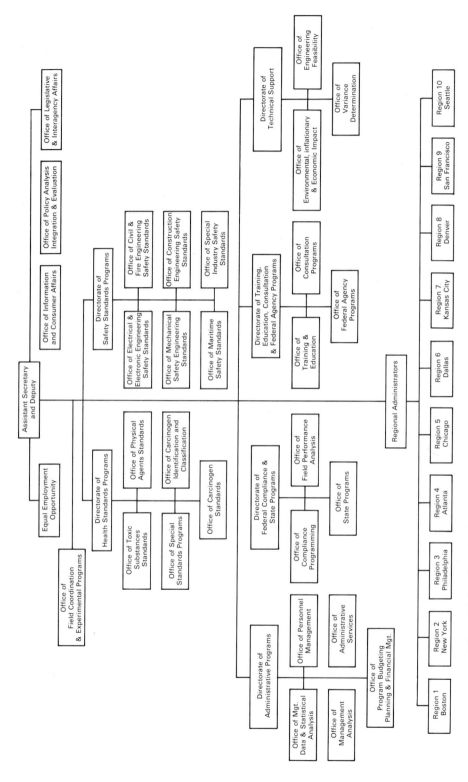

Figure 29-2. Organization of the Occupational Safety and Health Administration (November 1976).

complaint may represent an idiosyncratic reaction. However, similar complaints from several people may be significant. It is clear that Congressional conferees intended that the requirement to maintain records err on the side of safety.

Records of adverse effects on employee health must be retained for 30 years. In the case of some materials, such as asbestos, records must be retained for 40 years. It can be seen that the surveillance and record-keeping requirements stimulated by regulation of toxic substances are extensive.

The substance-by-substance approach of the regulatory agencies has recently come into question. A move is being made to deal with generic standards, such as the generic standard for carcinogens proposed by the Occupational Safety and Health Administration in October 1977 (Identification, Classification, and Regulation of Occupational Carcinogens, 1977). This approach embodies the treatment of chemicals by class, rather than by individual substance. A generic standard includes a framework for regulation, rather than extensive material on a single substance. The OSHA generic standard for carcinogens establishes four categories of carcinogens or potentially carcinogenic substances and specifies the evidence on which the agency will assign a substance to a category. The regulatory actions following substance categorization are specified. Table 29–6 briefly summarizes the OSHA proposal. On July 14, 1978, OSHA released a preliminary list of 269 chemicals it would assign to category I for regulation under its proposed rule for carcinogen classification (Table 29–6).

It is anticipated that the generic approach to toxic chemicals control will enable the regulatory agencies to deal more rapidly with chemicals scheduled for control under the due process of law (administrative procedures requirements) and will also lessen the reporting requirements of the regulatees. The generic approach requires only that a hearing be held on the data relevant to the assignment of a chemical to a category for regulation. At the time of this writing, OSHA Hearings on the Generic Standards for Carcinogens have been held. The outcome of this approach remains to be determined. However, the agency has revealed plans for a similar generic approach to pesticides and to labeling of chemicals. The Consumer Product Safety Commission has issued a tentative classification system for carcinogens, one similar to that of OSHA.

SUMMARY

A new term, "regulatory toxicology," has been introduced to describe governmental activities and procedures to ensure safe utilization of chemicals in our society. The enormous growth of the chemical industry and the ubiquitous nature of chemicals in our environment have stimulated a plethora of legislation related to the regulation of chemicals in the workplace, in the outdoor environment, and in commercial products. The enabling legislation specifies creation of a responsible agency to administer the statute and standards of performance for regulatees. The development of feasible, meaningful standards is a highly controversial and litigious activity that, under most statutes, adheres to the Federal Administrative Procedures Act. Standards can

Table 29–6. CLASSIFICATION OF SUBSTANCES ACCORDING TO PROPOSED OSHA RULE FOR CARCINOGENS*

CATEGORY	SCIENTIFIC EVIDENCE	MODEL STANDARD	EXPOSURE LIMIT
I. Confirmed carcinogen	Carcinogenic in humans, in 2 mammalian species, or in repeated tests in the same species	Emergency temporary standard; permanent standard in 6 months	Lowest feasible level, or banned if suitable substitute is available
II. Suspect carcinogen	Evidence from only one animal species or if evidence is inconclusive	Permanent standard	Low enough to prevent acute or chronic toxic effects
III.	Insufficient evidence to classify it in a higher category	No standard, but would be listed as needing more data	
IV.	Substances that could fall into the 3 higher categories, but not found in U.S. workplaces	No standard, listed to alert to potential danger	

* From Identification, Classification, and Regulation of Occupational Carcinogens. OSHA Proposed Rule, 42FR54148, Oct. 4, 1977.

include provisions for permissible exposure concentrations, engineering controls, work practices, medical and environmental surveillance, record keeping, and so forth. Civil, and in some cases criminal penalties are associated with violation of standards. It is recognized that the toxicologic basis for standards for potentially toxic substances is weak and that regulators must act prudently to ensure erring on the side of safety. The concept of standards is changing rapidly and the "generic standard," one applicable to classes of chemical agents, has been introduced in rule-making procedures. Undoubtedly, "regulatory toxicology" is in its infancy. Our present struggles to equitably, safely, and effectively regulate chemical usage will in the near future be viewed as pioneering, but clumsy initial encounters with the problem.

REFERENCES

Calabrese, E. J.: *Pollutants and High-Risk Groups. The Biological Basis of Increased Humans Susceptibility to Environmental and Occupational Pollutants.* Wiley-Interscience, New York, 1978.

Chemicals and Health. Report of the Panel on Chemicals and Health of the President's Science Advisory Committee, Science and Technology Policy Office, National Science Foundation, Washington, D.C., September 1973.

Chemical Dangers in the Workplace, 94th Congress, 2nd Session, House Report No. 94-1688, 34th Report by the Committee on Government Operations. U.S. Government Printing Office, Washington, D.C., 1976.

Commerce Clearing House, Inc.: *Guidebook to Occupational Safety and Health*, 1978 ed. 4025 Peterson Ave., Chicago, 1978.

Committee on Principles of Decision Making for Regulating Chemicals in the Environment: *Decision Making for Regulating Chemicals in the Environment.* National Academy of Sciences, Washington, D.C., 1975.

Corn, J. K.: Historical perspective to a current controversy on the clinical spectrum of plumbism. *Health and Society, MMMFQ*, Winter, 1975, pp. 93–114.

Corn, M.: The impact of federal regulations on engineers. *Chem. Eng. Prog.*, July, 1978.

Corn, M., and Corn, J. K.: Setting standards for the public: A historical perspective. *Proc. LASL Third Life Sciences Symposium on Impact of Energy Production on Human Health.* CONF-75-1022, Technical Information Center, Office of Public Affairs, ERDA, 1976, pp. 29–33.

Exposure to Coke Oven Emissions: Department of Labor, Occupational Safety and Health Administration, Occupational Safety and Health Standards. *Federal Register*, 41(No. 206):46742–90, Oct. 22, 1976.

Flowers, B. D. (chairman): *Royal Commission on the Environment, Sixth Report: Nuclear Power and the Environment.* Her Majesty's Stationery Office, London, Sept., 1976, p. 77.

Hatch, T. F.: Changing objectives in occupational health. *Am. Ind. Hyg. Assoc. J.*, 23:1–7, 1962.

Health and Safety at Work, Etc., Act 1974, Chapter 37. Her Majesty's Stationery Office, London, 1975.

House Interstate and Foreign Commerce Committee Report, *Toxic Substances Control Act*, 94th Congress, 2nd Session. Report No. 94-1341, July 14, 1976, Section 7.

Identification, Classification, and Regulation of Occupational Carcinogens. OSHA Proposed Rule. 42FR54148, Oct. 4, 1977.

Legislative History of the Occupational Safety and Health Act of 1970 (S. 2193, P.L. 91-596). Prepared by the Subcommittee on Labor, Committee on Labor and Public Welfare, U.S. Senate, 92nd Congress, 1st Session, June 1971.

Lowrance, W. W.: *Of Acceptable Risk—Science and the Determination of Safety.* William Kaufmann, Inc., Los Altos, CA, 1976.

Rosen, G.: *A History of Public Health.* M.D. Publications, Inc., New York, 1958.

Rowe, W. D.: *An Anatomy of Risk.* Wiley-Interscience, New York, 1977.

Sand, R.: *The Advance to Social Medicine.* Staples Press, New York, 1952.

Science Council of Canada, Report No. 28. *Policies and Poisons: The Containment of Long-Term Hazards to Human Health in the Environment and in the Workplace.* Thorn Press Ltd., Don Mills, Ont., Oct. 1977.

The Working Environment Act, Act No. 681, Ministry of Labor, Copenhagen, Denmark, 1975.

Weinberg, A. M.: Science and trans-science. *Minerva*, 10:209–22, 1972.

Wilson, R.: A rational approach to reducing cancer risk. *New York Times*, July 7, 1978.

Workers Protection Act and Law on Work Environment. Stockholm, Sweden, 1974. (N.B.: Law on Work Environment scheduled to take effect in 1978).

Workshop on the Assessment of Reproductive Hazards in the Workplace. Society of Occupational Health and National Institute of Occupational Safety and Health, Washington, D.C., April 19, 1978.

Chapter 30

TOXICOLOGY AND THE LAW

Rob S. McCutcheon

INTRODUCTION

Toxicology has aided us in establishing laws and in implementing regulations for our protection against all manner of poisonous substances. Our developing technology and growing population density aggravate existing environmental problems and create new ones. The growing unease regarding these problems was expressed in 1960 in a symposium on "Problems in Toxicology" (Coon and Maynard, 1960). The dangers discussed included the usual environmental problems and the possible interaction of the various pollutants. Lay attention was drawn to the growing seriousness of these matters by publications such as *Silent Spring* (Carson, 1962). In the years since, the public has become more aware and better informed so that a number of legislative steps have resulted in necessary control measures. This discussion will be concerned with laws and agencies designed to regulate and control chemicals and other substances having poisonous or dangerous qualities.

Many useful and common substances, frequently contacted in our daily lives, may not be recognized as hazards, yet they are the cause of many poisonings. A casual look at our surroundings, at home or at work, will illustrate the need for consciousness of these hazards. Examples include solvents, cleaners, detergents, paints, paint removers, and household and garden pesticides. They would also include insect repellents applied to the skin, rat poisons, moth killer, mildew preventive, fireproofing chemicals, waterproofing chemicals, and polishes. Many of these useful chemicals are sold in pressure containers for aerosol dispersal. Some propellant gases have proved harmful when misused and some are also considered a threat to the environment.

Many drugs kept in the home are distinct hazards and need more regulatory attention. For example, aspirin, sleeping pills, iron tablets, and reducing pills have produced many serious or fatal poisonings, particularly in children. Other potential sources of injury include flammable fabrics and explosives. Such dangers are cause for concern for improvement of consumer protection.

The widely distributed environmental poisons polluting our air and water are a serious problem requiring increased regulation. Air pollutants, including lead, CO, ozone, carbon solids, nitrogen oxides, and SO_2, increase with population and industrialization. However, earlier use of known techniques would have reduced our problems. The Environmental Protection Agency, in responding to these worsening problems, is emphasizing control. Beside industrial wastes, we have the growing problem of sewage disposal. These matters have received little previous attention because of apathy. Despite useful laws and a capable technology, progress has been made only as the result of strong public demand.

It is clear that we are constantly in contact with chemicals that are designed to serve a myriad of beneficial purposes. For example, products such as pesticides have made our lives easier and more comfortable, but we cannot have the benefits without accepting a degree of risk as well. Many of these products are highly toxic, even in low concentrations, and they often present difficulties in their application and disposal because of their persistent qualities and toxic breakdown substances. We have solutions for some questions of safety concerning these; other questions remain unanswered. Additional information must be sought through research and experiment before we attain adequate regulations (Crow, 1968).

REGULATORY DEVELOPMENT

The intense interest in the health hazards of our environment, emphasized by the news media in recent years, has resulted in more effective legislation for their control. But public concern has not always been such a powerful factor in the passage of regulatory legislation. Before 1900, neither the lawmakers, nor the manufacturers, nor others responsible for these problems felt much pressure to correct them. There was at that time practically no legislation for protecting either the worker or the public from exposure to toxic materials, and injured parties had only limited recourse even in the courts. Two factors were mainly responsible for the changes that took place around the turn of the century. The first was the development of chemical methods sensitive enough to detect the presence of traces of poisons in food or in other materials. These aided in establishing cause-effect relationships. The second factor was the recognition that workers are entitled to some protection against industrial hazards and that the responsibility for this protection rests with the employer.

Regulatory law has been developed over the years both by legislation and by administrative promulgation. Much of this law, however, lacks coordination and often fails to keep pace with current needs, but reforming the law is difficult. In attempting reform, new laws are passed often without relation to the existing law, thus creating further confusion.

REGULATORY AGENCIES

Of the many regulatory acts and agencies of the United States government a number are of minor importance from the standpoint of toxicology. These will be briefly described at the end of the chapter with adequate reference for further reading if desired.

The agency of greatest concern to most of us in recent years is the Environmental Protection Agency (EPA). It was established, by Executive Order, to govern matters concerning air and water pollution, the use of pesticides, and other matters affecting the environment (Reorganization Plan, 1970). One primary purpose of its formation was to consolidate the functions of the several agencies relating to the environment in order to improve regulatory performance. The creation of this agency is an example of law reform and simplification that should result in better control of environmental hazards. The powers of the former regulatory agencies to control pollution were weakened by fragmentation. The Mrak Commission cites an example in which the Food and Drug Administration was setting tolerance limits for pesticides, but had no power to prevent pesticide registration by the Department of Agriculture (Mrak, 1969). The Reorganization Plan of 1970 now assigns both of these tasks to EPA.

All activities of the Department of Interior relating to water quality, water pollution control, studies of the effects of pesticides on fish and wildlife resources, and the Gulf Breeze Biological Laboratory were moved to EPA. EPA now controls the former functions of the Department of Health, Education, and Welfare relating to the Air Pollution Control Administration and the Environmental Control Administration, and DHEW's provision of technical assistance to the states. The Bureau of Solid Waste Management, the Bureau of Water Hygiene, and, with some exceptions, the Bureau of Radiological Health are also included. In addition, EPA assumed the activities of the Council of Environmental Quality (CEQ) that pertain to ecologic systems; those tasks of the Department of Energy, administered through its Division of Radiation Protection Standards, establishing environmental standards for protection from radioactive material; and all functions of the Federal Radiation Council.

TOXIC SUBSTANCES CONTROL ACT

After the formation of EPA, the Toxic Substances Control Act (TOSCA) was added in an attempt to consolidate regulation of the chemical industry. Chemicals are all around us—in our air, our water, and our food, and in the things we touch. Many of these chemicals have become essential to our lives, and their production contributes significantly to our national economy. However, for many of these substances, we have little knowledge of the ill effects they might cause after many years of exposure. The Toxic Substances Control Act, which became effective January 1, 1977, regulates commerce and protects human health and the environment by requiring testing and the necessary use restrictions on certain chemical substances.

While we have enjoyed the extensive economic and social benefits of chemicals, we have not always realized the risks that may be associated with them. Many chemicals that have been commonly used and widely dispersed have been found to present significant health and environmental dangers. Vinyl chloride, which is commonly used in plastics, has caused the death of workers who were exposed to this chemical. Asbestos has long been known to cause cancer when inhaled. Mercury has caused debilitating effects in Japan. Perhaps the most vivid example was the careless dispersal into our environment of millions of pounds of polychlorinated biphenyls (PCB's), a highly persistent and toxic group of chemicals.

The new law promotes acquisition of adequate chemical data. It provides authority to regulate but says such authority shall not be used to create unnecessary economic barriers to innovation. It was passed following a five-year congressional effort. It is complex, and both enforcement and compliance will undoubtedly prove expensive. The Act requires the formation of the TOSCA

Interagency Testing Committee. This is made up of representatives from eight agencies, which include the National Science Foundation, the Occupational Safety and Health Administration, and the National Cancer Institute. There are also four nonvoting liaison agencies, including the Food and Drug Administration and the Department of Defense.

The primary purpose of TOSCA is to assure that chemical substances and mixtures do not present an unreasonable risk of injury to health or the environment. Yet when one considers that there are about 100,000 chemicals in commerce and that at least 1,000 new ones are added each year, it is obvious that the Agency faces a tremendous job. Think of the toxicologists needed! The early efforts of the Agency have resulted in a Toxic Substances List and four to eight chemical substances marked for study.

FOOD AND DRUG ADMINISTRATION

Another agency of great importance and interest to toxicologists is the Food and Drug Administration (FDA). In this consideration it is of interest to review briefly the background of the present law for protection of our food and drug supply. The first general food law was passed in Massachusetts in 1784, and in 1824 a Flour Inspection Act was passed in the District of Columbia. In 1848, when it was discovered that the quinine for our soldiers in the Mexican War was adulterated, the Import Drugs Act was passed. From that time until 1905, more than 100 food and drug acts were introduced but failed to pass the Congress. The many attempts do, however, show an increasing awareness of the need for such regulation. Early in this century a number of investigations of food and drug problems were carried out, including the effective efforts of Dr. Harvey Wiley and his so-called "poison squad," which operated mainly in Chicago. By exposing the indescribably filthy conditions existing in some of the food-processing industries of that time, Dr. Wiley and his group, together with such writings as *The Jungle* by Upton Sinclair, aroused great enough public demand that passage of effective laws resulted.

From 1906 until 1933 a number of improved food and drug laws were passed, but by 1933 it became clear that a stronger law was needed. A revised law, the Food, Drug and Cosmetic Act, was finally passed in 1938 following a drug-poisoning incident killing more than 100 persons. Besides establishment of the Food and Drug Administration, the new Act provided for (1) extension of coverage to cosmetics and medical devices; (2) requirement of predistribution clearance on safety of new drugs; (3) elimination of the Shirley Amendment requirement to prove intent to defraud in drug-misbranding cases; (4) provision for establishing tolerances for unavoidable or required poisonous substances; (5) authorization of standards of identity, quality, and fill of container for foods; (6) authorization of factory inspections; and (7) addition of the remedy of court injunction to previous remedies of seizure and prosecution.

The FDA was transferred from the Department of Agriculture to the Federal Security Agency in 1940, and this agency became the Department of Health, Education, and Welfare in 1953. It has since grown in both size and power. At present it is divided into six bureaus: Drugs, Foods, Radiological Health, Veterinary Medicine, Biologics, and Medical Devices. The Bureau of Foods is most closely associated with control of poisons and hazardous substances. There are also several National Centers: for Drug Analysis, for Microbiological Analysis, and for Antibiotics and Insulin Analysis. The newest of these, the National Center for Toxicological Research at Pine Bluff, Arkansas, is operated jointly with the Environmental Protection Agency.

Consumer protection against harmful food colorings began in 1907, when concern was expressed about the safety of the new coal tar colors just coming into use. Responsible food processors asked the government to set up a system for testing these colors and certifying them as pure and harmless. This voluntary system lasted until 1938, when certification was made compulsory by the passage of the new Food, Drug, and Cosmetic Act. As new testing techniques for colors, not available when they were first listed as "harmless," were developed, colors were reevaluated. This retesting showed that, in fact, some of the colors in use were not completely harmless if used in unlimited amounts. So in 1960, the Color Additive Amendments were passed, strengthening consumer protection in three ways.

First, the Amendments brought all colors (not just coal tar colors) under the jurisdiction of the law. Second, they required reevaluation—using new scientific tests—of all colors, even those previously listed and certified as harmless. (Any color that produces cancer in a test animal is automatically ruled out.) Finally, they allowed FDA to set limits on the amounts of color used.

The Act also provides for the control of food additives as defined by the FDA: "A food additive is any substance that becomes part of food, or affects the characteristics of food, through direct or indirect use and with useful intention." They may be intentionally added to food to preserve, emulsify, flavor, add nutritive value, color, or achieve other useful, desired purposes. Materials that might also get into foods while they are grown, processed, or packaged are called incidental additives. Before an additive can be used to improve a food product, it is subjected to toxicity studies by the food (or chemical) manufacturer, and it is evaluated and regulated by the FDA.

The Food, Drug, and Cosmetic Act, under the Miller Amendment of 1954, also provided that the FDA establish tolerances for those registered economic poisons that appeared as residues in food products, and that the FDA maintain surveillance for conformity with the law. Thus, before a pesticide residue can be allowed to remain in or on food, the use of the pesticide on food crops must be approved by the Environmental Protection Agency. The pesticide is subjected to toxicity studies by the manufacturer and is evaluated and regulated by the EPA.

Food products are labeled with the required information to guide and protect the consumer. An amendment to the Food, Drug, and Cosmetic Act was passed in 1958 prohibiting the use of new food additives until the sponsor established safety and the FDA issued regulations specifying the conditions of use.

In 1962, much publicity resulted from the action of Dr. Frances O. Kelsey in keeping thalidomide off the American market. This drug produced thousands of deformities in babies born in western Europe. The tragedy and attendant publicity created a great deal of public interest in drug problems. Subsequently, that year the Kefauver-Harris Drug Amendments strengthened new drug clearance procedures. As a result of this legislation, drug manufacturers had to prove effectiveness of drugs before marketing them. Further changes, including the amended versions of January 1971 and October 1976, have improved the law.

To summarize, the enactment of the modern Federal Food, Drug, and Cosmetic Act is aimed at assuring foods that are safe, pure, and wholesome; drugs and therapeutic devices that are safe and effective; and cosmetics that are harmless. All these products must be honestly and informatively labeled and packaged. The FDA also requires that dangerous household products carry adequate warnings for safe use and are properly labeled, and that there be no counterfeiting of drugs.

Also of interest to toxicologists is the establishment by the Food and Drug administration of a National Drug Code Directory (NDC System). The system provides a unique ten-digit, three-part number for every drug. The system is computerized, and among other things it will provide a prompt identification of drugs in poisoning cases. This computerized information will be available for "those needing identification of the drug product, by-product, or generic name, manufacturer or labeler name, dosage form, strength, route of administration, or legal status." It will also be of assistance for third-party reimbursement programs. This drug code system also has potential applications in hospitals for inventory control, billing, and medication records, and in government agencies for such diverse purposes as adverse reaction reporting systems, drug utilization reviews, poison control center operations, and drug product recalls.

The Drug Listing Act of 1972 dictated the expansion of the NDC System to include both human over-the-counter and veterinary drugs.

OCCUPATIONAL SAFETY AND HEALTH ACT

A new law with wide-ranging effect and of great concern to industry is the Occupational Safety and Health Act (OSHA) of 1970, designed to assure that no employee will suffer diminished health, functional capacity, or life expectancy as a result of his work experience. The Act is administered by the Secretary of Labor. He is authorized to set mandatory occupational safety and health standards for businesses in interstate commerce and to establish a review commission for carrying out adjudicatory functions under the Act. The Act calls for research in occupational safety and health to assist in the discovery of latent diseases, to establish the connection between diseases and the work environment where these exist, and to study other health problems. It also provides for training of personnel engaged in the field of occupational safety and health. It stipulates enforcement and encourages states to adequately administer state safety and health laws. It is clear that toxicologists will be extensively involved in both administrative and compliance aspects of this Act.

NATIONAL INSTITUTE FOR OCCUPATIONAL SAFETY AND HEALTH

The National Institute for Occupational Safety and Health (NIOSH) is the principal federal agency engaged in research in the national effort to eliminate on-the-job hazards to the health and safety of America's working men and women. The Institute was established within the Department of Health, Education, and Welfare under the provisions of the Occupational Safety and Health Act. Administratively, NIOSH is located within HEW's Center for Disease Control of the Public Health Service. The portion of OSHA administered by the Department of Labor is largely regulatory, but much of the Department's work will rest on the results of research conducted by NIOSH under HEW.

NIOSH is responsible for identifying occupational safety and health hazards and for recommending changes in the regulations limiting them. It also has obligations for training occupational health manpower and conducting research for new occupational safety and health standards. The recommended standards are transmitted to the Department of Labor, which then has the responsibility for their development, promulgation, and enforcement.

The Institute's main research laboratories are in Cincinnati, where studies include not only the effects of exposure to hazardous substances used in the workplace, but also the psychologic, motivational, and behavioral factors involved in occupational safety and health. Much of the Institute's research deals with specific hazards, such as asbestos and other fibers, beryllium, coal tar pitch volatiles, silica, noise, and stress.

The establishment of both TOSCA and NIOSH has resulted in a strong demand for toxicologists. The increased activity in industry in attempts to comply with the law and the research and enforcement activities under OSHA have been powerful stimulants to all facets of toxicology. Perhaps the area of research and training will be most greatly affected. In this connection a program of grants for both training and research has been instituted.

DRUG ABUSE

Of great concern to all citizens, as well as to toxicologists and to legislators, has been the great increase in drug abuse in recent years. In an attempt to control the problem the Comprehensive Drug Abuse Prevention and Control Act of 1970 was enacted to provide for increased research into the prevention of drug abuse and drug dependence, for treatment and rehabilitation of addicts, and to improve law enforcement. The law makes available rehabilitation programs, research, medical treatment, education, control, and enforcement. This is another instance of a law that is administered by more than one agency. The National Institute of Mental Health has been designated to carry out the medical, educational, and research aspects of the law. Extramural research is supported by both a grant and a contract program administered by the Institute. This Institute also conducts an extensive public relations program. Toxicologists are involved within the Institute and as outside consultants for developing appropriate methods of treatment of addicts and solution of other problems.

The Act combines federal controls over narcotic, stimulant, and depressant drugs into one statute with enforcement delegated to one other agency, the Bureau of Narcotics and Dangerous Drugs of the Drug Enforcement Administration, U.S. Department of Justice. To assist in enforcement, the law provides for a controlled substances list compiled by the Attorney General, following a scientific and medical evaluation and recommendation concerning such substances supplied by the Secretary of HEW. The Controlled Substances List classifies drugs into five categories on the basis of their established medical use and liability for causing addiction or dependence. Classification is the responsibility of HEW and again involves the work of government scientists as well as medical practitioners, pharmacologists, and toxicologists as consultants outside the government. Drugs can be added to or deleted from the classification list as necessary. The list is of interest to toxicologists because it gives at a glance the legal status of nearly every possible drug of abuse. Schedule I lists drugs of abuse with no acceptable medical use in the United States. The remaining schedules list drugs in descending order of importance from the standpoint of abuse liability. Of some toxicologic interest is the provision that practitioners may not prescribe, nor pharmacists dispense, a schedule II, III, or IV controlled substance in a quantity that exceeds a 34-day supply or 100 dosage units, whichever is less. Toxicologists will be interested to compare the legal definitions of drug, narcotic, or addict, and other items with the scientific terms with which he is familiar.

Toxicologists may also be encouraged to know that an Office of Drug Abuse Policy has been established in the Executive Office of the President to coordinate and speed the work of the Federal agencies involved in drug control or drug abuse programs. The Director is to set priorities for federal drug abuse control and related activities. The Office is to develop a comprehensive, coordinated, long-term federal strategy for all drug abuse programs conducted, directed, sponsored, or supported by any department or agency of the federal government.

CONSUMER PRODUCT SAFETY ACT

Another law that will have considerable impact on consumer safety and poisoning cases is the Consumer Product Safety Act, passed late in 1972 and amended in 1976. The principal purposes of the act are to protect the public against unreasonable risk of injury and assist in evaluating the comparative safety and uniform safety standards for consumer products. The Act is also intended to promote research of the causes and prevention of product-related deaths, illnesses, and injury. The term "consumer product" is defined as any article or part thereof for use, consumption, or enjoyment in or around a permanent or temporary household or residence, a school, in recreation or otherwise. The law specifically does not apply to tobacco, motor vehicles or their equipment, pesticides, aircraft or parts and appliances, boats, drugs, medical devices, cosmetics, food, or firearms, as all of these were controlled by law when the Act was passed.

The Act establishes an independent regulatory commission known as the Consumer Product Safety Commission (CPSC). The Commission is independent, not under a department of government. This relatively new law has proved something of a toothless cat in some danger of extinction. It is, however, the only agency of the government whose title contains the word "consumer." This, in the end, may save it. The exemptions from the Act noted above are considered by some to have been an emasculation. Nonetheless, the Act was given the responsibility for implementing several already existing laws, specifically:

The Flammable Fabrics Act (1972).
The Federal Hazardous Substances Act (1967).
The Poison Prevention Packaging Act of 1970.
The Refrigerator Safety Act of 1956.

FLAMMABLE FABRICS ACT

The Flammable Fabrics Act had formerly been administered in part by HEW, the Department of Commerce, and the Federal Trade Commission. The functions of each department as they related to flammable fabrics were transferred to the Consumer Product Safety Commission (CPSC). The Act prohibits the marketing or interstate transport of articles of clothing or fabrics that are so flammable that they are dangerous when worn or when used for interior furnishings in homes and public buildings.

The law defines terms that apply and specifies what transactions are prohibited. It is of interest to toxicologists that the requirements of this Act led to the treatment of children's sleep wear with tris (2,3-dibromopropyl)phosphate. The subsequent discovery of the carcinogenic properties of this chemical required the removal of treated garments from the market at a high cost both economically and in terms of confidence in the federal bureaucracy.

FEDERAL HAZARDOUS SUBSTANCES ACT

The Federal Hazardous Substances Act of 1967 was also transferred to CPSC as noted above. The intent of the Act is to regulate "toxic" substances, defined as any substance (other than a radioactive substance) that has the capacity to produce personal injury or illness to mankind through ingestion, inhalation, or absorption through any body surface.

Other terms are given a legal definition for the benefit of the toxicologist and others who must administer the law. The term "highly toxic" means any substance that (1) produces death within 14 days in half or more than half of a group of ten or more laboratory white rats each weighing between 200 and 300 g; (a) at a single dose of 50 mg or less per kilogram of body weight, when orally administered; or (b) when inhaled continuously for a period of one hour or less at an atmospheric concentration of 200 ppm by volume or less of gas or vapor, or 2 mg/1 by volume or less of mist or dust, provided such concentration is likely to be encountered when the substance is used in any reasonably foreseeable manner; or (2) produces death with 14 days in half, or more than half, of a group of ten or more rabbits tested in a dosage of 200 mg or less per kilogram of body weight, when administered by continuous contact with the bare skin for 24 hours or less. If it is found that available data on human experience with any substance indicate results different from those obtained on animals in the above-named dosages or concentrations, the human data shall take precedence.

"Corrosive" applies to any substance that in contact with living tissue will cause destruction of tissue by chemical action.

"Irritant" means any substance, not corrosive as defined above, that on immediate, prolonged, or repeated contact with normal living tissue will induce a local inflammatory reaction.

"Strong sensitizer" means a substance that will produce in a normal living tissue, by an allergic or photodynamic process, a hypersensitivity, evident on reapplication.

"Extremely flammable" shall apply to any substance that has a flash point at or below 20° F, as determined by the Tagliabue open cup tester.

"Flammable" applies to any substance that has a flash point of above 20° to and including 80° F, as determined by the Tagliabue open cup tester.

"Radioactive substance" means a substance that emits ionizing radiation.

"Label" means a display of written, printed, or graphic matter on the immediate container of any substance. Labeling requirements are specified in detail with provision for declaring an item misbranded. In this revision of the law, additions are made regulating substances and toys used primarily by children. Branding of such items must include adequate direction for the protection of children from hazard.

A new term, "banned hazardous substance," is introduced that, besides several other meanings, includes any toy or other article intended for use by children that is a hazardous substance or that bears or contains a hazardous substance that could be accessible to a child to whom such toy or article is entrusted.

The Act lists various prohibitions, penalties, and other provisions, and repeals the Federal Caustic Poison Act with certain stated exceptions.

POISON PREVENTION PACKAGING ACT

The Poison Prevention Packaging Act, as mentioned above, requires special packaging to protect children from serious personal injury or serious illness resulting from handling, using, or ingesting household substances, and for other purposes. One result of this law was the marketing of prescription and some over-the-counter drugs in containers having trick openings designed to prevent young children from opening them. Such common drugs as aspirin and iron compounds have been serious offenders in accidental poisonings.

TOY SAFETY

The Child Protection and Toy Safety Act of 1969 is not of much interest from a toxicologic standpoint except as it applies to the control of substances or objects that could leak or spray injurious material into an eye or be harmfully aspirated or ingested. Such toy or other article may be deemed to be a banned hazardous substance.

FEDERAL HAZARDOUS SUBSTANCES LABELING ACT

In 1962 this law replaced the Federal Caustic Poison Act except for any "dangerous caustic or corrosive substance," as defined by the Federal Caustic Poison Act subject to the federal Food, Drug, and Cosmetic Act. The Act is essentially a labeling law, which specifies the label required on certain caustic substances. It is designed to regulate the distribution and sale of certain dangerous caustic or corrosive acids, alkalies, and other substances in interstate and foreign commerce. The law is largely of interest to toxicologists who might be acting as advisors or consultants to a business or industry interested in distributing such substances.

LEAD-BASED PAINT POISONING PREVENTION ACT

This Act (January 1971) provides grants for detection and treatment of lead-based paint poisoning and for support of programs leading to the elimination of such poisoning. It prohibits the use of lead-based paints in any residential structures funded with federal assistance in any form. It is administered by HEW in conjunction with the Secretary of Housing and Urban Development. The Act has provided support for a number of toxicologic projects.

AIRCRAFT SPRAYING

The spraying of pesticides from aircraft is controlled by the Federal Aviation Administration under its regulations for agricultural aircraft operation. The operator must be certified; he must show by test that he is qualified in regard to safe handling of economic poisons. He must understand the proper disposal of used containers, the effects produced, and the symptoms of poisoning caused by the substances used and the appropriate measures to take in emergencies and the location of poison treatment centers in his locality. Other detailed specifications are given in the regulations for the safety of the operator and of the people on the ground.

REFERENCES

Buhler, D. R.; Rasmusson, M. E.; and Shanks, W. E.: Chronic oral DDT toxicity in juvenile Coho and Chinook salmon. *Toxicol. Appl. Pharmacol.* **14**:535–55, 1969.

Carson, R.: *Silent Spring*. Houghton-Mifflin Co., Boston, 1962.

Coon, J. M., and Maynard, E. A. (eds.): Problems in toxicology. *Fed. Proc. Suppl.*, **4**:1–52, Sept., 1960.

Crow, J. F.: *Scientist and Citizen*. Scientist's Institute for Public Information, St. Louis, June, July, 1968.

Dominquez, G. S.: *Guidebook: Toxic Substances Control Act*. CRC Press, Cleveland, 1977.

Environmental Quality. The Second Annual Report of the Council on Environmental Quality. U.S. Government Printing Office, Washington, D.C., August, 1968.

Gold, M. D.; Blum, A.; and Ames, B. N.: Another flame retardant, tris-(1,3-dichloro-2-propyl)phosphate, and its expected metabolites are mutagens. *Science*, **200**:785–87, 1978.

Mrak, E. M. (Chairman): *Report of the Secretary's Commission on Pesticides and Their Relationship to Environmental Health*, Parts I and II. U.S. Government Printing Office, Washington, D.C., 1969.

Reorganization Plan No. 3. H.R. Document No. 91-364, 1970.

Copies of most of the laws discussed are available in the following:
95th Congress 1st session Committee Print 95-6
    Federal Food, Drug, and Cosmetic Law
    Controlled Substances Act
    Special Action Office for Drug Abuse Prevention
95th Congress 1st session Committee Print 95-7
    Toxic Substances Control Act
    Lead-Based Paint Poisoning Prevention Act
    Occupational Safety and Health Act

INDEX*

Aatrex. *See* Atrazine
Abate, chemical structure, 367
Abrin, 584
Abrus precatorius, 584-85
ABS, chemical structure, 532
Absorption, **31-38**
  gastrointestinal tract, 31-33
  lungs, 33-35, 516
  skin, 35-37
Acacia, 72, 599-600
Acacia berlandieri, 588
Acceptable daily intake (ADI), 26,
  595
  conditional, 595
  temporary, 595
  unconditional, 595
Accessory cell function, **344**
Accidental deaths, 661
Acetaldehyde, 477
  as food additive, 599
Acetamide, 103, 122
  chemical structure, 91
  teratogenic effects, 168
5-Acetamido-3-(5-nitro-2-furyl)-6-
  H-1,2,4-oxadiazine, chemical
  structure, 95
Acetaminophen (paracetamol),
  682-83
  biotransformation, 682
  depletion of glutathione by, 682
  effect on kidney, 241
  effect on liver, 209, 223
  incidence of poisoning, 663
  pK_a, $t_{1/2}$, Vd, 678
  plasma levels, 682
  specific therapy with
    N-acetylcysteine, 678
  stages in poisoning by, 682
  treatment of poisoning, 682-83
Acetanilide, 76, 117
Acetate, effect on eye, 278
Acetazolamide (Diamox), 167, 285,
  695
  teratogenic effects, 168
Acetic acid, effect on eye, 284
  effect on lung, 614
  as food additive, 599-600
Acetic anhydride, 284
Acetohexamide, 210
Acetoin, 599
Acetone, analysis for, 668
  effect on eye, 278
  incidence of poisoning, 663
  potentiation of hepatotoxicity, 226
3-Acetoxyhexadecanoic acid, 558

Acetoxymethylnitrosamine, 101
2-Acetylaminofluorene, carcinogenic effects, 222
  chemical structure, 90, 93
  teratogenic effects, 163
Acetylaminofluorine. *See* 2-Acetyl-
  aminofluorene
Acetylcholine, 367
  chemical structure, 373
Acetylcholinesterase, inhibition by
  organophosphorus insecti-
  cides, 365, 369
Acetyl-coenzyme A, 61
N-Acetylcysteine (Mucomyst), 61,
  678, 683
Acetylesterases, 59
N-Acetyl-1-hydroxylaminofluorene,
  94
Acetylisoniazid, 224
N-Acetyl-*para*-aminophenol, 241
N-Acetyl-*D,L*-penicillamine, 428
3-Acetylpyridine, 168, 191, **199**
Acetylsalicylic acid. *See* Salicylates
N-Acetyl transferases, **64-65**
Acetyl tributyl citrate, 549
Acetyl triethyl citrate, 549
Achondroplasia, 458
Achondroplasia muscular dystro-
  phy, 143
Acidosis, 689
Acids, **275-77**, **683-84**
  effect on eye, 275-77
  as food additive, 600
  symptoms of poisoning, 683
  treatment of poisoning, 683-84
Aconite, 3
Aconitine, 588
Aconitum napellus, 588
Acquired tolerance, 415
Acriflavine, 164
Acrodynia, 426
Acrolein, **626**
  in air pollution, 614, 619, 626
  effect on liver, 224
Acroosteolysis, 533
Acrosome, 335
Acrylamide, 191, **194-95**
Acrylics, **546-47**, 703
Acrylonitrile, chemical structure,
  103
  OSHA standards, 721
  use as fumigant, 397-98
  use in plastics, 532
Acrylonitrilebutadiene styrene,
  chemical structure, 532

Actinide oxide, 518
Actinides, radiation effects, **521-22**
Actinolite, 270, 654
Actinomycins, 105. *See also* Dac-
  tinomycin
Active transport, 30
Acts. *See* Laws
Acute exposure, definition, 14
Acute lymphocytic leukemia, 315
Acute myelogenous leukemia, 315
Acute nonspecific upper respiratory
  disease, 610
Acylonium, 102
Adaptation, 415
Additive effect, 17, 671
Adenosine, 558
Adenosylethionine, 164
S-Adenosylmethionine (SAM), 64,
  216
ADH. *See* Alcohol dehydrogenase
ADI. *See* Acceptable daily intake
Adipic acid, 599
Adipic acid esters, **549**
Adjuvants, 71
Administrative Procedures Act, 722
Adrenal corticosteroids (glucocor-
  ticoids), effect on
  phagocytes, 314
  teratogenic effects, 167, 171
Adrenalectomy, effect on toxicity,
  78
Adriamycin, 105, 343
Adverse reactions, classification, 15
Aeralanol, 711
Aerodynamic diameter, equivalent,
  516
Aerodynamic diameter of particles,
  257, 261
Aerodynamic mass distribution,
  256
Aerosol particle size, aerodynamic
  diameter, 257
  count median diameter (CMD),
  257
  mass median diameter (MMD),
  257
Aerosols, 255
  deposition mechanisms, 257
Aerosol sprays, 468
A-esterase. *See* Aliesterase
AF-2, 96
Aflatoxin, carcinogenic effects, 105
  effect on liver, 209, 212
  effect on reproduction, 343
  as food contaminant, 605

---

*Page numbers in **boldface** type indicate primary discussion.